Oxford Textbook of

Paediatric Pain

Oxford Textbook of
Paediatric Pain

Edited by

Patrick J. McGrath

Bonnie J. Stevens

Suellen M. Walker
and

William T. Zempsky

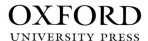

OXFORD
UNIVERSITY PRESS

OXFORD
UNIVERSITY PRESS

Great Clarendon Street, Oxford, OX2 6DP,
United Kingdom

Oxford University Press is a department of the University of Oxford.
It furthers the University's objective of excellence in research, scholarship,
and education by publishing worldwide. Oxford is a registered trade mark of
Oxford University Press in the UK and in certain other countries

First Edition published in 2014

Impression: 1

Published in the United States of America by Oxford University Press
198 Madison Avenue, New York, NY 10016, United States of America

British Library Cataloguing in Publication Data

Data available

Library of Congress Control Number: 2013945062

ISBN 978–0–19–964265–6

Printed in China by
C&C Offset Printing Co. Ltd

Contents

Abbreviations *ix*

Contributors *xi*

SECTION 1
Introduction

1. **History of pain in children** 3
   Anita M. Unruh and Patrick J. McGrath

2. **Prevalence and distribution of pain in children** 12
   Bonnie J. Stevens and William T. Zempsky

3. **Long-term effects of early pain and injury: animal models** 20
   Suellen M. Walker

4. **Long-term effects of pain in children** 30
   Ruth E. Grunau

5. **Prevention of the development and maintenance of paediatric chronic pain and disability** 39
   M. Gabrielle Pagé, Anna Huguet, and Joel Katz

SECTION 2
Biological basis of paediatric pain

6. **Nociceptive signalling in the periphery and spinal cord** 53
   Suellen M. Walker and Mark L. Baccei

7. **Neuroimmune interactions and pain during postnatal development** 65
   David Vega-Avelaira and Simon Beggs

8. **Central nociceptive pathways and descending modulation** 74
   Maria Fitzgerald

SECTION 3
Social and psychological basis of paediatric pain

9. **Psychological theories and biopsychosocial models in paediatric pain** 85
   Rebecca Pillai Riddell, Nicole M. Racine, Kenneth D. Craig, and Lauren Campbell

10. **Cognitive styles and processes in paediatric pain** 95
    Liesbet Goubert and Laura E. Simons

11. **Pain in cultural and communicative contexts** 102
    Ignasi Clemente

12. **Families and pain** 111
    Kathryn A. Birnie, Katelynn E. Boerner, and Christine T. Chambers

13. **Pain, social relationships, and school** 119
    Paula Forgeron and Sara King

14. **The effects of sex and gender on child and adolescent pain** 127
    Erin C. Moon and Anita M. Unruh

15. **Sleep and pain in children and adolescents** 135
    Bruce D. Dick, Penny Corkum, Manisha Witmans, and Christine T. Chambers

SECTION 4
Pain in specific populations and diseases

16. **Pain in children with intellectual or developmental disabilities** 147
    John L. Belew, Chantel C. Barney, Scott A. Schwantes, Dick Tibboel, Abraham J. Valkenburg, and Frank J. Symons

17. **Paediatric cancer pain** *157*
Jennifer Hickman, Jaya Varadarajan,
and Steven J. Weisman

18. **Pain management in major paediatric trauma and burns** *171*
Greta M. Palmer and Franz E. Babl

19. **Needle procedures** *184*
Anna Taddio

20. **Procedural sedation** *194*
Joseph P. Cravero

21. **Neuropathic pain in children** *205*
Suellen M. Walker

22. **Inflammatory arthritis and arthropathy** *215*
Peter Chira and Laura E. Schanberg

23. **Chronic pain syndromes in childhood: one trunk, many branches** *228*
Neil L. Schechter

24. **Non-inflammatory musculoskeletal pain** *237*
Jacqui Clinch

25. **Pain in sickle cell disease** *248*
Carlton Dampier and Lamia Barakat

26. **Pain and gastroenterological diseases** *257*
Akshay Batra, Amanda Bevan, and R. Mark Beattie

27. **Postoperative pain management** *269*
Richard F. Howard

28. **Pain in palliative care** *280*
Ross Drake and Renée McCulloch

29. **Recurrent abdominal pain** *289*
Jennifer Verrill Schurman, Amanda Drews Deacy,
and Craig A. Friesen

30. **Chronic pelvic pain in children and adolescents** *298*
Susan L. Sager and Marc R. Laufer

31. **Headaches** *307*
Andrew D. Hershey

32. **Persisting pain in childhood medical illness** *319*
Martha Mherekumombe and John J. Collins

33. **Common pain problems in the outpatient setting** *328*
F. Ralph Berberich and Neil L. Schechter

34. **Effective management of children's pain and anxiety in the emergency department** *338*
Robert M. (Bo) Kennedy

SECTION 5
Measurement of pain

35. **Neonatal and infant pain assessment** *353*
Grace Y. Lee and Bonnie J. Stevens

36. **Self-report: the primary source in assessment after infancy** *370*
Carl L. von Baeyer

37. **Behavioural measures of pain** *379*
Jill MacLaren Chorney and C. Meghan McMurtry

38. **Biomarkers of pain: physiological indices of pain reactivity in infants and children** *391*
Susanne Brummelte, Tim F. Oberlander,
and Kenneth D. Craig

39. **The neurophysiological evaluation of nociceptive responses in neonates** *401*
Ravi Poorun and Rebeccah Slater

40. **Sensory processing and neurophysiological evaluation in children** *407*
Christiane Hermann

41. **Measurement of health-related quality of life and physical function** *417*
See Wan Tham, Anna C. Wilson, and Tonya M. Palermo

SECTION 6
Pharmacological interventions

42. **Principles of pain pharmacology in paediatrics** *429*
Kim Chau and Gideon Koren

43. **The non-steroidal anti-inflammatory drugs and acetaminophen** *436*
Brian J. Anderson

44. **Developmental pharmacology of opioids** *449*
Gareth J. Hathway

45. **Opioids in clinical practice** *457*
Scott A. Strassels

46. **Interventional pain management techniques for chronic pain** *474*
Navil F. Sethna, Pradeep Dinakar, and Karen R. Boretsky

47. **Topical anaesthetics and analgesics** *486*
William T. Zempsky

48. **Drugs for neuropathic pain** *495*
Sachin Rastogi and Fiona Campbell

49. **Sucrose and sweet taste** 508
Denise Harrison, Vanessa C. Z. Anseloni,
Janet Yamada, and Mariana Bueno

SECTION 7
Psychosocial interventions

50. **Cognitive-behavioural interventions** 519
Deirdre E. Logan, Rachael M. Coakley,
and Brittany N. Barber Garcia

51. **Operant treatment** 531
Keith J. Slifer, Adrianna Amari, and
Cynthia Maynard Ward

52. **Child life interventions in paediatric pain** 543
Chantal K. LeBlanc and Christine T. Chambers

53. **Procedural pain distraction** 553
Lindsey L. Cohen, Laura A. Cousins, and Sarah R. Martin

54. **Hypnosis and relaxation** 560
Christina Liossi, Leora Kuttner, Chantal
Wood, and Lonnie K. Zeltzer

55. **New information and communication
technologies for pain** 569
Jennifer Stinson and Lindsay Jibb

SECTION 8
Physical interventions

56. **Physical therapy interventions for pain
in childhood and adolescence** 581
Susan M. Tupper, Mary S. Swiggum, Deborah
O'Rourke, and Michael L. Sangster

57. **Occupational therapy** 590
Liisa Holsti, Catherine L. Backman, and Joyce M. Engel

58. **Mother care for procedural pain in infants** 600
Celeste Johnston and Marsha Campbell-Yeo

SECTION 9
Special topics

59. **Complementary drugs—herbs, vitamins,
and dietary supplements for pain
and symptom management** 613
Joy A. Weydert

60. **Complementary therapy in paediatric pain** 623
Lonnie K. Zeltzer

61. **Theory-informed approaches to translating
pain evidence into practice** 633
Janet Yamada and Alison M. Hutchinson

62. **Organizational systems in paediatric pain** 642
Mark Embrett and Norman Buckley

63. **Education for paediatric pain** 653
Alison Twycross and Susan O'Conner-Von

64. **The ethics of pain control in
infants and children** 661
Gary A. Walco and Maureen C. Kelley

65. **Sociodemographic disparities in paediatric pain
management: relationships and predictors** 669
Miriam O. Ezenwa and Anna Huguet

Index 677

Abbreviations

ACC	anterior cingulate cortex
ACT	acceptance and commitment therapy
ADR	adverse drug reaction
AIDS	acquired immunodeficiency syndrome
ALL	acute lymphoblastic leukaemia
ANS	autonomic nervous system
AOE	acute otitis externa
AOM	acute otitis media
APS	acute pain service
ART	antiretroviral therapy
ASA	American Society of Anesthesiologists
BART	biofeedback-assisted relaxation training
BBB	blood–brain barrier
BDNF	brain-derived neurotrophic factor
BOLD	blood oxygen level-dependent
ca	corrected age
CAM	complementary and alternative medicine
CAMPIS	Child Adult Medical Procedure Interaction Scale
CARRA	Childhood Arthritis and Rheumatology Research Alliance
CBT	cognitive-behaviour therapy
CBT-I	cognitive-behavioural therapy for insomnia
CCBT	contextual cognitive-behavioural therapy
CD	Crohn's disease
CFA	complete Freund's adjuvant
CFCS	Child Facial Coding System
CHEOPS	Children's Hospital of Eastern Ontario Pain Scale
CHQ	Child Health Questionnaire
CI	confidence interval
CIBP	cancer-induced bone pain
CIHR	Canadian Institutes of Health Research
CIN	chemotherapy-induced neuropathy
CMV	cytomegalovirus
CNS	central nervous system
CO_2	carbon dioxide
COMT	catecholamine-O-methyltransferase
COPM	Canadian Occupational Performance Measure
COX	cyclooxygenase
CP	cerebral palsy or chronic prostatitis
CRPS	complex regional pain syndrome
CSF	cerebrospinal fluid
CT	computed tomography or complementary therapy
CTTH	chronic tension-type headache
CYP	cytochrome P450
DD	developmental disabilities
DEX	dexmedetomidine
DIP	diffuse idiopathic pain
DRG	dorsal root ganglion
DTI	diffusion tensor imaging
E	embryonic day
ED	emergency department
ECG	electrocardiography
EEG	electroencephalography
ELGA	extremely low gestational age
EM	erythromelalgia
EMG	electromyography
ERP	event-related potential
FAP	functional abdominal pain
fcMRI	functional connectivity magnetic resonance imaging
FD	functional dyspepsia
FDA	Food and Drug Administration
FDI	Functional Disability Inventory
FGID	functional gastrointestinal disorders
FLACC	Face, Legs, Activity, Cry, and Consolability scale
FM	fibromyalgia
fMRI	functional magnetic resonance imaging
GA	gestational age
GBS	Guillain–Barré syndrome
GCS	Glasgow coma scale
GI	gastrointestinal
GORD	gastro-oesophageal reflux disease
GVHD	graft-versus-host disease
GW	gestational weeks
h	hour/s
HIV	human immunodeficiency virus
HL	heel lance
HPA	hypothalamic–pituitary–adrenal
HR	heart rate
HRQOL	health-related quality of life
HRV	heart rate variability
IASP	International Association for the Study of Pain

IBD	inflammatory bowel disease
IC	interstitial cystitis
ICF	International Classification of Functioning, Disability and Health
ICF-CY	International Classification Framework for Children and Youth
ICT	information and communication technologies
ICU	intensive care unit
ID	intellectual disabilities
ifn	interferon
IM	intramuscular
IMg^{2+}	ionized magnesium
INF	intranasal fentanyl
INF	intranasal
IPM	interventional pain management
IV	intravenous
JIA	juvenile idiopathic arthritis
KT	knowledge translation
LA	local anaesthesia
LC	locus coeruleus
LCT	limited attentional capacity theory
LET	lidocaine-epinephrine-tetracaine
LPS	lipopolysaccharide
LTP	long-term potentiation
m-health	mobile-health
min	minute/s
MIDAS	Migraine Disability Assessment
MPC	multidisciplinary pain care
mPFC	medial prefrontal cortex
MRI	magnetic resonance imaging
MRT	multiple attentional resource theory
MS	multiple sclerosis
N_2O	nitrous oxide
NAA	N-acetylaspartate
NCCAM	National Center on Complementary and Alternative Medicine
NCCN	National Comprehensive Cancer Network
NCCPC	Non-communicating Children's Pain Checklist
NG	nasogastric
NICE	National Institute for Health and Clinical Excellence
NICU	neonatal intensive care unit
NIH	National Institutes of Health
NIRS	near-infrared spectroscopy
NMDA	N-methyl-D-aspartate
NNS	non-nutritive sucking
NNT	number needed to treat
NP	neuropathic pain
NRS	numerical rating scale
NS	nociceptive specific
NSAID	non-steroidal anti-inflammatory drug
OIH	opioid-induced hypersensitivity
OMRU	Ottawa Model of Research Use
OR	odds ratio
OSBD	Observation Scale of Behavioural Distress
P	postnatal day
PACU	post-anaesthesia care unit
PADS	pain-associated disability syndrome
PAG	periaqueductal grey

PARiHS	Promoting Action on Research Implementation in Health Services
PBn	parabrachial area
PBRS	Procedure Behavioural Rating Scale
PBS	painful bladder syndrome
PCA	patient-controlled analgesia
PedMiDAS	paediatric Migraine Disability Assessment
PedQL	Pediatric Quality of Life Inventory
PEPD	paroxysmal extreme pain disorder
PET	positron emission tomography
P-gp	P-glycoprotein
PHN	postherpetic neuralgia
PID	pelvic inflammatory disease
PMP	prescription monitoring programme
PNA	postnatal age
PNCA	parent/nurse-controlled analgesia
PNI	peripheral nerve injury
PO	per os (orally)
POTS	postural orthostatic tachycardia syndrome
PPC	Paediatric Pain Centre
PPI	proton pump inhibitor
PPPM	Parents' Postoperative Pain Measure
PROMIS	Patient Reported Outcomes Measurement Information System
PSA	procedural sedation and analgesia
PT	physical therapist
QST	quantitative sensory testing
RAP	recurrent abdominal pain
RBC	red blood cell
RCT	randomized controlled trial
RVM	rostroventral medulla
S1	primary somatosensory cortex
S2	secondary somatosensory cortex
SC	subcutaneous
SCD	sickle cell disease
SCM	social communication model
SD	standard deviation
SDH	superficial dorsal horn
sec	second/s
SES	socioeconomic status
SIB	self-injurious behaviour
SSNRI	selective serotonin and noradrenaline reuptake inhibitor
SSRI	selective serotonin re-uptake inhibitor
STT	spinothalamic tract
TCA	tricyclic antidepressant
TCM	traditional Chinese medicine
TDM	therapeutic drug monitoring
UC	ulcerative colitis
UGT	uridine diphosphate glucuronosyltransferase
VAS	visual analogue scale
VNS	verbal numeric scale
VPL	ventroposterolateral nucleus
VPn	ventroposterior nucleus
WDR	wide dynamic range
WHO	World Health Organization

Contributors

Adrianna Amari Pediatric Psychology Consultation Program, Department of Behavioral Psychology, Kennedy Krieger Institute and Assistant Professor, Department of Psychiatry and Behavioral Sciences, Johns Hopkins University School of Medicine, Baltimore, MD, USA

Brian J. Anderson Department of Anaesthesia and Intensive Care, Starship Children's Hospital, Auckland, New Zealand

Vanessa C. Z. Anseloni Department of Neural and Pain Sciences University of Maryland Baltimore, MD, USA

Franz E. Babl Emergency Department, Royal Children's Hospital and Murdoch Children's Research Institute, Melbourne, Australia and Associate Professor, University of Melbourne, Melbourne, Australia

Mark L. Baccei Pain Research Center, Department of Anesthesiology, University of Cincinnati, Cincinnati, OH, USA

Catherine L. Backman Department of Occupational Science and Occupational Therapy, The University of British Columbia, Vancouver, BC, Canada

Lamia Barakat Psychosocial Services, Division of Oncology, The Children's Hospital of Philadelphia, and Associate Professor of Clinical Psychology, Department of Pediatrics, Perelman School of Medicine, University of Pennsylvania, PA, USA

Brittany N. Barber Garcia Pain Treatment Service, Boston Children's Hospital, Boston, MA, USA

Chantel C. Barney Department of Educational Psychology, University of Minnesota, MN, USA

Akshay Batra Department of Paediatric Gastroenterology, Child Health Division, Southampton Children's Hospital, Southampton, UK

R. Mark Beattie Paediatric Medical Unit, Southampton General Hospital, Southampton, UK

Simon Beggs Program in Neurosciences and Mental Health, Hospital for Sick Children and University of Toronto, ON, Canada

John L. Belew Department of Nursing and Patient Services, Gillette Children's Specialty Healthcare, St Paul, MI, USA

F. Ralph Berberich Pediatric Medical Group, Berkeley, CA, USA

Amanda Bevan Paediatric Medical Unit, Southampton General Hospital, Southampton, UK

Kathryn A. Birnie Department of Psychology and Neuroscience, Dalhousie University, Halifax, NS, Canada

Katelynn E. Boerner Department of Psychology and Neuroscience, Dalhousie University, Halifax, NS, Canada

Karen R. Boretsky Perioperative Regional Anesthesia Service, Department of Anesthesiology, Perioperative and Pain Medicine, Boston Children's Hospital, MA, USA

Susanne Brummelte Department of Psychology, Wayne State University, Detroit, MI, USA

Norman Buckley Department of Anesthesia, Michael G DeGroote School of Medicine, McMaster University, Hamilton, ON, Canada

Mariana Bueno Department of Maternal-Child and Public Health, School of Nursing, Federal University of Minas Gerais, Belo Horizonte, Minas Gerais, Brazil

Fiona Campbell Department of Anesthesia and Pain Medicine, Hospital for Sick Children, University of Toronto, Toronto, ON, Canada

Lauren Campbell Department of Psychology, York University, Toronto, ON, Canada

Marsha Campbell-Yeo Department of Paediatrics, Division of Neonatal-Perinatal Medicine, IWK Health Centre and School of Nursing, Dalhousie University, Halifax, NS, Canada

Christine T. Chambers Departments of Pediatrics and Psychology, Dalhousie University and Centre for Pediatric Pain Research, IWK Health Centre, Halifax, NS, Canada

Kim Chau Division of Clinical Pharmacology & Toxicology, The Hospital for Sick Children and University of Toronto, Toronto, ON, Canada

Peter Chira Department of Pediatrics, Section of Pediatric Rheumatology, Indiana University, Riley Hospital for Children, IN, USA

Jill MacLaren Chorney Departments of Anesthesia, Pain Management and Perioperative Medicine and Psychology, Dalhousie University, and IWK Health Centre, Halifax, NS, Canada

Ignasi Clemente Department of Anthropology, Hunter College, City University of New York, NY, USA

Jacqui Clinch Department of Paediatric Rheumatology, Bristol Royal Hospital for Children, Bristol, UK

Rachael M. Coakley Departments of Anesthesia and Psychiatry, Boston Children's Hospital, Boston, MA, USA

Lindsey L. Cohen Department of Psychology, Georgia State University, Atlanta, GA, USA

John J. Collins Department of Pain Medicine and Palliative Care, The Children's Hospital at Westmead, Sydney, Australia

Penny Corkum Department of Psychology and Neuroscience Dalhousie University, Halifax, NS, Canada

Laura A. Cousins Department of Psychology, Georgia State University, Atlanta, GA, USA

Kenneth D. Craig Department of Psychology, University of British Columbia, Vancouver, BC, Canada

Joseph P. Cravero Department of Anesthesiology, Boston Children's Hospital, Boston, MA, USA

Carlton Dampier AFLAC Cancer and Blood Disorders Center, Children's Healthcare of Atlanta and Department of Pediatric, Emory University School of Medicine, Atlanta, GA, USA

Amanda Drews Deacy Division of Developmental and Behavioral Sciences, Children's Mercy Hospitals and Clinics, Kansas City, MO, USA

Bruce D. Dick Departments of Anesthesiology and Pain Medicine, Psychiatry, and Pediatrics, University of Alberta, Edmonton, AB, Canada

Pradeep Dinakar Department of Anesthesiology, Perioperative and Pain Medicine and Neurology, Boston Children's Hospital and Brigham and Women's Hospital, Harvard Medical School, Boston, MA, USA

Ross Drake Paediatric Palliative Care and Complex Pain Services, Starship Children's Hospital, Auckland District Health Board, Auckland, New Zealand

Mark Embrett Center for Health Economics and Policy Analysis, DeGroote School of Business, McMaster University, Hamilton, ON, Canada

Joyce M. Engel Department of Occupational Science and Technology, University of Wisconsin-Milwaukee, WI, USA

Miriam O. Ezenwa Department of Biobehavioral Health Science, College of Nursing, University of Illinois at Chicago, IL, USA

Maria Fitzgerald Developmental Neurobiology and Scientific Director of the Paediatric Pain Research Centre at UCL, London, UK

Paula Forgeron University of Ottawa, Faculty of Health Sciences, School of Nursing, Ottawa, ON, Canada

Craig A. Friesen Division of Gastroenterology, Hepatology, and Nutrition, Children's Mercy Hospitals and Clinics, Kansas City, MO, USA

Liesbet Goubert Department of Experimental-Clinical and Health Psychology, Ghent University, Ghent, Belgium

Ruth E. Grunau Department of Pediatrics, University of British Columbia, Developmental Neurosciences and Child Health, Child and Family Research Institute, Vancouver, BC, Canada

Denise Harrison Nursing Care of Children, Youth and Families, Children's Hospital of Eastern Ontario (CHEO) and University of Ottawa, ON, Canada

Gareth J. Hathway School of Biomedical Sciences, University of Nottingham, Nottingham, UK

Christiane Hermann Department of Clinical Psychology and Psychotherapy, Justus-Liebig University Giessen, Giessen, Germany

Andrew D. Hershey Neurology, Director, Headache Center, Cincinnati Children's Hospital Medical Center and Professor, Pediatrics and Neurology, University of Cincinnati, College of Medicine, Cincinnati, OH, USA

Jennifer Hickman Jane B. Pettit Pain Management Center, Children's Hospital of Wisconsin and Assistant Professor of Anesthesiology, Medical College of Wisconsin Milwaukee, WI, USA

Liisa Holsti Department of Occupational Science and Occupational Therapy, University of British Columbia, Vancouver, BC, Canada

Richard F. Howard Department of Anaesthesia and Pain Medicine, Great Ormond Street Hospital for Children NHS Trust, London, UK

Anna Huguet IWK Health Centre, Halifax, NS, Canada

Alison M. Hutchinson School of Nursing and Midwifery, Faculty of Health, Deakin University, Melbourne, Australia

Lindsay Jibb Division of Hematology and Oncology, Department of Pediatrics, Hospital for Sick Children, Toronto, ON, Canada

Celeste Johnston McGill Scientist, IWK Health Centre, Halifax, NS, Canada

Joel Katz Department of Psychology and School of Kinesiology & Health Science, York University, Toronto, ON, Canada

Maureen C. Kelley Department of Pediatrics, University of Washington School of Medicine, Seattle, WA USA

Robert M. (Bo) Kennedy Department of Pediatrics, Division of Emergency Medicine, Washington University in St. Louis School of Medicine, St. Louis, MI, USA

Sara King Mount Saint Vincent University, Halifax, NS, Canada

Gideon Koren Division of Clinical Pharmacology and Toxicology, Hospital for Sick Children and University of Toronto, Toronto, ON, Canada

Leora Kuttner Department of Paediatrics, BC Children's Hospital and University of British Columbia, Vancouver, BC, Canada

Marc R. Laufer Boston Children's Hospital, Gynecologist, Brigham and Women's Hospital and Professor of Obstetrics, Gynecology, and Reproductive Biology, Harvard Medical School, MA, USA

Chantal K. LeBlanc Child Life Services, IWK Health Centre, Halifax, NS, Canada

Grace Y. Lee Lawrence S. Bloomberg Faculty of Nursing, University of Toronto, ON, Canada

Christina Liossi School of Psychology, University of Southampton, Southampton, UK and Pain Control Service, Great Ormond Street Hospital for Children NHS Trust, London, UK

Deirdre E. Logan Departments of Anesthesia and Psychiatry, Boston Children's Hospital, Boston, MA, USA

Sarah R. Martin Department of Psychology, Georgia State University, Atlanta, GA, USA

Renée McCulloch Paediatric Palliative Care Consultant, Bayt Abdullah Children's Hospice, Kuwait City, State of Kuwait

Patrick J. McGrath Dalhousie University, Vice President Research, IWK Health Centre and Capital District Health Authority, Canada

C. Meghan McMurtry Department of Psychology, University of Guelph, ON, Canada

Martha Mherekumombe Department of Pain Medicine and Palliative Care, The Children's Hospital at Westmead, Sydney, Australia

Erin C. Moon Department of Psychology, British Columbia Children's Hospital, Vancouver, BC, Canada

Tim F. Oberlander Complex Pain Service, BC Children's Hospital; Professor, Department of Pediatrics, University of British Columbia, Vancouver, BC, Canada

Susan O'Conner-Von School of Nursing, Center for Children with Special Health Care Needs, University of Minnesota, Minneapolis, MN, USA

Deborah O'Rourke Department of Rehabilitation and Movement Science, University of Vermont, Burlington, VT, USA

M. Gabrielle Pagé PhD Candidate, Clinical Psychology, Department of Psychology, Faculty of Health, York University, Toronto, ON, Canada

Tonya M. Palermo Department of Anesthesiology and Pain Medicine, University of Washington, Seattle, WA, USA

Greta M. Palmer Department of Anaesthesia and Pain Management, Royal Children's Hospital and Murdoch Children's Research Institute, Melbourne, Australia and Associate Professor, University of Melbourne, Melbourne, Australia

Rebecca Pillai Riddell Department of Psychology, York University, Toronto, ON, Canada

Ravi Poorun Wellcome Trust MBPhD Student, The London Pain Consortium, Guy's, King's College, and St. Thomas' Hospitals Medical School, King's College London and Nuffield Department of Clinical Neurosciences University of Oxford, Oxford, UK

Nicole M. Racine Department of Psychology, York University, Toronto, ON, Canada

Sachin Rastogi Department of Anaesthesia and Pain Medicine, Royal Victoria Infirmary, Newcastle upon Tyne, UK

Susan L. Sager Department of Anesthesiology, Perioperative and Pain Medicine, Boston Children's Hospital, Boston, MA, USA

Michael L. Sangster Pediatric Complex Pain Service, IWK Health Centre, Halifax, NS, Canada

Laura E. Schanberg Department of Pediatrics, Duke University Medical Center, Durham, NC, USA

Neil L. Schechter Chronic Pain Program, Division of Pain Medicine, Department of Anesthesiology, Perioperative, and Pain Medicine, Boston Children's Hospital and Harvard Medical School, Boston, MA, USA

Jennifer Verrill Schurman Division of Developmental and Behavioral Sciences, Children's Mercy Hospitals and Clinics, Kansas City, MO, USA

Scott A. Schwantes Department of Paediatrics, Gillette Children's Specialty Healthcare, Saint Paul, MN, USA

Navil F. Sethna Mayo Family, Pediatric Pain Rehabilitation Center, Department of Anesthesiology, Perioperative and Pain Medicine, Boston Children's Hospital and Harvard Medical School, Boston Children's Hospital, MA, USA

Laura E. Simons Department of Anesthesiology, Perioperative and Pain Medicine, Boston Children's Hospital, Boston, MA, USA

Rebeccah Slater Department of Neuroscience, Physiology and Pharmacology, University College London, London, UK

Keith J. Slifer Pediatric Psychology Consultation Program, Department of Behavioral Psychology, Kennedy Krieger Institute and Johns Hopkins University School of Medicine, Baltimore, MD, USA

Bonnie J. Stevens Lawrence S. Bloomberg Faculty of Nursing, University of Toronto and Signy Hildur Eaton Chair in Paediatric Nursing Research, Senior Scientist, The Hospital for Sick Children, Toronto, ON, Canada

Jennifer Stinson Child Health Evaluative Sciences, The Hospital for Sick Children and Assistant Professor, Lawrence S. Bloomberg Faculty of Nursing, University of Toronto, Toronto, ON, Canada

Scott A. Strassels Department of Health Outcomes and Pharmacy Practice, University of Texas at Austin, Austin, TX, USA

Mary S. Swiggum Lynchburg College, Doctor of Physical Therapy Program, Lynchburg, VA, USA

Frank J. Symons Department of Educational Psychology, University of Minnesota, MN, USA

Anna Taddio Leslie Dan Faculty of Pharmacy, University of Toronto and Senior Associate Scientist, The Hospital for Sick Children, Toronto, ON, Canada

See Wan Tham Department of Anesthesiology and Pain Medicine, Seattle Children's Hospital, WA, USA

Dick Tibboel Erasmus MC, Sophia Children's Hospital, Rotterdam, the Netherlands

Susan M. Tupper Department of Pediatrics, University of Saskatchewan, Saskatoon, SK, Canada

Alison Twycross Department of Children's Nursing, London South Bank University, London, UK

Anita M. Unruh Faculty of Health Professions, Dalhousie University, Halifax, NS, Canada

Abraham J. Valkenburg Department of Pediatric Surgery, Erasmus University Medical Center-Sophia Children's Hospital, Rotterdam, the Netherlands

Jaya Varadarajan Jane B. Pettit Pain Management Center, Children's Hospital of Wisconsin and Medical College of Wisconsin Milwaukee, WI, USA

David Vega-Avelaira Departamento de Ciencias Biomédicas Básicas, Universidad Europea de Madrid, Madrid, Spain

Carl L. von Baeyer University of Saskatchewan, SK, Canada

Gary A. Walco University of Washington School of Medicine and Seattle Children's Hospital, Seattle, WA, USA

Suellen M. Walker Portex Unit, Pain Research and Department of Anaesthesia and Pain Medicine, UCL Institute of Child Health and Great Ormond St Hospital for Children NHS Foundation Trust, London, UK

Cynthia Maynard Ward Department of Behavioral Psychology, Kennedy Krieger Institute and Department of Psychiatry and Behavioral Sciences, Johns Hopkins University School of Medicine, Baltimore, MD, USA

Steven J. Weisman Jane B. Pettit, Children's Hospital of Wisconsin and Medical College of Wisconsin, Milwaukee, WI, USA

Joy A. Weydert Department of Pediatrics and Integrative Medicine, University of Kansas Medical Center, Kansas City, KS, USA

Anna C. Wilson Institute on Development and Disability, Department of Pediatrics, Oregon Health and Science University, Portland, OR, USA

Manisha Witmans Department of Pediatrics, University of Alberta, Edmonton, AB, Canada

Chantal Wood Pain and Palliative Centre, Robert Debré University Hospital, Paris, France

Janet Yamada The Hospital for Sick Children, Toronto, ON, Canada

Lonnie Zeltzer Pediatric Pain Program, Mattel Children's Hospital and David Geffen School of Medicine at the University of California at Los Angeles Los Angeles, CA USA

William T. Zempsky Connecticut Children's Medical Center, University of Connecticut School of Medicine, CT, USA

SECTION 1

Introduction

CHAPTER 1

History of pain in children

Anita M. Unruh and Patrick J. McGrath

Summary

The problem of pain has likely concerned humankind from the beginning as pain is a compelling call for attention and a signal to escape from its source. Early efforts to understand pain, and its origins, features, and treatment reflected the duality between spiritual conceptualizations of pain and physiological explanations depending on the predominance of such views in a given culture in any given historical period (McGrath and Unruh, 1987). In the absence of physiological or behavioural explanations to explain persistent pain without obvious injury, when spiritual perspectives dominated, prayer, amulets, supplication, and religious rites dominated approaches to pain treatment. Herbal remedies were often part of such strategies and might themselves have had potent properties (Unruh, 1992, 2007). In ancient writings about pain and disease, treatments for children were often given alongside discussions about the health issues of women. In this chapter, we trace early approaches to pain in children to the modern era highlighting points of transition and improvements in paediatric pain management.

A brief early history from ancient times to the mid nineteenth century

The earliest medical writings about the pain and diseases of children do not provide much information about symptoms of pain and disease in children but they do illustrate an understanding that children could not be treated medically as if they were adults. For example, the Atharva Veda of India (1500–800 BCE) provided paediatric incantations for headache, earache, and musculoskeletal pains (Garrison, 1923). The Susruta Samhita of India (second century BCE) gave dosages of drugs and herbal remedies for children separately from adults and advised administering them with milk, clarified butter, or in a plaster spread on the breasts of the nurse (Garrison, 1923). Hippocrates (about 460–357 BCE), Celsus (25 BCE–50 CE), Soranus (second century CE), Galen (130–200 CE), Oribasius (325–403 CE), Aurelianus (fifth century CE), Aetius (sixth century CE), and Aegineta (seventh century CE) all contributed to treatment of disease in infancy and childhood in their time period and beyond, in Greece and Rome, and in the Arab world. The Hippocratic writings of the fifth and fourth centuries BCE described constitutional differences between adults and children, and gave different doses of herbal remedies and means of administration

(Garrison, 1923; Still, 1931). Crying, restlessness, and sleeplessness were regarded as the primary symptoms of a child's pain and distress (Unruh, 1992).

One of the most reported pains of childhood prior to the eighteenth and nineteenth centuries was teething pain. The treatments for teething pain (Table 1.1) are fascinating to the modern reader and illustrate the underlying concern with which a child-specific pain was regarded throughout those centuries, and the ways in which remedies were passed down and modified over time. It was not uncommon for children to die in infancy and childhood when they were teething though illness and death were likely due to issues other than teething (McGrath and Unruh, 1987).

Determining whether a child was in pain was a challenge and not surprisingly generally determined by appeals to observation of changes in the child's behaviour. Aurelianus (fifth century CE) illustrates the emphasis on a child's behaviour as an indicator of pain:

> The child groans in its sleep, rolls about, gnashes its teeth, tends to lie prone, cries out suddenly, or falls silent, is seized with convulsions, sometimes becomes somnolent, the face becomes emaciated and loses its colour; the child gets cold and answers questions with difficulty; sometimes throws itself about with outstretched hands, working itself into perspiration. (Quoted in Garrison, 1923, p. 47)

Though changes in general behaviour were important, crying was usually regarded as the chief indicator of a child's pain. Some physicians, such as Omnibonus Ferrarius (1577) (an Italian physician), (Still 1931), and Starr (1895) and Holt (1897) (both American physicians), believed that children only cried if there was a reason associated with distress. Both Starr (1895) and Holt (1897, 1908) associated different features of cries with specific illnesses and severity of pain. For example, a sudden, very loud and paroxysmal shriek was described as hydrencephalic cry associated with headache (Starr, 1895, p. 6). Holt (1987) described acute pain as having a sharp and piercing cry that was usually accompanied by contracting facial features and drawing up the legs and sometimes falling into an exhausted sleep. He ascribed these pains to earache and colic. Starr (1895) may have been the first physician to describe facial expression of pain. He also used these features to identify the source of pain:

> The picture (of a healthy child) is altered by the onset of any illness, the change being in proportion to the severity of the attack. An expression of anxiety or suffering appears, or the features become pinched and the lines are seen about the eyes and mouth. Pain most of all sets its

Table 1.1 Historical treatments of children's teething pain

Source	Treatments
Soranus, 2nd century CE	'Before teething, the gums should be gently rubbed with oil or fats, and the child may be permitted to suck fat bacon without swallowing, but this should cease when the teeth appear. The gums should not be irritated by butter or acid substances, and if there is much inflammation, poulticing, and sponging are recommended' (quoted in Garrison, 1923, p. 46)
Oribasious, 325–403 CE	'If they are in pain, smear [the gums] with dog's milk or with hare's brain; this works also if eaten. But if a tooth is coming through with difficulty, smear cyperus with butter and oil-of-lilies over the part where it is erupting' (quoted in Still, 1931, p. 38)
Aetious, 6th century CE	'He advises the root of colocynth, hung on the child in a gold or silver case, or brambleroot, or the tooth of a viper, especially of a male viper, set in gold, or a green jasper suspended on the neck so as to hang down over the stomach' (quoted in Still, 1931, p. 40)
Rhazes, 859–932 CE	'And the treatment of it, when the gum is swollen, is that the gum should be rubbed a little with the finger, and afterwards with oil and hen's fat or hare's brain or dog's milk; and apply to the child's head water in which there have been boiled camomile and dill, and put plasters which have a dispersing effect on his jaws; and if the pain in the part increases after this, take butter and oil of laurels, mix together and apply over the part; or take cow's butter and marrow from the thigh, and apply; and if the points of the teeth have appeared, put over the whole head and neck clean wool, and let some tepid water be sprinkled on the wool each day' (quoted in Still 1931, pp. 46–47)
Avicenna, 980–1036 CE	'For burning pain in the gums apply oil and wax as an epitheme or use salted flesh which is a little "high"' (quoted in Gruner, 1930, p. 372)
Phaer, 1546 CE	'There be divers things that are good to procure as easy breeding of teeth, among them the chiefest is to anoint the gummes with the braynes of an hare nyxte with as much capons grece and hony, or any of these thynges alone is exceadynge good to supple the gummes and the synewes … And whan the peyne is greatte and intolerable with apostema or inflammacion of the gummes, it is good to make an ointment of oile of roses with the juyce of morelle otherwise called nightshade, and in lack of it annoint the jawes within with a little fresshe butter and honye' (quoted in Still, 1931, p. 121)
Sainte-Marthe, 1569 CE	'Hare's brain, honey and red coral ring as amulet' (cited in Ruhrah, 1925)
Ferrarius, 1577 CE	'A dead man's tooth in the opinion of some, through some particular virtue when hung on the neck of an infant, soothes and disperses the pain of teething' (quoted in Still, 1931, p. 156)
Primerose, 1659 CE	'Tooth of a dog, wolf or male viper hung around the neck to ease teething pain' (cited in Still, 1931)

mark upon the countenance, and by noting the features affected it is often possible to fix the seat of serious disease. Thus, contraction of the brow denotes pain in the head; sharpness of the nostrils, pain in the chest; and a drawing up of the upper lip, pain in the abdomen. (Starr 1895, pp. 3–4)

At least two surgical procedures, trepanation (a hole bored in the skull to treat headaches, mental illness, and convulsions) and circumcision, were performed on children in the ancient world throughout history (Liskowski, 1967). Other paediatric surgeries included repair of inguinal hernia, and harelip, tonsillectomy, and severance of the frenulum of the tongue (Mettler and Mettler, 1947). Opium, hyoscyamus, mandragora, and wine were used for pain relief during surgery (e.g. Celsus 25 BCE–50 CE and Avicenna 980–1036 CE) (McGrath and Unruh, 1987; Mettler and Mettler, 1947) but physical restraint was the more common approach. For children, surgical procedures were exceedingly painful and difficult for the patient and physician. Celsus' advice for the surgeon was:

A chirurgien must have a strong, stable and intrepid hand and a mind resolute and merciless; so that to heal him that he taketh in hand, he be not moved to make more haste than the thing requireth, or to cut less than is needful, but which doth all things as if he were nothing affected with their cries. (Quoted in Griffith, 1951, p. 127)

Children suffered when they had pain throughout this period (Newton, 2011). Although there is evidence that children were also cared about, and efforts made to manage their pain (McGrath and Unruh, 1987), it was anaesthesia that offered the first prospect of significant pain relief.

Early modern history starts with anaesthesia 1840–1950

The experience of pain was transformed by the development of anaesthesia in the nineteenth century. In 1842, Crawford Long used diethyl ether to excise a cyst from a patient's neck (Long, 1849), and then in 1846 William Morton gave a public demonstration of the use of ether for a dental procedure (Costarino and Downes, 2005). Children were involved in the earliest clinical applications of anaesthesia; the third patient who received ether from Long was an 8-year-old boy whose diseased toe was amputated on 8 July 1842 (Stewart, 1989). John Snow (1885), Queen Victoria's anaesthetist, started using diethyl ether for children in 1847 and 10 years later reported on his use of chloroform with several hundred children, 186 of whom were infants (Costarino and Downes, 2005). While children commonly received anaesthesia for surgery from the beginning, they were also perceived to have more problems associated with anaesthesia such as nausea and vomiting, hypotension, respiratory depression, and cardiac arrest, especially with chloroform (Costarino and Downes, 2005). The first recorded deaths due to anaesthesia occurred in children (Stewart, 1989). Some invasive procedures were considered so short or so minor that anaesthesia was thought not to be required. For example, Wharton (1895) did not consider a tracheotomy painful if there was marked dyspnoea, and thought that it was only the first incision that was painful. Similarly, Casselberry (1895) did not feel an anaesthetic was needed for a tonsillectomy because of the brevity of the procedure unless the adenoids were also to be removed. Pernick (1985) noted that procedures other than amputations of limbs were often considered minor.

In 1898, August Bier used cocaine to induce spinal anaesthesia in six patients, two of whom were children but he did not perceive spinal anaesthesia to be beneficial (Brown, 2012). By 1910, three papers had been published in *The Lancet* each referring to 100 or more paediatric cases in which spinal anaesthetics, rather than general anaesthesia, were used (Gray, 1909a, 1909b, 1910). Regional anaesthesia may have evolved due to the associated risks of general anesthesia in children but as paediatric general anaesthesia improved in the 1930s to 1950s, regional anaesthetics were less frequently used and are still not widespread (Brown, 2012).

The advancement of paediatric pain management during surgery was dependent on the development of anaesthetic agents, management of negative side effects of these agents, adequate training of physicians in the use of anaesthetics, and development of anaesthetic equipment that was appropriate for use with infants and children. Rendell-Baker (1992) described the historical evolution of paediatric anaesthesia equipment as having different developmental phases including: use of open drop mask for chloroform; introduction of tracheal intubation (beginning in 1909); development of various breathing systems (Magill's breathing system, Mapleson E T-piece breathing system, paediatric laryngoscopes, paediatric tracheal tubes, the Crowe–Davis mouth gag, the laryngeal mask airway); design of cyclopropane and carbon dioxide absorption systems (non-rebreathing valves); the T-piece system; specialization of paediatric anaesthesia as a medical subspecialty; use of halothane and low-dead space paediatric face masks and related equipment; introduction of standard breathing systems; and use of constant positive airway pressure and intermittent mandatory ventilation. The first paediatric anaesthetic textbook, *Anaesthesia in Children* by Langton Hewer, appeared in 1923, with a second textbook, Leigh and Belton's *Pediatric Anesthesia*, available in 1948.

The primary advantage of anaesthesia was the relief of pain with the secondary effect of permitting increasingly more complex (and invasive) surgical procedures. At the outset, in its earliest period, the beneficiaries were most likely to be women, white people, young children, and people from upper and middle classes (Jackson Rees, 1991). Children were viewed as more sensitive to pain, and more difficult to control if they were anxious and fearful about the procedure (Pernick, 1985). But with respect to the pain experience of infants, there was disagreement about the best approach. On the one hand, there were those physicians, like Eliza Thomas (1849), who regarded infants as hypersensitive to pain (cited in Pernick, 1985). There were other physicians whose views resonated with Henry Bigelow (1848) who wrote: 'The fact that it [infant] has neither the anticipation nor the remembrance of suffering, however severe, seems to render this stage of narcoticism [full anesthesia] unnecessary' (quoted in Pernick 1985, p. 172). Stewart (1989) wrote that infants were considered ideal patients for surgery by some because they were considered relatively insensitive to pain, unable to appreciate it, and even capable of sleeping through the surgery. In 1938, Thorek wrote: 'Often no anesthesia is required. A sucker consisting of a sponge dipped in some sugar will often suffice to calm a baby' (p. 2021).

This view of relative insensitivity to pain in infants seemed to be supported by studies that endeavoured to elicit pain. In 1917, Blanton reported on studies of the response of infants to procedures such

as blood draws, lancing of infections, and exposure to pin pricks during sleep. She observed crying and defensive escape behaviour but reported them as complex and advanced, reflexive and instinctive behaviours. In 1941, McGraw used pin pricks to examine the maturation of nerves in 75 children from infancy to 4 years. She maintained that the diffuse body movements of neonates with crying reflected a limited sensitivity to pain in the first 2 weeks of life and that it was unlikely for there to be any neural mediation above the thalamus.

But there continued to be opposing points of view. Charles Robson, anaesthetist at the Hospital for Sick Children in Toronto, perhaps the first paediatric anaesthesiologist (Mai and Yaster, 2011), vehemently rejected outright assumptions about infant insensitivity to pain:

> First, it has been stated that infants under seven days of age do not require anesthetics for operations—that their association tracts for pain are not fully established and that minor operations may be carried out without any damaging effects on the infant. Personally I do not believe this and it is simply vivisection to operate on a conscious screaming wriggling infant without using a general or local anesthetic. (Robson, 1925, p. 235)

Robson used open-drop ether and cyclopropane along with tracheal intubation for infant anaesthesia (Mai and Yaster, 2011).

Views such as Robson's were probably in the minority. There is little discussion about pain in early textbooks about paediatric anaesthesia, not even with respect to neonates. Smith's *The Physiology of the Newborn Infant* (1945) did not mention pain at all. Leight and Belton (1948) made only one substantive comment about pain:

> Newborn infants are not as sensitive to pain and some degree of analgesia is present without anesthetic. Most infants, however, do have some pain sensation even at birth and one cannot rely on the old adage that there is no pain sensation for the first three weeks of life. It is nearer the truth to say that sensitivity to pain is decreased. Since there is some basic analgesia, very low concentrations of anesthetic agent will produce complete analgesia. (p. 30)

By the mid twentieth century, the prevailing view, that infants had reduced sensitivity to pain, provided an accepted position for the use of minimal anaesthesia for surgery on infants. In the 1950s, Gordon Jackson Rees in Liverpool, England, introduced an approach that came to be known as the Liverpool technique. He modified a part of the paediatric anaesthetic equipment to permit better monitoring of respiratory movements of anaesthetized children and provide intermittent ventilation if needed (Costarino and Downes, 2005). He also introduced curare and other relaxants into practice and nitrous oxide and oxygen anaesthesia without ether (Jackson Rees, 1960). In his 1950 discussion about anaesthesia in the newborn, Jackson Rees argued that the newborn was substantially different from an adult in neuromuscular structure and physiology (mechanical differences, sensitivity of the respiratory system, muscle tone). While he supported using muscle relaxants to reduce the amount of anaesthetic agents, he believed that control of respiration was possible with light anaesthesia without muscle relaxants for infants because of these structural and physiological differences. He believed the 'operative risk' to full-term infants was slight because fetal cord blood levels of corticosteroids at birth paralleled those of the mother, hence surgical trauma was less at birth but then increased rapidly during the first week of life. The optimum operative period was regarded by Jackson Rees (1950) to be the first 24 hours of life. Jackson Rees (1950) noted that Leigh and Belton

(1948) had suggested premedication with morphine for very young infants with morphine but believed it was generally not necessary:

> This treatment appears to facilitate the smooth maintenance of anesthesia, and would seem to be desirable if respiration is not to be aided or controlled. It does, however, make the induction of anesthesia by inhalation agents—a tedious process at best—a very prolonged procedure. (p. 1421)

In his 1960 paper, Jackson Rees discussed in some detail the anaesthetic complications of paediatric anaesthesia such as the tendency for infants under 6 months to become hypothermic in response to anaesthesia whereas older infants became hyperthermic. Hypothermia was more readily managed but hyperthermia sometimes led to convulsions and death. Ether anaesthesia and atropine premedication contributed to this risk. In summarizing his views, Jackson Rees (1960) wrote:

> The respiratory deficiencies of the infant during early life and the hazards of hyperthermia in older children suggest that controlled ventilation during the maintenance of anaesthesia has special advantages. It should be regarded as an essential part of the technique for prolonged operations, and is highly desirable for shorter procedures. Anesthesia can be maintained at very light levels with nitrous oxide-oxygen and a relaxant drug, with the result that recovery is rapid…. There are, therefore, cogent practical and theoretical reasons for maintaining anaesthesia with controlled ventilation, a relaxant drug, nitrous oxide and oxygen. (p. 138–139)

Although Jackson Rees is said to have introduced nitrous oxide and oxygen anaesthesia without ether, it had already been in use for some years in the US by some physicians. Mary Botsford in San Francisco (1935) reported using this preparation over a 2-year period for children from 1 month to 4 years of age for procedures of 4 minutes to 1 hour and 40 minutes. However, for the youngest infants, Botsford regarded ether as the anaesthetic of choice. Botsford also noted that by the 1930s, chloroform had been almost completely discontinued for infants and children because of deleterious effects on the liver, cardiac depression, and postoperative acidosis. In the discussion section of Botsford's paper, where responses were provided from colleagues, two writers, Weeks and Delprat, commented, 'We are glad to see that she still allows us to use ether in babies, even though she so strongly favours nitrous oxid[e] and oxygen'. Weeks and Delprat maintained that for abdominal surgery nitrous oxide and oxygen provided too little relaxation of the tissues, and they were prepared to risk a less safe anaesthetic (ether).

Nitrous oxide and oxygen anaesthesia with a muscle relaxant was considered for many years a light anaesthetic that was sufficient for many paediatric procedures. It appeared to reduce a number of surgical risks, especially for infants, based on the knowledge in this period of the physiology of infants and children. Although there were some efforts to understand the responses of the paediatric patient to surgical procedures, evidence of informed decision-making was typically on the basis of published clinical series. Such papers provided clinical information but very limited data about an infant's physiological stress response to invasive procedures. Paediatric pain research during this period was limited and focused on the first epidemiological studies and not clinical care.

Scientific approaches to pain in children

The second half of the twentieth century can rightly be considered the modern era of paediatric pain research and management. Major developments occurred that brought scientific thinking to the area and widespread realization in the health system that paediatric pain was an important issue. Development of the field of paediatric pain was, and continues to be, uneven. Even in developed countries, the provision of services is not at all uniform. In the developing world, paediatric pain research is just beginning (e.g. Forgeron et al., 2009). Advances in science have not always resulted in advances in implementation of care. There were significant landmark events that led to the modern era of paediatric pain.

Recurrent pain in children certainly was known and written about earlier (e.g. Matthews, 1938), but programmes of research about pain in children developed primarily in post-war Europe. The seminal work in headache was by Bo Vahlquist (Vahlquist, 1955; Vahlquist and Hackzell, 1949) and later by his protégé Bo Bille (1962) in Sweden. Vahlquist defined criteria for diagnosis of headache in children and presented clinical series and described common features. Bille's doctoral dissertation, published as a monograph in *Acta Pediatrica*, was a large-scale epidemiological study of the children of Uppsala. He described the prevalence and correlates of migraine and provided a more detailed set of lab studies and interviews with a subgroup of children who had pronounced migraine. Bille personally followed the group of 73 children with pronounced migraine for 40 years (Bille 1997). This work was foundational for all subsequent studies of migraine and other headaches in children and adolescents.

John Apley and colleague (Naish and Apley, 1951) in Bristol, England, published epidemiological research on recurrent limb pains demonstrating that about 4% of children had such pain. This paper was followed by his groundbreaking epidemiological and aetiological studies on recurrent abdominal pain (Apley, 1959). Apley found that recurrent abdominal pain was common, affecting10.8% of children. Girls were more likely to have recurrent abdominal pain than boys. He linked recurrent abdominal pain to psychosocial problems and argued that overmedicalization of recurrent pain led to long-term consequences. Apley's studies still inform our understanding of recurrent limb and abdominal pain. While these studies on recurrent pains in children were well known in the paediatric literature, and stimulated clinical practice, they did not trigger much systematic research interest until the 1980s.

In 1965, Melzack and Wall introduced an imaginative and comprehensive theory, known as the gate control theory of pain, to account for horrific injuries that sometimes were not felt as pain, and minor injuries that were sometimes felt as severe pain. They used recently discovered physiological data and clinical data to suggest that a mechanism in the substantia gelatinosa of the dorsal horn of the spinal cord gated sensations of pain from pain receptors before they were interpreted or reacted to as pain. This theory changed how pain was conceptualized and united clinical observations with physiology. Although not specifically describing mechanisms of action for the role of attention, thoughts, and emotions in pain, Melzack and Wall included these phenomena by hypothesizing a central control trigger that could mediate specific central activities. The development of modern models of pain increased interest in pain research and in the integration of clinical observation with the biology of pain.

But drawing attention specifically to pain in children did not come easily. Interest was sporadic and research still almost nonexistent. Jo Eland was the first North American clinician scientist to bring pain in children to the forefront. In 1971, she was a faculty member supervising students on a paediatric oncology unit in Omaha, Nebraska. Children were typically diagnosed late, received ineffective treatment, and died in pain with little pain relief. In her President's Message at the American Society of Pain Management Nurses in 2012, Eland said of this experience:

> Watching so many children die in unrelieved pain caused me to begin reading everything I could about pain and soon found there was virtually nothing written about pediatric pain. The memories of so many children dying in unrelieved pain left a lasting impression that has never left me. (Reproduced with kind permission of Jo Eland)

Eland and Anderson (1977) noted that only 33 scientific articles had been published on pain in children by the mid 1970s and most of these papers were on paediatric recurrent pain. Their own important contribution to paediatric pain was a comparative chart review of the pain relief given to adults and children following similar surgical procedures. In the review of 25 children, aged 4–8 years, 21 children had been ordered analgesics but only 12 received any medication. Eighteen of the children were then matched with adults receiving similar surgery. The adult group were given 372 opioid analgesic doses and 299 non-opioid pain doses. There were methodological limitations to this review as a study: it was not experimentally well controlled, it used questionable matching, and did not measure pain. It is unknown whether the data from the adult sample came from a similar time period to that of the children or from the same institution. Nevertheless, the difference in the provision of pain relief between child and adult patients was startling and overwhelming in illustrating that children and adults were not treated similarly for pain. This study triggered two methodologically superior studies with similar though less extreme results. Beyer and colleagues (1983) compared 50 children with 50 adults on the postoperative analgesia they received following similar cardiac surgeries. The only patients who were not prescribed any analgesics at all were six children. Overall children received less than 50% of the analgesic doses given to adults. Schechter et al. (1986) reviewed charts for the postoperative analgesics received by 90 children and 90 adults who were randomly selected and matched for sex and diagnosis. Adults received an average of 2.2 doses of opioids narcotics per day, whereas children received half this amount. It is unknown whether the children in these studies were in more pain than adults, as pain was not measured. Nevertheless, these three studies critically established that children's pain was significantly undertreated in hospitals.

Along with these early studies which identified the problem of recurrent pains, abdominal pain, and headache in childhood, and undertreatment of postoperative pain in children, work was beginning to untangle the cry of infants, crying long being regarded as symptomatic of pain and distress in infants. In the 1960s, auditory and spectographic cry analysis of infants was systematized by Ole Wasz-Höckert and colleagues in Finland (Wasz-Höckert et al., 1968). This work was sophisticated and well respected, and dealt with pain and other types of cries, but did not influence the investigation of pain outside of cry analysis.

The most seminal developments to draw attention to pain in infants and children were two events in the 1980s. The first was a series of studies by Kanwaljeet Singh Anand as a PhD student at Oxford University. With support from a Rhodes Scholarship and the John Radcliffe Hospital, Anand began one of the first research programmes on pain in neonates. Anand developed sophisticated methods of measuring hormonal stress responses using very small samples of blood (Anand et al., 1985). He then demonstrated in clinical series and well-controlled, randomized trials, that term and preterm neonates mounted a major stress response following surgery for patent ductus repair (Anand and Hickey, 1987; Anand et al., 1987, 1988, 1990). These studies showed that neonates receiving minimal anaesthetic, the 'Liverpool' technique that had been standard care since the 1950s, compared to neonates receiving halothane anaesthesia, had significantly elevated levels of plasma epinephrine, norepinephrine, cortisol, glucagon, beta endorphins, and insulin, and as well as increased mortality in the postoperative period.

Anand's research was well received in the academic community. Anand won the 1986 Dr Michael Blacow prize for the best paper by a trainee at the annual meeting of the British Paediatric Society (Royal College of Paediatrics and Child Health, n. d.). For the public, the realization that infants were exposed to surgery with minimal anaesthesia came as a profound shock and was met with initial disbelief. In the media, Anand was viciously attacked in the *Daily Mail* (UK newspaper) in a story titled 'Pain killer shock in babies operation' (*Daily Mail*, 1987). Anand and colleagues were accused of experimenting on babies by withholding anaesthesia. The All Party Parliamentary Pro Life Group demanded that the General Medical Council investigate these experiments. Many distinguished medical scientists insisted that these studies were ethical, and methodologically rigorous challenges of then current standard of anaesthetic procedure for infants undergoing surgery, and would lead to better care. In 1988, Sir Bernard Braine, head of the All Party Group publicly apologized for his accusations (Anonymous, 1988).

The second seminal event was related to Anand's work but occurred in the US and was not research but one family's experience. Like Anand's research, the story of Jeffrey Lawson focused on neonatal anaesthesia and it too was debated in the public arena through the media. Jeffrey Lawson was born in February 1985, at 25–26 weeks gestational age, weighing 760 grams, and was admitted to the Washington National Children's Hospital for treatment of patent ductus arteriosus—a not uncommon problem in a premature infant. The ductus arteriosus is a blood vessel that permits blood to circulate through the baby's lungs before birth, closing a few days after birth. A patent ductus arteriosus leads to abnormal blood flow between the aorta and pulmonary artery, two major blood vessels that carry blood from the heart. After some medical attempts to correct this condition, Jeffrey Lawson underwent open heart surgery to correct this abnormality. His mother described Jeffrey's anaesthesia during the surgery in this way:

> Jeffrey was awake through it all. The anesthesiologist paralyzed him with pavulon, a drug that left him unable to move, but totally conscious. When I questioned the anesthesiologist later she said Jeffrey was too sick to tolerate powerful anesthetics. Anyway, she said, it had never been demonstrated to her that premature babies feel pain. (Lawson, 1986, pp. 124–125)

Following surgery, Jeffrey went into shock, catabolized, and suffered heart, kidney, and liver failure. He died on 31 March 1985, 5 weeks following surgery. Ms Lawson contacted many professional and social service agencies and other individuals to support her belief that babies should receive pain control for surgical procedures before her story was picked up by the media.

In writing the story of Jeffrey Lawson for *The Washington Post*, Sandy Rovner quoted Willis McGill, Chair of Anesthesia at the

Children's Hospital National Medical Centre. Dr McGill asserted that there were risks with anaesthesia and that 'it doesn't do any good to have a dead patient who doesn't feel pain' (Rovner, 1986, p. 7). The article in *The Washington Post* triggered other coverage emphasizing that babies were undergoing surgery without anaesthesia. The American Society of Anaesthesiologists (1987) and the American Academy of Pediatrics (1987) asserted that anaesthesia should not be routinely withheld from neonates. In 1996, the American Pain Society established the Jeffrey Lawson Award for Advocacy in Children's Pain Relief to honour Jeffrey Lawson and the contribution of his mother to the advancement of pain in infants and children.

The Anand story in England and the Lawson case in the US were compelling. They were followed by a dramatic increase in professional and scientific interest in pain in children. Between 1981 and 1990, there were 2966 articles on paediatric pain with a striking increase occurring in the 1980s (Guardiola and Baños, 1993) and an upsurge in articles on pain in neonates (Baños et al., 2001). Books on some specific pains in childhood, such as Apley's book on abdominal pain (1959), had already appeared, but now, the first books covering the broad area of childhood pain were published (Table 1.2). Most of these books have been directed to health professionals but some focused on helping parents to manage their children's pain (Table 1.3).

Table 1.2 Books for health professionals on pain in infants, children, or adolescents

Author(s)	Title	Year
Ross and Ross	*Childhood pain: Current issues, research and treatment*	1988
McGrath	*Pain in children: Nature, assessment, and treatment*	1989
Schechter and Berde	*Pain in infants, children and adolescents*	1993
Kuttner	*A child in pain: How to help, what to do*	1997
Yaster et al.	*Pediatric pain management and sedation handbook*	1997
Finley and McGrath (eds)	*Measurement of pain in infants and children*	1998
Dahlquist	*Pediatric pain management*	1999
Finley and McGrath	*Acute and procedure pain in infants and children*	2001
Anand et al. (eds)	*Pain in neonates and infants (three editions)*	2002, 2004, 2007
McGrath and Finley	*Pediatric pain: Biological and social contexts*	2003
Tobias and Deshpande	*Pediatric pain management for primary care (2nd edn)*	2004
Finley et al. (eds)	*Bringing pain relief to children: Treatment approaches*	2006
Oberlander	*Pain in children and adults with developmental disabilities*	2006
Rogers	*Managing persistent pain in adolescents*	2008
Walco and Goldschneider (eds)	*Pain in children: A guide for primary care*	2008
Twycross et al. (eds)	*Managing pain in children*	2009
Kuttner	*A child in pain: What health professionals can do to help*	2010
McClain and Suresh (eds)	*Handbook of pediatric chronic pain: Current science and integrative practice*	2011
Oakes	*Compact clinical guide to infant and child pain management: An evidence-based approach for nurses*	2011
Chambers et al.	*Pediatric pain: A clinical casebook*	2012
Palermo	*CBT for chronic pain in children and adolescents*	2012

Table 1.3 Books for parents on managing children's pain

Author(s)	Title	Year
Finley and Turner	*Making cancer less painful: A handbook for parents*	1992
McGrath et al.	*Pain, pain go away: Helping children with pain*	1994
Kuttner	*A child in pain: How to help, What to do*	1997
Krane and Sinberg	*Relieve your child's chronic pain: A doctor's program for easing headaches, abdominal pain, fibromyalgia, juvenile rheumatoid arthritis, and more*	2005
Zeltzer and Schlank	*Conquering your child's chronic pain: A pediatrician's guide to reclaiming a normal childhood*	2005

The International Association for the Study of Pain established a Special Interest Group on Pain in Childhood (<http://www.child-pain.org>) in the 1980s. One of its activities is the International Symposium on Pediatric Pain (<http://childpain.org/ispp.shtml>), the first was held in Seattle in 1988. The PEDIATRIC-PAIN electronic discussion list began in the 1990s (PEDIATRIC-PAIN@lists.dal.ca>). At present it has over 800 members and remains an active discussion forum. The Pediatric Pain Letter (<http://www.childpain.org.ppl>) began in 1996. The International Pediatric Pain Forum is another paediatric pain meeting. It is held every 2–3 years on a focused theme (<http://pediatric-pain.ca/content/IFPP>).

It is difficult to know how much of this increased attention on children's pain was due to the public attention and debate that surrounded the research of Anand, or the tragic story of Jeffrey Lawson. The research in this area was gaining sufficient momentum for the first paediatric pain books to appear and the first paediatric pain conference to be held. Nevertheless, there is no doubt that these events highlighted in undeniable ways the assumptions and misconceptions that prevailed and persisted in children's pain, their serious potential for harm, and lent urgency to the need for change.

The contributions of modern science to paediatric pain and the future

Science relies on assessment and measurement. Until the last three decades of the twentieth century, measurement of children's pain relied on unstandardized, largely descriptive approaches to determine whether a child was in pain. Empirical research confirmed that an infant's cry due to distress had specific spectrographic properties (Wasz-Höckert et al., 1968), and that cries due to pain, hunger, and fear could be distinguished from each other by trained observers and by spectrographic analysis (Anand and Hickey, 1987). Moreover, there are behavioural and spectrographic differences in the pain cries of healthy full-term neonates, preterm neonates, and neonates with neurological impairments (Anand and Hickey, 1987). Facial characteristics of a child in pain, the features noted by Starr in 1895 with respect to the brow, the nostrils, and the upper lip, are characteristics of the pain face now captured in paediatric pain measures such as the Neonatal Facial Action Coding System (Grunau and Craig, 1987). In the 1970s and 1980s, the first self-report measures of pain were developed and later, self-report measures based on facial characteristics—e.g. the Faces Pain Scale (Bieri et al., 1990) and the Faces Pain Scale—Revised (Hicks et al., 2001). In addition, observational measures of children's pain behaviour, particularly in the postoperative context, were constructed and validated. Measures were also developed for children with developmental disabilities and for pain in infants. Such tools provided the capacity to measure the effectiveness of pain intervention for infants, children, and adolescents. Much of this work is reviewed in the books mentioned in Table 1.2 and in Section 5 of this book.

In addition to pain measurement, attention was drawn to special areas of pain in infants, children, and adolescents and its treatment such as in burns, procedural pain, cancer pain, arthritis, and so on. There was greater appreciation of the immediate and long-term consequences of pain in childhood due to physical and sexual abuse. In the last 10 years there has been a more solid focus on the social and cultural context of children's pain and the role of parents in children's learning about pain. A great deal of work has focused on children's pain in the Western world. Recently, researchers have come to recognize that the pain of children in underdeveloped countries is even more greatly challenged by the lack of education about child pain and limited or no access to appropriate pain management.

Only fools try to predict the future but some emerging trends are evident. There will certainly be greater advances in our understanding of the biomedical, social, cultural, clinical, and health systems science of pain in children. The yet to be resolved problem of insufficient access to scientifically demonstrated treatments for pain for infants, children, and adolescents is slowly being recognized, and is leading to new ways of developing interventions such as Web-based alternatives (see Stinson and Jibb, Chapter 55, this volume). The need for personalized approaches to care is being understood. But will all of our progress in science make a difference in practice? Will the financial crisis that is gripping many parts of the world lead to less care for the most vulnerable who have the least ability to demand better care? Will there be better solutions to the inadequate management of pain in children in all parts of the world? We need to consider and take responsibility for narrowing the gap between the generation of evidence and its application in the real world where pain occurs.

Acknowledgements

McGrath's research is supported by grants from the Canadian Institutes of Health Research and his Canada Research Chair. This chapter is based on previous publications including McGrath (2011), McGrath and Unruh (1987), and (Unruh, 1992).

References

American Academy of Pediatrics Committee on Fetus and Newborn, Committee on Drugs, Section on Anesthesiology, Section on Surgery. (1987). Neonatal anesthesia. *Pediatrics*, 80, 446.

American Pain Society, Jeffrey Lawson Award for Advocacy in Children's Pain Relief. Available at: <http://www.americanpainsociety.org/about-aps/awards/jeffrey-lawson-award-past-award-winners.html>.

American Society of Anesthesiologists. (1987). Neonatal anesthesia. *ASA Newsletter*, December 15, p. 2.

Anand, K. J., Brown, M. J., Bloom, S. R., and Aynsley-Green, A. (1985). Studies on the hormonal regulation of fuel metabolism in the human newborn infant undergoing anaesthesia and surgery. *Horm Res*, 22(1–2), 115–128.

Anand, K. J., Hansen, D. D., and Hickey, P. R. (1990). Hormonal-metabolic stress response in neonates undergoing cardiac surgery. *Anesthesiology*, 73, 661–670.

Anand, K. J. and Hickey, P. R. (1987). Pain and its effects in the human neonate and fetus. *N Engl J Med*, 317(21), 1321–1329.

Anand, K. J., Sippell, W. G., and Aynsley-Green, A. (1987). Randomized trial of fentanyl anesthesia in preterm neonates undergoing surgery: effects on the stress response. *Lancet*, 1, 243–248.

Anand, K. J., Sippell, W. G., Schofield, N. M., and Aynsley-Green, A. (1988). Does halothane anesthesia decrease the metabolic and endocrine stress responses of newborn infants undergoing operation? *Br Med J*, 296, 668–672.

Anand, K. J. S., Stevens, B. J., and McGrath, P. J. (2007). *Pain in neonates and infants* (3rd edn). Amsterdam: Elsevier.

Anonymous. (1987). Pain killer shock in babies' operations. *Daily Mail*, July 28.

Anonymous. (1988). MP apologizes. *Br Med J*, 297, 865.

Apley, J. (1959). *The child with abdominal pains*. Springfield, IL: Charles C. Thomas.

Baños, J. E., Ruiz, G., and Guardiola, E. (2001). An analysis of articles on neonatal pain published from 1965 to 1999. *Pain Res Manag*, 6(1), 45–50.

Beyer, J. E., DeGood, D. E., Ashley, L. C., and Russell, G. A. (1983). Patterns of postoperative analgesic use with adults and children following cardiac surgery. *Pain*, 17(1), 71–81.

Bieri, D., Reeve, R., Champion, G. D., Addicoat, L., and Ziegler, J. (1990). The Faces Pain Scale for the self-assessment of the severity of pain experienced by children: Development, initial validation and preliminary investigation for ratio scale properties. *Pain*, 41, 139–150.

Bille, B. (1962). Migraine in school children. A study of the incidence and short-term prognosis, and a clinical, psychological and electroencephalographic comparison between children with migraine and matched controls. *Acta Paediatr Suppl*, 136, 1–151.

Bille, B. (1997). A 40-year follow-up of school children with migraine. *Cephalalgia*, 17(4), 488–491.

Blanton, M. G. (1917). The behaviour of the human infant in the first 30 days of life. *Psychol Rev*, 24, 456–483.

Botsford, M. E. (1935). Anesthesia in infant surgery. *Cal West Med*, 43(4), 271–273.

Brown, T. C. K. (2012). History of pediatric regional anesthesia. *Pediatr Anesth*, 22, 3–9.

Casselberry, W. E. (1895). Diseases of pharynx and the nasopharynx. In: L. Starr and T. S. Westcott (eds) *An American text-book of the diseases of children*, pp. 431–456. Philadelphia, PA: Saunders.

Chambers, C., Finley, G. A., and McGrath, P. J. (2012). *Pediatric pain: a clinical casebook*. Totowa, NJ: Humana.

Costarino, A. T. and Downes, J. T. (2005). Pediatric anesthesia historical perspective. *Anesthesiol Clin North America*, 23, 573–595.

Dahlquist, L. M. (1999). *Pediatric pain management*. New York: Plenum Press.

Eland, J. M. and Anderson, J. E. (1977). The experience of pain in children. In: A. Jacox (ed.) *Pain: a source-book for nurses and other health care professionals*, pp. 453–478. Boston, MA: Little, Brown & Co.

Finley, G. A. and McGrath, P. J. (1998). *Measurement of pain in infants and children*. Seattle, WA: IASP Press.

Finley, G. A. and McGrath, P. J. (2001). *Acute and procedure pain in infants and children*. Seattle, WA: IASP Press.

Finley, G. A., McGrath, P. J., and Chambers, C. T. (eds) (2006). *Bringing pain relief to children: treatment approaches*. Totowa, NJ: Humana Press.

Forgeron, P. A., Jongudomkarn, D., Evans, J., Finley, G. A., Thienthong, S., Siripul, P., *et al.* (2009). Children's pain assessment in northeastern Thailand: perspectives of health professionals. *Qual Health Res* 19(1), 71–81.

Garrison, F. H. (1923). *A system of pediatrics*. Philadelphia, PA: Saunders.

Gray, H. T. (1909a). A study of spinal anesthesia in children and infants. *Lancet*, 2, 913–917.

Gray, H. T. (1909b). A study of spinal anesthesia in children and infants. *Lancet*, 2, 991–996.

Gray, H. T. (1910). A further study on spinal anesthesia in children and infants. *Lancet*, 2, 1611–1616.

Griffith, E. F. (1951). *Doctors by themselves: an anthology*. London: Cassell.

Grunau, R. and Craig, K. (1987). Pain expression in neonates: facial action and cry. *Pain*, 28, 395–410.

Gruner, O. C. (1930). *A treatise on the canon of medicine of Avicenna incorporating a translation of the first book*. London: Luzac.

Guardiola, E. and Baños, J. E. (1993). Is there an increasing interest in pediatric pain? Analysis of the biomedical articles published in the 1980s. *J Pain Symptom Manag*, 8(7), 449–450.

Hewer, C. L. (1923). *Anaesthesia in children*. New York: Paul B. Hober.

Hicks, C. L., von Baeyer, C. L., Spafford, P., van Korlaar, I., and Goodenough, B. (2001). The Faces Pain Scale—Revised: toward a common metric in pediatric pain measurement. *Pain*, 93, 173–183.

Holt, L. E. (1897). *The diseases of infancy and childhood: for the use of students and practitioners of medicine*. New York: Appleton.

Holt, L. E. (1908). *The care and feeding of children. a catechism for the use of mothers and children's nurses* (4th edn). London: Appleton.

Jackson Rees, G. (1950). Anaesthesia in the newborn. *Br Med J*, 23, 1419–1422.

Jackson Rees, G. (1960). Paediatric anaesthesia. *Br J Anaesth*, 32, 132–40.

Jackson Rees, G. (1991). An early history of paediatric anaesthesia. *Paediatr Anaesthes*, 1, 3–11.

Krane, E. J. and Sinberg, L. (2005). *Relieve your child's chronic pain: a doctor's program for easing headaches, abdominal pain, fibromyalgia, juvenile rheumatoid arthritis, and more*. New York: Fireside.

Kuttner, L. (1997). *A child in pain: how to help, what to do*. Vancouver, BC: Hartley & Marks.

Kuttner, L. (2010). *A child in pain: what health professionals can do to help*. Bancyfelin, Wales: CrownHouse.

Lawson, J. R. (1986). Letter. *Birth*, 13, 124–125.

Lawson, J. R. (1988). Standards of practice and the pain of premature infants. *Zero to Three*, 9, 1–5.

Leigh, M. D. and Belton, M. K. (1948). *Pediatric anaesthesiology*. New York: Macmillan.

Liskowski, F. P. (1967). Prehistoric and early history of trepanation. In: D. Brothwell and A. T. Sandison (eds) *Diseases of antiquity: a survey of the diseases, injuries and surgery of early populations*, pp. 651–667. Springfield, IL: Charles T. Thomas.

Long, C. W. (1849). An account of the first use of sulphuric ether by inhalation as an anesthetic in surgical operation. *South Med Surg J*, 5, 705–713.

Mai, C. M. and Yaster, M. (2011). Pediatric anesthesia: a historical perspective. *Am Soc Anesthesiol*, 75, 10–13.

Matthews, J. S. (1938). Recurrent abdominal pain in children. *Ulster Med J*, 7(3), 179–206.

McClaine, B. C. and Suresh, S. (2011). *Handbook of pediatric chronic pain: current science and integrative practice*. New York: Springer.

McGrath, P. A. (1989). *Pain in children: nature, assessment, and treatment*. New York: Guilford Press.

McGrath, P. J. (2011). Science is not enough: the modern history of pediatric pain. *Pain*, 152, 2457–2459.

McGrath, P. J. and Finley, G. A. (2003). *Pediatric pain: biological and social contexts*. Seattle, WA: IASP Press.

McGrath, P. J., Finley, G. A., Ritchie, J. A., and Dowden, S. J. (2003). *Pain, pain go away: helping children with pain* (2nd edn). Available at: <http://www.rch.org.au/emplibrary/anaes/Pain_go_away.pdf>.

McGrath, P. J., Finley, G. A., and Turner, C. (1992). *Making cancer less painful*. Available at: <http://is.dal.ca/~pedpain/mclp/.html>.

McGrath, P. J. and Unruh, A. M. (1987). *Pain in children and adolescents*. Amsterdam: Elsevier.

McGraw, M. (1941). Neural maturation as exemplified in the changing reactions of the infant to pin prick. *Child Dev*, 12, 31–42.

Melzack, R. and Wall, P. D. (1965). Pain mechanisms: a new theory. *Science*, 150, 971–979.

Mettler, C. C. and Mettler, F. A. (1947). *History of medicine*. Philadelphia, PA: The Blakiston Co.

Naish, J. M. and Apley, J. (1951). 'Growing pains': a clinical study of non-arthritic limb pains in children. *Arch Dis Child*, 26, 134–140.

National Centre of Complementary and Alternative Medicine. (2010). *Traditional Chinese medicine: an introduction*. Available at: <http://nccam.nih.gov/health/whatiscam/chinesemed.htm>.

Newton, H. (2011). 'Very sore nights and days': the child's experience of illness in early modern England, c.1580–1720. *Med Hist*, 55, 153–182.

Oakes, L. L. (2011). *Compact clinical guide to infant and child pain management: an evidence-based approach for nurses*. New York: Springer.

Oberlander, T. (2006). *Pain in children and adults with developmental disabilities*. Baltimore, MD: Brookes Publishing.

Palermo, T. M. (2012). *CBT for chronic pain in children and adolescents.* Oxford: Oxford University Press.

Pernick, M. S. (1985). *A calculus of suffering: pain, professionalism, and anesthesia in nineteenth-century America.* New York: Columbia University Press.

Rendall-Baker, L. (1992). History and evolution of pediatric anesthesia equipment. *Int Anesthesiol Clin*, 30, 1–34.

Robson, C. (1925). Anesthesia in children. *Anesth Analg*, 4 August, 235–240.

Rogers, R. (2008). *Managing persistent pain in adolescents.* Milton Keyes: Radcliffe Publishing.

Ross, D. M. and Ross, S. A. (1988). *Childhood pain: current issues, research and management.* Munich: Urban & Schwartzenberg.

Rovner, S. (1986). Surgery without anesthesia: can preemies feel pain? *Washington Post*, August 13, pp. 7–8.

Royal College of Paediatrics and Child Health. Dr Michael Blacow Memorial Prize. Available at: <http://www.rcpch.ac.uk/what-we-do/fellowships-and-prizes/dr-michael-blacow-memorial-prize/dr-michael-blacow-memorial-prize> (accessed 23 April 2011).

Ruhrah, J. (1925). *Pediatrics of the past.* New York: Paul B. Hoeber.

Schechter, N. L., Allen, D. A., and Hanson, K. (1986). Status of pediatric pain control: a comparison of hospital analgesic usage in children and adults. *Pediatrics*, 77(1), 11–15.

Schechter, N. L., Berde, C., and Yaster, M. (1993). *Pain in infants, children and adolescents.* Baltimore, MD: Williams and Wilkins.

Snow, J. (1858). *On chloroform and other anesthetics: their action and administration.* London: John Churchill.

Starr, L. (1895). The clinical investigation of disease and the general management of children In: L. Starr and T. S. Westcott (eds) *An American text-book of the diseases of children*, pp. 3–4. Philadelphia, PA: Saunders.

Stewart, D. J. (1989). History of pediatric anesthesia. In: G. A. Gregory (ed.) *Pediatric anesthesia* (2nd edn), pp. 1–14. New York: Churchill Livingstone.

Still, G. F. (1931). *The history of pediatrics: the progress of the study of diseases of children up to the end of the XVIIIth century.* London: Oxford University Press.

Straus, S., Tetroe, J., and Graham I. (2009). *Knowledge translation in health care moving from evidence to practice.* London: Wiley-Blackwell BMJ Books.

Thorek, M. (1938). *Modern surgical technique.* Philadelphia, PA: Lippincott.

Tobias, J. D. and Deshpande, J. K. (2005). *Pediatric pain management for primary care* (2nd edn). Chicago, IL: American Academy of Pediatrics.

Unruh, A. M. (1992). Voices from the past: ancient views of pain in childhood. *Clin J Pain*, 8, 247–254.

Twycross, A., Dowden, S., and Bruce, L. (eds) (2009). *Managing pain in children: a clinical guide.* Mississauga, ON: Wiley-Blackwell.

Unruh, A. M. (2007). Spirituality, religion and pain. *Can J Nurs Res*, 39, 66–86.

Vahlquist, B. (1955). Migraine in children. *Int Arch Allergy*, 7, 348–355.

Vahlquist, B. and Hackzell, G. (1949). Migraine of early onset. *Acta Paediatr*, 38, 622–636.

Walco, G. A. and Goldschneider, K. R. (eds) (2008). *Pain in children: a guide for primary care.* New York: Humana Press.

Wharton, H. R. (1895). Tracheotomy. In L. Starr and T. S. Westcott (eds) *An American text-book of the diseases of children*, pp. 290–310. Philadelphia, PA: Saunders.

Yaster, Y., Cote, J. C., Krane, E. J., Kaplan, R. F., and Lappe, D. G. (1997). *Pediatric pain management and sedation handbook.* Maryland Heights, MI: Mosby.

Wasz-Höckert, O., Lind, J., Vuorenkoski, V., Partanen, T., and Valanne E. (1968). The infant cry: a spectrographic and auditory analysis. *Child Dev*, 49, 580–589.

Zeltzer, L. Z. and Schlank, C. B. (2005). *Conquering your child's chronic pain: a pediatrician's guide to reclaiming a normal childhood.* Scarborough, ON: Harper Collins.

CHAPTER 2

Prevalence and distribution of pain in children

Bonnie J. Stevens and William T. Zempsky

Introduction

There has been a paucity of studies that have attempted to determine the prevalence and distribution of pain (acute or chronic) in large groups of infants and children across multiple settings. Rather, there is a preponderance of single-site studies that report local prevalence and distribution of paediatric pain data. Although one could extrapolate these results to gain a broader sense of pain in children, this approach would garner only a general estimate at best. Furthermore, studies of pain prevalence vary as to the pain and prevalence definitions used, the reporting period (i.e. *point prevalence, period prevalence*), and stratification by duration of involvement, which makes comparison of findings challenging. In this chapter, definitions of prevalence and acute and chronic pain will be clarified and used to explore the prevalence and distribution of pain in hospitals and in community health care settings for infants and children. Recommendations for clinical practice and future research will be proposed.

Definitions

Prevalence is the proportion of a population found to have a condition (typically a disease) and is determined by comparing the number of individuals with the condition with the total number of people studied. 'Point prevalence' is the proportion of a population that has the condition at a specific point in time. 'Period prevalence' is the proportion of a population that has the condition at some time during a given period (e.g. neonatal period during the first year of life). Prevalence is different from incidence, which is a measure of *new* cases arising in a population over a given period.

Acute pain signals a specific nociceptive event, injury, or illness and is usually limited to a short period of time. Acute pain is frequently associated with sudden-onset, short, sharp, tissue-damaging procedures (e.g. heel lances, finger pricks, intravenous starts, intramuscular injections, lumbar punctures) for diagnostic or non-tissue-damaging procedures (e.g. suctioning) for therapeutic purposes. Acute pain typically subsides with effective management after the painful event (e.g. heel lance) or when the illness or injury resolves; however, it can be prolonged and reoccur in multiple episodes over time. *Acute prolonged pain* extends beyond that of the short-sharp, tissue damaging procedural pain but usually has

a predictable course that coincides with a 'usual' healing time and subsides within a few hours or days (e.g. postoperative pain).

Chronic pain is frequently defined as pain without apparent biological value that has persisted beyond the normal tissue healing time. Chronic pain promotes an extended and maladaptive stress response that includes neuroendocrine dysregulation, fatigue, dysphoria, myalgia and impaired psychological and social functioning. The temporal delineation of 'healing time' is frequently debated but is usually stated as somewhere between 3 and 6 months. The International Association for the Study of Pain (IASP) defines chronic pain as pain that lasts longer than 3 months (<http://www.iasp-pain.org/Content/NavigationMenu/GeneralResourceLinks/PainDefinitions/>). The temporal delineation presents additional dilemmas when considering prolonged pain in infants and young children and in those with disabilities who either are incapable of or may have difficulty in reporting their pain. For further discussion on assessment of pain in vulnerable populations, see Lee and Stevens (Chapter 35, this volume) and Below et al. (Chapter 16, this volume). Chronic pain can either be recurrent or persistent. *Recurrent pain* includes episodic acute pains such as headaches and stomach aches; more *persistent pain* is more enduring pains includes backaches.

Pain in hospitalized infants and children

Acute pain

Neonates and infants

Acute pain during infancy was ignored until approximately three decades ago due to biases and misconceptions regarding the maturity of the infant's developing nervous system, their inability to verbally report pain, and their perceived inability to remember pain. Many infants endured frequent invasive medical procedures such as repetitive heel sticks and even surgery without benefit of anaesthesia or analgesia. More recently, these beliefs and misconceptions are rarely stated or acknowledged due to enhanced understanding of the developmental neurobiology of infant pain pathways and supraspinal processing. However, infants, and particularly hospitalized neonates, continue to be exposed to multiple painful procedures for diagnostic and treatment purposes and persistent, prolonged, or even chronic pain.

Several researchers have documented the incidence, prevalence, and frequency of procedural pain in infants hospitalized in the neonatal intensive care unit (NICU). Johnston and colleagues (2011) conducted a prospective observational study in 14 Canadian NICUs documenting both tissue-damaging (e.g. heel lance) and non-tissue-damaging (e.g. suctioning) procedures over a 1-week period. A total of 3508 tissue-damaging (mean = 5.8, standard deviation (SD) = 15) and 14 085 (mean = 25.6, SD = 15) non-tissue-damaging procedures were recorded for 582 infants. Twelve years earlier, Johnston and colleagues (1997) reported that the average number of painful procedures per infants was 14, similar to other prevalence surveys of infant procedural pain at the time (Anand and Selankio, 1996; Barker and Rutter, 1995; Fernandez and Rees, 1994; Porter et al., 1997; Simons et al., 2003).

In Johnston et al.'s 2011 study, the mean of 5.8 (SD 15, range 0–89) tissue-damaging procedures per infant appears to be a significant improvement. In 1996, no infants received pharmacological interventions for heel lancing—the most common of the tissue-damaging procedures—whereas in 2011, of the 46% of infants who were exposed to tissue-damaging procedures, 14.5% were administered opioids and 14.3% received sweet-tasting solutions such as sucrose or glucose. Johnston et al. concluded that although the prevalence of painful procedures was lower in the more recent survey, pain management of procedures had generally not improved significantly.

In other countries, hospitalized infants were reported to experience an average of 12 tissue-damaging procedures per day (Carbajal et al., 2008). Carbajal and colleagues reported that, of 42 413 painful procedures performed on 430 infants, 79.2% of patients received no preprocedural analgesia, 2.1% received pharmacological interventions, while 18.2% painful procedures were managed using non-pharmacological strategies.

These data continue to support that there are a significant number of painful procedures performed on hospitalized infants and a gross undertreatment of procedural pain in infants.

Children and adolescents

Several surveys have also been conducted to evaluate the prevalence of acute pain in hospitalized children and adolescents. In a recent audit of the epidemiology of procedural pain and pain management in 32 hospital units in eight paediatric hospitals in Canada, 2987 of 3822 children in the study had undergone at least one painful procedure in the preceding 24 hours with a mean of 6.3 painful procedures per child (Stevens et al., 2011). Of those who had a painful procedure, 78.1% had a pain management intervention recorded; however, only 28.3% had one or more pain management interventions administered and documented specifically for the painful procedure (Stevens et al., 2011).

Other researchers have focused specifically on acute pain intensity that is moderate to severe (e.g. >3 or 4 on a 10-point scale). Generally, prevalence rates from these studies are consistent and high; for example, Ellis et al. (2002) and Cummings et al. (1996) in cross-sectional studies reported a prevalence rate of 20–21% of clinically significant pain in hospitalized children in Canada. More recently, Groenewald et al. (2012) reported a prevalence rate of 27% of moderate to severe pain in hospitalized children in the USA. Adolescents and infants exhibited higher prevalence rates (38% and 32% respectively) than other children (17%). In addition, those hospitalized on surgical units demonstrated much higher rates of

moderate to severe pain (44%) than those on medical units (13%). Other studies described even higher prevalence rates of moderate to severe pain intensity; Taylor et al. (2008) stated that approximately 50% of hospitalized children from one tertiary level academic paediatric hospital reported moderate to severe pain during their stay with 23% reporting persistent pain.

Several studies indicate that child risk factors (e.g. age) and hospital service (e.g. surgical) are associated with the highest levels of moderate to severe pain (e.g. Groenewald et al., 2012; Stevens et al., 2011).

Chronic pain

Neonates and infants

As with acute pain, health professionals responsible for the care provision of infants and parents may harbour misconceptions or lack understanding of prolonged, persistent, or chronic pain in infancy. In a recent study by Pillai Riddell et al. (2009), two types of prolonged pain were described by the health professionals for hospitalized infants including 'chronically pained' (a pain state that involved prolonged exposure of the infant to repetitive painful procedures, which was characterized by overlap with recovery from a previous painful procedure) and 'chronic pain' (related to the aftermath of acute pain that is prolonged and has not resolved due to unknown cause) in infants. Examples of infants exhibiting chronic pain include: (1) a subgroup of postsurgical gastrointestinal patients ('short-gut babies') who continue to be distressed weeks after the completion of painful surgeries and reductions, (2) infants with chronic intestinal problems who suffer repetitive bouts of abdominal discomfort due to an inability to tolerate feeds and a distended abdomen, (3) infants who suffer from osteogenesis imperfecta, (4) infants who have sickle cell disease, (5) infants who have invasive malignant tumours, and (6) extremely low birth weight babies seen months/years later in follow-up clinics who would not weight bear or walk on their scarred heels (i.e. from repetitive heel lancing).

Anecdotal evidence from professional and parental caregivers suggests that there are significant numbers of medically comprised infants that are potentially experiencing chronic pain; however, there are no precise estimates of prevalence. These infants and young children may be even more vulnerable to the consequences of chronic pain and suffering as management strategies that are geared for the acute pain context may be ineffective. The longer untreated chronic pain continues in infancy, the more likely that maladaptive responses will develop later in life (Buskila et al., 2003; Hamilton and Zeltzer, 1994). Potential responses could include central nervous system sensitization, increased functional disability (Campo et al., 2001; Kashikar-Zuck et al., 2001), dysfunctional cognitive or emotional processes, (Eccleston and Crombez, 1999; Taddio, 1999; Taddio et al., 2002), and disrupted family functioning.

Children and adolescents

Chronic pain has serious developmental and functional implications for children and adolescents (King et al., 2011). Chronic pain is common within chronic disease states (e.g. juvenile idiopathic arthritis (JIA), cancer) as well as outside disease states. As chronic pain may be associated both with children who are hospitalized, as well as those in the community, these two areas will be discussed together in this section, although chronic pain may also occur in children and adolescents cared for at home or in the community.

The first comprehensive review on the epidemiology of pain was published by Goodman and McGrath over two decades ago (Goodman and McGrath, 1991). Prevalence rates, time periods, measures utilized, and approaches to measurement are variable:

- Perquin et al. (2000), in school and population studies, evaluated 6000 Dutch children (aged 0–18 years) and found that 54% had experienced pain in the previous 3 months and a quarter had pain which lasted greater than 3 months with about 8% suffering from severe chronic pain. Chronic pain increased with age and was more common in girls.

- Abu-Saad (2010) noted that chronic pain is more likely in girls than boys and increases with advancing age.

- In a Greek study of over 8000 7-year-olds, recurrent complaints of pain (headache, abdominal pain, or limb pain which occurred at least once a week) occurred in 7.2% of the sample (8.8% of girls, 5.7% of boys; p <0.001) (Bakoula et al., 2006).

- In a Spanish point prevalence study of 561 8- to 16-year-olds, chronic pain (pain lasting more than 3 months experienced continuously or at least once or twice each month) was reported by 37% of the sample although in only 5.1% of the sample was the pain problem moderate or severe (Huguet and Miro, 2008).

- In a national survey of children in Canada that included 2488 10- to 11-year-olds, up to five times, every 2 years, across 12 to 19 years of age, weekly or more frequent incident rates ranged from 26.1% to 31.8% for headache, 13.5% to 22.2% for stomach ache, and 17.5% to 25.8% for backache (Stanford et al., 2008).

- Within the community population, in a Canadian study of approximately 500 13-year-olds, 96% experienced acute pain over the previous month. The most common acute pains were headache (78%), sore muscles (73%), and toothache (45%) (Van Dijk et al., 2006).

- Dangel (2005) reported that approximately 5% of school-age children experience recurrent abdominal pain (RAP), 5% to 10% experience chronic headaches, and 15% experience musculoskeletal pains with many receiving inadequate treatment.

King et al. (2011) used a comprehensive and rigorous approach to systematically review all of the existing literature, which included 41 studies. The prevalence of headache ranged from 8% to 83%; abdominal pain: 4% to 53%; back pain: 14% to 24%; musculoskeletal pain: 4% to 40%; multiple pains: 4% to 49%; and other pains: 5% to 88%. Prevalence of chronic pain was higher in girls and increased with age for most pain types. Lower socioeconomic status (SES) was associated with higher pain prevalence, especially for headache.

Acute and recurrent pain in community health care settings

In addition to hospitalized children with a broad array of illnesses, children across the health-illness spectrum also experience a variety of acute and chronic pains. Although there is some overlap of acute, recurrent, and chronic pain, these entities will be loosely divided into pain of a more acute nature and those of a more chronic or persistent nature. Disease-related chronic pain will be discussed separately.

Injection pain

Needle procedures, including injections, venous access procedures, heel sticks, and finger lances, are likely to be the most prevalent causes of iatrogenic pain. A child's interactions with medical providers are often coloured by the child's fear that s/he will get a shot or a poke. In the USA, healthy children undergo over three dozen separate vaccine injections by the time they reach adulthood (<http://www.immunize.org/catg.d/p4050.pdf>). A recent study demonstrated that approximately two-thirds of children have a fear of needles (Taddio et al., 2012). This problem persists into adulthood as approximately 25% of adults are afraid of needles (Taddio et al., 2012) and 10% meet the criteria for needle phobia (Hamilton 1995). For further discussion of pain associated with needle procedures see Taddio (Chapter 19, this volume).

Dental/oral pain

Oral and dental pain is a frequent experience in children. Lifetime prevalence of oral pain in 5-year-olds is 25% (Moura-Leite et al., 2008) and in 8- to 10-year-olds is reported in 48% to 88% (Ratnayake and Ekanayake, 2005) with ranges for prevalence in the preceding 2 months of 24% to 70%. Up to 40% to 59% of children in prevalence studies report having had severe dental pain in the past. Pain impacted the child's ability to eat, sleep, play, and brush their teeth. Not surprisingly, dental caries are responsible for the majority of oral pain in children (Slade, 2001). Prevalence of oral pain is consistently higher in lower SES groups (Slade, 2001).

Growing pains

The prevalence of growing pains varies widely between 2.6% and 49.4%. This disparity is likely to be because of the varying ages and definitions for this condition used in these studies. Recent studies using more rigorous methodology, larger sample size (532 and 596 children), and standard criteria which include only patients with pain that is intermittent, bilateral, not involving joints, occurring in the late afternoon or evening, with normal physical exam/and laboratory studies (Petersen et al., 2003) have found the incidence to be 24.5% and 36.9% respectively (Evans and Scutter, 2004; Kaspiris and Zafiropoulou, 2009).

Musculoskeletal pain

Musculoskeletal pain is commonly reported by children of all ages. Studies vary as to the sites of pain evaluated (i.e. as a subset of all pain, all musculoskeletal pain, limb pain, or specific joint pain) as well as the reporting period (i.e. point prevalence, weekly, monthly, or more than monthly) and stratification by duration of involvement, which makes it difficult to compare findings. Musculoskeletal pain once a week occurs in 32%, and once a month in 38.9% of 9- to 11-year-old Finnish children (Mikkelson et al., 1997) but once a week in 8.5% of Swedish 9- to 15-year-olds (Brun Sundblad et al., 2006), 40% of Brazilian children aged 10-to-18-years within the last 6 months (Zapata at al., 2006), and 45.1% of Italians aged 12 to 16 years had musculoskeletal pain with in the last 12 months (34.4% of who had pain which lasted longer than 3 months) (Masiero et al., 2010). Six per cent of 1000 consecutive visits to an urban paediatric clinic in the USA were for musculoskeletal pain (de Inocencio, 1998). The most common sites of pain include the knee, lower extremities, neck, and spine (de Inocencio, 1998; Masiero et al., 2010; Mikkelsson et al., 1997). Most studies found that musculoskeletal pain prevalence increases with age and is more common in girls (King et al., 2011). Widespread musculoskeletal pain and lower limb pain both persist at a rate of about 30% of the initial population at 1- and 4-year follow-up (El-Metwally et al., 2005; Mikkelsson et al., 2008). For further discussion on inflammatory arthritis and arthropathies, see Chira and Schanberg (Chapter 22, this volume) and for non-inflammatory musculoskeletal pain, see Clinch (Chapter 24, this volume).

Abdominal pain

Epidemiological studies of abdominal pain in youth vary by how abdominal pain, or more typically RAP, is defined. Some researchers use the definition by Apley and Naish (1958) of three episodes of abdominal pain over the previous 3 months that limit function; however, this is not universal. With the updating of the Rome criteria, differentiation of functional abdominal pain syndromes further into functional dyspepsia, irritable bowel syndrome, functional abdominal pain syndrome, and abdominal migraine further clouds this picture (Drossman, 2006).

In a USA study of 507 adolescents, 73% to 78% experienced abdominal pain in the past year, while it occurred weekly in 13% to 24% and impacted function in 17% to 24% of those surveyed (Hyams et al., 1996). Another US study of adolescent girls found a similar weekly prevalence with 20.7% reporting weekly stomach aches (Ghandour et al., 2004), while in a Canadian adolescent longitudinal sample the prevalence of weekly abdominal pain ranged from 13.5% to 22.2% (Stanford et al., 2008). In Iceland, over 2000 11- to 12- and 15- to 16-year-old children were surveyed. It was found that 18.4% of the sample had at least weekly abdominal pain, and there was a higher prevalence of pain in the younger group and in girls (Kristjánsdóttir, 1996). An Irish study evaluating epigastric pain symptoms in 1133 adolescents found 6% experienced epigastric pain at least once a week (Murray et al., 2007). In a Malaysian sample of 11- to 16-year-olds using Apley's criteria, the prevalence of pain was 10.2% (Boey et al., 2000).

Studies of younger children also use a variety of methodologies to evaluate the epidemiology of abdominal pain. In a Swedish study of 1155 6- to 13-year-olds, 39% experienced abdominal pain monthly, 19% experienced abdominal pain weekly, and an additional 8% had it more than once per week. Again girls experienced pain more often than boys (Petersen et al., 2003). In a population-based, retrospective birth cohort study conducted with 5700 children less than 5 years of age in Rochester, Minnesota, 11% of the sample sought care for abdominal pain at least three times within the first 5 years of life (Chitkara et al., 2007). Finally a British study that defined RAP as five or more episodes of pain over the previous year evaluated a cohort of almost 14 000 children. The prevalence of RAP increased from 3.8% at 2.5 years, to 6.9% at 3.5 years, to 11.8% at 6.5 years (Ramchandani et al., 2005). For further discussion on recurrent abdominal pain, see Schurman (Chapter 29, this volume).

Headache

Headache is one of the most common pain complaints in children. Population studies of headache prevalence report that headache is frequently experienced by children and adolescents. Stanford et al.'s (2008) study of almost 2500 Canadian adolescents found that prevalence rates for weekly headache ranged from 26% to 31.8%, while 24.0% of American adolescent girls experienced headache weekly (Ghandour et al., 2004).

In younger children, Kroner-Herwig et al.'s (2007) study of German children aged 7 to 14, showed that headache prevalence in the last 6 months increased from 38.6% in 7- to 8-year-olds to 63.4% in 13- to 14-year-olds. The prevalence of weekly headache increased from 2.6% to 9.6%, while weekly prevalence was 23% in Swedish children (Petersen et al., 2003). Aromaa et al. (1998) found that 21.7% of 6-year-old Finnish children had a headache which impacted their daily activities within their lifetime.

Some studies differentiate the prevalence of migraine headache within larger headache samples using criteria defined by the International Headache Society by questionnaire or direct interview (Headache Classification Subcommittee of the International Headache Society, 2004). In Bille's prevalence study of 9000 Swedish children, 1.4% had migraine at 7 years of age increasing to 5.3% at 15 years of age (Bille, 1962). In a long-term follow-up of 73 of the children with migraine, 23% were migraine free by 25 years of age and 47% were migraine free by age 50 (Bille, 1997). Migraine prevalence was 9.9% in a cohort of Brazilian children aged 10-18 years (Barea et al., 1996), 10.4% in Turkish children aged 8-16 years (Bugdayci et al., 2005), and 10.6% in British children aged 5 to 15 years (Abu-Arefeh and Russell, 1994). For more on headache see Hershey (Chapter 31, this volume).

Pain and obesity

Obesity is increasingly prevalent in children and adolescents though few studies have addressed pain in this population. Almost two-thirds of 270 overweight and obese children reported pain in a 1-month period (Lim et al., 2012). Obesity was a risk factor for musculoskeletal pain in a population-based cohort of over 3000 English children (Deere et al., 2012). Furthermore, being obese increased the odds of any pain (odds ratio (OR) 1.33), regional pain (OR = 2.04), and knee pain (OR = 1.87) (Deere et al., 2012). Obese patients' average pain was also more severe than their non-obese counterparts (Deere et al., 2012). Obesity was observed at a higher rate among youth presenting to a chronic pain clinic than a normative sample (20.8% versus 9.6%), and youth with back pain in this sample had a rate of obesity of 57% (Wilson et al., 2010).

Contextual factors influencing chronic recurrent pain

As indicated in many of the previously discussed studies, there are several factors connected with the child and family that are associated with chronic and recurrent pain in children. These include: (1) age (e.g. where infants and adolescents often have higher prevalence and lower pain management strategies implemented), (2) sex (e.g. where girls often have higher pain prevalence and intensity than boys), and (3) diagnosis (e.g. JIA and number of joints evaluated). Factors such as SES also influence pain with greater prevalence of pain associated with lower SES in some situations (e.g. oral/dental pain).

Differences in definitions of pain (e.g. acute, chronic, persistent, prolonged, recurrent), in criteria for establishing pain diagnoses (e.g. International Headache Society criteria, Apley and Naish criteria), research methods (retrospective chart review, prospective survey or interview), data collection measures (whether validated or not), time or prevalence point, and reporting period also influence reported prevalence and paediatric pain distribution rates.

Chronic disease-related pain

Sickle cell disease

Pain is the most common symptom of sickle cell disease (SCD), and can begin early in the first year of life as levels of fetal haemoglobin decline in susceptible individuals, but remains poorly characterized. The frequency of pain episodes is consistently higher in the children who have hemoglobin SS or SB^0 thalassaemia compared with other genotypes. Most children with SCD have increasing pain episodes as well as pain-associated disability as they mature into adolescence and young adulthood. In a cohort of over 500 adults with SCD, 30% of respondents reported pain in greater than 95% of diary days. While 70% of emergency department visits in children with SCD are for pain, the large majority of these painful episodes continue to be managed at home (Dampier et al., 2002a, 2002b). Pain episode frequency is correlated with mortality (Platt et al., 1991). The average pain episode is 2 to 9 days in duration. For further discussion on sickle cell disease, see Dampier and Barakat (Chapter 25, this volume).

Juvenile idiopathic arthritis/juvenile rheumatoid arthritis

The intensity of pain in JIA is quite variable; however, pain is frequent. Children with JIA report pain on 70% of days (Schanberg et al., 2003). Most children reported mild to moderate pain, but 25% of children reported pain in the severe range. Disease status typically predicts only a small to medium proportion of the variance in children's pain ratings (8–28%) (Malleson et al. 2004; Schanberg et al. 1997; Thompson, 1987; Vandvik and Eckblad, 1990). Other variables such as demographic variables (possibly older age), psychological variables (such as coping and mood), and environmental factors (parent pain history) also determine pain report. For more on juvenile rheumatoid arthritis/JIA, see Chira and Schanberg (Chapter 22, this volume).

Cancer pain

Pain is an almost universal symptom of childhood cancer, whether because of the disease itself, pain associated with treatment (mucositis, abdominal pain, surgery, neuropathic pain), or procedural pain from procedures such as venous access, lumbar puncture, and bone marrow aspiration. In interviews with children, Ljungman et al. (1999) found treatment-related pain to be the most severe pain problem associated with cancer (49%) with fewer reporting procedure-related pain (39%) and disease-related pain (13%) as the most severe pain problem. In a study of hospitalized children with cancer, more than half (27 of 49 patients) indicated they were experiencing pain. Eleven patients (22.4%) had mild pain, ten (20.4%) had moderate pain, and six (12.2%) had severe pain (Jacob et al., 2007). In a study of 164 youth dying from cancer, 92% experienced pain (Goldman et al., 2006). For cancer survivors, risk of reporting pain conditions and using prescription analgesics in adulthood were higher than sibling controls (Lu et al., 2011). For more on cancer pain, see Hickman et al. (Chapter 17, this volume).

Infants and children with disabilities

In general, pain is common in children with disabilities due to the underlying disease state, under-recognition of pain, and association with medical care needs. Stevens and colleagues (Stevens et al., 2003) reported that all neonates underwent more than ten painful procedures per day; those at the highest risk for neurological impairment had more procedures and received the least amount of analgesia during the first days of life.

In a pain diary study recorded of children with severe cognitive impairments over 2 weeks (n = 34), 73% of the children had a painful experience on at least 1 day (Stallard et al., 2001). In a longitudinal study, children with moderate to profound intellectual disability (n = 94) were found to experience pain for an average of 9 hour per week (Breau et al., 2003).

The majority of epidemiological studies in children with disability have been performed in children with cerebral palsy (CP). The prevalence of pain with CP is between 50% and 75% (Doralp and Bartlett, 2010; Parkinson et al., 2009; Tüzün et al., 2010). In a European study of 490 8- to 12-year-old children who could self-report and parents of 806 children (those who could and could not self-report), self-reported pain in the last week was 60% with parent-reported pain in the last 4 weeks of 73% (Parkinson et al., 2009). Self-reported pain was more frequent in older children but was not associated with disability severity, though parent-reported pain was associated with severity of disability. Other studies in CP have also found pain to be associated with severity of motor impairment (Houlihan et al., 2004). In 68 children with spina bifida, 56% experienced pain at least once a week, including headache in 88% with shunted hydrocephalus and 79% without hydrocephalus (Clancy et al., 2005).

The most common type of pain among children with CP is musculoskeletal pain. The most common sites of pain include feet, legs, back, hips, hands, and arms (Engel et al., 2005). Maximal pain is in the lower extremities in 70% of children (Ramstad et al., 2011). In addition, pain can result from commonly found secondary conditions including pressure ulcers and constipation.

Implications for clinical practice, education, knowledge translation, and future research

Although considerable variability and inconsistency exist amongst definitions for various types of pain, measures and approaches to determining the prevalence of pain, and factors that influence pain, overall acute and chronic pain is common, and often under-recognized and undertreated in infants, children, and adolescents. This issue persists in clinical and community settings and includes hospitalized children who receive significant numbers of painful procedures during their hospital stay, healthy children in the community who are subjected to painful procedures associated with preventative/primary care (e.g. immunizations), and children with chronic illness who experience pain both while receiving care in the community and during repeated periods of hospitalization.

Decreasing the prevalence of pain requires increased efforts in prevention and implementation of better pain assessment and management strategies in all health care settings. Success in these areas requires behavioural change on behalf of both health care professional and parent care providers. Furthermore, awareness of the prevalence of paediatric pain and implementation of effective knowledge translation (KT) strategies is required and needs to be specifically targeted to particular audiences. Effective implementation of KT strategies requires a strong basis of evidence, a positive context where evidence is implemented (e.g. culture), and strategically planned methods of facilitating the translation of evidence into useful products for users (e.g. clinical practice guidelines for health care professionals and tips or fact sheets for parents). Champions for change and a wide array of KT strategies including reminders, education, and audit and feedback for use in quality improvement initiatives are also required. An in-depth discussion of KT is provided by Yamada and Hutchinson (Chapter 61, this volume).

Research and evaluation form the basis for determining and reporting prevalence and distribution of paediatric pain and treatment. The research generally suffers from both methodological and interpretation problems. From a methodological perspective, samples are often inadequate and limited to single settings or clinical sites. Additionally, approaches to assessing prevalence and reporting period vary considerably and often non-validated/untested measures are used. Consistency in definition of types of pain, evaluation criteria, approach, measures, and timing of prevalence ratings would greatly enhance research in this area. Interpretation of results is often difficult due to methodological issues and inconsistent or wide-ranging prevalence estimates, which impact on potential changes in practice. Further efforts to critically evaluate

the quality of existing research (such as by King et al., 2011), standardize prevalance and pain definigions, and address areas which have received inadequate attention will assist in making interpretation of research results more meaningful and useful for both clinicians and researchers.

References

Abu-Arefeh, I. and Russell, G. (1994). Prevalence of headache and migraine in schoolchildren. *BMJ*, 309(6957), 765–769.

Abu-Saad, H. H. (2010). Chronic pain in children and adolescents: a review. *J Med Leban*, 58(2), 5–110.

Anand, K. J. S. and Selankio, J. D. (1996). SOPAIN Study Group: routine analgesia practices in 109 neonatal intensive care units (NICUs). *Pediatr Res*, 39, 192A.

Apley, J. and Naish, N. (1958). Recurrent abdominal pains: a field survey of 1000 school children. *Arch Dis Child*, 33, 165–170.

Aromaa, M., Sillanapaa, M. L., Rautava, P., and Helenius, H. (1998). Childhood headache at school entry- controlled clinical trial. *Neurology*, 50(6), 1729–1736.

Bakoula, C., Kapi, A., Veltsista, A., Kavadias, G., and Kolaitis, G. (2006). Prevalence of recurrent complaints of pain among Greek schoolchildren and associated factors: a population-based study. *Acta Paediatr*, 95(8), 947–951.

Barea, L. M., Tannhauser, M., and Rotta, N. T. (1996). An epidemiologic study of headaches among children and adolescents of southern Brazil. *Cephalalgia*, 16(8), 545–549.

Barker, D. and Rutter, N. (1995). Heel pricks were unnecessarily painful. *BMJ*, 311(7007), 747.

Bille, B. (1997). A 40-year follow-up of school children with migraine. *Cephalalgia*, 17, 488–91.

Bille, B. S. (1962). Migraine in school children. A study of the incidence and short-term prognosis, and a clinical, psychological and electroencephalographic comparison between children with migraine and matched controls. *Acta Paediatr Suppl*, 136, 1–151.

Boey, C. C. M., Yap, S. B., and Goh, K. L. (2000). The prevalence of recurrent abdominal pain in 11- to 16-year-old Malaysian schoolchildren. *J Paediatr Child Health*, 36(2), 114–116.

Breau, L. M., Camfield, C. S., McGrath, P. J., and Finley, G. A. (2003). The incidence of pain in children with severe cognitive impairments. *Arch Pediatr Adolesc Med*, 157(12), 1219–1226.

Brun Sundblad, G. M., Saartok, T., and Engström, L. M. T. (2007). Prevalence and co-occurrence of self-rated pain and perceived health in schoolchildren: age and gender differences. *Eur J Pain*, 11(2), 171–180.

Bugdayci, R., Ozge, A., Sasmaz, T., Oner Kurt, A., Kaleagasi, H., Karakelle, A., *et al.* (2005). Prevalence and factors affecting headache in Turkish schoolchildren. *Pediatr Int*, 47(3), 316–322.

Buskila, D., Neumann, L., Zmora, E., Feldman, M., Bolotin, A., and Press, J. (2003). Pain sensitivity in prematurely born adolescents. *Arch Pediatr Adolesc Med*, 157(11), 1079–82.

Campo, J. V., Di Lorenzo, C., Chiappetta, L., Bridge, J., Colborn, D. K., Gartner, J. C., *et al.* (2001). Adult outcomes of pediatric recurrent abdominal pain: do they just grow out of it? *Pediatrics*, 108(1), E1.

Carbajal, R., Rousset, A., Danan, C., Coquery, S., Nolent, P., Ducrocq, S., *et al.* (2008). Epidemiology and treatment of painful procedures in neonates in intensive care units. *JAMA*, 300(1), 60–70.

Chitkara, D. K., Talley, N. J., Weaver, A. L., Katusic, S. K., De Schepper, H., Rucker, M. J., *et al.* (2007). Incidence of presentation of common functional gastrointestinal disorders in children from birth to 5 years: a cohort study. *Clin Gastroenterol Hepatol*, 5(2), 186–191.

Clancy, C. A., McGrath, P. J., and Oddson, B. E. (2005). Pain in children and adolescents with spina bifida. *Dev Med Child Neurol*, 47, 481–91.

Cummings, E. A., Reid, G. J., Finley, G. A., McGrath, P. J., and Ritchie, J. A. (1996). Prevalence and source of pain in pediatric inpatients. *Pain*, 68(1), 25–31.

Case example

Jackson is a 13-year-old boy who presents to his paediatrician with a 6-month history of episodic abdominal pain. The pain started the previous autumn. It comes on about 20 to 30 minutes after eating and is sometimes associated with diarrhoea. There is no blood in his stools; he has no fevers, or weight loss. His parents separated earlier this year. While his pain doesn't wake him from sleep he does have trouble falling asleep and will lie in bed for an hour or more several nights a week. Jackson has avoided going to friends' houses because he is afraid he will have pain or diarrhoea. He has missed over 2 weeks of school this year for abdominal complaints.

In a review of Jackson's pain history with his mother she describes several issues of pain in the past. As an infant Jackson had colic which resulted in several middle-of-the-night phone calls to his paediatrician. His parents learned to sooth him through these episodes by running the vacuum cleaner in his room.

When he was 3 years old, Jackson woke several times in the middle of the night with pain in his knees. He would cry out for his parents, they would give him ibuprofen, massage his back, or, on occasion, put him in a warm bath. By his fifth birthday these episodes had resolved.

Prior to starting school Jackson had developed a fear of receiving his immunizations—a problem which persists to the present day. For his yearly flu vaccination Jackson receives lidocaine prilocaine cream, and learned some guided imagery techniques from a family friend. His fear of needles extended to his interactions with his dentist and he required general anaesthesia to have three cavities filled.

At age 11 Jackson collided with a teammate while playing soccer. He landed on his back. He complained about pain in his lower back for several weeks before his parents sought medical treatment. He was diagnosed with a muscular strain and received physical therapy for 2 months before he could return to full activity without pain.

Dampier, C., Ely, B., Brodecki, D., and O'Neal, P. (2002a). Characteristics of pain managed at home in children and adolescents with sickle cell disease by using diary self-reports. *J Pain*, 3(6), 461–470.

Dampier, C., Ely, E., Brodecki, D., and O'Neal, P. (2002b). Home management of pain in sickle cell disease: a daily diary study in children and adolescents. *J Pediatr Hematol Oncol*, 24(8), 643–647.

Dangel, T. (2005). Management of chronic pain in children. *Curr Paediatr*, 15, 69–74.

De Inocencio, J. (1998). Musculoskeletal pain in primary pediatric care: analysis of 1000 consecutive general pediatric clinic visits. *Pediatrics*, 102(6), e63–e66.

Deere, K. C., Clinch, J., Holliday, K., McBeth, J., Crawley, E. M., Sayers, A., *et al.* (2012). Obesity is a risk factor for musculoskeletal pain in adolescents: findings from a population cohort. *Pain*, 153, 1932–1938.

Doralp, S. and Bartlett, D. J. (2010). The prevalence, distribution, and effect of pain among adolescents with cerebral palsy. *Pediatr Phys Ther*, 22(1), 26–33.

Drossman, D. A. (2006). The functional gastrointestinal disorders and the Rome III. *Gastroenterology*, 130, 1377–1390.

Eccleston, C. and Crombez, G. (1999). Pain demands attention: a cognitive-affective model of the interruptive function of pain. *Psychol Bull*, 125(3), 356–66.

Ellis, J. A., O'Connor, B. V., Cappelli, M., Goodman, J. T., Blouin, R., and Reid, C. W. (2002). Pain in hospitalized pediatric patients: how are we doing? *Clin J Pain*, 18(4), 262–269.

El-Metwally, A., Salminen, J. J., Auvinen, A., Kautiainen, H., and Mikkelsson, M. (2005). Lower limb pain in a preadolescent population: prognosis and risk factors for chronicity—a prospective 1- and 4-year follow-up study. *Pediatrics*, 116(3), 673–681.

Engel, J. M., Petrina, T. J., Dugeon, B. J., and McKearnan, K. A. (2005). Cerebral palsy and chronic pain: a descriptive study of children and adolescents. *Phys Occup Ther Pediatr*, 25(4), 73–84.

Evans, A. M. and Scutter, S. D. (2004). Prevalence of 'growing pains' in young children. *J Pediatr*, 145(2), 255–8.

Fernandez, C. V. and Rees, E. P. (1994). Pain management in Canadian level 3 neonatal intensive care units. *CMAJ*, 150(4), 469–470.

Ghandour, R. M., Overpeck, M. D., Huang, Z. J., Kogan, M. D., and Scheidt, P. C. (2004). Headache, stomachache, backache, and morning fatigue among adolescent girls in the United States: associations with behavioral, sociodemographic, and environmental factors. *Arch Pediatr Adolesc Med*, 158(8), 797–803.

Goldman, A., Hewitt, M., Collins, G. S., Childs, M., and Hain, R. (2006). Symptoms in children/young people with progressive malignant disease: United Kingdom Children's Cancer Study Group/Paediatric Oncology Nurses Forum survey. *Pediatrics*, 117(6), e1179–e1186.

Goodman, J. E. and McGrath, P. J. (1991). The epidemiology of pain in children and adolescents: a review. *Pain*, 46(3), 247–264.

Groenewald, C. B., Rabbitts, J. A., Schroeder, D. R., and Harrison, T. E. (2012). Prevalence of moderate-severe pain in hospitalized children. *Pediatr Anaesth*, 22(7), 661–668.

Hamilton, A. B. and Zeltzer, L. K. (1994). Visceral pain in infants. *J Pediatr*, 125(6II), S95–S102.

Headache Classification Subcommittee of the International Headache Society (2004). The International Classification of Headache Disorders: 2nd edition. *Cephalalgia*, 24(S1), 9–160.

Houlihan, C., O'Donnell, M., Conaway, M., and Stevenson, R. D. (2004). Bodily pain and health-related quality of life in children with cerebral palsy. *Dev Med Child Neurol*, 46, 305–310.

Huguet, A. and Miro, J. (2008). The severity of chronic pediatric pain: an epidemiological study. *J Pain*, 9(3), 226–236.

Hyams, J., Burke, G., Davis, P., Rzepski, B., and Andrulonis, P. A. (1996). Abdominal pain and irritable bowel syndrome in adolescents: a community-based study. *J Pediatr*, 129(2), 220–226.

Jacob, E., Hesselgrave, J., Sambuco, G., and Hockenberry, M. (2007). Variations in pain, sleep, and activity during hospitalization in children with cancer. *J Pediatr Oncol Nurs*, 24(4), 208–219.

Johnston, C. C., Collinge, J. M., Henderson, S., and Anand, K. J. (1997). A cross sectional survey of pain and analgesia in Canadian neonatal intensive care units. *Clin J Pain*, 3(4), 1–5.

Johnston, C. C., Barrington, K. J., Taddio, A., Cabajal, R., and Filion, F. (2011). Pain in Canadian NICUs. Have we improved over the past 12 years? *Clin J Pain*, 27(3), 225–232.

Kashikar-Zuck, S., Goldschneider K. R., Powers, S. W., Vaught, M. H., and Hershey, A. D. (2001). Depression and functional disability in chronic pediatric pain. *Clin J Pain*, 17(4), 341–9.

Kaspiris, A. and Zafiropoulou, C. (2009). Growing pains in children: epidemiological analysis in a Mediterranean population. *Joint Bone Spine*, 76, 486–490.

King, S., Chambers, C. T., Huguet, A., MacNevin, R. C., McGrath, P. J., Parker, L., *et al.* (2011). The epidemiology of chronic pain in children and adolescents revisited: a systematic review. *Pain*, 152(12), 2729–2738.

Kristjánsdóttir, G. (1996). Sociodemographic differences in the prevalence of self-reported stomach pain in school children. *Eur J Pediatr*, 155(11), 981–983.

Kroner-Herwig, B., Heinrich, M., and Morris, L. (2007). Headache in German children and adolescents: a population-based epidemiological study. *Cephalalgia*, 27(6), 519–527.

Lim, C. S., Mayer-Brown, S. J., and Janicke, D. M. (2012). The impact of pain on physical activity and quality of life in obese children. Presented at the American Psychological Association Annual Convention, presidential track poster session, Orlando, FL, August.

Ljungman, G., Gordh, T., Sorensen, S., and Kreuger, A. (1999). Pain in paediatric oncology: interviews with children, adolescents and their parents. *Acta Paediatr*, 88(6), 623–630.

Lu, Q., Krull, K. R., Leisenring, W., Owen, J. E., Kawashima, T., Tsao, J. C., *et al.* (2011). Pain in long-term adult survivors of childhood cancers and their siblings: a report from the Childhood Cancer Survivor Study. *Pain*, 152(11), 2616–2624.

Malleson, P. N., Oen, K., Cabral, D. A., Petty, R. E., Rosenberg, A. M., and Cheang, M. (2004). Predictors of pain in children with established juvenile rheumatoid arthritis. *Arthritis Rheum*, 51(2), 222–227.

Masiero, S., Carraro, E., Sarto, D., Bonaldo, L., and Ferraro, C. (2010). Healthcare service use in adolescents with non-specific musculoskeletal pain. *Acta Pædiatr*, 99, 1224–1228.

Mikkelsson, M., El-Metwally, A., Kautiainen, H., Auvinen, A., Macfarlane, G. J., and Salminen, J. J. (2008). Onset, prognosis and risk factors for widespread pain in schoolchildren: a prospective 4-year follow-up study. *Pain*, 138, 681–687.

Mikkelsson, M., Salminen, J. J., and Kautiainen, H. (1997). Non-specific musculoskeletal pain in preadolescents. Prevalence and 1-year persistence. *Pain*, 73(1), 29–35.

Moura-Leite, F. R., Ramos-Jorge, M. L., Bonanato, K., Paiva, S. M., Vale, M. P., and Pordeus, I. A. (2008). Prevalence, intensity and impact of dental pain in 5-year-old preschool children. *Oral Health Prev Dent*, 6(4), 295–301.

Murray, L. J., McCarron, P., Boreham, C. A., McGartland, C. P., and Johnston, B. T. (2007). Prevalence of epigastric pain, heartburn and acid regurgitation in adolescents and their parents: evidence for intergenerational association. *Eur J Gastroenterol Hepatol*, 19(4), 297–303.

Parkinson, K. N., Gibson, L., Dickinson, H. O., and Colver, A.F. (2009). Pain in children with cerebral palsy: a cross-sectional multicentre European study. *Acta Paediatr*, 99(3), 446–451.

Perquin, C. W., Hazebroek-Kampschreur, A. A., Hunfeld, J. A., Bohnen, A. M., Van Suijlekom-Smit, L. W., Passchier J., *et al.* (2000). Pain in children and adolescents: a common experience. *Pain*, 87(1), 51–58.

Petersen, S., Bergstrom, E., and Brulin, C. (2003). High prevalence of tiredness and pain in young schoolchildren. *Scand J Public Health*, 31, 367–374.

Pillai Riddell, R., Stevens, B., McKeever, P., Gibbins, S., Asztalos, E., Katz, J., *et al.* (2009). Chronic pain in hospitalized infants: health professionals' perspectives. *J Pain*, 10(12), 1217–1225.

Platt, O. S., Thorington, B. D., Brambilla, D. J., Milner, P. F., Rosse, W. F., Vichinsky, E., *et al.* (1991). Pain in sickle cell disease. Rates and risk factors. *N Engl J Med*, 325(1), 11–16.

Porter, F. L., Wolf, C. M., Gold, J., Lotsoff, D., and Miller, J.P. (1997). Pain and pain management in newborn infants: a survey of physicians and nurses. *Pediatrics*, 100(104), 626–632.

Ramchandani, P. G., Hotopf, M., Sandhu, B., and Stein, A. (2005). The epidemiology of recurrent abdominal pain from 2 to 6 years of age: results of a large, population-based study. *Pediatrics,* 116(1), 46–50.

Ramstad, K., Jahnsen, R., Skjeldal, O. H., and Diseth, T. H. (2011). Characteristics of recurrent musculoskeletal pain in children with cerebral palsy aged 8 to 18 years. *Dev Med Child Neurol,* 53, 1013–1018.

Ratnayake, N. and Ekanayake, L. (2005). Prevalence and impact of oral pain in 8-year-old children in Sri Lanka. *Int J Paediatr Dent,* 15(2), 105–112.

Schanberg, L. E., Lefebvre, J. C., Keefe, F. J., Kredich, D. W., and Gil, K. M. (1997). Pain coping and the pain experience in children with juvenile chronic arthritis. *Pain,* 73(2), 181–189.

Schanberg, L. E., Anthony, K. K., Gil, K. M. and Maurin, E. C. (2003). Daily pain and symptoms in children with polyarticular arthritis. *Arthritis Rheum*, 48(5), 1390–1397.

Simons, S. H., Van Dijk, M., Anand, K. J. S. Roofthooft, D., Van Lingen, R., and Tibboel, D. (2003). Do we still hurt newborn babies? A prospective study of procedural pain and analgesia in neonates. *Arch Pediatri Adolesc Med*, 157(11), 1058–1064.

Slade, G. D. (2001). Epidemiology of dental pain and dental caries among children and adolescents. *Community Dent Health,* 18, 219–227.

Stallard, P., Williams, L., Lenton, S., and Vellemn, R. (2001). Pain in cognitively impaired, non-communicating children. *Arch Dis Child,* 85(6), 460–462.

Stanford, E. A., Chambers, C. T., Biesanz, J. C., and Chen, E. (2008). The frequency, trajectories and predictors of adolescent recurrent pain: a population-based approach. *Pain,* 138, 11–21.

Stevens, B., McGrath, P., Gibbins, S., Beyene, J., Breau, L., Camfield, C., et al. (2003). Procedural pain in newborns at risk for neurologic impairment. *Pain,* 105(1–2), 27–35.

Stevens, B. J., Abbott, L. K., Yamada, J. Harrison, D., Stinson, J., Taddio, A., et al. (2011). Epidemiology and management of painful procedures in children in Canadian hospitals. *CMAJ,* 183(7), e403–e410.

Taddio, A. (1999). Effects of early pain experience: the human literature. In P. J. McGrath and G. A. Finley (eds) *Chronic and Recurrent Pain in Children and Adolescents*, pp. 57–74. Seattle: IASP Press.

Taddio, A., Shah, V., Gilbert-Macleod, C., and Katz, J. (2002). Conditioning and hyperalgesia in newborns exposed to repeated heel lances. *JAMA*, 288, 857–61.

Taddio, A., Ipp, M., Thivakaran, S., Jamal, A., Parikh, C., Smart, S., et al. (2012). Survey of the prevalence of immunization non-compliance due to needle fears in children and adults. *Vaccine*, 30, 4807–4812.

Taylor, E. M., Boyer, K., and Campbell, F. A. (2008). Pain in hospitalized children: a prospective cross-sectional survey of pain prevalence, intensity, assessment and management in a Canadian pediatric teaching hospital. *Pain Res Manag*, 13, 25–32.

Thompson, K. L., Varni, J. W., and Hanson, V. (1987). Comprehensive assessment of pain in juvenile rheumatoid arthritis: an empirical model. *J Pediatr Psychol,* 12(2), 241–255.

Tüzün, E. H., Guven, D. K., and Eker, L. (2010). Pain prevalence and its impact on the quality of life in a sample of Turkish children with cerebral palsy. *Disabil Rehabil,* 32(9), 723–728.

Vandvik, I. H. and Eckblad, G. (1990). Relationship between pain, disease severity and psychosocial function in patients with juvenile chronic arthritis (JCA). *Scand J Rheumatol,* 19(4), 295–302.

Van Dijk, M. A., McGrath, P.A., Pickett, W., and Van Den Kerkhof, E. G. (2006). Pain prevalence in nine- to 13-year-old school children. *Pain Res Manag,* 11(4), 234–240.

Wilson, A. C., Samuelson, B., and Palermo, T. M. (2010). Obesity in children and adolescents with chronic pain: associations with pain and activity limitations. *Clin J Pain,* 26(8), 705–711.

Zapata, A. L., Moraes, A. J. P., Leone, C., Doria-Filho, U., and Silva, C. A. A. (2006). Pain and musculoskeletal pain syndromes in adolescents. *J Adolesc Health*, 38(6), 769–771.

CHAPTER 3

Long-term effects of early pain and injury: animal models

Suellen M. Walker

Summary

Nociceptive pathways are functional following birth and acute responses to noxious stimuli have been documented from early development in both clinical and laboratory studies. The ability of noxious afferent input to alter the level of sensitivity of nociceptive pathways in the adult nervous system, with, for example the development of central sensitization, is well established (Woolf, 2011). However, the developing nervous system has additional susceptibilities to alterations in neural activity, and increases due to pain and injury in early life may produce effects not seen following the same input at older ages. As a result, early tissue injury may lead to persistent changes in somatosensory processing and altered sensitivity to future noxious stimuli. The impact of early pain and injury cannot be simply viewed as increasing or decreasing sensitivity as results vary depending on the type and severity of injury and the outcomes used for assessment. Laboratory studies allow evaluation of different forms of injury, potential confounding factors, underlying mechanisms, and potential for modulation by analgesia.

Introduction

Persistent alterations in pain sensitivity following early pain experience in neonates and infants are outlined by Grunau (Chapter 4, this volume). Clinical evaluations vary in their methodology, and it is clear that early pain experience does not simply either increase or decrease pain sensitivity. Preclinical studies similarly document differing long-term consequences of early pain and injury (Fitzgerald and Walker, 2009), and allow further evaluation of:

+ The impact of different types and severity of early injury.

+ Responses at different developmental stages to determine if there are critical periods during which alterations in normal development produce long-term effects.

+ The mechanisms underlying persistent sensory changes.

+ The degree to which the impact of early injury can be modulated by analgesia.

This chapter will firstly summarize factors that influence long-term effects in animal models with examples from different studies, and secondly, describe in more detail the specific effects of different forms of injury. In line with clinical reports, the majority of studies focus on injuries sustained within the neonatal period and early life. Laboratory studies allow evaluation of neural processes underlying the encoding and processing of noxious stimuli (i.e. 'nociception'), whereas the term 'pain' may be reserved for the human experience which encompasses cognitive and emotional dimensions; but for the purposes of this chapter 'pain' will also be used in association with behavioural and tissue responses to injury in animals.

Evaluating the long-term impact of early pain: general principles

A number of different variables and outcomes can be assessed in preclinical studies evaluating the long-term impact of early pain, and as seen with clinical evidence, studies vary in their design and methodology.

Extrapolation across species

Understanding the potential clinical significance of early life injury in animal models requires extrapolation to a similar developmental stage in humans. While direct translation of developmental age from rodents to humans, and the specific timing of events after birth, continues to be debated, the *sequence* of development of sensory and reflex systems in rodents correlate with those of human infants (Wood et al., 2003). Statistical models have been developed to translate development across species (Clancy et al., 2007b; Nagarajan et al., 2010), but are predominantly based on structural measures, and acknowledge that they cannot account for activity-dependent modification following birth (Clancy et al., 2007a). Maturation varies in different regions of the peripheral and central nervous systems, but in terms of spinal processing many approximate a postnatal day (P)3 rat with a preterm human neonate, P7 with an infant, P21 with an adolescent, and P35 with young adulthood (Brambrink et al., 2010; Fitzgerald and Walker, 2009; McCutcheon and Marinelli, 2009; see also Walker and Baccei, Chapter 6, and Fitzgerald, Chapter 8, this volume for further details of the developmental changes in nociceptive signalling).

An additional difficulty relates to evaluating the potential 'effect size' of observations in animals models. For example, what degree of change in baseline sensory thresholds is likely to correlate with a clinically significant effect? Enhanced responses to future pain, which can result in alterations in the degree and duration of hyperalgesia, are more quantifiable and perhaps easier to translate to the clinical setting.

Ideally, effects in several species would be evaluated, and although primate studies are being performed to evaluate potential adverse effects of general anaesthesia in early development (Brambrink et al., 2010), resources for primate studies are limited. The majority of pain studies are performed in rats or mice, and the rodent has several advantages as a developmental model:

- Rodents are born at a relatively immature stage, thus allowing evaluation of effects that correlate with the preterm human infant. Mice and rats have similar gestation periods (19 and 21 days respectively) and then mature at similar rates.

- Rat pups are weaned at P21 and reach adulthood by 6 to 8 weeks of age, so persistent effects can be followed across a relatively compressed lifespan.

- Control animals in the same litter can be used to assess potential confounding effects due to handling and maternal separation.

- The ability of analgesics to modify persistent effects can be studied in a standardized comparative manner.

Type of injury

A range of injuries can be utilized to model the many different sources of pain that may be experienced in early life, including: surgical injury, inflammation, repeated needle sticks, and visceral insults (see later sections for specific details). This allows evaluation of the response to specific components of various injuries, underlying mechanisms, and also allows comparison of the differential sensitivity to analgesic interventions.

Impact on sensory function and/or response to future injury

Changes in baseline sensory sensitivity or in the response to a subsequent noxious stimulus in adulthood are the primary outcomes for assessing the long-term impact of prior pain and injury. Evaluation methods may include, but are not limited to, the following:

- Changes in behavioural sensory threshold, such as the threshold for hindlimb withdrawal from a mechanical stimulus applied to the hindpaw or the latency to withdraw from a thermal stimulus. A decrease in the mechanical threshold or thermal latency for withdrawal indicates increased sensitivity or *hyper*algesia, and conversely an increase in threshold or latency indicates decreased sensitivity or *hypo*algesia.

- *In vivo* electrophysiological recordings. Electromyography (EMG) can further quantify reflex sensitivity to threshold and suprathreshold stimuli. Extracellular recordings from cells in the dorsal horn assess responses to physical, chemical, or electrical stimuli or drugs; these may be applied to peripheral tissue

(e.g. hindpaw or gut), directly on the spinal cord, or by injection in other sites within the central nervous system (CNS).

- Detailed evaluation of activity in different ion channels at a cellular level. Patch clamp techniques on neurons within nociceptive pathways may be performed in slices of CNS tissue, including spinal cord, or *in vivo*.

Responses to stimuli of varying intensity can reveal differences in the distribution, time course, and underlying mechanisms of altered sensory processing. For example, neonatal inflammation produces late-onset generalized baseline hypoalgesia, as noted earlier in this section. In addition, an enhanced segmental hyperalgesia is unmasked by subsequent inflammation or incision in the previously injured, but not the contralateral paw (Chu et al., 2007; Ren et al., 2004).

The degree of hyperalgesia following injury in later life is frequently assessed. This may be in response to the same form of injury, such as repeat surgical incision (Beggs et al., 2012b) or re-inflammation of the hindpaw (Ren et al., 2004). Alternatively, different stimuli may be used to assess specific mechanisms (e.g. evaluation of C-fibre mediated responses by subsequent injection of capsaicin; Hohmann et al., 2005) or to evaluate the generalizability of altered sensitivity to different forms of injury (e.g. initial somatic injury and subsequent visceral sensitivity).

Age at time of injury

The majority of current clinical and laboratory research focuses on long-term effects following pain experienced in the neonatal period and/or early infancy. An important feature of injury is early life is that effects in the developing nervous system may differ from those seen following the same injury at older ages. There are 'critical periods' when changing levels of neural activity can alter neural development (Hensch, 2004), but this period of vulnerability differs in different regions of the nervous system, and is also dependent on the type of injury.

To confirm specific developmental or age-dependent responses, the same injury must be performed and compared across a number of postnatal ages. In addition, the same *intensity* of stimulus should be delivered at each age. For example, the volume of inflammatory agent or irritant solution injected at different ages needs to be standardized for the rapidly changing size and weight of the animal, to confirm that enhanced effects following early injury are not due to a more severe injury or more intense acute stimulus in the youngest animals. The volume of the C-fibre stimulant mustard oil applied to the hindpaw has been adjusted according to the size or 'volume' of the paw at different ages (Jiang and Gebhart, 1998), the volume of capsaicin altered to produce comparative local responses (S. M. Walker et al., 2007), and anatomical landmarks used to produce incision of the same relative proportion of hindpaw at different ages (S. M. Walker et al., 2009).

Time interval before evaluation

The impact of neonatal injuries on different outcomes may change with time. Ideally the time course of response should be evaluated by regular assessments until the animal or the system being evaluated is fully mature, as rodents may be considered 'adult' at different ages (McCutcheon and Marinelli, 2009). Peripheral nociceptive mechanisms mature relatively early, but spinal cord processing, and particularly modulation by descending pathways from the brainstem (Hathway et al., 2009, 2012) is not mature until the 3rd to 4th postnatal week (see Fitzgerald, Chapter 8, this volume). Following neonatal inflammation, a clear change is seen as the animal matures, with generalized hypoalgesia or decreased baseline sensitivity emerging only after P30 (Ren et al., 2004), potentially due to alterations in descending modulation (Zhang et al., 2010).

Non-sensory behavioural outcomes

The effect of early injury on anxiety in adulthood has been assessed using established paradigms, but results vary with the type and intensity of initial stimulus. A low anxiety trait in adulthood (P50–55) followed early inflammation (0.25% carrageenan at P3) as assessed by: more time spent in the open arms of an elevated plus maze; enhanced ability to cope with stress related to a forced swim test; and reduced basal and stress-related neuroendocrine markers at rest and following the swim test (Anseloni et al., 2005). Conversely, more severe hindpaw inflammation (10 mcl of complete Freund's adjuvant (CFA) in P1 mice) *increased* anxiety behaviours in adulthood (fewer entries into open arms of elevated plus maze at P90; Roizenblatt et al., 2010). Formalin in P1 rats (10 mcl 4% into right forepaw and hindpaw) reduced exploratory behaviour in males and increased anxiety (reduced time in open arm of elevated plus maze) in females (Negrigo et al., 2011). Similarly, daily formalin injections (5 mcl of 4%) into each hindpaw from P1 to P4 reduced exploratory behaviour and impaired learning in a radial arm maze test (Anand et al., 2007; Rovnaghi et al., 2008). Repeated hindpaw needle pricking from P0 to P7 was also postulated to increase vulnerability to stress and anxiety-mediated behaviours, as deficits in exploratory and defensive withdrawal behaviour were found at P65, but without differences in stress hormones (Anand et al., 1999).

An early visceral insult (repeated colorectal distension from P8 to P21) also reduced exploratory activity in adulthood (J. Wang et al., 2008). Interestingly, most models associated with increased anxiety also produced long-term *increased* pain sensitivity (reduced hindlimb withdrawal sensory thresholds); whereas carrageenan inflammation produces generalized *hypo*algesia and reduced anxiety. This potential link between the pattern of pain and anxiety outcomes requires further evaluation.

As central pathways involved in pain and reward processing are linked, the long-term impact of repeated neonatal hindpaw incision (at P3, P10, and P17) on motivational behaviour in adulthood was tested. Exploratory behaviours in adulthood were not altered by neonatal incisions or anaesthesia. Following a subsequent incision in adulthood, motivational behaviours were similar, but activity in orexin neurons in the lateral hypothalamus (an important region for reward signalling) was increased (Low and Fitzgerald, 2012).

For some behaviours the link with pain signalling is less clear. For example, ethanol preference was reduced after repeat formalin injection (Bhutta et al., 2001), but was increased following repeat needle stick injury (Anand et al., 1999).

Tissue analysis and mechanisms

An obvious advantage of laboratory studies is the ability to analyse tissue at various sites to evaluate both the impact of the initial injury and any long-term consequences in structure and/or function. Examples include:

- Assessing the localized response to injury in the peripheral tissue (e.g. degree of persistent inflammation or changes in innervation).

- Evaluating changes in receptor expression in the cell bodies of peripheral afferents in the dorsal root ganglion (DRG) or spinal cord or other CNS regions using antibodies to the receptor (immunohistochemistry) or measuring receptor protein levels (Western blot).

- Alterations in gene expression which indicate neuronal activation (e.g. c-fos) or which relate to specific mechanisms mediating long-term consequences (e.g. upregulation or downregulation of genes controlling receptors, transmitters, or signalling pathways involved in nociceptive function). Use of genetically modified mice can also provide further insights by comparison of wild-type strains with animals in which a portion of the gene is permanently non-functional (knockout), inactivated in a tissue- or time-specific manner (conditional knockout), or briefly silenced (knockdown).

Pharmacological interventions

Pharmacological strategies may be used to further define mechanisms associated with the effects of early pain and injury. For example, in addition to immunohistochemistry studies showing altered microglial morphology and increased reactivity, a reduction in hyperalgesia by administration of an inhibitor of microglia (e.g. minocycline) further established the role of microglia in mediating effects of prior neonatal incision (Beggs et al., 2012b). Similarly, prevention of long-term consequences by local anaesthetic blockade of peripheral nerves supplying the area of injury (S. M. Walker et al., 2009), not only confirms that activity within primary afferent fibres has a mechanistic role, but also suggests a potential therapeutic intervention. Administration of drugs by different routes can more closely evaluate the site of action: comparing responses following intrathecal administration rather than systemic (oral, subcutaneous, intraperitoneal, intravenous) administration identifies selective spinal cord effects; and localized small volume injections into the brain can evaluate the impact of altering function in different brain regions.

Assessing modulation of long-term effects by analgesics has important clinical implications. Two different aspects may be evaluated: (1) the ability of different forms of analgesia at the time of the initial insult to modify or prevent long-term consequences; and/or (2) the ability of different analgesics to effectively manage any alterations in pain response at the time of injury in later life.

Sex differences

The degree to which male or female sex influences the susceptibility to long-term consequences of early injury varies, both with the type of initial injury and with the outcome being assessed. Although not all studies include comparison of female and male animals, alterations in either the degree or type of long-term impact of neonatal interventions have been reported in some, but not all, studies and warrant further evaluation (Cataldo et al., 2010; LaPrairie and Murphy, 2007, 2010; Negrigo et al., 2011). At this stage, it is not possible to reliably conclude whether males or females are more susceptible.

Maternal separation, handling, and neonatal stress

As developmental studies involve experiments on young animals that are dependent on maternal care, it is necessary to control for non-injury related effects due to handling and separation or interactions with the mother (Sternberg and Ridgway, 2003).

Repeated and often prolonged maternal separation, for up to 3 hours a day across the first 2 postnatal weeks, increases visceral sensitivity in adulthood (Chung et al., 2007; Schwetz et al., 2005; Tjong et al., 2010). Alterations in subsequent stress-induced analgesia (Sternberg and Ridgway, 2003) and opioid tolerance (Kalinichev et al., 2002) suggest changes in endogenous pain inhibitory systems. This degree of handling and duration of separation is predominantly utilized to assess changes in stress-related behaviour mediated via the hypothalamic–pituitary–adrenal axis (Chung et al., 2007; Faturi et al., 2010), and is greater than required for most neonatal injury models. However, control groups with the same degree of handling and separation in the absence of the noxious stimulus are required to confirm that effects seen in later life are specific for the injury itself.

The impact of maternal–pup interactions is complex, as injury in the pups may also alter maternal behaviour and outcomes. An initial increase in maternal contact but later neglect was reported after hindpaw inflammation in rat pups (Anseloni et al., 2005), but no change in maternal behaviour was seen following laparotomy in newborn mice (Sternberg and Ridgway, 2003; Sternberg et al., 2005). Maternal care may modulate adverse effects: increased grooming was noted after P6 and was postulated to decrease the impact of repeated heel prick from P2 to P14 in rats (C. D. Walker et al., 2003). In a subsequent study, varying levels of grooming by different mothers influenced thermal withdrawal latency in adulthood, but had no impact on long-term effects following repeated formalin injection (twice daily from P3 to P14; C. D. Walker et al., 2008). The need to care for injured pups may also alter maternal outcomes, with one study reporting long-term alterations in pain threshold, anxiety, and sleep fragmentation in the dams of pups with CFA-induced hindpaw inflammation (Roizenblatt et al., 2010).

Evaluating the long-term impact of early pain: specific injury models

A large number of different injury models have evaluated the impact of early pain, and responses vary both with the type and severity of initial injury (Fitzgerald and Walker, 2009) (Figure 3.1).

Peripheral inflammation

Initial injury

Different agents can induce a peripheral inflammatory response, are commonly injected in the hindpaw, and changes in hindlimb reflex sensitivity assess the degree of subsequent sensitivity. CFA comprises inactivated mycobacteria emulsified in mineral oil, and carrageenan contains polysaccharides extracted from seaweeds.

Long-term effects following neonatal inflammation vary with the type and severity of stimulus. An early model documenting persistent changes in sensory processing utilized 25 mcl CFA on P1 (Ruda et al., 2000), however this is a relatively large volume in the neonatal paw, producing chronic inflammation rather than a specific neonatal insult (Lim et al., 2009; S. M. Walker et al., 2003). Hindpaw injection of carrageenan in different volumes and concentrations (0.5–2 mcl/g of 0.25–2%) produces a robust but shorter duration acute inflammatory hyperalgesia (Ren et al., 2004; Torsney and Fitzgerald, 2002; S. M. Walker et al., 2003), and doses as low as 1 mcgl/g of 0.25% lambda carrageenan produce persistent effects (Anseloni et al., 2005; Ren et al., 2004; G. Wang et al., 2004).

Impact on sensory thresholds

Large volumes of CFA in neonatal rodents (25 mcl in P1 rat or 20 mcl in P1 mouse) have been associated with either no change (Lim et al., 2009; Ruda et al., 2000; S. M. Walker et al., 2003) or a reduction in sensory thresholds (i.e. increased sensitivity) (Blom et al., 2006; Roizenblatt et al., 2010) in adulthood. By contrast, carrageenan (1 mcl/g 0.25%) has been consistently associated with higher thresholds (i.e. decreased sensitivity) from P30 until adulthood (Anseloni et al., 2005; Lidow et al., 2001; Ren et al., 2004; G. Wang et al., 2004). In addition to a generalized hypoalgesia in all paws, neonatal carrageenan also decreased the visceromotor response to colorectal distension in adulthood, suggesting a modulatory impact on both somatic and visceral processing (G. Wang et al., 2004).

Response to subsequent noxious stimulus

Neonatal hindpaw inflammation increases the response to noxious stimuli in adulthood. CFA 25 mcl at P1 enhanced the response to different stimuli in the previously injured paw including: increased behavioural hyperalgesia following repeat CFA (Lim et al., 2009; Ruda et al., 2000) or capsaicin (Hohmann et al., 2005); earlier onset of response to formalin; and increased dorsal horn neuronal response to peripheral brush or pinch (Ruda et al. 2000). Prior CFA inflammation did not alter the response to nerve injury in adulthood (Lim et al., 2009). Neonatal carrageenan inflammation also increases the degree of behavioural hyperalgesia to subsequent inflammation (Ren et al., 2004) or incision (Chu et al., 2007) of the previously injured paw.

Critical period

The first postnatal week is the critical period for persistent effects following inflammation. Persistent changes follow CFA 25 mcl at P1, but not 50 mcl CFA at P14 in rats (Hohmann et al., 2005; Ruda et al., 2000) and CFA 20 mcl at P1 but not 40 mcl at P14 in mice (Blom et al., 2006). However, it is difficult to determine if these volumes produced the same degree of inflammation at the two ages. Carrageenan in doses adjusted for body weight (1 mcl/g) at P0, P1, P3, and P5 but not at P8 and older was associated with long-term alterations in threshold (Ren et al., 2004), and the pattern of gene expression in the dorsal horn also differed if injury occurred at P3 rather than at P12 (Ren et al., 2005). Similarly, altered behaviours indicative of a low anxiety trait in adulthood were seen following carrageenan inflammation at P3 but not P12 (Anseloni et al., 2005).

Mechanisms

Injection of CFA 25 mcl in newborn rat pups produces long-term increases in paw diameter (not seen after carrageenan or smaller volumes or CFA) and histological signs of chronic inflammation (Lim et al., 2009; S. M. Walker et al., 2003). This may contribute to the persistent reductions in sensory threshold that have been reported following this stimulus (Blom et al., 2006; Roizenblatt et al., 2010).

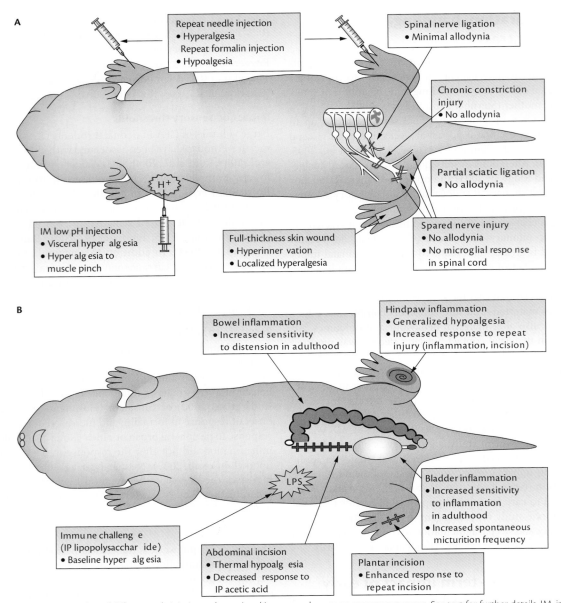

Figure 3.1 Diagramatic representation of different early injuries and associated impact on long-term sensory outcomes. See text for further details. IM, intramuscular; IP, intraperitoneal.
Reprinted by permission from Macmillan Publishers Ltd. From Fitzgerald, M. and Walker, S. M., Infant pain management: a developmental neurobiological approach, *Nature Clinical Practice Neurology*, Volume 5, Issue 1, pp. 35–50, Copyright © 2009, http://www.nature.com/nrneurol/index.html

As the baseline *hypo*algesia following carrageenan is generalized to all paws and emerges later in development (after P30), brain-stem-mediated alterations in descending modulation have been postulated (G. Wang et al., 2004). Enhanced inhibition from the rostroventral medulla (RVM; Zhang et al., 2010) and alterations in opioid-mediated response in the periaqueductal grey (PAG; Laprairie and Murphy, 2009) have been noted in adults following neonatal hindpaw carrageenan. Increased expression of several subtypes of serotonin (5HT) receptor in the PAG has also followed early inflammation (Anseloni et al., 2005).

Different mechanisms are likely to underlie the enhanced hyper-algesic response to noxious stimuli in adulthood, which differs in both time course and distribution from changes in baseline threshold.

Enhanced re-injury responses are apparent from soon after the initial injury and are segmentally restricted to the previously inflamed paw (Chu et al., 2007; Ren et al., 2004). Following CFA 25 mcl at P1 (Ruda et al., 2000) (but not CFA 5 mcl or 25 mcl carrageenan; S. M. Walker et al., 2003), the terminal field of sciatic nerve afferents was expanded in the ipsilateral spinal cord, with increased calcitonin gene-related peptide-positive terminals. This likely contributes to an enhanced central response to a noxious peripheral stimulus, as supported by increased c-fos expression in response to repeat CFA (Tachibana et al., 2001) or capsaicin in adulthood (Hohmann et al., 2005). Long-term alterations in the spinal cord expression of genes related to nociceptive transmitter systems (Ren et al., 2005), and in the function and/or structure of N-methyl-D-aspartate receptors in the spinal cord

(Chu et al., 2007) and in the thalamus and other brain regions (Blom et al., 2006) may also contribute to enhanced responses to subsequent injury.

Modulation by analgesia

The long-term impact of neonatal carrageenan inflammation was reduced by morphine at the time of the initial insult (Laprairie et al., 2008; Rahman et al., 1997).

Formalin injection

Initial injury

Injection of formalin (0.5–15%) into the hindpaw is used as a model of acute nociception and produces a biphasic behavioural response with licking, twitching, flicking, and elevation of the paw in adult rats (Le Bars et al., 2001). Although responses differ in neonatal rat pups, formalin does produce specific nociceptive behaviours that are reduced by morphine (Abbott and Guy, 1995; Barr et al., 2003; McLaughlin et al., 1990).

Impact on sensory thresholds

Repeated injection of 5 mcl of 10% formalin (all four paws at P1 and forepaws or hindpaws on alternate days from P2 to P7; Bhutta et al., 2001) or daily injections into each hindpaw from P1 to P4 (5 mcl of 4%; Anand et al., 2007; Rovnaghi et al., 2008) decreased thermal sensitivity in adulthood. As responses were compared to undisturbed controls, the impact of repeated injection versus the formalin injectate itself cannot be determined. By contrast, formalin at a single time point (10 mcl of 4% into right forepaw and hindpaw on P1) had no impact on thermal latency in adulthood (Negrigo et al., 2011). Twice-daily injections of a lower concentration of formalin (10 mcl 0.2–0.4%) in alternating hindpaws from P3 to P14 also had no impact on thermal sensitivity in adulthood (C. D. Walker et al., 2008).

Response to subsequent noxious stimulus

Repeated formalin from P3 to P14 increased the area under the behavioural response curve following subsequent hindpaw formalin in adulthood (C. D. Walker et al., 2008).

Critical period and mechanisms

There has been limited comparison of age-dependent susceptibility for persistent effects following formalin, as many protocols include repeated injections across the first 1 to 3 postnatal weeks. Histological evaluation of the effect of repeated formalin injection on the peripheral tissue would be beneficial to exclude chronic injury. The pattern of gene expression in the spinal cord differed following hindpaw formalin injection at P3 (5 mcl or 20 mcl of 2%) versus P21 (200 mcl of 2%; Barr et al., 2005).

Response to analgesia

Long-term behavioural changes in adults were reduced by morphine administration prior to neonatal formalin injection (Bhutta et al., 2001). Ketamine reduced the thermal hypoalgesia in adult females, but not in males (Anand et al., 2007).

Repeat needle injury

Initial injury

Repeated needle injection in the paws of rat pups has been performed to model repeated heel lance for clinical blood sampling in neonates. However, the relative size of the needle and depth of penetration may be relatively greater in the rodent paw.

Impact on sensory responses

A 25-gauge needle was inserted through each paw, once, twice, or four times daily from P0 to P7. Thermal sensitivity was increased in the four-times daily injection group at P16 and P22. This may reflect residual inflammation, as there was no significant difference from controls by P65 (Anand et al., 1999).

Repeated unilateral injections in the gastrocnemius muscle on alternate days from P8 to P20 were performed with a needle alone or combined with injection of 100 mcl of an acidic pH 4 or physiological pH 7.4 saline solution. No intervention altered reflex sensitivity to a hindpaw mechanical stimulus in adulthood (Miranda et al., 2006).

Response to subsequent noxious stimulus

Although there were no detectable changes in muscle histology, the response to deep muscle pinch was enhanced following repeated muscle injection of the pH 4, but not pH 7, solution. Additionally, the pH 4 group had an increased visceromotor response (EMG response in abdominal muscles) and spinal dorsal horn neuron response (in areas of viscerosomatic convergence) to colonic distension in adulthood, which may reflect more generalized alterations in descending modulation (Miranda et al., 2006).

Full-thickness skin wound

Initial injury

Neonatal skin is thin and sensitive to injury (Fox, 2011). In the laboratory, long-term effects have been evaluated following removal of a small full-thickness skin flap on the dorsal hindpaw (Reynolds and Fitzgerald, 1995).

Impact on sensory responses

Neonatal skin wounding produces localized hyperalgesia that persists well beyond the period of wound healing (Alvares et al., 2000; Reynolds and Fitzgerald, 1995; Young et al., 2008).

Critical period

Persistent hyperalgesia follows full-thickness skin wounding in the first postnatal week, but not at older ages, and the degree of hyperinnervation is much greater than seen following the same injury in adulthood (Reynolds and Fitzgerald, 1995).

Mechanism

Full-thickness skin wounds result in both peripheral changes in innervation density and central changes in the spinal cord. Marked peripheral hyperinnervation due to collateral sprouting from adjacent axons, and from distant intact neurons (Alvares and Fitzgerald, 1999), occurs within the wounded area, mediated by local release of neurotrophic factors including NGF and NT-3 (Beggs et al., 2012a; Constantinou et al., 1994; Reynolds et al., 1997). In addition, there are changes in short-range neural inhibitory cues (Moss et al., 2005). Ephrins act as contact-mediated guidance molecules during development and repair, and ephrin-A4 inhibits neurite outgrowth. However, following neonatal skin wounding this inhibition is reduced as ephrin-A4 expression is downregulated, allowing an increase in innervation density (Moss et al., 2005). NK-1 expressing neurons in the spinal cord are involved as ablating these neurons with intrathecal substance P-saporin at the time of neonatal injury or in adulthood reduced injury-related effects (Young et al., 2008). In addition, the receptive field size of dorsal horn neurons is significantly greater 3 and 6 weeks following neonatal skin wounding when compared with control animals (Torsney and Fitzgerald, 2003).

Modulation by analgesia

A single sciatic block with bupivacaine prior to skin wounding produced an acute sensory and motor block but did not prevent hyperinnervation or persistent hyperalgesia (De Lima et al., 1999). Intra-articular injection of lidocaine in the medial and lateral ankle reduced acute vocalizations following stimulation of the injured hindpaw, although it is not clear how frequently injections were performed, and there was no impact on persistent effects (Young et al., 2007).

Surgical incision

Initial injury

Surgical injury produces inflammation, skin wounding, and peripheral nerve injury (Kehlet et al., 2006). The plantar hindpaw incision model comprises skin incision plus elevation and incision of the underlying plantaris muscle, and produces acute hyperalgesia and increased hindlimb reflex sensitivity at all postnatal ages in the rat (Ririe et al., 2003; S. M. Walker et al., 2009). A midline abdominal incision in mice on the day of birth has also evaluated the impact of neonatal laparotomy (Sternberg et al., 2005).

Impact on sensory responses and future injury

Neonatal laparotomy in mice was associated with a generalized decrease in baseline sensitivity to thermal and visceral stimuli in adulthood (Sternberg et al., 2005). Similarly, and as seen following carrageenan inflammation, neonatal hindpaw incision decreases baseline sensitivity to mechanical and thermal stimuli in adulthood, but a subsequent injury unmasks segmental hyperalgesia. Both the degree and duration of hyperalgesia are increased when the same paw is re-injured, either 2 weeks later or in adulthood (P60) (Beggs et al., 2012b; S. M. Walker et al., 2009). A series of three hindpaw incisions performed at P3, P10, and P17 also increased the degree of incision-related hyperalgesia at P90 (Low and Fitzgerald, 2012).

Critical period

Hindpaw incision in the first postnatal week (P3 or P6) but not at older (P10, P21, P40) ages enhanced the response to future incision (S. M. Walker et al., 2009).

Mechanism

Prior neonatal incision primes the spinal neuroimmune response to repeat incision in adulthood. The enhanced incision-related hyperalgesia in adults with prior neonatal incision is associated with an earlier onset, and increased duration and degree of microglial reactivity in the spinal cord (Beggs et al., 2012b).

Modulation by analgesia

Administration of systemic morphine at the time of neonatal laparotomy prevented long-term changes in sensory responses (Sternberg et al., 2005). The effect of neonatal incision on later incision-related hyperalgesia was prevented by repeated perioperative sciatic blocks (four 2-hourly blocks) but not by a single preoperative block, suggesting that more prolonged primary afferent blockade is required to modify persistent effects. In adults with prior neonatal incision, intrathecal minocycline selectively prevents the enhanced hyperalgesic response, confirming a functional role for microglial reactivity (Beggs et al., 2012b; see Vega-Avelaira and Beggs, Chapter 7, this volume, for further details of neuroimmune interactions in nociceptive pathways).

Visceral injury

Initial injury

Visceral injury is modelled in rodents by exposing the bladder or to bowel to chemical irritants, such as mustard oil or zymosan, or repeated mechanical stimuli (e.g. rectal distension).

Impact on sensory responses and future injury

Early visceral injury has been associated with visceral hyperalgesia in adulthood. Daily mechanical distension or chemical (mustard oil 0.2 ml 5%) colonic irritation from P8 to P21 increased behavioural (Al-Chaer et al., 2000) and abdominal muscle EMG responses to subsequent colonic distension, and also altered food consumption and faecal output (J. Wang et al., 2008). Shorter exposures to intracolonic mustard oil (2% 10 mcl from P8 to P10; Christianson et al., 2010) or infusion of acetic acid at P10 (Winston et al., 2007) also increased sensitivity to mechanical colonic distension in adulthood.

Bladder inflammation (daily intravesical injections of zymosan P14–P16) increased spontaneous micturition frequency and the response to subsequent inflammation in adulthood (Randich et al., 2006).

Spinal neurons receive convergent input from both somatic and visceral afferents, and neonatal visceral injury increased somatic reflex sensitivity to hindpaw thermal (J. Wang et al., 2008) or mechanical stimuli (Christianson et al., 2010), in some but not all models (Randich et al., 2006). Neonatal somatic insults also have an impact on visceral sensitivity in adulthood, as noted in previous sections (Miranda et al., 2006; G. Wang et al., 2004).

Critical period

Visceral insults in the first 2 to 3 postnatal weeks, but not at older ages, have been associated with persistent changes in sensitivity, including: repeat colonic stimulus from P1 to P20 but not P21 to P42 (Al-Chaer et al., 2000); daily bladder injections from P14 to P16 but not P28 to P30 (Randich et al., 2006); intracolonic acetic acid at P10 but not 8 weeks of age (Winston et al., 2007).

Mechanism

Neonatal colonic irritation increased electrophysiological responses in adult spinal cord viscerosensitive neurons, in the absence of any demonstrable changes in peripheral bowel histology (Al-Chaer et al., 2000; Christianson et al., 2010; Lin and Al-Chaer, 2003). Changes in receptor expression in the DRG may reflect the nature of the initial insult. Increased TRPV1 expression in cell bodies of colon afferents in the DRG followed acetic acid irritation at P10 (Winston et al., 2007); whereas P8 to P10 mustard oil (which stimulates TRPA-1 receptors), increased expression of TRPA-1 but not TRPV1 (Christianson et al., 2010).

Immune challenge

Initial injury

Early life immune challenges are modelled by various stimuli, such as injection of the bacterial endotoxin lipopolysaccharide (LPS) or endothelin-1, and can have a significant impact on the immune response in later life (McKelvy and Sweitzer, 2009; Spencer et al., 2011).

Impact on sensory responses and mechanisms

Intraperitoneal LPS at P14 had persistent effects on sensory function, as hindpaw sensitivity to mechanical and thermal stimuli and spinal expression of cyclo-oxygenase 2 was increased in adulthood (Boisse et al., 2005). Similarly, intracerebral injection of LPS at P5 produced persistent hyperalgesia and increased microglial reactivity in the brain, which was attenuated by administration of an interleukin-1 receptor antagonist (K. C. Wang et al., 2011). As severe inflammation may be associated with a significant immune response, and increased microglial reactivity in the spinal cord has been associated with persistent alterations in pain sensitivity, interactions between the immune system and nociceptive processing can have a significant impact on the long-term consequences of early injury.

Peripheral nerve injury

Several different models have been used to investigate the pathophysiology of traumatic nerve injury and ontogeny of neuropathic pain (Sorkin and Yaksh, 2009). In rodents, injury to the sciatic nerve or its branches or related central spinal nerves allows evaluation of changes in hindlimb reflex responses to hindpaw sensory stimuli, and comparison both with baseline and the contralateral side. Spared nerve injury, chronic constriction injury, partial sciatic ligation, and spinal nerve ligation performed in the first 2 to 3 weeks of postnatal life do not produce the same degree of acute allodynia as seen in adults (Howard et al., 2005; Lee and Chung, 1996; Ririe and Eisenach, 2006). Less commonly, nerves innervating the tail are injured and tail flick responses are used to evaluate sensitivity (Back et al., 2008). Age-related differences in the glial response to nerve injury contribute to the lack of neuropathic allodynia in early life. The effects and mechanisms of nerve injury are discussed by Vega-Avelaira and Beggs (Chapter 7, this volume).

Conclusion

Both clinical and preclinical studies demonstrate the complexity and diversity of persistent changes in pain responses following early pain and injury. It is too simplistic to expect that pain experience will reliably either increase or decrease sensitivity, as multiple contributory factors may interact to influence nociceptive processing and/or the behavioural response to pain. Evaluation in animal models is essential to investigate age-dependent changes in both the acute and persistent effects of different forms of injury, understand underlying mechanisms, and ultimately how effects may be modified or prevented by clinically applicable analgesic interventions.

References

Abbott, F. V. and Guy, E. R. (1995). Effects of morphine, pentobarbital and amphetamine on formalin-induced behaviours in infant rats: sedation versus specific suppression of pain. *Pain*, 62, 303–312.

Al-Chaer, E. D., Kawasaki, M., and Pasricha, P. J. (2000). A new model of chronic visceral hypersensitivity in adult rats induced by colon irritation during postnatal development. *Gastroenterology*, 119, 1276–1285.

Alvares, D. and Fitzgerald, M. (1999). Building blocks of pain: the regulation of key molecules in spinal sensory neurones during development and following peripheral axotomy. *Pain* (Suppl. 6), S71–85.

Alvares, D., Torsney, C., Beland, B., Reynolds, M., and Fitzgerald, M. (2000). Modelling the prolonged effects of neonatal pain. *Prog Brain Res*, 129, 365–373.

Anand, K. J., Coskun, V., Thrivikraman, K. V., Nemeroff, C. B., and Plotsky, P. M. (1999). Long-term behavioral effects of repetitive pain in neonatal rat pups. *Physiol Behav*, 66, 627–637.

Anand, K. J., Garg, S., Rovnaghi, C. R., Narsinghani, U., Bhutta, A. T., and Hall, R. W. (2007). Ketamine reduces the cell death following inflammatory pain in newborn rat brain. *Pediatr Res*, 62, 283–290.

Anseloni, V. C., He, F., Novikova, S. I., Turnbach Robbins, M., Lidow, I. A., Ennis, M., et al. (2005). Alterations in stress-associated behaviors and neurochemical markers in adult rats after neonatal short-lasting local inflammatory insult. *Neuroscience*, 131, 635–645.

Back, S. K., Kim, M. A., Kim, H. J., Lee, J., Sung, B., Yoon, Y., et al. (2008). Developmental characteristics of neuropathic pain induced by peripheral nerve injury of rats during neonatal period. *Neurosci Res*, 61, 412–419.

Barr, G. A., Gao, P., Wang, S., Cheng, J., Qin, J., Sibille, E. L., et al. (2005). Microarray analysis of gene expression following the formalin test in the infant rat. *Pain*, 117, 6–18.

Barr, G. A., Limon, E., Luthmann, R. A., Barr, G. A., Cheng, J., and Wang, S. (2003). Analgesia induced by local plantar injections of opiates in the formalin test in infant rats. *Dev Psychobiol*, 42, 111–122.

Beggs, S., Alvares, D., Moss, A., Currie, G., Middleton, J., Salter, M.W., and Fitzgerald, M (2012a). A role for NT-3 in the hyperinnervation of neonatally wounded skin. *Pain*, 153, 2133-2139.

Beggs, S., Currie, G., Salter, M. W., Fitzgerald, M., and Walker, S. M. (2012b). Priming of adult pain responses by neonatal pain experience: maintenance by central neuroimmune activity. *Brain*, 135, 404–417.

Bhutta, A. T., Rovnaghi, C., Simpson, P. M., Gossett, J. M., Scalzo, F. M., and Anand, K. J. (2001). Interactions of inflammatory pain and morphine in infant rats: long-term behavioral effects. *Physiol Behav*, 73, 51–58.

Blom, J. M., Benatti, C., Alboni, S., Capone, G., Ferraguti, C., Brunello, N., et al. (2006). Early postnatal chronic inflammation produces long-term changes in pain behavior and N-methyl-D-aspartate receptor subtype gene expression in the central nervous system of adult mice. *J Neurosci Res*, 84, 1789–1798.

Boisse, L., Spencer, S. J., Mouihate, A., Vergnolle, N., and Pittman, Q. J. (2005). Neonatal immune challenge alters nociception in the adult rat. *Pain*, 119, 133–141.

Brambrink, A. M., Evers, A. S., Avidan, M. S., Farber, N. B., Smith, D. J., Zhang, X., et al. (2010). Isoflurane-induced neuroapoptosis in the neonatal rhesus macaque brain. *Anesthesiology*, 112, 834–841.

Cataldo, G., Bernal, S. Y., Rozengurtel, S., Medina, K., and Bodnar, R. J. (2010). Neonatal and adult gonadal hormone manipulations enhance morphine analgesia elicited from the ventrolateral periaqueductal gray in female rats. *Int J Neurosci*, 120, 265–272.

Christianson, J. A., Bielefeldt, K., Malin, S. A., and Davis, B. M. (2010). Neonatal colon insult alters growth factor expression and TRPA1 responses in adult mice. *Pain*, 151, 540–549.

Chu, Y. C., Chan, K. H., Tsou, M. Y., Lin, S. M., Hsieh, Y. C., and Tao, Y. X. (2007). Mechanical pain hypersensitivity after incisional surgery is enhanced in rats subjected to neonatal peripheral inflammation: effects of N-methyl-D-aspartate receptor antagonists. *Anesthesiology*, 106, 1204–1212.

Chung, E. K., Zhang, X., Li, Z., Zhang, H., Xu, H., and Bian, Z. (2007). Neonatal maternal separation enhances central sensitivity to noxious colorectal distention in rat. *Brain Res*, 1153, 68–77.

Clancy, B., Finlay, B. L., Darlington, R. B., and Anand, K. J. (2007a). Extrapolating brain development from experimental species to humans. *Neurotoxicology*, 28, 931–937.

Clancy, B., Kersh, B., Hyde, J., Darlington, R. B., Anand, K. J., and Finlay, B. L. (2007b). Web-based method for translating neurodevelopment from laboratory species to humans. *Neuroinformatics*, 5, 79–94.

Constantinou, J., Reynolds, M. L., Woolf, C. J., Safieh-Garabedian, B., and Fitzgerald, M. (1994). Nerve growth factor levels in developing rat skin: upregulation following skin wounding. *Neuroreport*, 5, 2281–2284.

De Lima, J., Alvares, D., Hatch, D. J., and Fitzgerald, M. (1999). Sensory hyperinnervation after neonatal skin wounding: effect of bupivacaine sciatic nerve block. *Br J Anaesth*, 83, 662–664.

Faturi, C. B., Tiba, P. A., Kawakami, S. E., Catallani, B., Kerstens, M., and Suchecki, D. (2010). Disruptions of the mother-infant relationship and stress-related behaviours: altered corticosterone secretion does not explain everything. *Neurosci Biobehav Rev*, 34, 821–834.

Fitzgerald, M. and Walker, S. M. (2009). Infant pain management: a developmental neurobiological approach. *Nat Clin Pract Neurol*, 5, 35–50.

Fox, M. D. (2011). Wound care in the neonatal intensive care unit. *Neonatal Netw, 30*, 291–303.

Hathway, G. J., Koch, S., Low, L., and Fitzgerald, M. (2009). The changing balance of brainstem-spinal cord modulation of pain processing over the first weeks of rat postnatal life. *J Physiol, 587*, 2927–2935.

Hathway, G. J., Vega-Avelaira, D., and Fitzgerald, M. (2012). A critical period in the supraspinal control of pain: opioid-dependent changes in brainstem rostroventral medulla function in preadolescence. *Pain, 153*, 775–783.

Hensch, T. K. (2004). Critical period regulation. *Annu Rev Neurosci, 27*, 549–579.

Hohmann, A. G., Neely, M. H., Pina, J., and Nackley, A. G. (2005). Neonatal chronic hind paw inflammation alters sensitization to intradermal capsaicin in adult rats: a behavioral and immunocytochemical study. *J Pain, 6*, 798–808.

Howard, R. F., Walker, S. M., Mota, P. M., and Fitzgerald, M. (2005). The ontogeny of neuropathic pain: postnatal onset of mechanical allodynia in rat spared nerve injury (SNI) and chronic constriction injury (CCI) models. *Pain, 115*, 382–389.

Jiang, M. C. and Gebhart, G. F. (1998). Development of mustard oil-induced hyperalgesia in rats. *Pain, 77*, 305–313.

Kalinichev, M., Easterling, K. W., and Holtzman, S. G. (2002). Early neonatal experience of Long-Evans rats results in long-lasting changes in reactivity to a novel environment and morphine-induced sensitization and tolerance. *Neuropsychopharmacology, 27*, 518–533.

Kehlet, H., Jensen, T. S., and Woolf, C. J. (2006). Persistent postsurgical pain: risk factors and prevention. *Lancet, 367*, 1618–1625.

LaPrairie, J. L., Johns, M. E., and Murphy, A. Z. (2008). Preemptive morphine analgesia attenuates the long-term consequences of neonatal inflammation in male and female rats. *Pediatr Res, 64*, 625–630.

LaPrairie, J. L. and Murphy, A. Z. (2007). Female rats are more vulnerable to the long-term consequences of neonatal inflammatory injury. *Pain, 132* (Suppl. 1), S124–133.

LaPrairie, J. L. and Murphy, A. Z. (2009). Neonatal injury alters adult pain sensitivity by increasing opioid tone in the periaqueductal gray. *Front Behav Neurosci, 3*, 31.

LaPrairie, J. L. and Murphy, A. Z. (2010). Long-term impact of neonatal injury in male and female rats: Sex differences, mechanisms and clinical implications. *Front Neuroendocrinol, 31*, 193–202.

Le Bars, D., Gozariu, M., and Cadden, S. W. (2001). Animal models of nociception. *Pharmacol Rev, 53*, 597–652.

Lee, D. H. and Chung, J. M. (1996). Neuropathic pain in neonatal rats. *Neurosci Lett, 209*, 140–142.

Lidow, M. S., Song, Z. M., and Ren, K. (2001). Long-term effects of short-lasting early local inflammatory insult. *Neuroreport, 12*, 399–403.

Lim, E. J., Back, S. K., Kim, M. A., Li, C., Lee, J., Jeong, K. Y., et al. (2009). Long-lasting neonatal inflammation enhances pain responses to subsequent inflammation, but not peripheral nerve injury in adult rats. *Int J Dev Neurosci, 27*, 215–222.

Lin, C. and Al-Chaer, E. D. (2003). Long-term sensitization of primary afferents in adult rats exposed to neonatal colon pain. *Brain Res, 971*, 73–82.

Low, L. A. and Fitzgerald, M. (2012). Acute pain and a motivational pathway in adult rats: influence of early life pain experience. *PLoS ONE, 7*, e34316.

McCutcheon, J. E. and Marinelli, M. (2009). Age matters. *Eur J Neurosci, 29*, 997–1014.

McKelvy, A. D. and Sweitzer, S. M. (2009). Endothelin-1 exposure on postnatal day 7 alters expression of the endothelin B receptor and behavioral sensitivity to endothelin-1 on postnatal day 11. *Neurosci Lett, 451*, 89–93.

McLaughlin, C. R., Lichtman, A. H., Fanselow, M. S., and Cramer, C. P. (1990). Tonic nociception in neonatal rats. *Pharmacol Biochem Behav, 36*, 859–862.

Miranda, A., Peles, S., Shaker, R., Rudolph, C., and Sengupta, J. N. (2006). Neonatal nociceptive somatic stimulation differentially modifies the activity of spinal neurons in rats and results in altered somatic and visceral sensation. *J Physiol, 572*, 775–787.

Moss, A., Alvares, D., Meredith-Middleton, J., Robinson, M., Slater, R., Hunt, S. P., et al. (2005). Ephrin-A4 inhibits sensory neurite outgrowth and is regulated by neonatal skin wounding. *Eur J Neurosci, 22*, 2413–2421.

Nagarajan, R., Darlington, R. B., Finlay, B. L., and Clancy, B. (2010). ttime: an R package for translating the timing of brain development across mammalian species. *Neuroinformatics, 8*, 201–205.

Negrigo, A., Medeiros, M., Guinsburg, R., and Covolan, L. (2011). Long-term gender behavioral vulnerability after nociceptive neonatal formalin stimulation in rats. *Neurosci Lett, 490*, 196–199.

Rahman, W., Fitzgerald, M., Aynsley-Green, A., and Dickenson, A. (1997). The effects of neonatal exposure to inflammation and/or morphine on neuronal responses and morphine analgesia in adult rats. In T. S. Jensen, J. A. Turner, and Z. Wiesenfeld-Hallin (eds) *Proceedings of the 8th World Congress on Pain. Progress in Pain Research and Management. Vol 8*, pp. 783–794. Seattle: IASP Press.

Randich, A., Uzzell, T., Deberry, J. J., and Ness, T. J. (2006). Neonatal urinary bladder inflammation produces adult bladder hypersensitivity. *J Pain, 7*, 469–479.

Ren, K., Anseloni, V., Zou, S. P., Wade, E. B., Novikova, S. I., Ennis, M., et al. (2004). Characterization of basal and re-inflammation-associated long-term alteration in pain responsivity following short-lasting neonatal local inflammatory insult. *Pain, 110*, 588–596.

Ren, K., Novikova, S. I., He, F., Dubner, R., and Lidow, M. S. (2005). Neonatal local noxious insult affects gene expression in the spinal dorsal horn of adult rats. *Mol Pain, 1*, 27.

Reynolds, M., Alvares, D., Middleton, J., and Fitzgerald, M. (1997). Neonatally wounded skin induces NGF-independent sensory neurite outgrowth in vitro. *Brain Res Dev Brain Res, 102*, 275–283.

Reynolds, M. L. and Fitzgerald, M. (1995). Long-term sensory hyperinnervation following neonatal skin wounds. *J Comp Neurol, 358*, 487–498.

Ririe, D. G. and Eisenach, J. C. (2006). Age-dependent responses to nerve injury-induced mechanical allodynia. *Anesthesiology, 104*, 344–350.

Ririe, D. G., Vernon, T. L., Tobin, J. R., and Eisenach, J. C. (2003). Age-dependent responses to thermal hyperalgesia and mechanical allodynia in a rat model of acute postoperative pain. *Anesthesiology, 99*, 443–448.

Roizenblatt, S., Andersen, M. L., Bignotto, M., D'almeida, V., Martins, P. J., and Tufik, S. (2010). Neonatal arthritis disturbs sleep and behaviour of adult rat offspring and their dams. *Eur J Pain, 14*, 985–991.

Rovnaghi, C. R., Garg, S., Hall, R. W., Bhutta, A. T., and Anand, K. J. (2008). Ketamine analgesia for inflammatory pain in neonatal rats: a factorial randomized trial examining long-term effects. *Behav Brain Funct, 4*, 35.

Ruda, M. A., Ling, Q. D., Hohmann, A. G., Peng, Y. B., and Tachibana, T. (2000). Altered nociceptive neuronal circuits after neonatal peripheral inflammation. *Science, 289*, 628–631.

Schwetz, I., McRoberts, J. A., Coutinho, S. V., Bradesi, S., Gale, G., Fanselow, M., et al. (2005). Corticotropin-releasing factor receptor 1 mediates acute and delayed stress-induced visceral hyperalgesia in maternally separated Long-Evans rats. *Am J Physiol Gastrointest Liver Physiol, 289*, G704–7012.

Sorkin, L. S. and Yaksh, T. L. (2009). Behavioral models of pain states evoked by physical injury to the peripheral nerve. *Neurotherapeutics, 6*, 609–6019.

Spencer, S. J., Galic, M. A., and Pittman, Q. J. (2011). Neonatal programming of innate immune function. *Am J Physiol Endocrinol Metab, 300*, E11–118.

Sternberg, W. F. and Ridgway, C. G. (2003). Effects of gestational stress and neonatal handling on pain, analgesia, and stress behavior of adult mice. *Physiol Behav, 78*, 375–383.

Sternberg, W. F., Scorr, L., Smith, L. D., Ridgway, C. G., and Stout, M. (2005). Long-term effects of neonatal surgery on adulthood pain behavior. *Pain, 113*, 347–353.

Tachibana, T., Ling, Q. D., and Ruda, M. A. (2001). Increased Fos induction in adult rats that experienced neonatal peripheral inflammation. *Neuroreport*, 12, 925–957.

Tjong, Y. W., Ip, S. P., Lao, L., Wu, J., Fong, H. H., Sung, J. J., Berman, B., and Che, C. T. (2010). Neonatal maternal separation elevates thalamic corticotrophin releasing factor type 1 receptor expression response to colonic distension in rat. *Neuro Endocrinol Lett*, 31, 215–220.

Torsney, C. and Fitzgerald, M. (2002). Age-dependent effects of peripheral inflammation on the electrophysiological properties of neonatal rat dorsal horn neurons. *J Neurophysiol*, 87, 1311–1317.

Torsney, C. and Fitzgerald, M. (2003). Spinal dorsal horn cell receptive field size is increased in adult rats following neonatal hindpaw skin injury. *J Physiol*, 550, 255–261.

Walker, C. D., Kudreikis, K., Sherrard, A., and Johnston, C. C. (2003). Repeated neonatal pain influences maternal behavior, but not stress responsiveness in rat offspring. *Brain Res Dev Brain Res*, 140, 253–261.

Walker, C. D., Xu, Z., Rochford, J., and Johnston, C. C. (2008). Naturally occurring variations in maternal care modulate the effects of repeated neonatal pain on behavioral sensitivity to thermal pain in the adult offspring. *Pain*, 140, 167–176.

Walker, S. M., Meredith-Middleton, J., Cooke-Yarborough, C., and Fitzgerald, M. (2003). Neonatal inflammation and primary afferent terminal plasticity in the rat dorsal horn. *Pain*, 105, 185–195.

Walker, S. M., Meredith-Middleton, J., Lickiss, T., Moss, A., and Fitzgerald, M. (2007). Primary and secondary hyperalgesia can be differentiated by postnatal age and ERK activation in the spinal dorsal horn of the rat pup. *Pain*, 128, 157–168.

Walker, S. M., Tochiki, K. K., and Fitzgerald, M. (2009). Hindpaw incision in early life increases the hyperalgesic response to repeat surgical injury: critical period and dependence on initial afferent activity. *Pain*, 147, 99–106.

Wang, G., Ji, Y., Lidow, M. S., and Traub, R. J. (2004). Neonatal hind paw injury alters processing of visceral and somatic nociceptive stimuli in the adult rat. *J Pain*, 5, 440–449.

Wang, J., Gu, C., and Al-Chaer, E. D. (2008). Altered behavior and digestive outcomes in adult male rats primed with minimal colon pain as neonates. *Behav Brain Funct*, 4, 28.

Wang, K. C., Wang, S. J., Fan, L. W., Cai, Z., Rhodes, P. G., and Tien, L. T. (2011). Interleukin-1 receptor antagonist ameliorates neonatal lipopolysaccharide-induced long-lasting hyperalgesia in the adult rats. *Toxicology*, 279, 123–129.

Winston, J., Shenoy, M., Medley, D., Naniwadekar, A., and Pasricha, P. J. (2007). The vanilloid receptor initiates and maintains colonic hypersensitivity induced by neonatal colon irritation in rats. *Gastroenterology*, 132, 615–627.

Wood, S. L., Beyer, B. K., and Cappon, G. D. (2003). Species comparison of postnatal CNS development: functional measures. *Birth Defects Res B Dev Reprod Toxicol*, 68, 391–407.

Young, E. E., Baumbauer, K. M., Hillyer, J., and Joynes, R. L. (2007). Local anesthetic treatment significantly attenuates acute pain responding but does not prevent the neonatal injury-induced reduction in adult spinal behavioral plasticity. *Behav Neurosci*, 121, 1073–1081.

Young, E. E., Baumbauer, K. M., Hillyer, J. E., Patterson, A. M., Hoy, K. C., Jr., Mintz, E. M., *et al.* (2008). The neonatal injury-induced spinal learning deficit in adult rats: central mechanisms. *Behav Neurosci*, 122, 589–600.

Zhang, Y. H., Wang, X. M., and Ennis, M. (2010). Effects of neonatal inflammation on descending modulation from the rostroventromedial medulla. *Brain Res Bull*, 83, 16–22.

CHAPTER 4

Long-term effects of pain in children

Ruth E. Grunau

Introduction

Major advances in high-technology medical care have led to greatly increased survival of medically fragile infants born extremely preterm, or with major congenital anomalies or other life-threatening conditions. These infants are exposed to procedural, surgical, and post-surgical pain. For millennia human infancy was a prolonged period of adult protection, with pain rarely encountered early in life. While the biological mechanisms for perception of pain develop during the fetal period, endogenous capacities to dampen pain mature later. Until relatively recently, this biological substrate was a good fit, matching the environment of infancy. However, the revolution in medical care has led to unforeseen challenges to understand and manage infant pain. In full-term infants, the primary concern is whether early pain alters later pain sensitivity. In contrast, due to the immaturity of the developing nervous system, the greatest impact of pain is likely to occur in the least maturely born infants. Therefore, in infants born very preterm who undergo lengthy hospitalization, pain may affect multiple aspects of development. This chapter focuses on long-term effects of early pain on subsequent pain perception, neurodevelopment, brain development, and programming of stress systems in the context of clinical studies, and whether caregiving factors may ameliorate potential long-term adverse effects.

Full-term infants: early pain and later pain thresholds

Stimulation of peripheral nociceptors can trigger long-term changes in circuitry of the central nervous system (CNS; Fitzgerald and Walker, 2009). To better understand the potential long-lasting changes associated with early pain in infants born full-term, studies of the effects of circumcision, major surgery and burns on tactile and pain thresholds later in childhood have been conducted.

Circumcision

One line of investigation to evaluate whether neonatal pain has long-term effects in healthy infants born full-term, has been follow-up of subsequent pain sensitivity in boys circumcised early in life. In a post hoc analysis of behavioural response to immunization

pain, boys who had been circumcised (regardless of analgesia) displayed greater pain behaviour to immunization at age 4 to 6 months, compared to uncircumcised boys (Taddio et al., 1995). Then a prospective randomized controlled study was conducted in which boys underwent neonatal circumcision with either local anaesthetic lidocaine-prilocaine 5% cream (EMLA®) or placebo, or were not circumcised. These three groups of boys were studied later during immunization at age 4 to 6 months (Taddio et al., 1997). Circumcised boys who had received placebo showed higher facial actions, cry duration, and observer visual analogue scale (VAS) pain ratings in response to immunization compared to the uncircumcised group.

Importantly, using quantitative sensory testing, adult penile sensitivity did not differ in men who had or had not been circumcised as neonates (Bleustein et al., 2005). Long-term effects of circumcision on pain threshold may be transitory. There is scant research on this question, given that placebo studies for neonatal circumcision studies are no longer ethical by current standards. Further studies are needed that compare later pain thresholds among infants that receive varying pain relief for circumcision (e.g. lidocaine-prilocaine 5% cream versus penile block). Moreover, caregiver behaviours during immunization should be measured to rule out possible confounding factors between parents who choose to circumcise their newborn boys, compare to those who do not.

Major surgery

Long after surgery early in life, there appear to be changes in later tactile sensitivity that vary depending on the type of surgery, and whether in the region of surgery or elsewhere, indicating both local and global effects. In a combined sample of children born full-term or preterm, skin sensitivity was tested at age 9 to 12 years in a group of children who had chest surgery in infancy, and compared with children who had no surgery (Schmelzle-Lubiecki et al., 2007). Those who had surgery showed hyposensitivity to touch, cold, and heat in the region of the surgery, and subtle abnormalities in everyday sensations. In contrast to these long-term changes, Andrews and Fitzgerald (2002) found that infants who had abdominal surgery showed *hyper*sensitivity to touch, both in the wound area and the contralateral side of the body in the first 24 postoperative hours. In another study, infants who underwent surgery in the first 3 months of life, and then subsequent surgery in the same dermatome 15 (range 8–70; median: 10th–90th percentile) weeks later, needed more intraoperative fentanyl, had higher behavioural pain scores, had greater noradrenaline plasma concentrations, and needed more postoperative morphine than infants with no prior surgery (Peters et al., 2005). In contrast, in that study, infants who previously underwent surgery in a different dermatome had only higher postoperative analgesic requirements and noradrenaline plasma concentrations. These studies suggest spinal and supraspinal changes following early surgery. The long-term consequences of surgery in early infancy appear to be greater in areas of prior tissue damage, suggesting neurobiological changes with clinical implications for subsequent pain management. However, importantly no differences were found in heart rate, cortisol, or behavioural responses to vaccination in toddlers who had surgery early in life (Peters et al., 2003).

It is likely that effects of surgery will be related to age at surgery, the severity of the intervention, provision of effective pain management, how well surgery and the hospital stay were managed emotionally and cognitively for the young child, as well as the type and timing of subsequent evaluation. Taken together, it appears that early surgery can induce changes in peripheral and central tactile and pain processing; however, the direction, magnitude, and nature of the functional impact depend on multiple factors. In some of these studies samples of infants born preterm and full-term were combined. It is unknown whether physiological and brain maturity at the time of surgery (i.e. varying duration of gestation) contributes to the long-term impact on later pain threshold. Moreover, very preterm infants who undergo neonatal surgery also have been exposed to multiple other invasive procedures due to their prematurity, Studies on effects of early surgery on sensitivity to pain later in childhood that account for multiple sources of early pain experience during hospitalization are needed to uncover differences between infants born preterm and full-term.

Burns

Children who had suffered burns early in life (at 6–24 months), displayed altered mechanical and pain sensitivity later in childhood at age 9 to 16 years, that varied by severity of the initial injury (Wollgarten-Hadamek et al., 2009). Compared to controls, children with moderate burns in infancy showed higher mechanical detection thresholds (hyposensitivity), lower mechanical pain thresholds (hypersensitivity), and greater sensitization to repetitive mechanical stimuli; however, no significant changes were found for thermal stimuli. In contrast, compared to controls, severely burned children showed elevated thermal pain thresholds, whereas mechanical pain sensitivity was not consistently different. The authors concluded that this differential pattern of altered sensory and pain sensitivity may reflect differences in stress, pain, and analgesic treatment between moderately and severely burned infants. Importantly, early traumatic and painful injuries, such as burns, can induce global long-term alterations in tactile and pain processing.

Neonatal pain in preterm infants

Very preterm infants born 2 to 4 months before their due date spend weeks to months in the neonatal intensive care unit (NICU), outside the protective intrauterine environment. During this time the synaptic connections, integrated circuits, and descending modulatory endogenous controls are immature (Fitzgerald and Walker, 2009), and pain induces diffuse activation across multiple brain regions (Fabrizi et al., 2011) therefore preterm infants are potentially most susceptible to pain and long-term effects of pain during the developmental period corresponding to the late second and entire third trimester of fetal life. Preterm neonates display lower thresholds (i.e. are more sensitive) and greater reflex responses to peripheral stimuli compared to full-term infants (Fitzgerald and Beggs, 2001). With repeated stimulation, reflex thresholds may drop even further (see Walker and Baccei, Chapter 6, this volume, for details of peripheral and central mechanisms of reflex sensitization). Importantly, sensitization to repeated tactile stimulation is greatest below 33 weeks postconceptional age (Andrews and Fitzgerald, 1994). Due to altered touch thresholds and sensitization, even non-invasive handling such as diaper change can elicit pain-like behavioural and autonomic responses in very premature infants, if the diaper change follows blood collection even after a 30-min rest period in between the procedures (Holsti et al., 2005). Similarly, when diaper change preceded blood collection, pain response to heel lance was heightened compared to blood collection after at least 1 h undisturbed (Holsti et al., 2006). In this way, sensitization may provide one mechanism whereby repetitive pain and handling lays the groundwork for ongoing pain and discomfort during neonatal intensive care.

Later pain thresholds

Evidence for long-term effects of neonatal pain on later tactile and pain perception has now been demonstrated in multiple studies. Whereas the early work on long-term effects of neonatal pain on later pain sensitivity utilized parent report (Grunau et al., 1994a) or pictures (Grunau et al., 1998), more recent studies have directly compared behavioural and autonomic pain responses in infants born very preterm compared to healthy infants born at full-term. Findings differ depending on age at testing. Contrary to expectation, after hospital discharge, preterm infants showed little difference in reactivity to pain at 4 months corrected age (CA), either to a pain-naïve site of finger lance (Oberlander et al., 2000), or to more intense pain of immunization injections (Grunau et al., 2010). However, at 8 months CA, pain responses diverged in that the preterm group showed brief initial facial hyperresponsiveness to a finger lance, followed by faster behavioural and heart-rate recovery (Grunau et al., 2001). This rapid dampening evident at 8 months CA may underlie the appearance of reduced pain response to everyday bumps, scrapes, and falls reported by parents of preterms born at 800g or less compared to full-term toddlers (Grunau et al., 1994a). Differences may emerge across time, as reported in animal studies (e.g. Ren et al., 2004; see also Walker, Chapter 3, this volume).

At later ages, detection and pain thresholds for thermal, mechanical, and pressure stimuli have been studied, providing converging evidence of altered sensation in children born preterm. Pressure points were tested with a dolorimeter to measure later pain threshold, revealing that adolescents born preterm had more tender points and lower pain threshold (Buskila et al., 2003). Using quantitative sensory testing, both hyperreactivity (enhanced sensitivity) and hyporeactivity (reduced sensitivity) to pain have been reported at ages 9 to 14 years in children born preterm compared to full-term. The direction and the extent of effects varied depending on the type of pain stimulus and whether the pain was short-lasting or ongoing (Hermann et al., 2006; S. M. Walker et al., 2009). Preterms and full-terms exposed to NICU care both differed from full-term healthy controls displaying increased baseline thermal thresholds (i.e. reduced sensitivity), but a greater degree of sensitization following prolonged heat at non-injured sites, suggestive of central changes. Findings of both baseline hyporeactivity but hyperreactivity to a noxious stimulus in these human studies are consistent with the animal literature on long-term effects of early pain (Ren et al., 2004; see also Walker, Chapter 3, this volume).

Importantly, the study of preterm infants born at less than 26 weeks of gestation (S. M. Walker et al., 2009) was the first to differentiate those who had neonatal surgery. While there were generalized differences between the children born preterm compared to full-term in heat and cold thresholds and also in response to mechanical stimulation adjacent to scars, it was the preterms that had neonatal surgery that primarily accounted for those findings. While the extent of tissue damage may be the most salient difference in those extreme preterms micropremies exposed to surgery, it is also possible that those requiring surgery may have been sicker and may have been exposed to more cumulative procedural pain during their NICU care. Further research is needed to elucidate the role of neonatal surgery in the long-term effects of altered pain thresholds in children born extremely preterm.

Using functional magnetic resonance imaging (fMRI) while children were exposed to pain stimulation, children born preterm showed greater cortical and subcortical brain activation (Hohmeister et al., 2010). In response to heat stimuli of moderate pain intensity, preterm but not full-term children that had required NICU care as neonates, exhibited significant activations in a number of brain regions (thalamus, anterior cingulate cortex, cerebellum, basal ganglia, and periaqueductal grey) that were not significantly activated in non-NICU exposed full-term controls. Moreover, the preterms showed significantly greater activation than controls in primary somatosensory cortex, anterior cingulate cortex, and insula. This exaggerated brain response in preterms was pain-specific.

Recurrent pain in the long run: children, adolescents, and young adults

Self-report is considered the 'gold standard' for pain assessment. Surprisingly, given the altered sensory thresholds described earlier, there have been several reports that adolescents and young adults born preterm report few if any differences in recurrent pain in daily life compared to their peers born healthy at full-term (Buskila et al., 2003; Saigal et al., 1996, 2007; Schmelzle-Lubiecki et al., 2007; S. M. Walker et al., 2009). However, given the high prevalence of abdominal pain, headaches, limb pain, and other non-specific pain complaints in children in the general population, it is difficult to evaluate differences in these relatively small studies. Similarly, by parent report, greater somatization (functional pain complaints with no medical explanation) was more common in young preterm children at age 5 years (Grunau et al., 1994b; Sommerfelt et al., 1996); however, in a longitudinal cohort these differences were no longer apparent in later childhood at age 9 years (Whitfield et al., 1997) or in late adolescence at 17 years (Grunau et al., 2004a). Thus, although touch and pain thresholds differ in children born preterm, and brain activity in response to pain differs in preterms, contrary to expectations, there is little evidence at this point for long-term functional pain problems that impact daily life. However, further research is needed to evaluate gender differences in the emergence of pain problems in adulthood, and the role that environmental life stresses may play in this population.

Neurodevelopment

Infants born very preterm spend weeks to months in the NICU during a period of extremely rapid brain development and programming of stress systems, rendering them far more vulnerable to environmental perturbations such as neonatal pain, than infants born at term. For the tiniest, most fragile infants, the period of pain exposure is prolonged, during the last trimester of 'fetal' life, a time of very complex and rapid brain development. Neurodevelopmental problems including cognitive, language, visual-perceptual, visual-motor, attention and learning deficits as well as motor dysfunction are common in children born prematurely (e.g. Allen, 2008; Grunau et al., 2002), persisting to adulthood (e.g. Hack et al., 2002; Grunau et al., 2004a). Two mechanisms have been identified that may potentially link neonatal pain exposure to altered neurodevelopment in this vulnerable population, namely changes to the developing brain and programming of stress systems. It is known that immature neurons are more sensitive to neurotoxic environmental influences (see Lagercrantz et al., 2010). Atypicalities in structural and functional brain development are evident in preterm infants (e.g. Ment et al., 2009, S. P. Miller and Ferriero, 2009), however the causes are unclear.

Greater neonatal pain exposure, defined as the cumulative number of skin-breaking procedures from birth to term equivalent, was found to be associated with poorer motor and cognitive development to 18 months CA, after adjusting for medical neonatal confounders (Grunau et al., 2009). This is consistent with evidence in another longitudinal cohort that repeated neonatal pain was associated with alterations in the developing preterm brain (Brummelte et al., 2012). Furthermore, prolonged exposure to repeated neonatal pain in preterm infants appears to contribute to altered programming of the hypothalamic–pituitary–adrenocortical (HPA) axis across the first 2 years of life (Grunau et al., 2004b, 2007), which has important implications for brain function.

Pain and the immature developing brain
Brain reactivity to procedures

The brain undergoes very rapid developmental changes in macrostructure, microstructure, and connectivity during the time that infants born extremely preterm are undergoing neonatal intensive care. An example of the progression of structural brain maturation from 28 weeks of gestation to term-equivalent age is shown in Figure 4.1. Magnetic resonance imaging (MRI) studies have revealed atypical brain development in neonates born very preterm, e.g. smaller volume of the brain and specific regions, abnormalities in white matter microstructure, reduced cortical thickness, disturbances of the thalamocortical system, and altered development of the cerebellum and other structures (e.g. see Ball et al., 2011; Volpe 2009; see also Poorun and Slater, Chapter 39, this volume).

There has been long-standing concern that procedures conducted as part of life-saving care of preterm neonates may adversely affect brain development. Thirty years ago, Perlman and Volpe (1983) reported that endotracheal suctioning affected neonatal cerebral blood flow. In recent years there have been a number of important studies of cortical activity during procedural intervention in the NICU, utilizing near infrared spectroscopy to examine cerebral blood flow and electroencephalography (EEG) to measure electrical

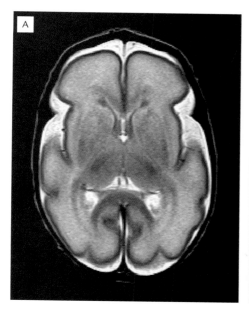
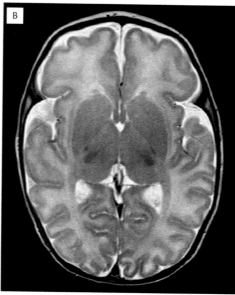

Figure 4.1 Structural maturation of the developing brain in one preterm infant from 28 weeks (A) to term equivalent age (B) MRI images courtesy of Dr Steven Miller.

activity, demonstrating that blood collection evokes responses in the cortex (Bartocci et al., 2006; Fabrizi et al., 2011; Slater et al., 2006, 2010; Tombini et al., 2009; Vanhatalo et al., 2009). Fabrizi et al. (2011) reported increased incidence of widely dispersed non-specific neuronal bursts of EEG activity in response to touch and pain in preterm infants, rather than the typical focused-evoked somatosensory potentials, maximal at the central electrodes that were evident in full-term neonates. This study is very important for understanding the vulnerability of preterm neonates, as it underscores the sensitivity of the preterm neonate to both mechanical and nociceptive stimulation. This phenomenon of responses widespread across the brain contributes to understanding why diaper change can evoke as much behavioural and autonomic reactivity as blood collection in preterm neonates while in the NICU (Holsti et al., 2005). It is challenging to record specific brain activity in response to painful procedures in young infants, since even after excluding overt movement artefacts, tensing of muscles in the face and limbs may affect the signal, given the proximity of the motor and somatosensory regions of the cortex (Maimon et al., 2013).

In the only fMRI study of the brain during pain stimulation, at age 9 to 14 years children born preterm showed greater activation in the somatosensory cortex and several other brain regions compared to children born full-term with or without early hospitalization (Hohmeister et al., 2010; see also Hermann, Chapter 40, this volume). More research is needed to explicate relationships between brain, behaviour, and autonomic reactivity in the preterm neonate under various conditions across post-conceptional age in the NICU.

Neonatal pain and brain development

Utilizing state-of-the-art brain imaging techniques to study microstructure development from early in life to term equivalent age, Grunau and colleagues found an association between greater exposure to pain-related stress in preterm infants in the NICU and poorer neonatal brain development (Brummelte et al., 2012). In a longitudinal design, serial MRI and diffusion tensor imaging was carried out shortly after birth and again at term equivalent age in neonates born at 24 to 32 weeks of gestation. After adjusting for multiple clinical confounding factors, such as gestational age at birth, infections, brain injury, and surgery, higher exposure to procedural pain was associated with reduced development of white matter (indexed by fractional anisotropy (FA)) and subcortical grey matter (measured by N-acetylaspartate to choline ratio (NAA/choline)—a marker of cerebral metabolism and density). Reduced FA was predicted by early pain prior to the first brain scan, whereas lower NAA/choline was predicted by pain exposure throughout the neonatal course, suggesting a primary and early effect on subcortical structures with secondary white matter changes. This study appears to be the first in human infants to show that neonatal pain is associated with adverse brain development. Until now, relationships between pain and brain development in preterm infants were speculative.

In the first study to examine whether neonatal pain is associated with brain activity later in childhood, in a different longitudinal cohort of preterm infants followed from birth to school age, Grunau and colleagues found an association between greater cumulative neonatal pain and spontaneous oscillatory brain activity under resting conditions using magnetoencephalography at age 7 years (Doesburg et al., 2013). In turn, the cortical activity was associated with cognitive function. Importantly, in this study the link between neonatal pain and brain function was evident in infants born extremely preterm at 24 to 28 weeks, but not in more mature preterm infant born 29 to 32 weeks. It is well established that there are progressive changes in the maturation of oscillatory brain activity throughout the preterm period, as shown in the spectral composition of EEG recordings (Okumura et al., 2003). The finding that neonatal pain was associated with brain activity in infants born at 24 to 28 weeks, but not later, may reflect the distinct phases of development occurring within thalamocortical systems within the 24- to 28- and 29- to 32-week gestational periods, and the implications for how pain is processed within the developing CNS (Kostovic and Judas, 2010).

Furthermore, the findings described are consistent with reports that adverse early stress beyond pain exposure, such as maternal separation, is implicated in altered brain structure and function (Als et al., 2004; Milgrom et al., 2010; Smith et al., 2011). In one study (Als et al., 2004), preterm neonates were randomized to receive the Neonatal Individualized Developmental Care and Assessment Program (NIDCAP; Als, 1982) or standard care during their NICU stay. The NIDCAP programme involves recognition of infant stress cues and provision of supportive care. At 2 weeks CA, the infants that received the intervention programme displayed significantly better motor system functions and self-regulatory behaviours, as well as increased coherence between frontal and a broad spectrum of primarily occipital brain regions on electrophysiological testing (Als et al., 2004). Furthermore improved behavioural function was still apparent at 9 months CA. In another randomized controlled trial, effectiveness of training parents to reduce stressful experiences for their very preterm infants in the NICU was evaluated (Milgrom et al., 2010). At term equivalent, the stress sensitivity training was associated with fewer atypicalities in cerebral white matter microstructure and connectivity on advanced MRI, compared to infants that received standard care.

Taken together, these studies on brain reactivity to procedures, as well as associations between pain and brain development, begin to address the role that pain might play in contributing to altered spontaneous cortical oscillatory activity (within functionally distinct frequency ranges, theta (46–7 Hz), alpha (8–14 Hz), beta (15–29 Hz), and gamma (30–60 Hz) neuromagnetic activity (Doesburg et al., 2011a)) and atypical long-range neuromagnetic synchronization during visual short-term and working memory maintenance associated with alteration and reorganization of functional connectivity in children born very preterm (Doesburg et al., 2011b), as well as a host of atypicalities in structural and functional brain development revealed by MRI in children born very preterm (see Ment et al., 2009 for review). There is now converging evidence that the developing brain is exquisitely sensitive to ongoing procedural perturbations during a 'critical window' in early life, suggesting that the long-term effects of pain are potentially greatest in extremely preterm infants during hospitalization in the NICU.

Programming of stress systems

Altered programming of stress systems, including the HPA axis, due to both fetal and neonatal stress is well established in the animal literature (e.g. Matthews, 2002), and in humans in studies of posttraumatic stress disorder (G. E. Miller et al., 2007) or early adversity such as institutional care in orphanages (Loman and Gunnar, 2010). Unexpectedly, in animal studies of long-term effects of early pain, no changes were found in HPA responses later in adult rats (Anand et al., 1999; C. D. Walker et al., 2003). Importantly, C. D. Walker et al. (2003) showed that following pain, maternal licking and grooming increased, thus preventing changes to the stress hormone system. In preterm infants, exposure to repeated neonatal pain in the NICU is typically combined with the stress of maternal separation. The developmental trajectory of the expression of cortisol (the endpoint of HPA axis activity) appears to be altered across the first 2 years of life in infants born at extremely low gestational age (24–28 weeks), with downregulation extending from the NICU period (Grunau et al., 2005) switching to upregulation at 8 and 18 months CA (Grunau et al., 2004b, 2007), associated with greater exposure to procedural pain.

Sleep

Sleep–waking states develop during the third trimester of fetal life, and thus are emerging during the period that preterm infants are exposed to repeated procedural pain in the NICU. There is long-standing interest in effects of sleep disruption on the developing CNS (e.g. Anders and Roffwarg, 1973; Scher et al., 2005). Sleep plays an essential role in brain development (Blumberg and Seelke, 2010). Shifts in sleep state occur in response to pain in the NICU, thus have become a key part of pain assessment (e.g. Holsti et al., 2008; Stevens et al., 2010), however little is known about effects of pain and pain management on sleep in preterm neonates. Importantly, opioids for pain management affect sleep structure, for example, decreasing rapid eye movement sleep (Axelin et al., 2010). Fabrizi et al. (2011) reported that the occurrence of noxious-specific EEG potentials was not state dependent, since the proportion of awake infants was the same for those who did and did not exhibit the noxious-specific EEG response. However, very preterm infants typically spend little time awake in the NICU. Further EEG and behavioural studies of effects of pain on sleep are needed, to elucidate the role of pain in preterm infants on brain development via disruption of sleep.

Sex and gender

Sex refers to biological and physiological characteristics, whereas gender is defined as the socially constructed roles, behaviours, activities, and attributes that a given society considers appropriate for men and women (World Health Organization, 2012). Sex differences in long-term effects of early pain and stress are widely reported in the animal literature (Laprairie and Murphy, 2007), and gender differences in adult pain experience are well-established (Unruh, 1996). However, in human clinical studies of long-term effects of early pain, sex and gender differences have rarely been examined. In a longitudinal cohort no differences were found between boys and girls in cortisol levels during infancy and toddlerhood (Grunau et al., 2004b, 2007). Contradictory findings have been reported, for example, in one study girls displayed greater pain sensitivity than boys among both preterm and full-term adolescents (Buskila et al., 2003). In a cohort of micropremies (S. M. Walker et al., 2009) term control boys were more sensitive than girls to cold and heat stimulation, but no gender differences were found in the preterm group. More research with larger sample sizes is needed to explicate the role of gender, and possible interactions with environmental caregiver factors.

Caregiver behaviour and long-term effects of neonatal pain

Setting the foundation for optimal infant support to minimize pain-related stress begins in the NICU. Nursing interventions during procedures, and teaching parents how to read their infant's cues and how to provide environmental support such as skin-to-skin contact, swaddling, and facilitated tucking is likely to be fundamental in helping the infant to gradually self-regulate stress (Feldman et al., 2002; Maroney, 2003; Symington and Pinelli, 2006). Importantly, parent involvement to reduce infant stress in the NICU led to improved behaviour and EEG coherence (Milgrom et al., 2010).

Social modelling, family factors, child temperament, culture, and gender affect pain expression and thereby pain threshold later in childhood and beyond. This body of work has been conducted primarily on full-terms (e.g. Braarud and Stormak 2006; Moon et al., 2008; Piira et al., 2007; Pillai Riddell and Chambers, 2007). Parent soothing is associated with greater reactivity, not less, whereas verbalizations that promoted coping reduce pain responses in infants undergoing immunization. Little research after NICU discharge has addressed whether parent behaviours across infancy and childhood may ameliorate or exacerbate effects of early pain on later pain sensitivity or on neurodevelopment in children born preterm exposed to prolonged pain early in life. Greater parenting stress appears to compound the association between higher neonatal pain exposure and poorer cognitive development at 18 months in children born very preterm (Grunau et al., 2009). However, since poorer neurodevelopment in preterm children is in turn associated with persisting parenting stress (Brummelte et al., 2011), it is difficult to disentangle these effects. Among infants with extensive history of exposure to neonatal pain in the NICU due to extremely preterm birth, child and family factors predicted somatization at age 4 years (Grunau et al., 1994b). In another study, at age 9 to 14 years, maternal factors in relation to responses to quantitative sensory testing of pain thresholds were compared in three groups of children: those born preterm who had been in the NICU, full terms who had been in the NICU, and full-term healthy controls (Hohmeister et al., 2009). Threshold testing was conducted with and without the infant's mother present. Only former preterms displayed more catastrophizing and elicited greater maternal solicitous responses to pain. Importantly, mother presence led to higher pain thresholds (reduced sensitivity) in all groups.

Major gaps in knowledge include whether parent involvement in NICU care can prevent effects of neonatal pain on brain development, and whether in the long term, parent stress, anxiety, and other factors across childhood may exacerbate effects of pain exposure early in life in vulnerable infants. The extent to which sensitive parenting may ameliorate effects of neonatal pain, and whether gender has differential effects, is also unknown.

Conscious awareness and adverse effects of pain

Accepted definitions of pain as a phenomenon involving a complex interplay of sensation and cognition are adult focused, and may not capture fundamental characteristics of the developing organism. Based on this adult orientation, attempts to understand when the fetus and neonate might become consciously aware have been used to determine when pain might be perceived. Conditioned learning is evident early in life even during sleep (Fifer et al., 2010)—implying memory presumably without conscious recall. Moreover, behavioural evidence of conditioning, as well as evoked EEG and physiological responses after pain underlie 'biological memory'. Thus, although infants cannot recall early experiences, the CNS appear to retain 'memory' that is manifested later in altered responses to pain in new situations (Grunau, 2003; Taddio et al., 1997).

Recent evidence suggests that the long-term impact of pain on later brain function differs depending on the biological maturity of the infant and the stage of underlying brain development at the time of hospitalization (Doesburg et al., 2013). In the case of extremely premature birth (see case example), effects of repetitive procedural pain-related stress on the vulnerable developing brain and stress

systems likely occur irrespective of conscious awareness. Thus, consideration of the distinction between *nociception* and *pain* may be helpful in elucidating long-term impacts on different systems.

It has been proposed that conscious perception of pain is required for pain to impact the individual (e.g. Lee et al., 2005). This has led to a focus on the topic of when consciousness emerges in during fetal life, which has implications for intrauterine interventions as well as treatment of infants born very preterm. However, biological processes initiated by nociception stimuli can impact the organism regardless of conscious awareness. Even extremely preterm neonates born at 24 weeks of gestation display sensitization to skin-breaking stimulation, which is a basic physiological phenomenon of the immature organism's hypersensitivity to tactile inputs, together with limited capacity to regulate excitatory and inhibitory systems (Andrews and Fitzgerald, 1994; Fitzgerald, 2005). Thus, nociceptive reactivity can be altered due to changes at the spinal cord level. Similarly, altered stress hormone levels associated with repetitive exposure to neonatal procedures do not have to involve higher order consciousness to induce short- and long-term effects. These altered systems are signs of implicit biological memory, and the processes engaged can alter the CNS and stress physiology without any conscious perception of pain. Pain, on the other hand, is defined as a complex response engaging both emotional and nociceptive responses. This distinction between nociception and pain is important in considering long-term effects of procedural events in neonates and young infants. This distinction does not rule out the possibility that higher-order cortical regions of the brain may be engaged in relation to procedures early in infancy, but rather removes the idea that conscious perception of pain is a requirement for a long-term impact to take place. Specifically, nociceptive response can initiate a physiological cascade of events that directly or indirectly impacts the brain and stress development of very preterm neonates, *regardless of whether they perceive pain consciously*.

Conclusion

Long-term effects of early pain on later pain and tactile sensitivity are complex, and depend on multiple factors such as age at pain stimulation, extent of tissue damage, type of noxious insult, intensity, duration, and age. Recent studies show that neonatal pain evokes changes in brain activity, providing important clinical evidence that the behavioural, autonomic, and hormonal responses to procedures in infants go beyond defensive reflexes. Advanced imaging techniques have revealed that neonatal pain in preterm infants is associated with altered brain development during the neonatal period in very preterm infants, for the first time providing clinical evidence of mechanisms that may underlie the emerging association between cumulative procedural pain exposure and neurodevelopment and behaviour in children born very preterm.

Probably the most unexpected finding in recent years has been convergent evidence from several countries showing that, despite the impact of early pain on somatosensory processing and pain sensitivity, self-reported everyday pain problems do not appear to be more pronounced in late adolescence or early adulthood following exposure to extensive pain in the neonatal period. However, long-term studies are needed to evaluate whether under life stresses over time, differentially by gender, pain syndromes may develop later.

Case example: long-term impact of pain in preterm twin girls

As part of a longitudinal programme of research in long-term effects of neonatal pain in preterm infants born at 24 to 32 weeks of gestation, non-identical twin girls (here referred to as Iris and Betty—not their real names) participated in studies in the NICU, and at ages 3 months, 8 months, 18 months, and 7 years. The twins were born at 29 weeks of gestation with birthweight appropriate for their gestational age, and similar size at birth, but had different neonatal experiences that illustrate divergent trajectories of early pain and outcomes. Betty had 75 skin-breaking procedures from birth to term equivalent while Iris had 111; neither girl underwent surgery. The most striking discrepancy in outcome between the sisters was that at age 7 years, when Betty's cognitive functioning was above average with verbal comprehension and perceptual reasoning at the 95th and 97th percentiles respectively, whereas Iris had scores significantly lower than her sister, with verbal comprehension at the 45th percentile and a deficit in perceptual reasoning at the 4th percentile. In addition, Iris was below age expectation in planning and problem solving aspects of executive functioning. Despite these low scores, in second grade Iris copes with early reading and arithmetic, displaying compensation for her difficulties with aspects of cognitive abstraction. This capacity to compensate is consistent with the finding that very preterm children engage different brain networks reflecting brain plasticity over time (Doesburg et al., 2012), despite the association between neonatal pain and early brain development while in the NICU from birth to term (Brummelte et al., 2012). There are numerous confounding factors that obscure potential effects of neonatal pain per se in hospitalized infants, therefore it is important that neither of the children had any infections in the neonatal period, received no postnatal steroids, and that Betty underwent no mechanical ventilation and Iris only needed it for 4 days. Given that the twins grew up in the same family and broader social environment, the difference in skin-breaking neonatal events appears to be a salient factor that may have contributed to their differences in cognitive outcomes; however, clinical research alone can only establish associations, not causality. In addition, as non-identical twins, their genetic make-up differs. Another avenue of future investigation is to uncover what genetic factors may render some infants more vulnerable to pain-related stress early in life, and what genetic factors may be protective.

Acknowledgements

Dr Grunau's research is supported by operating grants from the National Institute for Child Health and Human Development (R01 HD39783) and the Canadian Institutes for Health Research (MOP-86489; MOP-79262). She is supported by a Senior Scientist award from the Child & Family Research Institute.

References

Allen, M. C. (2008). Neurodevelopmental outcomes of preterm infants. *Curr Opin Neurol*, 21, 123–128.

Als, H. (1982). Toward a synactive theory of development: Promise for the assessment of infant individuality. *Inf Mental Health J*, 3, 229–243.

Als, H., Duffy, F. H., McAnulty, G. B., Rivkin, M. J., Vajapeyam, S., Mulkern, R.V., *et al.* (2004). Early experience alters brain function and structure. *Pediatrics*, 113, 846–857.

Anand, K. J. S, Coskun, V., Thrivikraman, K. V., Nemeroff, C. B., and Plotsky, P. M. (1999). Long-term behavioural effects of repetitive pain in neonatal rat pups. *Physiol Behav*, 66, 627–637.

Anders, T. F. and Roffwarg, H. P. (1973). The effects of selective interruption and deprivation of sleep in the human newborn. *Dev Psychobiol*, 6, 77–89.

Andrews, K. and Fitzgerald, M. (1994). The cutaneous withdrawal reflex in human neonates: sensitization, receptive fields, and the effects of contralateral stimulation. *Pain*, 56, 95–101.

Andrews, K. and Fitzgerald, M. (2002). Wound sensitivity as a measure of analgesic effects following surgery in human neonates and infants. *Pain*, 99, 185–95.

Axelin, A., Kirjavainen, J., Salanterä, S., and Lehtonen, L. (2010). Effects of pain management on sleep in preterm infants. *Eur J Pain*, 14, 752–758.

Ball, G., Boardman, J. P., Rueckert, D., Aljabar, P., Arichi, T., Merchant, N., *et al.* (2011). The effect of preterm birth on thalamic and cortical development. *Cereb Cortex*, 21, 300–306.

Bartocci, M., Bergzvist, L. L., Lagercrantz, H., and Anand, K.J. (2006). Pain activates cortical areas in the preterm newborn brain. *Pain*, 122, 109–117.

Bleustein, C. B., Fogarty, J. D., Eckholdt, H., Arezzo, J. C., and Melman, A. (2005). Effect of neonatal circumcision on penile neurologic sensation. *Urology*, 65, 773–777.

Blumberg, M. S. and Seelke, A. M. (2010). The form and function of infant sleep: from muscle to cortex. In M. S. Blumberg, J. H. Freeman, and S. R Robinson (eds) *The Oxford handbook of developmental and behavioural neuroscience*, pp. 391–423. New York: Oxford University Press.

Braarud, H. C. and Stormark, K. M. (2006). Maternal soothing and infant stress responses: soothing, crying and adrenocortical activity during inoculation. *Infant Behav Dev*, 29, 70–79.

Brummelte, S., Grunau, R. E., Chau, V., Poskitt, K. J., Brant, R., Vinall, J., *et al.* (2012). Procedural pain and brain development in premature newborns. *Ann Neurol*, 71(3), 385–396. doi: 10.1002/ana.22267.

Brummelte, S., Grunau, R. E., Synnes, A. R., Whitfield, M. F., Petrie-Thomas, J. (2011). Declining cognitive development from 8 to 18 months in preterm children predicts persisting higher parenting stress. *Early Hum Dev*, 87, 273–280.

Buskila, D., Neumann, L., Zmora, E., Feldman, M., Bolotin, A. and Press, J. (2003) Pain sensitivity in prematurely born adolescents. *Arch Pediatr Adolesc Med*, 157, 1079–1082.

Doesburg, S. M., Chau, C. M., Cheung, T. P., Moiseev, A., Ribary, U., Herdman, A. T., *et al.* (2013). Neonatal pain-related stress, functional cortical activity and visual-perceptual abilities in school-age children born at extremely low gestational age. *Pain*, 10 April [Epub ahead of print.]

Doesburg, S. M., Moiseev, A., Ribary, U., Herdman, A. T., Miller, S. P., Poskitt, K. J., *et al.* (2012). Magnetic source imaging reveals atypical cortical network dynamics in very preterm children during visual short-term memory processing. Poster symposium, Pediatric Academic Societies Annual Meeting, 28 April–1 May, Boston, MA, USA. E-PAS20122830.7.

Doesburg, S. M., Ribary, U., Herdman, A. T., Moiseev, A., Cheung, T., Miller, S. P., *et al.* (2011a). Magnetoencephalography reveals slowing of resting peak oscillatory frequency in children born very preterm. *Pediatr Res*, 70, 171–175.

Doesburg, S. M., Ribary, U., Herdman, A. T., Miller, S. P., Poskitt, K. J., Moiseev, A., *et al.* (2011b). Altered long-range alpha-band synchronization during visual short-term memory retention in children born very preterm. *Neuroimage*, 54, 2330–2339.

Fabrizi, L., Slater, R., Worley, A., Meek, J., Boyd, S., Olhede, S., *et al.* (2011). A shift in sensory processing that enables the developing human brain to discriminate touch from pain. *Curr Biol*, 21, 1552–1558.

Feldman, R., Eidelman, A. I., Sirota, L., and Weller, A. (2002). Comparison of skin-to-skin (kangaroo) and traditional care: parenting outcomes and preterm infant development. *Pediatrics*, 110, 16–26.

Fifer, W. P., Byrd, D. L., Kaku, M., Eigsti, I. M., Isler, J. R., Grose-Fifer, J., *et al.* (2010). Newborn infants learn during sleep. *Proc Natl Acad Sci U S A*, 107, 10320–10323.

Fitzgerald, M. (2005). The developmental of nociceptive circuits. *Nat Rev Neurosci*, 6, 507–520.

Fitzgerald, M. and Beggs, S. (2001). The neurobiology of pain: developmental aspects. *Neuroscientist*, 7, 246–257.

Fitzgerald, M. and Walker, S. M. (2009). Infant pain management: a developmental neurobiological approach. *Nat Clin Pract Neuro,* 5, 35–50.

Grunau, R. E. (2003). Self-regulation and behaviour in preterm children: Effects of early pain. In: P. J. McGrath and A. Finley (eds) *Pediatric pain: biological and social context, progress in pain research and management. Volume 26*, pp. 23–55. Seattle, WA: IASP Press.

Grunau, R. E., Haley, D. W., Whitfield, M. F., Weinberg, J., Yu, W., and Thiessen, P. (2007). Altered basal cortisol levels at 3, 6, 8 and 18 months in infants born at extremely low gestational age. *J Pediatr*, 150, 151–156.

Grunau, R. E., Holsti, L., Haley, D. W., Oberlander, T., Weinberg, J., Solimano, A., *et al.* (2005). Neonatal procedural pain exposure predicts lower cortisol and behavioural reactivity in preterm infants in the NICU. *Pain*, 113, 293–300.

Grunau, R. E., Oberlander, T. F., Whitfield, M. F., Fitzgerald, C., Morison, S. J., and Saul, J. P (2001). Pain reactivity in former extremely low birth weight infants at corrected age 8 months compared with term born controls. *Infant Behav Dev*, 24, 41–55.

Grunau, R. E., Tu, M. T., Whitfield, M. F., Oberlander, T. F., Weinberg, J., Yu, W., *et al.* (2010). Cortisol, behaviour, and heart rate reactivity to immunization pain at 4 months corrected age in infants born very preterm. *Clin J Pain*, 26, 698–704.

Grunau, R. E., Whitfield, M. F., and Davis, C. (2002). Pattern of learning disabilities in children with extremely low birth weight and broadly average intelligence. *Arch Pediat Adol Med*, 156, 615–620.

Grunau, R. E., Whitfield, M. F., and Fay, T. B. (2004a). Psychosocial and academic characteristics of extremely low birth weight (800 g) adolescents who are free of major impairment compared with term-born control subjects. *Pediatrics*, 114, e725–732.

Grunau, R. E., Whitfield, M. F., and Petrie, J. (1998). Children's judgements about pain at age 8–10 years: do extremely low birthweight (≤ 1000 g) children differ from full birthweight peers? *J Child Psychol Psyc*, 39, 587–594.

Grunau, R. E., Whitfield, M. F., and Weinberg, J. (2004b). Neonatal procedural pain exposure and preterm infant cortisol response to novelty at 8 months. *Pediatrics*, 114, e77–e84.

Grunau, R. E., Whitfield, M. F., Petrie-Thomas, J., Synnes, A. R., Cepeda, I. L., Keidar, A., *et al.* (2009). Neonatal pain, parenting stress and interaction, in relation to cognitive and motor development at 8 and 18 months in preterm infants. *Pain,* 143, 138–146.

Grunau, R. V. E., Whitfield, M. F., and Petrie, J. H. (1994a). Pain sensitivity and temperament in extremely-low-birth-weight premature toddlers and preterm and full-term controls. *Pain*, 58, 341–346.

Grunau, R. V. E., Whitfield, M. F., Petrie, J. H., and Fryer, E. L. (1994b). Early pain experience, child and family factors, as precursors of somatization: a prospective study of extremely premature and fullterm children. *Pain*, 56, 353–359.

Hack, M., Flannery, D. J., Schluchter, M., Cartar, L., Borawski, E. and Klein N. (2002). Outcomes in young adulthood for very-low-birth-weight infants. *New Engl J Med*, 346, 149–157.

Hermann, C., Hohmeister, J., Demirakça, S., Zohsel, K., and Flor, H. (2006). Long-term alteration of pain sensitivity in school-aged children with early pain experiences. *Pain,* 125, 278–285.

Hohmeister, J., Demirakça, S., Zohsel, K., Flor, H., and Hermann, C. (2009). Responses to pain in school-aged children with experience in a neonatal intensive care unit: cognitive aspects and maternal influences. *Eur J Pain*, 13, 94–101.

Hohmeister, J., Kroll, A., Wollgarten-Hadamek, I., Zohsel, K., Demirakça, S., Flor, H., *et al.* (2010). Cerebral processing of pain in school-aged children with neonatal nociceptive input: An exploratory fMRI study. *Pain*, 150, 257–267.

Holsti, L., Grunau, R. E., Oberlander, T. F., and Osiovich, H. (2008). Is it painful or not? Discriminant validity of the Behavioural Indicators of Infant Pain (BIIP) scale. *Clin J Pain*, 24, 83–88.

Holsti, L., Grunau, R. E., Oberlander, T. F., and Whitfield, M. F. (2005). Prior pain induces heightened motor responses during clustered care in preterm infants in the NICU. *Early Hum Dev*, 81, 293–302.

Holsti, L., Grunau, R. E., Whitfield, M. F., Oberlander, T. F., and Lindh, V. (2006). Behavioural responses to pain are heightened after clustered care in preterm infants born between 30 and 32 weeks gestational age. *Clin J Pain*, 22, 757–764.

Kostovic, I. and Judas, M. (2010). The development of the subplate and thalamocortical connections in the human foetal brain. *Acta Paediatr*, 99, 1119–1127.

Lagercrantz, H., Hanson, M. A., Ment, L. R., and Peebles, D. M. (2010). *The newborn brain: neuroscience and clinical applications* (2nd edn). Cambridge: Cambridge University Press.

LaPrairie, J. L. and Murphy, A. Z. (2007). Female rats are more vulnerable to the long-term consequences of neonatal inflammatory injury. *Pain*, 132(Suppl.1) S124–133.

Lee, S. J., Ralston, H. J., Drey, E. A., Partridge, J.C., and Rosen, M. A. (2005). Fetal pain: a systematic multidisciplinary review of the evidence. *JAMA*, 294, 947–954.

Loman M. M. and Gunnar, M. R. (2010). Early experience and the development of stress reactivity and regulation in children. *Neurosci Biobehav Rev,* 34, 867–876.

Maimon, N., Grunau, R. E., Cepeda, I. L., Friger, M., Selnovik, L., Gilat, S., *et al.* (2013). Electroencephalographic activity in response to procedural pain in infants born at 28 and 33 weeks gestational age. *Clin J Pain*, 26 February. [Epub ahead of print.]

Maroney, D. I. (2003). Recognizing the potential effect of stress and trauma on premature infants in the NICU: How are outcomes affected? *J Perinatol*, 23, 679–683.

Matthews, S. G. (2002). Early programming of the hypothalamo-pituitary-adrenal axis. *Trends Endocrin Met*, 13, 373–380.

Ment, L. R., Hirtz, D., and Hüppi, P. S. (2009). Imaging biomarkers of outcome in the developing preterm brain. *Lancet Neurol*, 8, 1042–1055.

Milgrom, J., Newnham, C., Anderson, P. J., Doyle, L. W., Gemmill, A. W., Lee, K., *et al.* (2010). Early sensitivity training for parents of preterm infants: impact on the developing brain. *Pediatr Res*, 67, 330–335.

Miller, G. E, Chen, E., and Zhou, E.S. (2007). If it goes up, must it come down? Chronic stress and the hypothalamic-pituitary-adrenocortical axis in humans. *Psychol Bull*, 133, 25–45.

Miller, S. P. and Ferriero, D. M. (2009). From selective vulnerability to connectivity: insights from newborn brain imaging. *Trends Neurosci*, 32, 496–505.

Moon, E. C., Chambers, C. T., Larochette, A. C., Hayton, K., Craig, K. D., and McGrath, P. J. (2008). Sex differences in parent and child pain ratings during an experimental child pain task. *Pain Res Manag*, 13, 225–230.

Oberlander, T. F., Grunau, R. E., Whitfield, M. F., Fitzgerald, C., Pitfield, S. and Saul, J. P. (2000). Biobehavioural pain responses in former extremely low birth weight infants at four months corrected age. *Pediatrics*, 105, e6.

Okumura, A., Kubota, T., Toyota, N., Kidokoro, H., Maruyama, K., Kato, T., *et al.* (2003). Amplitude spectral analysis of maturational changes in delta waves in preterm infants. *Brain Dev*, 25, 406–410.

Perlman, J. M. and Volpe, J. J. (1983). Suctioning in the preterm infant: effects on cerebral blood flow velocity, intracranial pressure, and arterial blood pressure. *Pediatrics*, 72, 329–334.

Peters, J. W. B., Koot, H. M., de Boer, J. B., Passchier, J., Bueno-de-Mesquita, J. M., de Jong, F. H., *et al.* (2003). Major surgery within the first 3 months of life and subsequent biobehavioural pain responses to immunization at later age: A case comparison study. *Pediatrics*, 111, 129–135.

Peters, J. W. B., Schow, R., Anand, K. J. S., van Dijk, M., Duivenvoorden, H. J. and Tibboel, D. (2005). Does neonatal surgery lead to increased pain sensitivity in later childhood? *Pain*, 114, 444–454.

Piira, T., Champion, G. D., Bustos, T., Donnelly, N., and Lui, K. (2007). Factors associated with infant pain response following an immunization injection. *Early Hum Dev*, 83, 319–326.

Pillai Riddell, R. R. and Chambers, C. T. (2007). Parenting and pain during infancy. In K. J. S. Anand, B. Stevens, and P. J. McGrath (eds) *Pain in neonates and infants* (3rd edn), pp. 289–298. Amsterdam: Elsevier.

Ren, K., Anseloni, V., Zou, S. P., Wade, E. B., Novikova, S. I., Ennis, M., *et al.* (2004). Characterization of basal and re-infalmmation-associated long-term alteration in pain rewsponsivity following short-lasting neonatal local inflammatory insult. *Pain*, 110, 588–596.

Saigal, S., Feeny, D., Rosenbaum, P., Furlong, W., Burrows, E., and Stoskopf, B. (1996). Self-perceived health status and health-related quality of life of extremely low-birth-weight infants at adolescence. *JAMA*, 276, 453–459.

Saigal, S., Stoskopf, B., Boyle, M., Paneth, N., Pinelli, J., Streiner, D., *et al.* (2007). Comparison of current health, functional limitations, and health care use of young adults who were born with extremely low birth weight and normal birth weight. *Pediatrics*, 119, e562–753.

Scher, M. S., Johnson, M. W., and Holditch-Davis, D. (2005). Cyclicity of neonatal sleep behaviours at 25 to 30 weeks' postconceptional age. *Pediatr Res*, 57, 879–882.

Schmelzle-Lubiecki, B. M., Campbell, K. A., Howard, R. H., Franck, L. and Fitzgerald, M. (2007). Long-term consequences of early infant injury and trauma upon somatosensory processing. *Eur J Pain*, 11, 799–809.

Slater, R., Cantarella, A., Gallella, S., Worley, A., Boyd, S., Meek, J., *et al.* (2006). Cortical pain responses in human infants. *J Neurosci*, 26, 3662–3666.

Slater, R., Fabrizi, L., Worley, A., Meek, J., Boyd, S., and Fitzgerald, M. (2010). Premature infants display increased noxious-evoked neuronal activity in the brain compared to healthy age-matched term-born infants. *Neuroimage*, 52, 583–89.

Smith, G. C., Gutovich, J., Smyser, C., Pineda, R., Newnham, C., Tjoeng, T. H., *et al.* (2011). Neonatal intensive care unit stress is associated with brain development in preterm infants. *Ann Neurol*, 70, 541–549.

Sommerfelt, K., Troland, K., Ellertsen, B., and Markestad, T. (1996). Behavioural problems in low-birthweight preschoolers. *Dev Med Child Neurol*, 38, 927–940.

Stevens, B., Johnston, C., Taddio, A., Gibbins, S., and Yamada, J. (2010). The premature infant pain profile: evaluation 13 years after development. *Clin J Pain*, 26, 813–830.

Symington, A. and Pinelli, J. (2006). Developmental care for promoting development and preventing morbidity in preterm infants. *Cochrane Database Syst Rev*, 2, CD001814.

Taddio, A., Goldbach, M., Ipp, M., Stevens, B., and Koren, G. (1995). Effect of neonatal circumcision on pain responses during vaccination in boys. *Lancet*, 345, 291–292.

Taddio, A., Katz, J., Ilersich, A. L., and Koren, G. (1997). Effect of neonatal circumcision on pain response during subsequent routine vaccination. *Lancet*, 349, 599–603.

Tombini, M., Pasqualetti, P., Rizzo, C., Zappasodi, F., Dinatale, A., Seminara, M., *et al.* (2009). Extrauterine maturation of somatosensory pathways in preterm infants: a somatosensory evoked potential study. *Clin Neurophysiol*, 120, 783–789.

Unruh, A. M. (1996). Gender variations in clinical pain experience. *Pain*, 65, 123–167.

Vanhatalo, S., Jousmäki, V., Andersson, S., and Metsäranta, M. (2009). An easy and practical method for routine, bedside testing of somatosensory systems in extremely low birth weight infants (ELBW). *Pediatr Res*, 66, 710–713.

Volpe, J. J. (2009). The encephalopathy of prematurity-brain injury and impaired brain development inextricably intertwined. *Semin Pediatr Neurol*, 16, 167–178.

Walker, C. D., Kudreikis, K., Sherrard, A., and Johnston, C. C. (2003). Repeated neonatal pain influences maternal behaviour, but not stress responsiveness in rat offspring. *Dev Brain Res*, 140, 253–261.

Walker, S. M., Franck, L. S., Fitzgerald, M., Myles, J., Stocks, J., and Marlow, N. (2009). Long-term impact of neonatal intensive care and surgery on somatosensory perception in children born extremely preterm. *Pain*, 141, 79–87.

Whitfield, M. F., Grunau, R. E. and Holsti, L. (1997). Extreme prematurity (< 800 g) at school age: Multiple areas of hidden disability. *Arch Dis Child*, 77, F85–90.

Wollgarten-Hadamek, I., Hohmeister, J., Demirakça, S., Zohsel, K., Flor, H., and Hermann, C. (2009). Do burn injuries during infancy affect pain and sensory sensitivity in later childhood? *Pain*, 141, 165–172.

World Health Organization. (2012). *What do we mean by "sex" and "gender"?* Available at: <http://www.who.int/gender/whatisgender/en/> (accessed 23 February 2012).

CHAPTER 5

Prevention of the development and maintenance of paediatric chronic pain and disability

M. Gabrielle Pagé, Anna Huguet , and Joel Katz

Summary

Understanding the predisposing factors that confer a greater risk of developing chronic pain is an essential step in pain prevention and management. This chapter focuses on current theoretical models that can inform prevention of paediatric pain and disability. We review the literature on known risk/protective factors, markers, correlates, and prognostic factors for the transition to chronic pain and disability across a variety of pain conditions. We distinguish between primary, secondary, and tertiary levels of pain prevention and discuss the clinical implications of this distinction.

Introduction

Estimates of paediatric chronic pain (i.e. pain that continues past the usual tissue healing time—typically 3 months) range between 15% and 30% (Bandell-Hoekstra et al., 2001; Perquin et al., 2003). The consequences of poorly managed acute and chronic pain are potentially quite significant. Unrelieved pain is associated with medical (medical complications, longer hospital stay, higher risk of infections), physiological (neuroplasticity, sensitization, increased risk of chronic pain), psychological (distress), and socioeconomical (increased health care costs) consequences (Aasvang and Kehlet, 2007; Anand et al., 1987; McCaffery, 1977). Among children who report experiencing chronic pain for more than 3 months, between one-half and two-thirds continue to report chronic pain 1 and 2 years later, respectively (Perquin et al., 2003).

The mechanisms underlying the transition from acute to chronic pain are not fully understood. It is likely that they involve a combination of biopsychosocial, behavioural, and physiological components (Priest and Hoggart, 2002). Identifying risk factors for the development of chronic pain can lead to preventive programmes including treatment before the pain begins, or before it has become chronic. This would help prevent the processes that are involved in the development and maintenance of chronic pain.

In this chapter, we focus on the biological and psychological factors associated with the development of paediatric chronic pain. We define and identify risk/protective factors, predictors, correlates, markers, and prognostic factors across pain conditions, describe three types of pain prevention, review current theoretical models of the development and persistence of pain, and describe prevention strategies associated with identified correlates, markers, risk/protective, and prognostic factors.

Correlated factors, risk/protective factors, markers, and prognostic factors

Preventing paediatric pain necessitates the identification of risk and protective factors from which risk levels for a child to develop pain can be determined. It also requires the identification of prognostic factors to better understand a child's probability of recovering from a chronic pain state. A risk factor is defined as a 'measurable characterization of each subject in a specified population that precedes the outcome of interest and can be used to divide the population into … high-risk and … low-risk groups' (Kraemer et al., 1997, p. 338). The temporal criterion of precedence is essential for a variable to qualify as a risk factor; otherwise it is a correlate. Similarly, a protective factor predicts a lower risk of the outcome (i.e. it protects against the risk). Risk and protective factors are both called predictors (i.e. without reference to sign). Predictors that cannot be modified are referred to as fixed markers (e.g. sex, race; Kraemer et al., 1997). A prognostic factor is a variable that provides information about the chances of recovery from, or recurrence of, a disease or condition. Thus, a risk or protective factor predicts the chances of developing or contracting a disease, whereas a prognostic factor predicts the outcome of a disease (recovery or recurrence once the disease has developed; Laupacis et al., 1994).

Primary, secondary, and tertiary prevention of paediatric pain

Prevention of paediatric pain not only focuses on effectively managing and averting acute pain due to iatrogenic causes (e.g. from medical and surgical origins), but also on ensuring that acute pain

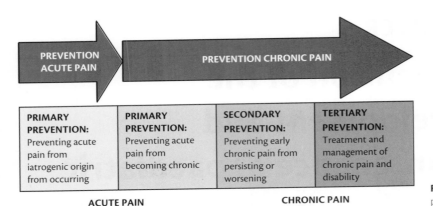

Figure 5.1 Primary, secondary, and tertiary prevention of paediatric pain.

does not become chronic and disabling. It is essential to develop intervention strategies that target these various forms of prevention, namely primary, secondary, and tertiary (see Figure 5.1).

Preventing acute pain of iatrogenic origin

Preventing acute pain generally refers to the anticipation and avoidance of pain onset. Complete prevention of acute pain is not desirable; children learn coping skills and safety behaviours from experiencing minor cuts, bruises, scrapes, etc. Many efforts have been made, through programmes such as Safe Kids USA and Safe Kids Canada to prevent serious injuries and traumas and indirectly prevent children from experiencing pain. While these programmes are examples of primary prevention, they will not be reviewed here given the lack of a pain-specific focus. Rather, the focus will be on acute pain from invasive medical and surgical procedures, as it can have long-lasting consequences including preprocedural anxiety, hyperalgesia, avoidance of health care, development of chronic pain, and disability. Prevention of acute pain of iatrogenic origin relies on neutralizing the risk factors associated with the onset of acute pain. Interventions that decrease the risk of developing acute pain are amongst the most cost-effective in managing pain.

Preventing the development and maintenance of chronic pain

Primary prevention refers to the early identification of acute pain and management strategies to ensure the pain does not become chronic. Identification of risk factors for chronic pain and intervention strategies aimed at modifying these factors when the pain is acute are strategies associated with primary prevention of chronic pain.

Secondary prevention consists of preventing early chronic pain states from worsening or persisting. Identification and modification of prognostic factors with the aim of reducing or eliminating the chronic pain experience are examples of secondary prevention strategies.

Tertiary prevention refers to the reduction of pain-related disability and impairment, as well as the improvement of quality of life. Tertiary prevention also focuses on identifying and removing barriers to treatment, facilitating treatment adherence, and improving adaptive daily functioning.

Until recently, the lack of a paediatric pain-related disability or pain interference tool has hindered research on tertiary prevention. The Functional Disability Index (FDI; Walker and Green,

1991) is widely used to evaluate functional disability in children with chronic pain; however, the source of disability is not specified in the FDI. This lack of specificity may impede efforts aimed at reducing pain-related disability or at validating theoretical models of paediatric pain-related disability. Other pain-specific and often population-specific scales, such as the Child Activity Limitations Interview (CALI; Palermo et al., 2004), the PROMIS Pediatric Pain Interference Scale (Varni et al., 2010), the Pediatric Migraine Disability Assessment (PedMIDAS; Hershey et al., 2001) can be used by clinicians and researchers to assess the extent to which the pain per se contributed to the child's disability. Future research directions include the evaluation of theoretical models of pain-related disability using these scales as well as examination of the convergent validity of global functional and pain-related disabilities.

Theoretical models and theories

Prevention of chronic paediatric pain relies on the identification and appropriate modification of empirically validated causal risk, protective, and prognostic factors. A critical examination of current theoretical models may help in the search for factors that can ultimately be used in preventing paediatric chronic pain (see also Pillai Riddell et al., Chapter 9, this volume).

The causal risk and protective factors, and hence, the mechanisms underlying the transition from acute to chronic pain and the maintenance of chronic pain likely involve a combination of various components (e.g. biological, psychological, sociocultural, genetic). Although some researchers have proposed theoretical models of the development and persistence of paediatric pain (Palermo and Chambers, 2005) most have been developed either for adult pain populations or are paediatric models not specific to chronic pain. The dominant models are summarized as follows.

The *operant conditioning model* (Fordyce et al., 1968) posits that pain behaviours are influenced by a system of punishment, reinforcement, and extinction. It also stipulates that pain behaviours may become independent of physiological and sensory elements and occur in response to external reinforcement contingencies. The *fear-avoidance models of pain* (Asmundson et al., 2004; Leeuw et al., 2007; Vlaeyen et al., 1995) illustrate the relationships among pain-related catastrophic thinking, pain-related fear/anxiety, and pain perception. In the absence of pain-related fear, symptoms of pain are confronted, leading to recovery. Alternatively, when pain symptoms are interpreted catastrophically, pain-related fear and anxiety reactions ensue, followed by avoidance behaviours and hypervigilance of somatic symptoms, in particular pain, followed by disuse, disability, and depression, which in turn feed back into the pain experience to fuel pain-related fears in a never-ending cycle. The recently developed *paediatric fear-avoidance model of chronic pain* (Asmundson et al., 2012) adds to the adult fear-avoidance model child/adolescent factors and parental variables that contribute to the development and maintenance of chronic pain. More specifically, parental pain management behaviours (e.g. protectiveness, solicitousness) and child psychological responses (e.g. catastrophizing, acceptance) will interact and influence child psychological response and escape/avoidance behaviours (Asmundson et al., 2012). The *diathesis-stress model of chronic pain and disability* (Turk, 2002) explains the progression from acute pain following an injury/trauma to chronic disabling pain in adults. The model stresses several constructs as major predictors of the development of chronic pain and the maintenance of disability: (1) a predisposing factor: anxiety sensitivity; (2) cognitive processes: fear of further pain and harm, catastrophizing cognitions, and low self-efficacy; and (3) operant processes. A modification of the model to include symptoms of post-traumatic stress disorder has received empirical support in patients before (Martin et al., 2010) and after (Kleiman et al., 2011) surgery.

The *integrative model of parent and family factors in paediatric chronic pain and associated disability* (Palermo and Chambers, 2005) emphasizes the importance of parents and family to understand the child's pain experience and specifically suggests three interrelated levels of factors that influence pain and disability: (1) individual factors (e.g. parental behaviours), (2) parent–child interactions, and (3) family-related variables (e.g. familial environment).

The *biopsychosocial model of pain* (Engel 1977; Gatchel et al., 2007; Turk, 1996) posits that 'pain' is a subjective idiosyncratic experience that includes biological (e.g. autonomic, endocrine, and immune systems, genetic predispositions), psychological (e.g. fear, anxiety, previous pain experiences), and social (e.g. cultural and familial) aspects. The *perceived self-efficacy model of chronic pain* (Bursch et al., 2006; Vuorimaa et al., 2008) states that beliefs about one's ability to cope with pain and to maintain everyday life activities despite pain will impact one's regards towards pain control, pain coping, and daily functioning, which in turn regulates pain and associated disability. The *modelling/social learning theory* (Bandura, 1986; Craig and Prkachin, 1978) emphasizes the important role of modelling; that is, the capacity to learn a wide range of behaviours, such as complex pain behaviour patterns, through observation of pain behaviours of others. The potency of modelling as a method of learning can be enhanced by the consequences (reinforcement or punishment) of the modelled behaviour, the consequences that meet the imitative behaviour adopted from the model, the expectancies of one's abilities to execute the modelled behaviour, and the outcome expectancies of future consequences. Last, the *attachment theory* (Bowlby, 1973) when applied to pain suggests that pain serves as a signal of threat and consequently activates a sequence of attachment behaviours, which in turn will influence the pain experience.

Specificity of pain models

Most models described have not been evaluated in children although there is support for various components (see Table 5.1).

Taken together, these results suggest the models are relevant to the paediatric population but important components remain to be tested in children and adolescents.

Research has been slow to identify factors responsible for the development and maintenance of chronic pain and disability in children. This is in part because of: (1) the relative absence of theoretical models conceptualized (or adapted) specifically for paediatric populations, (2) the heterogeneity of pain outcomes assessed by current adult theoretical pain models, and (3) the absence of empirically validated questionnaires to measure constructs relevant to specific models. While it is clear that factors identified in the following section are associated with paediatric pain, they have been mainly examined in isolation from one another. Remediating this lack of an integrative framework might be a necessary subsequent step through which underlying mechanisms can be identified (Huguet et al., 2011).

Importantly, as mentioned earlier, the primary outcome of interest differs from one model to the other (e.g. pain behaviours, pain experience, chronic pain, and disability). Predictor variables in one study are commonly used as outcome measures in other studies and vice versa, reflecting the complexity of the problem and the variety in hypothesized mechanisms (Katz, 2012). As such, these differences must be taken into account when creating integrative models of chronic pain. One of the challenges is to develop sufficiently broad models of the factors hypothesized to be associated with chronic pain outcomes. Recent advances in the quality of clinical research are due in large part to recommendations regarding assessment of core domains of functioning (Turk et al., 2003); the issue of the most appropriate measure with a given domain however, remains to be determined (Turk et al., 2008). Core outcome domains that have been recommended to be included in paediatric clinical trials include pain, physical functioning/physical recovery, emotional functioning, role functioning, patients' satisfaction with treatment, symptoms and adverse events, sleep, and economic factors (McGrath et al., 2008). This type of integrative research is essential to the elaboration of testable hypotheses about underlying mechanisms of paediatric chronic pain and disability, leading to the elaboration of prevention strategies.

Common correlates, predictors, markers, and prognostic factors of chronic pain and disability

The literature has focused mostly on finding correlates of chronic paediatric pain using cross-sectional studies and only more recently on finding risk/protective and prognostic factors associated with the onset and course of paediatric chronic pain. The factors that have been more commonly explored through a cross-sectional or longitudinal design are: (1) demographic characteristics (i.e. gender and age; Egger et al., 1998; Sjolie, 2002; Vikat et al., 2000), (2) health status (e.g. Vikat et al., 2000), (3) anthropometric characteristics (Kovacs et al., 2003; Sjolie, 2002), (4) physical conditions (Kovacs et al., 2003), (5) mechanical characteristics (Bejia et al., 2005; Jones et al., 2003), (6) sleep problems and physical activity (Laurell et al., 2005; Vikat et al., 2000), and (8) smoking (Kovacs et al., 2003).

In addition, the following factors have been studied as potential correlates, predictors, markers or prognostic factors of paediatric pain-related disability: (1) demographic characteristics (i.e. age and sex; Konijnenberg et al., 2005; Logan and Scharff, 2005);

Table 5.1 Empirical support for pain and pain-related disability models in paediatric populations

Outcome	Predictors						
	Person-centred models			**Systemic models**			
	Operant	**Diathesis**	**Fear-avoidance**	**Biopsychosocial**	**Perceived self-efficacy**	**Social learning**	**Attachment theory**
Chronic pain		**Anxiety sensitivity** (Tsao et al., 2009) **Pain-related fear and pain anxiety** (Simons et al., 2011) **Pain catastrophizing** (Crombez et al., 2003; Vervoort et al., 2006) **Self-efficacy** (Bursch et al., 2006; Vuorimaa et al., 2008)		**Biological** (e.g. age, gender, genetic factors) (El-Metwally et al., 2008; Hechler et al., 2010; Martin et al., 2007b) **Psychological** (e.g. coping, distress) (Gauntlett-Gilbert and Eccleston, 2007) **Social** (e.g. family, parental response) (Logan and Scharff, 2005)	**Perceived self-efficacy** (Bursch et al., 2006; Vuorimaa et al., 2008)	**Punishment reinforcement expectancies of modelling** (Allen and Shriver, 1998; Minuchin et al., 1975)	**Attachment style**
Disability/ disuse			**Pain catastrophizing** (Crombez et al., 2003; Lynch et al., 2006; Vervoort et al., 2006) **Pain-related fear and anxiety** (Martin et al., 2007a) **Pain-related fear and avoidance** (Wilson et al., 2011)		**Perceived self-efficacy** (Bursch et al. 2006)		
Pain behaviours	**Punishment reinforcement** (Allen and Shriver, 1998; Minuchin et al., 1975)						**Attachment style** (Walsh et al., 2008)

(2) general health status (Claar et al., 1999; Konijnenberg et al., 2005); (3) psychological characteristics such as depression, vulnerability, or psychological distress (Logan et al., 2006; Vervoort et al., 2006); (4) pain coping responses (Kashikar-Zuck et al., 2001; Sawyer et al., 2005); (5) catastrophic thinking (Kashikar-Zuck et al., 2001; Vervoort et al., 2006); (6) environmental contingencies to pain behaviours (Craig and Pillai Riddell, 2003; Van Slyke and Walker, 2006); and (7) parental or family characteristics including parental pain, parental distress, parental stress (Logan and Scharff, 2005). Recently, pain unpleasantness has been found to be associated with the transition from acute to chronic pain while anxiety sensitivity has been associated with the maintenance of chronic pain after surgery (Pagé et al., 2013).

Systematic reviews and meta-analyses will make it possible to identify the most important evidence-based factors that contribute to the development and course of paediatric pain and determine the specific and common factors associated with particular pain conditions (Huguet et al., 2011). At the moment, the most common factors that are considered to be correlates, predictors, markers or prognostic factors of paediatric pain are highlighted in Table 5.2, based on published reviews. The majority of these reviews, however, are non-systematic.

Prevention strategies for paediatric pain

Prevention strategies can be classified into the following three domains: physical, psychosocial, and pharmacological. A combination of more than one approach will be optimal in preventing the development and/or maintenance of pain in children. As highlighted in the theoretical models previously described, sensory, cognitive, and affective factors are thought to interact to predict paediatric pain and disability. It follows, then, that pain prevention will also involve a multidisciplinary approach which will vary according to the level of intervention.

Whereas clinical pain management relies increasingly on multimodal approaches (e.g. pain management in neonates; Allegaert, 2009; Parry, 2011), research typically focuses on unidimensional aspects of pain prevention and management. A good example of this disconnect between clinical practice and research can be found in the literature on recurrent abdominal pain (RAP). Three Cochrane reviews focus on the tertiary prevention of RAP: one focuses on dietary management (Huertas-Ceballos et al., 2009), a second focuses on pharmacological interventions (Huertas-Ceballos et al., 2008a), and the third examines psychosocial interventions (Huertas-Ceballos et al., 2008b). Individually, these reviews provide important

Table 5.2 Reviews of predictors of paediatric pain (systematic and non-systematic)

Pain condition	Authors	Outcome	Findings	
Recurrent abdominal pain	(Gieteling et al., 2011)[a]	Persistence of RAP	Predictors: prognostic factors, markers Non-significant predictors, prognostic factors, markers: Unclear/still unknown:	High levels of negative life events High levels of functional gastrointestinal complaints in family Illness perception Female sex Behavioural disturbances Psychological disorders Severe abdominal pain. Young age Low educational level Depressive/anxiety disorders Self-perceived academic competence Long duration of abdominal pain History of two or more surgeries Presence of other associated symptoms (nausea, vomiting, headaches) High levels of functional disability Low socioeconomic status Attitude towards health care
	(Scharff, 1997)	RAP	Correlates, predictors, prognostic factors, markers:	Underlying physiological predisposition Dietary influences Anxiety Recent stressful events and coping abilities Family issues
	(Schulte et al., 2010)	Development of RAP	Predictors, prognostic factors, markers:	Abdominal inflammation processes Familiar genetic vulnerability to gastrointestinal symptoms and psychopathology Temperament Life events and stressors Psychopathological comorbidity
		Maladaptation to RAP	Predictors, prognostic factors, markers:	Maladaptive pain processing Maladaptive pain communication in the family Maladaptive coping style Psychopathological comorbidity
	(Chogle and Saps, 2009)	RAP	Correlates, predictors, prognostic factors, markers:	Stress, school-related stress Parent-related factors psychological factors Family demographics Seasonal variations Infectious agents Altered intestinal flora Antibiotics Diet
Recurrent paediatric headache	(Martin and Smith, 1995)	Recurrent paediatric headache	Correlates, predictors, prognostic factors, markers:	Depressive and symptoms Stress Multiple somatic symptoms Exposure to pain models Internalizing behaviours (+ externalizing behaviours for boys)

(Continued)

Table 5.2 *(Continued)*

Pain condition	Authors	Outcome	Findings	
Musculoskeletal pain	(Malleson et al., 2001)	Development of musculoskeletal pain/fibromyalgia and disability	Predictors, prognostic factors, markers:	*Intrinsic factors:* Low pain thresholds Female gender Hypermobility Poor perceived control over pain and maladaptive pain coping strategies Difficult temperament *Extrinsic factors:* Previous pain experiences Social deprivation Physical or sexual abuse Parenting modelling of pain behaviours Sleep disturbance Exercise
	(Prins et al., 2008)[a]	Development of the upper quadrant musculoskeletal pain	Predictors, prognostic factors, markers:	Static sitting posture Depression Stress Psychosomatic symptoms Gender Age

[a] Systematic reviews.

prevention and treatment approaches to childhood RAP, but they do not provide a comprehensive, multidisciplinary approach to the treatment of RAP nor do they provide insight into the effectiveness of combining, or the optimal combination of, various approaches. Methodological challenges and realistic constraints and costs associated with conducting multidisciplinary, multiple group studies may, in part, explain this lack of integrative research. Investigating the efficacy of separate interventions is a good first step in designing prevention and treatment programmes. But it is important to keep in mind that the outcome of such research results in isolated islands of knowledge and a lack of understanding of the optimal multidisciplinary treatment combination that would be most effective. The next step would be to conduct outcome research combining multiple interventions consisting of those that have been shown to be the most effective.

The non-modifiable factors identified earlier (e.g. age, sex) can help in identifying children at higher risk of developing pain and engage them in early prevention treatments. Most of the prognostic factors, predictors, and risk factors, however, are modifiable and intervention strategies should focus on minimizing the risk of developing pain or maintaining pain and pain-related disability associated with these factors.

Primary prevention of acute pain of iatrogenic origin

Significant efforts have been deployed to prevent or reduce pain during hospitalization. A forerunner of this type of prevention was the implementation of the 'ouchless place model' in the 1990s (Schechter, 2008). The goals of this programme were to provide a better integration of research into clinical practice and focused specifically on postoperative pain control, pain assessment, needle-related pain, and encouraging parental involvement in children's pain management. This type of model is essential to knowledge translation and the implementation of systematic programmes aimed at preventing and reducing acute pain in hospital.

Two important areas targeted by this model are procedural pain and postoperative pain. Because the timing and nature of these procedures are known in advance, it is possible to conduct longitudinal studies beginning prior to the procedures in order to identify risk and protective factors associated with the acute pain experience.

Systematic reviews of the literature on procedural pain have supported development of clinical practices guidelines that outline effective pharmacological and non-pharmacological interventions (including contextual, behavioural and cognitive strategies) to reduce procedural pain (e.g. Taddio et al., 2010) (see Table 5.3).

Research has also focused on reducing acute postoperative pain. One randomized controlled trial on the effectiveness of behavioural interventions on post-operative pain in children showed that behavioural preparation reduces anxiety before surgery and during induction of anaesthesia, and leads to lower frequency of emergence delirium, lower consumption of analgesic in the recovery room, and shorter stay in the recovery room (Kain et al., 2007). Guided imagery has also been found to reduce levels of pain and anxiety hours, but not 1 day after surgery when used 1 week and a few hours before surgery (Huth et al., 2004).

Table 5.3 Evidence-based interventions to reduce procedural-related pain (i.e. immunization and injection pain) in infants, children, and adolescents

			Systematic reviews evaluating the effect of these interventions
Non-pharmacological management	Infants	Breastfeeding Kangaroo care (skin-to-skin contract) A sweet-testing solution Swaddling/facilitated tucking Rocking/holding Sucking-related interventions	(Pillai Riddell et al., 2011; Stevens et al., 2010)
	Children and adolescents	Psychological interventions: ◆ Distraction (e.g. music, cartoon movies) ◆ Relaxation breathing ◆ Information/preparation ◆ Combined cognitive-behavioural interventions Physical interventions/injection technique: ◆ Injecting the least painful brand during vaccination ◆ Having the child sit up ◆ Stroking the skin or applying pressure close to the injection site before and during injection; ◆ Injecting the most painful vaccine last when 2 vaccines are being administered sequentially during a single office visit; ◆ Performing a rapid intramuscular injection without aspiration.	(Cepeda et al., 2006; Chambers et al., 2009; Uman et al., 2006)
Pharmacological interventions		Topical anaesthetics (e.g. EMLA™)	(Taddio et al., 2009)

Primary prevention of chronic pain

Very little is known about primary prevention of chronic pain mainly because most research is conducted when the pain is already present or chronic. One area that has received some empirical attention involves perioperative pain. Intervention strategies that aim to minimize acute postoperative pain intensity have the potential to play an important role in preventing the development of chronic post-operative pain. These interventions include pharmacological and psychosocial approaches to minimizing pain.

Pre-emptive/preventive analgesia

Pre-emptive analgesia involves blocking pre- or intraoperative versus postoperative nociceptive inputs with the aim of preventing a state of central sensitization; thereby leading to less intense postoperative pain and lower analgesic consumption (Katz, 1995; Kissin, 2000). Preventive analgesia is a broader concept that aims to prevent the development of sensitization (peripheral and central) by blocking noxious inputs perioperatively (pre-, intra-, and postoperatively). Systematic reviews of the efficacy of pre-emptive analgesia are equivocal (Katz, 2003, Ong et al., 2005).

In contrast, more recent reviews suggest that preventive analgesia is more effective than the more narrow, classical view of pre-emptive analgesia in large part due to the blockade of nociceptive inputs across the perioperative phases of surgery (Katz and McCartney, 2002; Katz et al., 2011) and the use of more effective agents such as the alpha 2 delta ligands (Clarke et al., 2012). The focus of preventive analgesia is not on the relative timing of analgesic or anaesthetic interventions as is pre-emptive analgesia, but on attenuating the impact of the peripheral nociceptive barrage associated with

noxious preoperative, intraoperative, and/or postoperative stimuli. These stimuli induce peripheral and central sensitization, which increase postoperative pain intensity and analgesic requirements. Preventing sensitization reduces pain and analgesic requirements.

The reason why pre-emptive analgesic interventions have been equivocal is because the classic, two-group, pre- versus post-surgery design assumes that the intraoperative nociceptive barrage contributes to a greater extent to postoperative pain than does the postoperative nociceptive barrage. However, some studies have since shown that central sensitization is induced to an equal (or greater) extent by incision and intraoperative trauma, on the one hand (i.e. in the post-surgical treatment group), and postoperative inflammatory inputs and/or ectopic neural activity, on the other (i.e. in the preoperative treatment group), which would lead to non-significant intergroup differences in pain and analgesic consumption. The absence of significant differences in postoperative pain or analgesic consumption between the groups may point to the relative efficacy in reducing central sensitization of post incisional or postsurgical blockade, and not to the inefficacy of preoperative blockade (Katz et al., 2011).

The literature on paediatric pre-emptive/preventive analgesia (Yaster, 2010) is at best equivocal. Some studies have found that pre-emptive analgesia significantly reduces postoperative pain scores (Giannoni et al., 2001; Kundra et al., 1998) whereas similar studies fail to show a benefit (Giannoni et al., 2002; Ozcengiz et al., 2001).

Psychosocial interventions

Researchers have examined the effectiveness of interventions aimed at reducing psychological distress and/or pain intensity during the perioperative period. In a randomized controlled trial of cognitive behavioural therapy (information, coping skills training, combined information and coping skills training, or control group) administered once before and once after surgery, the combined intervention group showed reduced levels of pre- and post-surgical anxiety, whereas the coping skills group showed significantly reduced levels of postoperative anxiety and pain intensity (LaMontagne et al., 2003). As well, the control group exhibited the highest levels of postoperative pain 4 days after surgery compared to the treatment groups. Finally, the information-only group significantly increased their level of usual activities at 6 versus 3 months after surgery whereas younger children in the control or combined groups were more engaged in social activities compared to children in the coping group (LaMontagne et al., 2004). Similarly, a randomized controlled trial examining the effectiveness of behavioural interventions (family-centred behavioural preparation versus parental presence at induction versus oral midazolam versus control) found that children who received family-centred behavioural preparation before surgery exhibited lower preoperative anxiety, had a lower frequency of emergence delirium, consumed less analgesic in the recovery room, and were discharged faster from the recovery room compared to children in the other groups (Kain et al., 2007).

Secondary and tertiary prevention of chronic pain

Psychological interventions including cognitive behavioural treatment, biofeedback, and/or relaxation can be effective in managing a wide array of pain problems, whereas pharmacological interventions appear to be more pain-condition specific. A Cochrane review has shown that psychological treatments are effective at reducing pain, but not disability, in children with headaches, fibromyalgia, and recurrent abdominal pain (Eccleston et al., 2009). A review of complementary and alternative medicine approaches has reported that children with recurrent headaches benefit significantly from hypnosis and guided imagery whereas other approaches, such as acupuncture, massage therapy, homeopathy, biofeedback, arts, and herbal therapy were found to be 'possibly efficacious' or 'promising' for other paediatric chronic pains (Tsao and Zeltzer, 2005).

One area of tertiary prevention that has received significant attention is headache. Chronic daily headaches and migraines are among the most frequent paediatric pain conditions. Reviews of pharmacological interventions show that acetaminophen, ibuprofen, and a sumatriptan nasal spray (Damen et al., 2005) as well as propranolol and flunarizine (Victor and Ryan, 2003) significantly reduce paediatric migraine-related symptoms. More high-quality randomized control trials are needed to establish the effect of additional drugs for which no trials of sufficient quality have been conducted (Damen et al., 2005; Victor and Ryan, 2003) in addition to examining the long-term potential of these drugs in preventing pain and related disability. Moreover, reviews have found that psychological therapies (Cvengros et al., 2007; Kroner-Herwig, 2011) are effective in treating paediatric headaches, but this effect was moderated by other variables, such as demographic and treatment characteristics.

Together, these results suggest that psychological and pharmacological factors play an important role in the secondary and tertiary prevention of chronic pain. More research is needed to examine the long-term benefits of using these interventions.

Recent adult chronic pain research indicates that the risk and protective factors involved in the transition to chronicity differ from those involved in the maintenance of already established chronic pain (Katz, 2012). For example, a prospective, longitudinal study of patients after lateral thoracotomy, showed that perioperative factors (i.e. preoperative pain disability, preoperative emotional numbing symptoms, and acute postoperative pain intensity) failed to predict the transition to chronic pain disability 6 months after surgery, but the very same variables measured 6 months later were highly significant predictors of the maintenance of 12-month chronic pain disability (Katz et al., 2009). Seebach et al. (2012) reported a similar pattern of findings in their prospective, longitudinal study of the psychosocial recovery trajectory in patients after spine surgery. The results indicate the risk factors that predict the maintenance of established chronic postsurgical pain disability or pain intensity, pain interference, and functional status are different from those that predict the initial transition to chronicity. Evidence for the distinction between triggering and maintaining factors in paediatric chronic post-surgical pain has been provided by Pagé et al. (2013) who showed that pain unpleasantness ratings 24 to 48 hours after surgery predicted the transition to moderate/severe CPSP at 6 months (but not 12 months), whereas 6-month anxiety sensitivity scores predicted the maintenance of moderate/severe CPSP (i.e. from 6 to 12 months after surgery). Implications of these findings for the design and conduct of paediatric studies and for pain prevention are discussed in the following section.

Future research directions and clinical implications

The field of paediatric pain prevention, particularly chronic pain, is in its infancy. The search for risk and protective factors would be aided by well-designed, prospective, longitudinal epidemiological studies. These studies would: (1) assess participants prior to the onset of the procedure or as early as possible after injury or illness, (2) follow them until chronic pain has developed (i.e. 3–6 months), and (3) include a sufficient number of follow-ups to capture the critical window during which relevant processes and factors contribute to the transition to chronicity. It is crucial to assess outcomes at multiple time points because the transition to chronic pain and related psychosocial dysfunction is a dynamic process that evolves over time (Katz, 2012; Katz and Seltzer, 2009; Kehlet and Rathmell, 2010).

Such research would build on current observational studies of individual factors associated with the pain experience. This will lead to the development of integrative theoretical models of pain and disability adapted to paediatric populations, to a better understanding of the risk and protective factors involved in the transition of acute to chronic pain, and ultimately to clearer guidelines and recommendations for chronic pain prevention.

Current research on factors associated with the presence of chronic pain in children and mechanisms associated with the transition from acute to chronic pain can help further our understanding of the physical, pharmacological, and psychosocial correlates of paediatric chronic pain and provide important information for tertiary pain prevention. Prospective studies of the development of chronic pain and the transition from acute to chronic pain will help identify important risk factors, which can lead to the development of primary and secondary prevention strategies.

In addition, few randomized controlled trials have examined the effectiveness of psychological treatments in the treatment of paediatric chronic pain and disability and little is known about recent intervention strategies (e.g. acceptance and commitment therapy; Wicksell et al., 2009) that successfully reduce pain-related disability. Systematic reviews show psychological treatment is effective for pain, but little evidence to support an effect on pain disability. Clinical trials are needed to extend the support of psychological treatment for pain to pain-related disability and other pain-related outcomes.

Many factors and mechanisms that affect the development and course of paediatric pain. Although there has been a growing body of literature over the last 15 years that explore the role of some factors influencing pain and pain-related disability, systematic reviews and meta-analyses are needed to identify the most important evidence-based factors and determine the specific and common factors associated with particular pain conditions. This will has enormous implications for the development of strategies to prevent unnecessary pain and suffering.

References

Aasvang, E. K. and Kehlet, H. (2007). Chronic pain after childhood groin hernia repair. *J Pediatr Surg,* 42, 1403–1408.

Allegaert, K. (2009). Clinical pharmacology of systemic analgesics in neonates. *Curr Drug Ther,* 4, 152–158.

Allen, D. and Shriver, M. D. (1998). Role of parent-mediated pain behavior management strategies in biofeedback treatment of childhood migraines. *Behav Ther,* 29, 477–490.

Anand, K. J. S., Carr, D. B., and Hickey, P. R. (1987). Randomized trial of high-dose anesthesia in neonates undergoing cardiac surgery: Hormonal and hemodynamic stress responses. *Anesthesiology,* 67, A502.

Asmundson, G. J. G., Noel, M., Petter, M., and Parkerson, H. (2012). Pediatric fear-avoidance model of chronic pain: foundation, application and future directions. *Pain Res Manag,* 17, 397–405.

Asmundson, G. J. G., Norton, P. J., and Vlaeyen, J. W. (2004). Fear-avoidance models of chronic pain: an overview. In G. J. G. Asmundson, J. W. S. Vlaeyen, and G. Crombez (eds) *Understanding and treating fear of pain,* pp. 3–24. Oxford: Oxford University Press.

Bandell-Hoekstra, I. E., Abu-Saad, H. H., Passchier, J., Frederiks, C. M., Feron, F. J., and Knipschild, P. (2001). Prevalence and characteristics of headache in Dutch schoolchildren. *Eur J Pain,* 5, 145–153.

Bandura, A. (1986). *Social foundations of thought and action. a social cognitive theory.* Englewood Cliffs, NJ: Prentice-Hall.

Bejia, I., Abid, N., Ben Salem, K., Letaief, M., Younes, M., Touzi, M., et al. (2005). Low back pain in a cohort of 622 Tunisian schoolchildren and adolescents: an epidemiological study. *Eur Spine J,* 14, 331–336.

Bowlby, J. (1973). *Attachment and loss. Vol II Attachment.* New York: Basic Books.

Bursch, B., Tsao, J. C., Meldrum, M., and Zeltzer, L. K. (2006). Preliminary validation of a self-efficacy scale for child functioning despite chronic pain (child and parent versions). *Pain,* 125, 35–42.

Cepeda, M. S., Carr, D. B., Lau, J., and Alvarez, H. (2006). Music for pain relief. *Cochrane Database Syst Rev,* 2, CD004843.

Chambers, C. T., Taddio, A., Uman, L. S., and McMurtry, C. M. (2009). Psychological interventions for reducing pain and distress during routine childhood immunizations: a systematic review. *Clin Ther,* 31(Suppl 2), S77–S103.

Chogle, A. and Saps, M. (2009). Environmental factors of abdominal pain. *Pediatr Ann,* 38, 398–401, 404.

Claar, R. L., Walker, L. S., and Smith, C. A. (1999). Functional disability in adolescents and young adults with symptoms of irritable bowel syndrome: the role of academic, social, and athletic competence. *J Pediatr Psychol,* 24, 271–280.

Clarke, H., Bonin, R. P., Orser, B. A., Englesakis, M., Wijeysundera, D. N., and Katz, J. (2012). The prevention of chronic postsurgical pain using gabapentin and pregabalin: a combined systematic review and meta-analysis. *Anesth Analg,* 115(2), 428–442.

Craig, K. D. and Pillai Riddell, R. (2003). Social influences, culture and ethnicity. In G. A. Finley and P. J. McGrath (eds) *The context of pediatric pain: biology, family, society and culture,* pp. 159–182. Seattle, WA: IASP Press.

Craig, K. D. and Prkachin, K. M. (1978). Social modeling influences on sensory decision theory and psychophysiological indexes of pain. *J Pers Soc Psychol,* 36, 805–815.

Crombez, G., Bijttebier, P., Eccleston, C., Mascagni, T., Mertens, G., Goubert, L., and Verstraeten, K. (2003). The child version of the pain catastrophization scale (PCS-C): a preliminary validation. *Pain,* 104, 639–646.

Cvengros, J. A., Harper, D., and Shevell, M. (2007). Pediatric headache: an examination of process variables in treatment. *J Child Neurol,* 22, 1172–1181.

Damen, L., Bruijn, J. K., Verhagen, A. P., Berger, M. Y., Passchier, J., and Koes, B. W. (2005). Symptomatic treatment of migraine in children: a systematic review of medication trials. *Pediatrics,* 116, e295–302.

Eccleston, C., Palermo, T. M., Williams, A. C., Lewandowski, A., and Morley, S. (2009). Psychological therapies for the management of chronic and recurrent pain in children and adolescents. *Cochrane Database Syst Rev,* 2, CD003968.

Egger, H. L., Angold, A., and Costello, E. J. (1998). Headaches and psychopathology in children and adolescents. *J Am Acad Child Adolesc Psychiatry,* 37, 951–958.

El-Metwally, A., Mikkelsson, M., Stahl, M., Macfarlane, G. J., Jones, G. T., Pulkkinen, L., et al. (2008). Genetic and environmental influences on non-specific low back pain in children: a twin study. *Eur Spine J,* 17, 502–508.

Engel, G. L. (1977). The need for a new medical model: a challenge for biomedicine. *Science,* 196, 129–136.

Fordyce, W. E., Fowler, R., Lehman, J., and Delateur, B. (1968). Some implications of learning in problems of chronic pain. *J Chronic Dis,* 21, 179–190.

Gatchel, R. J., Peng, Y. B., Peters, M. L., Fuchs, P. N., and Turk, D. C. (2007). The biopsychosocial approach to chronic pain: scientific advances and future directions. *Psychol Bull,* 133, 581–624.

Gauntlett-Gilbert, J. and Eccleston, C. (2007). Disability in adolescents with chronic pain: Patterns and predictors across different domains of functioning. *Pain,* 131, 132–141.

Giannoni, C., White, S., and Enneking, F. K. (2002). Does Dexamethasone with preemptive analgesia improve pediatric tonsillectomy pain? *Otolaryngol Head Neck Surg,* 126, 307–315.

Giannoni, C., White, S., Enneking, F. K., and Morey, T. (2001). Ropivacaine with or without clonidine improves pediatric tonsillectomy pain. *Arch Otolaryngol Head Neck Surg,* 127, 1265–1270.

Gieteling, M. J., Bierma-Zeinstra, S. M., Van Leeuwen, Y., Passchier, J., and Berger, M. Y. (2011). Prognostic factors for persistence of chronic abdominal pain in children. *J Pediatr Gastroenterol Nutr,* 52, 154–161.

Hechler, T., Blankenburg, M., Dobe, M., Kosfelder, J., Hubner, B., and Zernikow, B. (2010). Effectiveness of a multimodal inpatient treatment for pediatric chronic pain: a comparison between children and adolescents. *Eur J Pain,* 14, 97.e1–9.

Hershey, A. D., Powers, S. W., Vockell, A. L., Lecates, S., Kabbouche, M. A., and Maynard, M. K. (2001). PedMIDAS: development of a questionnaire to assess disability of migraines in children. *Neurology,* 57, 2034–2039.

Huertas-Ceballos, A., Logan, S., Bennett, C., and MacArthur, C. (2008a). Pharmacological interventions for recurrent abdominal pain (RAP) and irritable bowel syndrome (IBS) in childhood. *Cochrane Database Syst Rev,* 1, CD003017.

Huertas-Ceballos, A., Logan, S., Bennett, C., and MacArthur, C. (2008b). Psychosocial interventions for recurrent abdominal pain (RAP) and irritable bowel syndrome (IBS) in childhood. *Cochrane Database Syst Rev*, 1, CD003014.

Huertas-Ceballos, A. A., Logan, S., Bennett, C., and Macarthur, C. (2009). Dietary interventions for recurrent abdominal pain (RAP) and irritable bowel syndrome (IBS) in childhood. *Cochrane Database Syst Rev*, 1, CD003019.

Huguet, A., McGrath, P. J., Stinson, J., Chambers, C. T., and Miro, J. (2011). Shaping the future of research on chronic pain in children. *Pediatr Pain Lett*, 13, 7–12.

Huth, M. M., Broome, M. E., and Good, M. (2004). Imagery reduces children's post-operative pain. *Pain*, 110, 439–448.

Jones, G. T., Watson, K. D., Silman, A. J., Symmons, D. P., and MacFarlane, G. J. (2003). Predictors of low back pain in British schoolchildren: a population-based prospective cohort study. *Pediatrics*, 111, 822–828.

Kain, Z. N., Caldwell-Andrews, A. A., Mayes, L. C., Weinberg, M. E., Wang, S. M., Maclaren, J. E., *et al.* (2007). Family-centered preparation for surgery improves perioperative outcomes in children: a randomized controlled trial. *Anesthesiology*, 106, 65–74.

Kashikar-Zuck, S., Goldschneider, K. R., Powers, S. W., Vaught, M. H., and Hershey, A. D. (2001). Depression and functional disability in chronic pediatric pain. *Clin J Pain*, 17, 341–349.

Katz, J. (1995). Pre-emptive analgesia: evidence, current status and future directions. *Eur J Anaesthesiol Suppl*, 10, 8–13.

Katz, J. (2003). Timing of treatment and preemptive analgesia. In A. S. C. Rice, C. A. Warfield, D. Justins, and C. Eccleston (eds) *Clinical pain management*, pp. 113–162. London: Arnold.

Katz, J. (2012). One man's risk factor is another man's outcome: difference in risk factor profiles for chronic postsurgical pain maintenance vs transition. *Pain*, 153, 505–506.

Katz, J., Asmundson, G. J., Mcrae, K., and Halket, E. (2009). Emotional numbing and pain intensity predict the development of pain disability up to one year after lateral thoracotomy. *Eur J Pain*, 13, 870–878.

Katz, J., Clarke, H., and Seltzer, Z. (2011). Review article: Preventive analgesia: quo vadimus? *Anesth Analg*, 113, 1242–1253.

Katz, J. and McCartney, C. J. (2002). Current status of preemptive analgesia. *Curr Opin Anaesthesiol*, 15, 435–441.

Katz, J. and Seltzer, Z. (2009). Transition from acute to chronic postsurgical pain: risk factors and protective factors. *Expert Rev Neurother*, 9, 723–744.

Kehlet, H. and Rathmell, J. P. (2010). Persistent postsurgical pain: the path forward through better design of clinical studies. *Anesthesiology*, 112, 514–515.

Kissin, I. (2000). Preemptive analgesia. *Anesthesiology*, 93, 1138–1143.

Kleiman, V., Clarke, H., and Katz, J. (2011). Sensitivity to pain traumatization: a higher-order factor underlying pain-related anxiety, pain catastrophizing and anxiety sensitivity among patients scheduled for major surgery. *Pain Res Manag*, 16, 169–177.

Konijnenberg, A. Y., Uiterwaal, C. S., Kimpen, J. L., Van Der Hoeven, J., Buitelaar, J. K., and De Graeff-Meeder, E. R. (2005). Children with unexplained chronic pain: substantial impairment in everyday life. *Arch Dis Child*, 90, 680–686.

Kovacs, F. M., Gestoso, M., Gil Del Real, M. T., Lopez, J., Mufraggi, N., and Mendez, J. I. (2003). Risk factors for non-specific low back pain in schoolchildren and their parents: a population based study. *Pain*, 103, 259–268.

Kraemer, H. C., Kazdin, A. E., Offord, D. R., Kessler, R. C., Jensen, P. S., and Kupfer, D. J. (1997). Coming to terms with the terms of risk. *Arch Gen Psychiatry*, 54, 337–343.

Kroner-Herwig, B. (2011). Psychological treatments for pediatric headache. *Expert Rev Neurother*, 11, 403–410.

Kundra, P., Deepalak Shmi, K., and Ravishankar, M. (1998). Preemptive caudal bupivicaine and morphine for postoperative analgesia in children. *Anesth Analg*, 87, 52–56.

Lamontagne, L. L., Hepworth, J. T., Cohen, F., and Salisbury, M. H. (2003). Cognitive-behavioral intervention effects on adolescents' anxiety and pain following spinal fusion surgery. *Nurs Res*, 52, 183–190.

Lamontagne, L. L., Hepworth, J. T., Cohen, F., and Salisbury, M. H. (2004). Adolescent scoliosis: effects of corrective surgery, cognitive-behavioral interventions, and age on activity outcomes. *Appl Nurs Res*, 17, 168–177.

Laupacis, A., Wells, G., Richardson, W. S., and Tugwell, P. (1994). Users' guides to the medical literature. V. How to use an article about prognosis. Evidence-Based Medicine Working Group. *JAMA*, 272, 234–237.

Laurell, K., Larsson, B., and Eeg-Olofsson, O. (2005). Headache in schoolchildren: association with other pain, family history and psychosocial factors. *Pain*, 119, 150–158.

Leeuw, M., Goossens, M. E., Linton, S. J., Crombez, G., Boersma, K., and Vlaeyen, J. W. (2007). The fear-avoidance model of musculoskeletal pain: current state of scientific evidence. *J Behav Med*, 30, 77–94.

Logan, D. E., Guite, J. W., Sherry, D. D., and Rose, J. B. (2006). Adolescent-parent relationships in the context of adolescent chronic pain conditions. *Clin J Pain*, 22, 576–583.

Logan, D. E. and Scharff, L. (2005). Relationships between family and parent characteristics and functional abilities in children with recurrent pain syndromes: an investigation of moderating effects on the pathway from pain to disability. *J Pediatr Psychol*, 30, 698–707.

Lynch, A. M., Kashikar-Zuck, S., Goldschneider, K. R., and Jones, B. A. (2006). Psychosocial risks for disability in children with chronic back pain. *J Pain*, 7, 244–251.

Malleson, P. N., Connell, H., Bennett, S. M., and Eccleston, C. (2001). Chronic musculoskeletal and other idiopathic pain syndromes. *Arch Dis Child*, 84, 189–192.

Martin, A. L., Halket, E., Asmundson, G. J., Flora, D. B., and Katz, J. (2010). Posttraumatic stress symptoms and the diathesis-stress model of chronic pain and disability in patients undergoing major surgery. *Clin J Pain*, 26, 518–527.

Martin, A. L., McGrath, P. A., Brown, S. C., and Katz, J. (2007a). Anxiety sensitivity, fear of pain and pain-related disability in children and adolescents with chronic pain. *Pain Res Manag*, 12, 267–272.

Martin, A. L., McGrath, P. A., Brown, S. C., and Katz, J. (2007b). Children with chronic pain: impact of sex and age on long-term outcomes. *Pain*, 128, 13–19.

Martin, S. E. and Smith, M. S. (1995). Psychosocial factors in recurrent pediatric headache. *Pediatr Ann*, 24, 464–474.

McCaffery, M. (1977). Pain relief for the child. *Pediatr Nurs*, 3, 1–16.

McGrath, P. J., Walco, G. A., Turk, D. C., Dworkin, R. H., Brown, M. T., Davidson, K., *et al.* (2008). Core outcome domains and measures for pediatric acute and chronic/recurrent pain clinical trials: PedIMMPACT recommendations. *J Pain*, 9, 771–783.

Minuchin, S., Baker, L., Rosman, B. L., Liebman, R., Milman, L., and Todd, T. C. (1975). A conceptual model of psychosomatic illness in children. Family organization and family therapy. *Arch Gen Psychiatry*, 32, 1031–1038.

Ong, C. K., Lirk, P., Seymour, R. A., and Jenkins, B. J. (2005). The efficacy of preemptive analgesia for acute postoperative pain management: a meta-analysis. *Anesth Analg*, 100, 757–773.

Ozcengiz, D., Gunduz, M., Ozbek, H., and Isik, G. (2001). Comparison of caudal morphine and tramadol for postoperative pain control in children undergoing inguinal herniorrhaphy. *Paediatr Anaesth*, 11, 459–464.

Pagé, M. G., Stinson, J., Campbell, F., Isaac, L., and Katz, J. (2013). Identification of pain-related psychological risk factors for the development and maintenance of chronic pediatric post-surgical pain. *J Pain Res*, 6, 167–180.

Palermo, T. M. and Chambers, C. T. (2005). Parent and family factors in pediatric chronic pain and disability: an integrative approach. *Pain*, 119, 1–4.

Palermo, T. M., Witherspoon, D., Valenzuela, D., and Drotar, D. D. (2004). Development and validation of the Child Activity Limitations Interview: a measure of pain-related functional impairment in school-age children and adolescents. *Pain*, 109, 461–70.

Parry, S. (2011). Acute pain management in the neonate. *Anaesth Intensive Care*, 12, 121–125.

Perquin, C. W., Hunfeld, J. A., Hazebroek-Kampschreur, A. A., Van Suijlekom-Smit, L. W., Passchier, J., Koes, B. W., et al. (2003). The natural course of chronic benign pain in childhood and adolescence: a two-year population-based follow-up study. *Eur J Pain*, 7, 551–559.

Pillai Riddell, R. R., Racine, N. M., Turcotte, K., Uman, L. S., Horton, R. E., Din Osmun, L., et al. 2011. Non-pharmacological management of infant and young child procedural pain. *Cochrane Database Syst Rev*, 10, CD006275.

Priest, T. D. and Hoggart, B. (2002). Chronic pain: mechanisms and treatment. *Curr Opin Pharmacol*, 2, 310–315.

Prins, Y., Crous, L., and Louw, Q. A. (2008). A systematic review of posture and psychosocial factors as contributors to upper quadrant musculoskeletal pain in children and adolescents. *Physiother Theory Pract*, 24, 221–242.

Sawyer, M. G., Carbone, J. A., Whitham, J. N., Roberton, D. M., Taplin, J. E., Varni, J. W., et al. (2005). The relationship between health-related quality of life, pain, and coping strategies in juvenile arthritis—a one year prospective study. *Qual Life Res*, 14, 1585–1598.

Scharff, L. (1997). Recurrent abdominal pain in children: a review of psychological factors and treatment. *Clin Psychol Rev*, 17, 145–166.

Schechter, N. L. (2008). From the ouchless place to comfort central: the evolution of a concept. *Pediatrics*, 122(Suppl 3), S154–160.

Schulte, I. E., Petermann, F., and Noeker, M. (2010). Functional abdominal pain in childhood: from etiology to maladaptation. *Psychother Psychosom*, 79, 73–86.

Seebach, C. L., Kirkhart, M., Lating, J. M., Wegener, S. T., Song, Y., Riley, L. H., 3rd et al. (2012). Examining the role of positive and negative affect in recovery from spine surgery. *Pain*, 153, 518–525.

Simons, L. E., Sieberg, C. B., Carpino, E., Logan, D., and Berde, C. (2011). The Fear of Pain Questionnaire (FOPQ): assessment of pain-related fear among children and adolescents with chronic pain. *J Pain*, 12, 677–686.

Sjolie, A. N. (2002). Psychosocial correlates of low-back pain in adolescents. *Eur Spine J*, 11, 582–588.

Stevens, B., Yamada, J., and Ohlsson, A. (2010). Sucrose for analgesia in newborn infants undergoing painful procedures. *Cochrane Database Syst Rev*, 1, CD001069.

Taddio, A., Appleton, M., Bortolussi, R., Chambers, C., Dubey, V., Halperin, S., et al. (2010). Reducing the pain of childhood vaccination: an evidence-based clinical practice guideline (summary). *CMAJ*, 182, 1989–1995.

Taddio, A., Ilersich, A. L., Ipp, M., Kikuta, A., and Shah, V. (2009). Physical interventions and injection techniques for reducing injection pain during routine childhood immunizations: systematic review of randomized controlled trials and quasi-randomized controlled trials. *Clin Ther*, 31 Suppl 2, S48–76.

Tsao, J. C., Evans, S., Meldrum, M., and Zeltzer, L. K. (2009). Sex differences in anxiety sensitivity among children with chronic pain and non-clinical children. *J Pain Manag*, 2, 151–161.

Tsao, J. C. and Zeltzer, L. K. (2005). Complementary and alternative medicine approaches for pediatric pain: a review of the state-of-the-science. *Evid Based Complement Alternat Med*, 2, 149–159.

Turk, D. C. (1996). Biopsychosocial perspective on chronic pain. In R. J. Gatchel and D. C. Turk (eds) *Psychological approaches to pain management: a practitioner's handbook*, pp. 6–23. New York: Guilford Press.

Turk, D. C. (2002). A diathesis-stress model of chronic pain and disability following traumatic injury. *Pain Res Manag*, 7, 9–19.

Turk, D. C., Dworkin, R. H., Allen, R. R., Bellamy, N., Brandenburg, N., Carr, D. B., et al. (2003). Core outcome domains for chronic pain clinical trials: IMMPACT recommendations. *Pain*, 106, 337–345.

Turk, D. C., Dworkin, R. H., Revicki, D., Harding, G., Burke, L. B., Cella, D., et al. (2008). Identifying important outcome domains for chronic pain clinical trials: an IMMPACT survey of people with pain. *Pain*, 137, 276–285.

Uman, L. S., Chambers, C. T., McGrath, P. J., and Kisely, S. (2006). Psychological interventions for needle-related procedural pain and distress in children and adolescents. *Cochrane Database Syst Rev*, 4, CD005179.

Van Slyke, D. A. and Walker, L. S. (2006). Mothers' responses to children's pain. *Clin J Pain*, 22, 387–391.

Varni, J. W., Stucky, B. D., Thissen, D., Dewitt, E. M., Irwin, D. E., Lai, J. S., et al. (2010). PROMIS Pediatric Pain Interference Scale: an item response theory analysis of the pediatric pain item bank. *J Pain*, 11, 1109–1119.

Vervoort, T., Goubert, L., Eccleston, C., Bijttebier, P., and Crombez, G. (2006). Catastrophic thinking about pain is independently associated with pain severity, disability, and somatic complaints in school children and children with chronic pain. *J Pediatr Psychol*, 31, 674–683.

Victor, S. and Ryan, S. W. (2003). Drugs for preventing migraine headaches in children. *Cochrane Database Syst Rev*, 4, CD002761.

Vikat, A., Rimpela, M., Salminen, J. J., Rimpela, A., Savolainen, A., and Virtanen, S. M. (2000). Neck or shoulder pain and low back pain in Finnish adolescents. *Scand J Public Health*, 28, 164–173.

Vlaeyen, J. W., Kole-Snijders, A. M., Boeren, R. G., and Van Eek, H. (1995). Fear of movement/(re)injury in chronic low back pain and its relation to behavioral performance. *Pain*, 62, 363–372.

Vuorimaa, H., Tamm, K., Honkanen, V., Konttinen, Y. T., Komulainen, E., and Santavirta, N. (2008). Empirical classification of children with JIA: a multidimensional approach to pain and well-being. *Clin Exp Rheumatol*, 26, 954–961.

Walker, L.S. and Greene, J.W. (1991). The functional disability inventory: measuring a neglected dimension of child health status. *J Pediatr Psychol*, 16; 39–58.

Walsh, T. M., McGrath, P. J., and Symons, D. K. (2008). Attachment dimensions and young children's response to pain. *Pain Res Manag*, 13, 33–40.

Wicksell, R. K., Melin, L., Lekander, M., and Olsson, G. L. (2009). Evaluating the effectiveness of exposure and acceptance strategies to improve functioning and quality of life in longstanding pediatric pain—a randomized controlled trial. *Pain*, 141, 248–257.

Wilson, A. C., Lewandowski, A. S., and Palermo, T. M. (2011). Fear-avoidance beliefs and parental responses to pain in adolescents with chronic pain. *Pain Res Manag*, 16, 178–282.

Yaster, M. (2010). Multimodal analgesia in children. *Eur J Anaesthesiol*, 27, 851–857.

SECTION 2

Biological basis of paediatric pain

CHAPTER 6

Nociceptive signalling in the periphery and spinal cord

Suellen M. Walker and Mark L. Baccei

Summary

Responses to painful or noxious stimuli are functional at birth. However, postnatal changes in the transmitters, receptors, and pathways involved in nociceptive signalling result in significant age-related changes in the nature and degree of response.

Noxious mechanical, thermal, and chemical stimuli are detected by peripheral nociceptors, transduced into electrical stimuli, and transmitted to the spinal cord. Within the spinal cord, there are significant postnatal changes in the balance of inhibitory and excitatory signalling, that not only influence the acute response to afferent input, but can also underlie long-term alterations in sensory processing following tissue injury in early life.

Evaluating age-related changes in nociceptive signalling is essential not only for understanding acute behavioural responses to noxious stimuli, but also for identifying the most appropriate and effective pain management interventions at different developmental ages.

Introduction

Throughout postnatal development, there are significant functional and structural changes in the developing nervous system that influence nociceptive transmission. Patterns of innervation, receptor expression and distribution, and synaptic function within nociceptive pathways vary with age and influence the sensitivity and nature of response. This chapter describes the peripheral and spinal cord components of nociceptive processing, and outlines important age-related changes that influence the transmission and modulation of pain signalling in early life. Issues related to fetal nociception will not be discussed, as the marked differences between *in utero* and postnatal physiology also influence nociceptive signalling (Mellor et al., 2005).

The ability to detect and respond to potentially damaging environmental stimuli is an essential function that is maintained across species (Smith and Lewin, 2009). Infant rodents provide an established model for assessment of mammalian development and are frequently utilized to assess age-dependent changes in nociceptive mechanisms, with structural and functional methods that are not possible in clinical studies (Fitzgerald and Walker, 2009). The rat pup is born at a relatively immature stage, and data collected from human fetal tissue and rat pups suggest that the development of peripheral and spinal somatosensory function during the first postnatal week in the rat pup corresponds to preterm development from 24 weeks until full-term birth at 40 post-conceptional weeks (Fitzgerald, 1991a). Pups mature relatively rapidly and can be considered infants by postnatal day (P) 7, and as children or young adolescents when they are weaned at P21. Rather than representing absolute correlations, these timelines provide a framework for assessing progressive changes in function throughout development, and it is important to note that different regions of the nervous system mature at different rates. Subsequent chapters will extend this discussion to: interactions between neurons and immune cells in nociceptive processing (Vega-Avelaira and Beggs, Chapter 7) and transmission to higher centres and modulation by brainstem centres (Fitzgerald, Chapter 8) (Figure 6.1). Visceral pain processing is discussed by Batra et al. (Chapter 27).

Peripheral nociceptive pathways

'Nociception' refers to the physiological and pathophysiological component of sensory processing (which is the focus of the current chapter), whereas 'pain' encompasses sensory, emotional, and cognitive components. However, the terms are often used interchangeably, and will be for the purposes of this chapter.

One role of the peripheral nervous system is to sense and transduce potentially or actually damaging stimuli into electrical signals that are then transmitted along the axon to the central nervous system (CNS). Peripheral nociceptive pathways have four functional components (Woolf and Ma, 2007):

1. A nociceptor is a high-threshold sensory receptor of the peripheral somatosensory nervous system that is capable of transducing and encoding noxious stimuli. A stimulus is noxious if it is damaging or threatens damage to normal tissues (Merskey and Bogduk, 1994; see also updated IASP definitions <http://www.iasp-pain.org/Content/NavigationMenu/GeneralResourceLinks/PainDefinitions/>).

2. A peripheral branch of the axon that conducts the action potential and transports receptors/proteins from the cell body to the site of transduction. Two main groups of cutaneous afferents terminate as free nerve endings in the epidermis:

   ♦ Myelinated Aδ fibres associated with high-threshold, slowly adapting mechanoreceptors, and in addition a proportion respond to heat and cold.

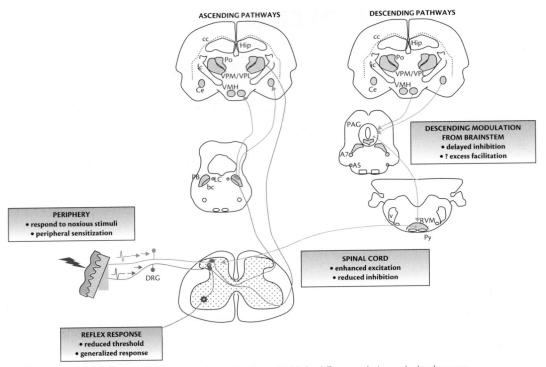

Figure 6.1 Diagrammatical representation of major nociceptive pathways. Textboxes highlight differences during early development.
Adapted by permission from Macmillan Publishers Ltd: *Nature Reviews Neuroscience*, Stephen P. Hunt and Patrick W. Mantyh, The molecular dynamics of pain control, Volume 2, Issue 2, p. 85, Copyright © 2001, http://www.nature.com/nrn/index.html.

- Unmyelinated C fibres, the majority of which are polymodal and respond to noxious mechanical, thermal and chemical stimuli. 'Silent' nociceptors become responsive to mechanical and/or heat stimuli after inflammation (Smith and Lewin, 2009).

3. The neuronal cell body in the dorsal root ganglion (DRG) is the major site for transcription and protein synthesis. In addition to sensory neurons, satellite glial cells are present in the DRG (see Vega-Avelaira and Beggs, Chapter 7, this volume, for further details). The small cell bodies of nociceptors are divided into two groups (Woolf and Ma, 2007):

  - Those that express tyrosine receptor kinase A (TrkA) and respond to nerve growth factor (NGF). These peptidergic nociceptors express calcitonin gene-related peptide (CGRP) and substance P (SP) and project to lamina I and lamina II outer in the superficial dorsal horn of the spinal cord.

  - Those that express Ret, the transmembrane signalling component of the receptor for glial cell-line derived neurotrophic factor (GDNF). These non-peptidergic neurons bind isolectin B4 (IB4), express the $P2X_3$ purine receptor, and project to lamina II inner in the dorsal horn (Hunt and Mantyh, 2001).

4. The central branch of the axon that projects from the DRG to the superficial dorsal horn and forms synaptic contacts with the second-order neuron. Presynaptic release of neurotransmitter (i.e. glutamate, substance P, brain-derived neurotrophic factor (BDNF)) is regulated by modulating calcium influx in the primary afferent terminal.

Peripheral nociceptive function has been evaluated by multiple experimental techniques, some of which have been conducted both in laboratory animals and in human experimental or clinical studies (Smith and Lewin, 2009). These include:

- Electrophysiology/microneurography recordings from sensory afferent fibres. This can be performed *in vitro* from isolated skin-nerve preparations (Koltzenburg et al., 1997; Reeh, 1986), or by *in vivo* studies in animals and humans (Koltzenburg and Handwerker, 1994).

- Analysis of receptor function and channel properties in cultured DRG neurons using patch clamp recordings and Ca^{2+}-imaging techniques.

- Evaluating the organism's behaviour in response to noxious stimuli (e.g. changes in spinal reflex sensitivity).

An important protective function of the nervous system is its ability to detect and localize noxious stimuli and produce rapid reflex motor responses, which draw the affected area away from the potential injury. Evaluating spinal reflex sensitivity to peripheral stimuli allows quantification of the impact of both injury and/or analgesia (Le Bars et al., 2001; Walker et al., 2009). Although thresholds for eliciting reflex responses vary with age, correlations between stimulus intensity and reflex response have been demonstrated at all ages in laboratory animals (Holmberg and Schouenborg, 1996), and in human neonates (Andrews and Fitzgerald, 1999) and adults (Willer, 1983).

Peripheral innervation

Nociceptive neurons are derived from neural crest cells in the dorsal part of the neural tube (Fitzgerald, 2005; Woolf and Ma, 2007). During embryonic development, sensory axons extend down the developing limbs to innervate the epidermis (Jackman and Fitzgerald, 2000). Larger-diameter A-fibre innervation occurs first, but by birth in the rat and by the second trimester in man, both A and C sensory fibres are distributed to all body regions (Fitzgerald, 2005). In rodent skin, fibres initially penetrate up to the epidermal surface but then retract to form a subepidermal plexus that becomes more organized over the first 2 postnatal weeks and innervates end organs, such as sweat glands and hair follicles (Jackman and Fitzgerald, 2000). Navigation of sensory terminals to their target tissue is controlled by long- and short-range guidance cues that permit or inhibit axon growth (i.e. they are attractive or repulsive; Kolodkin and Tessier-Lavigne, 2011). Ephrins are a family of cell-surface signalling molecules involved in short-range axon guidance during development that includes class A ephrins interacting with multiple class A ephrin (Eph) receptors. Neural growth cones are inhibited by ephrin-A4, which is localized to the upper epidermis postnatally, thus restricting skin terminals to lower epidermal regions, and levels decrease as innervation stabilizes postnatally. However, levels of ephrin-A4 are also influenced by injury, and downregulation following neonatal full-thickness skin wounds contributes to persistent hyperinnervation (Moss et al., 2005; see Walker, Chapter 3, this volume for further details).

Neurotrophins

In addition to established roles in modulating nociceptive sensitivity in adulthood (Pezet and McMahon, 2006), neurotrophins regulate multiple aspects of the development of sensory nerves (Fitzgerald, 2005), including:

- Neuronal survival. Neurotrophins promote the survival of specific types of neurons during development. NGF is present in the skin of the rat from birth (Constantinou et al., 1994), and is essential for nociceptor survival (Kirstein and Farinas, 2002). BDNF produced within sensory ganglia also plays a role in survival of nociceptive neurons responsive to NGF and GDNF (Valdes-Sanchez et al., 2010).

- Innervation. The pattern and density of skin innervation is regulated by access to local neurotrophic factors.

- Nociceptor differentiation. Levels of NGF and neurotrophin-3 (NT3) regulate the differentiation of Aδ high-threshold mechanoreceptors and C-fibre nociceptors.

- DRG neuronal phenotype. During embryonic development, 70% to 80% of DRG neurons and almost all that project to the superficial dorsal horn express trkA and are NGF dependent. A subpopulation of neurons downregulate expression of trkA around the time of birth, and begin to express Ret, the signalling component for GDNF, leading to a postnatal increase in this IB4+ve population (Beland and Fitzgerald, 2001; Fitzgerald, 2005). Neurons that continue to express trkA remain as the peptidergic population and express CGRP and SP (Guo et al., 2001).

Nociceptors and transduction

In adulthood, nociceptors have high thresholds for activation and respond to stimuli of sufficient intensity to cause damage. In addition, repeated stimuli can result in sensitization of the peripheral terminal, and release of neuropeptides from the terminal contributes to local vasodilation and erythema. DRG neurons respond to a range of peripheral mechanical, thermal, and chemical stimuli at birth (Fitzgerald, 1987b, 1987c). Age-related changes in receptor function and distribution, and in firing frequency, can alter sensitivity to different stimuli, but nociceptors are responsive to noxious stimuli and respond to tissue damage after birth (Fitzgerald and Walker, 2009).

Thermal and chemical stimuli

Transient receptor potential (TRP) ion channels comprise a large family of receptors that transduce varying stimuli into electrical potentials (Wang and Woolf, 2005). Receptors expressed in sensory neurons or skin which respond in specific temperature ranges include TRPV1 to TRPV4, TRPM8, and TRPA1 (Patapoutian et al., 2009). Messenger RNA (mRNA) levels of the different receptors in the DRG, and neuronal responses to temperature and specific chemical ligands, change during postnatal development (Hjerling-Leffler et al., 2007).

- *TRPV1* is activated by temperatures greater than 43°C, but also by a range of chemicals including capsaicin, and its function is modulated by low pH. Changes in TRPV1 receptor expression and function, many of which are mediated by NGF, contribute to inflammatory hyperalgesia. Post-translational changes, which alter channel kinetics, and increased insertion of the receptor into the membrane, also contribute to increased sensitivity (Linley et al., 2010; Patapoutian et al., 2009). TRPV1 mRNA is present in the DRG prior to and after birth, and the receptors are functional as these neurons respond to capsaicin (Hjerling-Leffler et al., 2007). The delivery of TRPV1 to both peripheral and central terminals is developmentally regulated. TRPV1-positive nerve terminals are present in cutaneous structures at P10, but at a reduced density compared with adult animals (Guo et al., 2001) and the degree of sensitization to capsaicin by NGF is lower (Zhu et al., 2004).

- *TRPA1* is activated by noxious cold (<18°C in some but not all studies), and by pungent compounds such as horseradish, mustard, and formalin (Patapoutian et al., 2009). Responses to mustard oil have been recorded from DRG neurons in early development (Fitzgerald, 1987b, 1987c), but there is limited direct activation of spinal reflex responses in the first postnatal week (Fitzgerald and Gibson, 1984; Walker et al., 2007) when levels of TRPA1 mRNA are low in DRG neurons (Hjerling-Leffler et al., 2007) and central C-fibre connections are immature.

- *TRPM8* is activated by innocuous cold and cooling compounds such as menthol (Wang and Woolf, 2005). TRPM8 mRNA is present in DRG neurons at levels similar to the adult at P0, and although levels are reduced at P7 and P14, responses to menthol are present (Hjerling-Leffler et al., 2007).

- *Purinergic receptors* comprise a P2X family of ionotropic channels and a P2Y family of G-protein coupled receptors. The $P2X_3$ receptor and $P2X_{2/3}$ heteromultimers have the highest level of expression in sensory neurons. $P2X_3$ receptors on the sensory terminals of IB4+ve subpopulation of nociceptive neurons respond to adenosine triphosphate (ATP) that has been released from endothelial and Merkel cells and from sympathetic neurons. $P2X_7$ receptors also play an important role in inflammatory hyperalgesia (Burnstock, 2006). In early development, a higher proportion of DRG neurons express $P2X_3$ receptors, and this gradually becomes limited to IB4+ve neurons. In addition, $P2X_3$ agonists evoke a greater degree of depolarization and more marked behavioural response. There is also a reciprocal relationship with $P2X_7$ receptor expression on satellite glial cells, which increases as $P2X_3$ receptor expression decreases throughout postnatal development (Chen et al., 2012).

Mechanical stimuli

Mechanoreceptors detect pressure stimuli at a range of intensities, and *in vivo* may be classified according to their threshold. A range of additional mechanical stimuli (e.g. light brush, texture, vibration, touch) can be detected via specialized nerve endings in skin and in association with specialized structures such as hair follicles, Meissner corpuscles, or Pacinian corpuscles (Delmas et al., 2011). Glabrous skin in the distal extremities (e.g. soles of feet/hindpaws) is more densely innervated than hairy skin, with a higher proportion of high threshold and faster conducting mechanosensitive fibres (Boada et al., 2010).

Low threshold mechanoreceptors (LTMs) respond to innocuous levels of pressure and are generally associated with Aβ nerve endings. High-threshold mechanoreceptors (HTMs) are activated by noxious or injurious mechanical forces, and are associated with Aδ and polymodal C fibres. Mechanosensitive neurons can also be differentiated by their firing frequency which encodes features of the mechanical stimulus (i.e. rapidly, intermediately, slowly, or ultra-slowly adapting), with nociceptive responses predominantly mediated by slowly and ultra-slowly adapting currents (Delmas et al., 2011). Transduction is thought to be the result of an ion channel that is opened directly by mechanical force, and candidate ion channels include acid-sensing ion channels (ASICs) and members of the TRP family (Woolf and Ma, 2007).

Sodium channels

Voltage-gated sodium channels not only play an important role in transmission of the action potential along the axon, but different subtypes can modulate sensitivity, and are expressed along axons as well as in the peripheral intra-epidermal nerve endings (Dib-Hajj et al., 2010; Persson et al., 2010). Voltage-gated sodium channels (Na_v) may be either sensitive or resistant to tetrodotoxin (designated as TTX-S and TTX-R respectively). The TTX-S subtypes Na_v 1.3 and 1.7 and TTX-R subtypes Na_v 1.8 and 1.9 are expressed by nociceptors. Post-translational modifications enhance the excitability of TTX-R channels and contribute to peripheral nociceptor sensitization, and alterations in expression of Na_v channels may occur in persistent pain states in adulthood (Lai et al., 2004; Liu and Wood, 2011).

Both TTX-S and TTX-R Na channels can be identified from birth in rat DRG (Ogata and Tatebayashi, 1992). Na_v 1.3 is expressed at higher levels during embryonic development. The TTX-R sodium channels Na_v1.8 and Na_v 1.9 are expressed on C-fibres at birth and reach adult levels by P7 (Benn et al., 2001).

Peripheral sensitization

The response to a given nociceptive stimulus can change with time, and sensitization of nociceptive pathways provides further warning and encourages protection of the injured part (Woolf and Ma, 2007). *Hyperalgesia* refers to an increased response to a noxious stimulus (increased response to suprathreshold stimuli) and *allodynia* refers to pain or nociceptor firing in response to a previously non-noxious stimulus (reduction in threshold and spontaneous activity). *Primary hyperalgesia* or peripheral sensitization is the result of altered nociceptor sensitivity, with an increased response to thermal and mechanical stimuli within the area of tissue damage. By contrast, *secondary hyperalgesia* refers to increased sensitivity in the area surrounding the injured tissue, and is centrally-mediated.

Although initially advantageous, ongoing sensitization of nociceptive responses can become maladaptive and contribute to persistent pain states (Hucho and Levine, 2007; Woolf and Ma, 2007). It has recently been suggested that nociceptive pathways may be described not just as being in a naïve or a sensitized state, but that prior injury may induce a 'primed' state, in which the system is more responsive to future injury, such that lower concentrations of mediators can elicit enhanced and prolonged hyperalgesia (Hucho and Levine, 2007).

In early life, peripheral sensory fibres are also responsive to changing levels of activity in two different manners:

◆ Repeated stimuli can produce acute peripheral sensitization or hyperalgesia as seen at older ages (see later).

◆ Activity is required for strengthening synaptic connections and pathway development. During normal physiological development, activation of nociceptors is rare, and low threshold A-fibre input contributes to shaping of nociceptive circuits (Waldenstrom et al., 2003). Altering this balance of activity during critical periods in early life impairs normal development. Excessive *reductions* in afferent activity can alter synaptic function, structural and somatotopic organization in the spinal cord, and increase neuronal apoptosis resulting in long-term decreases in sensory thresholds (Beggs et al., 2002; Fitzgerald, 2005; Granmo et al., 2008; Walker et al., 2010). Excessive *increases* in activity as a result of pain and injury at specific developmental stages can also alter future sensitivity in a manner that is not seen following the same injury at older ages (Walker et al., 2009; for further details see Walker, Chapter 3, this volume).

C-fibre stimuli

Sensitization of peripheral afferents following noxious or repeated stimuli can be demonstrated from early development, but the degree of activation by different stimuli can vary (Fitzgerald, 1987c, 1991b; Koltzenburg and Lewin, 1997). Mustard oil, which acts on TRPA1 receptors, produces only weak afferent responses in neonatal rat DRG recordings (Fitzgerald, 1987c), but does sensitize the nociceptor to subsequent stimuli within the area of injury, i.e. primary hyperalgesia (Fitzgerald, 1991b), although to a lesser degree than at older ages (P3 < P10 < P21; Walker et al., 2007). By contrast, secondary hyperalgesia, which is dependent on central mechanisms, is not induced by C-fibre stimuli (capsaicin or mustard oil) in the first postnatal week, but has reached adult levels by the third postnatal week (i.e. approximately late childhood; Jiang and Gebhart, 1998; Walker et al., 2007).

Inflammation

Peripheral inflammation results in pain, heat, and redness (due to vasodilation), and swelling (due to plasma extravasation). An 'inflammatory soup' that is 'tasted' by receptors on nerve terminals (Woolf and Ma, 2007) is made up of multiple mediators including: prostaglandins (Kawabata, 2011), leukotrienes (Noguchi and Okubo, 2011), substance P, nitric oxide, cytokines, chemokines, bradykinin, serotonin, histamine, tumour necrosis factor (TNFα) and neurotrophic factors (e.g. NGF). Following release from the nerve terminal, or from inflammatory cells or damaged tissue, these mediators activate and/or sensitize the nociceptor terminal by acting on specific sensory receptors that include (Woolf and Ma, 2007; Linley et al., 2010):

* G protein-coupled receptors (e.g. bradykinin B1 and B2; protease-activated receptors, PAR 1–3; histamine receptors).

* Receptor tyrosine kinases (e.g. growth factor receptors such as trkA).

* Ionotropic receptors/ion channels, such as TRP channels (Patapoutian et al., 2009), purinergic receptors (Burnstock, 2006), and acid-sensitive channels.

Inflammatory mediators initiate intracellular signalling cascades, involving activation of a range of protein kinases (Bhave and Gereau, 2004; Hucho and Levine, 2007) and mediate increased sensitivity by:

* Rapid response post-translational changes which directly modulate ion channel activity, change membrane potential, or increase insertion of receptors into the membrane (Bhave and Gereau, 2004).

* Alterations in transcriptional programmes and changes in gene expression resulting in longer-term altered sensitivity (Linley et al., 2010), such as changes in the expression and transport of pro-nociceptive molecules (e.g. substance P, NGF) and ion channels.

Inflammatory hyperalgesia occurs from early development. Responses to thermal stimuli are enhanced following application of inflammatory mediators in skin-nerve preparations from embryonic chick (Koltzenburg and Lewin, 1997). Inflammatory stimuli, such as carrageenan and complete Freund's adjuvant (CFA), produce hyperalgesia in neonatal rat pups, and the degree and duration of response varies with the dose and type of agent (Ren et al., 2004; Walker et al., 2003). Hindpaw inflammation also accelerates the postnatal upregulation of IB4+ve neurons in the DRG (Beland and Fitzgerald, 2001). Although the pattern of response changes with age, hindpaw formalin injection also produces a significant behavioural response in rat pups (Guy and Abbott, 1992).

The acute and potential long-term effects of neonatal injury in different laboratory models are further discussed by Walker (Chapter 3, this volume).

Nociceptive processing in the spinal cord

The processing of noxious information by the CNS begins in the superficial dorsal horn (SDH) of the spinal cord (laminae I–II), which receives direct projections from nociceptive primary afferent neurons (Aδ and C fibres) with cell bodies in the DRG. The vast majority (>95%) of neurons within the SDH correspond to propriospinal and local circuit interneurons (Bice and Beal, 1997a, 1997b). As a result, the SDH network has the ability to integrate sensory inputs, which vary in modality, intensity, and location, and transform them into an output signal, which ascends to the brain. This output of the SDH circuit is conveyed by a small percentage of lamina I neurons (c.5%) which project to multiple supraspinal sites (Spike et al., 2003) and are known to be instrumental for the generation of chronic pain following tissue or nerve injury (Mantyh

et al., 1997; Suzuki et al., 2002). Importantly, the functional properties of the SDH network are highly age-dependent. As a result, understanding how the immature SDH is organized at a cellular and molecular level may yield new insight into novel approaches to regulate the ascending flow of noxious information to the brain, and resultant pain perception, in infants and children.

Electrophysiological properties of neonatal dorsal horn neurons

Extracellular single-unit recordings in intact, anesthetized rodents clearly demonstrated that immature dorsal horn neurons are characterized by low thresholds, large peripheral receptive fields, and prolonged action potential after-discharges compared to adult dorsal horn cells (Fitzgerald, 1985; Torsney and Fitzgerald, 2002). Repetitive low-threshold stimulation also leads to a progressive sensitization of neonatal dorsal horn neurons, which disappears by P21 (Jennings and Fitzgerald, 1998). Notably, these same functional properties also characterize nociceptive withdrawal reflexes in the newborn rodent (Schouenborg, 2003), kitten (Ekholm, 1967), and human (Andrews and Fitzgerald, 1994; Andrews et al., 2002). The developmental alterations in the response of dorsal horn neurons following stimulation of their peripheral receptive fields may be explained by three factors:

* Developmental changes in sensory transduction and/or the functional properties of primary afferent neurons.

* Age-dependent changes in the intrinsic membrane properties of dorsal horn cells which influence the level of neuronal excitability.

* The maturation of excitatory and inhibitory synaptic inputs onto dorsal horn neurons. This section of the chapter will focus on the last two factors.

Intrinsic excitability of developing SDH neurons

An important feature of developing CNS networks is spontaneous activity (SA), which can be generated by a variety of mechanisms (Blankenship and Feller, 2010) and contributes to both early circuit formation (Tritsch et al., 2007) and the subsequent establishment of appropriate sensory maps (Kandler et al., 2009). SA in the newborn SDH is predominantly localized to lamina I, and is then downregulated with age (J. Li and Baccei, 2011a). During early life, a subset of glutamatergic interneurons within lamina I function as 'pacemaker' neurons that are capable of generating oscillatory burst-firing. This is independent of synaptic transmission within the network and instead relies on a combination of intrinsic voltage-gated conductances (including persistent Na^+ currents and high-threshold N-type and L-type Ca^{2+} channels). As these pacemaker neurons are innervated by nociceptive afferents and project throughout the dorsal–ventral axis of the immature spinal cord, they may provide an endogenous source of activity to the developing sensorimotor circuits mediating spinal nociceptive reflexes (J. Li and Baccei, 2011a). Alternatively, they may serve to synchronize the firing of ascending spinal projection neurons in the neonate. In this context, burst-firing also characterizes somatosensory processing in the developing human brain (Fabrizi et al., 2011).

The morphological and intrinsic membrane properties of SDH neurons appear to be developmentally regulated in a cell-type dependent manner.

- Supraspinal projection neurons undergo their axonal and dendritic development prior to birth (Bicknell and Beal, 1984), but ascending spinothalamic tract neurons increase in diameter during the first postnatal week (Davidson et al., 2010).

- Presumptive interneurons within the SDH exhibit extensive growth and reorganization of their dendritic trees during early life (Bicknell and Beal, 1984).

- The general population of laminae I and II neurons (mostly corresponding to interneurons) demonstrates an age-dependent hyperpolarization of the resting potential, decrease in membrane resistance and elevation in rheobase (amount of current needed to evoke an action potential), contributing to a decrease in excitability with maturation (J. Li and Baccei, 2011a; Walsh et al., 2009).

- Lamina I neurons projecting to the parabrachial nucleus and periaqueductal grey (PAG) differ from surrounding interneurons as their passive membrane properties and levels of spontaneous activity are stable during the first 3 weeks of life (J. Li and Baccei, 2012).

While the intrinsic firing properties of a neuron clearly depend on the expression of both voltage-gated and voltage-independent (i.e. 'leak') ionic conductances, surprisingly little is known about how age influences the expression of the underlying ion channels within developing spinal nociceptive circuits. Voltage-gated Na^+ currents are upregulated postnatally in the axonal (but not somatic) membrane of laminae I and II neurons (Safronov et al., 1999). This may occur in the absence of a significant shift in the Na^+ channel isoforms expressed within the region, as $Na_v1.2$ and $Na_v1.3$ are the dominant isoforms in rat laminae I and II neurons at both P6 to P9 and P25 to P30 (Hildebrand et al., 2011). In addition, these neurons demonstrate an age-dependent increase in the levels of fast, A-type voltage-gated K^+ currents, which may contribute to the observed rise in the prevalence of SDH neurons which exhibit delayed firing in response to intracellular current injection (Walsh et al., 2009). Meanwhile, although 'leak' currents (which can result from any ion channel open at the resting membrane potential) strongly modulate neuronal excitability in many areas of the CNS and can be regulated by a host of factors such as neurotransmitters, pH or anaesthetics (Goldstein et al., 2001), there are no data currently available regarding the molecular basis for these currents in developing SDH neurons.

Understanding how the expression of voltage-dependent and 'leak' channels in the SDH varies as a function of both age and specific cell type (i.e. GABAergic versus glutamatergic, interneuron versus projection neuron, etc.) could allow novel pharmacological strategies to target the output of spinal pain pathways in an age-specific manner.

Maturation of primary afferent input to the developing SDH

Large myelinated A-fibre primary afferents penetrate the rat dorsal horn in a somatotopically appropriate manner at embryonic day (E) 15 (Mirnics and Koerber, 1995), and make functional synaptic contacts in the SDH during early life (Coggeshall et al., 1996; Fitzgerald et al., 1994). Over the first 3 postnatal weeks, the majority of A fibres gradually retract to occupy deeper laminae in the dorsal horn, via activity-dependent mechanisms (Beggs et al., 2002). Some controversy exists regarding the extent to which these exuberant A-fibre terminals reflect low-threshold Aβ-fibre inputs; at least some correspond to myelinated high-threshold mechanoreceptors (Woodbury and Koerber, 2003), and a proportion continue to project into lamina I-II throughout life (Boada and Woodbury, 2008). Regardless of whether Aβ fibres make direct synaptic contacts onto laminae I and II neurons or communicate with these cells via polysynaptic pathways, significant evidence points to enhanced Aβ input to the SDH during the early postnatal period:

- Aβ fibre stimulation evokes the expression of c-fos (a marker of neuronal activation) in laminae I and II at P3 but not at P21 (Jennings and Fitzgerald, 1996).

- Patch clamp studies, which allow assessment of synaptic currents at a cellular level, have demonstrated an increased prevalence of polysynaptic Aβ-input to neonatal GABAergic neurons within the SDH (Daniele and MacDermott, 2009).

- Repetitive stimulation of Aβ fibres prior to P21 sensitizes neonatal dorsal horn neurons (Jennings and Fitzgerald, 1998).

As a result, less intense or low-threshold stimuli can elicit activation of neurons in the spinal cord in early life.

Small-diameter sensory afferents (Aδ and C fibres) grow into the rat dorsal horn at E19 (Fitzgerald, 1987a) and likely have established a mature pattern of projections to the substantia gelatinosa (SG) by birth (Fitzgerald and Swett, 1983). However, the maturation of C-fibre synaptic connections within the developing dorsal horn is delayed:

- Electrical activation of high-threshold afferents fails to produce significant spike discharge in many newborn dorsal horn neurons (Fitzgerald, 1985, 1988).

- Chemical stimulation of C-fibres fails to evoke nociceptive withdrawal reflexes or neurogenic oedema until the second postnatal week (Fitzgerald and Gibson, 1984).

- Ultrastructural studies demonstrate increasing numbers of central terminals corresponding to fine-diameter primary afferents from P5 to P20 (Pignatelli et al., 1989).

- Capsaicin elevates glutamatergic signalling within the SDH to a greater extent at P10 compared to P0 (Baccei et al., 2003).

Excitatory synapses in the developing SDH

All sensory neurons release glutamate from their central terminals in the spinal cord. Activation of ionotropic (AMPA, NMDA and kainate ion channel receptors) and/or metabotropic (mGluR, which signal via coupling with G-proteins), glutamate receptors results in membrane depolarization and increased excitability in dorsal horn neurons (H. J. Hu et al., 2007; P. Li et al., 1999; Yoshimura and Jessell, 1990). The functional properties of glutamate receptors depend on their subunit composition, and the relative expression of mGluR (Berthele et al., 1999; Valerio et al., 1997) and AMPAR subunits (Jakowec et al., 1995) within the dorsal horn vary according to postnatal age.

- GluR2 reduces the Ca^{2+}-permeability of AMPARs (Hollmann et al., 1991; Washburn et al., 1997). As neonatal rat SG neurons express a lower ratio of GluR2 to GluR1, 3, and 4 (Jakowec et al., 1995), AMPAR-dependent Ca^{2+} influx may be increased in neonatal spinal neurons, increasing excitability (Hartmann et al., 2004).

- NMDARs expressed by neonatal SDH neurons have a higher Mg^{2+} sensitivity and greater affinity for NMDA (Hori and Kanda, 1994; Green and Gibb, 2001). This suggests a distinct NMDAR composition during early life, but direct evidence is presently lacking.

- Synapses expressing only NMDARs (referred to as 'silent' synapses due to the block of the NMDAR by extracellular Mg^{2+} at resting membrane potentials) are present in laminae I and II at early postnatal ages (Baba et al., 2000; Bardoni et al., 1998; P. Li and Zhuo, 1998). 'Silent' synapses have been observed at high-threshold Aδ fibre synapses onto NK1R-expressing lamina I neurons as late as P19 to P24 (Torsney, 2011). However, since 93% to 94% of glutamatergic synapses within laminae I and II of the neonatal rat express AMPAR subunits (Yasaka et al., 2009), the overall importance of 'silent' synapses for nociceptive processing within the developing SDH remains unclear.

Synaptic inhibition within the developing SDH

GABA and glycine

GABA and glycine serve as the major inhibitory neurotransmitters in the spinal dorsal horn via activation of two ligand-gated Cl^- channels (the $GABA_AR$ and glycine receptor), and are predominantly released from local interneurons, although descending inhibitory pathways from the brainstem may also include GABAergic and glycinergic projections (Kato et al., 2006). The number of GABAergic neurons within the rodent SDH peaks during the first two postnatal weeks (Dougherty et al., 2009; Ma et al., 1992; Schaffner et al., 1993) before declining to approximately 30% of the overall population during adulthood (Todd and Sullivan, 1990). Glycinergic neurons represent a subset of GABAergic neurons throughout embryonic and postnatal development (Berki et al., 1995; Huang et al., 2008; Todd and Sullivan, 1990). GABA and glycine are transported into the same synaptic vesicles by the vesicular inhibitory amino acid transporter (VIAAT) and co-released in the spinal cord, resulting in mixed $GABA_AR$-GlyR miniature inhibitory post-synaptic currents (IPSCs; Jonas et al., 1998).

GABAergic signalling dominates within lamina II of the neonatal spinal cord (Baccei and Fitzgerald, 2004). Glycinergic mIPSCs are absent in these cells during the first postnatal week, but these neurons respond robustly to exogenous glycine, suggesting that functional glycine receptors (GlyRs) are present but are not yet clustered at appropriate synaptic locations. This may reflect a reduced expression of gephyrin, a membrane protein known to interact with both GlyRs and the cytoskeleton in order to 'trap' the GlyR at synaptic sites in the membrane (Charrier et al., 2010; Kirsch et al., 1993).

From P8, mixed $GABA_AR$-GlyR mIPSCs are apparent in lamina I-II but are subsequently modulated in a regionally-specific manner. Within lamina I, the mixed responses are replaced by pure GlyR-mediated mIPSCs by P23, while in mature lamina II neurons either $GABA_AR$-only or GlyR-only mIPSCs are observed. This shift results from an age-dependent reorganization of receptors in the postsynaptic membrane (Keller et al., 2001).

Inhibition versus excitation

In mature neurons, the activity of the potassium-chloride (K^+-Cl^-) co-transporter KCC2 maintains low levels of intracellular Cl^-. Following activation of the $GABA_AR$ or GlyR and opening of the associated chloride channel, Cl^- flows into the cell, the membrane is hyperpolarized, and the neuron inhibited (Rivera et al., 1999). However, in many parts of the CNS, a low level of KCC2 during the neonatal period results in high levels of intracellular Cl^- and a reversal potential for Cl^- ions (E_{Cl}) that is more positive than both the resting potential and action potential (AP) threshold (Ben-Ari, 2002). As a result, following $GABA_AR$ (or GlyR) activation, Cl^- moves out of the cell (down its concentration gradient), spike discharges can be evoked, and excitation (rather than inhibition) results in the developing network (Ben-Ari et al., 1989). Neonatal SDH neurons can depolarize in response to $GABA_AR$ activation (Baccei and Fitzgerald, 2004), and do not attain a mature Cl^- extrusion capacity until the third postnatal week (Cordero-Erausquin et al., 2005). This raises a critical question of whether GABAergic signalling within newborn spinal pain circuits is excitatory or inhibitory in nature.

Intrathecal administration of $GABA_AR$ antagonists (gabazine and bicuculline) at P3 significantly increased mechanical and thermal withdrawal thresholds, while the same antagonists at P21 decreased thresholds (Hathway et al., 2006). The $GABA_AR$ agonist midazolam sensitized nociceptive withdrawal reflexes in the neonate, but increased threshold at older ages (Koch et al., 2008). At first glance, these results appear to support the notion that GABA acts as an excitatory neurotransmitter within the newborn SDH. However, other evidence suggests that GABA has inhibitory actions in the SDH from birth. *In vitro* patch clamp studies demonstrated that E_{Cl} was consistently more negative than spike threshold even in neonatal SDH cells that depolarized in response to GABA, suggesting that $GABA_AR$ activation would ultimately limit action potential discharge and inhibit these neurons (Baccei and Fitzgerald, 2004). *In vivo* recordings from neonatal SDH neurons show that spinal application of gabazine enlarges receptive fields and enhances afferent-evoked discharge from the first days of life (Bremner et al., 2006) although spinal inhibitory circuits may be poorly tuned in the neonate (Bremner and Fitzgerald, 2008). Collectively, these results suggest that GABAergic synaptic inhibition in the SDH is functional from birth.

This apparent discrepancy can be explained if the excitatory actions of GABA on reflex sensitivity are not the direct result of its actions in the dorsal horn, but also involve modulation by supraspinal activity. Following transection of the neonatal spinal cord, intrathecal $GABA_AR$ antagonists facilitate nociceptive withdrawal reflexes in a similar manner as at P21, and gabazine also enhances primary afferent-evoked ventral root potentials in the isolated neonatal spinal cord (Hathway et al., 2006). This supports a role for supraspinal structures in modulation of neonatal cutaneous reflex sensitivity. While reflex behaviour undoubtedly provides insight into how the nervous system processes noxious information, measuring only the motor output of the spinal cord network may not specifically indicate the level of excitability within the ascending sensory pathways that project to the cortex.

Signal processing in the developing SDH under pathological conditions

Understanding pain mechanisms in early life requires additional knowledge of how tissue and nerve damage modulate both the intrinsic membrane properties of immature dorsal horn neurons as well as their synaptic inputs.

Peripheral inflammation significantly increases spontaneous firing and receptive field size in neonatal dorsal horn neurons within hours after the injury (Ririe et al., 2008; Torsney and Fitzgerald, 2002), which at least in part results from an injury-evoked enhancement in the intrinsic excitability of immature dorsal horn cells (Rivera-Arconada and Lopez-Garcia, 2010). However, inflammation may evoke biphasic changes in the membrane properties of developing SDH neurons, as this short-term enhancement in intrinsic excitability is followed (at *c*.20 hours post-injury) by an upregulation of sustained voltage-gated K^+ currents and *reduction* in excitability (Rivera-Arconada and Lopez-Garcia, 2010). Meanwhile, neonatal sciatic nerve injury failed to alter neuronal excitability in the SDH, although it did unmask increased sensitivity to the pro-inflammatory cytokine TNFα (J. Li et al., 2009b).

The effects of peripheral tissue and nerve damage on synaptic function within spinal nociceptive networks are highly age-dependent. Tissue damage during early postnatal development evokes an activity-dependent elevation in glutamate release within the SDH (J. Li and Baccei, 2009; J. Li et al., 2009a). Synaptic inhibition was not significantly affected (J. Li and Baccei, 2009), which is in contrast to the adult dorsal horn where a reduction in the efficacy of glycinergic inhibition is thought to make a key contribution to inflammatory hyperalgesia (Harvey et al., 2004; Hosl et al., 2006; Muller et al., 2003). Similarly, while peripheral nerve injury compromises GABAergic inhibition in the adult (Moore et al., 2002; Scholz et al., 2005), it had no significant effects on synaptic transmission within lamina II in the neonate (J. Li et al., 2009b). However, it remains possible that injury-evoked changes in the expression of KCC2 (and thus Cl^- homeostasis) occur within the neonatal SDH, as reported previously in the adult (Coull et al., 2003; Zhang et al., 2008), which could reduce the functional strength of synaptic inhibition within immature spinal nociceptive circuits.

Injury-induced facilitation of excitatory signalling is also associated with an increased efficacy of nociceptive synapses within the immature SDH. Surgical incision selectively enhanced glutamatergic responses mediated by high-threshold (i.e. Aδ- and C-fibre) primary afferent neurons in a manner consistent with an elevated number of nociceptive synapses in the region (J. Li and Baccei, 2011b). Sensory neurons expressing TRPV1 contribute to this nociceptive synaptic plasticity, as selective destruction of these fibres by prior systemic capsaicin prevented the injury-evoked increase in spontaneous glutamate release (J. Li and Baccei, 2011b). In addition, peripheral inflammation in the neonate, but not adult, leads to a proliferation of nociceptive primary afferent projections to the SDH (Ruda et al., 2000; Walker et al., 2003). While the mechanisms underlying this strengthening of nociceptive synaptic input are not fully understood, NGF signalling at the trkA receptor is likely to play a role (J. Li and Baccei, 2011b).

Persistent effects of early tissue injury on SDH network function

Tissue damage during a critical period of early life can evoke long-term changes in pain sensitivity in rodents, with many studies reporting a baseline hypoalgesia accompanied by an exaggerated hyperalgesia following re-injury during adulthood (see Walker, Chapter 3, this volume). These prolonged changes in nociceptive processing could, in part, reflect long-term alterations in the function of spinal pain circuits, as brief inflammation of the neonatal hindpaw is known to result in significant changes in gene expression within the adult dorsal horn (Ren et al., 2005). However, the extent to which early tissue damage modulates intrinsic membrane properties and synaptic function within the mature SDH network remains unclear.

The majority of behavioural studies have identified the first postnatal week as the 'critical period' during which tissue damage is capable of altering pain sensitivity throughout life (LaPrairie and Murphy, 2007; Ren et al., 2004; Walker et al., 2009). This correlates well with the ages at which tissue damage elevates glutamatergic signalling within the SDH (J. Li and Baccei, 2009; J. Li et al., 2009a). Nonetheless, the mechanistic basis for the critical period within the developing SDH currently remains unknown. One possibility is that the gradual maturation of inhibitory synaptic transmission within the SDH (Baccei and Fitzgerald, 2004; Cordero-Erausquin et al., 2005; Ingram et al., 2008; Keller et al., 2001) is involved in terminating the critical period (Hensch, 2004). Closure of the critical period also coincides with the onset of myelination in the spinal cord (Kapfhammer and Schwab, 1994). CNS myelin contains proteins that potently inhibit axonal growth (F. Hu and Strittmatter, 2004), and enhanced collateral sprouting of nociceptive fibres has been observed in the mature dorsal horn in the presence of reduced myelination (Schwegler et al., 1995); and experience-dependent plasticity in the visual cortex persists throughout life in mice lacking normal myelin-derived signalling at the Nogo receptor (McGee et al., 2005). Future identification of factors responsible for closing the critical period for plasticity within developing spinal pain circuits may identify potential strategies to limit the long-term effects of neonatal tissue damage.

Conclusions and clinical implications

Nociceptive signalling in the periphery and spinal cord in early life has the following features:

- Peripheral nociceptors are functional and respond to a range of chemical, thermal and mechanical stimuli.
- Prolonged noxious stimuli or inflammation produce peripheral sensitization.
- The structure and function of spinal cord nociceptive pathways continues to mature across the first 2 to 3 postnatal weeks in the rodent, a period which may extend throughout infancy and early childhood in humans.
- Spinal cord signalling is initially characterized by an excess of excitatory effects and delayed development of inhibitory mechanisms.
- Spinal reflex responses have low thresholds and are poorly localized in early life.

Clinical studies evaluating peripheral nociceptive function in neonates and infants show parallels with the patterns of reflex response and changes in sensitivity described. Spinal reflex thresholds are lower in neonates and infants, but a clear relationship between the degree of response and intensity of the stimulus is maintained (Andrews and Fitzgerald, 1999). Sensitization of reflex responses has clearly been demonstrated following repeated mechanical stimuli (Andrews and Fitzgerald, 1994), repeated heel lance for blood tests (Fitzgerald et al., 1988), and surgery (Andrews and Fitzgerald, 2002) in neonates and infants.

An early study evaluating the response of neonates to skin scratch allergy tests demonstrated histamine-induced erythema even in preterm neonates (Matheson et al., 1952), and along with clinical observations following surgery, suggests that localized inflammatory responses are functional in early life.

Clinical investigations of genetic disorders also demonstrate the importance of nociceptive mechanisms throughout early life. Mutations affecting genes encoding the trkA receptor for NGF can result in congenital insensitivity to pain and anhidrosis (Indo, 2002). Loss-of-function mutations affecting Na_v 1.7 channels on nociceptive afferents result in congenital insensitivity to pain, while gain of function mutations produce episodic severe pain syndromes (paroxysmal extreme pain disorder or erythromelalgia) that may present in infancy or childhood (Fischer and Waxman, 2010; see also Walker, Chapter 21, this volume).

Integration of data from laboratory studies is essential to improve our understanding of the changing impact of pain and injury throughout development, interpret clinical observations, and ultimately improve the management of pain for neonates, infants, and children of all ages.

References

Andrews, K. and Fitzgerald, M. (1994). The cutaneous withdrawal reflex in human neonates: sensitization, receptive fields, and the effects of contralateral stimulation. *Pain*, 56, 95–101.

Andrews, K. and Fitzgerald, M. (1999). Cutaneous flexion reflex in human neonates: a quantitative study of threshold and stimulus-response characteristics after single and repeated stimuli. *Dev Med Child Neurol*, 41, 696–703.

Andrews, K. and Fitzgerald, M. (2002). Wound sensitivity as a measure of analgesic effects following surgery in human neonates and infants. *Pain*, 99, 185–195.

Andrews, K. A., Desai, D., Dhillon, H. K., Wilcox, D. T., and Fitzgerald, M. (2002). Abdominal sensitivity in the first year of life: comparison of infants with and without prenatally diagnosed unilateral hydronephrosis. *Pain*, 100, 35–46.

Baba, H., Doubell, T. P., Moore, K. A., and Woolf, C. J. (2000). Silent NMDA receptor-mediated synapses are developmentally regulated in the dorsal horn of the rat spinal cord. *J Neurophysiol*, 83, 955–962.

Baccei, M. L., Bardoni, R., and Fitzgerald, M. (2003). Development of nociceptive synaptic inputs to the neonatal rat dorsal horn: glutamate release by capsaicin and menthol. *J Physiol*, 549, 231–242.

Baccei, M. L. and Fitzgerald, M. (2004). Development of GABAergic and glycinergic transmission in the neonatal rat dorsal horn. *J Neurosci*, 24, 4749–4757.

Bardoni, R., Magherini, P. C., and MacDermott, A. B. (1998). NMDA EPSCs at glutamatergic synapses in the spinal cord dorsal horn of the postnatal rat. *J Neurosci*, 18, 6558–6567.

Beggs, S., Torsney, C., Drew, L. J., and Fitzgerald, M. (2002). The postnatal reorganization of primary afferent input and dorsal horn cell receptive fields in the rat spinal cord is an activity-dependent process. *Eur J Neurosci*, 16, 1249–1258.

Beland, B. and Fitzgerald, M. (2001). Influence of peripheral inflammation on the postnatal maturation of primary sensory neuron phenotype in rats. *J Pain*, 2, 36–45.

Ben-Ari, Y. (2002). Excitatory actions of gaba during development: the nature of the nurture. *Nat Rev Neurosci*, 3, 728–739.

Ben-Ari, Y., Cherubini, E., Corradetti, R., and Gaiarsa, J. L. (1989) Giant synaptic potentials in immature rat CA3 hippocampal neurones. *J Physiol*, 416, 303–325.

Benn, S. C., Costigan, M., Tate, S., Fitzgerald, M., and Woolf, C. J. (2001). Developmental expression of the TTX-resistant voltage-gated sodium channels Nav1.8 (SNS) and Nav1.9 (SNS2) in primary sensory neurons. *J Neurosci*, 21, 6077–6085.

Berki, A. C., O'Donovan, M. J., and Antal, M. (1995). Developmental expression of glycine immunoreactivity and its colocalization with GABA in the embryonic chick lumbosacral spinal cord. *J Comp Neurol*, 362, 583–596.

Berthele, A., Boxall, S. J., Urban, A., Anneser, J. M., Zieglgansberger, W., Urban, L., *et al.* (1999). Distribution and developmental changes in metabotropic glutamate receptor messenger RNA expression in the rat lumbar spinal cord. *Brain Res Dev Brain Res*, 112, 39–53.

Bhave, G. and Gereau, R. W. (2004). Posttranslational mechanisms of peripheral sensitization. *J Neurobiol*, 61, 88–106.

Bice, T. N. and Beal, J. A. (1997a). Quantitative and neurogenic analysis of the total population and subpopulations of neurons defined by axon projection in the superficial dorsal horn of the rat lumbar spinal cord. *J Comp Neurol*, 388, 550–564.

Bice, T. N. and Beal, J. A. (1997b). Quantitative and neurogenic analysis of neurons with supraspinal projections in the superficial dorsal horn of the rat lumbar spinal cord. *J Comp Neurol*, 388, 565–574.

Bicknell, H. R., Jr. and Beal, J. A. (1984). Axonal and dendritic development of substantia gelatinosa neurons in the lumbosacral spinal cord of the rat. *J Comp Neurol*, 226, 508–522.

Blankenship, A. G. and Feller, M. B. (2010). Mechanisms underlying spontaneous patterned activity in developing neural circuits. *Nat Rev Neurosci*, 11, 18–29.

Boada, M. D., Houle, T. T., Eisenach, J. C., and Ririe, D. G. (2010). Differing neurophysiologic mechanosensory input from glabrous and hairy skin in juvenile rats. *J Neurophysiol*, 104, 3568–3575.

Boada, M. D. and Woodbury, C. J. (2008). Myelinated skin sensory neurons project extensively throughout adult mouse substantia gelatinosa. *J Neurosci*, 28, 2006–2014.

Bremner, L., Fitzgerald, M., and Baccei, M. (2006). Functional GABA(A)-receptor-mediated inhibition in the neonatal dorsal horn. *J Neurophysiol*, 95, 3893–3897.

Bremner, L. R. and Fitzgerald, M. (2008). Postnatal tuning of cutaneous inhibitory receptive fields in the rat. *J Physiol*, 586, 1529–1537.

Burnstock, G. (2006). Purinergic P2 receptors as targets for novel analgesics. *Pharmacol Ther*, 110, 433–454.

Charrier, C., Machado, P., Tweedie-Cullen, R. Y., Rutishauser, D., Mansuy, I. M., and Triller, A. (2010). A crosstalk between beta1 and beta3 integrins controls glycine receptor and gephyrin trafficking at synapses. *Nat Neurosci*, 13, 1388–1395.

Chen, Y., Li, G., and Huang, L. Y. (2012). P2X7 receptors in satellite glial cells mediate high functional expression of P2X3 receptors in immature dorsal root ganglion neurons. *Mol Pain*, 8, 9.

Coggeshall, R. E., Jennings, E. A., and Fitzgerald, M. (1996). Evidence that large myelinated primary afferent fibers make synaptic contacts in lamina II of neonatal rats. *Brain Res Dev Brain Res*, 92, 81–90.

Constantinou, J., Reynolds, M. L., Woolf, C. J., Safieh-Garabedian, B., and Fitzgerald, M. (1994). Nerve growth factor levels in developing rat skin: upregulation following skin wounding. *Neuroreport*, 5, 2281–2284.

Cordero-Erausquin, M., Coull, J. A., Boudreau, D., Rolland, M., and De Koninck, Y. (2005) Differential maturation of GABA action and anion reversal potential in spinal lamina I neurons: impact of chloride extrusion capacity. *J Neurosci*, 25, 9613–9623.

Coull, J. A., Boudreau, D., Bachand, K., Prescott, S. A., Nault, F., Sik, A., et al. (2003). Trans-synaptic shift in anion gradient in spinal lamina I neurons as a mechanism of neuropathic pain. *Nature*, 424, 938–942.

Daniele, C. A. and MacDermott, A. B. (2009). Low-threshold primary afferent drive onto GABAergic interneurons in the superficial dorsal horn of the mouse. *J Neurosci*, 29, 686–695.

Davidson, S., Truong, H., and Giesler, G. J. Jr. (2010). Quantitative analysis of spinothalamic tract neurons in adult and developing mouse. *J Comp Neurol*, 518, 3193–3204.

Delmas, P., Hao, J., and Rodat-Despoix, L. (2011). Molecular mechanisms of mechanotransduction in mammalian sensory neurons. *Nat Rev Neurosci*, 12, 139–153.

Dib-Hajj, S. D., Cummins, T. R., Black, J. A., and Waxman, S. G. (2010). Sodium channels in normal and pathological pain. *Annu Rev Neurosci*, 33, 325–347.

Dougherty, K. J., Sawchuk, M. A., and Hochman, S. (2009). Phenotypic diversity and expression of GABAergic inhibitory interneurons during postnatal development in lumbar spinal cord of glutamic acid decarboxylase 67-green fluorescent protein mice. *Neuroscience*, 163, 909–919.

Ekholm, J. (1967). Postnatal changes in cutaneous reflexes and in the discharge pattern of cutaneous and articular sense organs. A morphological and physiological study in the cat. *Acta Physiol Scand Suppl*, 297, 1–130.

Fabrizi, L., Slater, R., Worley, A., Meek, J., Boyd, S., Olhede, S., et al. (2011). A shift in sensory processing that enables the developing human brain to discriminate touch from pain. *Curr Biol*, 21, 1552–1558.

Fischer, T. Z. and Waxman, S. G. (2010). Familial pain syndromes from mutations of the NaV1.7 sodium channel. *Ann N Y Acad Sci*, 1184, 196–207.

Fitzgerald, M. (1985). The post-natal development of cutaneous afferent fibre input and receptive field organization in the rat dorsal horn. *J Physiol*, 364, 1–18.

Fitzgerald, M. (1987a). Prenatal growth of fine-diameter primary afferents into the rat spinal cord: a transganglionic tracer study. *J Comp Neurol*, 261, 98–104.

Fitzgerald, M. (1987b). Spontaneous and evoked activity of fetal primary afferents in vivo. *Nature*, 326, 603–605.

Fitzgerald, M. (1987c). Cutaneous primary afferent properties in the hind limb of the neonatal rat. *J Physiol*, 383, 79–92.

Fitzgerald, M. (1988). The development of activity evoked by fine diameter cutaneous fibres in the spinal cord of the newborn rat. *Neurosci Lett*, 86, 161–166.

Fitzgerald, M. (1991a). The developmental neurobiology of pain. In M. Bond, J. E. Charlton, and C. J. Woolf (eds) *Proceedings of the VIth World Congress on Pain. Pain research and clinical management*, volume 4, pp 253–261. Amsterdam: Elsevier.

Fitzgerald, M. (1991b). A physiological study of the prenatal development of cutaneous sensory inputs to dorsal horn cells in the rat. *J Physiol*, 432, 473–482.

Fitzgerald, M. (2005). The development of nociceptive circuits. *Nat Rev Neurosci*, 6, 507–520.

Fitzgerald, M., Butcher, T., and Shortland, P. (1994). Developmental changes in the laminar termination of A fibre cutaneous sensory afferents in the rat spinal cord dorsal horn. *J Comp Neurol*, 348, 225–233.

Fitzgerald, M. and Gibson, S. (1984). The postnatal physiological and neurochemical development of peripheral sensory C fibres. *Neuroscience*, 13, 933–944.

Fitzgerald, M., Millard, C., and MacIntosh, N. (1988). Hyperalgesia in premature infants. *Lancet*, 1, 292.

Fitzgerald, M. and Swett, J. (1983). The termination pattern of sciatic nerve afferents in the substantia gelatinosa of neonatal rats. *Neurosci Lett*, 43, 149–154.

Fitzgerald, M. and Walker, S. M. (2009). Infant pain management: a developmental neurobiological approach. *Nat Clin Pract Neurol*, 5, 35–50.

Goldstein, S. A., Bockenhauer, D., O'Kelly, I., and Zilberberg, N. (2001). Potassium leak channels and the KCNK family of two-P-domain subunits. *Nat Rev Neurosci*, 2, 175–184.

Granmo, M., Petersson, P., and Schouenborg, J. (2008). Action-based body maps in the spinal cord emerge from a transitory floating organization. *J Neurosci*, 28, 5494–5503.

Green, G. M. and Gibb, A. J. (2001). Characterization of the single-channel properties of NMDA receptors in laminae I and II of the dorsal horn of neonatal rat spinal cord. *Eur J Neurosci*, 14, 1590–1602.

Guo, A., Simone, D. A., Stone, L. S., Fairbanks, C. A., Wang, J., and Elde, R. (2001). Developmental shift of vanilloid receptor 1 (VR1) terminals into deeper regions of the superficial dorsal horn: correlation with a shift from TrkA to Ret expression by dorsal root ganglion neurons. *Eur J Neurosci*, 14, 293–304.

Guy, E. R. and Abbott, F. V. (1992). The behavioral response to formalin in preweanling rats. *Pain*, 51, 81–90.

Hartmann, B., Ahmadi, S., Heppenstall, P. A., Lewin, G. R., Schott, C., Borchardt, T., et al. (2004) The AMPA receptor subunits GluR-A and GluR-B reciprocally modulate spinal synaptic plasticity and inflammatory pain. *Neuron*, 44, 637–650.

Harvey, R. J., Depner, U. B., Wassle, H., Ahmadi, S., Heindl, C., Reinold, H., et al. (2004). GlyR alpha3: an essential target for spinal PGE2-mediated inflammatory pain sensitization. *Science*, 304, 884–887.

Hathway, G., Harrop, E., Baccei, M., Walker, S., Moss, A., and Fitzgerald, M. (2006). A postnatal switch in GABAergic control of spinal cutaneous reflexes. *Eur J Neurosci*, 23, 112–118.

Hensch, T. K. (2004). Critical period regulation. *Annu Rev Neurosci*, 27, 549–579.

Hildebrand, M. E., Mezeyova, J., Smith, P. L., Salter, M. W., Tringham, E., and Snutch, T. P. (2011). Identification of sodium channel isoforms that mediate action potential firing in lamina I/II spinal cord neurons. *Mol Pain*, 7, 67.

Hjerling-Leffler, J., Alqatari, M., Ernfors, P., and Koltzenburg, M. (2007). Emergence of functional sensory subtypes as defined by transient receptor potential channel expression. *J Neurosci*, 27, 2435–2443.

Hollmann, M., Hartley, M., and Heinemann, S. (1991). Ca2+ permeability of KA-AMPA—gated glutamate receptor channels depends on subunit composition. *Science*, 252, 851–853.

Holmberg, H. and Schouenborg, J. (1996). Postnatal development of the nociceptive withdrawal reflexes in the rat: a behavioural and electromyographic study. *J Physiol* 493 (Pt 1), 239–252.

Hori, Y. and Kanda, K. (1994). Developmental alterations in NMDA receptor-mediated [Ca2+]i elevation in substantia gelatinosa neurons of neonatal rat spinal cord. *Brain Res Dev Brain Res*, 80, 141–148.

Hosl, K., Reinold, H., Harvey, R. J., Muller, U., Narumiya, S., and Zeilhofer, H. U. (2006). Spinal prostaglandin E receptors of the EP2 subtype and the glycine receptor alpha3 subunit, which mediate central inflammatory hyperalgesia, do not contribute to pain after peripheral nerve injury or formalin injection. *Pain*, 126, 46–53.

Hu, F. and Strittmatter, S. M. (2004). Regulating axon growth within the postnatal central nervous system. *Semin Perinatol*, 28, 371–378.

Hu, H. J., Alter, B. J., Carrasquillo, Y., Qiu, C. S., Gereau, R. W. (2007). Metabotropic glutamate receptor 5 modulates nociceptive plasticity via extracellular signal-regulated kinase-Kv4.2 signaling in spinal cord dorsal horn neurons. *J Neurosci*, 27, 13181–13191.

Huang, M., Huang, T., Xiang, Y., Xie, Z., Chen, Y., Yan, R., et al. (2008). Ptf1a, Lbx1 and Pax2 coordinate glycinergic and peptidergic transmitter phenotypes in dorsal spinal inhibitory neurons. *Dev Biol*, 322, 394–405.

Hucho, T. and Levine, J. D. (2007). Signaling pathways in sensitization: toward a nociceptor cell biology. *Neuron*, 55, 365–376.

Hunt, S. P. and Mantyh, P. W. (2001). The molecular dynamics of pain control. *Nat Rev Neurosci*, 2, 83–91.

Indo, Y. (2002). Genetics of congenital insensitivity to pain with anhidrosis (CIPA) or hereditary sensory and autonomic neuropathy type IV. Clinical, biological and molecular aspects of mutations in TRKA(NTRK1) gene encoding the receptor tyrosine kinase for nerve growth factor. *Clin Auton Res*, 12(Suppl 1), I20–32.

Ingram, R. A., Fitzgerald, M., and Baccei, M. L. (2008). Developmental changes in the fidelity and short-term plasticity of GABAergic synapses in the neonatal rat dorsal horn. *J Neurophysiol*, 99, 3144–3150.

Jackman, A. and Fitzgerald, M. (2000). Development of peripheral hindlimb and central spinal cord innervation by subpopulations of dorsal root ganglion cells in the embryonic rat. *J Comp Neurol*, 418, 281–298.

Jakowec, M. W., Yen, L., and Kalb, R. G. (1995). In situ hybridization analysis of AMPA receptor subunit gene expression in the developing rat spinal cord. *Neuroscience*, 67, 909–920.

Jennings, E. and Fitzgerald, M. (1996). C-fos can be induced in the neonatal rat spinal cord by both noxious and innocuous peripheral stimulation. *Pain*, 68, 301–306.

Jennings, E. and Fitzgerald, M. (1998). Postnatal changes in responses of rat dorsal horn cells to afferent stimulation: a fibre-induced sensitization. *J Physiol*, 509(Pt 3), 859–868.

Jiang, M. C. and Gebhart, G. F. (1998). Development of mustard oil-induced hyperalgesia in rats., *Pain* 77, 305–313.

Jonas, P., Bischofberger, J., and Sandkuhler, J. (1998). Corelease of two fast neurotransmitters at a central synapse. *Science*, 281, 419–424.

Kandler, K., Clause, A., and Noh, J. (2009). Tonotopic reorganization of developing auditory brainstem circuits. *Nat Neurosci*, 12, 711–717.

Kapfhammer, J. P. and Schwab, M. E. (1994). Inverse patterns of myelination and GAP-43 expression in the adult CNS: neurite growth inhibitors as regulators of neuronal plasticity? *J Comp Neurol*, 340, 194–206.

Kato, G., Yasaka, T., Katafuchi, T., Furue, H., Mizuno, M., Iwamoto, Y., et al. (2006). Direct GABAergic and glycinergic inhibition of the substantia gelatinosa from the rostral ventromedial medulla revealed by in vivo patch-clamp analysis in rats. *J Neurosci*, 26, 1787–1794.

Kawabata, A. (2011). Prostaglandin E2 and pain—an update. *Biol Pharm Bull*, 34, 1170–1173.

Keller, A. F., Coull, J. A., Chery, N., Poisbeau, P., and De Koninck, Y. (2001). Region-specific developmental specialization of GABA-glycine cosynapses in laminas I-II of the rat spinal dorsal horn. *J Neurosci*, 21, 7871–7880.

Kirsch, J., Wolters, I., Triller, A., and Betz, H. (1993). Gephyrin antisense oligonucleotides prevent glycine receptor clustering in spinal neurons. *Nature*, 366, 745–748.

Kirstein, M. and Farinas, I. (2002). Sensing life: regulation of sensory neuron survival by neurotrophins. *Cell Mol Life Sci*, 59, 1787–1802.

Koch, S. C., Fitzgerald, M., and Hathway, G. J. (2008). Midazolam potentiates nociceptive behavior, sensitizes cutaneous reflexes, and is devoid of sedative action in neonatal rats. *Anesthesiology*, 108, 122–129.

Kolodkin, A. L. and Tessier-Lavigne M. (2011). Mechanisms and molecules of neuronal wiring: a primer. *Cold Spring Harb Perspect Biol*, 3(6).

Koltzenburg, M. and Handwerker, H. O. (1994). Differential ability of human cutaneous nociceptors to signal mechanical pain and to produce vasodilatation. *J Neurosci*, 14, 1756–1765.

Koltzenburg, M. and Lewin, G. R. (1997). Receptive properties of embryonic chick sensory neurons innervating skin. *J Neurophysiol*, 78, 2560–2568.

Koltzenburg, M., Stucky, C. L., and Lewin, G. R. (1997). Receptive properties of mouse sensory neurons innervating hairy skin. *J Neurophysiol*, 78, 1841–1850.

Lai, J., Porreca, F., Hunter, J. C., and Gold, M. S. (2004). Voltage-gated sodium channels and hyperalgesia. *Annu Rev Pharmacol Toxicol*, 44, 371–397.

LaPrairie, J. L. and Murphy, A. Z. (2007). Female rats are more vulnerable to the long-term consequences of neonatal inflammatory injury. *Pain* 132(Suppl 1), S124–133.

Le Bars, D., Gozariu, M., and Cadden, S. W. (2001). Animal models of nociception. *Pharmacol Rev*, 53, 597–652.

Li, J. and Baccei, M. L. (2009). Excitatory synapses in the rat superficial dorsal horn are strengthened following peripheral inflammation during early postnatal development. *Pain*, 143, 56–64.

Li, J. and Baccei, M. L. (2011a). Pacemaker neurons within newborn spinal pain circuits. *J Neurosci*, 31, 9010–9022.

Li, J. and Baccei, M. L. (2011b). Neonatal tissue damage facilitates nociceptive synaptic input to the developing superficial dorsal horn via NGF-dependent mechanisms. *Pain*, 152, 1846–1855.

Li, J. and Baccei, M. L. (2012). Developmental regulation of membrane excitability in rat spinal lamina I projection neurons. *J Neurophysiol*, 107, 2604–2614.

Li, J., Walker, S. M., Fitzgerald, M., and Baccei, M. L. (2009a). Activity-dependent modulation of glutamatergic signaling in the developing rat dorsal horn by early tissue injury. *J Neurophysiol*, 102, 2208–2219.

Li, J., Xie, W., Zhang, J. M., and Baccei, M. L. (2009b). Peripheral nerve injury sensitizes neonatal dorsal horn neurons to tumor necrosis factor-alpha. *Mol Pain*, 5, 10.

Li, P. and Zhuo, M. (1998). Silent glutamatergic synapses and nociception in mammalian spinal cord. *Nature*, 393, 695–698.

Li, P., Wilding, T. J., Kim, S. J., Calejesan, A. A., Huettner, J. E., and Zhuo, M. (1999). Kainate-receptor-mediated sensory synaptic transmission in mammalian spinal cord. *Nature*, 397, 161–164.

Linley, J. E., Rose, K., Ooi, L., and Gamper, N. (2010). Understanding inflammatory pain: ion channels contributing to acute and chronic nociception. *Pflugers Arch*, 459, 657–669.

Liu, M. and Wood, J. N. (2011). The roles of sodium channels in nociception: implications for mechanisms of neuropathic pain. *Pain Med*, 12(Suppl 3), S93–99.

Ma, W., Behar, T., and Barker, J. L. (1992). Transient expression of GABA immunoreactivity in the developing rat spinal cord. *J Comp Neurol*, 325, 271–290.

Mantyh, P. W., Rogers, S. D., Honore, P., Allen, B. J., Ghilardi, J. R., Li, J., et al. (1997). Inhibition of hyperalgesia by ablation of lamina I spinal neurons expressing the substance P receptor. *Science*, 278, 275–279.

Matheson, A., Nierenberg, M., and Greengard, J. (1952). Reactivity of the skin of the newborn infant. *Pediatrics*, 10, 181–197.

McGee, A. W., Yang, Y., Fischer, Q. S., Daw, N. W., and Strittmatter, S. M. (2005). Experience-driven plasticity of visual cortex limited by myelin and Nogo receptor. *Science*, 309, 2222–2226.

Mellor, D. J., Diesch, T. J., Gunn, A. J., and Bennet, L. (2005). The importance of 'awareness' for understanding fetal pain. *Brain Res Brain Res Rev*, 49, 455–471.

Merskey H, and Bogduk N (1994). *Classification of chronic pain syndromes and definitions of pain terms* (2nd edn). Seattle, WA: IASP Press.

Mirnics, K. and Koerber, H. R. (1995). Prenatal development of rat primary afferent fibers: II. Central projections. *J Comp Neurol*, 355, 601–614.

Moore, K. A., Kohno, T., Karchewski, L. A., Scholz, J., Baba, H., and Woolf, C. J. (2002). Partial peripheral nerve injury promotes a selective loss of GABAergic inhibition in the superficial dorsal horn of the spinal cord. *J Neurosci*, 22, 6724–6731.

Moss, A., Alvares, D., Meredith-Middleton, J., Robinson, M., Slater, R., Hunt, S. P., et al. (2005). Ephrin-A4 inhibits sensory neurite outgrowth and is regulated by neonatal skin wounding. *Eur J Neurosci*, 22, 2413–2421.

Muller, F., Heinke, B., and Sandkuhler, J. (2003). Reduction of glycine receptor-mediated miniature inhibitory postsynaptic currents in rat spinal lamina I neurons after peripheral inflammation. *Neuroscience*, 122, 799–805.

Noguchi, K. and Okubo, M. (2011). Leukotrienes in nociceptive pathway and neuropathic/inflammatory pain. *Biol Pharm Bull*, 34, 1163–1169.

Ogata, N. and Tatebayashi, H. (1992). Ontogenic development of the TTX-sensitive and TTX-insensitive Na+ channels in neurons of the rat dorsal root ganglia. *Brain Res Dev Brain Res*, 65, 93–100.

Patapoutian, A., Tate, S., and Woolf, C. J. (2009). Transient receptor potential channels: targeting pain at the source. *Nat Rev Drug Discov*, 8, 55–68.

Persson, A. K., Black, J. A., Gasser, A., Cheng, X., Fischer, T. Z., and Waxman, S. G. (2010). Sodium-calcium exchanger and multiple sodium channel isoforms in intra-epidermal nerve terminals. *Mol Pain*, 6, 84.

Pezet, S. and McMahon, S. B. (2006). Neurotrophins: mediators and modulators of pain. *Annu Rev Neurosci*, 29, 507–538.

Pignatelli, D., Ribeiro-da-Silva, A., and Coimbra, A. (1989). Postnatal maturation of primary afferent terminations in the substantia gelatinosa of the rat spinal cord. An electron microscopic study. *Brain Res*, 491, 33–44.

Reeh, P. W. (1986). Sensory receptors in mammalian skin in an in vitro preparation. *Neurosci Lett*, 66, 141–146.

Ren, K., Anseloni, V., Zou, S. P., Wade, E. B., Novikova, S. I., Ennis, M., *et al.* (2004). Characterization of basal and re-inflammation-associated long-term alteration in pain responsivity following short-lasting neonatal local inflammatory insult. *Pain*, 110, 588–596.

Ren, K., Novikova, S. I., He, F., Dubner, R., and Lidow, M. S. (2005). Neonatal local noxious insult affects gene expression in the spinal dorsal horn of adult rats. *Mol Pain*, 1, 27.

Ririe, D. G., Bremner, L. R., and Fitzgerald, M. (2008). Comparison of the immediate effects of surgical incision on dorsal horn neuronal receptive field size and responses during postnatal development. *Anesthesiology*, 109, 698–706.

Rivera, C., Voipio, J., Payne, J. A., Ruusuvuori, E., Lahtinen, H., Lamsa, K., *et al.* (1999). The K+/Cl– co-transporter KCC2 renders GABA hyperpolarizing during neuronal maturation. *Nature*, 397, 251–255.

Rivera-Arconada, I. and Lopez-Garcia, J. A. (2010). Changes in membrane excitability and potassium currents in sensitized dorsal horn neurons of mice pups. *J Neurosci*, 30, 5376–5383.

Ruda, M. A., Ling, Q. D., Hohmann, A. G., Peng, Y. B., and Tachibana, T. (2000). Altered nociceptive neuronal circuits after neonatal peripheral inflammation. *Science*, 289, 628–631.

Safronov, B. V., Wolff, M., and Vogel, W. (1999). Axonal expression of sodium channels in rat spinal neurones during postnatal development. *J Physiol*, 514(Pt 3), 729–734.

Schaffner, A. E., Behar, T., Nadi, S., Smallwood, V., and Barker, J. L. (1993). Quantitative analysis of transient GABA expression in embryonic and early postnatal rat spinal cord neurons. *Brain Res Dev Brain Res*, 72, 265–276.

Scholz, J., Broom, D. C., Youn, D. H., Mills, C. D., Kohno, T., Suter, M. R., *et al.* (2005). Blocking caspase activity prevents transsynaptic neuronal apoptosis and the loss of inhibition in lamina II of the dorsal horn after peripheral nerve injury. *J Neurosci*, 25, 7317–7323.

Schouenborg, J. (2003). Somatosensory imprinting in spinal reflex modules. *J Rehabil Med*, 73–80.

Schwegler, G., Schwab, M. E., and Kapfhammer, J. P. (1995). Increased collateral sprouting of primary afferents in the myelin-free spinal cord. *J Neurosci*, 15, 2756–2767.

Smith, E. S. and Lewin, G. R. (2009). Nociceptors: a phylogenetic view. *J Comp Physiol A Neuroethol Sens Neural Behav Physiol*, 195, 1089–1106.

Spike, R. C., Puskar, Z., Andrew, D., and Todd, A. J. (2003). A quantitative and morphological study of projection neurons in lamina I of the rat lumbar spinal cord. *Eur J Neurosci*, 18, 2433–2448.

Suzuki, R., Morcuende, S., Webber, M., Hunt, S. P., and Dickenson, A. H. (2002). Superficial NK1-expressing neurons control spinal excitability through activation of descending pathways. *Nat Neurosci*, 5, 1319–1326.

Todd, A. J. and Sullivan, A. C. (1990). Light microscope study of the coexistence of GABA-like and glycine-like immunoreactivities in the spinal cord of the rat. *J Comp Neurol*, 296, 496–505.

Torsney, C. (2011). Inflammatory pain unmasks heterosynaptic facilitation in lamina I neurokinin 1 receptor-expressing neurons in rat spinal cord. *J Neurosci*, 31, 5158–5168.

Torsney, C. and Fitzgerald, M. (2002). Age-dependent effects of peripheral inflammation on the electrophysiological properties of neonatal rat dorsal horn neurons. *J Neurophysiol*, 87, 1311–1317.

Tritsch, N. X., Yi, E., Gale, J. E., Glowatzki, E., and Bergles, D. E. (2007). The origin of spontaneous activity in the developing auditory system. *Nature*, 450, 50–55.

Valdes-Sanchez, T., Kirstein, M., Perez-Villalba, A., Vega, J. A., and Farinas, I. (2010). BDNF is essentially required for the early postnatal survival of nociceptors. *Dev Biol*, 339, 465–476.

Valerio, A., Paterlini, M., Boifava, M., Memo, M., and Spano, P. (1997). Metabotropic glutamate receptor mRNA expression in rat spinal cord. *Neuroreport*, 8, 2695–2699.

Waldenstrom, A., Thelin, J., Thimansson, E., Levinsson, A., and Schouenborg, J. (2003). Developmental learning in a pain-related system: evidence for a cross-modality mechanism. *J Neurosci*, 23, 7719–7725.

Walker, S. M., Meredith-Middleton, J., Cooke-Yarborough, C., and Fitzgerald, M. (2003). Neonatal inflammation and primary afferent terminal plasticity in the rat dorsal horn. *Pain*, 105, 185–195.

Walker, S. M., Meredith-Middleton, J., Lickiss, T., Moss, A., and Fitzgerald, M. (2007). Primary and secondary hyperalgesia can be differentiated by postnatal age and ERK activation in the spinal dorsal horn of the rat pup. *Pain*, 128, 157–168.

Walker, S. M., Tochiki, K. K., and Fitzgerald, M. (2009). Hindpaw incision in early life increases the hyperalgesic response to repeat surgical injury: critical period and dependence on initial afferent activity. *Pain*, 147, 99–106.

Walker, S. M., Westin, B. D., Deumens, R., Grafe, M., and Yaksh, T. L. (2010). Effects of intrathecal ketamine in the neonatal rat: evaluation of apoptosis and long-term functional outcome. *Anesthesiology*, 113, 147–159.

Walsh, M. A., Graham, B. A., Brichta, A. M., and Callister, R. J. (2009). Evidence for a critical period in the development of excitability and potassium currents in mouse lumbar superficial dorsal horn neurons. *J Neurophysiol*, 101, 1800–1812.

Wang, H. and Woolf, C. J. (2005). Pain TRPs. *Neuron*, 46, 9–12.

Washburn, M. S., Numberger, M., Zhang, S., and Dingledine, R. (1997). Differential dependence on GluR2 expression of three characteristic features of AMPA receptors. *J Neurosci*, 17, 9393–9406.

Willer, J. C. (1983). Nociceptive flexion reflexes as a tool for pain research in man. *Adv Neurol*, 39, 809–827.

Woodbury, C. J. and Koerber, H. R. (2003). Widespread projections from myelinated nociceptors throughout the substantia gelatinosa provide novel insights into neonatal hypersensitivity. *J Neurosci*, 23, 601–610.

Woolf, C. J. and Ma, Q. (2007). Nociceptors—noxious stimulus detectors. *Neuron*, 55, 353–364.

Yasaka, T., Hughes, D. I., Polgar, E., Nagy, G. G., Watanabe, M., Riddell, J. S., *et al.* (2009). Evidence against AMPA receptor-lacking glutamatergic synapses in the superficial dorsal horn of the rat spinal cord. *J Neurosci*, 29, 13401–13409.

Yoshimura, M. and Jessell, T. (1990). Amino acid-mediated EPSPs at primary afferent synapses with substantia gelatinosa neurones in the rat spinal cord. *J Physiol*, 430, 315–335.

Zhang, W., Liu, L. Y., and Xu, T. L. (2008). Reduced potassium-chloride co-transporter expression in spinal cord dorsal horn neurons contributes to inflammatory pain hypersensitivity in rats. *Neuroscience*, 152, 502–510.

Zhu, W., Galoyan, S. M., Petruska, J. C., Oxford, G. S., and Mendell, L. M. (2004). A developmental switch in acute sensitization of small dorsal root ganglion (DRG) neurons to capsaicin or noxious heating by NGF. *J Neurophysiol*, 92, 3148–3152.

CHAPTER 7

Neuroimmune interactions and pain during postnatal development

David Vega-Avelaira and Simon Beggs

Summary

The immune system is essential for identifying and mounting defensive responses to tissue damage and infection. In addition, it is increasingly recognized that interactions between immune cells and nociceptive pathways can modulate pain sensitivity. The role and function of immune cells in the central nervous system changes during postnatal development, and as a result, the impact of neuroimmune interactions on pain signalling varies with both age and the type of injury.

Introduction

Interactions between nociceptive pathways and the immune system are important for detecting and responding to potential harm from tissue damage and infection, and involve multiple different cell types in different regions (Figure 7.1). In the periphery, nociceptors release a range of mediators which not only contribute to peripheral sensitization, but also attract and activate immune cells (mast cells, dendritic cells, T lymphocytes) to facilitate removal of pathogens and wound healing (Chiu et al., 2012). Macrophages are T lymphocytes which are present in the dorsal root ganglion (DRG), and increased activity and recruitment following nerve injury can contribute to pain sensitivity (Hu et al., 2007). In the spinal cord, microglia are no longer thought of as having only immune surveillance and supportive roles. Following noxious afferent input, microglial reactivity is increased, and the released proinflammatory cytokines, chemokines, and extracellular proteases, interact with neurons and contribute to central sensitization (Beggs and Salter, 2010; Clark et al., 2011). Astrocytes, another subtype of glial cells, are also activated in the spinal cord following inflammation, plantar incision, and nerve injury, but the degree and time course differ from microglia, and varies with the type of injury (Chiang et al., 2012). Modulators of glial activity reduce pain sensitivity associated with injury, but have little effect on normal or baseline pain processing, suggesting that the main role of glial activation is in pathological pain states (Chiang et al., 2012).

Peripheral nerve injury

Neuropathic pain can be severe and difficult to treat (see also Walker, Chapter 21; Rastogi and Campbell, Chapter 49, this volume). Despite considerable effort the conditions that initiate and maintain neuropathic pain are as yet not fully understood. Peripheral nerve injury (PNI) activates multiple cellular and molecular pathways in both the peripheral and central nervous systems. Of considerable interest now is parsing these cellular and molecular pathways; PNI will evoke a nerve regeneration response and a stress response associated with interrupted metabolic pathways (Costigan et al., 2009). Clearly, explicit damage to the peripheral nervous system is countered by responses in multiple systems, and it is the interaction between immune system reactivity and injury-driven changes in nociceptive signalling that is now under scrutiny.

PNI in experimental animals under 3 weeks of age does not result in the development of pain hypersensitivity, although evidence suggests that the onset is delayed (Howard et al., 2005; Vega-Avelaira et al., 2012). This developmental anomaly is due, at least in part, to differences between the early postnatal and adult immune systems (Moss et al., 2007; Vega-Avelaira et al., 2007, 2009).

Microglia

Microglia are the resident macrophages of the central nervous system (CNS). Their complex repertoire of functions in the adult includes maintaining homeostasis, detecting and responding to infection, and promoting or suppressing neuroinflammation. These actions also link microglia inextricably to neurodegenerative diseases such as Alzheimer's disease, Parkinsonism, and neuropathic pain (Beggs et al., 2012b; Kettenmann et al., 2011). Microglia respond to potentially damaging injury or disease to the CNS by adopting any of several reactive phenotypes. Morphological changes can be identified by changes in expression of the microglial marker, ionized calcium binding adaptor molecule1 (Iba-1; Beggs and Salter, 2007; Suter et al., 2009; Vega-Avelaira et al., 2007). Where once the concept of a monolithic microglial 'activation' was widely accepted, evidence now suggests there are different subpopulations

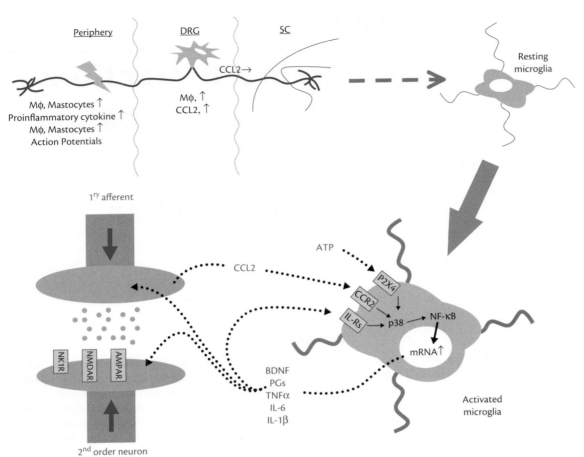

Figure 7.1 Neuroimmune interactions in neuropathic pain. Peripheral nerve injury provokes activation of innate immune cells such as macrophages and mastocytes proximal to the damaged area (Hu and McLachlan, 2002, 2003; Watkins and Maier, 2002). As a consequence, both immune cells and Schwann cells secrete pro-inflammatory cytokines to prevent further injury and repair the damage. This promotes physiological, cellular, and molecular changes in the DRG neurons and macrophages which result in neuronal aberrant electrical discharges, macrophage activation and pro-inflammatory cytokine release (Gabay et al., 2011; Hu and McLachlan, 2002; Ozaktay et al., 2006; Suter et al., 2009). Cytokines, such as CCL2 are anterogradely transported from the ganglia to the primary afferents terminals in the spinal cord (Thacker et al., 2009). Acting through CCR2 and interleukin receptors they activate intracellular pathways (e.g. P38 mak kinase pathway) promote translocation of transcription factors like NF-kB to microglia nuclei, and become activated (Capiralla et al., 2012; Chang and Waxman, 2010; Ren and Dubner, 2007; Schäfers et al., 2003; Svensson et al., 2003). As part of the activation process, microglia produce and release cytokines with an autocrine and paracrine activity which create a feedback positive loop that will sensitize second-order neurons and initiate the neuropathy (X. Gao et al., 2005; Y.-J. Gao and Ji, 2009, 2010).

with different reactive response profiles and capabilities (Scheffel et al., 2012).

Microglia are sensors for damage or disease in the CNS, capable of detecting pathogen-associated molecular patters (PAMPs) and damage-associated molecular patterns (DAMPs). One of the many classes of receptors expressed by microglia are the Toll-like receptors (TLRs). TLRs are part of the complex molecular sensor framework for detecting both PAMPs and DAMPs (Stewart et al., 2010; Zhang and Mosser, 2008) and members of this family of receptors have been implicated in the pathogenesis of neuropathic and inflammatory pain in adult animals (Sorge et al., 2011; Tanga et al., 2005).

Microglial function during development

Microglia are of haematopoietic origin, and first appear as primitive macrophages in the yolk sac in early embryogenesis from where they migrate into the CNS (Ginhoux et al., 2010). This process occurs throughout embryonic and into early postnatal life (Pont-Lezica et al., 2011). The actions of microglia during development are complex with a dual function as: (1) immune effectors in the removal of excess and exuberant axonal projections, and (2) a more classical glial role as cytotropic and cytotrophic factors (Schlegelmilch et al., 2011). Given the extensive remodelling and refining of connectivity throughout the CNS in the early postnatal period, it is clearly necessary for microglia to differentiate between normal physiology and pathology.

The induction of cytokines and chemokines resulting from TLR4 activation varies with postnatal age and the pattern is the same across the TLR family members, with a general *hypo*responsivity that peaks at postnatal day (P) 21. The transient changes and hyporesponsivity of some TLRs may be a reflection of the substantial reorganization and refinement of connectivity within the dorsal horn (and CNS generally) that occurs postnatally. Normal developmental synaptic elimination and pruning of exuberant axonal projections would provide a temporary increase in DAMPs and provoke an unwanted immune response.

This time point marks the end of a critical period of maturation of both the nervous and immune systems, and also the point at which central neuroimmune interactions stimulated by PNI are capable of driving neuropathic behavioural pain behaviours (Howard et al., 2005; Moss et al., 2007). Intriguingly, this postnatal maturation is also marked by a switch in gene expression such that gene transcripts associated with the classical, pro-inflammatory M1 phenotype are downregulated while those of the alternative anti-inflammatory M2 phenotype start to predominate (Gordon and Taylor, 2005; Mosser and Edwards, 2008; Scheffel et al., 2012).

T lymphocytes

T cells, also known as T lymphocytes, play an important role in cell-mediated immunity, but there is also increasing evidence for a role of T cells in the responses to PNI that produce pain. Helper T cells can be divided into two broad subtypes; Th1 and Th2, classified as such by the array of cytokines they produce. Th1 is generally pro-inflammatory and released cytokines include interferon gamma (IFNγ), which is heavily implicated in neuropathic pain pathogenesis (Costigan et al., 2009; Masuda et al., 2012; Tsuda et al., 2009). Th2 is generally anti-inflammatory, and ideally a balance of Th1 and Th2 exists. In early life, the Th1 pro-inflammatory response is weak (Fadel and Sarzotti, 2000), and the balance is shifted to a Th2 predominance, with Th1 gradually strengthening with exposure to allergens.

The complex developmental regulation of the immune system is occurring at the same time as the nervous system is undergoing extensive postnatal refinement (Beggs et al., 2002; Fitzgerald, 2005; Fitzgerald et al., 1994), it is not surprising that interactions of the immune system with the CNS following PNI differ significantly in the early postnatal period from those seen in the adult. Taken together, these observations indicate that the immune system in the immediate postnatal period does not react to PNI in the same way as in the mature adult animal. The pattern of T-cell activation and infiltration following PNI differs significantly in young animals. The predominance of Th2 T cells in the neonate underlies this, imbuing the immature immune system with a tolerance for the new antigens exposed by normal developmental changes within the CNS (Costigan et al., 2009).

Neuroimmune interactions in dorsal root ganglia

Macrophages are phagocytic immune cells, capable of engulfing and digesting cellular debris and pathogens, and act to maintain the cellular environment and protect against potential infection in the DRG (Watkins and Maier, 2002). In keeping with resident microglia in the CNS, macrophages in the DRG adopt a ramified surveillance state and are homogenously distributed between neuronal cell bodies and projecting fibres (Beggs et al., 2012b; Hu and McLachlan, 2002, 2003; Vega-Avelaira et al., 2009). PNI provokes both a reactive response of the resident macrophages as well as infiltration of new macrophages from the circulation (Hu and McLachlan, 2002, 2003). Macrophages in the DRG are characterized by expression of the 'macrophage scavenger receptor' CD163, and can also be identified by expression of CD68, which is increased 3 days following experimental PNI in adult animals (Hu et al., 2007). CD168-positive cell number remains the same, suggesting a reactive phenotypic switch in the normal resident macrophage population. Macrophage reactivity peaks at 7 days post injury, as shown by the adoption of

an amoeboid morphology and maximal proliferation, and persists for at least 3 months (Hu and McLachlan, 2002). Retrograde labelling studies have shown that these reactive macrophages cluster around damaged neurons and in particular the large cell bodies of myelinated afferents (Vega-Avelaira et al., 2009).

The injury-induced reactive phenotype of DRG macrophages is determined in part by their molecular phenotype. Increased expression of membrane receptors such as purinergic receptors (e.g. $P2X_4$) and chemokine receptors (e.g. IL6R, TNFαR, CCR2) activate intracellular second-messenger pathways (e.g. MAP kinases pathway; Gao and Ji, 2010; Ji et al., 2003, 2009; Scholz and Woolf, 2007), leading to increased expression of molecules that drive a phagocytic phenotype. This is accompanied by the release of chemokines (Hu and McLachlan, 2003) which maintain this adaptive phenotype through both autocrine and paracrine positive feedback loops and by macrophage recruitment from the circulation. Chemokines also act directly to influence neuronal excitability (Scholz and Woolf, 2007), thereby modulating afferent signal transduction from the dorsal root ganglia to the spinal cord.

Signalling molecules

MCP-1/CCL2

Macrophage chemo-attractant protein 1 (MCP-1, now CCL2) and its receptor CCR2 have been associated with several models of nerve injury (Thacker et al., 2009; Vega-Avelaira et al., 2009). MCP-1 is expressed in small DRG neurons and is transported anterogradely to the spinal cord after PNI where it has chemotactic effects on both glia and neurons (Thacker et al., 2009) (Figure 7.1). Genetically modified CCR2 null or 'knock-out' mice do not exhibit enhanced pain behaviour after PNI (Abbadie et al., 2003; Zhang et al., 2007). Taken together, these studies directly implicate macrophage-neuronal interactions in pain behaviour.

Tumour necrosis factor α (TNFα)

TNFα is a pro-inflammatory cytokine and one of many factors released following PNI (Jeon et al., 2011; Kim et al., 2011). Macrophages are the main source of TNFα but *de novo* expression is also evident in small-diameter nociceptive cells after nerve injury. TNFα activates the MAP kinase p38 intracellular pathway which instigates a feed-forward mechanism to increase further production of TNFα. Pharmacological blockade of TNFα is sufficient to ameliorate pain behaviour in animals with partial axotomy (Schäfers et al., 2003).

Interleukin-6 (IL-6)

IL-6 is a pleiotropic cytokine (Simpson et al., 1997) with roles in neuronal survival, growth and differentiation (Grothe et al., 2000). It is synthesized and released by macrophages and Schwann cells. The IL-6 receptor (IL-6R or CD126) is expressed in the DRG (Brázda et al., 2009; Watkins and Maier, 2002; Zhang et al., 2007) and there is evidence for IL-6 involvement in both the hyperalgesia and allodynia associated with neuropathic pain (DeLeo et al., 1996). IL-6 production is increased in neurons and satellite glial cells in DRGs within 24 h of PNI and persists for at least 2 weeks (Brázda et al., 2009). Furthermore, IL-6 has roles in multiple independent pathways mediating processes including nerve regeneration (Qiu et al., 2005) and TNFα-induced apoptosis of DRG neurons (Murata et al., 2011). As contradictory evidence exists for both beneficial and detrimental effects of IL-6 after PNI, further investigation is warranted.

Interleukin-1β (IL-1β)

IL-1β is intimately associated with the initiation and maintenance of neuropathic pain (Gabay et al., 2011; Wolf et al., 2006). It is constitutively expressed in primary sensory neurons (Copray et al., 2001) and has pro-excitatory effects in small and medium non-peptidergic neurons (Stemkowski and Smith, 2012) via a G protein-coupled receptor mediated mechanism (von Banchet et al., 2011). PNI induces a rapid increase in IL-1β in DRG macrophages (Thacker et al., 2007), sensitizing DRG neurons and contributing to increased mechanosensitivity (Ozaktay et al., 2006).

Prostaglandins

Prostaglandins, such as cyclo-oxygenase (COX)-2 dependent PGE_2, have an important role in the pathogenesis of neuropathic pain (Ma and Quirion, 2008; Ma et al., 2010). At the spinal cord level, COX-2 is upregulated within the first 3 days after injury (O'Rielly and Loomis, 2006), and in the periphery, COX-2 and PGE_2 production is upregulated in Schwann cells and macrophages infiltrating damaged nerves. PGE_2 receptors, such as EP_1 receptors, are expressed on DRG neurons, and nerve injury causes the upregulation of EP_1 in human and rat DRG neurons (Durrenberger et al., 2006; Ma et al., 2010). PGE_2 sensitizes damaged axons to mechanical and heat stimuli (Ma and Quirion, 2008; Michaelis et al., 1998), and increases production of substance P and calcitonin gene-related peptide in DRG neurons (Segond von Banchet et al., 2003).

Nitric oxide (NO)

Macrophages are a main source of nitric oxide (NO) after nerve injury (Moalem and Tracey, 2006), induced by TNFα via inducible NO synthase (iNOS) (Lowenstein et al., 1994). NO upregulates prostaglandin production and contributes to neuronal sensitization (Mollace et al., 1997; Purwata, 2011).

Nerve injury and spinal microglial reactivity

Increased microglial reactivity has been demonstrated in several animal models of PNI associated with chronic pain (Coull et al., 2005; Tsuda et al., 2003; Vega-Avelaira et al., 2009; Zhuang et al., 2005). Initiation of the microglial response after peripheral nerve damage is triggered by increased neural activity of sensory afferent fibres (Suter et al., 2009). Nociceptive stimuli are predominantly transmitted by Aδ- and C-fibres (see Walker and Baccei, Chapter 6, this volume). However, following nerve injury, activity in Aβ-fibres which normally transduce innocuous tactile sensation can contribute to persistent pain (Matsumoto et al., 2008). Afferent blockade with the local anaesthetic bupivacaine, which blocks conduction in all sensory neurons (C, Aδ, and Aβ fibres) prevented nerve injury-induced spinal microglial activation; but resiniferatoxin, which selectively blocks peripheral input from C and Aδ nociceptive fibres (Mitchell et al., 2010) had no effect (Suter et al., 2009). This suggests that the large myelinated fibres have an important role in the switch of microglia to a reactive phenotype after nerve injury. It has also been suggested that a small proportion of microglia are activity-independent, responding to retrograde axonal transport and cytokine stimulation (Abe and Cavalli, 2008; O'Brien and Nathanson, 2007). Microglia also respond to chemotactic factors and migrate towards the area in the spinal cord that receives the projections of degenerating C-fibre primary afferents (Beggs and Salter, 2007; Davalos et al., 2005; Nimmerjahn et al., 2005; Shehab et al., 2008; Shields et al., 2003).

Microglia express multiple receptors that may be involved in altering reactivity (Beggs and Salter, 2010) that include: P2X and P2Y purinergic receptors (Trang et al., 2009; Tsuda et al., 2003), TLR-4 receptors (Ji and Strichartz, 2004; Lehnardt et al., 2003), and chemokine receptors such as the fractalkine receptor CX3CR1 (Clark et al., 2011; Hughes et al., 2002), the CCR2 receptor for MCP-1/CCL2 (Thacker et al., 2009), and the IFNγ receptor (Tsuda et al., 2009). Release of ATP, which acts via purinergic receptors, contributes to microglia changing to a reactive phenotype (Haynes et al., 2006). This is accompanied by morphological changes, increased proliferative capacity, and increased expression of membrane molecules such as complement receptor 3 (CD11b; Kreutzberg, 1996; Nakajima and Kohsaka, 1998) and Iba1 (Beggs and Salter, 2010).

Pro-inflammatory cytokines sensitize neurons by enhancing excitatory AMPA/NMDA currents and reducing inhibitory gamma-aminobutyric acid (GABA)/glycine currents (Kawasaki et al., 2008; Reeve et al., 2000; Sweitzer et al., 2001; Wang et al., 2005), but also contribute to neuropathic pain by stimulating microglia. Microglia are the main source of pro-inflammatory cytokines in the CNS (Hanisch, 2002) and increased functional microglial reactivity increases production and release of proinflammatory mediators (fractalkine IL-1β, IL-4, TNFα), prostaglandins, and ATP (Giaume et al., 2007; Kreutzberg, 1996; Segond von Banchet et al., 2003; Watkins et al., 2001). Following receptor activation, an increase in the intracellular concentration of Ca^{2+} activates signalling pathways, such as those mediated by the mitogen-activated protein kinase (MAPK) p38 (Ji and Suter, 2007) (Figure 7.1). p38 MAPK is a key factor in regulating the expression of proinflammatory cytokines, PGE2 and COX-2 (Jana et al., 2003; Ji and Suter, 2007; Wilms et al., 2003), and is involved in the recruitment of microglia to areas of injury (Tsuda et al., 2005). p38 activation is increased following nerve damage, whereas its inhibition suppresses mechanical allodynia (Ji and Suter, 2007; Jin et al., 2003; Svensson et al., 2003). Activation of the transcription factor NF-kB also promotes the production of proinflammatory cytokines, chemokines, COX-2 and other molecules related to immune activity (Y.-J. Gao and Ji, 2010).

IL-6 is upregulated in both the DRG and the spinal cord after nerve injury (Raghavendra et al., 2003), and also has a dual function by stimulating microglia (Galiano et al., 2001; Klein et al., 1997) and neuronal responses to injury (Latrémolière et al., 2008).

TLR4 receptor

The metabotropic receptor TLR-4 is important for pathogen recognition, and is activated by various substances, such as lipopolysaccharide from Gram-negative bacteria (H. Cao and Zhang, 2008; Capiralla et al., 2012). It is expressed on microglia and activation induces intracellular signalling cascades resulting in increased NF-κB signalling and subsequent expression of numerous genes regulating proinflammatory cytokines and other immunological molecules (Capiralla et al., 2012). Deficiency of this receptor or its blockade attenuates microglial reactivity, decreases levels of IFNγ,

IL-1β, and TNF, and reduces pain behaviours associated with PNI (Tanga et al., 2005).

P2X$_4$ receptor

P2X$_4$ receptors are expressed by microglia following PNI (Tsuda et al., 2003). Blockade of this receptor prevents and reverses mechanical allodynia in animal models of PNI, and mice deficient in P2X$_4$ do not develop mechanical hypersensitivity after nerve injury (Ulmann et al., 2008). P2X$_4$R expression is increased through the activation of other microglial receptors such us IFNγ and fibronectin receptors (Masuda et al., 2012; Tsuda et al., 2008, 2009). P2X$_4$R activation induces the synthesis and release of brain-derived neurotrophic factor (BDNF) by microglia (Coull et al., 2005; Trang et al., 2009) via a p38 MAPK-dependent pathway (Beggs and Salter, 2010; Jin et al., 2003). BDNF activates its neuronal receptor tyrosine kinase B (TrkB) on lamina I neurons in the spinal cord dorsal horn (Slack et al., 2005). This reduces the expression of the chloride transporter KCC2 leading to intracellular accumulation of Cl$^-$. The net effect of this is disinhibition; reducing the inhibitory action of GABA, and facilitating further neuronal sensitization (Coull et al., 2003, 2005). BDNF signalling in neurons also activates kinase pathways leading to phosphorylation of the NMDA receptor NR1 subunit, which also contributes to enhanced sensitivity (Ren and Dubner, 2007; Suen et al., 1997).

CX3CR1 receptor

Fractalkine (CX3CL1) is released by neurons and its receptor CX3CR1 is expressed on microglia, making it a prime candidate for neuronal-microglial signalling (Verge et al., 2004). The increased activity of primary afferents after nerve injury releases fractalkine into the extracellular space (Zhuang et al., 2007) and creates a chemotactic gradient for microglia (Chapman et al., 2000). Intrathecal injection of fractalkine upregulates expression of CX3CR1 and induces thermal hyperalgesia, which can be prevented by blocking fractalkine activity with CX3CR1 antibodies (Sun et al., 2007). Inhibiting microglial function with minocycline also prevents the appearance of mechanical allodynia and thermal hyperalgesia induced by injection of fractalkine (Milligan et al., 2005).

Lymphocyte infiltration and central sensitization

In addition to increased macrophage and microglial reactivity following PNI, other immunocompetent cells, such as T-lymphocytes also play a role. T lymphocytes can release excitatory cytokines, generating ectopic impulse activity in sensory neurons after nerve injury (L. Cao and DeLeo 2008; L. Cao et al., 2009; Costigan et al., 2009; Hu and McLachlan 2002). The dorsal root ganglia have a small population of lymphocytes which perform an immune surveillance function (Hu and McLachlan 2002). Peripheral nerve damage causes infiltration of CD8+ lymphocytes into the DRG and spinal cord (Costigan et al., 2009; Hu and McLachlan 2002) which suggests that PNI triggers an adaptive immune response. Moreover, this lymphocyte infiltration contributes to microglia reactivity via CD40 (a member of the TNF-receptor superfamily) (L. Cao et al., 2009) and mechanical hypersensitivity (Costigan et al., 2009; Hu and McLachlan 2002). The role of T cells is also demonstrated by the reduction in pain behaviours after nerve injury exhibited by the lymphocyte deficient Rag1-null mice (Costigan et al., 2009).

Postnatal differences in immune system activation after nerve injury

The role of neuroimmune interactions as mediators of neuropathic pain has focused on experimental models in adult animals. However, clinical studies suggest that traumatic nerve injury is less likely to produce neuropathic pain in early life; brachial plexus avulsion, which causes intense neuropathic pain in adults, is not painful when the injury is sustained at birth (Anand and Birch, 2002; see also Walker, Chapter 21, this volume). Laboratory studies conducted in animals throughout postnatal development are consistent with this: in nerve injury models of neuropathic pain, persistent mechanical allodynia does not develop if the injury is performed in the first 3 weeks of life, a developmental period which has parallels with human development from the neonate to adolescence (Howard et al., 2005; Ririe and Eisenach, 2006). Since infant rats and humans clearly respond to acute noxious stimuli and display both acute and chronic inflammatory pain behaviour from an early neonatal age, it appears that the mechanisms underlying neuropathic pain are differentially regulated over a prolonged postnatal period. Important differences include:

- Microglia in the neonatal spinal cord are capable of being activated by exogenous stimuli (e.g. intraspinal NMDA), but nerve injury in young rats fails to induce either the spinal microgliosis or macrophage accumulation in the DRG, that are hallmarks of PNI in the adult (Moss et al., 2007; Vega-Avelaira et al., 2007).
- Microarray analysis of gene expression in the DRG following nerve injury demonstrate changes associated with pro-inflammatory cytokines such us IL-6, CSF-1, and MCP-1 being upregulated in adult but not in young rats (Vega-Avelaira et al., 2009).
- In the spinal cord, many genes are differentially regulated in the adult compared with the infant rat, and the majority of these are involved in immune function (Costigan et al., 2009).
- Activation and infiltration of T-cells associated with the Th1 pro-inflammatory response in the dorsal horn is much greater in adult rats than in young animals after nerve injury (Costigan et al., 2009).

Neonatal incision and long-term priming of microglial response

The mechanisms and effectors previously described, that are in place to mute the postnatal immune response as part of the normal developmental process, would at first suggest that early postnatal peripheral injury does not result in persistent neuropathic pain. While the incidence of neuropathic pain following traumatic nerve injury is lower in infants and young children, the concept that an absence of pain to early life injury indicates a lack of a response, whether CNS or immune, is simplistic. A key function that unites all sensory systems is that adult connectivity is shaped by the balance of sensory input in early postnatal life. In much the same way that auditory and visual system connectivity in the brain is driven by sound and light, tactile sense is driven by touch (Bourne, 2010; Sanes and Bao, 2009). Neural activity during critical postnatal periods can influence normal development (Hensch, 2004) and this is also true for nociceptive pathways (Beggs et al., 2002; Ren et al., 2004). A considerable canon of evidence from both laboratory and clinical studies now shows that exposure to nociceptive stimuli in early life can produce long-term changes in sensory processing and the response to future injury (see Walker, Chapter 3; Grunau, Chapter 4, this volume). Importantly, priming of neuroimmune signalling by neonatal injury can contribute to persistent effects. 'Priming' or 'neonatal programming' of adult immune responses by early life immune stressors has been described (Boisse et al., 2004; Spencer et al., 2011), and an early immune challenge can alter pain sensitivity in adulthood (Boisse et al., 2005). As microglia are long-lived cells and can retain an innate immune memory (Perry, 2010) they are well suited to a role in persistent alterations. Plantar hindpaw incision, an established model of postoperative pain, performed during the first postnatal week, but not at older ages, enhances the response to subsequent injury 2 weeks later (Walker et al., 2009). The impact of neonatal injury persists until adulthood, with increases in both the degree and duration of incision-related hyperalgesia (Beggs et al., 2012a). These functional changes are mirrored by alterations in the time course and degree of microglial reactivity in the dorsal horn. The primed state arises from centrally-mediated changes in dorsal horn sensitivity or connectivity as:

- Hyperalgesia is selectively reversed by intrathecal minocycline, which reduces microglial reactivity in the spinal cord.

- The increased sensitivity and microglial reactivity following neonatal incision is also seen following direct electrical stimulation of the tibial nerve, which bypasses peripheral nociceptors (Beggs et al., 2012a).

Conclusion

Interactions between the immune system and nociceptive pathways play an important role in modulating pain sensitivity. Throughout postnatal development, neuroimmune interactions have a significant impact on age-related changes in the response to PNI, and also play a role in persistent changes in future pain response following neonatal surgical injury. Evaluating the relative risks and benefits of modulating microglial activity to prevent long-term changes in nociceptive pathways, or to manage enhanced pain sensitivity states, requires further research.

References

Abbadie, C., Lindia, J. A., Cumiskey, A. M., Peterson, L. B., Mudgett, J. S., Bayne, E. K., et al. (2003). Impaired neuropathic pain responses in mice lacking the chemokine receptor CCR2. Proc Natl Acad Sci U S A, 100(13), 7947–7952. doi:10.1073/pnas.1331358100.

Abe, N. and Cavalli, V. (2008). Nerve injury signaling. Curr Opin Neurobiol, 18(3), 276–283. doi:10.1016/j.conb.2008.06.005.

Anand, P. and Birch, R. (2002). Restoration of sensory function and lack of long-term chronic pain syndromes after brachial plexus injury in human neonates. Brain, 125(Pt 1), 113–122.

Beggs, S., Currie, G., Salter, M. W., Fitzgerald, M., and Walker, S. M. (2012a). Priming of adult pain responses by neonatal pain experience: maintenance by central neuroimmune activity. Brain, 135, 404–417.

Beggs, S. and Salter, M. W. (2007). Stereological and somatotopic analysis of the spinal microglial response to peripheral nerve injury. Brain Behav Immun, 21(5), 624–633. doi:10.1016/j.bbi.2006.10.017.

Beggs, S. and Salter M. W. (2010). Microglia-neuronal signalling in neuropathic pain hypersensitivity 2.0. Curr Opin Neurobiol, 20(4), 474–480. doi:10.1016/j.conb.2010.08.005.

Beggs, S., Torsney C., Drew L. J., and Fitzgerald, M. (2002). The postnatal reorganization of primary afferent input and dorsal horn cell receptive fields in the rat spinal cord is an activity-dependent process. Eur J Neurosci, 16(7), 1249–1258.

Beggs, S., Trang, T., and Salter, M. W. (2012b). P2X4R+ microglia drive neuropathic pain. Nat Neurosci, 15, 1068–1073.

Boisse, L., Mouihate, A., Ellis, S., and Pittman, Q. J. (2004). Long-term alterations in neuroimmune responses after neonatal exposure to lipopolysaccharide. J Neurosci, 24, 4928–4934.

Boisse, L., Spencer, S. J., Mouihate, A., Vergnolle, N., and Pittman, Q. J. (2005). Neonatal immune challenge alters nociception in the adult rat. Pain, 119, 133–141.

Bourne, J. A. (2010). Unravelling the development of the visual cortex: implications for plasticity and repair. J Anat, 217(4), 449–468. doi:10.1111/j.1469-7580.2010.01275.x.

Brázda, V., Klusáková, I., Svízenská, I., Veselková, Z., and Dubový, P. (2009). Bilateral changes in IL-6 protein, but not in its receptor Gp130, in rat dorsal root ganglia following sciatic nerve ligature. Cell Mol Neurobiol, 29(6–7), 1053–1062. doi:10.1007/s10571-009-9396-0.

Cao, H. and Zhang, Y.-Q. (2008). Spinal glial activation contributes to pathological pain states. Neurosci Biobehav Rev, 32(5), 972–983. doi:10.1016/j.neubiorev.2008.03.009.

Cao, L. and DeLeo, J. A. (2008). CNS-infiltrating CD4+ T lymphocytes contribute to murine spinal nerve transection-induced neuropathic pain. Eur J Immunol, 38(2), 448–458. doi:10.1002/eji.200737485.

Cao, L., Palmer, C. D., Malon J. T., and DeLeo, J. A. (2009). Critical role of microglial CD40 in the maintenance of mechanical hypersensitivity in a murine model of neuropathic pain. Eur J Immunol, 39(12), 3562–3569. doi:10.1002/eji.200939657.

Capiralla, H., Vingtdeux, V., Zhao, H., Sankowski, R., Al-Abed, Y., Davies, P., et al. (2012). Resveratrol mitigates lipopolysaccharide- and Aβ-mediated microglial inflammation by inhibiting the TLR4/NF-κB/STAT signaling cascade. J Neurochem, 120(3), 461–472. doi:10.1111/j.1471-4159.2011.07594.x.

Chang, Y.-W. and Waxman S. G. (2010). Minocycline attenuates mechanical allodynia and central sensitization following peripheral second-degree burn injury. J Pain, 11(11), 1146–1154. doi:10.1016/j.jpain.2010.02.010.

Chapman, G. A., Moores, K., Harrison, D., Campbell, C.A., Stewart, B. R., and Strijbos, P. J. (2000). Fractalkine cleavage from neuronal membranes represents an acute event in the inflammatory response to excitotoxic brain damage. J Neurosci, 20(15), RC87.

Chiang, C. Y., Sessle, B. J., and Dostrovsky, J. O. (2012). Role of astrocytes in pain. Neurochem Res, 37, 2419–2431.

Chiu, I. M., Von Hehn, C. A., and Woolf, C. J. (2012). Neurogenic inflammation and the peripheral nervous system in host defense and immunopathology. Nat Neurosci, 15, 1063–1067.

Clark, A. K., Staniland, A. A., and Malcangio, M. (2011). Fractalkine/CX3CR1 signalling in chronic pain and inflammation. Curr Pharm Biotechnol, 12(10), 1707–1714.

Copray, J. C., Mantingh, I., Brouwer, N., Biber, K., Küst, B. M., Liem, R. S., et al. (2001). Expression of interleukin-1 beta in rat dorsal root ganglia. Curr Pharm Biotechnol, 118(2), 203–211.

Costigan, M., Moss, A., Latremoliere, A., Johnston, C., Verma-Gandhu, M., Herbert T. A., et al. (2009). T-cell infiltration and signaling in the adult dorsal spinal cord is a major contributor to neuropathic pain-like hypersensitivity. J Neurosci, 29(46), 14415–14422. doi:10.1523/JNEUROSCI.4569-09.2009.

Costigan, M., Scholz, J., and Woolf, C. J. (2009). Neuropathic pain: a maladaptive response of the nervous system to damage. Annu Rev Neurosci, 32, 1–32. doi:10.1146/annurev.neuro.051508.135531.

Coull, J. A. M., Beggs, S., Boudreau, D., Boivin D., Tsuda, M., Inoue, K., et al. (2005). BDNF from microglia causes the shift in neuronal anion gradient underlying neuropathic pain. Nature, 438(7070), 1017–1021. doi:10.1038/nature04223.

Coull, J. A. M., Boudreau, D., Bachand, K., Prescott, S. A, Nault, F., Sík, A., et al. (2003). Trans-synaptic shift in anion gradient in spinal lamina I neurons as a mechanism of neuropathic pain. *Nature*, 424(6951), 938–942. doi:10.1038/nature01868.

Davalos, D., Grutzendler, J., Yang, G., Kim, J. V., Zuo, Y., Jung, S., et al. (2005). ATP mediates rapid microglial response to local brain injury in vivo. *Nat Neurosci*, 8(6), 752–758. doi:10.1038/nn1472.

DeLeo, J. A., Colburn, R. W., Nichols, M., and Malhotra, A. (1996). Interleukin-6-mediated hyperalgesia/allodynia and increased spinal IL-6 expression in a rat mononeuropathy model. *J Interferon Cytokine Res*, 16(9), 695–700.

Durrenberger, P. F., Facer, P., Casula, M. A., Yiangou, Y., Gray, R. A., Chessell, I. P., et al. (2006). Prostanoid receptor EP1 and Cox-2 in injured human nerves and a rat model of nerve injury: a time-course study. *BMC Neurol*, 6, 1. doi:10.1186/1471-2377-6-1.

Fadel, S. and Sarzotti, M. (2000). Cellular immune responses in neonates. *Int Rev Immunol*, 19(2–3), 173–193.

Fitzgerald, M. (2005). The development of nociceptive circuits. *Nat Rev Neurosci*, 6(7), 507–520. doi:10.1038/nrn1701.

Fitzgerald, M., Butcher, T., and Shortland, P. (1994). Developmental changes in the laminar termination of a fibre cutaneous sensory afferents in the rat spinal cord dorsal horn. *J Comp Neurol*, 348(2), 225–233. doi:10.1002/cne.903480205.

Gabay, E., Wolf, G., Shavit, Y., Yirmiya, R., and Tal, M. (2011). Chronic blockade of interleukin-1 (IL-1) prevents and attenuates neuropathic pain behavior and spontaneous ectopic neuronal activity following nerve injury. *Eur J Pain*, 15(3), 242–248. doi:10.1016/j.ejpain.2010.07.012.

Galiano, M., Liu Z. Q., Kalla, R., Bohatschek, M., Koppius, A., Gschwendtner, A., et al. (2001). Interleukin (IL6) and cellular response to facial nerve injury: effects on lymphocyte recruitment, early microglial activation and axonal outgrowth in IL6-deficient mice. *Eur J Neurosci*, 14(2), 327–341.

Gao, X., Kim, H. K., Chung, J. M., and Chung, K. (2005). Enhancement of NMDA receptor phosphorylation of the spinal dorsal horn and nucleus gracilis neurons in neuropathic rats. *Pain*, 116(1–2), 62–72. doi:10.1016/j.pain.2005.03.045.

Gao, Y.-J., and Ji, R.-R. (2009). c-Fos and pERK, which is a better marker for neuronal activation and central sensitization after noxious stimulation and tissue injury? *Open Pain J*, 2, 11–17. doi:10.2174/1876386300902010011.

Gao, Y.-J., and Ji, R.-R. (2010). Chemokines, neuronal-glial interactions, and central processing of neuropathic pain. *Pharmacol Ther*, 126(1), 56–68. doi:10.1016/j.pharmthera.2010.01.002.

Giaume, C., Kirchhoff, F., Matute, C., Reichenbach, A., and Verkhratsky, A. (2007). Glia: the fulcrum of brain diseases. *Cell Death Differ*, 14(7), 1324–1335. doi:10.1038/sj.cdd.4402144.

Ginhoux, F., Greter, M., Leboeuf, M., Nandi, S., See, P., Gokhan, S., et al. (2010). Fate mapping analysis reveals that adult microglia derive from primitive macrophages. *Science*, 330(6005), 841–845. doi:10.1126/science.1194637.

Gordon, S. and Taylor, P. R. (2005). Monocyte and macrophage heterogeneity. *Nat Rev Immunol*, 5(12), 953–964. doi:10.1038/nri1733.

Grothe, C., Heese, K., Meisinger, C., Wewetzer, K., Kunz, D., Cattini, P., et al. (2000). Expression of interleukin-6 and its receptor in the sciatic nerve and cultured schwann cells: relation to 18-kD fibroblast growth factor-2. *Brain Res*, 885(2), 172–181.

Hanisch, U.-K. (2002). Microglia as a source and target of cytokines. *Glia*, 40(2), 140–155. doi:10.1002/glia.10161.

Haynes, S. E., Hollopeter, G., Yang, G., Kurpius, D., Dailey, M. E., Gan, W.-B., et al. (2006). The P2Y12 receptor regulates microglial activation by extracellular nucleotides. *Nat Neurosci*, 9(12), 1512–1519. doi:10.1038/nn1805.

Hensch, T. K. (2004). Critical period regulation. *Annu Rev Neurosci*, 27, 549–579. doi:10.1146/annurev.neuro.27.070203.144327.

Howard, R. F., Walker, S. M., Mota, P. M., and Fitzgerald, M. (2005). The ontogeny of neuropathic pain: postnatal onset of mechanical allodynia in rat spared nerve injury (SNI) and chronic constriction injury (CCI) models. *Pain*, 115(3), 382–389. doi:10.1016/j.pain.2005.03.016.

Hu P., Bembrick, A. L., Keay, K. A., and McLachlan, E. M. (2007). Immune cell involvement in dorsal root ganglia and spinal cord after chronic constriction or transection of the rat sciatic nerve. *Brain Behav Immun*, 21(5), 599–616.

Hu, P. and McLachlan, E. M. (2002). Macrophage and lymphocyte invasion of dorsal root ganglia after peripheral nerve lesions in the rat. *Neuroscience*, 112(1), 23–38.

Hu, P. and McLachlan, E. M. (2003). Distinct functional types of macrophage in dorsal root ganglia and spinal nerves proximal to sciatic and spinal nerve transections in the rat. *Exp Neurol*, 184(2), 590–605. doi:10.1016/S0014-4886(03)00307-8.

Hughes, P. M., Botham, M. S., Frentzel, S., Mir, A., and Perry, V. H. (2002). Expression of fractalkine (CX3CL1) and its receptor, CX3CR1, during acute and chronic inflammation in the rodent CNS. *Glia*, 37(4), 314–327.

Jana, M., Dasgupta, S., Saha, R. N., Liu, X., and Pahan, K. (2003). Induction of tumor necrosis factor-alpha (TNF-alpha) by interleukin-12 P40 monomer and homodimer in microglia and macrophages. *J Neurochem*, 86(2), 519–528.

Jeon, S.-M., Sung, J.-K., and Cho, H.-J. (2011). Expression of monocyte chemoattractant protein-1 and its induction by tumor necrosis factor receptor 1 in sensory neurons in the ventral rhizotomy model of neuropathic pain. *Neuroscience*, 190, 354–366. doi:10.1016/j.neuroscience.2011.06.036.

Ji, R.-R., Gereau 4th, R. W., Malcangio, M., and Strichartz, G. R. (2009). MAP kinase and pain. *Brain Res Rev*, 60(1), 135–148. doi:10.1016/j.brainresrev.2008.12.011.

Ji, R.-R. and Strichartz, G. (2004). Cell signaling and the genesis of neuropathic pain. *Sci STKE*, 2004(252), reE14. doi:10.1126/stke.2522004re14.

Ji, R.-R. and Suter, M. R. (2007). P38 MAPK, microglial signaling, and neuropathic pain. *Mol Pain*, 3, 33. doi:10.1186/1744-8069-3-33.

Jin, S.-X., Zhuang, Z.-Y., Woolf, C. J., and Ji, R.-R. (2003). P38 mitogen-activated protein kinase is activated after a spinal nerve ligation in spinal cord microglia and dorsal root ganglion neurons and contributes to the generation of neuropathic pain. *J Neurosci*, 23(10), 4017–4022.

Kawasaki, Y., Zhang, L., Cheng, J.-K., and Ji, R.-R. (2008). Cytokine mechanisms of central sensitization: distinct and overlapping role of interleukin-1beta, interleukin-6, and tumor necrosis factor-alpha in regulating synaptic and neuronal activity in the superficial spinal cord. *J Neurosci*, 28(20), 5189–5194. doi:10.1523/JNEUROSCI.3338-07.2008.

Kettenmann, H., Hanisch, U.-K., Noda, M., and Verkhratsky, A. (2011). Physiology of microglia. *Physiol Rev*, 91(2), 461–553. doi:10.1152/physrev.00011.2010.

Kim, D., You, B., Lim, H., and Lee, S. J. (2011). Toll-like receptor 2 contributes to chemokine gene expression and macrophage infiltration in the dorsal root ganglia after peripheral nerve injury. *Mol Pain*, 7, 74. doi:10.1186/1744-8069-7-74.

Klein, M. A., Möller, J. C., Jones, L. L., Bluethmann, H., Kreutzberg, G. W., and Raivich, G. (1997). Impaired neuroglial activation in interleukin-6 deficient mice. *Glia*, 19(3), 227–233.

Kreutzberg, G. W. (1996). Microglia: a sensor for pathological events in the CNS. *Trends Neurosci*, 19(8), 312–318.

Latrémolière, A., Mauborgne, A., Masson, J., Bourgoin, S., Kayser, V., Hamon, M., et al. (2008). Differential implication of proinflammatory cytokine interleukin-6 in the development of cephalic versus extracephalic neuropathic pain in rats. *J Neurosci*, 28(34), 8489–8501. doi:10.1523/JNEUROSCI.2552-08.2008.

Lehnardt, S., Massillon, L., Follett, P., Jensen, F. E., Ratan, R., Rosenberg, P. A., et al. (2003). Activation of innate immunity in the CNS triggers neurodegeneration through a toll-like receptor 4-dependent pathway. *Proc Natl Acad Sci U S A*, 100(14), 8514–8519. doi:10.1073/pnas.1432609100.

Lowenstein, C. J., Dinerman, J. L., and Snyder, S. H. 1994. Nitric oxide: a physiologic messenger. *Ann Intern Med*, 120(3), 227–237.

Ma, W., Chabot, J.G., Vercauteren, F., and Quirion, R. (2010). Injured nerve-derived COX2/PGE2 contributes to the maintenance of neuropathic pain in aged rats. *Neurobiol Aging*, 31(7), 1227–1237. doi:10.1016/j.neurobiolaging.2008.08.002.

Ma, W. and Quirion, R. (2008). Does COX2-dependent PGE2 play a role in neuropathic pain? *Neurosci Lett*, 437(3), 165–169. doi:10.1016/j.neulet.2008.02.072.

Masuda, T., Tsuda, M., Yoshinaga, R., Tozaki-Saitoh, H., Ozato, K., Tamura, T., *et al.* (2012). IRF8 is a critical transcription factor for transforming microglia into a reactive phenotype. *Cell Rep*, 1(4), 334–340. doi:10.1016/j.celrep.2012.02.014.

Matsumoto, M., Xie, W., Ma, L., and Ueda, H. (2008). Pharmacological switch in Abeta-fiber stimulation-induced spinal transmission in mice with partial sciatic nerve injury. *Mol Pain*, 4, 25. doi:10.1186/1744-8069-4-25.

Michaelis, M., Vogel, C., Blenk, K. H., Arnarson, A., and Jänig, W. (1998). Inflammatory mediators sensitize acutely axotomized nerve fibers to mechanical stimulation in the rat. *J Neurosci*, 18(18), 7581–7587.

Milligan, E., Zapata, V., Schoeniger, D., Chacur, M., Green, P., Poole, S., *et al.* (2005). An initial investigation of spinal mechanisms underlying pain enhancement induced by fractalkine, a neuronally released chemokine. *Eur J Neurosci*, 22(11), 2775–2782. doi:10.1111/j.1460-9568.2005.04470.x.

Mitchell, K., Bates, B. D., Keller, J. M., Lopez, M., Scholl, L., Navarro, J., *et al.* (2010). Ablation of rat TRPV1-expressing Adelta/C-fibers with resiniferatoxin: analysis of withdrawal behaviors, recovery of function and molecular correlates. *Mol Pain*, 6, 94. doi:10.1186/1744-8069-6-94.

Moalem, G. and Tracey, D. J. (2006). Immune and inflammatory mechanisms in neuropathic pain. *Brain Res Rev*, 51(2), 240–264. doi:10.1016/j.brainresrev.2005.11.004.

Mollace, V., Muscoli, C., Rotiroti, D., and Nisticó, G. (1997). Spontaneous induction of nitric oxide- and prostaglandin E2-release by hypoxic astroglial cells is modulated by interleukin 1 beta. *Biochem Biophys Res Commun*, 238(3), 916–919. doi:10.1006/bbrc.1997.7155.

Moss, A., Beggs, S., Vega-Avelaira, D., Costigan, M., Hathway, G. J., Salter, M. W., *et al.* (2007). Spinal microglia and neuropathic pain in young rats. *Pain*, 128(3), 215–224. doi:10.1016/j.pain.2006.09.018.

Mosser, D. M. and Edwards, J. P. (2008). Exploring the full spectrum of macrophage activation. *Nat Rev Immunol*, 8(12), 958–969. doi:10.1038/nri2448.

Murata, Y., Rydevik, B., Nannmark, U., Larsson, K., Takahashi, K., Kato, Y., *et al.* (2011). Local application of interleukin-6 to the dorsal root ganglion induces tumor necrosis factor-α in the dorsal root ganglion and results in apoptosis of the dorsal root ganglion cells. *Spine*, 36(12), 926–932. doi:10.1097/BRS.0b013e3181e7f4a9.

Nakajima, K. and Kohsaka, S. (1998). [Microglia: function in the pathological state]. *Nō to Shinkei*, 50(1), 5–16.

Nimmerjahn, A., Kirchhoff, F., and Helmchen, F. (2005). Resting microglial cells are highly dynamic surveillants of brain parenchyma in vivo. *Science*, 308(5726), 1314–1318. doi:10.1126/science.1110647.

O'Brien, J. J. and Nathanson, N. M. (2007). Retrograde activation of STAT3 by leukemia inhibitory factor in sympathetic neurons. *J Neurochem*, 103(1), 288–302. doi:10.1111/j.1471-4159.2007.04736.x.

O'Rielly, D. D. and Loomis, C. W. (2006). Increased expression of cyclooxygenase and nitric oxide isoforms, and exaggerated sensitivity to prostaglandin E2, in the rat lumbar spinal cord 3 days after L5-L6 spinal nerve ligation. *Anesthesiology*, 104(2), 328–337.

Ozaktay, A. C., Kallakuri, S., Takebayashi, T., Cavanaugh, J. M., Asik, I., DeLeo, J. A., *et al.* (2006). Effects of interleukin-1 beta, interleukin-6, and tumor necrosis factor on sensitivity of dorsal root ganglion and peripheral receptive fields in rats. *Eur Spine J*, 15(10), 1529–1537. doi:10.1007/s00586-005-0058-8.

Perry, V. H. (2010). Contribution of systemic inflammation to chronic neurodegeneration. *Acta Neuropathol*, 120, 277–286.

Pont-Lezica, L., Béchade, C., Belarif-Cantaut, Y., Pascual, O., and Bessis, A. (2011). Physiological roles of microglia during development. *J Neurochem*, 119(5), 901–908. doi:10.1111/j.1471-4159.2011.07504.x.

Purwata, T. E. (2011). High TNF-alpha plasma levels and macrophages iNOS and TNF-alpha expression as risk factors for painful diabetic neuropathy. *J Pain Res*, 4, 169–175. doi:10.2147/JPR.S21751.

Qiu, J., Cafferty, W. B. J., McMahon, S. B., and Thompson, S. W. N. (2005). Conditioning injury-induced spinal axon regeneration requires signal transducer and activator of transcription 3 activation. *J Neurosci*, 25(7), 1645–1653. doi:10.1523/JNEUROSCI.3269-04.2005.

Raghavendra, V., Tanga, F., and DeLeo, J. A. (2003). Inhibition of microglial activation attenuates the development but not existing hypersensitivity in a rat model of neuropathy. *J Pharmacol Exp Ther*, 306(2), 624–630. doi:10.1124/jpet.103.052407.

Reeve, A. J., Patel, S., Fox, A., Walker, K., and Urban, L. (2000). Intrathecally administered endotoxin or cytokines produce allodynia, hyperalgesia and changes in spinal cord neuronal responses to nociceptive stimuli in the rat. *Eur J Pain*, 4(3), 247–257. doi:10.1053/eujp.2000.0177.

Ren, K., Anseloni, V., Zou, S.-P., Wade, E.-B., Novikova, S.-I., Ennis, M., *et al.* (2004). Characterization of basal and re-inflammation-associated long-term alteration in pain responsivity following short-lasting neonatal local inflammatory insult. *Pain*, 110(3), 588–596. doi:10.1016/j.pain.2004.04.006.

Ren, K. and Dubner, R. (2007). Pain facilitation and activity-dependent plasticity in pain modulatory circuitry: role of BDNF-TrkB signaling and NMDA receptors. *Mol Neurobiol*, 35(3), 224–235.

Ririe, D. G. and Eisenach, J. C. (2006). Age-dependent responses to nerve injury-induced mechanical allodynia. *Anesthesiology*, 104(2), 344–350.

Sanes, D. H. and Bao, S. (2009). Tuning up the developing auditory CNS. *Curr Opin Neurobiol*, 19(2), 188–199. doi:10.1016/j.conb.2009.05.014.

Schäfers, M., Svensson, C. I., Sommer, C., and Sorkin, L. S. (2003). Tumor necrosis factor-alpha induces mechanical allodynia after spinal nerve ligation by activation of P38 MAPK in primary sensory neurons. *J Neurosci*, 23(7), 2517–2521.

Scheffel, J., Regen, T., Van Rossum, D., Seifert, S., Ribes, S, Nau, R., *et al.* (2012). Toll-like receptor activation reveals developmental reorganization and unmasks responder subsets of microglia. *Glia*, 60(12), 1930–1943. doi:10.1002/glia.22409.

Schlegelmilch, T., Henke, K., and Peri, K. (2011). Microglia in the developing brain: from immunity to behaviour. *Curr Opin Neurobiol*, 21(1), 5–10. doi:10.1016/j.conb.2010.08.004.

Scholz, J. and Woolf, C. J. (2007). The neuropathic pain triad: neurons, immune cells and glia. *Nat Neurosci*, 10(11), 1361–1368. doi:10.1038/nn1992.

Segond von Banchet, G., Scholze, A., and Schaible, H.-G. (2003). Prostaglandin E2 increases the expression of the neurokinin1 receptor in adult sensory neurones in culture: a novel role of prostaglandins. *Br J Pharmacol*, 139(3), 672–680. doi:10.1038/sj.bjp.0705278.

Shehab, S. A. S., Al-Marashda, K., Al-Zahmi, A., Abdul-Kareem, A., and Al-Sultan, M. A. H. (2008). Unmyelinated primary afferents from adjacent spinal nerves intermingle in the spinal dorsal horn: a possible mechanism contributing to neuropathic pain. *Brain Res*, 1208, 111–119. doi:10.1016/j.brainres.2008.02.089.

Shields, S. D., Eckert, W.A. 3rd, and Basbaum, A. I. (2003). Spared nerve injury model of neuropathic pain in the mouse: a behavioral and anatomic analysis. *J Pain*, 4(8), 465–470.

Simpson, R. J., Hammacher, A., Smith, D. K., Matthews, J. M., and Ward, L. D. (1997). Interleukin-6: structure-function relationships. *Protein Sci*, 6(5), 929–955. doi:10.1002/pro.5560060501.

Slack, S. E., Grist, J., Mac, Q., McMahon, S. B., and Pezet, S. (2005). TrkB expression and phospho-ERK activation by brain-derived neurotrophic factor in rat spinothalamic tract neurons. *J Comp Neurol*, 489(1), 59–68. doi:10.1002/cne.20606.

Sorge, R. E., LaCroix-Fralish, M. L., Tuttle, A.H., Sotocinal, S. G., Austin, J.-S., Ritchie, J., *et al.* (2011). Spinal cord toll-like receptor 4 mediates inflammatory and neuropathic hypersensitivity in male but not female mice. *J Neurosci*, 31(43), 15450–15454. doi:10.1523/JNEUROSCI.3859-11.2011.

Spencer, S. J., Galic, M. A. and Pittman, Q. J. (2011). Neonatal programming of innate immune function. *Am J Physiol Endocrinol Metab*, 300, E11–8.

Stemkowski, P. L. and Smith, P. A. 2012. Long-term IL-1β exposure causes subpopulation-dependent alterations in rat dorsal root ganglion neuron excitability. *J Neurophysiol*, 107(6), 1586–1597. doi:10.1152/jn.00587.2011.

Stewart, C. R., Stuart, L. M., Wilkinson, K., van Gils, J. M., Deng, J., Halle, A., et al. (2010). CD36 ligands promote sterile inflammation through assembly of a toll-like receptor 4 and 6 heterodimer. *Nat Immunol*, 11(2), 155–161. doi:10.1038/ni.1836.

Suen, P. C., Wu, K., Levine, E. S., Mount, H. T., Xu, J. L., Lin, S. Y., et al. (1997). Brain-derived neurotrophic factor rapidly enhances phosphorylation of the postsynaptic N-methyl-D-aspartate receptor subunit 1. *Proc Natl Acad Sci U S A*, 94(15), 8191–8195.

Sun, S., Cao, H., Han, M., Li, T.-T., Pan, H.-L., Zhao, Z.-Q., et al. (2007). New evidence for the involvement of spinal fractalkine receptor in pain facilitation and spinal glial activation in rat model of monoarthritis. *Pain*, 129(1–2), 64–75. doi:10.1016/j.pain.2006.09.035.

Sung, C.-S., Wen, Z.-H., Chang, W.-K., Chan, K.-H., Ho, S.-T., Tsai, S.-K., et al. (2005). Inhibition of P38 mitogen-activated protein kinase attenuates interleukin-1beta-induced thermal hyperalgesia and inducible nitric oxide synthase expression in the spinal cord. *J Neurochem*, 94(3), 742–752. doi:10.1111/j.1471-4159.2005.03226.x.

Suter, M. R., Berta, T., Gao, Y.-J., Decosterd, I., and Ji, R.-R. (2009). Large A-fiber activity is required for microglial proliferation and P38 MAPK activation in the spinal cord: different effects of resiniferatoxin and bupivacaine on spinal microglial changes after spared nerve injury. *Mol Pain*, 5, 53. doi:10.1186/1744-8069-5-53.

Svensson, C. I., Marsala, M., Westerlund, A., Calcutt, N. A., Campana, W. M., Freshwater, J. D., et al. (2003). Activation of P38 mitogen-activated protein kinase in spinal microglia is a critical link in inflammation-induced spinal pain processing. *J Neurochem*, 86(6), 1534–1544.

Sweitzer, S., Martin, D., and DeLeo, J. A. (2001). Intrathecal interleukin-1 receptor antagonist in combination with soluble tumor necrosis factor receptor exhibits an anti-allodynic action in a rat model of neuropathic pain. *Neuroscience*, 103(2), 529–539.

Tanga, F. Y., Nutile-McMenemy, N., and DeLeo, J. A. (2005). The CNS role of toll-like receptor 4 in innate neuroimmunity and painful neuropathy. *Proc Natl Acad Sci U S A*, 102(16), 5856–5861. doi:10.1073/pnas.0501634102.

Thacker, M. A., Clark, A. K., Bishop, T., Grist, J., Yip, P. K., Moon, L. D. F., et al. (2009). CCL2 is a key mediator of microglia activation in neuropathic pain states. *Eur J Pain*, 13(3), 263–272. doi:10.1016/j.ejpain.2008.04.017.

Thacker, M. A., Clark, A. C., Marchand, F., and McMahon, S. B. (2007). Pathophysiology of peripheral neuropathic pain: immune cells and molecules. *Anesth Analg*, 105(3), 838–847. doi:10.1213/01.ane.0000275190.42912.37.

Trang, T., Beggs, S., Wan, X., and Salter, M. W. (2009). P2X4-receptor-mediated synthesis and release of brain-derived neurotrophic factor in microglia is dependent on calcium and P38-mitogen-activated protein kinase activation. *J Neurosci*, 29(11), 3518–3528. doi:10.1523/JNEUROSCI.5714-08.2009.

Tsuda, M., Inoue, K., and Salter, M. W. (2005). Neuropathic pain and spinal microglia: a big problem from molecules in 'small' glia. *Trends Neurosci*, 28(2), 101–107. doi:10.1016/j.tins.2004.12.002.

Tsuda, M., Masuda, T., Kitano, J., Shimoyama, H., Tozaki-Saitoh, H., and Inoue, K. (2009). IFN-gamma receptor signaling mediates spinal microglia activation driving neuropathic pain. *Proc Natl Acad Sci U S A*, 106(19), 8032–8037. doi:10.1073/pnas.0810420106.

Tsuda, M., Shigemoto-Mogami, Y., Koizumi, S., Mizokoshi, A., Kohsaka, S., Salter, M. W., et al. (2003). P2X4 receptors induced in spinal microglia gate tactile allodynia after nerve injury. *Nature*, 424(6950), 778–783. doi:10.1038/nature01786.

Tsuda, M., Toyomitsu, E., Komatsu, T., Masuda, T., Kunifusa, E., Nasu-Tada, K., et al. (2008). Fibronectin/integrin system is involved in P2X(4) receptor upregulation in the spinal cord and neuropathic pain after nerve injury. *Glia*, 56(5), 579–585. doi:10.1002/glia.20641.

Ulmann, L., Hatcher, J. P., Hughes, J. P., Chaumont, S., Green, P. J., Conquet, F., et al. (2008). Up-regulation of P2X4 receptors in spinal microglia after

peripheral nerve injury mediates BDNF release and neuropathic pain. *J Neurosci*, 28(44), 11263–11268. doi:10.1523/JNEUROSCI.2308-08.2008.

Vega-Avelaira, D., Géranton, S., and Fitzgerald, M. (2009). Differential regulation of immune responses and macrophage/neuron interactions in the dorsal root ganglion in young and adult rats following nerve injury. *Mol Pain*, 5(1), 70. doi:10.1186/1744-8069-5-70.

Vega-Avelaira, D., McKelvey, R., Hathway, G., and Fitzgerald, M. (2012). The emergence of adolescent onset pain hypersensitivity following neonatal nerve injury. *Mol Pain*, 8, 30. doi:10.1186/1744-8069-8-30.

Vega-Avelaira, D., Moss, A., and Fitzgerald, M. (2007). Age-related changes in the spinal cord microglial and astrocytic response profile to nerve injury. *Brain Behav Immun*, 21(5), 617–623. doi:10.1016/j.bbi.2006.10.007.

Verge, G. M., Milligan, E. D., Maier, S. F., Watkins, L. R., Naeve, G. S., and Foster, A. C. (2004). Fractalkine (CX3CL1) and fractalkine receptor (CX3CR1) distribution in spinal cord and dorsal root ganglia under basal and neuropathic pain conditions. *Eur J Neurosci*, 20(5), 1150–1160. doi:10.1111/j.1460-9568.2004.03593.x.

Von Banchet, G. S., Fischer, N., Uhlig, B., Hensellek, S., Eitner, A., and Schaible, H.-G. (2011). Molecular effects of interleukin-1β on dorsal root ganglion neurons: prevention of ligand-induced internalization of the bradykinin 2 receptor and downregulation of G protein-coupled receptor kinase 2. *Moll Cell Neurosci*, 46(1), 262–271. doi:10.1016/j.mcn.2010.09.009.

Walker, S. M., Tochiki, K. K., and Fitzgerald, M. (2009). Hindpaw incision in early life increases the hyperalgesic response to repeat surgical injury: critical period and dependence on initial afferent activity. *Pain*, 147, 99–106.

Wang, X.-J., Kong, K.-K., Qi, W.-L., Ye, W.-L., and Song, P.-S. (2005). Interleukin-1 beta induction of neuron apoptosis depends on P38 mitogen-activated protein kinase activity after spinal cord injury. *Acta Pharmacol Sin*, 26(8), 934–942. doi:10.1111/j.1745-7254.2005.00152.x.

Watkins, L. R., Milligan, E. D., and Maier, S. F. (2001). Glial activation: a driving force for pathological pain. *Trends Neurosci*, 24(8), 450–455.

Watkins, L. R. and Maier, S. F. (2002). Beyond neurons: evidence that immune and glial cells contribute to pathological pain states. *Physiol Rev*, 82(4), 981–1011. doi:10.1152/physrev.00011.2002.

Wilms, H., Rosenstiel, P., Sievers, J., Deuschl, G., Zecca, L., and Lucius, R. (2003). Activation of microglia by human neuromelanin is NF-kappaB dependent and involves P38 mitogen-activated protein kinase: implications for Parkinson's disease. *FASEB J*, 17(3), 500–502. doi:10.1096/fj.02-0314fje.

Wolf, G., Gabay, E., Tal, M., Yirmiya, R., and Shavit, Y. (2006). Genetic impairment of interleukin-1 signaling attenuates neuropathic pain, autotomy, and spontaneous ectopic neuronal activity, following nerve injury in mice. *Pain*, 120(3), 315–324. doi:10.1016/j.pain.2005.11.011.

Zhang, J., Shi, X. Q., Echeverry, S., Mogil, J. S., De Koninck, Y., and Rivest, S. (2007). Expression of CCR2 in both resident and bone marrow-derived microglia plays a critical role in neuropathic pain. *J Neurosci*, 27(45), 12396–12406. doi:10.1523/JNEUROSCI.3016-07.2007.

Zhang, P.-L., Levy, A. M., Ben-Simchon, L., Haggiag, S., Chebath, J., and Revel, M. (2007). Induction of neuronal and myelin-related gene expression by IL-6-receptor/IL-6: a study on embryonic dorsal root ganglia cells and isolated schwann cells. *Exp Neurol*, 208(2), 285–296. doi:10.1016/j.expneurol.2007.08.022.

Zhang, X. and Mosser, D. M. (2008). Macrophage activation by endogenous danger signals. *J Pathol*, 214(2), 161–178. doi:10.1002/path.2284.

Zhuang, Z.-Y., Gerner, P., Woolf, C. J., and Ji, R.-R. (2005). ERK is sequentially activated in neurons, microglia, and astrocytes by spinal nerve ligation and contributes to mechanical allodynia in this neuropathic pain model. *Pain*, 114(1–2), 149–159. doi:10.1016/j.pain.2004.12.022.

Zhuang, Z.-Y., Kawasaki, Y., Tan, P.-H., Wen, Y.-R., Huang, J., and Ji, R.-R. (2007). Role of the CX3CR1/p38 MAPK pathway in spinal microglia for the development of neuropathic pain following nerve injury-induced cleavage of fractalkine. *Brain Behav Immun*, 21(5), 642–651. doi:10.1016/j.bbi.2006.11.003.

CHAPTER 8

Central nociceptive pathways and descending modulation

Maria Fitzgerald

Summary

Infants and children respond to noxious stimulation from birth, but these responses arise from neural activity at different levels of the central nervous system. Nociceptive activity at the level of the spinal cord or brainstem can produce reflex movements, autonomic and metabolic responses that may parallel pain, but cannot be equated with true pain experience. The key to pain experience lies in neural activation of central regions of the brain responsible for sensory discrimination and emotional responses. Thus higher centres in the brain allow noxious events to be discriminated from innocuous ones and create a sense of unpleasantness and threat. Laboratory and clinical studies are building up a picture of the functional connections in regions of the brain concerned with sensory and emotional aspects of pain at different stages of infant and child development. There is also increasing understanding of the maturation of endogenous control systems generated by the brain, which are likely to determine a child's ability to cope with pain. Furthermore, evidence is increasing that excess noxious stimulation in early life can alter the course of development of both central nociceptive pathways and descending modulation of pain.

Introduction

Pain has many dimensions and is processed at multiple different levels of the nervous system. When tissue is injured in young individuals, it is essential that nociceptive pathways in the peripheral and central nervous system (CNS) are activated to stimulate protective behaviour and alert the attention of caregivers. Thus noxious stimulation stimulates reflex motor responses through circuits in the spinal cord and brainstem to ensure that the affected body region is protected from harm. In addition, autonomic circuits in the brainstem and hypothalamus are activated, to produce appropriate changes in the cardiovascular, respiratory, and endocrine systems and maintain homeostatic control of the body. It is these reactions that form the basis of paediatric clinical pain scores that measure movement, facial expression, cry, and other physiological indicators.

However, of great importance is not only the sensory discriminative, but also the emotional or affective component of pain, and the fact that it has a uniquely unpleasant and stressful quality and the potential to cause great suffering. As soon as a child is old enough for self-report, researchers and clinicians attempt to score the unpleasantness as well as the intensity of pain experience in order to better understand and alleviate the pain. The key to the maturation of this complete pain experience lies in neural activation of central subcortical and cortical regions of the brain and neuroscientists aim to map the nociceptive output from the spinal cord as it projects through ascending pathways, brainstem, and subcortical structures to the cerebral cortex and to investigate how different regions of the brain concerned with sensory and emotional aspects of pain become activated at different stages of infant and child development.

Another key determinant of pain experience is the activation of endogenous control mechanisms within the CNS that can modulate nociceptive activity through the release of endogenous opioids and a powerful system of pathways descending from the brainstem to the spinal cord. These descending and endogenous pain modulatory pathways are themselves controlled by subcortical and cortical networks and are the route by which factors such as attention and distraction, suggestion and expectation, stress and anxiety, context and past experience, can influence pain experience. Understanding the neural basis of developing endogenous descending pain control is as important as understanding ascending pain pathways, as this will influence a child's ability to cope with pain and the extent to which it may be manipulated.

Finally, the plasticity of these CNS pain pathways in infants and children is of great clinical importance. The formation of correct connections in sensory regions of the brain is highly dependent on an appropriate balance of sensory input from the periphery, and excessive noxious stimulation in childhood may alter the formation of cortical pain connections through neural activity-dependent mechanisms. Importantly, it may also change the normal balance of descending endogenous pain control, leaving an individual less able to cope with pain in the future.

In this chapter, the current state of knowledge of the development of central nociceptive pathways and descending controls is reviewed. Information has been gathered from laboratory studies in animal models and clinical and experimental investigations in infants and children. The picture is far from complete but this is a fast moving and important area of research.

The developmental anatomy and physiology of central pain pathways

The development and maturation of neural connections in the brain are commonly mapped in the laboratory animals using anatomical, electrophysiological and behavioural techniques, and more recently, optogenetic stimulation of genetically controlled light-sensitive neurons. Knowledge gained from the laboratory can be combined with human data, from traditional autopsy studies and more recently, neurophysiological recording and imaging of the living human brain using structural and functional magnetic resonance imaging (fMRI) to provide an overall picture of the maturation of a particular pathway.

Changing output from the spinal dorsal horn

Nociceptive information from the periphery is first integrated in the dorsal horn of the spinal cord (for the body) and trigeminal nuclei (for the head and neck). Multiple sensory afferent nerve fibres, carrying information from the skin, muscle, joints, deep tissues, and organs synapse onto single dorsal horn neurons resulting in spatial and modality convergence. Receptive fields of single dorsal horn neurons are larger and more overlapping than those of primary afferents, and multiple sensory modalities, such as touch and pinch, are processed by single 'wide dynamic range' (WDR) cells. However, there are also a smaller number of 'nociceptive-specific' (NS) cells in the dorsal horn that receive information only from nociceptive afferents. The vast majority of dorsal horn neurons are interneurons, connecting locally with other neurons in the same segment of the spinal cord, but a small percentage (c.5%), both WDR and NS, are 'projection' cells, that have long axons that travel up the spinal cord to higher centres in the CNS. Thus nociceptive information is transmitted partly by so-called 'labelled lines' devoted solely to nociception, and partly by multimodal pathways, where nociceptive information is coded by spatial and temporal patterns of neuronal activity.

Importantly, the proportion of WDR and NS neurons changes substantially with postnatal age (Fitzgerald and Jennings, 1999). The neonatal dorsal horn is dominated by low-threshold, tactile inputs and although WDR and NS cells responding to nociceptive input can be recorded in the newborn rat dorsal horn, numbers are low in the first week and build up slowly (see Table 8.1).

Activity in dorsal horn networks ensure that spinal projection neurons transmit information to higher centres that is already substantially altered from the original afferent nociceptive input. Thus noxious information may have already been dampened down or amplified in magnitude and duration, through local interneuronal activity and central sensitization mechanisms both of which differ in young and adult animals (see Walker and Baccei, Chapter 6, this volume). It may also be modulated by descending inhibitory or excitatory influences arising in the brainstem that also change through postnatal development (see 'The development of descending brainstem modulation of nociception' section).

Ascending spinal nociceptive projection pathways and cortical pain processing in adults

The cell bodies of dorsal horn projection neurons are found in superficial lamina I and deeper laminae VI to V and their long axons travel up the spinal cord in the contralateral spinothalamic tract (STT). Since the STT arises from WDR and NS cells, this tract does not exclusively transmit nociceptive information but also low-threshold tactile information and temperature sense. The thalamus is a major sensory integration centre and the information that thalamic neurons receive and send on to the cerebral cortex through thalamocortical tracts is essential for the awareness of pain. Nevertheless, it should be remembered that only 10% of STT axons directly terminate in the thalamus. Thus, while the classic termination site of STT axons in the ventral posterior nucleus (VPn) and other sensory nuclei in the thalamus (collectively called the ventrobasal complex) are commonly emphasized, most STT fibres also project to the brainstem reticular formation including the periaqueductal grey (PAG), the parabrachial nucleus (PBn), the locus coeruleus, and the hypothalamus (Gauriau and Bernard, 2004; Todd 2010).

The importance of these different pathways lies in the information that they subserve. Thus it appears that there is an anatomical basis for separating the sensory or nociceptive aspects of pain from its emotional or unpleasant aspects. Recent research has focused upon the projections of NS neurons in lamina I. Direct projections to thalamus are thought to mediate the sensory discriminative aspects of pain, while projections to the PAG and to the PBn, which in turn project to the hypothalamus and amygdala, are thought to mediate the emotional and autonomic aspects of pain.

Table 8.1 Postnatal change in the proportion of rat dorsal horn cell responding to cutaneous noxious pinch, non-noxious brush or both (P = postnatal days).

Age	Dorsal horn cell response		
	Brush	Pinch	Brush and pinch
P3 (n = 22)	20 (91%)	1 (4.5%)	1 (4.5%)
P6 (n = 65)	54 (83%)	7 (11%)	4 (16%)
P10 (n = 53)	22 (42%)	12 (22%)	19 (36%)
P21 (n = 35)	10 (29%)	5 (14%)	20 (57%)

The output from the thalamus also appears to divide into two projections, a lateral and medial stream. While the lateral stream emanates from the thalamic ventroposterolateral nucleus (VPL) and projects directly to the primary somatosensory cortex (SI), a key cortical region for the sensory aspects of pain experience, the medial stream arises in the medial dorsal thalamic nuclei and projects to the secondary somatosensory cortex (SII) and the anterior cingulate and may contribute to the emotional aspects of pain (Willis et al., 2002).

Importantly, there is no 'pain' cortex, analogous to the visual or auditory cortex, rather noxious stimulation evokes a characteristic pattern of activity in many brain areas, including somatosensory, insular, and cingulate areas, as well as frontal and parietal areas. Coordinated activity in a collection of brain regions, none of which are unique to pain, are proposed to result in the multidimensional perception of pain. Other brain regions may be recruited to increase or reduce the intensity and unpleasantness of the pain in certain circumstances or in certain individuals (Apkarian et al., 2005; Tracey and Mantyh, 2007; Tracey and Johns, 2010). This is a rapidly changing area of pain research, however, with some controversy (LeGrain et al., 2011).

The development of ascending spinal nociceptive projection pathways to brainstem and thalamus

STT neurons develop before birth in rodents: embryonic-day (E)-18, 2-day-old, and 1-week-old mice do not differ from adults in the number or distribution of STT neurons back-labelled from the thalamus although they significantly increase in size over the first postnatal week. Arborizations and boutons of STT neurons can also be observed within the ventrobasal complex of neonatal thalamus, suggesting that synaptic connections are formed with thalamic cells at this very early age (Davidson et al., 2010).

However, while anatomical connections to the thalamus may be present early in development, the functional maturation of nociceptive inputs to these regions is slower. The neural activity in subcortical brain areas has been mapped following formalin-induced injury to the paw using the neural activity marker, fos, in the brain of fetal and infant rats. By day 3, formalin evoked fos expression in the ventral lateral medulla (the site of origin of descending control pathways to the spinal cord), but not in subcortical areas responsible for signalling sensory and emotional information (namely the paraventricular and medial dorsal nuclei of the thalamus, the hypothalamus, and the PAG) which were all clearly labelled by 14 days of age (Barr, 2011). This developmental pattern may be related not only to the maturation of pain perception but also to development of autonomic and defensive reactions to pain in the infant (Chan et al., 2011).

Little is known about the development of the ascending STTs to the brainstem and thalamus in man although their presence is inferred from cortical activity in preterm infants (see later). Changes in facial expression in response to noxious stimulation are observed in extremely preterm infants, even in the presence of cerebral injury, suggesting direct functional nociceptive connections from the spinal cord to the brainstem at a very early age (Oberlander et al., 2002). Non-invasive diffusion tensor MRI and tractography in 1-to 4-month-old healthy infants show the spinothalamic tract and the corticospinal tract to be among the most mature bundles, while the most immature tracts are the internal capsule and cingulum (Dubois et al., 2008).

The development of thalamocortical connections—rodents

While nociceptive activity in the spinal cord, brainstem, and subcortical midbrain structures are sufficient to generate reflex behaviours, autonomic and hormonal responses, they are not sufficient to support pain perception and awareness. Understanding the maturation of pain perception requires the study of supraspinal brain centres especially at the cortical level during early life.

A key step in the cortical processing of noxious stimuli is the development of thalamocortical projections. In rodents, thalamic axons leave the thalamus at E13.5 and begin to grow towards the subplate (SP) neurons, which are among the first born cortical neurons and reside at the white matter/cortical plate boundary. The SP zone, marginal zone, and cortical plate represent the early structures from which the layers of the cerebral cortex develop; the SP is largely transient, and the marginal zone forms layer I and cortical plate neurons form layers II to VI. Thalamocortical projections appear to exit the thalamus by E16 and form their first functional synaptic connections in the SP region around E18 to E19. By birth, thalamic axons are extending into layers IV, V, and VI of the developing cortex in a topographically precise manner and thalamocortical afferents and cortical sensory areas settle into place in the first week after birth. The refinement of topographical projections from the thalamus to the cortex is thought to arise through an activity-dependent process in which thalamic axons compete for cortical targets. If activity is altered during a critical period in early development, normal connectivity is disrupted. Synaptic connections are strengthened during development by correlated pre- and postsynaptic activity, and a likely mechanism for this process is N-methyl-D-aspartate receptor-dependent long-term potentiation (Li and Crair 2011). Cortical synaptic circuitry develops rapidly in the second postnatal week, simultaneous with experience-dependent turnover of dendritic spines. Patterned neuronal activity, such as spindle bursts in the neonatal cortex, promote the maturation of cortical synapses and neuronal circuits. Selective removal of SP neurons in the limb region of the somatosensory S1 cortex abolishes endogenous and sensory-evoked spindle burst activity and weakens thalamocortical inputs to layer 4 neurons. Thus, SP neurons are crucially involved in the generation of early network activity in the neonatal cortex, which is an important feature of cortical development (Tolner et al., 2012).

The maturation of transmission from thalamocortical connections takes place over a prolonged postnatal period. Thus a clear somatosensory-evoked potential from stimulation of the forepaw is not recorded until the end of the first week of life in rats and does not acquire a recognizably adult pattern until postnatal day (P) 12 (Thairu, 1971). An investigation of single cells in 7-day-old rat primary somatosensory cortex revealed low levels of spontaneous activity compared to adults and diminished excitability and longer latencies to cutaneous stimulation than in adults. In addition, receptive fields were considerably larger at 7 days, which reduces spatial discrimination. In contrast to adult cells, the immature cells commonly responded cyclically, with alternating phases of increased and decreased firing rate for periods of up to 3 s following punctate stimulation (Armstrong-James, 1975).

More complex functions in the cortex require linked activity in several areas, such as the pain matrix, carried out by large-scale neuronal networks integrating several cortical areas. Little is known about the functional development of these networks and the maturational processes by which distant networks become functionally connected. Recordings across the whole cortical surface together with intracortical electrodes, reveals that sensory evoked cortical responses mature continuously throughout the first 3 weeks with the strongest developmental changes occurring in a very short time around postnatal day 13 (P13) (Quairiaux et al., 2011). This period, at the end of the second postnatal week coincides with the onset of mature pain behaviour (Fitzgerald, 2005), as well as major synaptic and functional changes within the S1 cortex.

The neural circuitry of the medial prefrontal cortex (mPFC), an area of the brain that is key to assessing the threat of sensory stimuli and generating defensive responses, progressively develops more capacities as the animal matures. When rats are exposed to a threatening stimulus at P14, the mPFC is neither active nor responsive, but becomes responsive in processing aversive sensory stimulation at P26, and only finally regulates freezing in adolescence at P38 to P42 days (Chan et al., 2011).

The development of thalamocortical connections—humans

The growth of thalamocortical afferents has been well documented in the human brain (Kostovic and Judas, 2010). In infants younger than 24 gestational weeks (GW), thalamocortical afferents are 'waiting' in a transient SP zone. These axons then penetrate the cortical plate between 24 and 26 GW and form functional synapses with layer IV cortical neurons beginning at 29 GW. The SP region gradually dissolves between 33 to 35 GW and after 36 GW there is a substantial growth and maturation of associative and callosal connections in the cortex (see Figure 8.1).

Results from a systematic fMRI study on mainly sedated preterm infants are consistent with the anatomical data and demonstrate well-localized blood oxygen level-dependent (BOLD) signal activity in the SI in response to balloon inflation of the hand in infants aged 25.5 to 34 GW. In this preterm group, positive BOLD activity to this proprioceptive and tactile stimulus was seen in the contralateral hemisphere only, while in preterm infants studied at term-corrected gestational age (36.5–41.5 weeks GA), the spatial distribution of the response was more complex with bilateral activity, and additional adjacent areas of negative BOLD signal change in the contralateral primary somatosensory and motor cortices. The results suggest that thalamocortical synapses carrying tactile information are functional by 25.5 weeks but more complex intra- and interhemispheric projections are not active until after 34 weeks GA (Arichi et al., 2010).

Functional connectivity magnetic resonance imaging (fcMRI) utilizes spontaneous, low-frequency (<0.1 Hz), coherent fluctuations in the BOLD signal to identify networks of functional cerebral connections and promises to be useful for mapping the development of key connections in the brain. Such mapping indicates that cortical hubs of connectivity in the newborn infant brain are largely targeted in the primary sensorimotor, auditory, and visual systems and only to a small extent in higher-order frontal, associative cortex (Fransson et al., 2011). However, the immature brain displays spontaneous patterns of electrical activity not seen in adults which may not be precursors of the spontaneous neuronal activity that forms

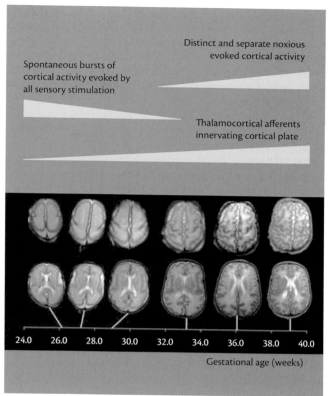

Figure 8.1 The development of thalamocortical input and the changing pattern of somatosensory evoked activity in the human infant cortex over 24 to 40 weeks' gestation.

resting state networks in the adult; therefore fcMRI in this age group should be interpreted with care (Colonnese and Khasipov, 2012; see also Poorun and Slater, Chapter 39, this volume).

The development of cortical pain processing

Advances in our knowledge of the onset of cortical pain processing in human infants and children have come through the application of imaging and electroencephalographic (EEG) measurements during clinical noxious procedures or in the presence of chronic pain.

Measurements of cerebral oxygenation have demonstrated that brief noxious stimulation (in the form of a heel lance for routine blood sampling) evokes a clear response in the contralateral somatosensory cortex of infants from 25 weeks postmenstrual age. Importantly, this cortical response is modality-specific, as non-noxious stimulation of the heel failed to evoke the response even when accompanied by a withdrawal reflex (Slater et al., 2006). Noxious inputs of longer duration may result in bilateral activation of the somatosensory cortex (Bartocci et al., 2006). These haemodynamic responses, which reflect a localized increase in total haemoglobin concentration, are caused by increased neuronal activity within the same area, as time-locked EEG recordings have demonstrated that the heel lance also evokes a clear nociceptive-specific potential in the infant cortex (Slater et al., 2010a). Furthermore EEG recording of noxious-evoked activity in infants of different gestational ages has revealed how the brain begins to distinguish noxious information from innocuous tactile stimulation in early life (Fabrizi et al., 2011). Recording the brain neuronal activity in response to time-locked touches and clinically essential noxious lances of the heel in infants aged 28 to 45 weeks' gestation reveals a transition in brain response following tactile and noxious stimulation from non-specific, evenly dispersed neuronal bursts to modality-specific, localized, evoked potentials (see Figure 8.1). These recordings suggest that the haemodynamic recordings in very young infants reflect an increase in spontaneous burst responses, which is greater with noxious than tactile stimulation, but that the specific neural circuits necessary to distinguish the qualitative difference between touch and nociception emerge from 35 to 37 weeks' gestation in the human brain (Fabrizi et al., 2011).

The measurement of noxious-evoked brain activity in human infants has provided a valuable opportunity to determine the extent to which the clinical tools used to assess paediatric pain are correlated to the level of cortical activation following noxious stimulation. For example, facial expression correlates better with cortical haemodynamic activity than physiological responses such as heart rate, but cortical pain responses were observed in some infants in the absence of any change in facial expression following heel lance (Slater et al., 2008). In a double-blind, randomized controlled trial of oral sucrose, commonly used to reduce the behavioural response to painful procedures in neonatal intensive care, EEG and electromyographic recording revealed that sucrose does not significantly affect activity in neonatal brain or spinal cord nociceptive circuits (Slater et al., 2010a). This study suggests that the ability of sucrose to reduce clinical observational scores after noxious events in newborn infants is mediated at brainstem level.

Little information is available about the development of cortical pain processing in older infants and children. Childhood is a time of great change in the cerebral cortex: the highest number of dendritic spines in the dorsal prefrontal cortex is reached at 2.5 to 7 years and dendritic spine density in childhood exceeds adult values by two- to threefold and begins to decrease during puberty (Petanjek et al., 2011), but very little is known about how this influences the pain experience. The explosion of brain imaging studies examining the functional anatomy of pain processing in adults is gradually being extended to the paediatric population. A first, exploratory fMRI study of nociceptive processing in the cerebral cortex of thirteen 11- to 16-year-olds to tonic mild to moderately painful heat showed significant activation in somatosensory cortex, the anterior insula, the premotor cortex, and the prefrontal cortex (Hohmeister et al., 2010), all brain regions known to be activated by pain in adults (Apkarian, 2005). Activation of the anterior insula has been associated with pain affect while the prefrontal cortex activation has been related to cognitive aspects of pain processing, such as anticipation, attention, stimulus evaluation, and memory. Prefrontal cortex activation can modulate the pain experience and the premotor cortex has been linked to pain-evoked motor planning. Interestingly, these children did not show activation in the anterior cingulate, a region primarily involved in affective pain processing and modulation in adults (Hohmeister et al., 2010; see also Hermann, Chapter 40, this volume).

The development of descending brainstem modulation of nociception

It has long been appreciated that the activation of descending pathways from brainstem regions, such as rostroventral medulla (RVM), can exert both inhibitory and facilitatory effects on spinal excitability and pain sensitivity in the adult (Heinricher et al., 2009). The RVM has strong inputs from the PAG which in turn is driven from the amygdala and other parts of the limbic system (see Figure 8.1). This is therefore the pathway that mediates top-down control of nociceptive input and pain, as has been elegantly demonstrated in man in imaging studies (Eippert et al., 2009; Tracey and Mantyh, 2007). However, laboratory studies have demonstrated that the maturation of this descending control is relatively late in development. Hence, in young animals, in the resting state, descending facilitation of spinal nociceptive processing dominates during the first weeks of life, with the typical biphasic descending facilitation and inhibition observed in adults not apparent until P28 (Hathway et al., 2009, 2012). The RVM, which is the main output nucleus for brainstem descending control, undergoes a remarkable maturational switch after P21: both lesioning and electrical stimulation of RVM at different postnatal ages reveal that RVM control over spinal nociceptive circuits switches from being entirely facilitatory before P21 to inhibitory at older ages. Between P25 and P35, descending inhibition begins to dominate, but it is not as powerful as in the adult until P40. Thus, the influence of the RVM over spinal nociceptive reflexes and dorsal horn neuronal activity gradually changes over this critical developmental period (Hathway et al., 2009). The delayed maturation of these inhibitory pathways from the RVM could explain why activating the PAG region (which sends extensive projections to the RVM) does not produce analgesia until P21 (van Praag and Frenk, 1991) or why stimulating the dorsolateral funiculus is unable to inhibit the firing of dorsal horn neurons or c-fos activation until at least P10 (Boucher et al., 1998; Fitzgerald and Koltzenburg, 1986).

The mechanism of change is likely to lie in the maturation of RVM and PAG circuitry, rather than in lack of descending connections, neurotransmitter levels, or receptor expression in the spinal cord. Interestingly, the postnatal development of inhibitory GABAergic neurons in the rat PAG matter mirrors the development of descending controls: very few such neurons are found from P0 to P5, with a small increase from P5 to P10, a marked maturation beginning at P14 and the adult pattern of GABA immunoreactivity only established between P20 to P30 (Barbaresi, 2010). The maturation of brainstem opioidergic signalling is also an important factor contributing to this developmental switch, as the switch also occurs when μ-opioid receptor agonists are microinjected into the RVM suggesting that the descending facilitation of spinal nociception in young animals is mediated by μ-opioid receptor pathways within the RVM. Furthermore, the developmental transition from descending facilitation to inhibition of pain is determined by activity in central opioid networks at a critical period of periadolescence (Hathway et al., 2012). Blockade of tonic opioidergic activity from P21 to P28, but not at earlier or later ages, prevents the normal development of descending RVM inhibitory control of spinal nociceptive reflexes, while enhancing opioidergic activity with chronic morphine over P7 to P14 accelerates this development. This change in control of supraspinal centres over spinal nociceptive reflexes and dorsal horn neuronal activity over a critical periadolescent developmental period is likely to be of key importance in setting future pain sensitivity in adulthood.

Plasticity of developing central nociceptive pathways

Evidence in rodent brain

While it is well known that the development of central sensory pathways, such as the visual and auditory systems, is dependent upon a balance of sensory activity arising in the periphery, the absence of a clear 'pain' cortex and the complexity of regions activated during pain experience has meant that the influence of peripheral nociceptive activity in shaping the maturation of central pain pathways has been harder to establish, but evidence is rapidly emerging. Thus, rat pups that have received skin incisions in early life, not only have greater pain sensitivity to a repeat injury when they reach adulthood but also show differences in reward-related neural activity. Following exposure to a novelty-induced hypophagia paradigm (a test of motivation), fos activity in lateral hypothalamic orexin neurons, part of a specific reward seeking pathway in the brain, in acutely injured rats was the same as in uninjured naive animals but in those rats with a 'neonatal pain history', orexinergic activity was significantly increased and highly correlated with their motivational behaviour. Thus neonatal pain experience can cause long-term changes in brain motivational orexinergic pathways, known to modulate mesolimbic dopaminergic reward circuitry (Low et al., 2012).

Neonatal pain has also been shown to influence the generation of new neurons in the dentate gyrus region of the hippocampus. Rat pups receiving intraplantar injections of the painful inflammatory agent complete Freund's adjuvant, on P8, had more BrdU-labelled cells and a higher density of cells expressing doublecortin, both measures of newborn neurons, in the subgranular zone of the dentate gyrus, thought to be involved in memory formation (Leslie et al., 2011).

Descending pain control systems in the brainstem can also be influenced by early pain experience. Inflammatory pain induced by intraplantar carrageenan at birth induces significant changes in the brainstem endogenous opioid system into adulthood, namely increased beta-endorphin and met/leu-enkephalin protein levels and decreased opioid receptor expression in the PAG. These long-lasting alterations in endogenous opioid tone are likely to affect later pain sensitivity (Laprairie and Murphy, 2009). This is supported by the observation that focal electrical stimulation of the RVM in adult animals treated neonatally with carrageenan produced significantly greater descending inhibition of nociceptive responses to noxious thermal stimuli applied to the hindpaws and the tail, indicating that neonatal tissue injury and inflammation produces lasting alterations in descending modulatory systems that modify nociceptive processing (Zhang et al., 2010).

Evidence in human brain—effects of neonatal intensive care

The developmental plasticity observed in laboratory animals is supported by structural and functional evidence of changes in the human infant brain following repeated noxious stimulation. Structural MRI studies suggest that procedural pain in the neonatal intensive care unit can affect early brain development in preterm infants. Infants born very preterm (24–32 weeks GA) have been followed prospectively from birth and the number of skin-breaking events quantified to search for structural changes in their brain scans. After adjusting for clinical confounders such as illness severity, morphine exposure, brain injury, and surgery, the results show that greater neonatal procedural pain is associated with reduced measures of white matter and of subcortical grey matter. Reduced white matter was predicted by early pain, whereas grey matter changes were predicted by pain exposure throughout the neonatal course, suggesting a primary early effect on subcortical structures, such as the thalamus, followed by secondary white matter reductions (Brummelte et al., 2012; see also Grunau, Chapter 4, this volume).

Infants who are born prematurely and who have experienced at least 40 days of intensive or special care also have increased brain neuronal responses to noxious stimuli compared to healthy newborns at the same postmenstrual age. Evoked potentials generated by noxious clinically-essential heel lances are significantly larger in prematurely-born infants, while responses to non-noxious touch stimuli are unaffected, suggesting a functional change in pain processing in the brain (Slater et al., 2010b). FMRI of cerebral pain responses in a similar cohort of preterm infants when they have reached school-age (11–16 years) show that aside from more general neurodevelopmental consequences, repeated neonatal nociceptive input may result in continued increased sensitivity in central pain pathways into adolescence. Tonic heat stimuli (of individually adjusted moderate pain intensity) applied to the ex-preterm children causes significant activation in the thalamus, anterior cingulate cortex, cerebellum, basal ganglia, and PAG that is not observed in full-term hospitalized children or controls. The preterms also show significantly higher activation in the S1, anterior cingulate cortex, and insula than controls. This exaggerated brain response is pain specific and is not observed during non-painful warmth stimulation (Hohmeister et al., 2010)

There is also evidence that neonatal intensive care can alter endogenous descending control systems. Children, aged between 7 and 11 years, divided into term, preterm exposed to numerous painful interventions, or preterm exposed to few painful interventions, have comparable pain thresholds but differ in their responses to conditioning cold stimulation. Thus while cold stimulation significantly increases heart rate and decreases thermal pain sensitivity of term-born children and 'preterm less pain' children, changes in heart rate and pain sensitivity in response to conditioning cold stimulation were not observed in 'preterm more pain' children. These results suggest that endogenous pain modulatory mechanisms are not as well developed as those of children not exposed to noxious insult at birth (Goffaux et al., 2008; Wollgarten-Hadamek et al., 2011)

Evidence in human brain—paediatric chronic pain

Evidence suggests that central changes in the brain can occur in older children who develop chronic pain syndromes. Children with migraine when undertaking an experimental attentional task, display EEG activity associated with an automatic attentional bias towards painful and potentially painful somatosensory stimuli, perhaps due to alterations in connectivity within the limbic system (Zohsel et al., 2008).

CNS activation to sensory stimulation in paediatric patients (9–18 years) with complex regional pain syndrome (CRPS) affecting the lower extremity also reveals changes. In an fMRI study each patient underwent two scanning sessions: once during an active period of pain (CRPS(+)), and once after symptomatic recovery (CRPS(−). In each session, mechanical (brush) and thermal (cold) stimuli were applied to the affected region of the involved limb and the corresponding mirror region of the unaffected limb. Several interesting observations were made in this study but notably in the CRPS(−) state, significant activation differences persist despite nearly complete elimination of evoked pain suggesting prolonged changes in CNS pain circuitry in paediatric patients with CRPS that outlast the illness itself (Lebel et al., 2008).

There is an urgent need for more investigative studies of pain processing in the brains of children. Despite the ethical and practical challenges that such studies present, it is important to allow children to participate in well-designed research studies so that they can benefit from research advances to the same degree as adult populations (Sava et al., 2009).

References

Apkarian, A. V., Bushnell, M. C., Treede, R.-D., and Zubieta, J.-K. (2005). Human brain mechanisms of pain perception and regulation in health and disease. *Eur J Pain*, 9, 463–484.

Arichi, T., Moraux, A., Melendez, A., Doria, V., Groppo, M., Merchant, N., et al. (2010). Somatosensory cortical activation identified by functional MRI in preterm and term infants. *Neuroimage*, 49(3), 2063–2071.

Armstrong-James, M. (1975). The functional status and columnar organization of single cells responding to cutaneous stimulation in neonatal rat somatosensory cortex S1. *J Physiol*, 246(3), 501–538.

Barbaresi, P. (2010). Postnatal development of GABA-immunoreactive neurons and terminals in rat periaqueductal gray matter: a light and electron microscopic study. *J Comp Neurol*, 518(12), 2240–2260.

Barr, G. A. (2011). Formalin-induced c-fos expression in the brain of infant rats. *J Pain*, 12(2), 263–271.

Boucher, T., Jennings, E., and Fitzgerald, M. (1998). The onset of diffuse noxious inhibitory controls in postnatal rat pups: a C-Fos study. *Neurosci Lett*, 257(1), 9–12.

Brummelte, S., Grunau, R. E., Chau, V., Poskitt, K. J., Brant. R., Vinall, J., et al. (2012). Procedural pain and brain development in premature newborns. *Ann Neurol*, 71(3), 385–396.

Chan, T., Kyere, K., Davis, B. R., Shemyakin, A., Kabitzke, P. A., Shair, H. N., et al. (2011). The role of the medial prefrontal cortex in innate fear regulation in infants, juveniles, and adolescents. *J Neurosci*. 31(13), 4991–4999.

Colonnese, M. and Khazipov, R. (2012). Spontaneous activity in developing sensory circuits: implications for resting state fMRI. *Neuroimage*, 62(4), 2212–2221.

Davidson, S., Truong, H., and Giesler, G. J. Jr. (2010). Quantitative analysis of spinothalamic tract neurons in adult and developing mouse. *J Comp Neurol*, 518(16), 3193–3204.

Dubois, J., Dehaene-Lambertz, G., Perrin, M., Mangin, J. F., Cointepas, Y., Duchesnay, E., et al. (2008). Asynchrony of the early maturation of white matter bundles in healthy infants: quantitative landmarks revealed noninvasively by diffusion tensor imaging. *Hum Brain Mapp*, 29(1), 14–27.

Eippert, F., Finsterbusch, J., Bingel, U., and Büchel, C. (2009). Direct evidence for spinal cord involvement in placebo analgesia. *Science*, 326(5951), 404.

Fabrizi, L., Slater, R., Worley, A., Meek, J., Boyd, S., Olhede, S., et al. (2011). A shift in sensory processing that enables the developing human brain to discriminate touch from pain. *Curr Biol*, 21(18), 1552–1558.

Fitzgerald, M. (2005). The development of nociceptive circuits. *Nat Rev Neurosci*, 6(7), 507–520.

Fitzgerald, M. and Jennings, E. (1999). The postnatal development of spinal sensory processing. *Proc Natl Acad Sci U S A*, 96(14), 7719–7722.

Fitzgerald, M. and Koltzenburg, M. (1986). The functional development of descending inhibitory pathways in the dorsolateral funiculus of the newborn rat spinal cord. *Brain Res*, 389, 261–270.

Fransson, P., Aden, U., Blennow, M., and Lagercrantz, H. (2011). The functional architecture of the infant brain as revealed by resting-state fMRI. *Cereb Cortex*, 21(1), 145–154.

Gauriau, C. and Bernard, J. F. (2004). A comparative reappraisal of projections from the superficial laminae of the dorsal horn in the rat: the forebrain. *J Comp Neurol*, 468(1), 24–56.

Goffaux, P., Lafrenaye, S., Morin, M., Patural, H., Demers, G., and Marchand, S. (2008). Preterm births: can neonatal pain alter the development of endogenous gating systems? *Eur J Pain*, 12(7), 945–951.

Hathway, G. J., Koch, S., Low, L., and Fitzgerald, M. (2009). The changing balance of brainstem-spinal cord modulation of pain processing over the first weeks of rat postnatal life. *J Physiol*, 587(Pt 12), 2927–2935.

Hathway, G. J., Vega-Avelaira, D., and Fitzgerald, M. (2012). A critical period in the supraspinal control of pain: opioid-dependent changes in brainstem rostroventral medulla function in preadolescence. *Pain*, 153(4), 775–783.

Heinricher, M. M., Tavares, I., Leith, J. L., and Lumb, B. M. (2009). Descending control of nociception: specificity, recruitment and plasticity. *Brain Res Rev*, 60(1), 214–225.

Hohmeister, J., Kroll, A., Wollgarten-Hadamek, I., Zohsel, K., Demirakça, S., Flor, H., et al. (2010). Cerebral processing of pain in school-aged children with neonatal nociceptive input: an exploratory fMRI study. *Pain*, 150(2), 257–267.

Laprairie, J. L. and Murphy, A. Z. (2009). Neonatal injury alters adult pain sensitivity by increasing opioid tone in the periaqueductal gray. *Front Behav Neurosci*, 3, 31.

Lebel, A., Becerra, L., Wallin, D., Moulton, E. A., Morris, S., Pendse, G., et al. (2008). fMRI reveals distinct CNS processing during symptomatic and recovered complex regional pain syndrome in children. *Brain*, 131, 1854–1879.

Legrain, V., Iannetti, G. D., Plaghki, L., and Mouraux, A. (2011). The pain matrix reloaded: a salience detection system for the body. *Prog Neurobiol*, 93(1), 111–124.

Leslie, A. T., Akers, K. G., Martinez-Canabal, A., Mello, L. E., Covolan, L., and Guinsburg, R. (2011). Neonatal inflammatory pain increases hippocampal neurogenesis in rat pups. *Neurosci Lett*, 501(2), 78–82.

Li, H. and Crair, M. C. (2011). How do barrels form in somatosensory cortex? *Ann N Y Acad Sci*, 1225, 119–129.

Low, L. A. and Fitzgerald, M. (2012). Acute pain and a motivational pathway in adult rats: influence of early life pain experience. *PLoS ONE*, 7(3), e34316.

Oberlander, T. F., Grunau, R. E., Fitzgerald, C., and Whitfield, M. F. (2002). Does parenchymal brain injury affect biobehavioral pain responses in very low birth weight infants at 32 weeks' postconceptional age? *Pediatrics*, 110(3), 570–576.

Quairiaux, C., Mégevand, P., Kiss, J. Z., and Michel, C. M. (2011). Functional development of large-scale sensorimotor cortical networks in the brain. *J Neurosci*, 31(26), 9574–9584.

Sava, S., Lebel, A. A., Leslie, D. S., Drosos, A., Berde, C., Becerra, L., et al. (2009). Challenges of functional imaging research of pain in children. *Mol Pain*, 5, 30.

Slater, R., Cantarella, A., Franck, L., Meek, J., and Fitzgerald, M. (2008). How well do clinical pain assessment tools reflect pain in infants? *PLoS Med*, 5(6), e129.

Slater, R., Cantarella, A., Gallella, S., Worley, A., Boyd, S., Meek, J., et al. (2006). Cortical pain responses in human infants. *J Neurosci*, 26(14), 3662–3666

Slater, R., Cornelissen, L., Fabrizi, L., Patten, D., Yoxen, J., Worley, A., et al. (2010a). Oral sucrose as an analgesic drug for procedural pain in newborn infants: a randomised controlled trial. *Lancet*, 376(9748), 1225–1232.

Slater, R., Fabrizi, L., Worley, A., Meek, J., Boyd, S., and Fitzgerald, M. (2010b). Premature infants display increased noxious-evoked neuronal activity in the brain compared to healthy age-matched term-born infants. *Neuroimage*, 52(2), 583–589.

Thairu, B. K. (1971). Post-natal changes in the somaesthetic evoked potentials in the albino rat. *Nat New Biol*, 231(18), 30–31.

Todd, A. J. (2010). Neuronal circuitry for pain processing in the dorsal horn. *Nat Rev Neurosci*, 11(12), 823–836.

Tolner, E. A., Sheikh, A., Yukin, A. Y., Kaila, K., and Kanold, P. O. (2012). Subplate neurons promote spindle bursts and thalamocortical patterning in the neonatal rat somatosensory cortex. *J Neurosci*, 32(2), 692–702.

Tracey, I. and Johns, E. (2010). The pain matrix: reloaded or reborn as we image tonic pain using arterial spin labelling. *Pain*, 148(3), 359–360.

Tracey, I. and Mantyh, P. W. (2007). The cerebral signature for pain perception and its modulation. *Neuron*, 55(3), 377–391.

van Praag, H. and Frenk, H. (1991). The development of stimulation-produced analgesia (SPA) in the rat. *Brain Res Dev Brain Res*, 64, 71–76.

Willis, W. D. Jr, Zhang, X., Honda, C. N., and Giesler, G. J. Jr. (2002). A critical review of the role of the proposed VMpo nucleus in pain. *J Pain*, 3(2), 79–94.

Wollgarten-Hadamek, I., Hohmeister, J., Zohsel, K., Flor, H., and Hermann, C. (2011). Do school-aged children with burn injuries during infancy show stress-induced activation of pain inhibitory mechanisms? *Eur J Pain*, 15(4), 423.e1–e10.

Zhang, Y. H., Wang, X. M., and Ennis, M. (2010). Effects of neonatal inflammation on descending modulation from the rostroventromedial medulla. *Brain Res Bull*, 83(1–2), 16–22.

Zohsel, K., Hohmeister, J., Flor, H., and Hermann, C. (2008). Altered pain processing in children with migraine: an evoked potential study. *Eur J Pain*, 12(8), 1090–1101.

SECTION 3

Social and psychological basis of paediatric pain

CHAPTER 9

Psychological theories and biopsychosocial models in paediatric pain

Rebecca Pillai Riddell, Nicole M. Racine, Kenneth D. Craig, and Lauren Campbell

Summary

The purpose of this chapter is to review existing biopsychosocial models of paediatric pain and to examine common key factors across different theoretical conceptualizations. Critical gaps in the empirical and theoretical literature are elucidated. In particular, lack of specific attention to developmental factors in biological, behavioural, and social functioning and the need for models that examine gaps in different types of pain responding (e.g. immediate acute pain response, acute pain responding in the context of chronic pain) are highlighted. Moreover, the need for comprehensive, conceptual models, representative of current knowledge, that readily generate specific hypotheses confirmable by experimentation are also discussed as ways of moving the field of paediatric pain forward, both conceptually and pragmatically.

Introduction

Except in very rare cases of congenital insensitivity, pain is inevitable and ubiquitous in the lives of children. Despite its universality, the complexity of any child or adult's actual experience of pain remains elusive to others, given its subjective nature. Nevertheless, the established deleterious impact of unmanaged pain during childhood on biological, psychological, and social well-being (Anand, 2000; Fitzgerald, 2005; Grunau, 2006; Hohmeister et al., 2010; Taddio et al., 1997) dictates a necessity to better understanding of not only the 'ever-elusive' pain experience but also how the more easily quantifiable 'pain expression' contributes to understanding the experience, assessment, and management of paediatric pain.

The complexity of different pain experiences (e.g. acute, acute-prolonged, chronic) and the varying importance of both broader system factors (medical staff, cultural norms) and more narrow system factors (such as parents and peers) have led to diverse frameworks in understanding the interplay of biopsychosocial factors in paediatric pain. Having biopsychosocial models help scientists and clinicians attempt to discern and integrate the multifaceted pieces to approximate an understanding of the complex enigma of another's pain. In addition to comprehensiveness of bio-, psycho-, and social variables, ideally good models should represent current scientific knowledge in the field and generate new ideas that can be subjected to empirical validation. This chapter will review key models in the field and discuss their content in terms of comprehensiveness, representativeness, and potential for novel hypothesis generation.

The first biopsychosocial model of pain: gate control theory

A review of theoretical models would be incomplete without mentioning the road the gate control theory of pain paved for modern transdisciplinary models of pain. Moving away from antiquated dualistic conceptualizations of pain as existing in the mind or the body and building upon current knowledge in the field, Melzack and Wall (1965) proposed a groundbreaking model that included testable mechanisms bridging the interplay between psychosocial and biological features of the pain experience. One of the key landmark implications of gate control theory and the subsequent neuromatrix theory for researchers and clinicians was the central role of the brain in processing and representing noxious stimuli (Melzack, 1996, 1999). Ushering pain research into the modern age, the realization that 'without the brain there would not be pain' became a fundamental principle of pain research. Moreover, with recognition that pain is substantially more than mere sensory experience, theoretical models broadened their scope to include diverse factors implicated in pain experience, i.e. biological substrates, internal cognitive/affective/biological schema, social, and environmental (Craig et al., 1996). Despite minor criticisms that have been put forward including that pain inhibition is much more complicated than laid out in gate control, by recognizing the primacy of the brain as the *active* recipient of noxious input and by specifying testable mechanisms that addressed both biological and psychosocial dimensions, these models set the stage for research proliferation in the field of pain that continues to this day. In addition, it also fostered the development of more targeted biopsychosocial models of pain. It was recently asserted that the prospects of advances in clinical assessment and management of children's pain are best served by comprehensive models that are inclusive of all determinants (Hadjistavropoulos et al., 2011).

While not biopsychosocial in scope, two other theories should be discussed at the outset due to their integral role in modern theories of paediatric pain. Both operant conditioning and social learning models have set a foundation in which to help operationalize the psychological and the social aspects for current biopsychosocial conceptualizations.

Operant and social learning models of paediatric pain

Operant models of pain have been extensively used to understand chronic pain in the adult pain literature (Fordyce, 1976). The application to paediatric pain came onto the scene later. Turk and colleagues (1987) conducted one of the first reviews on the involvement of the family on child chronic pain. They discussed the concept of 'painful families', which are families where there is an increased incidence of chronic pain problems. Ultimately, they concluded that the family plays a major role as an agent of positive and negative reinforcement. The child's pain behaviours (e.g. crying, moaning) can be strengthened or extinguished depending on environmental responses. Reinforcement may be particularly salient for children with chronic pain since parent behaviours, such as attending to pain behaviours and granting permission to avoid daily activities, are related to higher levels of illness behaviours in children with recurrent abdominal pain (Walker and Zeman, 1992). A more recent review has also highlighted the contribution of operant conditioning on paediatric chronic pain and put forward an integrative model (discussed fully later in this chapter) of factors impacting on paediatric chronic pain, including individual variables such as parental reinforcement and solicitousness (Palermo and Chambers, 2005).

While reinforcement and punishment are key aspects to understanding how paediatric pain responses develop and are maintained, by nature the theory tends to focus on more narrow contributors that are temporally linked to the pain response without expounding other aspects of environmental learning such as through observation and modelling. Social learning theory is a broader approach to learning emphasizing not only child factors related to their appraisal of a painful situation but also familial/larger system influences on how to think about and act when in pain (Williams et al., 2011).

Social learning theory puts forward that children learn within a social context, which is facilitated by modelling and observation (Bandura, 1977). According to social learning theory children learn behaviour by observing others and imitating what they have observed. Moreover, whether the behaviour is imitated and learned depends on the salience of the model and the consequence of the behaviour. The child is also more likely to exhibit the learned behaviour if he or she believes that the pain behaviour will lead to a specific response from their support network (Osborne et al., 1989). An example of social learning was demonstrated in a study that found that children of chronic low-back pain patients exhibited a higher frequency of similar pain behaviours when they had a parent with a chronic pain condition versus when they had parents who were healthy or diabetic (Rickard, 1988).

While much social learning literature has focused on paediatric chronic pain, Page and Blanchette argue that social learning theory is also a useful perspective from which to understand paediatric procedural pain (2009). For example, work by Chambers and colleagues demonstrated that positive reinforcement and modelling of pain behaviours by parents during an acute pain task had an impact on child pain behaviour, particularly for girls. Girls whose mothers demonstrated pain-promoting behaviours reported more pain than girls whose mothers did not react in the same manner (Chambers et al., 2002). Social learning theory is also relevant to paediatric procedural pain because of the roles anticipatory anxiety and avoidance play in pain responses (Page and Blanchette, 2009). Children may display anticipatory anxiety or avoidance because they believe they will be unable to manage the procedure. Social learning theory is a useful model through which to understand the development and maintenance of child pain behaviour in both acute and chronic pain contexts. As will become apparent, social learning contributes, either overtly or covertly, to the psychosocial foundation for all biopsychosocial models presented in this chapter.

The current review found that biopsychosocial models of paediatric pain fell into two broad categories: (1) a small and relatively recent literature specifically addressing chronic pain and (2) a much more developed literature examining acute procedural pain. The following examines these two broad categories, including a more detailed section on the social communication model (SCM) of pain as this model is one of the most widely cited explanatory models in the field of paediatric pain. We begin our discussion of biopsychosocial models by tackling paediatric chronic pain.

Biopsychosocial models of paediatric chronic pain: theoretical beginnings

Rather than defining chronic pain in terms of duration, current conceptualizations base the distinction between chronic and acute pain on functionality (Woolf, 2010). Acute nociceptive pain serves to warn the organism of real or imminent tissue damage, whereas persistent pain diminishes or prevents movement and can promote healing. Within the broad domain of persistent pain one can identify chronic pain that is pathological because it serves neither function and would appear to be the consequence of an abnormally functioning or damaged nervous system. Neuropathic pain best illustrates the latter. A recent epidemiological review of chronic pain during childhood and adolescence described many different types of chronic pain (e.g. headache, back pain, musculoskeletal pain), with median reports of prevalence ranging between 11% and 38% of the populations studied (King et al., 2011). However, most of the studies reviewed used 'duration of pain' to classify children's reports of pain as chronic. A commentary on this review suggested that probably 5% to 15% of children suffer from chronic pain that is disabling and requires professional intervention (von Baeyer, 2011).

Clearly significant numbers of children suffer from chronic pain, thus, models of this pain type need to assist clinicians and researchers in understanding why a subsample of children come to report disabling chronic pain when others do not. One must turn to formulations of how biological endowment and maturation interact with the physical and social environment to appreciate the emergence of individual differences in the experience and expression of pain and disability.

An integrative conceptual model for understanding paediatric chronic pain and disability

There have been recent attempts to describe interactions among biological, psychological, and social features and/or determinants of children's chronically painful conditions. In their 'integrative model of parent and family factors in paediatric chronic pain and associated disability', Palermo and Chambers (2005) focused on the psychosocial component of the biopsychosocial perspective. They describe operant-behavioural perspectives of parent–child interaction within the broader framework of family systems theories. Individual parenting variables, such as parenting style or parental reinforcement of child pain behaviours, are recognized as important within the context of dyadic interactions with the child. For example, the quality of the parent–child interactions, which in turn are nested within broader family-level variables, such as family cohesion or overall functioning, were outlined. Specific child variables, such as the level or nature of pain or disability, or moderating/mediating variables, such as the child's gender, age, emotional status, and coping, are hypothesized to influence the family, dyadic, and individual variables. In this model, complex bidirectional relationships are proposed between the aforementioned nested variables and paediatric chronic pain, such that not only do parenting, dyadic, and family-level variables influence paediatric chronic pain, but paediatric pain would have an impact on family dyadic interactions and overall functioning. This model emphasizes the developmental context of these complex and bidirectional relationships and the dynamic, progressive nature of changes in relationships. Thus, there is an emphasis on recognizing that the specific variables of interest would vary with the developmental status of the child and contribute to developmentally appropriate care. Ultimately, the model emphasizes the mutually influencing relationship between the family unit's functioning (both the whole system and multiple subsystems within) and the child's pain, functional disability and the variables that moderate or mediate the relationship between the two. In this model, psychosocial factors within the narrow family system are handled well because the model accurately reflects current knowledge on this topic. This is clearly seen in the specification of potential mediators/moderators that may influence the relationship between pain and functional disability. However, although not its set out purpose, in terms of comprehensiveness, it does not go beyond immediate family factors (such as medical systems and cultural norms) and does not look at the interplay with biological factors within the child. Moreover, the actual relative relationships among individual, parent, and family factors on chronic pain/functional disability are vague.

Palermo (2012) extended the theoretical foundation proposed by Palermo and Chambers (2005) by explicitly adding in new components to the model, namely: (1) biological processes, (2) the dimension of psychological factors influencing health habits, and (3) social factors that go beyond consideration of parents and the family. The 'guiding conceptual model for understanding paediatric chronic pain and disability' (see Figure 9.1) is therefore more comprehensive in its scope. In terms of the biological levels of influence, consideration was given to ontogenetic maturation, including genetic factors, central nervous system functioning, sex, and pubertal status. Psychological variables proposed as important in paediatric chronic pain include individual beliefs, coping, mood/affect, anxiety, and fear. Broader social variables, such as culture,

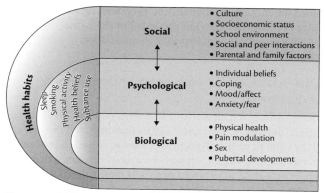

Figure 9.1 Guiding conceptual model for understanding paediatric chronic pain and disability.

Reproduced from Tonya M. Palermo, *Cognitive-Behavioral Therapy for Chronic Pain in Children and Adolescents*, Oxford University Press, Inc., New York, USA, p. 13, Copyright © 2012, by permission of Oxford University Press.

socioeconomic status, school environment, and characteristics of the health care system, were recognized as providing context for the more proximal family and parent social factors. A novel aspect of this model is close examination of the role of health habits (such as sleep, physical activity, substance use) play in paediatric chronic pain and disability. Explicitly making stable health habits salient highlights the importance of assessing these peripheral but fundamental behaviours because of their potential role in moderating pain and disability, particularly in older children and adolescents. This model posits bidirectional relationships among biological, psychological, and social factors with biological factors nested within the psychological context of the child, which in turn is nested within social contexts. Health habits would develop on the basis of the interplay of all three factors. Developmental considerations are advanced in this model, with the biology of pubertal development highlighted as particularly important. Reflective of current research in the broader field of paediatric psychology, the innovation of including health habits are noted as particularly relevant in adolescent populations. The model is broad in scope and describes an interplay of different aspects of the systems. However, while the comprehensiveness and representativeness of the model facilitates a broad inventory of potential factors in chronic pain, this appears to come at the cost of its specific predictive power. Specific hypotheses about how factors within different systems interact for empirical validation purposes (e.g. mood, culture, and puberty) and the directionality of these relationships are not readily evident from the model descriptions.

As discussed earlier, integrative models in the area of paediatric chronic pain are still in their early stages, with modelling typically representing the product of a particular investigative group. In contrast, paediatric models of acute pain began proliferating about a decade earlier and have had the benefit of diverse viewpoints on the topic. The following section addresses a number of recent models.

Biopsychosocial models of paediatric acute pain

Contrary to the dearth of theoretical literature on paediatric chronic pain, several models that specifically address acute or procedural paediatric pain have been advanced in the paediatric pain literature. In all of these models, the proposed relationships and interplay between variables are presented in the context of a particular painful episode (e.g. a specific immunization or other painful medical procedure).

A social-ecological framework for understanding procedure pain

Informed and laid out similarly to Bronfenbrenner's (1977) social-ecological framework, Kazak and Kunin-Batson's (2001) model situated the child in pain at the centre of a series of nested concentric circles representing the increasingly broad social settings that have an impact on a child in pain and that exert bidirectional influences on the child. Contained in the first circle of influence, the microsystem, are child-specific, or intrapersonal, factors such as age, biology, coping, health, and the pain experience itself. In the mesosystem, or second circle of influence, are social factors in the child's immediate life contexts, such as those relating to family, peers, school staff, and hospital staff, and the interrelationships between these social units. Finally, broader social environments are represented by the largest circle of influence or the exosystem, such as social networks of parents, ethnocultural influences, including cultural beliefs and practices, health care systems, and public policy. The interpersonal meso- and exosystems are hypothesized to exert a direct and indirect impact on the child in pain (the microsystem) and all three systems are expected to interact, a position this perspective shares with other models discussed. Once again, the model, while comprehensive in its scope and grounded in current research, has limited impact beyond providing a comprehensive description of potential variables related to procedural pain. In essence, specific hypothesis testing of the dynamic interplay of nested spheres is impossible because of the large number of interactive possibilities that different factors within different spheres present.

Stimulus–response model of (paediatric) pain

The 'stimulus–response model of (paediatric) pain' (Cohen et al., 2008) takes a different perspective by structuring the model around a linear sequence of events that follow a specific painful stimulus (e.g. injection, inflammation). First, there is a short-term response phase in which pain, distress, and anxiety can be experienced, but also in which the opportunity to learn, practice, cope, or be coached exists. The link between the painful stimulus and the short-term response is hypothesized to be modulated by child factors (e.g. coping behaviours, prior experiences), parent factors (e.g. coaching behaviours, parent anxiety), medical staff factors (e.g. coaching behaviours, staff anxiety), and contextual factors (e.g. environmental factors, culture). Following this short-term response phase is the long-term response phase in which health attitudes/behaviours, distress memories, and expectations can develop, physiological changes can occur, and the opportunity to cope or be coached exists. Similar to the link between the painful stimulus and the short-term response phase, the link between the short-term response phase and the long-term response phase is hypothesized to be modulated by the same child, parent, medical staff, and contextual factors discussed earlier. In line with a biopsychosocial approach to understanding paediatric pain, this model addresses biological, psychological, and social spheres of influence, as well as the interplay between the specific variables that subsume these three levels. Compared to earlier models discussed previously, this model does not overtly hypothesize a transactional, or bidirectional, relationship

among features and determinants of the pain experience choosing rather to specifically outlay the directionality of certain relationships. However, with this model we see a different type of limitation in that while specific mechanisms are readily identifiable and testable, potential gaps in the conceptualization of relationships between variables are evident. For example, whereas it is hypothesized that child factors (such as coping behaviours) or parent factors (such as anxiety) can modulate the child's short-term pain response or long-term distress memories, the model does not explicitly propose that the child's short-term pain response or long-term distress memories would exert influence on the child's coping behaviours or the parent's anxiety. Moreover, it provides only a surface treatment of biological variables and a more comprehensive integration of biological factors would improve its conceptual value.

Young's model of paediatric procedural pain

Similarly to Cohen's model, Young's (2005; see Figure 9.2) biopsychosocial model contextualizes paediatric procedural acute pain by first breaking the time sequence of a procedural pain event into three phases: (1) pre-procedure, (2) procedure, and (3) post-procedure. This framework acknowledges that while acute pain occurs in a distinct episode of time (procedure), it is substantially influenced by pre-procedural factors, such as the mindset the child brings to the procedure (memories of past pain, fear/anxiety, temperament), unique biological dispositions (such as pain receptor density, endogenous opioids), and social influences (such as parental modelling, cultural beliefs, media attention, peer influences). Furthermore, the cumulative impact of both pre-procedural and procedural factors would continue to influence the child after the procedure has been completed. Similar observations must apply to acute pain arising from injury. Importantly, this model stands alone from models reviewed thus far by including a specific feedback loop postulating that after the procedural pain response, long-term effects of pain and distress (such as memories of the acutely painful experience) will in turn directly impact on an individual's cognitive control and coping skills in the next painful experience.

In addition, the model explicitly incorporates Melzack and Wall's (1965) gate control theory by noting that both individual (such as age, sex, development, and temperament) and other systemic factors (such as ethnicity/psychobiological factors, cultural/familial factors, and societal/environmental factors) impact on central cortical control processes and descending inhibitory mechanisms of the pain gate, which in turn determine the pain response (sensory, affective, and physiological).

Given such a broad array of factors and clearly laid out interrelationships, the potential for contributing to the development of the field becomes readily apparent. When critically appraising the model, questions quickly arise regarding interactions among specific subunits of the model. For example, why is a child's pain and distress presumed to only impact on individual factors but not psychobiological factors such as pain thresholds? Additionally, given the integral role of ongoing threat appraisals in the actual pain response, pain responding (in particular physiological responding) would also be directly impacted upon by pre-procedural factors such as previous pain experiences, rather than solely being mediated by a child's cognitive abilities and schemas. It is notable that the various mechanisms and constructs describing the pain response are laid out explicitly. Hence, this model provides clear avenues for empirical validation and its in-depth empirical basis is clearly

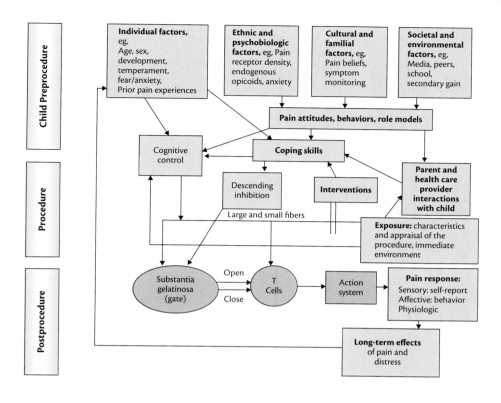

Figure 9.2 Model for conceptualizing and studying paediatric procedural pain (Young, 2005). Reprinted from *Annals of Emergency Medicine*, Volume 45, Issue 2, Kelly D. Young, Pediatric Procedural Pain, pp. 160–171, Copyright © 2005, with permission from Elsevier, http://www.sciencedirect.com/science/journal/01960644

laid out in the paper. One conceptual criticism of the model is that the caregiver of child in pain appears to be relegated to a peripheral role during the procedural phase and is not acknowledged as having a direct impact on the child's construction of previous pain experiences.

The social communication model of pain

In a hybrid approach that incorporates the sequencing of events in acute pain and yet acknowledges larger spheres of both inter- and intrapersonal influence, Craig and colleagues have taken a broader perspective that emphasizes social learning theory in how the child, the caregiver, and the relationship function in the pain context (see Figure 9.3). The focus is upon dyadic interactions between the child and others, but consideration is given to the broader social ecological systems within which child pain is suffered. Having had the benefit of over a decade of development, including exploration of its empirical and theoretical ramifications (e.g. Craig, 2009; Craig et al., 1996; Hadjistavropoulos et al., 2011), the conceptual framework now provides by far the most developed biopsychosocial formulation of paediatric acute pain. It predates other models described here with the first paediatric version released in the early 1990s when the importance of the social context to understanding children in pain was only beginning to be established.

Important and relatively unique features of the SCM include the impact of socialization on child pain experience and expression as well as the inclusion of persons other than the individual experiencing the pain, caregivers in particular. This is particularly important in paediatric pain because vulnerable infants and children are heavily reliant on family, other adults, and professionals for caregiving, including assessment and relief from pain (Pillai Riddell and Racine, 2009). The SCM as it relates to paediatric pain includes processes whereby the subjective pain experience of the child is transduced into a pain expression that can be assessed by

caregivers who, when deemed necessary, will take action to manage the pain.

These transactions between the child and persons in the social environment are explicitly examined during four sequenced, conceptually distinct but interactive stages following an initial painful event: (1) the child's pain experience, (2) the child's pain expression, (3) assessment of pain by a caregiver, and (4) and actions taken (or not taken) by others that would impact on the child's pain.

Thus, when tissue damage or trauma occurs, the noxious input is transduced into the child's perception of pain. The biological dispositions triggered are the outcome of the biological, personal, and social history of the child, not only the nociceptive sensory input. The experience includes both automatic/reflexive features as well as higher level processing reflecting the learning history of the child. Thus, an understanding of the reaction to a noxious event, whether acute tissue trauma or exacerbation of chronic pain, requires consideration of both immediate and personal history events.

The second stage concerns the complexities of how painful experience becomes manifest in the expression of pain. Pain expression may be observed in infants vocally through crying or screaming, as well as through non-vocal expression, including facial expression and body actions. Depending on the developmental stage of the child, they may be able to use language to communicate pain. There are bidirectional relationships between pain experience and pain expression, whereby the child's pain experience will impact on pain expression, and a child's expression of pain will impact on how it is experienced. The distinction between the experience and expression of pain implicitly acknowledges they may be discordant. This complicates the challenge caregivers confront when attempting to assess a child's distress, with decisions about an appropriate course of action depending upon this judgement.

Pain expression and caregiver assessments mutually influence each other. Pain expression primarily, but not exclusively,

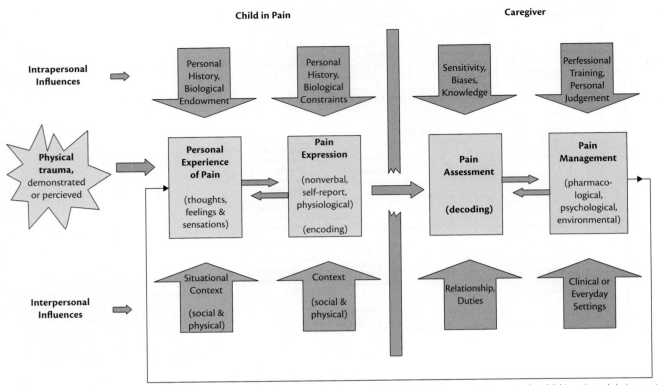

Figure 9.3 The social communication model of pain. A conceptual biopsychosocial model depicting the interaction between the child in pain and their caregiver. Reprinted with permission from Craig, K. D., The social communication model of pain, *Canadian Psychology*, Volume 50, pp. 22–32, Copyright © 2009, American Psychological Association. DOI: 10.1037/a0014772.

determines the observer's pain assessment, and this reaction in turn will have an impact on the pain expression (and experience) depending upon the reaction. The component of the model encompassing child expression and caregiver assessment is at the heart of the model and exemplifies the belief that pain is fundamentally a social experience. Pain was evolutionarily conserved as a biological adaptation, with expression and adult reactions to the child playing no small part. Children modulate signals of pain and distress contingent upon perception of the immediate context, including receptivity of the caregiver, and the caregiver would also attune sensitivity to signals based on their interpretation of the child's expressivity. Parental and health practitioner sensitivity as social determinants of children's pain expression seem obvious and would not seem to require further illustration here.

Finally, the caregiver's assessment of the urgency, intensity, and necessity of the pain signal determine whether the caregiver will take action and attempt to control pain. As with all phases of the process, caregiver judgements and decisions to provide care are mutually influential. The actions a caregiver takes may also impact on their assessment (e.g. if the actions are effective, the assessment might be that the pain is lower). Moreover, how a caregiver manages a child's pain will also feed back to the beginning of the sequence and impact on how a child's pain experience is constructed. These four steps delineate the dynamic interaction between children and caregivers in the paediatric pain context.

Upon review, four key features of the model contribute to its explanatory value. First, the model characterizes important interactions between the child in pain and her/his caregivers. Social learning approaches to child development in a pain context, including both operant (e.g. Gatzounis et al., 2012) and observational learning (e.g. Goubert et al., 2011) processes have proven particularly useful in model refining. Second, the model examines a progression of four stages following onset of painful events that first concern the child and then the caregiver (see later). Third, the SCM recognizes dynamic reciprocal relationships between the infant's or child's experience and communication of pain and the caregiver's interpretation and reaction to the pain-related distress. Finally, as the model developed, intrapersonal and interpersonal factors unique to the biological and environmental history and current status of the individual child and caregiver were shown to be crucial to understanding the child and the caregiver, separately and interactively.

As aforementioned, the SCM has provided rich fodder for empirical work in the field trying to elucidate the psychosocial influences on paediatric pain. However, in contrast to more focused models of paediatric procedural acute pain (such as Young's model), the SCM is not ideally suited to provide detailed guidance regarding specific mechanisms subsuming the interplay between components. It provides broader conceptual guidance postulating the general sequence of acute pain from painful trigger to caregiver management and outlining the spheres of influence with specific mention of potential variables on each step of the sequence. The differing approaches, while overlapping, tend to generate different types of hypotheses. For example, while both models suggest previous pain history impacts on a child's pain response, the SCM postulates that it impacts on the experience of pain which in turn impacts on expression, while the Young model suggests a more specified feedback loop such that previous experience impacts on current experience via the child's cognitive control exerted over the pain gate pathways and via the child's coping skills, which both in turn impact on current pain experience and then, subsequently, future pain experience. One final criticism of all paediatric pain models presented to date, whether they focus on the sequence of events, the larger spheres of influence, or both, is the lack of specific attention to the developmental stage of the child—a key variable in understanding paediatric pain.

A biopsychosocial model specifically for infant pain: the DIAPR model

An appreciation of the unique developmental stage of infancy in terms of both the inter- and intrapersonal influences inspired the creation of a new biopsychosocial model specifically constructed to provide a framework for understanding acute pain over the first year of life: The 'development of infant acute pain responding' or DIAPR model (Pillai Riddell, 2009; see Figure 9.4). Acknowledging the SCM innovation of the primary role of the dynamics between caregiver and child, this new model incorporates novel components that have not been seen in other models of paediatric acute pain to date, including the separate conceptualization of the initial pain reaction and ongoing pain regulation, the *indirect* influence of larger social contexts, and the hypothesis of three specific feedback loops involving either the infant, the caregiver, or both. The model is based on evidence gathered from a growing literature base generated by the OUCH cohort (e.g. Ahola Kohut 2012; Pillai Riddell et al., 2011, 2013; Racine et al., 2012). The OUCH cohort is an ongoing cohort sequential sample of over 750 healthy children and parents being followed through routine immunization injections at 2, 4, 6, 12 months and/or most recently preschool age (with a subsample of 130 infants that was also followed at 12–18 months during a non-painful yet distressing parent–child interaction procedure).

The model begins with the chain of events arising from an acutely painful incident, typically conceptualized in terms of triggering biological processes related to a nociceptive threshold. The tissue stress

or damage is then transduced into an initial pain reaction via nociceptive afferents exceeding noxious sensory thresholds. Rather than pursuing the infinite challenge of operationalizing the non-verbal infant's subjective experience of the noxious stimulus, the model focuses on overtly measurable pain behaviours. After an immediate automatic/reflexive peak response is manifest following the painful event (observable via measures such as physiological or overt behavioural pain responses like cry, facial actions, or body movements), the infant begins the process of self-regulation towards re-establishing homeostasis (measurable via the decrease in overt pain responding as the immunization appointment progresses). Using complex, multifactorial modelling, emerging research on the OUCH cohort has clearly shown that the largest studied determinant of infant initial pain reactivity and pain regulation is the infant's earlier pain behaviour, either earlier in the specific immunization appointment or earlier in the life of the child.

Accordingly, over the first year of life in a standard immunization setting where almost all younger infants were immunized on an examining table and older infants were being held during immunization, specific caregiver factors (e.g. verbal reassurance, emotional availability, proximal soothing) have no to small relationships with infant pain behaviour, thus, the relegation of caregiver factors to peripheral determinant roles (compared to actual infant behaviour) in this infant-specific model. Moreover, all larger spheres of social influence, such as the family (e.g. the spouse or siblings), hospital ecology, or culture are speculated to exert influence *indirectly* through influencing the primary caregiver at the time the infant is in pain. For example, during an immunization, the parent's internal cognitive schema for pain will be influenced by cultural beliefs, availability/acceptability of pharmaceuticals, general pain knowledge and beliefs, skills for coping with the child's pain, and societal expectations for an infant's pain response. This schema in turn will influence caregiver pain assessment and management which then directly influences infant pain regulation and reactivity. Previous work confirming that a parent's recall of their child's painful immunization experiences was significantly determined by potential cultural stress (Pillai Riddell et al., 2007) add credence to this hypothesis regarding the influence of larger spheres on pain assessment.

There are three feedback loops inherent in the model. Consideration of the infant responding self-regulatory loop (see interrelationships between boxes in the model in Figure 9.4) suggests that within an appointment, the actual stimulus and the infant's sensory thresholds (influenced by previous pain experiences and genetic nociceptive thresholds) triggers an infant's initial pain reaction and that the initial pain reaction will contribute to determining regulation from the initial pain reaction. Moreover, it is postulated that future pain responding, through modification of pain thresholds, will be impacted upon by past pain responding (both initial pain reaction and the infant's regulation from it). Examination of the infant–caregiver regulatory feedback loop (see interrelationships *between* the boxes and the ovals in Figure 9.4) suggests that not only will a caregiver's initial assessment and management of an infant's acute pain be predicted by immediate pain reactivity, a feedback loop occurs relating to infant regulation and subsequent caregiver assessment and management. Thus, how an infant is regulating following the pain event will impact ongoing assessment and management in a cyclical fashion until the distress is no longer evident (i.e. infant regulation re-establishes homeostatic balance).

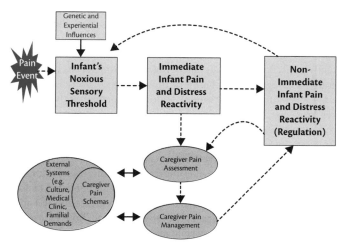

Figure 9.4 The development of infant acute pain responding model (the DIAPR model).

Finally, unique consideration must be given to the broader psychosocial systems of infancy. A parent feedback loop (see relations between ovals in the model in Figure 9.4) acknowledges that while an infant's pain responding (i.e. initial reactivity and regulation) contributes to caregiver assessment and management of the infant's pain, information arising directly from the infant is accommodated within existing parental schemas of the situation, based on influences such as cultural norms, medical institution guidelines, and the familial demands.

Finally, to attempt to bring further awareness to the steep trajectory of development during infancy, in Figure 9.4 dashed lines were used to portray those relationships that are hypothesized to change in strength over the course of infancy. For example, simply comparing infants at 2 months versus 12 months, OUCH cohort research indicated that the influence of parental factors, such as sensitivity or verbal reassurance, on pain responding was stronger at 12 months of age than at 2 months of age. Moreover, the transition and relationships between pain responses (i.e. pain reactivity and pain regulation) changes according to developmental stages within infancy. Solid arrows suggest that while changes may occur over time, this is likely to be not as strongly linked to the infant's development. Thus, the model attempts to capture the interplay between and among infant and caregiver factors as they change over the first year of life.

While attempting to capture observable inter- and intrapersonal factors to generate specific testable hypotheses regarding the infant, the model does not yet specifically outlay specific caregiver schemas that may be filtering influences from larger spheres of culture, medical norms, etc. Understanding patterns regarding how these larger systems influence the parental schemas which in turn impact on their behaviour towards their child in pain is crucial in trying to target interventions.

Critical review of paediatric pain models to date and future directions

Paediatric pain emerged as a distinct area of study in its own right relatively recently. There has been a proliferation of conceptual models over the past two decades. Generally speaking, these models share similar explanatory purposes in trying to understand the interplay among biological, psychological, and social processes during children's painful events. They postulate and emphasize different dimensions in seeking features of children's pain that are potentially modifiable to reduce pain and suffering in this vulnerable sector of society. Rather than conflicting with each other, the models reflect a remarkable degree of concordance concerning the key factors involved. However, one stark difference is the primacy of the caregiver. Most models embed the influence of the caregiver in a social dimension—only the SCM assigns caregivers a central role.

Interestingly, the biopsychosocial models presented here have chosen by design to either focus on acute or chronic pain. However, the formulations overlap. The models that examine the sequence of events involved in an acute pain episode acknowledge that previous pain experiences impact on current pain experiences. This provides an opportunity to examine relationships between acute and chronic pain. As Palermo and colleagues' models of chronic pain (2005, 2012) suggest, very similar aspects of the biology, psychology, and social environment (such as physical health, coping mechanisms, and culture) come into play, yet no models to date have attempted to explicitly bridge the theoretical gap that currently separates acute and chronic pain. The opportunity may be available in the study of biopsychosocial factors that are involved with the transition from acute to chronic pain. In children this must give consideration to the developing nervous system.

A problematic tendency of most paediatric models has been to treat pain expression as a unitary construct. Yet, as others have acknowledged in the more adult-centric theoretical literature (e.g. Hadjistavropoulos et al. 2011), there are both automatic-reflexive components and more controlled-cognitively mediated components to pain, with both reflecting ontogenetic and socialization features of pain experience and expression. Pragmatically, one also could acknowledge this divide using a similar dichotomy based on pain reactivity (a child's immediate response to a painful event) versus pain regulation (a child's pain and distress temporally distal to the actual painful event as the child moves toward re-establishing homeostasis). It would follow that the strength of impact of biopsychosocial factors would vary, with more innate/reflexive factors (e.g. pain receptor density, temperament) likely more prominent with pain reactivity and psychosocial factors (such as attachment, cultural beliefs about the value of pain, gender biases) likely more important determinants of how the child self-regulates subsequent to the painful event.

The most important limitation of existing biopsychosocial models of paediatric pain arises from how development is handled. With a few focused exceptions, we know little about the developmental transformations in biological, psychological, and social bases of pain through infancy, childhood, and adolescence, particularly through longitudinal study. While all existing models acknowledge the importance of development, it is argued here that in biopsychosocial models the interplay of these dimensions must be recognized as different across childhood (defined here as from birth to adolescence).

Taken from the larger field of child development, Arnold Sameroff's unified theory of development (2010) provides an exemplar for this position. At the core of this model is the tenet that while biological, psychological, and social factors are important in understanding all stages of the developing child, the magnitude of influence varies through infancy, childhood, adolescence, and adulthood. Factors external to the child increase in prominence with age and exposure to ecological systems, such as those provided by parents, the family, peers, and the community (including health care system and geopolitical contexts). One can then discern that to the newborn infant larger psychosocial contexts (culture, community norms, institutional practices, etc.) outside the self are not directly consequential (they likely indirectly impact on the infant through a caregiver's mediation of these factors). These influences change over time as attachment bonds are formed with primary caregivers over early infancy and childhood and then as the child enters into new systems of psychosocial influence such as daycare, elementary, or university spheres.

Although challenging, given the crucial nature that developmental stage plays in paediatric pain, it is imperative that this role is acknowledged more specifically because the relative weight of related factors change over time. One alternative would be to create models specific to unique stages of life as in the DIAPR model. Biopsychosocial models could then be more explicit and clearly elaborate on key factors involved within the specified age range, without fear of becoming convoluted. Potential developmental 'phases', based on key

Case example

Leah is 4 years old and her parents would describe her as being 'sensitive' to tactile and noxious stimulation. She is about to have her preschool immunization. Her mother and 1-year-old brother are waiting with her in the examination room. She told her mother earlier that she did not want to go to the doctor today because she hates needles. Her mother reminded her to behave because 'good girls don't make a fuss'. Her mother also reminded her that when she was a young girl her mother gave her a spanking if she embarrassed the family by overreacting in public. Adding to her dismay about the appointment, Leah had to miss her favourite period in junior kindergarten, music, to come to the doctor. The minute the doctor entered the room Leah started crying, which triggered her younger brother's tears. Her mother soothed her young son and apologized to the doctor for Leah's outburst. By the time the doctor could restrain Leah and quickly insert the immunization needle, Leah expressed maximal pain behaviours and took a long time to calm down after the needle.

Acute immunization pain is just one type of pain that children face over the span of childhood. As Leah's case helps illustrate, to best understand her pain experience and responding, one must take a biopsychosocial perspective.

areas of development (e.g. reliance on parents versus peers, ability to self-report, biological/physical changes), could be birth through infancy (0–2 years), early childhood (3–6 years), middle childhood (7–12 years), and adolescence (13–18 years). This would allow for models that more precisely outline the relative contributions of features and roles of biology, psychology and the social environment.

Conclusion

A child's experience of pain is an important area of focus within the broader pursuit of understanding human suffering. Developing biological and psychological capacities and social interactions distinguish infant, children, and adolescent experiences from those of the mature adult. The social contexts of pain, which interact with the child's biological and psychological action tendencies, are defined strongly by the impact of direct caregivers such as parents. Existing models in the field primarily describes these relationships separately for acute and chronic pain—integration is necessary. Future models could benefit by careful consideration of developmental stage factors.

Key recommendations

Having reviewed current biopsychosocial models of paediatric pain, key recommendations stemming from this work can be made:

(1) Biological, psychological, and social dimensions are useful constructs that encapsulate the key factors influencing paediatric pain.

(2) These dimensional influences are not static, but rather are dynamic, not only over the child's development, but also over the course of a discrete painful event or episode.

(3) More work that acknowledges how factors within a dimension impact on the child differentially over different developmental stages will prove theoretically and pragmatically beneficial.

References

Ahola Kohut, S., Pillai Riddell, R. R., Flora, D., and Oster, H. (2012). A longitudinal analysis of the development of infant facial expressions in responses to acute pain: immediate and regulatory expressions. *Pain*, 153(12), 2458–2465.

Anand, K. J. (2000). Pain plasticity and premature birth: a prescription for permanent suffering. *Nat Med*, 6, 971–973. doi:10.1038/79658

Bandura, A. (1977). *Social learning theory*. Englewood Cliffs, NJ: Prentice-Hall.

Bronfenbrenner, U. (1977). Toward an experimental ecology of human development. *Am Psychol*, 32(7), 513–531. doi:10.1037/0003-066X.32.7.513

Chambers, C. T., Craig, K. D., and Bennett, S. M. (2002). The impact of maternal behavior on children's pain experiences: an experimental analysis. *J Pediatr Psychol*, 27, 293–301. doi:10.1093/jpepsy/27.3.293

Cohen, L. L., MacClaren, J. E., and Lim, C. S. (2008). Pain and pain management. In R. G. Steele, D. T. Elkin, and M. C. Roberts (eds), *Handbook of evidence-based therapies for children and adolescents*, pp. 281–295. New York: Springer.

Craig, K. D. (2009). The social communication model of pain. *Can Psychol*, 50, 22–32. doi:10.1037/a0014772

Craig, K. D., Lilley, C. M., and Gilbert, C. A. (1996). Social barriers to optimal pain management in infants and children. *Clin J Pain*, 12, 232–242.

Fitzgerald, M. (2005). The development of nociceptive circuits. *Nat Rev Neurosci*, 6, 507–520.

Fordyce, W. (1976). *Behavioural methods for chronic pain and illness*. St. Louis, MI: Mosby.

Gatzounis, R., Schrooten M. G., Crombez G., and Vlaeyen, J. W. (2012). Operant learning theory in pain and chronic pain rehabilitation. *Curr Pain Headache Rep*, 16, 117–126. doi:10.1007/s11916-012-0247-1

Goubert L., Vlaeyen, J. W. S., Cromvez, G., and Craig, K. D. (2011). Learning about pain from others: an observational leaning account. *J Pain*, 12, 167–174.

Grunau, R. E. (2006). Long-term consequences of pain in human neonates. *Semin Fetal Neonatal Med*, 11(4), 268–275.

Hadjistavropoulos, T., Craig, K. D., Duck, S., Cano, A., Goubert, L., Jackson, P. L., *et al*. (2011). A biopsychosocial formulation of pain communication. *Psychol Bull*, 137(6), 910–939. doi:10.1037/a0023876

Hohmeister, J., Kroll, A., Wollgarten-Hadamek, I., Zohsel, K., Demirakça, S., Flor, H., *et al*. (2010). Cerebral processing of pain in school-aged children with neonatal nociceptive input: an exploratory fMRI study. *Pain*, 150(2), 257–267. doi:10.1016/j.pain.2010.04.004

Kazak, A. E. and Kunin-Batson, A. (2001). *Psychological and integrative interventions in pediatric procedure pain in infants and children*, pp. 77–100. Seattle, WA: IASP Press.

King, S., Chambers, C. T., Huguet, A., MacNevin, R. C., McGrath, P. J., Parker, L., *et al*. (2011). The epidemiology of chronic pain in children and adolescents revisited: a systematic review. *Pain*, 152, 2729–2138. doi:10.1016/j.pain.2011.07.016

Melzack, R. (1996). Gate control theory: on the evolution of pain concepts. *Pain Forum*, 5, 128–138. doi:10.1016/S1082-3174(96)80050-X

Melzack, R. (1999). From the gate to the neuromatrix. *Pain* (Suppl. 6), S121–126.

Melzack, R. and Wall, P. D. (1965). Pain mechanisms: a new theory. *Science*, 150, 971–979.

Osborne, R. B., Hatcher, J. W., and Richtsmeler, A. J. (1989). The role of social modeling in unexplained pediatric pain. *J Pediatr Psychol*, 14, 43–61. doi:10.1093/jpepsy/14.1.43

Page, L. and Blanchette, J. A. (2009). Social learning theory: toward a unified approach of pediatric procedural pain. *Int J Behav Consult Ther*, 5, 124–141.

Palermo, T. M. (2012). The problem of chronic pain in children and adolescents. In T. Palermo (ed.) *Cognitive-behavioral therapy for chronic pain in children and adolescents*, pp. 5–16. New York: Oxford University Press.

Palermo, T. M. and Chambers, C. T. (2005). Parent and family factors in pediatric chronic pain and disability: an integrative approach. *Pain*, 119, 1–4.

Pillai Riddell, R. (2009). Keynote award address to Canadian pain society 2009 annual meeting: dependent yet developing: new theorizing on the unique social context of infant pain. *Pain Res Manag*, 14(2), 143.

Pillai Riddell, R., Campbell, L., Flora, D., Racine, N., Din Osmun, L., Greenberg, S., *et al.* (2011). Caregiver sensitivity and infant pain: the relative relationships between infant behaviors and caregiver sensitivity over the first year of life. *Pain*, 152, 2673–2896.

Pillai Riddell, R. and Racine, N. (2009). Assessing pain in infancy: the caregiver context. *Pain Res Manag*, 14, 27–32.

Pillai Riddell, R., Stevens, B. J., Cohen, L. L., Flora, D. B., and Greenberg, S. (2007). Predicting maternal and behavioral measures of infant pain: the relative contribution of maternal factors. *Pain*, 133(1–3), 138–149. doi:10.1016/j.pain.2007.03.020

Pillai Riddell, R. R., Flora, D. B., Stevens, S. A., Stevens, B. J., Cohen, L. L., Greenberg, S., *et al.* (2013). Variability in infant acute pain responding meaningfully obscured by averaging pain responses. *Pain*, 154, 714–721.

Racine, N., Pillai Riddell, R., Flora, D., Garfield, H., and Greenberg, S. (2012). A longitudinal examination of verbal reassurance during infant immunization. *J Pediatr Psychol*, 37(8), 935–944.

Rickard, K. (1988). The occurrence of maladaptive health-related behaviours and teacher-rated conduct problems in children of chronic low back pain patients. *J Behav Med*, 11, 107–116. doi:10.1007/BF00848259

Sameroff, A. (2010). A unified theory of development: a dialectic integration of nature and nurture. *Child Dev*, 81, 6–22.

Taddio, A., Katz, J., Ilersich, A. L., and Koren, G. (1997). Effect of neonatal circumcision on pain response during subsequent routine vaccination. *Lancet*, 349, 599–603.

Turk, D., Flor, H., and Rudy, T. (1987). Pain and family. I. Etiology, maintenance and psychosocial impact. *Pain*, 30, 3–27.

von Baeyer, C. (2011). Interpreting the high prevalence of pediatric chronic pain revealed in community surveys. *Pain*, 152, 2683–2684. doi: 10.1016/j.pain.2011.08.023

Walker, L. S., and Zeman, J. L. (1992). Parental response to child illness behavior. *J Pediatr Psychol*, 17(1), 49–71. doi:10.1093/jpepsy/17.1.4

Williams, S., Blount, R. and Walker, L. (2011). Children's pain threat appraisal and catastrophizing moderate the impact of parent verbal behavior on children's symptom complaints. *J Pediatr Psychol*, 36(1), 55–63. doi: 10.1093/jpepsy/jsq043

Woolf, C. (2010). What is this thing called pain? *J Clin Invest*, 120(11), 3742–3744. doi:10.1172/JCI45178

Young, K. D. (2005). Pediatric procedural pain. *Ann Emerg Med*, 45, 160–171. doi: 10.1016/j.annemergmed.2004.09.019

CHAPTER 10

Cognitive styles and processes in paediatric pain

Liesbet Goubert and Laura E. Simons

Summary

Chronic pain is prevalent in children and adolescents. The current chapter outlines an interpersonal perspective on child pain, demonstrating the central role of child and parent pain-related cognitions in the development and maintenance of chronic pain in childhood. Pain takes place within a social context: children's expressions of pain (e.g. facial pain displays) are observed and decoded by others (parents), eliciting emotional and behavioural responses. Parents' responses may impact child outcomes in two ways, directly by imposing activity limitations/encouraging activity engagement or indirectly through observational learning. Although personality and temperamental factors may predispose children and parents to perceive pain as more or less threatening to deal with, the model presented in this chapter focuses on proximal pain-related cognitive processes and associated behaviours that contribute to pain-related disability in children. Recent evidence suggests that perceptions of pain as highly threatening (i.e. catastrophizing) may lead to fearful reactions to pain, activity avoidant behaviours, and more disability. In parents, catastrophizing thoughts about child pain are associated with higher levels of child disability, with recent evidence implicating parent protective behaviours as a mediating mechanism.

Introduction

Chronic and recurrent pain is prevalent in children and adolescents, with median prevalence rates ranging from 11% to 38% (King et al., 2011). A study in 987 children recruited from the general population showed that one-third of children and adolescents who were experiencing chronic pain at baseline reported chronic pain at 1-year and 2-year follow-up (Perquin et al., 2003). Most children seem to function well despite pain, although a minority (5%) are moderately or severely disabled across several domains of functioning (Huguet and Miro, 2008). The central question is why some children easily recover from pain and resume daily activities, while others seem to experience it as a major burden, hindering them in pursuing daily activities. This chapter will outline an interpersonal perspective on the development and maintenance of child chronic pain complaints, describing the role of cognitive processes in children and parents. Additionally, challenges for future research will be discussed.

Setting the stage: personality and temperament

Since the introduction of the gate control theory of pain, it has been increasingly acknowledged that the way individuals perceive and interpret pain is a determinant of pain outcomes. Early studies demonstrated that people's personality or characteristic ways of thinking impact how they process pain. Most studies focused upon the role of neuroticism—i.e. the trait-like tendency to experience a broad range of negative feelings such as distress or worry—which has been associated with a heightened experience of bodily sensations (Watson and Pennebaker, 1989), and, in particular, pain (Charles et al., 2008). In the context of paediatric pain, a fearful temperament has been identified as a predictor of somatic complaints 1 year later (Wolff et al., 2010) and 7 years later (Rocha and Prkachin, 2007). Furthermore, adolescents suffering from chronic pain have been found to be more vulnerable than healthy peers in terms of neuroticism (Merlijn et al., 2003). Originating from the positive psychology movement, the concept of optimism—i.e. the generalized expectancy of positive outcomes—has received increasing attention in the context of pain. In particular, optimism has been linked with lower pain reports in adults (Geers et al., 2008) and adolescents (Mannix et al., 2009; Williams et al., 2010). In children with cancer, Williams et al. (2010) demonstrated that optimism primarily related to lower self-report of pain and better emotional functioning, while pessimism was linked to poorer mental health.

Although these studies indicate that temperament and personality traits have a direct effect upon pain outcomes, other research has suggested that personality variables are better viewed as vulnerability or resilience factors, impacting on pain outcomes through more proximal variables involving pain-specific cognitive processes (Goubert et al., 2004; Hood et al., 2012; Leeuw et al., 2007; Muris et al., 2007; Vervoort et al., 2006).

Pain-specific cognitive processes

A cognitive process which has received ample attention in the pain literature is catastrophic thinking about pain, characterized by an individual's tendency to focus on, and exaggerate, the threat value of painful stimuli and negatively evaluate one's own ability to deal with pain (Sullivan et al., 2001). Extensive evidence is available that catastrophizing about pain relates to more intense pain and higher disability (Leeuw et al., 2007), and also is predictive of the persistence of pain and disability (e.g. Linton et al., 2000). Catastrophic thinking has been shown to give rise to an excessive fear of pain/injury (Goubert et al., 2004), which, in turn motivates individuals to escape or avoid activities thought to induce pain. Numerous studies have shown that catastrophizing thoughts about pain and pain-related fear (i.e. fear-avoidance beliefs) exert their effects upon pain experience and pain-related disability through longstanding avoidance behaviours and physical inactivity (Leeuw et al., 2007).

In line with the vulnerability hypothesis, several studies have demonstrated that neuroticism impacts on pain outcomes through catastrophizing about pain, in adults (Goubert et al., 2004) and children (Vervoort et al., 2006). Furthermore, a study in young adolescents showed that reactive temperament traits (involving fear and anger-frustration) were positively associated with pain catastrophizing, whereas regulative traits (i.e. attention and inhibitory control) were negatively associated with catastrophizing about pain (Muris et al., 2007). Interestingly, a recent study in healthy adults demonstrated that the protective link between optimism and pain perception operates through lower catastrophizing thoughts about pain, suggesting that individuals who are lower in optimism are more likely to ruminate, magnify or feel helpless about their pain experience, resulting in higher pain (Hood et al., 2012). Given the bulk of evidence supporting the proximal link of pain-specific cognitive processes on outcomes, the remainder of the chapter will primarily focus upon the role of fear-avoidance beliefs in children and parents.

Fear-avoidance beliefs in children: catastrophizing and pain-related fear

In recent years research has accumulated demonstrating the importance of fear-avoidance beliefs in the context of paediatric pain. Although the available evidence is markedly smaller than in adults, the findings are consistent with the adult literature. Child pain catastrophizing has been found to be related to higher pain intensity in samples of healthy school children and children with chronic pain (e.g. Hermann et al., 2007) and to lower pain tolerance (Piira et al., 2002). High catastrophizing children with chronic pain also report having more difficulty performing daily activities in home, school, recreational and social domains (Crombez et al., 2003; Guite et al., 2011). To our knowledge, only one prospective study of pain catastrophizing is available in children (Vervoort et al., 2010), indicating that it contributes to increased pain and disability 6 months later.

Research examining the theorized consequent of pain catastrophizing, pain-related fear, has gained support in relation to pain-related outcomes. In a small pilot study, Martin and colleagues (2007) found that pain-related fear accounted for 40% of the variance in pain-related disability. In another study, child pain-related fear predicted physical activity limitations beyond the influence of pain and depressive symptoms (Wilson et al., 2011). Furthermore, in a recent study among paediatric patients experiencing acute post-surgical pain, pain-related fear was associated with pain unpleasantness and functional disability 2 weeks after surgery (Page et al., 2011). In paediatric patients with persistent pain, Simons et al. (2011) found higher levels of pain-related fear to be associated with more frequent physician visits and higher levels of functional disability. In addition, a decrease in pain-related fear over a 1-month period

was associated with a decrease in functional disability, suggesting that a decline in pain-related fear corresponds with a resumption of daily activities. This study also examined the relationship between pain catastrophizing and pain-related fear. As expected, these sequentially linked variables were highly related to one another. At present, no studies have examined the sequential predictive role of pain catastrophizing to pain-related fear to pain-related outcomes in children. Proceeding from a cognitive-behavioural model of pain (see Leeuw et al., 2007), pain-related fear and escape or avoidance behaviours are expected to mediate the association between catastrophizing and the chronification of pain.

Children's fear-avoidance beliefs in a social context

It has become increasingly clear that child pain does not exist in a social vacuum. The biopsychosocial model of pain communication of Hadjistavropoulos and colleagues (2011) outlines how pain becomes a social experience. Following a pain stimulus, a child encodes its internal experience of pain into an expressive display of pain (e.g. facial pain behaviour), observable to others (e.g. parents). These expressive displays demand attention from others, which are then decoded (i.e. discriminated and interpreted), and may elicit emotional (e.g. distress) and behavioural responses (e.g. comforting) in the parent (Goubert et al., 2005). In turn, parents' responses may impact the child's experience and expression of pain. A comprehensive understanding of pain as a *social* experience (i.e. the dynamic interplay between a child's pain experience and the social environment in which pain emerges) thus requires consideration of expressive (i.e. how is pain communicated to others) and receptive features (i.e. how is pain perceived by others) of pain (Hadjistavropoulos et al., 2011).

On the expressive side, studies have indicated that children are able to modulate their expression of pain. An important determinant of pain expression is the intensity of pain experienced. Yet, pain intensity only explains a small to moderate amount of the variance in children's pain expression (Vervoort et al., 2009). A child's display of pain may vary according to the way a child is socialized to think and behave when in pain. Studies have shown that children's expression of pain depends on the beliefs endorsed about pain and the child's perceived ability to cope with it. Specifically, in line with research in adults (e.g. Keefe et al., 2003), recent findings revealed that children who endorse high levels of catastrophizing about pain express high levels of pain, regardless of the intensity of pain experienced (Vervoort et al., 2009). Furthermore, contextual factors, such as the presence of others, may be critical in understanding varying levels of child pain expression (Hadjistavropoulos et al., 2011). Children may consider the potential response from the other when deciding to express or hide pain. For example, children as young as 9 years old report being less likely to express pain in front of a peer than in presence of their parent because they expect more negative reactions from peers compared to parents following pain disclosure (Zeman and Garber, 1996). Furthermore, the social context may interact with children's beliefs in the impact upon child's pain expression. Of interest in this regard are studies from Vervoort et al. (2008, 2011a), investigating the impact of different types of observers in the relationship between child pain catastrophizing and child's display of pain. An interesting finding from these studies is that children who perceive the pain as threatening (i.e. catastrophize) indiscriminately display their pain, regardless whether they are alone, with a stranger, or with a parent. In contrast, low-catastrophizing children modulated their expression depending on whether a solicitous response is more likely (e.g. higher expression in presence of parent compared with when alone or in presence of a stranger).

Yet, it is still largely unknown why children who catastrophize express more pain, and the impact upon others. The findings of Vervoort et al. (2008, 2011a) support the suggestion of Sullivan et al. (2001), that catastrophizing about pain has an interpersonal function. In particular, it has been suggested that, through a heightened display of distress, individuals who catastrophize may be maximizing the probability that potential caregivers will maintain proximity or offer support or assistance (Sullivan et al., 2001). To truly understand the dynamics of children's pain catastrophizing in a social context, understanding the nature of the interaction between the child in pain and those able to provide care is essential. It is still unclear what type of responses high catastrophizing children elicit in others and how, in turn, these responses influence the child's future pain experience. Research in adult populations has indicated that others' responses toward high catastrophizers can vary substantially; catastrophizing appears to elicit positive responses such as the provision of instrumental support as well as negative responses such as criticizing the sufferer in pain or responding punitively (Keefe et al., 2003). In the context of paediatric pain, a recent study suggests that child catastrophizing may not always elicit solicitous responses, but also discouraging responses (e.g. criticism), although this association was only found for mothers (Vervoort et al., 2011b). This study also indicated that the negative effects of child catastrophizing upon pain outcomes may be reduced when parents promote well behaviours in their child. Only one pilot study could be found that has examined the relationship between child pain-related fears and parent responses to pain. Wilson et al. (2011) found that child pain-related fear and parent protective responses to pain were significantly correlated, with child pain-related fear mediating the relationship between protective parent responses and child activity limitations.

In sum, the available evidence suggests that observing their child in pain may initially elicit positive attention or care in parents. Over time, however, repeated exposure to their catastrophizing child's pain complaints may become a source of frustration and distress. In addition, the way in which high-catastrophizing children communicate their distress and demand help may impact parent responses. Lastly, differences found between mothers and fathers underscore the importance of examining each parent, rather that restricting our understanding of this complex phenomena to only mothers (Hechler et al., 2011). Clearly more research is needed in this burgeoning area of inquiry.

Fear-avoidance beliefs in parents

Beyond investigating the type of responses pain catastrophizing in children elicits in others and how these responses impact upon the child's future pain experience, it is also important to investigate who is likely to be less or more sensitive and responsive to heightened pain displays in the child (i.e. the receptive side) (Goubert et al., 2005; Hadjistavropoulos et al., 2011). Not only characteristics of the child, such as the extent to which the child engages in pain expression, but also characteristics of the observer and contextual variations are important here. These different influences are clearly described within a recent model of empathy and pain (Goubert

et al., 2005, 2009, 2013). When a child displays an internal experience of pain, others attend to, discriminate, and interpret pain signals, which may give rise to emotional (e.g. distress) and behavioural responses (e.g. comforting), with strongest reactions elicited by more intense pain displays. Yet, child pain expression is not the only source of information for others. Both characteristics of the observer (such as beliefs about the pain) and characteristics of the context may be important here.

In line with the cognitive-affective model of pain (Leeuw et al., 2007), it is likely that parents who perceive their child's pain as highly threatening (i.e. have catastrophic thoughts) may experience high distress, and, accordingly, feel motivated to engage in behaviours aimed at the reduction or avoidance of pain in their child, at the expense of other important domains (e.g. school performance) in the child's life. For example, it is reasonable to assume that parents, who perceive the child's pain as highly threatening and dangerous, may keep their child home from school more frequently. Preliminary evidence is available. Studies have shown that more protective behaviours from parents are associated with higher child disability (Peterson and Palermo, 2004; Simons et al., 2008). Furthermore, it was found that higher parental catastrophizing about their child's pain is related to higher parental distress (Caes et al., 2011; Goubert et al., 2006), higher child disability and lower school attendance (Goubert et al., 2006), and a higher tendency to restrict their child's pain-inducing activity (Caes et al., 2011). When examining parent catastrophizing and protective parent behaviours together, protective behaviours mediated the relationship between parent catastrophizing and child school functioning (Logan et al., 2012) and partially mediated the relationship between catastrophizing and functional disability (Sieberg et al., 2011). Additionally, parent pain-related fears are related to higher levels of child functional disability and child healthcare utilization (Simons et al., 2011). More insight into these mechanisms is expected to be of crucial clinical significance, as it will enable us to identify those parents who negatively influence children's vulnerability to deal with pain, and, as such, increase children's risk for delays in academic or social skills due to persistent pain problems.

One might argue that some level of parental worry is necessary as children depend upon parental care and protection. In this context, it might be useful to redefine catastrophizing as (more) extreme levels of parental worry. Indeed, very low levels of parental worry may fail to elicit parental care. Very high levels of parental worry, on the other hand, may relate to 'catastrophizing', with its maladaptive consequences for child outcomes. Future research may disentangle which levels of worry are most adaptive with the possibility that moderate levels of parental worry are most adaptive and promote effective child self-regulation of distress, while at the same time facilitating empathic concern and attention for the needs of the child (Caes et al., 2011).

Parental beliefs about pain and parental behaviours may not only influence children's pain and disability in a direct way, but may also have an indirect impact by means of observational learning processes. Observational learning has been defined as changes in patterns of behaviour that are a consequence of observing the behaviour of others (Goubert et al., 2011). In the context of pain, a child may acquire information about a particular situation and about the consequences of specific actions in that situation through observation of another's behaviour (e.g. parent) in that particular situation. For example, children who observe their parents displaying fear and avoidance reactions to back-stressing activities, such as lifting heavy objects, may adjust their appreciation of that particular situation ('back-stressing activities are dangerous') and the behavioural consequences ('avoidance of back-stressing activities reduces pain'). This information may translate into changes in attitudes and behaviour immediately, e.g. acquisition of catastrophizing thoughts related to certain activities, or later when the child experiences pain him/herself. In this way, how parents perceive pain and cope with pain may impact children's beliefs and behavioural repertoire (Goubert et al., 2011). Although early studies have found evidence for social modelling effects, indicating that observational learning influences both observable expression of pain as well as subjective experience (Craig, 1986), the evidence in the context of paediatric pain is limited. Few available studies suggest that families may influence children's experiences of pain through family members' own experiences/history of pain and use of coping strategies in dealing with their own pain and their child's pain (e.g. Thastum et al., 1997). To our knowledge, only one experimental study in children and their mothers showed that children displayed lower pain thresholds for a cold water task when their mother had voluntarily exaggerated her pain (Goodman and McGrath, 2003). Further research is needed to investigate the role of observational learning processes in the development of catastrophizing thoughts and pain-related fear in children.

Interpersonal fear avoidance model of pain

Based upon current evidence, the present chapter proposes a model involving pain-specific cognitive processes to understand how acute paediatric pain may evolve into chronic problems. Recent evidence suggests that a key determinant of adverse child outcomes may be a child's prioritized focus upon pain relief resulting in avoidance of daily activities (e.g. school, hobbies), motivated by fearful and catastrophic thoughts about pain. Prolonged avoidance of daily activities may result in long-term disability, child depression, and even delays

in the normal child's development. Indeed, prioritized pursuit of pain control goals may hinder the pursuit of developmentally appropriate goals, such as the achievement of new academic and social skills. Children who endorse high levels of worrisome thoughts about pain (i.e. catastrophize) may be likely to become entrapped into a vicious cycle of pain, fear, and prolonged disability (see Figure 10.1).

Child pain, however, takes place in a social context, of which parents are most influential agents. On the expressive side, a child encodes its internal experience in an overt display of pain, with high catastrophizing children engaging in an indiscriminate display of pain. On the receptive side, a parent decodes the child's pain signals, which may give rise to their own emotional and behavioural responses. Parents' catastrophizing thoughts about their child's pain may impact the decoding of the child's pain, fuelling pain-related fears, and motivating toward (over)protective behaviours. These parental responses, may, in turn, impact the child's pain-related cognitions, fears, and behaviour, and may promote child disability. Furthermore, when the child's pain becomes chronic, parents may become continuously focused upon the goal of alleviating their child's pain, which might interfere with other personal goals they have (e.g. work performance). This may lead to frustration, feelings of incompetence, and eventually depressive feelings in parents, which might, in turn, impact the child (see Figure 10.1).

As mentioned previously, more research is needed to understand the differential influence of mothers and fathers. In some cases, fathers may counteract the impact of mothers, who have generally been found to ruminate more about their child's pain than fathers (Hechler et al., 2011). For example, while both mothers and fathers with high levels of catastrophizing have been found to report a stronger inclination to engage in solicitous behaviours, only catastrophizing fathers also reported a stronger tendency to engage in behaviours discouraging child's pain expression or distracting child's attention from pain (Goubert et al., 2012; Hechler et al.,

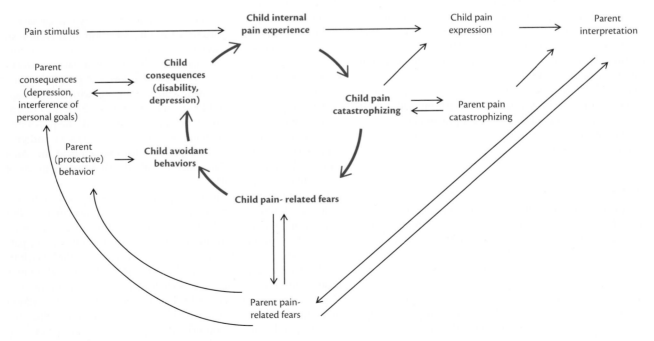

Figure 10.1 Interpersonal Fear Avoidance Model of Pain.

2011). Furthermore, given the impact of both child and parent variables in determining child outcomes, it is reasonable to assume that child and parent catastrophizing may have a cumulative impact; i.e. children who catastrophize about pain, and have pain-related fears, whose parents also have catastrophic thoughts about child pain might be at highest risk for longstanding problems.

Finally, contextual variables may modulate child and parent responses. A pertinent contextual variable may be the situational threat value of pain. For example, pain of unknown origin (i.e. functional pain) may be particularly threatening for parents (Williams et al., 2009), motivating parents (especially, those who already have catastrophizing thoughts about their child's pain) to engage in protective behaviours (Goubert et al., 2012). Furthermore, information a family receives regarding pain and its management (e.g. by a physician) may impact how child and parent cope with it. Research examining the role of contextual variables beyond child and parent pain-related cognitions/fears is an emerging and important area of inquiry.

Clinical implications

Extensive evidence points to the usefulness of cognitive-behavioural interventions in targeting catastrophic thoughts and pain-related fears in adults (Smeets et al., 2006). In children and adolescents, cognitive-behavioural approaches are also gaining support (Eccleston et al., 2002; Logan and Simons, 2010). Further research is needed to examine whether targeting catastrophic thoughts in parents is an efficient way to promote better pain outcomes in children. Furthermore, when families become trapped in a vicious cycle of pain, catastrophizing, fears, and disability, and the pain problem dominates family life at the cost of other important life goals, acceptance-based therapies may help families to give up the dominant search for a definitive cure for pain and reorient their attention toward positive everyday activities and other rewarding aspects of life (McCracken and Eccleston, 2003). Although most research on acceptance-based strategies has taken place in the context of adult pain (Veehof et al., 2011), two treatment studies among adolescents using an approach combining exposure and acceptance-based strategies support its effectiveness in adolescents (Wicksell et al., 2007, 2009). These studies found that pain-related fear, in addition to pain and disability, reduces following treatment.

To prevent the initiation of a vicious interpersonal cycle of fear-avoidance beliefs and the development of chronic pain problems, screening for vulnerability factors, such as high neuroticism may be useful. However, it has been suggested that individuals with an increased vulnerability may be less changeable in their fear-avoidance beliefs compared with individuals without pre-existing vulnerabilities (Leeuw et al., 2007).

Finally, further research is needed regarding variables that buffer against the development of catastrophizing thoughts and pain-related fear (e.g. optimism). Given that optimism may foster confidence to overcome stressful situations (Hood et al., 2012), interventions promoting positive optimistic beliefs in children and parents may have potential in the prevention or recovery from chronic pain problems.

Conclusion and future challenges

In this chapter, we outlined how child and parental cognitive styles and processes may impact the development and the maintenance of chronic pain complaints. Child and parent beliefs about pain and pain-related behaviours interact in determining child pain outcomes, with trait-like cognitive styles (e.g. neuroticism, optimism) acting as a vulnerability or resilience factor to developing catastrophic thoughts about pain and pain-related fears. Our understanding of childhood pain/disability may further benefit by focusing in future research on the motivational context of child and parent fear-avoidant behaviours. When pain persists, pain control may become the most dominant goal for children and parents who engage in catastrophic and fearful cognitions at the expense of other valuable life goals, resulting in persistent disability and/or depression (see Crombez et al., 2012). Child and parent may become frustrated because of experienced conflicts between pain-related goals (i.e. goals related to the reduction of pain) and other (e.g. social, academic/work) goals, potentially resulting in feelings of incompetence, and eventually depressive feelings. When attempts to solve the pain problem have repeatedly failed, adequate functioning and the successful attainment of developmental goals may depend upon the adjustment of unattainable goals (e.g. no exclusive focus on pain elimination) and the engagement in new goals (e.g. learning to function despite pain) by both child and parent. Evidence is accumulating that the ability to disengage from and adjust unattainable goals is positively associated with quality of life (Crombez et al., 2012). Future study is warranted regarding the goals parents and children pursue when faced with child pain, the concordance in the goals parent and child value, and the effect upon a child's functioning.

Case example

Molly is an athletic 13-year-old girl who suffered a hyperextension injury to her non-dominant left wrist when she fell backward trying to head a ball while playing in a soccer tournament. Working under the presumed diagnosis of a fracture, Molly underwent a series of castings, splints, and physical therapy. Notably, Molly reported intense pain throughout. Several months after her initial injury, she was diagnosed with complex regional pain syndrome, type II and underwent a left supraclavicular brachial plexus block and left ulnar nerve block. She reported only transient relief with this treatment. Shortly after the block Molly was evaluated in a multidisciplinary pain clinic by a physician, physical therapist, and clinical psychologist.

Molly and her mother presented for the evaluation in significant distress. Molly's mother indicated that in the past 6 months Molly's symptoms had only worsened and stated that 'something had to be done immediately' to help her daughter. Throughout the evaluation, Molly's mother would often quickly respond to questions directed at Molly. At the time of evaluation Molly described her pain as 7 to 8/10 in her left wrist and forearm. She described burning, sharp shooting, and throbbing pain from her fingers to her left shoulder. She also described pins and needles, weakness, and muscle twitching. She reported increased pain with activity and at rest. She described associated colour changes of her left hand and wrist to blue and purple, as well as increased oedema, sweating, and hair growth. Molly had significantly limited her involvement in sports, no longer participating in basketball or lacrosse (her favourite sport). She continued to play soccer, with a splint on the left wrist. Molly missed several days of school due to pain and her sleep was significantly disrupted. With regards to social history, Molly lives at home with her mother, father, and three younger siblings (brother aged 12, sister 10, sister 7). Prior to her injury, it was expected that Molly would regularly help to care for her three younger siblings. Her father is in sales and mother is a stay-at-home mom, who played lacrosse in college and coaches Molly's lacrosse team. Recommendations at the evaluation included continued medication management of gabapentin Neurontin, three times weekly physical therapy, and initiation of biofeedback/relaxation training.

For the next 9 months, Molly struggled with her pain symptoms with multiple follow-up medical appointments, medical tests, and three subsequent sympathetic blocks. She attended limited sessions of biofeedback training. Notably, Molly and her mother presented very distressed at appointments and expressed significant frustration that her pain did not seem to be resolving. Without physician direction, Molly's mother weaned her from all medications. Molly did experience periods of improved functioning during a spring vacation to Florida and multiple weeks in the summer while vacationing at the family's summer home.

After a period of improved symptoms, Molly experienced a flare in her symptoms approximately 18 months after her initial injury, shortly before the start of the lacrosse season. Molly presented frustrated and sad. Her sleep was significant disrupted and she was arriving to school late or missing the day entirely most days. She had almost completely stopped using her left arm and complained of intense, constant pain. After re-evaluation at the pain clinic, she underwent an additional sympathetic block and re-initiated psychological treatment. In addition to a focus on biofeedback and relaxation training, Molly set goals to: (1) attend a full week of school, (2) play in a soccer game, (3) deal with her frustration better with family members, (4) spend more time with friends, and (5) improve her mood. Molly was introduced to 'radical acceptance' of her pain symptoms versus the internal struggle with her pain in an effort to diffuse some of the anger and frustration that she had towards her pain and increase her ability to tolerate her physical discomfort. Molly also explored her values in each domain of her life and noted how little pain had to do with her valued life directions. The patient was able to eloquently describe the difference between 'acceptance' and 'giving up.' She talked about living a meaningful and enjoyable life regardless of the presence of pain. Although the pressure of performing in lacrosse was discussed and explored, Molly denied that this played any role in her symptoms. In collaboration with Molly's mother, Molly began attending school full-time again. This initially increased Molly's pain and frustration and Molly's mother struggled to tolerate her daughter's distress, leading her to question the treatment plan. Through multiple family meetings with Molly and her mother centred on re-emphasizing Molly's valued life directions, treatment alliance was re-strengthened and Molly continued to make gain in her functioning. At the conclusion of psychological treatment, Molly was able to increase the frequency and intensity of her physical therapy treatment and she was playing soccer (scoring the winning goal for her team at a recent game).

Acknowledgements

We would like to thank Melissa Pielech for her graphical work. Work was supported by the National Institutes of Health grant HD067202 (LS).

References

Caes, L., Vervoort, T., Eccleston, C., Vandenhende, M., and Goubert, L. (2011). Parental catastrophizing about child's pain and its relationship with activity restriction: the mediating role of parental distress. *Pain,* 152, 212–222.

Charles, S., Gatz, M., Kato, K., and Pedersen, N. L. (2008). Physical health 25 years later: the predictive ability of neuroticism. *Health Psychol,* 27, 369–378.

Craig, K. D. (1986). Social modelling influences on pain. In R. A. Sternbach (ed.) *The psychology of pain* (2nd edn), pp. 67–96. New York: Raven Press.

Crombez, G., Bijttebier, P., Eccleston, C., Mascagni, T., Mertens, G., Goubert, L., *et al.* (2003). The child version of the pain catastrophizing scale (PCS-C): a preliminary validation. *Pain,* 104, 639–646.

Crombez, G., Eccleston, C., Van Damme, S., Vlaeyen, J. W. S., and Karoly, P. (2012). The fear avoidance model of chronic pain: the next generation. *Clin J Pain,* 28(6), 475–483.

Eccleston, C., Morley, S., Williams, A., Yorke, L., and Mastroyannopoulou, K. (2002). Systematic review of randomized controlled trials of psychological therapy for chronic pain in children and adolescents, with a subset meta-analysis of pain relief. *Pain,* 99, 157–165.

Geers, A. L., Wellman, J. A., Heifer, S. G., Fowler, S. L., and France, C. R. (2008). Dispositional optimism and thoughts of well-being determine sensitivity to an experimental pain task. *Ann Behav Med,* 36, 304–313.

Goodman, J. E. and McGrath, P. J. (2003). Mothers' modelling influences children's pain during a cold pressor task. *Pain,* 104, 559–565.

Goubert, L., Craig, K. D., Vervoort, T., Morley, S., Sullivan, M. J. L., de C. Williams A., *et al.* (2005). Facing others in pain: the effects of empathy. *Pain,* 118, 285–288.

Goubert, L., Crombez, G., and Van Damme, S. (2004). The role of neuroticism, pain catastrophizing and pain-related fear in vigilance to pain: a structural equations approach. *Pain,* 107, 234–241.

Goubert, L., Eccleston, C., Vervoort, T., Jordan, A., and Crombez, G. (2006). Parental catastrophizing about their child's pain. The parent version of the Pain Catastrophizing Scale (PCS-P): a preliminary validation. *Pain,* 123, 254–263.

Goubert, L., Vervoort, T., and Craig, K. D. (2013). Empathy and pain. In R. F. Schmidt and G. F. Gebhart (eds) *Encyclopedia of pain* (2nd edn). Heidelberg: Springer-Verlag.

Goubert, L., Vervoort, T., De Ruddere, L., and Crombez, G. (2012). The impact of parental gender, catastrophizing, and situational threat upon parental behaviour to child pain: a vignette study. *Eur J Pain,* 16(8), 1176–1184.

Goubert, L., Vlaeyen, J. W. S., Crombez, G., and Craig, K. D. (2011). Learning about pain from others: an observational learning account. *J Pain,* 12, 167–174.

Goubert, L., Craig, K. D., and Buysse, A. (2009). Perceiving others in pain: experimental and clinical evidence on the role of empathy. In W. Ickes and J. Decety (eds) *The social neuroscience of empathy,* pp. 153–165. Cambridge, MA: The MIT Press.

Guite, J. W., McCue, R. L., Sherker, J. L., Sherry, D. D., and Rose, J. B. (2011). Relationships among pain, protective parental responses, and disability for adolescents with chronic musculoskeletal pain: the mediating role of pain catastrophizing. *Clin J Pain,* 27, 775–81.

Hadjistavropoulos, T., Craig, K. D., Duck, S., Cano, A. M., Goubert, L., Jackson, P., *et al.* (2011). A biopsychosocial formulation of pain communication. *Psychol Bull,* 137, 910–939.

Hechler, T., Vervoort, T., Hamann, M., Tietze, A. L., Vocks, S., Goubert, L., Hermann, C., *et al.* (2011). Parental catastrophizing about their child's chronic pain: are mothers and fathers different and does this matter for the child? *Eur J Pain,* 15, 515.e1–515.e9.

Hermann, C., Hohmeister, J., Zohsel, K., Ebinger, F., and Flor, H. (2007). The assessment of pain coping and pain-related cognitions in children and adolescents: current methods and further development. *J Pain,* 8, 802–813.

Hood, A., Pulvers, K., Carrillo, J., Merchant, G., and Thomas, M. D. (2012). Positive traits linked to less pain through lower pain catastrophizing. *Pers Indiv Diff,* 52, 401–405.

Huguet, A. and Miro, J. (2008). The severity of chronic pediatric pain: an epidemiological study. *J Pain,* 9, 226–236.

Keefe, F. J., Lipkus, I., Lefebvre, J. C., Hurwitz, H., Clipp, E., Smith, J., *et al.* (2003). The social context of gastrointestinal cancer pain: a preliminary study examining the relation of patient pain catastrophizing to patient perceptions of social support and caregiver stress and negative responses. *Pain,* 103, 151–156.

King, S., Chambers, C. T., Huguet, A., MacNevin, R. C., McGrath, P. J., Parker, L., *et al.* (2011). The epidemiology of chronic pain in children and adolescents revisited: a systematic review. *Pain,* 152, 2729–2738.

Leeuw, M., Goossens, M. E. J. B., Linton, S. J., Crombez, G., Boersma, K., and Vlaeyen, J. W. S. (2007). The fear-avoidance model of musculoskeletal pain: current state of scientific evidence. *J Behav Med,* 30, 77–94.

Linton, S. J., Buer, N., and Vlaeyen, J. W. S. (2000). Are fear-avoidance beliefs related to the inception of an episode of back pain? A prospective study. *Psychol Health,* 14, 1051–1060.

Logan, D. E., Simons, L. E., and Carpino, E. (2012). Too sick for school? Parent influences on school functioning among children with chronic pain. *Pain,* 153(2), 437–443.

Logan, D. E., and Simons, L. E. (2010). Development of a group intervention to improve school functioning in adolescents with chronic pain and depressive symptoms: a study of feasibility and preliminary efficacy. *J Ped Psychol,* 35, 823–36.

Mannix, M. M., Feldman, J. M., and Moody, K. (2009). Optimism and health-related quality of life in adolescents with cancer. *Child Care Health Dev,* 35, 482–488.

Martin, A. L., McGrath, P. A., Brown, S. C., and Katz, J. (2007). Anxiety sensitivity, fear of pain and pain-related disability in children and adolescents with chronic pain. *Pain Res Manag,* 12, 267–272.

Merlijn, V. P. B. M., Hunfeld, J. A. M., van der Wouden, J. C., Hazebroek-Kampschreur, A. A. J. M., Koes, B. W., and Passchier, J. (2003). Psychosocial factors associated with chronic pain in adolescents. *Pain,* 101, 33–43.

McCracken, L. M. and Eccleston, C. (2003). Coping or acceptance: what to do about chronic pain? *Pain,* 105, 197–204.

Muris, P., Meesters, C., van den Hout, A., Wessels, S., Franken, I., and Rassin, E. (2007). Personality and temperament correlates of pain catastrophizing in young adolescents. *Child Psychiatry Hum Dev,* 38, 171–181.

Page, M. G., Campbell, F., Isaac, L., Stinson, J., Martin-Pichora, A. L., and Katz, J. (2011). Reliability and validity of the Child Pain Anxiety Symptoms Scale (CPASS) in a clinical sample of children and adolescents with acute postsurgical pain. *Pain,* 152, 1958–1965.

Perquin, C. W., Hunfeld, J. A. M., Hazebroek-Kampschreur, A. A. J. M., van Suijlekom-Smit, L. W. A., Passchier, J., Koes, B. W., *et al.* (2003). The natural course of chronic benign pain in childhood and adolescence: a two-year population-based follow-up study. *Eur J Pain,* 7, 551–559.

Peterson, C. C. and Palermo, T. M. (2004). Parental reinforcement of recurrent pain: the moderating impact of child depression and anxiety on functional disability. *Pain,* 131, 132–141.

Piira, T., Taplin, J. E., Goodenough, B., and von Baeyer, C. L. (2002). Cognitive-behavioural predictors of children's tolerance of laboratory-induced pain: implications for clinical assessment and future directions. *Behav Res Ther,* 40, 571–584.

Rocha, E. M. and Prkachin, K. M. (2007). Temperament and pain reactivity predict health behavior seven years later. *J Ped Psychol,* 32, 393–399.

Sieberg, C. B., Williams, S., and Simons, L. E. (2011). Do parent protective responses mediate the relation between parent distress and child functional disability among children with chronic pain? *J Ped Psychol,* 36, 1043–1051.

Simons, L. E., Claar, R. L., and Logan, D. L. (2008). Chronic pain in adolescence: parental responses, adolescent coping, and their impact on adolescent's pain behaviors. *J Ped Psychol,* 33, 894–904.

Simons, L. E., Sieberg, C. B., Carpino, E., Logan, D., and Berde, C. (2011). The Fear of Pain Questionnaire (FOPQ): assessment of pain-related fear among children and adolescents with chronic pain. *J Pain,* 12, 677–686.

Smeets, R. J. E. M., Vlaeyen, J. W. S., Kester, A. D. M., and Andre-Knottnerus, J. (2006). Reduction of pain catastrophizing mediates the outcome of both physical and cognitive-behavioral treatment in chronic low back pain. *J Pain,* 7, 261–271.

Sullivan, M. J. L., Thorn, B., Haythornthwaite, J., Keefe, F., Martin, M., Bradley, L., and Lefebvre, J. C. (2001). Theoretical perspectives on the relation between catastrophizing and pain. *Clin J Pain,* 17, 52–64.

Thastum, M., Zachariae, R., Schøler, M., Bjerring, P., and Herlin, T. (1997). Cold pressor pain: comparing responses of juvenile arthritis patients and their parents. *Scand J Rheum,* 26, 272–279.

Veehof, M. M., Oskam, M., Schreurs, K. M. G., and Bohlmeijer, E. T. (2011). Acceptance-based interventions for the treatment of chronic pain: a systematic review and meta-analysis. *Pain,* 152, 533–542.

Vervoort, T., Caes, L., Trost, Z., Sullivan, M. J. L., Vangronsveld, K., and Goubert, L. (2011a). Social modulation of facial pain display in high-catastrophizing children: An observational study in schoolchildren and their parents. *Pain,* 152, 1591–1599.

Vervoort, T., Eccleston, C., Goubert, L., Buysse, A., and Crombez, G. (2010). Children's catastrophic thinking about their pain predicts pain and disability 6 months later. *Eur J Pain,* 14, 90–96.

Vervoort, T., Eccleston, C., Goubert, L., Vandenhende, M., Claeys, O., Clarke, J., *et al.* (2009). Pain catastrophizing and expressive dimensions of pain: an observational study in adolescents with chronic pain. *Pain,* 146, 170–176.

Vervoort, T., Goubert, L., Eccleston, C., Bijttebier, P., and Crombez, G. (2006). Catastrophic thinking about pain is independently associated with pain severity, disability, and somatic complaints in school children and children with chronic pain. *J Ped Psychol,* 31, 674–683.

Vervoort, T., Goubert, L., Eccleston, C., Verhoeven, K., De Clercq, A., and Crombez, G. (2008). The effects of parental presence upon the facial expression of pain: the moderating role of child pain catastrophizing. *Pain,* 138, 277–285.

Vervoort, T., Huguet, A., Verhoeven, K., and Goubert, L. (2011b). Mothers' and fathers' responses to their child's pain moderate the relationship between the child's pain catastrophizing and disability. *Pain,* 152, 786–793.

Watson, D. and Pennebaker, J. W. (1989). Health complaints, stress, and distress: exploring the central role of negative affectivity. *Psychol Rev,* 96, 234–54.

Wicksell, R. K., Melin, L., Lekander, M., and Olsson, G. L. (2009). Evaluating the effectiveness of exposure and acceptance strategies to improve functioning and quality of life in longstanding pediatric pain—a randomized controlled trial. *Pain,* 141, 248–257.

Wicksell, R. K., Melin, L., and Olsson. G. L. (2007). Exposure and acceptance in the rehabilitation of adolescents with idiopathic chronic pain—a pilot study. *Eur J Pain,* 11, 267–274.

Williams, N. A., Davis, G., Hancock, M., and Phipps, S. (2010). Optimism and pessimism in children with cancer and healthy children: confirmatory factor analysis of the Youth Life Orientation Test and relations with health-related quality of life. *J Ped Psychol,* 35, 672–682.

Williams, S. E., Smith, C. A., Bruehl, S. P., Gigante, J., and Walker, L. S. (2009). Medical evaluation of children with chronic abdominal pain: impact of diagnosis, physician practice orientation, and maternal trait anxiety on mothers' responses to the evaluation. *Pain,* 146, 283–292.

Wilson, A. C., Lewandowski, A. S., and Palermo, T. M. (2011). Fear-avoidance beliefs and parental responses to pain in adolescents with chronic pain. *Pain Res Manage,* 16, 178–182.

Wolff, N., Darlington, A. S., Hunfeld, J., Verhulst, F., Jaddoe, V., Hofman, *et al.* (2010). Determinants of somatic complaints in 18-month-old children: the Generation R study. *J Ped Psychol,* 35, 306–316.

Zeman, J. and Garber, J. (1996). Display rules for anger, sadness, and pain: it depends on who is watching. *Child Dev,* 67, 957–973.

Online supplementary materials

Figure 10.2 Example of interpersonal fear avoidance model of pain worksheet

Figure 10.3 Example of completed interpersonal fear avoidance model of pain worksheet

CHAPTER 11

Pain in cultural and communicative contexts

Ignasi Clemente

Summary

Pain and culture are complex and multifactorial phenomena. They defy objectification, isolation, and simplification. They can neither be defined nor measured easily, since they intersect with the biological, psychological, and social realms. Taking into account the intrinsic multidimensionality of each phenomenon, we are only beginning to understand the myriad of ways in which culture may influence pain. As a consequence, (1) the study of the relationship between culture and pain is fraught with methodological and theoretical challenges; and (2) there is no conclusive evidence to support specific guidelines on how to assess and treat pain of specific cultural groups.

Pain in children is too often underestimated and undermanaged (Craig and Riddell, 2003). The situation is worse for cultural–racial–ethnic minority children, who are marginalized, relegated to the lowest socioeconomic status, and with multiple barriers that reduce or block their access to health care. The significant health disparities that minority children experience aggravate ever further their vulnerability (Kristjansdottir et al., 2012): their pain is persistently underassessed and undertreated.

Evidence emerging from multiple methodological approaches reveals that cultural factors may influence specific aspects of pain experiences more than others. While it is unclear how the sensory aspects of pain may be affected by culture, the evidence illustrates how culture affects pain response, even at an early stage in an infant's life.

In addition to cultural factors across different settings, pain experiences are also affected by the communicative factors specific to a particular environment or situation in which pain responses, self-report assessments, and descriptions occur. Pain is highly susceptible to its immediate communicative environment in subtle ways. Clinicians need to become aware of their own cultural biases, assumptions, and beliefs. A place to start is to observe and talk to the paediatric patient and his/her family.

I begin the chapter by defining three key concepts (culture, ethnicity, and race), and by presenting the methodological and theoretical problems of the research on pain and culture. The chapter proceeds with an examination of the evidence on the relationship between paediatric pain and culture, organized by the methodology
used (experimental, interview, self-report, and observational). The examination of paediatric pain in cultural context is followed by a synoptic description of the sociomedical and socioeconomic contexts of paediatric pain, with a focus on professional cultures and health disparities. The chapter closes with a discussion of the communicative, environmental, or situational factors that impact children's acute and chronic pain experiences.

Introduction

Over the last 50 years we have learned that pain is a multidimensional, complex, and subjective (sensory and emotional) experience (Charlton, 2005; Merskey and Bogduk, 1994). Cultural and communicative factors are consistently acknowledged by pain research, yet elusively studied, perhaps because of the inherent complexity of the two phenomena.

Key concepts: culture, race, and ethnicity

Culture, often confused with the terms 'ethnicity' and 'race' (Edwards et al., 2001; Finley et al., 2009; Kagawa-Singer, 2001), is as complex and multifactorial as pain. Culture is 'an ethereal concept with a multitude of definitions' (Bernstein and Patcher, 2003, p. 142). Defining culture, ethnicity, and race is challenging. Operationalizing them is even more difficult, since these categories cannot be isolated and formulated into discrete independent variables (Clay, 2009; Craig and Pillai Riddell, 2003). They influence and are influenced by gender, age, and socioeconomic class to name a few. Furthermore, they are dynamic, socially and historically changing phenomena. Culture, ethnicity, and race are no different than definitions of pain and childhood, which have also changed historically (Bonica and Loeser, 2001; Edwards et al., 2001; James and James, 2004; Unruh, 1992).

Culture is 'the collection of malleable, adaptive strategies that groups of people have developed to survive in their ecologic niche' (Kagawa-Singer, 2001, p. 228). Culture is: (1) adaptive, dynamically ever-changing to meet social and environmental changes; and (2) heterogeneous: cultural groups have internal or intracultural variation in terms of socioeconomic class, gender, age, education, rural/urban setting, religion, and so forth. Such significant internal variation can be found throughout this chapter, for instance, regarding the differences within the label of the 'Asian' child between Japanese, Chinese, Isan Thai, central and southern Thai, and southern Taiwanese. Rigid and deterministic definitions of culture found in health and social policy research often ignore individuals' ability to act and change, as well as obscure similarities and emphasize differences between cultural groups (Ahmad, 1996).

Race is an ideological construct that has been associated with colonialism, inequality, and the imposition of a hierarchy of dominant people over dominated others. Race as a scientific category is a myth (Kagawa-Singer, 2001). The American Anthropological Association (1998) and the American Association of Physical Anthropology (1996) underscore that 'race' is not a scientific category based on clearly demarcated and consistently distinct 'racial' biological groupings. Phenotypic differences, for instance, differences in skin colour, do not match genetic differences (Craig and Pillai Riddell, 2003; Kagawa-Singer, 2001). Most genetic variation (94% of the human DNA) lies within the so-called racial groups, whereas only 6% occurs between racial groups (American Anthropological Association, 1998).

Ethnicity simply denotes differences between two groups. Ethnicity is not culture, since culture refers to ways of doing, thinking, feeling, and being. Unlike essentialist 'racial' differences based on purportedly biological differences, ethnic differences depend on nationality, tribe, religion, language, culture, history, experience, ancestry, and beliefs (Craig and Pillai Riddell, 2003; Edwards et al., 2001; Kagawa-Singer, 2001). The term ethnicity is misused when: (1) some kind of ethnic purity is assumed, without contemplating the possibility that an individual may self-identify with multiple ethnic groups or none; (2) it is applied ethnocentrically exclusively to others (i.e. the others are the ones with *weird* customs); and (3) it is used to mask a 'difference' that is in fact inequality, subjugation, and discrimination of minorities.

A significant problem in pain research is the stereotypical, methodologically inconsistent, and widely diverse use of racial–ethnic–cultural labels (Bernstein and Patcher, 2003; Finley et al., 2009; LeResche, 2001; McGrath and Finley, 2003; Zatzick and Dimsdale, 1990). In a critique of some 'classic' research studies on pain and culture, psychiatrist and anthropologist Kleinman and colleagues (1992, p. 2) argue that these labels are dehumanizing, create caricatures instead of people, and fail to address pain as 'an intimate feature of lived experience of individuals in the context of their local social world and historic epoch'. Widely used racial–ethnic–cultural labels are nation-state labels (e.g. 'Chinese' with 1.6 billion people), designating thousands of millions of individuals who have little in common other than politically and militarily drafted international borders. The same applies to pan-ethnic labels such as Hispanic or Latino, which are contested and yet used as political manoeuvres to provide health care to minorities that cannot afford them otherwise (Duany, 2011; Santiago-Irizarry, 2001). In addition to a general lack of theoretical frameworks in studies of culture and pain (Kristjansdottir et al., 2012), the difficulties in systematically delineating ethnic groups make it challenging to develop comparative meta-analyses of findings, synthetic summary statements, and clinical guidelines (Bernstein and Patcher, 2003; Finley et al., 2009; Garro, 1990; Zatzick and Dimsdale, 1990). Finally, because of its clinical orientation, this chapter is not representative of contemporary work on pain in the humanities and the social sciences, which has abandoned a cross-cultural comparative perspective and has instead focused on the deeply personal, subjective and intersubjective nature of pain experiences. For the interested clinician, a selected list of publications is included in the online supplementary materials, which also includes patients' own published accounts.

Paediatric pain in cultural context

As in research with adults, findings on the relationship of culture and pain in children are inconclusive and do not support specific clinical recommendations (Bernstein and Patcher, 2003; Finley et al., 2009; Pfefferbaum et al., 1990; Rosmus et al., 2000; Zeltzer and LeBaron, 1985). Determining cultural influences on paediatric pain is more complex because of the additional variability introduced by parent–child relationships (e.g. development, socialization, and family context). There is a scarcity of research studies examining the relationship between culture–ethnicity and pain in children, and a total dearth of work that examines culture–ethnicity among paediatric chronic pain patients, despite the importance of the social context for its treatment (Fortier et al., 2009). In addition, only one study has examined cross-cultural differences on children's pain perceptions with an experimental methodology (Evans et al., 2008). In what follows, for the sake of clarity and despite the reservations that I have raised, I use the ethnic–cultural–racial labels that the authors themselves use.

Children's pain perceptions and experimental pain

Regarding the influence of culture on pain perception in experimental and non-experimental pain research, our current understanding can be summarized as follows. First, numerous studies are plagued with theoretical and methodological problems. Second, no agreement exists on how culture may influence pain perception, and on what aspects of pain perception may be influenced. Third, adult experimental and clinical pain research show that non-sensory aspects of pain, such as unpleasantness, tolerance, and intensity, may be susceptible to ethnic–cultural influences, but no cross-cultural evidence has been found in the neurophysiologic detection of pain (Edwards et al., 2001; Green et al., 2003; Zatzick and Dimsdale, 1990: 554). Finally, despite the abundant literature with adults, only one study has examined ethnic–racial differences with children in a laboratory setting. In this study of three pain tasks with 123 healthy children (mean age was 12.9 years) in the US, Evans et al. (2008) found that African American children were no more or no less sensitive to pain than Caucasian American children, and no more likely to use a specific coping strategy. However, when coping (attending versus distracting) and race were considered together, significant differences emerged. For African American children, attending was associated with lower levels of pain and lower pain sensitivity, while for Caucasian Americans, distracting was associated with lower levels of pain and lower pain sensitivity.

Children's descriptions and understandings of pain elicited in interview studies

With the exception of Abu-Saad's research (1984a, 1984b, 1984c), most interview studies of children's pain descriptions and understandings in clinical and non-clinical contexts have taken a developmental perspective without consideration to cultural differences, despite the fact they have often been conducted in various countries. The lack of a cross-cultural perspective makes it unclear whether reported non-developmental differences are due to culture, context of the study, or the methods used. Gaffney and Dunne's study (1987) illustrates this difficulty: the authors reported that some Irish schoolchildren viewed pain as punishment. However, because such views of pain have not been found by other studies, researchers have speculated that it may have to do with the religious context of the schools in the study or with some aspect of the test procedure (Esteve and Marquina-Aponte, 2011; McGrath, 1995).

Abu-Saad's influential research has examined cross-cultural differences in children's pain descriptions and understandings with Arab American, Asian (Chinese) American, Latin American, and Dutch schoolchildren (Abu-Saad, 1984a, 1984b, 1984c, 1990; Abu-Saad et al., 1990). Overall, Abu-Saad and colleagues found that the range of physical and psychological causes of pain did not differ widely amongst cultural groups. Some cross-cultural differences were found in the use of sensory, affective and evaluative terms to describe pain; the description of the causes of pain; and the types of aches reported. Intracultural differences were also found, for instance, in the intensity scores assigned to pain descriptions by children with and without hospital experience. Revealing a more complex description, Abu-Saad also identified similar and recurring intracultural gender differences in several cultural–ethnic groups. Within their respective cultural–ethnic group, Arab and Asian American girls reported more frequently psychological causes of pain, different feelings when in pain (e.g. girls reported more often feeling embarrassed) and different pain coping mechanisms (e.g. girls preferred to be comforted).

Three recent studies of children's pain experiences and descriptions have focused on smaller populations and situations. As with previous research, they have revealed minor cultural differences. Cheng's (2003) study of southern Taiwanese children's pain experiences reports that crying does not necessarily involve vocalizations, but may be limited to facial expressions. Cheng relates this finding to cultural norms that vocal crying is inappropriate in southern Taiwan. Cheng also reports that some Taiwanese children perceived that their parents lied to them about the possibility of experiencing pain during hospitalization. Jongudomkarn and colleagues' (2006) study of north-eastern Thai-Isan children living with pain found that Thai-Isan children often described their pain as torturing, and that their pain experiences may not be extrapolated to children of different cultures in central and southern Thailand. Finally, and also involving Thai children but with a Thailand versus US cross-cultural comparative design, McCarty et al. (1999) analysed six stressful situations in terms of cultural differences, coping goals, and type of coping (overt versus covert). The authors reported that culture did not have a monolithic effect on child coping, but interacted with other variables such as stressor situation, gender, and age. The two groups differed in some situational contexts more than others, depending on the cultural salience of the situation.

Taken together, the evidence emerging from cultural studies of children's pain descriptions, experiences, and understanding of pain reveals more cross-cultural similarities than differences, and points to significant intracultural differences depending on gender, age, stressor, and situation. Culture is not a monolithic influence on the totality of the pain experience: specific cultural practices interact with other variables to influence particular components of the pain experience. In addition, these studies debunk the wrongly assumed internal cultural homogeneity within nation-states and ethnic groups, and expose the ease in which cultural diversity

may be acknowledged in Western countries but ignored in non-Western ones. They illustrate the importance of avoiding cultural stereotypes, such as 'Children from culture X feel Y pain no matter what situation, what happens, what is said, who is present, what age, what gender, and so on and so forth' (see the later discussion of situational factors in acute paediatric pain).

Children's clinical pain score scale rating self-report studies

Three studies reveal minor cultural differences: Zeltzer and LeBaron's (1985) study of Anglo American and Mexican American adolescents (ages 10–21) with cancer in the US, Pfefferbaum et al.'s (1990) study of Anglo and Hispanic children (ages 3–15) with cancer in the US, and Alwugyan et al.'s (2007) study of Kuwaiti children (ages 6–12) from countries in the Gulf (Kuwait and Kingdom of Saudi Arabia), Egypt, and the Levant (Lebanon, Syria, Jordan, and Palestine). At the same time, all three studies report intracultural differences: Zeltzer and LeBaron report differences between the two groups of Mexican Americans (e.g. rural versus urban lifestyles, and clinic differences between treatment centers); Pfefferbaum et al. report differences between Hispanic children and their parents; and Alwugyan et al. report differences according to socioeconomic factors, such as family income and educational level of the mother.

The intracultural differences in the three studies raise a critical issue that underlies much of the research on children's pain and culture, namely the need to provide a complex description of the social context in which children are socialized and acculturated (e.g. assimilation into the majority group). Child development does not occur in a social vacuum. From the moment of birth, an infant inhabits a sociocultural world (Pillai Riddell et al., 2007; Pillai Riddell and Racine, 2009), a fact illustrated by research showing that infants as young as 2 or 4 months old show cultural differences in acute pain responses (Lewis et al., 1993; Rosmus et al., 2000). Furthermore, children are not raised by parents within a self-contained family context, but within and in relation to social contexts such as the village/city, the school, the peer group, extended family, the state, and the socioeconomic forces that affect parents and families in terms of income, occupation, and education. Consequently, socialization/acculturation is not a unilineal process, but one that results from children interacting with parents, relatives, children and teachers in school, the public media, health practitioners, and other individuals and institutions (Craig and Pillai Riddell, 2003). In conclusion, these studies find no significant intercultural differences in clinical pain reports and instead identify intracultural differences, such as generational, rural/urban setting, socioeconomics, minority group membership, and the institutional culture of each clinic.

Children's pain responses and observational measures

Observational studies of children's pain responses provide similar findings. There are no significant overall cross-cultural differences, but minor differences emerge when an abstract definition of culture is abandoned, and culture is considered as interacting with other factors, such as the training of health care professionals, ethnicity of the observer/pain rater, parental socioeconomic class, parental level of literacy, and phase of the medical procedure.

Some cross-cultural design observational studies found no remarkable cultural differences, such as Pfefferbaum et al.'s (1990), while others have found some minor differences. In an study examining Dutch and US children with cancer undergoing bone marrow aspirations (age 8 months to 18 years 7 months) in their respective countries, van Aken et al. (1989) found subtle differences between the two groups according to phase of the medical procedure (preparatory, bone marrow aspiration, recovery). The authors discuss several explanations to account for these subtle differences, including cultural and contextual factors (i.e. differences in hospital setting, presence/absence of parents, and adult behaviours).

Bohannon (1995) examined pre- and post-surgery pain differences between African American and Anglo American children (ages 3–7) in the US using behavioural, self-assessment, and physiological measures. Bohannon found that African American children were significantly rated lower on observed pain behaviours, despite the fact that children rated their pain similarly. Bohannon discussed different interpretations: (1) non-linguistic based pain scores may be less subject to cultural–ethnic differences or may indicate universal aspects of pain; (2) African American children may express their pain differently when compared to Anglo American children; (3) the observational measure (Children's Ontario Pain Scale) may be better suited to detect pain behaviours of Anglo American children; (4) the examiners, whose ethnicity was not controlled, may have exhibited a bias.

Three studies relied on Blount et al.'s original or revised Child Adult Medical Procedure Interaction Scales (CAMPIS) (Blount et al., 1989, 1990, 1997) to examine procedural pain with children from different cultural backgrounds. However, the lack of a cross-cultural design requires caution when interpreting the results. Overall, authors found great consistency between their findings and previous research. Salmon and colleagues' (2002) study of Australian children (ages 2–7) of European, Middle Eastern, Asian, and Pacific Island descent undergoing voiding cystourethrograms found no cultural differences. Pedro et al.'s (2010) study of Portuguese children (ages 3–6) undergoing routine immunizations found some differences. However, underscoring the exploratory nature of their study, Pedro et al. contemplated that these differences could be due to cultural differences and/or lack of specific training of professionals and parents. Mahoney et al.'s (2010) study of venipunctures among mostly white European children (ages 7–16) in the UK found that humour and non-procedural talk were more common in the UK when compared to studies in the US. Furthermore, they found that adult behaviours such as apologizing, criticizing, and making empathic comments were rare; and children's verbalized pain and fear were common. Mahoney et al.'s findings raise an interesting issue: the possibility that cultural differences may not necessarily involve different behaviours, but different distributions and different frequencies of similar behaviours.

Finally, Rosmus et al.'s (2000) and Lewis et al.'s (1993) cross-cultural design observational studies of infant pain provide a new understanding of cultural difference and infant pain response. They highlight that cross-cultural variation may occur earlier in life than previously assumed. In a study of 4-month-old Japanese and American Caucasian infants undergoing routine immunizations in the US Lewis et al. (1993) found that Caucasian and Japanese infants did not differ in pre- and post-inoculation cortisol increase, but Caucasian American infants were more *behaviourally* reactive to pain than the Japanese counterparts. The authors emphasized

that Japanese infants are not less affected by stress. Instead, they suggested two potential explanations for the differences in pain reactivity, one biological (i.e. genetic basis of temperament) and one cultural explanation related to socialization (i.e. Japanese infants are kept in close proximity to the parents, which may lead to a smaller need of signalling of distress).

Rosmus et al.'s (2000) examination of the behavioural pain response of Chinese and non-Chinese Canadian 2-month-old infants undergoing routine immunizations found that Chinese Canadian infants showed a higher degree of behavioural reactivity than non-Chinese. Rosmus et al.'s findings go in the opposite direction of Lewis et al.'s findings (non-Japanese infants showed increased reactivity), demonstrating that a globalizing category of 'Asian' is unsuitable.

Rosmus et al. underscored that the Chinese/non-Chinese groups also differed significantly according to socioeconomic status (i.e. parental education and occupation). The authors conducted an impressive discussion that brings together cultural, socioeconomic, communication styles, and situational factors, to account for the differences in infant pain reactivity. For instance, infant arousal state may be influenced by the mother's communication style, which in turn, may be influenced by the mother's socioeconomic status. Since mothers may feel that their infant's behaviour reflects on how good/bad a mother she is, mothers of varying occupation and education will likely hold different values and expectations about how to present their infants to (unknown) others. Furthermore, parental education and occupation may interact with situational factors related to the logistics of the study, such as the ability (or lack thereof) to read, write, and give reports. In brief, Rosmus et al.'s study demonstrated that cultural differences are already present at a very early age, and, in line with studies discussed earlier, that culture does not have a monolithic effect on child pain behaviour, but intersects with other variables such socioeconomic status, communication style, and situational factors.

The sociomedical and socioeconomic contexts of paediatric pain

If culture is an ethereal concept that is difficult to define, the consequences of cultural differences are palpable in the specific sociomedical and socioeconomic contexts of paediatric pain. Specifically, I discuss the impact of professional and institutional cultures, as well as health care disparities, on children's pain.

Regarding its sociomedical context, the assessment and treatment of paediatric pain are contingent on parents' and health professionals' attitudes and beliefs (Post et al., 1996). Pain assessment varies according to whom is observing it, in clinical practice (Davitz et al., 1976) and in research (Bernstein and Patcher, 2003; Neuman, 1996; Post et al., 1996; Zatzick and Dimsdale, 1990). Furthermore, health professionals are not acultural beings, but have their own specific cultural–ethnic–religious background (Free, 2002). Finally, physicians and nurses are also members of specific professional cultures, having undergone a professional socialization process (Cicourel, 1987; Good, 1995), which makes them members of the particular subculture of a specific hospital/clinic/unit within the culture of a specific health care centre.

In Western and non-Western hospitals, institutional cultures and clinicians' beliefs often are the barriers to optimal pain management (Finley et al., 2009; McGrath and Unruh, 2007) in both developed and developing countries (Cohen and MacLaren, 2007; Craig et al., 1996; Finley et al., 2008; Forgeron et al., 2006, 2009; McCarthy et al., 2004; Pillai Riddell et al., 2008). As Finley et al. (2008) note on the erroneous misconceptions about pain and opioid addiction, there is nothing Arab or Middle Eastern specific to them.

In terms of the socioeconomic context of paediatric pain, cultural–ethnic–racial differences place minority children as a vulnerable population when it comes to pain assessment and treatment (Kristjansdottir et al., 2012). Minoritized communities face overlapping problems such as racism, poverty, limited education, low income, limited proficiency in the majority language, lack of health insurance, high mobility due to migrant patterns associated with temporary jobs, and legal/illegal immigrant status. Furthermore, they have to overcome significant difficulties in access to care, in terms of financial affordability, living far from health care centres, and/or lacking transportation. Health care disparities have been qualified as a national and pervasive problem in the US (Williams and Organizing Committee of the Pain Disparities Special Interest Group of the American Pain Society, 2005). Although studies of sociodemographic disparities in paediatric pain management have yielded inconsistent results (see Ezenwa and Huguet, Chapter 65, this volume), disparities in adult pain (Green et al., 2003) and general health care disparities for minority children have been documented. Thus, it is not far-fetched to assume that minority children share the health care disadvantages of their parents.

Disparities in children's health have been reported within three common paediatric health conditions: asthma, oral health, and obesity/type 2 diabetes (Fuemmeler et al., 2009). Access to health care is also an obstacle for uninsured children, who are disproportionally minority children. Fuemmeler et al. also report that Hispanic children are more than twice as likely to be non-insured in the US. Hispanic children are also the least likely to be insured with the numerous risk factors and consequences (Flores et al., 2006). In a review study of barriers to health care for Latino children in the US, Flores and Vegas (1998) reported that Latino children are more likely to be poor, the most uninsured, and have parents with the lowest education attainment. In addition, Latino children experienced provider-related barriers such as reduced screening, missed vaccination opportunities, decreased likelihood of receiving prescriptions, suboptimal management plans, inadequate communication and patient education, and perceptions of negative attitudes. It is fundamental then to acquiesce that social inequalities and racism, and not culture per se, are often the culprits of profoundly unjust health disparities.

Paediatric pain in communicative context

Paediatric acute pain and communication

In the same way that culture and ethnicity influence children's pain experiences, a number of contextual factors—also referred to as situational or environmental—influence pain experiences. Contextual factors are discussed elsewhere in this volume in chapters on distraction (Cohen et al., Chapter 53), pain and the family (Birnie et al., Chapter 12), and the various measurement chapters—especially with non-verbal populations (e.g. Lee and Stevens, Chapter 35; Chorney and McMurtry, Chapter 37). However, a way to remember key contextual factors includes using interrogatives (what, when, who, whom, where, and how). Adult (parent and staff) and child behaviours are highly interactive, affecting each other in subtle, susceptible, and almost-immediate ways. Because of this, current and future studies are moving beyond who is present during a painful procedure, to

examine also what they are communicating verbally and non-verbally, when, who, to whom, where, and how (Table 11.1).

Paediatric chronic pain and communication

Children with chronic pain often feel that clinicians do not hear, understand, or believe them (Carter, 2002; Nutkiewicz, 2008). In an interview study of 32 adolescents with non-malignant chronic pain (ages 14–18) in the US, Nutkiewicz (2008) remarked that clinicians ignore the experiential component of the pain and the child's lived experience, and are not attentive to information that may not be discernibly or explicitly clinical. In addition, adolescents find themselves continually re-telling their pain stories in multiple unrelated visits to different clinicians. Children's perceived lack of physician understanding reinforces their frustration, loss of potential, sense of isolation and difference from peers; and lowers even further their expectations that clinicians or parents can help them (Meldrum et al., 2009).

In a narrative study of children with chronic pain and their families in the UK, Carter (2002, 2004) described how children experience 'referral fatigue' in their 'diagnostic quest' (see also Lillrank, 2003; Ong et al., 2004), from one specialist to the next, as well as professional 'ventriloquism,' where 'the child's words are reinterpreted and mistranslated through the professionals' own paradigmatic understanding of the narrative' (Carter, 2002, p. 36).

Children's negative experiences of communication inside the clinic/hospital are missed opportunities to incorporate the richness of children's own pain narratives into clinical decisions. Based on a qualitative analysis of the narratives of 45 children with chronic pain attending a US multidisciplinary tertiary care specializing in pain, Meldrum et al. (2009) identified five common themes in children's narratives: hiding pain from parents and friends; a sense of isolation and difference from peers and classmates; pain as an obstacle to personal activities; fears about how pain will affect the future; and perceived lack of physician understanding. These themes are articulated in six different narratives or plotlines: the constant patient, the invalid, the weary soldier, the stoic, the positive thinker, and the decision-maker. Meldrum et al. (2008) also identified a functioning strategy developed by the children themselves, 'getting on with life', which involves ignoring the pain and trying to keep going. These authors also provide additional support to two self-developed strategies identified by Hunfeld et al. (2001): 'planning ahead,' which involves deliberately organizing activities while reducing stress, and 'body awareness,' which involves becoming aware of one's body while distracting oneself from the pain. A further discussion of persisting pain can be found in Chapter 32 by Mherekumombe and Collins.

Conclusion

In this chapter, the complexity of examining the relationships between culture and pain, and communication and pain has been highlighted. Neither pain nor culture and communication are amenable to 'easy answers and fixes.' Indeed, 'easy answers and fixes' lead to ignoring or stereotyping cultural and communicative differences. On the contrary, the variability of cultural and communicative contextual factors only adds to the variability of subjective and deeply personal pain experiences.

We are beginning to understand how cultural and communicative factors influence pain and what aspects of pain they influence. Cultural and communicative factors affecting pain are characterized

Table 11.1 Contextual variables based on interrogatives

What[a]	Praising the child is neither related to child coping nor distress
	Empathic and apologetic statements are positively related to child distress
	Reassurances fail to diminish displays of child and infant distress, and may magnify them
	Adult promoted attention manipulation (e.g. passive and active distraction) are beneficial in child coping and reducing pain
	When the distraction intervention requires too much attention, the distress may interfere with the child's ability to focus on the distraction
When	Children's distress is likely to be preceded and followed by adult distress promoting behaviours (e.g. reassurances) in what seems a circular relationship
	Children's engagement in coping behaviours, such talk unrelated to the painful procedure, humour and coping statements, is also preceded and followed by adult coping-prompting behaviours
	Child distress and coping, and adult behaviours change according to the phase of the medical procedure
	Type of adult coping promoting and child coping behaviours correlate within a specific phase, but not across phases
Who	Nurses' increased coping promoting behaviours are associated with an increase in parental coping promoting behaviours
	Whereas nurses' and physicians' behaviours are uniformly negatively associated with child distress, some parental behaviours are associated with child distress
Whom	Whereas the same behaviour of adult non-procedural talk to another adult is neutral, when addressed to the child, non-procedural talk is child coping promoting
	Despite the developmental changes in children's pain expression, it remains to be determined whether observational measures of children' procedural pain need to be aged-normed
	Observational measures have shown good evidence supporting their validity from early childhood through late adolescence
Where	(1) Physical setting:
	Needle procedures should not be conducted in the patient's own room to preserve the room as a refuge
	Noise and light have a negative effect in the context of neonatal pain
	(2) Psychosocial setting:
	The evidence is inconclusive regarding the influence of parental presence child distress and behavioural outcomes, without distinguishing whether the father or the mother is the parent present, or whether one or both are present
	What parents do is more relevant than whether they are in the room vis-à-vis child distress reduction
	(3) The body as a means to communicate:
	Caregivers' instrumental, task-fulfilling (e.g. to restrain the child) touch is correlated with child distress, whereas supportive touch is not
	Caregivers may stand at a close distance but provide no supportive touch to the distressed child
	Combinations of supportive touch, posture, and movement (e.g. skin-to-skin kangaroo, rocking, holding, and to a lesser degree, bouncing, patting, kissing, rubbing, and hugging) have been shown to reduce preterm, neonate, and infant distress
	The evidence of the efficacy of handholding is inconclusive, although some evidence points that it depends on who is holding (nurse versus parent) the child's hand
How	The production of a parental linguistic expression can vary widely in terms of tone, pitch, loudness as well as in terms of the non-verbal communication accompanying it
	The lack of attention to non-verbal communication may explain the contradictory findings regarding whether parental empathic supportive talk is related to increased or decreased child pain during painful procedures
	Ordering the child to relax with a forceful imperative like 'Relax!' and 'Breathe!' is a different action when compared to parents modelling deep breathing
	Facial expressions of emotion (happy versus fearful) may be more salient feature than vocal tone (rising versus falling final intonation) to children

[a] See Birnie et al. (Chapter 12) and Cohen et al. (Chapter 52) for further discussion.

by their *variability* (e.g. each cultural and communicative context is somewhat different), *specificity* (e.g. pain experience occurs to a specific individual, in a specific situated context, at a specific time in his/her life), *multiplicity* (e.g. multiple cultural and communicative factors are operating simultaneously, interacting with each other, and mediating pain experiences), and *time sensitivity* (e.g. immediately preceding talk may influence subsequent pain responses). Rather than creating checklist inventories, clinicians can develop observational and interview tools to consider the multiple and simultaneous factors that influence pain. It is fundamental that clinicians become aware of their own cultural biases, learn that culture, ethnicity, and race cannot be assumed just by looking at the patient, and that no cultural recipe can substitute observing the patient and listening to him/her.

Case example

In a biopsychosocial approach to paediatric pain, eliciting children's (and parents') pain accounts is fundamental but challenging. Clinicians have two interlocutors at any given time, parents can take over the conversation, and disagreements arise between parents and children. There are small, practical communicative strategies to overcome these challenges (Clemente, 2009; Clemente et al., 2008, 2012). In the following case, a 12-year-old girl with recurrent stomach pains produces an account. The clinician uses a variety of strategies to support and encourage her. The clinician uses a question preface (lines 1–11) and broad open-ended questions and prompts (lines 13,

16, 22, 28, 33). When broad questions are met with prolonged silence (lines 26 and 35), the clinician retains the girl as respondent by asking questions that require only a yes/no answer (lines 36, 39–41). Despite her many silences and pauses, the clinician has given the girl ample time to answer. At the same time, giving ample time and broad directions have the risk that the child may get lost, which occurs in lines 18 to 20. In eliciting children's pain accounts, a balance may be required between giving not enough guidance (e.g. using broad questions that do not constrain patients' accounts but may result in disoriented patients who do not know what the clinician wants to hear) and too much guidance (e.g. narrow questions that constrain patients' answers to merely 'yes/no') (Figure 11.1).

1	DOC:		Nice to meet you too.
2			(0.5)
3	DOC:		allo Madame?,
4			(0.3)
5	DOC:		nice to meet you, (1.1) so I read
6			through your medical records, and
7			reviewed your questionnaires,
8	MOM:		O:h okay.
9	DOC:		I wanted to know a little about whatís
10			been going on from your point of
11			view.
12			(0.6)
13	DOC:	->	what brings yout here.
14			(1.8)
15	PAT:		Um (that I donít feel good?)
16	DOC:	->	Okay, keep going.
17			(0.5)
18	PAT:		U::m (2.1) um (0.5) youíre gonna try
19			to help me?
20	DOC:		·hh yea thatís t [rue:.
21	MOM:		[h
22	DOC:	->	Tell me about not feeling good.
23			(0.7)
24	PAT:		·h um (0.5) I donít feel good a lotta
25			times?,
26			(1.5)
27	PAT:		uh:: (1.3)what else.
28	DOC:	->	Okay whaddya mean by not feeling
29		->	good.
30			(0.6)
31	PAT:		Uh my stomach hurts?,
32			(0.3)
33	DOC:	->	Oka:y, (0.6) tell me about your
34		->	stomach hurting.
35			(1.2)
36	DOC:	=>	·hh you have Crohnís. Correct,
37	PAT:		Yeah.
38			(0.6)
39	DOC:	=>	And you were diagnosed (1.0) you had
40		=>	stomach aches when you were three.
41			Right?
42	PAT:		Yeah.

Figure 11.1 Communication between the doctor (DOC), mother (MOM), and patient (PAT).

Reprinted from *Social Science and Medicine*, Volume 66, Issue 6, Ignasi Clemente, Seung-Hee Lee and John Heritage, Children in chronic pain: Promoting pediatric patients' symptom accounts in tertiary care, pp. 1418–1428, Copyright © 2008, with permission from Elsevier, http://www.sciencedirect.com/science/journal/02779536

Acknowledgements

I would like to express my gratitude to my postdoctoral advisor Dr Lonnie K. Zeltzer at the D. Geffen School of Medicine at UCLA, and to Dr Carl von Baeyer, my advisor in the PICH (Pain in Child Health) Research Strategic Training Program of the Canadian Institutes of Health. My participation as an international post-doctoral trainee in the PICH program was made possible by the generous support of the Mayday Fund. I also wish to thank Dr Bonnie Stevens for her many contributions to this chapter and to Dr Marcia Meldrum, Dr Maria Katz, Mary-Caitlyn Valentinsson, and Eugene Danyo for their meticulous reading of this chapter.

References

Abu-Saad, H. (1984a). Cultural components of pain: the Arab-American child. *Issues Compr Pediatr Nurs*, 7(2–3), 91–99.

Abu-Saad, H. (1984b). Cultural components of pain: the Asian-American child. *Child Health Care*, 13(1), 11–14.

Abu-Saad, H. (1984c). Cultural group indicators of pain in children. *Matern Child Nurs J*, 13(3), 187–196.

Abu-Saad, H. (1990). Toward the development of an instrument to assess pain in children: Dutch study. In D. C. Tyler and E. J. Krane (eds) *Pediatric pain. advances in pain research and therapy, vol. 15*, pp. 101–106. New York: Raven Press.

Abu-Saad, H. H., Kroonen, E., and Halfens, R. (1990). On the development of a multidimensional Dutch pain assessment tool for children. *Pain*, 43(2), 249–256.

Ahmad, W. I. U. (1996). The trouble with culture. In D. Kelleher and S. Hillier (eds) *Researching cultural differences in health*, pp. 190–219. London: Routledge.

Alwugyan, D., Alroumi, F., and Zureiqi, M. (2007). Expression of pain by children and its assessment in Kuwait. *Med Prin Pract*, 16(Suppl. 1), 21–26.

American Anthropological Association. (1998). American Anthropological Association statement on 'race'. (17 May 1998). Available at: <http://www.aaanet.org/stmts/racepp.htm> (accessed 1 February 2012).

American Association of Physical Anthropologists. (1996). AAPA statement on biological aspects of race. *Am J Phys Anthropol*, 101(4), 569–570.

Bernstein, B. A. and Patcher, L. M. (2003). Cultural considerations in children's pain. In N. Schechter, C. Berde, and M. Yaster (eds) *Pain in infants, children and adolescents (2nd edn)*, pp. 142–156. Philadelphia, PA: Lippincott, Williams & Wilkins.

Blount, R. L., Cohen, L. L., Frank, N. C., Bachanas, P. J., Smith, A. J., Manimala, M. R., *et al.* (1997). The Child-Adult Medical Procedure Interaction Scale—revised: an assessment of validity. *J Pediatr Psychol*, 22(1), 73–88.

Blount, R. L., Corbin, S. M., Sturges, J. W., Wolfe, V. V., Prater, J. M., and James, L. D. (1989). The relationship between adults' behavior and child coping and distress during BMA/LP procedures: a sequential analysis. *Behav Ther*, 20, 585–601.

Blount, R. L., Sturges, J. W., and Powers, S. W. (1990). Analysis of child and adult behavioral variations by phase of medical procedure. *Behav Ther*, 21, 33–48.

Bohannon, A. S. (1995). Physiological, self-report, and behavioral ratings of pain in three to seven year old African-American and Anglo-American children. Unpublished 9540967, University of Miami, United States—Florida.

Bonica, J. J., and Loeser, J. D. (2001). History of pain concepts and therapies. In J. D. Loeser (ed.) *Bonica's management of pain (3rd edn)*, pp. 3–16. Philadelphia, PA: Lippincott Williams & Wilkins.

Carter, B. (2002). Chronic pain in childhood and the medical encounter: professional ventriloquism and hidden voices. *Qual Health Res*, 12(1), 28–41.

Carter, B. (2004). Pain narratives and narrative practitioners: a way of working 'in-relation' with children experiencing pain. *J Nurs Manag*, 12, 210–216.

Charlton, J. (2005). *Pain in infants, children, and adolescents core curriculum for professional education in pain*. Seattle, WA: IASP Press.

Cheng, S.-F., Foster, R. L., Hester, N. O., and Chu-Yu Huang, N. O. (2003). A qualitative inquiry of Taiwanese children's pain experiences. *J Nurs Res*, 11(4), 241–249.

Cicourel, A. V. (1987). Cognitive and organizational aspects of medical diagnostic reasoning. *Discourse Process*, 10, 346–367.

Clay, D. L. (2009). Cultural and diversity issues in research and practice. In M. C. Roberts and R. G. Steele (eds) *Handbook of pediatric psychology (4th edn)*, pp. 89–98. New York: Guilford Press.

Clemente, I. (2009). Progressivity and participation: children's management of parental assistance in paediatric chronic pain encounters. *Sociol Health Ill*, 31(6), 872–888.

Clemente, I., Heritage, J., Meldrum, M. L., Tsao, J. C. I., & Zeltzer, L. K. (2012). Preserving the child as a respondent: initiating patient-centered interviews in a U.S. outpatient tertiary care pediatric pain clinic. *Commun Med*, 9(2), 203–213.

Clemente, I., Lee, S. H., and Heritage, J. (2008). Children in chronic pain: promoting pediatric patients' symptom accounts in tertiary care. *Soc Sci Med*, 66(6), 1418–1428.

Cohen, L. L. and MacLaren, J. E. (2007). Breaking down the barriers to pediatric procedural preparation. *Clin Psychol-Sci Pr*, 14(2), 144–148.

Craig, K. D., Lilley, C. M., and Gilbert, C. A. (1996). Social barriers to optimal pain management in infants and children. *Clin J Pain*, 12(3), 232–242.

Craig, K. D., and Pillai Riddell, R. R. (2003). Social influences, culture, and ethnicity. In P. J. McGrath and G. A. Finley (eds) *Pediatric pain: biological and social context, progress in pain research and management*, vol. 26, pp. 159–182. Seattle, WA: IASP Press.

Davitz, L. J., Sameshima, Y., and Davitz, J. R. (1976). Suffering as viewed in six different cultures. *Am J Nurs*, 76(8), 1296–1297.

Duany, J. (2011). *Blurred borders: transnational migration between the Hispanic Caribbean and the United States*. Chapel Hill, NC: University of North Carolina Press.

Edwards, C. L., Fillingim, R. B., and Keefe, F. (2001). Race, ethnicity and pain. *Pain*, 94, 133–137.

Esteve, R. and Marquina-Aponte, V. (2011). Children's pain perspectives. *Child Care Health Dev*, 38(3), 441–452.

Evans, S., Lu, Q., Tsao, J. C., and Zelter, L. K. (2008). The role of coping and race in healthy children's experimental pain responses. *J Pain Manag*, 1(2), 151–162.

Finley, G. A., Forgeron, P., and Arnaout, M. (2008). Action research: developing a pediatric cancer pain program in Jordan. *J Pain Symptom Manag*, 35(4), 447–454.

Finley, G. A., Kristjánsdóttir, O., and Forgeron, P. A. (2009). Cultural influences on the assessment of children's pain. *Pain Res Manag*, 14(1), 33–37.

Flores, G., Abreu, M., and Tomany-Korman, S. C. (2006). Why are Latinos the most uninsured racial/ethnic group of US children? A community-based study of risk factors for and consequences of being an uninsured Latino child. *Pediatrics*, 118(3), E730–E740.

Flores, G. and Vega, L. R. (1998). Barriers to health care access for Latino children: a review. *Fam Med*, 30(3), 196–205.

Forgeron, P. A., Finley, G. A., and Arnaout, M. (2006). Pediatric pain prevalence and parents' attitudes at a cancer hospital in Jordan. *J Pain Symptom Manage*, 31(5), 440–448.

Forgeron, P. A., Jongudomkarn, D., Evans, J., Finley, G. A., Thienthong, S., Siripul, P., et al. (2009). Children's pain assessment in northeastern Thailand: perspectives of health professionals. *Qual Health Res*, 19(1), 71–81.

Fortier, M. A., Anderson, C. T., and Kain, Z. N. (2009). Ethnicity matters in the assessment and treatment of children's pain. *Pediatrics*, 124(1), 378–380.

Free, M. M. (2002). Cross-cultural conceptions of pain and pain control. *Proc (Bayl Univ Med Cent)*, 15(143–145).

Fuemmeler, B. F., Moriarty, L., and Brown, R. T. (2009). Racial and ethnic health disparities and access to care. In M. C. Roberts and R. G. Steele (eds) *Handbook of pediatric psychology (4th edn)*, pp. 575–585. New York: Guilford Press.

Gaffney, A. and Dunne, E. A. (1987). Children's understanding of the causality of pain. *Pain*, 29(1), 91–104.

Garro, L. C. (1990). Culture, pain and cancer. *J Palliat Care*, 6(3), 34–44.

Good, M.-J. D. (1995). *American medicine: the quest for competence*. Berkeley, CA: University of California Press.

Good, M.-J. D., Brodwin, P. E., Good, B. J., and Kleinman, A. (1992). Pain as human experience: an introduction. In M.-J. D. Good, P. E. Brodwin, B. J. Good, and A. Kleinman (eds) *Pain as human experience: an anthropological perspective*, pp. 1–28. Berkeley, CA: University of California Press.

Green, C. R., Anderson, K. O., Baker, T. A., Campbell, L. C., Decker, S., Fillingim, R. B., et al. (2003). The unequal burden of pain: confronting racial and ethnic disparities in pain. *Pain Med*, 4(3), 277–294.

Hunfeld, J. A. M., Perquin, C. W., Duivenvoorden, H. J., Hazebroek-Kampschreur, A., Passchier, J., van Suijlekom-Smit, L. W. A., et al. (2001). Chronic pain and its impact on quality of life in adolescents and their families. *J Pediatr Psychol*, 26(3), 145–153.

James, A. and James, A. L. (2004). *Constructing childhood*. New York: Palgrave Macmillan.

Jongudomkarn, D., Aungsupakorn, N., and Camfield, L. (2006). The meanings of pain: a qualitative study of the perspectives of children living with pain in north-eastern Thailand. *Nurs Health Sci*, 8(3), 156–163.

Kagawa-Singer, M. (2001). From genes to social science: impact of the simplistic interpretation of race, ethnicity, and culture on cancer outcome. *Cancer*, 91(1), 226–232.

Kristjansdottir, O., Unruh, A. M., McAlpine, L., and McGrath, P. J. (2012). A systematic review of cross-cultural comparison studies of child, parent, and health professional outcomes associated with pediatric medical procedures. *J Pain*, 13(3), 207–219.

LeResche, L. (2001). Gender, cultural and environmental aspects of pain. In J. D. Loeser (ed.) *Bonica's management of pain (3rd edn)*, pp. 191–195. Philadelphia, PA: Lippincott Williams & Wilkins.

Lewis, M., Ramsay, D. S., and Kawakami, K. (1993). Differences between Japanese infants and caucasian American infants in behavioral and cortisol response to inoculation. *Child Dev*, 64(6), 1722–1731.

Lillrank, A. (2003). Back pain and the resolution of diagnostic uncertainty in illness narratives. *Soc Sci Med*, 57(6), 1045–1054.

Mahoney, L., Ayers, S., and Seddon, P. (2010). The association between parent's and healthcare professional's behavior and children's coping and distress during venepuncture. *J Pediatr Psychol*, 35(9), 985–995.

McCarthy, P., Chammas, G., Wilimas, J., Alaoui, F. M., and Harif, M. (2004). Managing children's cancer pain in Morocco. *J Nurs Scholars*, 36(1), 11–15.

McCarty, C. A., Weisz, J. R., Wanitromanee, K., Eastman, K. L., Suwanlert, S., Chaiyasit, W., et al. (1999). Culture, coping, and context: primary and secondary control among Thai and American youth. *J Child Psychol Psychiatry*, 40(5), 809–818.

McGrath, P. J. (1995). Annotation: aspects of pain in children and adolescents. *J Child Psychol Psychiatry*, 36(5), 717–730.

McGrath, P. J., and Finley, G. A. (2003). Preface. In P. J. McGrath and G. A. Finley (eds) *Pediatric pain: biological and social context, progress in pain research and management*, vol. 26, pp. ix–xi. Seattle, WA: IASP Press.

McGrath, P. J., and Unruh, A. M. (2007). Neonatal and infant pain in a social context. In K. J. S. Anand, B. J. Stevens, and P. J. McGrath (eds) *Pain in neonates and infants (3rd edn)*, pp. 219–224. Edinburgh: Elsevier.

Meldrum, M. L., Tsao, J. C., and Zeltzer, L. K. (2008). 'Just be in pain and just move on': functioning limitations and strategies in the lives of children with chronic pain. *J Pain Manag*, 1(2), 131–141.

Meldrum, M. L., Tsao, J. C.-I., and Zeltzer, L. K. (2009). 'I can't be what I want to be': children's narratives of chronic pain experiences and treatment outcomes. *Pain Med*, 10(6), 1018–1034.

Merskey, H., and Bogduk, N. (eds) (1994). *Classification of chronic pain, second edition, IASP Task Force on Taxonomy.* Seattle, WA: IASP Press.

Neuman, B. M. (1996). Relationships between children's descriptions of pain, self-care and dependent-care, and basic conditioning factors of development, gender, and ethnicity: 'Bears in my throat'. Unpublished 9628925, Wayne State University, Michigan.

Nutkiewicz, M. (2008). Diagnosis versus dialogue: oral testimony and the study of pediatric pain. *Oral History Rev,* 35(1), 11–21.

Ong, B. N., Hooper, H., Dunn, K., and Croft, P. (2004). Establishing self and meaning in low back pain narratives. *Sociol Rev,* 532–549.

Pedro, H., Barros, L. S., and Moleiro, C. (2010). Brief report: parents and nurses' behaviors associated with child distress during routine immunization in a portuguese population. *J Pediatr Psychol,* 35(6), 602–610.

Pfefferbaum, B., Adams, J., and Aceves, J. (1990). The influence of culture on pain in Anglo and Hispanic children with cancer. *J Am Acad Child Adolesc Psychiatry,* 29(4), 642–647.

Pillai Riddell, R. R., Stevens, B. J., Cohen, L. L., Flora, D. B., and Greenberg, S. (2007). Predicting maternal and behavioral measures of infant pain: the relative contribution of maternal factors. *Pain,* 133(1–3), 138–149.

Post, L. F., Blustein, J., Gordon, E., and Dubler, N. N. (1996). Pain: ethics, culture, and informed consent to relief. *J Law Med Ethics,* 24, 348–359.

Pillai Riddell, R. R., Horton, R. E., Hillgrove, J., and Craig, K. D. (2008). Understanding caregiver judgments of infant pain: contrasts of parents, nurses and pediatricians. *Pain Res Manag,* 13(6), 489–496.

Pillai Riddell, R. R., and Racine, N. (2009). Assessing pain in infancy: the caregiver context. *Pain Res Manag,* 14(1), 27–32.

Rosmus, C., Johnston, C. C. l., Chan-Yip, A., and Yang, F. (2000). Pain response in Chinese and non-Chinese Canadian infants: is there a difference? *Soc Sci Med,* 51(2), 175–184.

Salmon, K. and Pereira, J. K. (2002). Predicting children's response to an invasive medical investigation: the influence of effortful control and parent behavior. *J Pediatr Psychol,* 27(3), 227–233.

Santiago-Irizarry, V. (2001). *Medicalizing ethnicity: the construction of Latino identity in a psychiatric setting.* Ithaca, NY: Cornell University Press.

Unruh, A. M. (1992). Voices from the past: ancient views of pain in childhood. *Clin J Pain,* 8(3), 247–254.

van Aken, M. A. G., van Lieshout, C. F. M., Katz, E. R., and Heezen, T. J. M. (1989). Development of behavioral distress in reaction to acute pain in two cultures. *J Pediatr Psychol,* 14(3), 421–432.

Williams, D. A. and Organizing Committee of the Pain Disparities Special Interest Group of the American Pain Society (2005). Racial and ethnic identifiers in pain management: the importance to research, clinical practice, and public health policy. *Am Pain Soc Bull,* 15(2), 9–10.

Zatzick, D. F. and Dimsdale, J. E. (1990). Cultural variations in response to painful stimuli. *Psychosom Med,* 52, 544–557.

Zeltzer, L. K. and LeBaron, S. (1985). Does ethnicity constitute a risk factor in the psychological distress of adolescents with cancer? *J Adolesc Health Care,* 6, 8–11.

Supplementary online materials

Figure 11.2 Selected list of publications

CHAPTER 12

Families and pain

Kathryn A. Birnie, Katelynn E. Boerner,
and Christine T. Chambers

Introduction

The family has long been acknowledged as an important social context where children learn about and receive support for their pain. When a child is in pain, it is the family who is responsible for the initial pain assessment and seeking appropriate evaluation and care. Families may inadvertently encourage the expression of pain and play a critical role in influencing their children's ability to cope with pain, both positively and negatively. Having a child in pain can also pose significant personal, familial, and economic strains. Therefore, consideration of the family is absolutely critical in the understanding of factors involved in children's acute and chronic pain experiences (McGrath, 2008). A concentration of research has continued since the last comprehensive review on the topic was published (Chambers, 2003). This chapter considers relevant theoretical models and summarizes current major research themes regarding the role of the family in both acute and chronic paediatric pain. Two illustrative case examples are provided and key areas for future research are identified.

Theoretical frameworks: families and pain

Recent work has situated family factors and relationships as one of many important determinants in a biopsychosocial formulation of pain communication (Hadjistavropoulos et al., 2011). Other broader theories related to parent–child interactions and the family environment have been applied to the pain context and have also guided research in the field; most notably operant conditioning/social learning theory (Bandura, 1977), theories of family systems (Turk et al., 1987), and attachment (Porter et al., 2007). Several pain-specific theories have also been proposed, such as the empathy model for others' pain (Goubert et al., 2005).

An integrative model of parent and family factors in paediatric pain was proposed by Palermo and Chambers (2005). This model (Figure 12.1) emphasizes the importance of multiple levels of family assessment, and situates individual parenting variables (e.g. parenting style, parental reinforcement) within a broader context of dyadic variables (e.g. quality of parent–child interaction), embedded within the global familial environment (e.g. family functioning). The model highlights reciprocal interactions of individual child and parent factors, with dyadic (parent–child), and familial levels in influencing children's reported pain severity, associated

functioning, and successful coping. The model was expanded by Evans and colleagues to more clearly delineate the specific contributions of various child and parent pain and functioning variables (Evans et al., 2008ab). This theoretical framing provides a basis for empirical work on the role of the family described in the following sections.

Acute pain: families and pain

Case example

Ryan is an 8-year-old boy who requires frequent blood work for monitoring of an endocrine disorder. He experiences considerable distress in the days leading up to his blood work. In the past he has needed to be restrained by one of his parents and/or a member of the medical staff. During the procedure Ryan's mother is visibly very anxious and tries to comfort him by saying 'You'll be okay. It will be over soon'. At the last appointment, Ryan's resistance was so strong that the medical staff were unable to complete the procedure. Ryan's parents and medical staff have become increasingly frustrated with his behaviour and have begun to avoid telling him in advance when he will need blood work, further increasing Ryan's distress and distrust around procedures. Ryan's endocrinologist refers him and his family to the Paediatric Health Psychology Service, where Ryan receives instruction in cognitive-behavioural pain management coping strategies, including distraction and deep breathing. His parents learn how they can best coach Ryan during the procedure, including prompting him to use deep breathing and use of distracting talk. The family, in collaboration with Ryan and the psychologist, develop a plan for preparing him for procedures (i.e. deciding how much advance notice Ryan needs for procedures) and for rewarding him for his hard work after procedures (i.e. going to get an ice cream cone). The family also learns about the value of using topical anaesthetics, such as EMLA®, as part of his pain management plan.

Parental assessment of acute pain

Children experience numerous acute painful events across childhood, typically in the form of everyday minor injuries (Fearon et al., 1996). Often, it is the parent who assesses the child's pain and

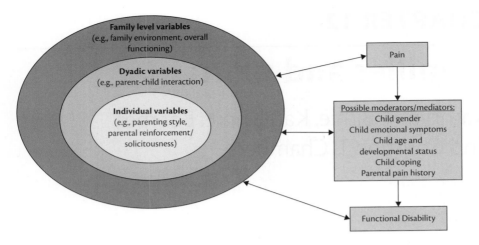

Figure 12.1 Integrative model of parent and family factors in pediatric pain. Reproduced from Palermo, T. M. and Chambers, C. T., Parent and family factors in pediatric chronic pain and disability: An integrative approach, *PAIN*®, Volume 119, Issues 1–3, pp. 1–4, 2005. This figure has been reproduced with permission of the International Association for the Study of Pain® (IASP). The figure may NOT be reproduced for any other purpose without permission.

makes decisions regarding management. Children also frequently experience painful medical procedures, either for routine immunizations or as a result of diagnostic and/or treatment procedures (Stevens et al., 2011). While health professionals are involved in assessing the child's pain in the medical setting, it is typically the parent who assumes the primary role in assessing their child's pain. Health professionals frequently rely on parents to provide information relevant to pain assessment, for example, the extent to which the child's current (pain) behaviour differs from their usual behaviour. This information is particularly important when child self-report is not available.

Parents are typically asked to provide observer ratings using self-report pain assessment tools used with children (Stinson et al., 2006). Parents generally underestimate their children's pain, although the reasons for this are not clear (Chambers and Craig 1999; Chambers et al., 1998; Goubert et al., 2009; Kelly et al., 2002; St Laurent-Gagnon et al., 1999). However, parents are generally more accurate in their estimation of children's pain as compared to health professionals, including physicians and nurses (Boerner et al., 2013). The extent that parents and children catastrophize about the child's pain may play an important role in parental pain assessment. In parents, higher levels of pain catastrophizing have been related to higher child-pain ratings by parents, and better agreement between parent and child pain ratings (Goubert et al., 2009). In children, lower levels of pain catastrophizing have been related to better agreement in parent–child pain ratings (Vervoort et al., 2009). Some situations may increase the challenge of pain assessment for parents. For example, while parents are relatively good at detecting when their children are genuinely experiencing or pretending to have pain, they have difficulty in accurately detecting when their children are suppressing pain (Larochette et al., 2006). More research is needed examining the various psychological and contextual factors that influence parent acute pain assessment and to distil this work into measures and approaches maximizing parents' ability to provide important information about pain assessment.

Parental behaviour and acute pain

Children's experiences during acute painful events can have an impact on their memories of the painful experience and their reactions to future painful events (Chen et al., 2000; Noel et al., 2010). Repeated negative interactions in the context of pain have the

potential to significantly impact children's later health care usage (Pate et al., 1996). Parent variables have played a critical role in children's coping and distress during painful medical procedures. It is now well accepted that parents should be present with their child during painful medical procedures, and the focus of research is on how and why parents' behaviours during medical procedures relates to their children's pain experiences.

Blount and colleagues (Blount et al., 1990, 1991, 1997) investigated the relationship between parent behaviours and child distress and coping by providing detailed coding of child and parent verbalizations during painful medical procedures. Specific parent behaviours are associated with decreases or increases in child distress, respectively classified as 'coping promoting' or 'distress promoting'. Behaviours classified as 'coping promoting' included non-procedural talk, suggestions on how to cope, and use of humour. A well-established, but seemingly, counterintuitive relationship between several parent behaviours and child distress was identified (e.g. empathy, reassurance). Reassurance is the most common parent behaviour exhibited during painful procedures (Cohen et al., 2002); yet it has consistently been linked to higher levels of child pain and distress, both in clinical and experimental research (Chambers et al., 2002; Taylor et al., 2011). The specific mechanisms through which reassurance promotes child distress and pain during acute painful medical procedures are not known; however, it appears that parental reassurance serves as a signal to the child that the parent is anxious, thereby triggering distress and pain in the child (McMurtry et al., 2006). Children report higher fear during parental reassurance than during parental distraction, and perceive their parents as being fearful or worried when they are providing reassurance to the child, especially when it is offered with a fearful facial expression and in a rising tone, indicative of uncertainty (McMurtry et al., 2010).

The tendency to catastrophize about pain has been proposed to play a role in parents' responses to their children's pain. Caes and colleagues (2011) found that parents' catastrophic thoughts about their child's pain were associated with a higher tendency by parents to restrict their child's behaviour (i.e. stop them from completing a painful experimental task). This relationship was mediated by parental distress, and was observed in parents of both healthy children and adolescents with chronic pain (Caes et al., 2011). Parental non-attending pain talk (i.e. utterances which did not focus on the child's pain or the painful stimulus) was associated with increased facial displays of pain and self-reported pain in high pain catastrophizing children, although this difference was not observed in low pain catastrophizing children (Vervoort et al., 2011). Child pain catastrophizing was related to parental responses to children's pain, and was moderated by parent–child attachment (Vervoort et al., 2010). Future research in this area needs to utilize more sophisticated statistical techniques, such as sequential analysis and dyadic analysis, as well as consideration of parent non-verbal as well as verbal behaviour.

The role of fathers

A major limitation of research on the role of the family in paediatric pain is the paucity of studies including fathers. Mothers are most often involved as they are accessible and are often identified as the primary caregiver. However, fathers play an increasingly important role in their children's lives and health care and, as such, are important to include (Phares et al., 2005). Moon and colleagues (2008) found that fathers showed better agreement with children's pain ratings than mothers. Moon and colleagues (2011) also examined parent's verbal behaviour while children completed the cold pressor task. Mothers and fathers generally did not differ in their proportions of attending and non-attending talk during children's pain; however, mothers used more non symptom-focused talk and commands, while fathers used more criticism (Moon et al., 2011). This work focused exclusively on comparing mother-father verbal behaviour; research is needed to also examine potential differences in use of non-verbal behaviour.

Sex differences exist in pain perception and responses to pain, which may be partially influenced by gender socialization (Myers et al., 2003). Gender socialization suggests that, through social learning processes such as modelling and reinforcement, children learn gender-specific behaviours that influence their responses to pain (Myers et al., 2003). Parents play an important role in teaching their children gender-specific behaviours (Langlois and Downs, 1980) and fathers tend to differentiate between male and female children more than mothers (Lytton and Romney, 1991). A survey of Finnish parents' perceptions of children's postoperative pain found that fathers were more likely than mothers to believe that their child should be able to independently cope with their pain, think that pain from surgery was acceptable, and believe that their children were capable of faking pain (Kankkunen et al., 2003). Additionally, boys were expected to tolerate more pain than girls. Researchers need to continue examining the unique role of fathers in paediatric pain, and avoid drawing conclusions about parent factors from research conducted primarily with mothers.

Parents' roles in acute pain management

The importance of appropriate pain management for medical procedures in children has continued to receive attention. Clinical practice guidelines identify evidence-based pharmacological, physical, and psychological strategies for management of immunization pain in children (Taddio et al., 2010a, 2010b). Systematic reviews of psychological interventions in paediatric procedural pain management (Chambers et al., 2009; Uman et al., 2006, 2008) identify a number of effective cognitive-behavioural strategies for reducing pain (e.g. distraction, deep breathing) that parents can encourage or direct. Involving parents in coaching their child to cope during painful

---

Box 12.1 Recommendations for parents for managing procedural pain in children

- Prepare yourself and stay calm.
- Prepare your child by using age-appropriate words and be honest; children 5 years old and older should be told about the procedure at least 1 day in advance.
- Distract your child using age-appropriate strategies (e.g. toys, books, music, or videos).
- Encourage your child to take slow, deep breaths (e.g. with bubbles or pinwheels).
- Avoid words that focus on the pain or the procedure (e.g. 'It'll be over soon' 'You'll be okay'); it's better to talk about things not related to the procedure.
- Use other age-appropriate pain-relieving interventions, such as breastfeeding or sucrose for infants or topical anaesthetic creams.
- After the procedure, praise your child for a job well done.

---

procedures is also effective for reducing parental anxiety (Cohen et al., 1997). Parents can be instructed in how to: (1) prepare themselves and their child in advance of the procedure, (2) distract their child during the procedure, (3) provide physical comfort and other pain-relieving interventions (e.g. breastfeeding, topical anaesthetics), and (4) praise the child after the procedure (Box 12.1).

Chronic pain: families and pain

Case example

Lauren is a 13-year-old girl with a 5-year history of recurrent stomach aches. When Lauren is seen by the Complex Pain Consultation Service, she has missed the past 6 weeks of school and reports daily stomach aches with an average pain intensity of 7 out of 10. Lauren's parents, Melissa and Doug, report considerable concern about her pain as well as frustration over how to best support Lauren. At the time Lauren's stomach aches worsened, Melissa was also home from work on disability as a result of a back injury she sustained in the work place. However, Melissa had recently returned to work, leaving Lauren unsupervised during the day. Lauren spends a typical day watching television, which she says helps to distract her from her pain. Melissa reported significant anxiety about Lauren's pain, and that she is frequently troubled by thoughts that perhaps Lauren will always have pain and never be able to return to school. Doug reports a strong family history of gastrointestinal symptoms, and acknowledged that he suffered from stomach aches as a child. The family reports considerable conflict about how to best manage Lauren's pain. Melissa feels that Lauren cannot return to school until her pain has improved or resolved, while Doug feels that Lauren just needs to 'tough it out' and return to school. Melissa reports waking up dreading the conversations they will have about Lauren's pain and whether Lauren will feel well enough to return to school that day.

Aggregation of pain in families

Research is mixed in understanding the relationship between parental and child pain with some showing an increased risk of chronic pain for children who have a parent with chronic pain (Groholt et al., 2003; Saunders et al., 2007). Associations between parent and child pain may be site specific. Two large population-based studies demonstrated that parental headache, abdominal pain, and back pain were predictive of the same pain sites in children (Groholt et al., 2003; Saunders et al., 2007). Additionally, a dose–response relationship in the number of pain sites reported by mothers was associated with a greater number of pain sites in children (Saunders et al., 2007). The influence of parental pain models may be sex specific with a higher concordance rate of parent–child pain among mothers and daughters; however, data for fathers were incomplete (Evans et al., 2010). A prospective study supported a relationship between parent and child pain experiences (Goodman et al., 1997); children of parents reporting four or more pain incidents over a 7-day period were at significantly increased risk for reporting a large number of total pain incidents, as well as clinically significant and disabling pain incidents. Together, these studies suggest a familial predisposition to pain sensitivity and reactivity.

Parent and child psychosocial and environmental factors may also account for associations between parent and child pain. Longitudinal examination over the first 6 years of life revealed that parent anxiety and child temperament during the child's first year were associated with later development of childhood recurrent abdominal pain (Ramchandani et al., 2006). Schanberg and colleagues (2001) reported associations between parental/familial pain history and current pain of children with chronic rheumatic disease were mediated by child pain catastrophizing. Maternal pain history has also been reported as a unique predictor of child functional impairment, although the impact of paternal pain history has not been examined (Kashikar-Zuck et al., 2008). Bruehl and colleagues (2005) found that children's recollections of parental pain significantly predicted the child's own chronic pain status and number of pain locations in adulthood, while objective parental history of chronic pain did not.

Altogether, findings from these studies demonstrate the potential role of risk factors contributing to parent and child pain, supporting the complex ways pain aggregates within families. Conclusions from these studies must be drawn cautiously as many are based on subjective retrospective report, employing varying definitions of intensity and frequency of parental and paediatric pain. Future research should continue focusing on longitudinal prospective designs that assess the possible influence of genetic, psychosocial, and environmental as risk factors for chronic pain.

Impact of child pain on the family

Paediatric chronic pain significantly impacts on the family. Parents of children with chronic pain report high levels of parental role stress, anxiety and depressive symptoms, and social impact (Palermo and Eccleston, 2009). Rates of anxiety, depression, and somatoform disorders are higher among mothers of children with chronic pain as compared to mothers of healthy children (Campo et al., 2007; Evans et al., 2008b; Kashikar-Zuck et al., 2008).

Several studies have qualitatively explored parents' experiences caring for a child with chronic pain (Jordan et al., 2007; Maciver et al., 2010; van Tilburg et al., 2006). These studies describe parents' experiences of fear, helplessness, and distress and describe parents as feeling powerless in attempts to help their child despite seeking resources and intervention. Parental adjustment is partially related to individual child and pain-related factors, with parents reporting higher levels of parenting stress with younger child age, pain chronicity, and child depression (Eccleston et al., 2004). Greater daily intensity of the child's chronic pain was predictive of greater maternal social restrictions, personal strain, and coping (Hunfeld et al., 2001). Parental factors, such as dispositional empathy and catastrophic thinking about their child's pain, also influenced parental distress in response to vignettes of children's pain experiences (Goubert et al., 2008). Addressing parents' psychological well-being is an area warranting greater research attention, as improved understanding of parental distress result in more effective management of children's pain and related disability (Palermo and Eccleston, 2009).

Siblings also worry about their sibling with chronic pain and became more considerate and compassionate toward them (Britton and Moore, 2002). Siblings reported confusion about their sick sibling's symptoms, wondering if they would develop chronic pain or what their own life would be like with chronic pain. Parents reported that siblings would sometimes compete for their attention. Research suggests that parents may alter their behaviour toward well siblings, excusing them from chores or offering special treats to assuage parental guilt associated with lessened attention (Jordan et al., 2007).

Influence of parental beliefs, psychological functioning, and behaviours

Parental beliefs, functioning, and behaviours reciprocally influence children's pain (Palermo and Chambers, 2005). Parental beliefs about the aetiology of the child's chronic pain have influenced child pain outcomes and parent behaviours. Children whose parents subscribed to a biopsychosocial model of pain were more likely to have successfully resolved recurrent abdominal pain than children whose parents cited physical cause only (Crushell et al., 2003). Children whose parents believed their pain was 'medical only' reported the highest pain and functional disability (Guite et al., 2009).

Substantial research has focused on parental responses to children's pain. The Adult Responses to Children's Symptoms questionnaire (Claar et al., 2010; Van Slyke and Walker 2006) categorizes parental responses to children's chronic pain on three factors: (1) protectiveness (e.g. limiting the child's activities and responsibilities), (2) minimization of pain (e.g. criticizing), and (3) encouraging and monitoring (e.g. reassuring, distracting the child). Parental protectiveness has been associated with increased pain-related disability, child depressive symptoms, and longer pain duration (Claar et al., 2010). Parental protectiveness predicted greater somatic complaints among adolescents with chronic pain; as well as greater physical disability for adolescents who reported infrequent use of passive coping strategies (Simons et al., 2008).

Parent–child interactions during painful activities provide additional support for the influence of parental behaviours on children's pain. Sequential analysis of adolescents with chronic pain and their parents during an exercise task revealed that when parents made statements that discouraged child coping, the child was less likely to remain on task, which was significantly associated with functional disability and school absences (Reid et al., 2005). Similarly to healthy children, children with chronic pain exhibited more symptom complaints during an experimental pain task when their parents attended to their pain, as opposed to when they distracted them (Walker et al., 2006). Clinical and experimental studies support the powerful influence of operant conditioning strategies of positive and negative reinforcement, whereby children's adoption of a sick role is continuously strengthened leading to increased disability and maladaptive coping.

Poorer psychological functioning of parents has been reported to negatively impact the child's reported pain and related disability (Logan and Scharff 2005; Palermo and Eccleston 2009), as well as influence parent behaviour. Mothers with greater psychological distress were more likely to seek physician consultation with child report of abdominal pain (Levy et al., 2006). Parental worry about the child's physical health was significantly related to child functional disability and parents' engagement in pain promoting behaviours (Guite et al., 2009). Additionally, greater maternal worry has been associated with higher perceived pain threat and limitations in family activities as a result of the child's pain (Lipani and Walker, 2006).

Parental pain catastrophizing strongly influences children's functioning. Mothers reported higher rates of pain catastrophizing than fathers, specifically a greater tendency to ruminate about their child's pain (Hechler et al., 2011). Negative consequences have been associated with parental catastrophic thinking about their child's pain, including increased parenting stress and parent psychological distress, as well as worsened child pain-related disability and school attendance (Goubert et al., 2006). As in acute pain, parent pain catastrophizing contributes significantly to parental responses to children's chronic pain (Hechler et al., 2011). Parental pain catastrophizing and protective responses to children's pain were unique predictors of school attendance and overall school impairment in adolescents with chronic pain, above the effects of adolescent pain intensity and depressive symptoms (Logan et al., 2012). Parental protectiveness mediated the relationship between parent pain catastrophizing and adolescent school functioning and attendance (Logan et al., 2012). Caes and colleagues (2011) demonstrated that parent distress mediated the relationship between parental catastrophic thinking and parents' tendency to restrict pain-inducing activity in children with chronic pain.

Children's psychological functioning and pain-related beliefs have repeatedly moderated the relationship between parent behaviours and child pain outcomes. The negative impact of maladaptive parent behaviours (i.e. solicitousness, protectiveness, minimization of the child's pain) on child's functional disability and somatic complaints were strongest for children with greater psychological distress (Claar et al., 2008; Peterson and Palermo, 2004). Furthermore, child pain catastrophizing moderated the relationship between parent symptom-related talk during a painful task and child symptom complaints; while the relationship between non-symptom talk and child symptom complaints was moderated by child perceived pain-related threat (Williams et al., 2010). Future research should continue integrating findings from experimental and clinic-based studies, and incorporate more complex multivariate analyses to allow stronger claims about the causal relationships between parental beliefs, functioning and behaviours, and child pain outcomes.

Role of the parent–child relationship

Despite its theorized relevance (Palermo and Chambers, 2005), limited research has expressly examined the parent–child relationship

in paediatric chronic pain. Child autonomy, in particular, has predicted greater functional impairment among adolescents with chronic pain after controlling for pubertal status, pain intensity, and depressive symptoms (Palermo et al., 2007). Greater parent–adolescent conflict, poorer family functioning, and less age-appropriate autonomy predicted greater depressive symptoms for adolescents with chronic headaches (Lewandowski and Palermo, 2009). Interviews with children with chronic pain and their mothers suggested that limited autonomy reduced the child's sense of self-efficacy for pain and non-pain related activities, as well as decreased the likelihood of regular attendance at school and other activities (Evans et al., 2010).

Greater parent–adolescent relationship distress was related to increased adolescent distress and lower pain intensity, but not to adolescent functional disability (Logan et al., 2006). Parents reported closer relationships with their adolescent than healthy norms (Logan et al., 2006), a finding supported by interviews with parents and children with chronic pain (Jordan et al., 2007). This intensive parenting role is more akin to parenting a younger child (Jordan et al., 2007) and is consistent with the lower levels of age-appropriate autonomy reported by adolescents with chronic headache (Lewandowski and Palermo, 2009).

Influence of family functioning

A recent systematic review revealed significant differences in family functioning between families of children with chronic pain and healthy controls (Lewandowski et al., 2010). Families of children with chronic pain generally reported poorer family functioning as exemplified through less family cohesion, less organization, greater conflict, and greater psychological distress. Poorer family functioning was also associated with increased child disability; however the relationship between family functioning and child pain was less consistent, possibly due to differences in how family functioning was measured across reviewed studies (Lewandowski et al., 2010). However, poor family functioning is not universal, as it appears to characterize a particular subgroup of children with chronic pain (Scharff et al., 2005) and is related to parental beliefs that the cause of the child's pain is 'medical only' (Guite et al., 2009). Altogether, these studies support the critical role of family factors in paediatric chronic pain and should be included as an important target for intervention.

Role of family in interventions for paediatric chronic pain

Research supports the effectiveness of parental involvement in treatment of chronic pain. Of 25 randomized controlled trials included in a recent meta-analytic review, seven described involvement of parents in psychological therapies for paediatric chronic pain (Palermo 2009); however, the influence of parent/family involvement on trial outcomes was not explored.

Cognitive-behaviour therapy (CBT) has received attention as an effective intervention for paediatric chronic pain, often with family involvement as an important component for achieving and maintaining treatment gains (Robins et al., 2005). Parent involvement in CBT is based on principles of operant conditioning and modelling, such that child pain and level of functioning by parent reinforcement of independent adaptive coping by the child and limiting parents' attention to child pain behaviours (Palermo and Eccleston, 2009; Noel et al., 2012b). Box 12.2 provides a summary

Box 12.2 Recommendations for parents for managing chronic pain in children

- Limit or remove attention from the pain.
- Be sure that your child goes to school each day.
- Help your child identify stress at home and at school.
- Provide attention and special activities on days when your child does *not* have stomach aches.
- Limit activities and interactions on sick days.
- Avoid talking about any pains or illness you have.
- Support your child in practising their pain coping strategies (e.g. relaxation, distraction).

of key messages to parents regarding behavioural pain management. Parents and children are engaged in a collaborative partnership where parents can both model and supportively 'coach' their child during treatment and for relapse prevention (Noel et al., 2012b; Palermo et al., 2009; Robins et al., 2005). CBT treatment protocols differ in the type and extent of parental involvement required, with some requiring joint attendance of the parent at a portion of treatment sessions (Robins et al., 2005) and others delivering content separately and concurrently to parents and children (Noel et al., 2012a; Palermo et al., 2009; for further discussion of CBT see Logan et al., Chapter 50, this volume). A randomized controlled trial comparing CBT to standard medical care for children with recurrent abdominal pain and their parents reported significantly reduced child pain and school absences for the CBT group immediately post-treatment and at 1-year follow-up (Robins et al., 2005). Significant reductions in parent pain-promoting behaviours were reported after a CBT intervention with parental involvement for children with recurrent abdominal pain (Noel et al., 2012a). Children with chronic pain and parents participating in an 8-week family CBT intervention online similarly reported significant reduced pain and activity limitations as compared with a wait-list control immediately post-treatment and maintained at 3-month follow-up (Palermo et al., 2009). Although some interventions address the importance of parents' own mental health (Noel et al., 2012a; Palermo et al., 2009), most do not assess parent psychosocial functioning. One study evaluating an interdisciplinary CBT programme reported significant improvements in parent anxiety, depression, and stress post-treatment that was maintained at 3-month follow-up (Eccleston et al., 2003). Children attending this programme also showed improvements in physical function and disability, anxiety, pain catastrophizing, somatic awareness, and school attendance (Eccleston et al., 2003).

Future research should explore the pathways through which family involvement exerts positive change on child pain outcomes. The role of parental involvement in more contemporary approaches to paediatric pain management, such as in acceptance-based treatments, is needed (Wicksell, 2007, 2008). Treatment studies should focus on the potential impact of changes in parent psychological functioning on children's pain-related outcomes, exploring the effectiveness of treatments for paediatric chronic pain designed to more directly address parents' emotional well-being (Palermo and Eccleston 2009).

Conclusion

A large body of research showcases the relevance of the family, particularly parents, in paediatric pain. Findings support the influence of parent behaviours, psychological functioning, and beliefs about pain (e.g. pain catastrophizing) on children's acute and chronic pain outcomes. Several studies have innovatively integrated clinical and experimental methods of inquiry, representing a promising trend in the field bringing both scientific rigour and external validity to research findings. Correspondingly, parent involvement in interventions is largely based on modifying parental responses to children's pain using principles of operant conditioning. Family relationships and the family environment are revealed as influential frameworks both moulded by and contributing to children's pain experience. Because of the expanding literature on sex differences in parent responding to children's pain, the inclusion of fathers in future research should be prioritized. Consideration of a developmental framework is often omitted from current theories of pain and the family. Diverging trends are noted in paediatric acute and chronic pain research. Investigations of the family in paediatric chronic pain are expanding in scope, exploring the influence of individual, dyadic and familial level factors. In contrast, studies examining the family in paediatric acute pain are narrowing in scope, seeking a more detailed understanding of parent–child interactions. Pain and the family remains a very active and innovative area of inquiry, offering continued insight into the broader context within which children experience pain.

References

Bandura, A. (1977). *Social learning theory.* Englewood Cliffs, NJ: Prentice-Hall Inc.

Blount, R. L., Cohen, L. L., Frank, N. C., Bachanas, P. J., Smith, A. J., Manimala, M. R., *et al.* (1997). The child-adult medical procedure interaction scale-revised: an assessment of validity. *J Pediatr Psychol,* 22, 73–88.

Blount, R. L., Landolffritsche, B., Powers, S. W., and Sturges, J. W. (1991). Differences between high and low coping children and between parent and staff behaviors during painful medical procedures. *J Pediatr Psychol,* 16, 795–809.

Blount, R. L., Sturges, J. W., and Powers, S. W. (1990). Analysis of child and adult behavioral variations by phase of medical procedure. *Behav Ther,* 21, 33–48.

Boerner, K. E., Chambers, C. T., Craig, K. D., Pillai Riddell, R. R., and Parker, J. A. (2013). Caregiver accuracy in detecting deception in facial expressions of pain in children. *Pain,* 154(4), 525–533.

Britton, C. and Moore, A. (2002). View from the inside, part 2: what the children with arthritis said, and the experiences of siblings, mothers, fathers and grandparents. *Br J Occup Ther,* 65, 413–419.

Bruehl, S., France, C. R., France, J., Harju, A., and al'Absi, M. (2005). How accurate are parental chronic pain histories provided by offspring? *Pain,* 115, 390–397.

Caes, L., Vervoort, T., Eccleston, C., Vandenhende, M., and Goubert, L. (2011). Parental catastrophizing about child's pain and its relationship with activity restriction: the mediating role of parental distress. *Pain,* 152, 212–222.

Campo, J. V., Bridge, J., Lucas, A., Savorelli, S., Walker, L., Di Lorenzo, C., *et al.* (2007). Physical and emotional health of mothers of youth with functional abdominal pain. *Arch Pediatr Adolesc Med,* 161, 131–137.

Chambers, C.T. (2003). The role of family factors in pediatric pain. In P. J. McGrath and G. A. Finley (eds) *Pediatric pain: biological and social context,* pp. 99–130. Seattle, WA: IASP Press.

Chambers, C. T. and Craig, K. D. (1999). Parents as judges of their children's pain: are they acccurate? *Pediatr Pain Lett,* 3, 14–17.

Chambers, C. T., Craig, K. D., and Bennett, S. M. (2002). The impact of maternal behavior on children's pain experiences: an experimental analysis. *J Pediatr Psychol*, 27, 293–301.

Chambers, C. T., Reid, G. J., Craig, K. D., McGrath, P. J., and Finley, G. A. (1998). Agreement between child and parent reports of pain. *Clin J Pain*, 14, 336–342.

Chambers, C. T., Taddio, A., Uman, L. S., and McMurtry, C. M. (2009). Psychological interventions for reducing pain and distress during routine childhood immunizations: a systematic review. *Clin Ther*, 31, S77–103.

Chen, E., Zeltzer, L. K., Craske, M. G., and Katz, E. R. (2000). Children's memories for painful cancer treatment procedures: implications for distress. *Child Dev*, 71, 933–947.

Claar, R. L., Guite, J. W., Kaczynski, K. J., and Logan, D. E. (2010). Factor structure of the adult responses to children's symptoms: validation in children and adolescents with diverse chronic pain conditions. *Clin J Pain*, 26, 410–417.

Claar, R. L., Simons, L. E., and Logan, D. E. (2008). Parental response to children's pain: the moderating impact of children's emotional distress on symptoms and disability. *Pain*, 138, 172–179.

Cohen, L. L., Bernard, R. S., Greco, L. A., and McClellan, C. B. (2002). A child-focused intervention for coping with procedural pain: are parent and nurse coaches necessary? *J Pediatr Psychol*, 27, 749–757.

Cohen, L. L., Blount, R. L., and Panopoulos, G. (1997). Nurse coaching and cartoon distraction: an effective and practical intervention to reduce child, parent, and nurse distress during immunizations. *J Pediatr Psychol*, 22, 355–370.

Crushell, E., Rowland, M., Doherty, M., Gormally, S., Harty, S., Bourke, B., *et al.* (2003). Importance of parental conceptual model of illness in severe recurrent abdominal pain. *Pediatrics*, 112, 1368–1372.

Eccleston, C., Crombez, G., Scotford, A., Clinch, J., and Connell, H. (2004). Adolescent chronic pain: patterns and predictors of emotional distress in adolescents with chronic pain and their parents. *Pain*, 108, 221–229.

Eccleston, C., Malleson, P. N., Clinch, J., Connell, H., and Sourbut, C. (2003). Chronic pain in adolescents: evaluation of a programme of interdisciplinary cognitive behaviour therapy. *Arch Dis Child*, 88, 881–885.

Evans, S., Meldrum, M., Tsao, J. C., Fraynt, R., and Zeltzer, L. K. (2010). Associations between parent and child pain and functioning in a pediatric chronic pain sample: a mixed methods approach. *Int J Disabil Hum Dev*, 9, 11–21.

Evans, S., Tsao, J. C. I., Lu, Q., Myers, C., Suresh, J., and Zeltzer, L. K. (2008a). Parent-child pain relationships from a psychosocial perspective: a review of the literature. *J Pain Manag*, 1, 237–246.

Evans, S., Tsao, J. C., and Zelter, L. K. (2008b). Relationship of child perceptions of maternal pain to children's laboratory and non-laboratory pain. *Pain Res Manag*, 13, 211–218.

Fearon, I., McGrath, P. J., and Achat, H. (1996). 'Booboos': the study of everyday pain among young children. *Pain*, 68, 55–62.

Goodman, J. E., McGrath, P. J., and Forward, S. P. (1997). Aggregation of pain complaints and pain-related disability and handicap in a community sample of families. In T. S. Jensen, J. A. Turner, and Z. Wiesenfeld-Hallin (eds) *Proceedings of the 8th World Congress on Pain: Progress in pain research and management*, pp. 673–682. Seattle, WA: IASP Press.

Goubert, L., Craig, K. D., Vervoort, T., Morley, S., Sullivan, M. J., de C Williams, A. C., *et al.* (2005). Facing others in pain: the effects of empathy. *Pain*, 118, 285–288.

Goubert, L., Vervoort, T., Cano, A., and Crombez, G. (2009). Catastrophizing about their children's pain is related to higher parent-child congruency in pain ratings: an experimental investigation. *Eur J Pain*, 13, 196–201.

Goubert, L., Vervoort, T., Crombez, G., Cano, A., Craig, K. D., and de C. Williams, A. C. (2006). Response to letter to the editor regarding our manuscript 'Facing others in pain: the effects of empathy'. *Pain*, 122, 328–330.

Goubert, L., Vervoort, T., Sullivan, M. J. L., Verhoeven, K., and Crombez, G. (2008). Parental emotional responses to their child's pain: the role of dispositional empathy and catastrophizing about their child's pain. *J Pain*, 9, 272–279.

Groholt, E., Stigum, H., Nordhagen, R., and Kohler, L. (2003). Recurrent pain in children, socio-economic factors and accumulation in families. *Eur J Epidemiol*, 18, 965–975.

Guite, J. W., Logan, D. E., McCue, R., Sherry, D. D., and Rose, J. B. (2009). Parental beliefs and worries regarding adolescent chronic pain. *Clin J Pain*, 25, 223–232.

Hadjistavropoulos, T., Craig, K. D., Duck, S., Cano, A., Goubert, L., Jackson P. L., *et al.* (2011). A biopsychosocial formulation of pain communication. *Psychol Bull*, 137, 910–939.

Hechler, T., Vervoort, T., Hamann, M., Tietze, A. L., Vocks, S., Goubert, L., *et al.* (2011). Parental catastrophizing about their child's chronic pain: are mothers and fathers different? *Eur J Pain*, 15(5), 515.e1–9.

Hunfeld, J. A. M., Perquin, C. W., Duivenvoorden, H. J., Hazebroek-Kampschreur, A. A., Passchier, J., van Suijlekom-Smit, L. W., *et al.* (2001). Chronic pain and its impact on quality of life in adolescents and their families. *J Pediatr Psychol*, 26, 145–153.

Jordan, A. L., Eccleston, C., and Osborn, M. (2007). Being a parent of the adolescent with complex chronic pain: an interpretative phenomenological analysis. *Eur J Pain*, 11, 49–56.

Kankkunen, P. M., Vehvilainen-Julkunen, K. M., Pietila, A. M. K., and Halonen, P. M. (2003). Parents' perceptions of their 1–6-year-old children's pain. *Eur J Pain*, 7, 203–211.

Kashikar-Zuck, S., Lynch, A. M., Slater, S., Graham, T. B., Swain, N. F., and Noll, R. B. (2008). Family factors, emotional functioning, and functional impairment in juvenile fibromyalgia syndrome. *Arthritis Rheum*, 59, 1392–1398.

Kelly, A. M., Powell, C. V., and Williams, A. (2002). Parent visual analogue scale ratings of children's pain do not reliably reflect pain reported by child. *Pediatr Emerg Care*, 18, 159–162.

Langlois, J. H. and Downs, A. C. (1980). Mothers, fathers, and peers as socialization agents of sex-typed play behaviors in young children. *Child Dev*, 51, 1237–1247.

Larochette, A., Chambers, C. T., and Craig, K. D. (2006). Genuine, suppressed and faked facial expressions of pain in children. *Pain*, 126, 64–71.

Levy, R. L., Langer, S. L., Walker, L. S., Feld, L. D., and Whitehead, W. E. (2006). Relationship between the decision to take a child to the clinic for abdominal pain and maternal psychological distress. *Arch Pediatr Adolesc Med*, 160, 961–965.

Lewandowski, A. S. and Palermo, T. M. (2009). Parent-teen interactions as predictors of depressive symptoms in adolescents with headache. *J Clinical Psychol Med Settings*, 16(4), 331–338.

Lewandowski, A. S., Palermo, T. M., Stinson, J., Handley, S., and Chambers, C. T. (2010). Systematic review of family functioning in families of children and adolescents with chronic pain. *J Pain*, 11, 1027–1038.

Lipani, T. A. and Walker, L. S. (2006). Children's appraisal and coping with pain: relation to maternal ratings of worry and restriction in family activities. *J Pediatr Psychol*, 31, 667–673.

Logan, D. and Scharff, L. (2005). Relationships between family and parent characteristics and functional abilities in children with recurrent pain syndromes: an investigation of moderating effects on the pathway from pain to disability. *J Pediatr Psychol*, 30, 698–707.

Logan, D. E., Guite, J. W., Sherry, D. D., and Rose, J. B. (2006). Adolescent–parent relationships in the context of adolescent chronic pain conditions. *Clin J Pain*, 22, 576–583.

Logan, D. E., Simons, L. E., and Carpino, E. A. (2012). Too sick for school? Parent influences on school functioning among children with chronic pain. *Pain*, 153, 437–443.

Lytton, H. and Romney, D. M. (1991). Parents' differential socialization of boys and girls: a meta-analysis. *Psychol Bull*, 109, 267–296.

Maciver, D., Jones, D., and Nicol, M. (2010). Parents' experiences of caring for a child with chronic pain. *Qual Health Res*, 20, 1272–1282.

McGrath, P. J. (2008). The family is the crucible. *Pain*, 137, 471–472.

McMurtry, C. M., Chambers, C. T., McGrath, P. J., and Asp, E. (2010). When 'don't worry' communicates fear: children's perceptions of parental reassurance and distraction during a painful medical procedure. *Pain*, 150, 52–58.

McMurtry, C. M., McGrath, P. J., and Chambers, C. T. (2006). Reassurance can hurt: parental behavior and painful medical procedures. *J Pediatr*, 148, 560–561.

Moon, E. C., Chambers, C. T., Larochette, A. C., Hayton, K., Craig, K. D., and McGrath, P. J. (2008). Sex differences in parent and child pain ratings during an experimental child pain task. *Pain Res Manag*, 13, 225–230.

Moon, E. C., Chambers, C. T., and McGrath, P. J. (2011). 'He says, she says': a comparison of fathers' and mothers' verbal behavior during child cold pressor pain. *J Pain*, 12, 1174–1181.

Myers, C. D., Riley, J. L., and Robinson, M. E. (2003). Psychosocial contributions to sex-correlated differences in pain. *Clin J Pain*, 19, 225–232.

Noel, M., Chambers, C. T., McGrath, P. J., Klein, R. M., and Stewart, S. H. (2012a). The influence of children's pain memories on subsequent pain experience. *Pain*, 153, 1563–1572.

Noel, M., McMurtry, C. M., Chambers, C. T., and McGrath, P. J. (2010). Children's memory for painful procedures: the relationship of pain intensity, anxiety, and adult behaviors to subsequent recall. *J Pediatr Psychol*, 35, 626–636.

Noel, M., Petter, M., Parker, J. A., and Chambers, C. T. (2012b). Cognitive behavioural therapy for pediatric chronic pain: the problem, research, and practice. *J Cog Psychother*, 25, 143–156.

Palermo, T. M. (2009). Assessment of chronic pain in children: current status and emerging topics. *Pain Res Manag*, 14, 21–26.

Palermo, T. M. and Chambers, C. T. (2005). Parent and family factors in pediatric chronic pain and disability: an integrative approach. *Pain*, 119, 1–4.

Palermo, T. M. and Eccleston, C. (2009). Parents of children and adolescents with chronic pain. *Pain*, 146, 15–17.

Palermo, T. M., Putnam, J., Armstrong, G., and Daily, S. (2007). Adolescent autonomy and family functioning are associated with headache-related disability. *Clin J Pain*, 23, 458–465.

Palermo, T. M., Wilson, A. C., Peters, M., Lewandowski, A., and Somhegyi, H. (2009). Randomized controlled trial of an Internet-delivered family cognitive-behavioral therapy intervention for children and adolescents with chronic pain. *Pain*, 146, 205–213.

Pate, J. T., Blount, R. L., Cohen, L. L., and Smith, A. J. (1996). Childhood medical experience and temperament as predictors of adult functioning in medical situations. *Child Health Care*, 25, 281–298.

Peterson, C. C. and Palermo, T. M. (2004). Parental reinforcement of recurrent pain: the moderating impact of child depression and anxiety on functional disability. *J Pediatr Psychol*, 29, 331–341.

Phares, V., Lopez, E., Fields, S., Kamboukos, D., and Duhig, A. M. (2005). Are fathers involved in pediatric psychology research and treatment? *J Pediatr Psychol*, 30, 631–643.

Porter, L. S., Davis, D., and Keefe, F. J. (2007). Attachment and pain: recent findings and future directions. *Pain*, 128, 195–198.

Ramchandani, P. G., Stein, A., Hotopf, M., Wiles, N. J., and ALSPAC Study Team (2006). Early parental and child predictors of recurrent abdominal pain at school age: results of a large population-based study. *J Am Acad Child Adolesc Psychiatry*, 45, 729–736.

Reid, G. J., McGrath, P. J., and Lang, B. A. (2005). Parent-child interactions among children with juvenile fibromyalgia, arthritis, and healthy controls. *Pain*, 113, 201–210.

Robins, P. M., Smith, S. M., Glutting, J. J., and Bishop, C. T. (2005). A randomized controlled trial of a cognitive-behavioral family intervention for pediatric recurrent abdominal pain. *J Pediatr Psychol*, 30, 397–408.

Saunders, K., Korff, M. V., Leresche, L., and Mancl, L. (2007). Relationship of common pain conditions in mothers and children. *Clin J Pain*, 23, 204–213.

Schanberg, L. E., Anthony, K. K., Gil, K. M., Lefebvre, J. C., Kredich, D. W., and Macharoni, L. M. (2001). Family pain history predicts child health status in children with chronic rheumatic disease. *Pediatrics*, 108, 1–7.

Scharff, L., Langan, N., Rotter, N., Scott-Sutherland, J., Schenck, C., Tayor, N., *et al.* (2005). Psychological, behavioral, and family characteristics of pediatric patients with chronic pain: a 1-year retrospective study and cluster analysis. *Clin J Pain*, 21, 432–438.

Simons, L. E., Claar, R. L., and Logan, D. L. (2008). Chronic pain in adolescence: parental responses, adolescent coping, and their impact on adolescent's pain behaviors. *J Pediatr Psychol*, 33, 894–904.

St Laurent-Gagnon, T., Bernard-Bonin, A. C., and Villeneuve, E. (1999). Pain evaluation in preschool children and by their parents. *Acta Paediatr*, 88, 422–427.

Stevens, B. J., Abbott, L. K., Yamada, J., Harrison, D., Stinson, J., Taddio, A., *et al.* (2011). Epidemiology and management of painful procedures in children in Canadian hospitals. *CMAJ*, 183, E403–410.

Stinson, J. N., Kavanagh, T., Yamada, J., Gill, N., and Stevens, B. (2006). Systematic review of the psychometric properties, interpretability and feasibility of self-report pain intensity measures for use in clinical trials in children and adolescents. *Pain*, 125, 143–157.

Taddio, A., Appleton, M., Bortolussi, R., Chambers, C., Dubey, V., Halperin, S., *et al.* (2010a). Reducing the pain of childhood vaccination: an evidence-based clinical practice guideline. *CMAJ*, 182, E843–855.

Taddio, A., Appleton, M., Bortolussi, R., Chambers, C., Dubey, V., Halperin, S., *et al.* (2010b). Reducing the pain of childhood vaccination: an evidence-based clinical practice guideline (summary). *CMAJ*, 182, 1989–1995.

Taylor, C., Sellick, K., and Greenwood, K. (2011). The influence of adult behaviors on child coping during venipuncture: a sequential analysis. *Res Nurs Health*, 34, 116–131.

Turk, D. C., Flor, H., and Rudy, T. E. (1987). Pain and families. I. Etiology, maintenance and psychosocial impact. *Pain*, 30, 3–27.

Uman, L. S., Chambers, C. T., McGrath, P. J., and Kisely, S. (2006). Psychological interventions for needle-related procedural pain and distress in children and adolescents. *Cochrane Database Syst Rev*, 4, CD005179.

Uman, L. S., Chambers, C. T., McGrath, P. J., and Kisely, S. (2008). A systematic review of randomized controlled trials examining psychological interventions for needle-related procedural pain and distress in children and adolescents: an abbreviated Cochrane review. *J Pediatr Psychol*, 33, 842–854.

Van Slyke, D. and Walker, L. S. (2006). Mothers' responses to children's pain. *Clin J Pain*, 22, 387–391.

Van Tilburg, M. A., Venepalli, N., Ulshen, M., Freeman, K. L., Levy, R., and Whitehead, W. E. (2006). Parents' worries about recurrent abdominal pain in children. *Gastroenterol Nurs*, 29(1), 50–55.

Vervoort, T., Caes, L., and Trost, Z. (2011). Social modulation of facial pain display in high-catastrophizing children: an observational study in schoolchildren and their parents. *Pain*, 152, 1591–1599.

Vervoort, T., Goubert, L., and Crombez, G. (2009). The relationship between high catastrophizing children's facial display of pain and parental judgment of their child's pain. *Pain*, 142, 142–148.

Vervoort, T., Goubert, L., and Crombez, G. (2010). Parental responses to pain in high catastrophizing children: the moderating effect of child attachment. *J Pain*, 11, 755–763.

Walker, L. S., Williams, S. E., Smith, C. A., Garber, J., Van Slyke, D. A., and Lipani, T. A. (2006). Parent attention versus distraction: impact on symptom complaints by children with and without chronic functional abdominal pain. *Pain*, 122, 43–52.

Wicksell, R. K. (2007). Values-based exposure and acceptance in the treatment of pediatric chronic pain: from symptom reduction to valued living. *Pediatr Pain Lett*, 9, 13–20.

Wicksell, R.K. (2008). Acceptance and commitment therapy for pediatric chronic pain. In L. A. Greco and S. C. Hayes (eds) *Acceptance and mindfulness treatments for children and adolescents: a practitioners guide*, pp. 89–113. Oakland, CA: New Harbinger Publications Inc.

Williams, S. E., Blount, R. L., and Walker, L. S. (2010). children's pain threat appraisal and catastrophizing moderate the impact of parent verbal behavior on children's symptom complaints. *J Pediatr Psychol*, 36, 55–63.

CHAPTER 13

Pain, social relationships, and school

Paula Forgeron and Sara King

Summary

Although recurrent and chronic pain impacts the whole life of a child and or adolescent, little research has been conducted on social consequences of chronic pain for children and adolescents. Emerging research suggests that (1) peer relationships, including close friendships, of children and adolescents with chronic pain may be negatively impacted by pain and (2) social reactions from others can negatively impact the child or adolescent's pain experience. School functioning may also be impaired as a result of chronic pain. Clinicians should understand the challenges experienced by children with chronic pain and should attend to the social and school consequences of pain when working with this population. Although little research has examined interventions to manage the effects of chronic pain on school and social functioning, researchers have identified helpful strategies that may mitigate the negative consequences to social and school functioning associated with chronic pain.

Introduction

Peer relationships and close friendships are a fundamental part of child development and become increasingly important as children approach adolescence. Peer relationships provide a milieu through which adolescents develop self-identity and values in the absence of adult monitoring (Rubin et al., 2005). Indeed, positive peer relationships and close friendships are associated with lower levels of depression and loneliness (Nangle et al., 2003), and positive school adjustment (Ladd et al., 1997). Close friendships can buffer the negative effects of peer victimization (Hodges et al., 1999) and negative family environments (Gauze et al., 1996).

School functioning is essential for positive development, as it has been linked to both academic and social success. Peer acceptance and close friendships have an impact on social functioning regardless of context, whereas teacher acceptance plays a critical role in school functioning for children and adolescents? Although typically developing children and adolescents often experience challenges in both school and social functioning, difficulties can be compounded for children and adolescents with chronic pain. Despite the importance of the relations between and among peers, friends, and school functioning for positive development, little is known about the impact of recurrent and chronic pain on these areas of functioning.

The goals of this chapter are: (1) to review the literature on social and school functioning for children and adolescents with chronic pain; (2) discuss strategies to ameliorate difficulties; and (3) highlight directions for future research.

Social communication model of pain

The social communication model (SCM) of pain (Craig 2002, 2009) suggests that pain is a social phenomenon that is experienced within a social context. This model underscores the relationship between a child's or adolescent's chronic pain experience and their relationship with peers, friends, and school functioning. According to this model, the individual's pain expression is an iterative social process. Thus, peer, friend, and teacher responses to an adolescent's pain expression may impact either positively or negatively on the adolescent's pain experience. Conversely, the expression of pain by the child or adolescent may have an impact on his or her peers', friends', and teachers' interpretation and response to pain. This cycle of pain expression, interpretation, and subsequent pain expression may be as influential in the social interactions of children and adolescents with chronic pain as individual pain factors such as pain intensity. The SCM is reviewed in depth by Pillai Riddell et al. (Chapter 9, this volume).

Background
Peers and friends

Research examining the relationship between peers, friends, and pain experience is in its infancy. Most research is based on general peer relationships (i.e. peer acceptance) as opposed to close friendships. When examining peer relationships of children and adolescents, it is necessary to differentiate between peer acceptance and close friendships. Peer acceptance (also defined as popularity) is a measure of general peer relationships based on unilateral liking and results in a feeling of belonging and inclusion (Buhrmester and Furman, 1986). Close friendships are based on mutual liking and provide one with intimacy and reliable alliance (Bagwell et al., 2001). Sullivan (1953) suggests that the need for peer acceptance is stronger for younger children, whereas the need for close friendships surpasses the need for general peer acceptance in adolescence. Thus, psychosocial adjustment in children may be linked more to peer acceptance whereas for adolescents it may be linked more to close friendships (Erdley et al., 2001).

Pain first begins to interfere with social functioning by interrupting regular physical activities, leisure activities, and school attendance (Logan et al., 2008; Roth-Isigkeit et al., 2005). Missing physical and leisure activities in addition to missing school presents challenges for establishing and maintaining friendships, as these venues provide most of the opportunities for children and adolescents to interact with peers. Interruptions to activities and school absence can be problematic from a social functioning perspective, but the extent to which this is the case is not clear, as impact varies between individuals. Indeed, children and adolescents with chronic pain have fewer friends compared to healthy peers, but it is not clear whether this difference is significant (see Forgeron et al., 2010 for a review). Typically developing children and adolescents have an average of three to four close friends (Berndt and Hoyle, 1985). Although children and adolescents with chronic pain have been found to have fewer friends the actual number of friends they have compared to typically developing peers remains unknown (Forgeron et al., 2010). Perhaps more important is that it is not clear whether children and adolescents with chronic pain are at higher risk for having no close friends.

Although spending time with peers is necessary to foster friendships, time spent together may not be sufficient for good social functioning or the development of close friendships. For example, structured leisure activities have been linked to lower levels of aggressive behaviour (Mahoney and Stattin, 2000) and assist in the development of self-identity (Coatsworth et al., 2005). Therefore, adolescents with chronic pain who have withdrawn from structured leisure and sport activities may struggle with self-identification in relation to their friends and peers. Chronic ponain was found to be a catalyst for adolescents to rethink their identity (Forgeron et al., 2011a). For example, children and adolescents with chronic pain may no longer identify themselves as a 'dancer' or 'football player', which may have a negative effect on self-identity. Recent research lends credence to this argument, as adolescents with chronic pain report lower self-esteem scores, increased loneliness, and depressed mood scores compared to healthy peers. However, the precise reasons are somewhat unclear (Forgeron et al., 2011b). It is possible that having a negative self-image contributes to feeling unequal to others in a group and to decreased participation in sport and leisure activities. Even when these adolescents spend time with friends, they may feel different and unequal to their friends, which can disrupt the establishment of close friendships.

Close friends

The majority of the research on close friendships and pain has been conducted with adolescent populations. This is understandable, as the prevalence of chronic pain tends to increase around or after puberty (King et al., 2011; Stanford et al., 2008). Adolescents with chronic pain have identified close friends as being both helpful and unhelpful in coping with chronic pain (Forgeron and McGrath, 2008). In a recent study, Forgeron and colleagues (2011b) found that adolescents with chronic pain rated narrative vignettes depicting a non-supportive social interaction between an adolescent with chronic pain and a close friend as more unsupportive compared to healthy peers. Although adolescents with chronic pain had higher rates of loneliness and depressed mood and lower self-esteem, scores on these measures did not contribute to the variance explained in the interpretation of non-supportive social situations. Adolescents with chronic pain may have a heightened sensitivity to negative social situations, as these situations may have the potential to negatively impact their pain experience. According to the SCM, adolescents with chronic pain who have experienced unsupportive social situations involving their friends may try to avoid these situations to avoid feeling uncared for by their friends. These situations may then be interpreted with heightened sensitivity in the future, due to the possibility of experiencing negative consequences. In other studies, adolescents with chronic pain described their friends as unable to understand their pain condition, alluding to the notion that their friends were unsupportive (Carter et al., 2002; Forgeron and McGrath, 2008). One of the reasons that friends might not fully understand an adolescent's pain condition is the unpredictable nature of pain. There are times when adolescents with chronic pain are able to socially engage much like their healthy peers and other times when pain interferes significantly with physical and social functioning. Additionally, as most chronic pain conditions are not visible, healthy friends may not always provide the level of support desired by the adolescent with chronic pain. Thus, adolescents with chronic pain may experience feelings of loneliness, even when they do engage with friends, if they feel they cannot fully share their pain experience with others.

Carter and colleagues (2002) reported that adolescents with chronic pain often describe 'sunny day friends' as friends who are only present when pain is not problematic. Interestingly, adolescents with chronic pain described some of their friends as having changed, as opposed to changing themselves. This finding points to a potential dichotomy between adolescents with chronic pain and their friends. Healthy friends may perceive the adolescent with chronic pain as the one who has changed. Not only does pain interfere with leisure and sport activities, but it can also contribute to disrupted sleep and irritability. One participant in a study by Sällfors and colleagues (2002) described classmates being shocked as she became more irritable when she was in pain. Thus, fatigue and irritability (a form of pain expression) may explain why some healthy friends only wish to interact with the adolescent with chronic pain when pain expression is minimal. Children and adolescents with chronic pain expressed difficulty when their friends did not believe them, and felt as though they were being blamed for their condition (Forgeron and McGrath, 2008; Sällfors et al., 2002).

Friends of children and adolescents with chronic pain continue to have friendship needs, regardless of whether the child or adolescent with chronic pain is able or willing to engage in various social activities. Healthy children and adolescents may develop additional friendships to buffer their own loneliness when their friend with chronic pain is not in school or unable to participate in social activities. It is not clear if or how friendships change over time when a child or adolescent has chronic pain. Healthy friends may be more understanding when the pain first begins but over time may need to find alternative friends to fill their own friendship needs.

Support from friends has a self-reported positive impact on social functioning (Carter et al., 2002; Forgeron and McGrath, 2008; Sällfors et al., 2002). Friends have been described as providing distraction, understanding, companionship (Carter et al., 2002; Forgeron and McGrath, 2008; Sällfors et al., 2002), and emotional and academic support to adolescents with chronic pain. Although close friends can provide positive support, it is unlikely that they provide support in every situation. In the narrative vignette study described earlier (Forgeron et al., 2011b), adolescents with chronic pain and healthy controls listed alternative responses to the healthy character's response depicted in the vignettes. The responses were coded as inclusive/helpful or not inclusive/helpful. There were no differences between the two groups with respect to the number of inclusive/helpful alternatives that were listed across the 12 vignettes. However, adolescents with chronic pain endorsed significantly more inclusive/helpful alternatives when asked to describe what they would have done if they had been the healthy character in the vignette. Even when healthy peers know what might be supportive to a friend with chronic pain, they may not feel skilled or prepared to provide that support in all situations. Alternatively, adolescents with chronic pain may have expectations that are above and beyond what another adolescent is capable of providing.

There are several caveats that should accompany the research previously described. First, positive alternative behaviours were coded as supportive if they ensured the inclusion/help for the adolescent with chronic pain. It remains unclear, however, if providing such support would improve the social functioning of an adolescent with chronic pain. Being overly solicitous may result in less competent social functioning, as it may enforce the belief that the adolescent with chronic pain believes his or her needs have priority over others. Nevertheless, even if participation in social activities is not increased by supportive friendship behaviours, perceived support may help an adolescent with chronic pain feel valued as a friend. Additionally, close friends are reciprocal in nature, therefore it may be important to ensure that adolescents with chronic pain remain empathic to the needs of their healthy friends. Second, sex differences in friendships exist in typically developing children and adolescents. Specifically, male friendships are characterized by more physical presence and female friendships are characterized by more emotional sharing (Benenson and Christakos, 2003). Although the vignettes included both physical activity situations and emotional sharing situations, there were not sufficient numbers of both to analyse separately. It is unclear if there are differences in the types of situations perceived by adolescents with chronic pain as non-supportive based on their sex. There is no research that examines the types of support offered by a friend and the pain coping and social functioning of children and adolescents with chronic pain.

In contrast to their healthy friends, adolescents with chronic pain may develop a different perspective on how they view friendships, support, and their place within relationships as a result of their pain. Adolescents in several qualitative studies described pain as interrupting their ability to be 'normal' (Carter et al., 2002; Forgeron and McGrath 2008; Sällfors et al., 2002) and making them feel different from their 'normal' healthy friends. Adolescents who have not experienced chronic pain may not appreciate the challenges of living with a chronic condition. Chronic pain does not always have an identifiable cause and there are no diagnostic tests that confirm the existence of pain. Additionally, although most healthy children and adolescents have experienced some form of acute pain, these experiences would not prepare them with the knowledge and understanding that adolescents with chronic pain feel they need from their friends. Not only could this difference in perspective lead to misunderstandings, but the invisible nature of chronic pain can add to confusion for healthy friends who do not understand how functioning can vary so much in their friend with chronic pain (Forgeron and McGrath, 2008; Sällfors et al., 2002).

Peers

Peer acceptance (unilateral liking/popularity) has been studied more extensively than close friendships in children and adolescents with chronic pain; however, results of studies completed to date have been inconclusive. Some researchers suggest there are no differences in peer acceptance of children and adolescents with chronic pain (Guite et al., 2000; Noll et al., 2008, 2010), whereas others suggest that there are differences (Kashikar-Zuck et al., 2007; Vanetta et al., 2008). Kashikar-Zuck and colleagues, using a classroom rating approach compared likeability ratings of adolescents with juvenile fibromyalgia with age-matched controls from the same class, found that peers rated the adolescent with juvenile fibromyalgia as less likeable than classmates (Kashikar-Zuck et al., 2007). However, Noll and colleagues using the same classroom rating approach did not find any differences in likeability between adolescents with juvenile arthritis and age-matched classmates (Noll et al., 2000). It remains uncertain which factors may contribute to the contrasting findings reported in these two studies.

One factor may be explained versus unexplained pain. Recurrent and ongoing pain from juvenile fibromyalgia is not as well understood compared to the pain from juvenile arthritis. In a hypothetical vignette study, 4th and 5th grade children in the US rated same age peers with both explained and unexplained abdominal pain as equally likeable as playmates (Guite et al., 2000). Older children and adolescents may perceive unexplained pain more negatively compared to younger children. Younger children may not have a biological understanding of illness and therefore do not make judgements based on the underlying aetiology of illness condition of a friend. Conversely, for older children and adolescents, the complexity of unexplained pain may not fit with their biological understanding of illness, which then contributes to judging children and adolescents with chronic pain as different than peers and hence less compatible.

Alternatively, peer likability of children or adolescents with unexplained chronic pain may not be related to age but instead related to the difference between actual versus hypothetical experiences of interacting with an adolescent with a chronic pain condition. In actual *in vivo* interactions with peers, there may be a negative iterative process between the pain behaviours expressed by the adolescent with chronic pain, the interpretation of these behaviours by peers, and further expression of pain that negatively impact peers' perception of the adolescent with unexplained recurrent or chronic pain.

There also are inherent limitations to the studies that compare peer relationships of children and adolescents with pain conditions with healthy peers (Kashikar-Zuck et al., 2007; Noll et al., 1996, 2000, 2007; Vannatta et al., 2008). The majority of the previously discussed studies examined perceptions of children and adolescents with various chronic pain conditions using a variety of sociometric measures. All researchers used classroom peers as the only measure of acceptance or likeability and did not examine other friendships the child or adolescent might have outside the classroom or school. Limiting research to classroom sociometric measures may be problematic when studying adolescents in junior high and high school, as class composition generally changes from class to class, and adolescents have increased opportunities to make friends in other settings. Most of these researchers also focused on quantity compared to the quality or characteristics of the friendship; therefore, it is unclear whether being viewed as accepted by classmates translates into deeper friendships for children and adolescents with chronic pain. Finally, most of the researchers explored peer relationships for a wide age range (i.e. 8–18 years); this is problematic, as patterns of peer relationships change as children age. Therefore, the inclusion of both children and adolescents may not have provided the necessary power in these studies to find subgroup differences. Since there were some interactions between pain and age of the child or adolescent, the separation of these developmental groups may be especially important.

Some studies used standardized quantitative measures to examine peer relationships of children and adolescents with chronic pain compared to healthy children and adolescents (Noll et al., 2000, 2007; Vannatta et al., 2008). Although using standardized measures is advisable, these measures may not be robust for children with chronic illness, as they may lack construct validity for this population (e.g. Perrin et al., 1991). Adams and colleagues (2002) note that a lack of normative data exists for some measures and clinical measures of child social functioning are generally designed to differentiate psychopathology versus a continuum of function. For example, if a child with chronic illness is not picked as often for a sport team, does this truly represent classmates' negative perception of the child or is this a reflection of classmates' recognition of the child's limitations? These measures also may not capture the true sense of perception of their peer relationships by the child or adolescent with a chronic pain condition.

Several researchers report that children and adolescents with chronic pain are subjected to more peer victimization than healthy children (Greco et al., 2007; Natvig et al., 2001). However, no causal link has been established between peer victimization and recurrent or chronic pain. Children and adolescents who experience recurrent or chronic pain may be viewed by their peers as more vulnerable than healthy children and therefore be preferred targets for more frequent bullying. The stress that results following peer victimization may subsequently increase a child's or adolescent's pain from a manageable to an unmanageable level. Relational victimization (i.e. aggression that impacts one's social status) can result in children and adolescents with chronic pain feeling stigmatized for having pain. In a focus group study exploring the self-identified needs of adolescents with chronic pain, one male participant described the experience of being asked personal questions from a non-friend peer and then subjected to cursing when he ignored her questions (Forgeron and McGrath, 2008). There also may be sex differences in the types of victimization children and adolescents with chronic pain are exposed to. For example, boys with abdominal pain who reported peer victimization experienced both overt and relational forms of victimization whereas girls with abdominal pain only reported relational forms of victimization (Greco et al., 2007). The significance of this sex difference regarding victimization is unclear, but relational victimization may be more difficult to recognize. As already noted, no research describes the consequences of having fewer friends compared to typically developing peers. However, given that positive friendships have been found to buffer the negative effects of peer victimization (Hodges et al., 1999) it is essential to understand the relationship between chronic pain and the actual number of close friends as having fewer friends suggests that they may be more impacted by peer victimization actions.

School functioning

School is central to the life of children and adolescents. Not only is school essential for academic learning, it also provides opportunities for children and adolescents to engage in social activities and relationships. Being exposed to different types of social relationships helps children develop social knowledge and practise a broad range of social skills, thereby leading to competent social functioning. However, school can also be a place of stigma and discrimination for children and adolescents with chronic pain. Chronic pain can negatively impact on academic performance and change relationships with teachers.

Academic achievement

Pain can negatively impact school attendance, which can contribute to academic and social sequelae. Youth with chronic pain may miss 1 to 5 days of school per month (Konijnenberg et al., 2005 Logan et al., 2008; Roth-Isigkeit et al., 2005); 20% of children and adolescents with chronic pain recruited from a pain clinic, can be absent from school more than 50% of the time (Logan et al., 2008) and 14% may be totally absent from school (Konijnenberg et al., 2005). However, absences alone do not account for all of the academic challenges faced by children and adolescents with chronic pain.

Ho and colleagues (2008) found that children and adolescents with chronic pain did not differ on standard cognitive tests in comparison to healthy children and adolescents, suggesting that intelligence is not negatively affected by the presence of a chronic pain condition. What may be affected, however, is an adolescent's ability to sustain the necessary focus and concentration to study and reach his or her academic potential. Logan and colleagues (2008) found 44.3% of adolescents with chronic pain and their parents reported a decrease in their grades since the onset of pain. The decline in grades ranged from one to four levels (i.e. a four-level change would mean that a student who generally achieves 'As' would now mostly achieve 'Cs'). Adolescent participants in other studies have reiterated experiencing difficulty in their academic ability due to chronic pain (Forgeron and McGrath, 2008).

Chronic pain can have a significant negative effect on academic achievement, and perhaps academic self-efficacy. Bandura (1993) suggests that a student's perceived self-efficacy in terms of ability to manage their learning and develop proficiency in academic activities affects motivation, goals, and academic success. Chronic pain may change an adolescent's self-efficacy in the academic realm as a result of the decrease in grades that often accompanies chronic pain.

Logan and Curran (2005) note that that teachers face many challenges when working with students experiencing chronic pain and subsequently need more information about chronic pain conditions from health care professionals, as well as guidance on how to manage pain symptoms and pain-related behaviours in school. In our experience, teachers indicate that they desired ongoing dialogue with health professionals in addition to receiving a formal letter informing them of the student's pain condition, similar to what has been supported by others (Logan and Curran, 2005).

Stress may add to school challenges for children and adolescents with chronic pain. Although both healthy children and children with recurrent abdominal pain experience more stress at school than outside of school, children with recurrent abdominal pain report greater daily stressors and a stronger association between stressors and pain symptoms than healthy children (Walker et al., 2001). Pain has also been associated with unhappiness at school (van Dijk et al., 2008), but the specific causes of school unhappiness are not entirely clear. Classmates and teachers may not understand an adolescent's pain and thus do not make necessary allowances for challenges that may arise in the school setting (Forgeron and McGrath, 2008). Classmates are often confused when children and adolescents with chronic pain are able to participate in physical activities one day but not another (Sällfors et al., 2002). Additionally, teachers may question the validity of an adolescent's pain condition (Logan and Curran, 2005). For example, Logan and Curran (2005) examined teacher perceptions of students with chronic pain and found that some teachers were sceptical of the validity of these students' pain report based on the association between context factors and pain expression. Specifically, teachers were concerned that adolescents might use pain as an excuse (fake pain) to be excused from tests or to receive attention from peers. Thus, negative perceptions and reactions from others may be a factor contributing to inability to concentrate in the classroom, as well as overall school unhappiness in children and adolescents with chronic pain.

There is no evidence to suggest that students with pain fake their pain to reduce school assignments or to avoid tests and exams. Interestingly, there is evidence that parents are able to easily detect when their child is faking pain but have more difficulty detecting when their child or adolescent is suppressing pain (Larochette et al., 2006). Thus, teachers may actually under-detect pain in the classroom, especially if a child or adolescent is suppressing his or her pain expression to blend in with classmates. When a student with chronic pain encounters a teacher who gives the impression that he or she believes the student is 'faking' he or she may feel stigmatized by the school experience.

Social context of school

When children and adolescents with chronic pain are absent from school, they are also absent from their primary social environment and risk falling behind in the social knowledge and exchanges that take place during the school day. Specifically, they may not be aware of the social events from previous days and the topic of conversation, which may contribute to feeling alone despite being among peers. Thus, the process of returning to school after a period of absence can be challenging because of the negative impact of their absence on academic skills and on their social knowledge.

Children and adolescents with chronic pain may feel singled out and different from their classmates (Forgeron and McGrath, 2008). This can be due to teachers and other students asking questions upon their return that make them feel unsupported and judged. These questions may include asking for reasons for their absences, details about their medical conditions, justification for academic or physical accommodations, and being outwardly teased by classmates. Additionally, in a study by Sällfors et al. (2002), adolescents have noted that it was often difficult to sit out of certain classes (i.e. physical education) and complete academic assignments while their classmates were having fun. Clearly, being separated from classmates would serve to highlight their pain condition and the differences between adolescents with a pain condition and their healthy peers. Although children and adolescents with pain conditions may not be able to participate in classes such as physical education, they may prefer to either take part in a modified version of the physical activity (e.g. walking rather than running, if possible)

or complete academic assignments elsewhere (e.g. the library or an empty classroom) so as to protect themselves from standing out from their healthy peers.

Adolescents describe feeling punished for their pain condition when teachers are unwilling to grant them academic accommodations (Forgeron and McGrath, 2008). These reactions (a response to their pain expression) may increase their stress and perhaps even their pain intensity (due to the relationship between stress and pain), which, in turn, affects their ability to attend school. However, when teachers modified academic requirements, adolescents with chronic pain reported feeling supported and perceived these accommodations as acknowledgement of their pain as real (Forgeron and McGrath, 2008).

Many schools have restrictions on participation in committees, sports, and special school events based on either school attendance or grades. Adolescents with chronic pain feel further punished when they are unable to participate in these extracurricular events. Having these restrictions waived for children and adolescents with chronic pain has a positive effect on how they feel in the social context of school, which then has a positive effect on how these students feel in the academic context. Collaboration and dialogue is necessary to obtain a waiver of these restrictions and to help teachers understand how their reaction to a student with chronic pain can either result in the student feeling supported or add to the student's stress.

Recommendations

Although there are no intervention studies to date that identify the most useful strategies to help children and adolescents with chronic pain manage peer relationships and friendships, we propose intervention strategies that are informed by the research reviewed in this chapter.

Clinical recommendations

Clinicians must recognize that chronic pain may present challenges to peer relationships and friendships. Children and adolescents may be reticent to speak negatively about their friends, as they acknowledge that many of their friends were supportive at times. Thus, ensuring a safe environment to discuss concerns is needed.

Improving peer perceptions of children and adolescents with chronic pain is important, as positive peer relationships have been positively correlated with more positive perceptions of social abilities of adolescents with chronic pain (Eccleston et al., 2008). Exploring situations in which peers and close friends have not been supportive may help the child or adolescent with chronic pain, as non-supportive situations tend to be the most troubling for this population and may lead to disengagement from friends. The clinician should work with the child or adolescent with chronic pain to determine an approach so the child or adolescent could take control of the situation. For example, they could practise the types of conversations that may occur with their friends and learn the types of actions that are helpful and non-helpful in conversations with friends. Helping a child or adolescent understand that some of their pain behaviours may be difficult for their friends to understand may also be needed. These discussions, along with activities such as role playing, may help the adolescent practise how to take control and advocate for their friendship needs. However, the adolescent with chronic pain must also understand that his or her needs should be balanced with a willingness to listen to their friends' needs, as friendships are reciprocal. Taking control of these situations may improve friendship quality by not only securing the friendship needs of adolescents with chronic pain but also allowing friends to discuss their friendship needs when the adolescent with chronic pain disengages from activities.

Understanding one's pain condition has been linked to acceptance and engagement in treatment; therefore, pain education is often offered to children and adolescents with chronic pain to help them understand their condition. However, pain education targeted at helping the child or adolescent develop language to help explain their condition to others has not been developed. It is necessary for a child or adolescent to understand his or her pain condition in a way that they could translate to their friends to decrease the scepticism they encounter. Future research should attempt to develop and evaluate interventions that focus on developing appropriate language to describe pain to others.

Given the regularity that some adolescents with chronic pain are absent from school, their friends may not find their absences unusual. Children and adolescents who miss school due to pain may need to be proactive in contacting their friends to fill them in on the social activities of the day. This approach may help a child or adolescent with chronic pain who is absent from school regularly to remain informed of the social context and perhaps a feeling of belonging when they do go back to school. Technology such as webcams and real-time chatting over the Internet could be offered as helpful tools to allow children and adolescents with chronic pain to continue interacting with their peers remotely.

School accommodations

Academic accommodations may help adolescents with chronic pain to view their teachers as taking a more positive attitude towards them and believing in their pain condition. Student perceptions of positive teacher regard have been linked to increases in academic values, achievement, and feelings of academic competency (Roeser and Eccles, 1998). Many of the adolescents in a study by Logan and colleagues (2008) had some form of accommodation in place; teachers rated students with more accommodations as being better adjusted to school compared to typical peers. Therefore, even when chronic pain negatively impacts academic performance the implementation of accommodations may help students perceive themselves as valued competent students.

The following academic accommodations have been identified as helpful either from clinical experience or the literature. First, regular communication between and among the health care professionals, school, and family is needed (Logan and Curran, 2005). Second, teachers are more apt to provide requested academic accommodations if the health professional provides these suggestions in writing (Forgeron and McGrath, 2008; Logan and Curran, 2005). Third, academic accommodations that offset the negative cognitive consequences of chronic pain need to be individualized, as not all patients require every accommodation. Such accommodations may include a combination of the following: (1) class notes (i.e. for missed work or to reduce motor demand when in class), (2) spacing out of projects and tests to allow for the increase length of time to complete tasks, and (3) decreased workload (i.e. the quality should be the same but amount may need to be reduced). Finally, in our clinical experience, having one teacher (or guidance counsellor) to act as a student advocate within the school has been helpful.

This member of the teaching staff is someone the student can go to have issues resolved instead of having to negotiate with several teachers at once.

Some children and adolescents may require physical accommodations such as the ability to leave their desk and walk around, have a private place outside of class (e.g. guidance or nurse office) to use non-pharmacological pain-reducing strategies (e.g. relaxation exercises such as deep breathing and guided imagery), or the use of an elevator pass or access to water in class (i.e. especially for children or adolescents on certain medications). These physical accommodations are aimed at helping to reduce pain in the moment so that the child or adolescent is able to remain in the school even if he or she must miss a class. In our clinical experience, once a child or adolescent leaves school due to their pain it is unlikely that the student will return to school that day.

A formal request for the child or adolescent to be exempt from the attendance or grade requirements to participate in school social life is also important. When excluded from school social life due to their pain condition, children and adolescents may feel as though they are being punished as a result of their condition. The more excluded socially, the more likely they are to experience loneliness, and other associated psychosocial sequelae (e.g. anxiety or depression). Children and adolescents with chronic pain may benefit from health professionals having a discussion with teachers regarding the best ways to communicate with a student challenged by chronic pain. Children and adolescents do not want to stand out and appear different from their peers; therefore, it is important to remind school personnel to keep conversations about pain and health confidential. A template of a school letter, developed and used at our clinic (IWK Health Centre, Halifax, Nova Scotia—where the first author was the clinical nurse specialist) is part of the online supplement of this chapter. An important component is a basic explanation of the physiology of chronic pain that may help teachers to reinforce the legitimacy of chronic pain to school personnel. We encourage other clinicians to use or modify this letter if they feel it would be useful in advocating for children and adolescents with chronic pain.

Research recommendations

There is limited research on the social consequences of chronic pain for children and adolescents. Little is known about the processes of how peer relationships or friendships impact the chronic pain experience and functioning of children and adolescents, or the processes through which pain impacts friendships. It appears that withdrawal from activities and school absences are important factors but further research examining the relationship between pain expression and pain interpretation are needed to understand the impact of these factors. To date, most of the research focuses on peer relationships and needs to expand to include close friendships. Additionally, examining the relationships of adolescents separately from children would allow developmental differences to be revealed. Studies are also needed that account for differences between male and female friendships. Finally, intervention studies to determine the best ways to maintain and strengthen close friendships are needed.

Although chronic pain may negatively affect subjective reports of academic performance (Dick and Pillai-Riddell, 2010), the exact processes remain elusive. Pain may negatively impact concentration and focus. However, negative academic performance may also be related to other pain related factors such as sleep disturbances.

Changes in social relationships in the school setting (both with peers and teachers) may contribute to a decline in overall school performance and school absence may intensify or be a consequence of these factors. Research is needed to examine the processes that interfere with specific aspects of school performance (academic performance, social relationships, restrictions on school involvement) along with designing and testing strategies that improve overall school performance.

Conclusion

A clear understanding of the social and school functioning of children and adolescents with chronic pain is an essential part of their clinical care. We have suggested strategies on to support improved social functioning and school performance-based current research. However, more research is needed to understand the processes underlying social functioning and school performance so that more specific interventions can be designed and implemented, thereby allowing children and adolescents challenged by chronic pain to be as successful as possible in the academic and social spheres.

Case example

Jill is a 16-year-old girl who developed widespread body pain at the end of the school year and her pain intensity progressively increased over the summer months. She has seen several specialists and all her diagnostic tests come back within normal limits. She rates her pain as 7 out of 10 most days with exacerbations up to 10 out of 10 at least once a week. The pain is keeping her from sleeping well; she finds it hard to fall asleep and wakes frequently thought the night because of pain. She started 10th grade 2 months ago, which meant a change in schools. She is missing about 2 to 3 days of school a week. Her classmates from last year are attending the same school but most are not in her classes.

In grade 9 Jill was on the volleyball team and achieved straight As. Her parents are supportive but wonder why the doctors cannot find anything wrong with Jill. Jill used to go out with her friends regularly and is described by her parents as being popular. However, since developing the widespread pain, she has been home much more, hardly goes out with her friends on the weekend, did not try out for the volleyball team, and her marks are now in the Bs. Jill reports that getting up from her seat and going for a walk is helpful when her pain becomes unbearable in class, but some of her teachers do not allow her to leave the classroom citing that she has missed so much time that she cannot afford to miss any more instruction. In private Jill mentions to you that she does not like to go out as she may have pain when she is out socializing. She also mentions that her friends called a lot when she first became ill but have stopped calling her.

Is Jill experiencing school avoidance?

What would you suggest from an academic perspective?

What would you suggest form a social perspective in terms of school?

Why do you think Jill's friends are no longer contacting her?

References

Bagwell, C. L., Schmidt, M. E., Newcomb, A. F., and Bukowski, W. M. (2001). Friendship and peer rejection as predictors of adult adjustment. In D. W. Nagle and C. A. Erdley (eds) *The role of friendship in psychological adjustment*, pp. 25–50. San Francisco, CA: Jossey-Bass.

Bandura, A. (1993). Perceived self-efficacy in cognitive development and functioning. *Educ Psychol*, 28, 117–148.

Benenson, J. and Christakos, A. (2003). The greater fragility of females' versus males' closest same-sex friendships. *Child Dev*, 74, 1123–1129.

Berndt, T. J. and Hoyle, S. G. (1985). Stability and change in childhood and adolescent friendships. *Dev Psychol*, 21, 1007–1015.

Buhrmester, D. and Furman, W. (1986). The changing functions of friends in childhood: a neo-Sullivanian perspective. In V. J. Derlega and B. A. Winstead (eds) *Friendship and social interaction*, pp. 41–45. New York: Springer-Verlag.

Carter, B., Lambrenos, K., and Thursfield, J. (2002). A pain workshop: an approach to eliciting the views of young people with chronic pain. *J Clin Nurs*, 11, 753–762.

Coatsworth, J. D., Sharp, E. H., Palen, A., Darling, N., Cumsille, P., and Marta, E. (2005). Exploring adolescent self-defining leisure activities and identity experiences across three countries. *Int J Behav Dev*, 29, 361–370.

Craig, K. (2009). The social communication model of pain. *Can Psychol*, 50, 22–32.

Craig, K. D. (2002). Pain in infants and children: socio developmental variations on the theme. In M. A. Giamberardino (ed), *Pain 2002—an updated review, refresher course syllabus, 10th World Congress on Pain, San Diego, CA*, pp. 305–314. Seattle, WA: IASP Press.

Dick, B. and Pillai Riddell, R. (2010). Cognitive and school functioning in children and adolescents with chronic pain: a critical review. *Pain Res Manag*, 15, 238–244.

Erdley, C. A., Nangle, D. W., Newman, J. E., and Carpenter, E. M. (2001). Children's friendship experiences and psychological adjustment: theory and research. In D. W. Nagle and C. A. Erdley (eds) *The role of friendship in psychological adjustment*, pp. 5–24. San Francisco, CA: Jossey-Bass.

Eccleston, C., Wastell, S., Crombez, G., and Jordan, A. (2008). Adolescent social development and chronic pain. *Eur J Pain*, 12, 765–774.

Forgeron, P. A., King, S., Stinson, J., McGrath, P. J., MacDonald, A. J., and Chambers, C. T. (2010). Social functioning and peer relationships in children and adolescents with chronic pain: a systematic review. *Pain Res Manag*, 15, 27–41.

Forgeron, P., and McGrath, P. J. (2008). Self-identified needs of adolescents with chronic pain. *J Pain Manag*, 1, 163–172.

Forgeron, P. A., McGrath, P., Evans, J., Stevens, B., and Finley, A. (2011a). My friends don't really understand me: examining close friendships of adolescents with chronic pain. PhD dissertation, Dalhousie University, Halifax.

Forgeron, P. A., McGrath, P. J., Stevens, B., Evans, J., Dick, B., Finley, G. A., *et al.* (2011b). Social information processing in adolescents with chronic pain: my friends don't really understand me. *Pain*, 152, 2771–2780.

Gauze, C., Bukowski, W. M., Aquan-Assee, J., and Sippola, L. K. (1996). Interactions between family environment and friendship and associations with self-perceived well-being during early adolescence. *Child Dev*, 67, 2201–2216.

Greco, L. A., Freeman, K. E., and Dufton, L. M. (2007). Overt and relational victimization among children with frequent abdominal pain: links to social skills, academic functioning, and health service use. *J Pediatr Psychol*, 32, 319–329.

Guite, J. W., Walker, L. S., Smith, C. A., and Garber, J. (2000). *Children's perceptions of peers with somatic symptoms: the impact of gender, stress, and illness. J Pediatr Psychol*, 25, 125–135.

Hodges, E. V. E., Boivin, M., Vitaro, F., and Bukowshi, W. M. (1999). The power of friendship: protection against an escalating cycle of peer victimization. *Dev Psychol*, 35, 94–101.

Kashikar-Zuck, S., Lynch, A., Graham, B., Swain, N., and Mullen, S. A. (2007). Social functioning and peer relationships of adolescents with juvenile fibromyalgia syndrome. *Arthritis Rheum*, 57, 474–480.

King, S., Chambers, C. T., Huguet, A., MacNevin, R. C., McGrath, P. J., Parker, L., et al. (2011). The epidemiology of chronic pain in children and adolescents revisited: a systematic review. *Pain*, 152, 2729–2738.

Konijnenberg, A. Y., Uiterwaal, C. S. P. M., Kimpen, J. L. L., van der Hoeven, J., Buitelaar, J. K., and de Graeff-Meeder, E. R. (2005). Children with unexplained chronic pain: substantial impairment in everyday life. *Arch Dis Child*, 90, 680–686.

Ladd, G. W., Kochenderfer, B. J., and Coleman, C. C. (1997). Classroom peer acceptance, friendship, and victimization: distinct relational systems that contribute uniquely to children's school adjustment? *Child Dev*, 68, 1181–1197.

Larochette, A. C., Chambers, C. T., and Craig, K. D. (2006). Genuine, suppressed and faked facial expression of pain in children. *Pain*, 126, 64–71.

Logan, D. E. and Curran, J. A. (2005). Adolescent chronic pain problems in the school setting: exploring the experiences of selected school personnel through focus group methodology. *J Adolescent Health*, 37, 281–288.

Logan, D. E., Simmons, L. E., Stein, M. J., and Chastain, L. (2008). School impairment in adolescents with chronic pain. *J Pain*, 9, 407–416.

Mahoney, J. L., and Stattin, H. (2000). Leisure activities and adolescent antisocial behavior: the role of structure and social context. *J Adolescences*, 23, 113–127.

Nangle, D., Erdley, C. A., Newman, J. E., Mason, C. A., and Carpenter, E. M. (2003). Popularity, friendship quantity, and friendship quality: interactive influences on children's loneliness and depression. *J Clin Child Adolesc Psychol*, 52, 546–555.

Natvig, G. K., Albrektsen, G., and Qvarnstrom, U. (2001). Psychosomatic symptoms among victims of school bullying. *J Health Psychol*, 6, 365–377.

Noll, R. B., Kiska, R., Reiter-Purtill, J., Gerhardt, C. A., and Vannatta, K. (2010). A controlled, longitudinal study of the social functioning of youth with sickle cell disease. *Pediatrics*, 125, e1453–1459.

Noll, R. B., Kozlowski, K., Gerhardt, C., Vannatta, K., Taylor, J., and Passo, M. (2000). Social, emotional and behavioral functioning of children with juvenile rheumatoid arthritis. *Arthritis Rheum*, 46, 1387–1396.

Noll, R. B., Reiter-Purtill, J., Vannatta, K., Gerhardt, C. A., & Short, A. (2007). Peer relationships and emotional well-being of children with sickle cell disease: a controlled replication. *Child Neuropsychol*, 13, 173–187.

Noll, R. B., Vannatta, K., Koontz, K., and Kalinyak. K. (1996). Peer relationships and emotional well being of youngsters with sickle cell disease. *Child Dev*, 67, 423–436.

Perrin, E. C., Stein, R. E. K., and Drotar, D. (1991). Cautions in using the Child Behavior Checklist: observations based on research about children with a chronic illness. *J Pediatr Psychol*, 16, 411–421.

Roeser, R. W., and Eccles, J. S. (1998). Adolescents' perceptions of middle school: relation to longitudinal changes in academic and psychological adjustment. *J Rese Adolesc*, 8, 123–158.

Roth-Isigkeit, A., Thyen, U., Stöven, H., Schwarzenberger, J., and Schmucker, P. (2005). Pain among children and adolescents: restrictions in daily living and triggering factors. Pediatrics, 11, 3152–3162.

Rubin, K. H., Chen, X., Coplan, R., Buskirk, A., and Wojslawowicz, J. C. (2005). Peer relationships in childhood. In M. H. Bornstein and M. E. Lamb (eds) *Developmental science: an advanced textbook* (5th edn), pp. 469–512. Mahwah, NJ: Erlbaum.

Sällfors, C., Fasth, A., and Hallberg, L.R. (2002). Oscillating between hope and despair—a qualitative study. *Child: Care, Health, Dev*, 28, 495–505.

Stanford, E. A., Chambers, C. T., Biesanz, J. C., and Chen, E. (2008). The frequency, trajectories and predictors of adolescent recurrent pain: a population-based approach. *Pain*, 138, 11–21.

Sullivan, H. S. (1953). *The interpersonal theory of psychiatry*. New York: W.W. Norton & Company.

Van Dijk, A., McGrath, P. A., Pickett, W., and Van Den Kerkhof, E. (2008). Pain and self reported health in Canadian children. *Pain Res Manag*, 13, 407–411.

Vannatta, K. Getzoff, E. A., Gilman, D. K., Noll, R. B., Gerhardt, C. A., Powers, S. W., et al. (2008). Friendships and social interactions of school-aged children with migraine. *Cephalalgia*, 28, 734–743.

Walker, L. S., Garber, J., Smith, C. A., Van Slyke, A., and Claar R. L. (2001). The relation of daily stressors to somatic and emotional symptoms in children with and without recurrent abdominal pain. *J Consult Clin Psychol*, 69, 85–91.

Online supplementary materials

Figure 13.1 Example letter.

Reproduced with permission from Forgeron, P. A. and McGrath, P. J, Distance Management of Pediatric Pain, in G. A. Walco and K. R. Goldschneider (eds), *Pediatric Pain Management in Primary Care: A Practical Guide*, Humana Press, Totowa, New Jersey, USA, Copyright © 2007.

CHAPTER 14

The effects of sex and gender on child and adolescent pain

Erin C. Moon and Anita M. Unruh

Summary

As women enter adulthood, they are at an increased risk for a number of clinical pain conditions and show higher experimental pain sensitivity relative to men (e.g. Fillingim et al., 2009). The feminine gender role encourages the expression of pain in both children and adults whereas the masculine gender role encourages stoicism in response to pain (e.g. Robinson et al., 2001; Zeman and Garber, 1996). The earlier work of Unruh (1996), Berkeley (1992, 1997), and LeResche (1997), demonstrated that sex and gender shaped the experience of pain and a subsequent body of research has continued to articulate their influence.

Before examining this literature, it is important to distinguish between the terms sex and gender. Sex usually refers to biological aspects and gender to the social or cultural dimensions of being male or female (Owen Blakemore et al., 2009). The World Health Organization defines sex as 'the biological and physiological characteristics that define men and women' and gender as 'the socially constructed roles, behaviours, activities, and attributes that a given society considers appropriate for men and women' (World Health Organization, n.d., para. 1).

This chapter will begin with a brief overview of sex and gender differences in adult pain to provide a context for then examining sex and gender differences in child and adolescent pain. The chapter will continue with a discussion of the biological, family, and socio-cultural factors thought to contribute to sex and gender differences in child and adolescent pain.

Sex and gender differences in adult pain

Much of the early research on sex differences in adult pain focused on experimental paradigms. A 1998 meta-analysis of these studies concluded that women were more likely to report lower pain threshold and tolerance than men, with effect sizes of $d = 0.55$ for threshold and $d = 0.57$ for tolerance (Riley et al., 1998). In an updated meta-analysis, Fillingim et al. (2009) concluded that there are reliable sex differences in pressure and electrical pain, with women reporting greater sensitivity than men. The largest study to date to assess sex differences in pain threshold using multiple experimental modalities found that women have significantly lower pain thresholds than men (Rolke et al., 2006).

In epidemiological studies worldwide, Fillingim et al. (2009) reported that neuropathic pain, chronic musculoskeletal pain, abdominal pain, headache, and migraine were more prevalent in women compared to men, and women had pain in more anatomical sites. Similarly, Tsang et al. (2008), in a study spanning 17 countries, found that women reported a higher prevalence of common chronic pain conditions.

Though sex differences are evident in experimental and epidemiological studies, in adult clinical pain samples they are equivocal. In a study of pain ratings in five samples of patients at chronic pain clinics, women were slightly more likely to give higher pain severity ratings than men (Robinson et al., 1998). Other studies have not reported sex differences (e.g. arthritis: Lander et al., 1990; temporomandibular pain: Bush et al., 1993; Wilson et al., 1994).

Findings on adult sex differences in medical procedure and postoperative pain are also inconsistent. In a study of needle procedures, women reported higher pain intensity (Ring et al., 2009). In a review of 15 studies of postoperative pain, Fillingim and colleagues (2009) concluded that women gave higher pain intensity ratings but noted that conflicting outcomes were also reported in some studies.

Men and women may cope differently with pain. The most robust findings are that women use more social support to cope with pain and a greater number of pain coping strategies compared to men (Unruh, 1997). Although not all studies find sex differences in catastrophizing (e.g. Unruh et al., 1999), there is evidence that women do catastrophize about pain more than men (Edwards et al., 2004; Jensen et al., 1994; Keefe et al., 2000).

Fewer studies have considered the impact of gender on adult pain. Existing studies show that higher scores on measures of masculine gender role stress increase systolic blood pressure reactivity to pain (indicating stress; e.g. Lash et al. 1990). Higher masculinity scores have also predicted higher pain tolerance and lower pain ratings (Otto and Dougher, 1985; Thorn et al., 2004).

There is no critical age marking the onset of sex and gender differences in adult pain. A number of studies suggest that the socialization mechanisms that shape gender role expectations of pain begin in childhood and that puberty is the biological catalyst for the onset of the physiological mechanisms that contribute to sex differences in pain (Unruh and Campbell, 1999).

Sex differences in child and adolescent pain

In 1999, Unruh and Campbell concluded that sex differences in studies of experimental pain in childhood and adolescence were not consistent but when they occurred, they were in the same direction as in adult studies. Girls generally reported similar or lower pain thresholds and tolerance compared to boys. The experimental studies of child and adolescent pain published since 1999 are summarized in Tables 14.1 and 14.2.

Two of these experimental studies used quantitative sensory testing (QST), a battery of somatosensory processing tests that provide reliable and valid measures of sensory thresholds in children (Meier et al., 2001), with different outcomes. Walker et al. (2009) used QST in a study of the long-term impact of early pain and injury on sensory perception. There were no sex differences in mechanical (pressure) detection thresholds between children born premature (and now 11 years of age) and a control group of children born full-term. Nevertheless, in the control group, boys were significantly more sensitive to heat and cold detection than girls. In contrast, with a healthy sample of 6- to 16-year-olds, Blankenburg and colleagues (2010) found that girls were more sensitive to heat and cold detection, as well as heat and cold pain stimuli, than boys. The wider age range of the participants in the Blankenburg et al. study may help account for these divergent findings.

In a sample of 244 children, Lu and colleagues (2005) found no sex differences in heat pain tolerance, but girls had a significantly

Table 14.1 Summary of recent child and adolescent experimental pain studies (paradigms other than cold pressor task) reporting on sex differences

Authors, year	Age range	Sex difference findings
Quantitative sensory testing		
Walker et al., 2009	11 years	Mechanical detection threshold: no differences
		Heat detection threshold: in control group, boys more sensitive
		Cold detection threshold: in control group, boys more sensitive
Blankenburg et al., 2010	6–16 years	Mechanical detection threshold: no differences
		Heat detection threshold: girls more sensitive
		Cold detection threshold: girls more sensitive
		Mechanical pain threshold: no differences
		Heat pain threshold: girls more sensitive
		Cold pain threshold: girls more sensitive
Pressure pain		
Lu et al., 2005	8–18 years	Pain tolerance: boys > girls
Lu et al., 2007	8–18 years	Pain intensity: no differences
		Pain unpleasantness: no differences
Heat pain		
Lu et al., 2005	8–18 years	Pain tolerance: no differences
Lu et al., 2007	8–18 years	Pain intensity: no differences
		Pain unpleasantness: no differences

Table 14.2 Summary of recent child and adolescent cold pressor task studies reporting on sex differences

Authors, year	Age range	Sex difference findings
Chambers et al., 2002	8–12 years	Pain intensity: no differences
		Pain affect: no differences
		Pain tolerance: no differences
		Heart rate: no differences
		Facial activity: boys > girls
Coldwell et al., 2002	8–11 years	Pain intensity: no differences (sex not predictor in regression)
Evans et al. 2008	8–18 years	Pain intensity: no differences
Goodman and McGrath, 2003	10–14 years	Pain intensity: no differences
		Pain tolerance: no differences
		Pain threshold: no differences
		Facial activity: no differences
Jaaniste et al., 2007	7–12 years	Pain intensity: no differences
		Pain tolerance: no differences
Larochette et al., 2006	8–12 years	Facial activity: no differences
Moon et al., 2008	4–12 years	Pain intensity: no differences
		Heart rate: no differences
		Facial activity: no differences
Myers et al., 2006	8–18 years	Pain intensity: more boys than girls in 'low pain' group
		Pain affect: no differences
		Pain tolerance: no differences
Pepino and Mennella, 2005	5–10 years	Pain intensity: no differences
		Pain tolerance: no differences
Piira et al., 2002	7–14 years	Pain tolerance: no differences (age by sex interaction)
Piira et al., 2006	7–14 years	Pain intensity: no differences
		Pain tolerance: no differences
Trapanotto et al., 2008	8–12 years	Pain intensity: no differences
		Pain affect: no differences
		Pain tolerance: no differences
Tsao et al., 2002	8–10 years	Pain intensity: no differences
		Pain tolerance: no differences
Tsao et al., 2006a	8–18 years	Pain intensity: no differences
Tsao et al., 2006b	8–18 years	Pain intensity: no differences
Tsao et al., 2004	8–18 years	Pain intensity: more boys than girls in 'low-pain' group

lower pressure pain tolerance than boys. A mediation analysis indicated that this sex difference was due to a higher pre-trial heart rate in girls (an indication of autonomic arousal). With the same sample of children, Lu et al. (2007) reported no sex differences in pressure or heat pain intensity or pain unpleasantness.

Since the review by Unruh and Campbell (1999), 16 studies of cold pressor pain in children and adolescents have examined sex differences (see Table 14.2). With a few exceptions, most of these studies do not identify sex differences in pain intensity, pain tolerance, pain affect, or facial response to pain.

Girls are at an increased risk of chronic pain. Based on data from population-based studies conducted in America (Stewart et al., 1991) and Germany (Kroner-Herwig et al., 2007), Fillingim et al. (2009) concluded that while boys have an earlier onset of both migraine and non-migraine headache, as adolescence approaches, incidence and prevalence rises more quickly in girls. Sex differences in the prevalence of child musculoskeletal pain are not as clear. For example, a Finnish study (Mikkelsson et al., 1997) indicated an increased prevalence of chest and upper back pain in girls whereas a nationwide study of musculoskeletal pain in Swedish students (Brun Sundblad et al., 2007) did not detect sex differences. In this Swedish study, girls were twice as likely to have weekly abdominal pain as boys. Other epidemiological studies of child abdominal pain support the increased prevalence of abdominal pain in girls (Kristjansdottir, 1996; Oh et al., 2004; Ramchandani et al., 2005; Stanford et al., 2008). In a study of Canadian adolescents, girls had higher rates of all types of pain (e.g. headaches, stomach aches, and backaches) than boys (Stanford et al. 2008) and in a European study, girls also reported more frequent chronic pain (Huguet and Miró, 2008).

Sex differences in clinical child pain have been explored in various studies but have not yet been the subject of systematic review. In two clinical studies, girls reported higher current pain (Keogh and Eccleston, 2006) and more continuing pain and utilization of health care services (Martin et al., 2007). In a sample of adolescent cancer patients, Hechler and colleagues (2009) found that girls reported higher pain intensity in the past week and month, but boys and girls were similar in present pain intensity ratings. In two other studies, present pain intensity ratings were comparable in girls and boys aged 8 to 18 years (Kaczynski et al., 2009; Lynch et al., 2007).

Otherwise healthy children frequently endure pain from medical procedures such as immunizations and blood draws. Unruh and Campbell (1999) concluded that findings on sex differences in children's needle pain were inconsistent. Since 1999, evidence continues to be mixed. Five recent studies that compared boys' and girls' immunization and venepuncture pain found no differences (Caprilli et al., 2007; Cohen et al., 2000, 2004; Goodenough et al., 1999a; Kleiber et al., 2007). In contrast, Chambers and colleagues (1999) found that girls aged 5 to 12 years gave higher pain intensity ratings following venepuncture than boys. Similarly, sex differences were reported with older children (11–17 years; von Baeyer et al., 2009) and younger children (4–6 years; Sparks 2001) undergoing immunizations. In another study of venepuncture pain, Goodenough et al. (1999b) discovered that girls gave significantly higher pain unpleasantness ratings than boys from the age of 8 years onwards. These authors suggested that boys over the age of 8 years may be increasingly influenced by gender role expectations that boys should be stoic about pain.

Data on sex differences in child postoperative pain have not been systematically reviewed. The available evidence suggests that similar to research with adults, sex differences in child postoperative pain are not clear. In one study, conducted with adolescents and young adults aged 12 to 20 years who had undergone elective surgery, girls gave higher pain intensity ratings than boys (Gillies et al., 1999). In addition, more girls in this study requested pain medication than boys in the first 24 hours after surgery. Another study, of children aged 5 to 13 years who had undergone minor surgery, found no sex differences in children's self-reports or parents' and nurses' reports of child pain intensity (Chambers et al., 2005). Similarly, in a study of children and young adults aged 8 to 21 years who had spinal fusion surgery, girls and boys gave similar postoperative pain intensity ratings and displayed similar levels of pain behaviour (Kotzer, 2000).

Regarding sex differences in coping with pain, data collected with child and adolescent samples parallels the findings from adult samples (Unruh and Campbell, 1999). Like women, girls aged 8 to 18 years use more social support in response to pain than boys (Keogh and Eccleston, 2006; Lynch et al., 2007). Boys in this age group use more behavioural distraction (e.g. doing something enjoyable to take their mind off pain; Lynch et al., 2007; Reid et al., 1998). The finding that boys are more likely than girls to distract themselves from pain has been interpreted as a way for boys to minimize pain and thereby act in accordance with the male gender role (Reid et al., 1998). Similar to studies in the adult literature, some studies with children and adolescents have not found sex differences in catastrophizing (Lynch et al., 2007; Reid et al., 1998) whereas other studies report that adolescent girls are more likely than boys to catastrophize in response to pain (Keogh and Eccleston, 2006).

Gender differences in child and adolescent pain

The impact of gender on child pain outcomes has not been extensively studied but existing research suggests that masculinity may have an impact on some pain outcomes. Myers and colleagues (2006) measured the relationship between self-reported gender-stereotyped personality traits and pain ratings in children aged 8 to 18 years using the Child Sex Role Inventory (CSRI; Boldizar, 1991). Children underwent three pain tasks: pressure, cold, and thermal. Masculinity scores for boys were unrelated to pain tolerance on all three tasks but significantly inversely related to heat pain intensity and pain affect ratings. For boys and girls aged 14 to 18 years, higher masculinity relative to femininity scores predicted lower cold and heat pain ratings. Surprisingly, for boys and girls aged 8 to 13 years, higher masculinity relative to femininity scores predicted higher cold pain ratings.

In a second study using the CSRI, Moon (2010) examined the relationship between parents' ratings of their children's gender-stereotyped personality traits and cold pressor pain outcomes in children aged 8 to 12 years. Similar to the findings of Myers and colleagues (2006), child gender was not associated with cold pressor pain intensity, pain affect, pain tolerance, or pain complaints. Nevertheless, for children under the age of 13 years, Myers and colleagues found that higher femininity, relative to masculinity, was predictive of lower cold pressor pain intensity ratings. They interpreted these findings to mean that responses to cold pressor pain that are in keeping with gender-role stereotypes (i.e. higher masculinity being associated with lower pain ratings) may only emerge after the age of 13 years. The findings of the study by Moon are in keeping with this interpretation.

Factors that contribute to sex and gender differences in child and adolescent pain

In order to better understand sex and gender differences in pain, researchers have begun to consider the relative contributions and interactions of biological, family, and sociocultural factors.

Biological factors

Sex hormones (mainly oestradiol, progesterone, and testosterone) play a role in men's and women's responses to experimental pain (e.g. Fillingim and Edwards, 2001; Riley et al., 1999) and have an impact on pain across the menstrual cycle (Unruh, 1996). Furthermore, sex differences in some pain conditions such as migraine headaches (Stewart et al., 1992) and temporomandibular disorders (LeResche, 1997) emerge only after puberty. There are also sex and hormonally determined differences in neuroactive substances such as gamma-aminobutyric acid, opioid and non-opioid analgesia, nerve growth factor (involved in pain perception), and the sympathetic nervous system that may help explain sex differences in experimental pain (Berkley, 1997).

Rodent models have been used to reduce the influence of sociocultural variables inherent in studies of human sex differences in pain. Findings of this animal research have led to the generally-held conclusion that female rodents have a lower pain threshold (Hurley and Adams, 2008). Nevertheless, in a review of the literature on sex differences in both human and animal pain, Hurley and Adams noted that the animal models with the most clinical relevance for human pain (e.g. the Brennan et al. model of post-incisional pain in rodents; Brennan et al., 1996) have not uncovered significant differences between male and female animals.

Some researchers have used brain imaging techniques such as positron emission tomography to study sex differences in human response to pain. Women have shown greater regional brain activation of the thalamus, contralateral prefrontal cortex, and contralateral insula than men following painful thermal stimulation (Paulson et al., 1998); however, in another study, men had greater regional brain activation (Derbyshire et al., 2002). No significant difference in brain activation has been reported using functional magnetic resonance imaging following thermal pain (Moulton et al., 2006). At present, it is premature to conclude that there are sex differences in brain activation in response to pain, and no studies have included child or adolescent samples.

Family factors

Parental behaviour has a powerful effect on child pain (Chambers et al., 2003; see also Birnie et al., Chapter 12, this volume). A handful of studies support the hypothesis that sex differences in child pain may be partly explained by familial socialization histories. These studies provide evidence that the expression of pain in girls is encouraged whereas the expression of pain in boys is discouraged by neutral or negative parental reactions (e.g. Kankkunen et al., 2003; Schechter et al., 1991; Walker et al., 1995).

According to the operant model of chronic pain (Fordyce, 1976), receiving attention from others about pain reinforces pain expression. Applying this model to child pain, Zeman and Shipman (1996) suggested that parents may teach their children to behave in accordance with gender-role stereotypes for pain by giving their daughters more attention when they express pain compared to their sons. This position was supported by an experimental pain study with 8- to 16-year-old children in which parents tended to use more attention with their daughters and more distraction with their sons (Walker et al., 2006). These findings were not replicated in a more recent experimental pain study with 8- to 12-year-olds (Moon et al., 2011).

Until very recently, there have been few studies comparing and contrasting the socialization influence of mothers and fathers on child pain, but those that exist point to the importance of comparing these parental roles. Kangaroo care (providing skin-to-skin care by the parent holding a nappy-clad infant against the bare chest) has a significant impact on reducing an infant's response to painful procedures (Johnston et al., 2011). Johnston and colleagues (2011) have shown that this effect is marginally but significantly stronger for the mother than the father. (See Johnston and Campbell-Yeo, Chapter 58, this volume, for further discussion of mother care pain interventions.) Moon (2010) found that higher femininity scores, relative to masculinity scores, were associated with fewer pain complaints when girls underwent a cold pressor task with their fathers present, but not with their mothers present. In an intriguing study of the relationship between parental catastrophizing and pain intensity and disability in a children's pain clinic, Hechler et al. (2011) found that maternal, not paternal, catastrophizing was related to child pain intensity. Surprisingly, in this study, child disability was not significantly related to maternal or paternal catastrophizing. In another recent study, parental catastrophizing and child pain intensity were associated with the perceived threat inherent in the child's pain and the parent's need to control the child's pain, with the relationship stronger for mothers than fathers (Caes et al., 2012). Mothers have reported more use of non-pharmacological methods than fathers to manage pain in their children (Gorodzinsky et al. 2011). Future studies in this domain will be important in determining the complex relationship between familial socialization processes and gender differences in child and adolescent pain.

Sociocultural factors

Research indicates that social roles support or permit pain expression for women but discourage it for men. Robinson and colleagues (2001) found that men and women expected men to have a higher level of pain endurance and a lower level of pain sensitivity than women. Pool et al. (2007) also reported that men and women believed that the ideal man should tolerate more pain than the ideal woman. Results from cross-cultural research indicate that such gender-role expectations are not unique to North American samples (e.g. Nayak et al., 2000; see also Clemente, Chapter 11, this volume).

Gender-role expectations for pain expression in children and adolescents have not been studied in detail. Still, a number of studies suggest that children, like adults, may behave according to gender-role expectations that encourage girls and discourage boys from expressing pain. In a widely cited early paper, Mechanic (1964) found that boys were significantly more likely to report that they were not afraid of getting hurt and that they did not pay attention to pain. Zeman and Garber (1996) found that girls reported they would be significantly more likely than boys to express pain in response to common pains. Girls were also more likely than boys to report that other people would understand and accept their expressions of pain. These findings were echoed in a qualitative study of Canadian adolescents (Hatchette et al., 2008). Girls reported feeling free to discuss their pain with peers whereas boys reported being reluctant to express their pain to peers.

Gender-stereotyped beliefs about pain help explain findings that girls (Keogh and Eccleston, 2006; Lynch et al., 2007) and women (Unruh et al., 1999) are more likely to seek social support when they experience pain and that women show increased health care utilization for pain compared to men (e.g. Chang et al., 2006; Gibbs et al., 2003). Robinson and colleagues (2001) suggested that there may be a greater response cost involved when men report their pain because men are expected to be stoic in response to pain. Acting in a way that is incongruent with this expectation may cause men anxiety and embarrassment. It is possible that the pattern of observed adult sex differences in experimental but not clinical pain settings may be because the relatively mild experimental pain makes it easier for men to conform to male gender-role expectations (Myers et al., 2003). Clinical pain that is intense enough for men to seek medical treatment may override the desire to conform to the stereotypical male gender role.

There has been substantial criticism that pain in women is more likely to be interpreted as a psychological problem (e.g. Hoffmann and Tarzian, 2001; Unruh, 1996) but this issue has not been examined in studies of child or adolescent pain. The greater willingness of girls to express their pain to others may increase this risk.

Clinical implications of sex and gender

The ways in which sex and gender may be manifested in children and adolescents in a pain clinic are illustrated in the following three case scenarios. The cases have been modified but reflect issues that have been clinically presented.

Case example: Matthew

Matthew was 17 when he came to the pain clinic with his mother. He seemed to be coping well with his pain and was generally disinterested in treatment. His mother was more concerned about his pain than he was. Nevertheless, when he was later seen by the school guidance counsellor for behaviour problems at school, it was apparent that Matthew was extremely distressed by his severe pain and did not know what to do with his anger and frustration about it.

Case example: Sonia

At 15, Sonia was seen by an orthopaedic surgeon for widespread pain that had originated 1 year earlier with back pain. As the imaging results were all negative, the surgeon told Sonia's parents that there was nothing wrong with Sonia. He told Sonia that if she found a nice boyfriend she would get better. By the time Sonia was seen at the pain clinic she had missed 8 months of school due to severe pain. As non-steroidal anti-inflammatory drugs (NSAIDs) had been ineffective in the past, and her sleep was poor, Sonia was started on gabapentin and amitriptyline. The psychologist saw her for pain-specific cognitive-behavioural therapy. A very slow pacing programme was initiated. Over the

next 4 years, Sonia progressed from no attendance at school to full attendance. By 5 years, she was pain-free and off pain medications. Sonia had many friends but in fact no boyfriend during these 5 years.

Case example: Maggie

Maggie was 14 and had a long history of abdominal pain, but not menstrual cramps or menstrual pain. She was referred to the pain clinic from gastroenterology. Maggie was started on gabapentin and amitriptyline following an unsuccessful trial of NSAIDs. At a follow-up assessment, it was observed that Maggie's abdominal pain increased about the time of her menses. When NSAIDs were added to her regimen for the several days before its onset, her ongoing abdominal pain and its flare at menses improved.

These cases illustrate the way in which sex and gender may interact with pain in the clinical setting. Mathew hid his pain and his emotional reaction to it under a stoic demeanour. Clinicians initially interpreted his reticence to engage clinically as disinterest in treatment. Sonia's pain was interpreted as a social and probably psychological problem when there was no physical finding to point to a cause. Maggie's abdominal pain was due to other issues than menstruation, but her menstrual cycle produced flares that changed treatment needs. For clinicians, it is important to consider that gender role expectations may shape the way in which a child or adolescent will communicate about their pain, as well as their own perceptions of this communication. Similarly, biological factors may intersect with gender and affect pain in clinical settings, particularly after puberty.

Recommendations for future research

Sex and gender differences are not usually the focus of pain research. Instead, sex is typically included as a demographic variable that may or may not be examined and reported. As noted by Unruh (1996), the results of studies that do not identify sex as a variable of primary interest a priori must be interpreted with caution because the power of these studies to detect sex differences is unclear. Pain researchers need to look beyond descriptive sex differences to examine how the psychosocial variable of gender affects child and adult pain responses. To date, only a handful of studies have examined gender differences in child and adult pain. This area is in great need of expansion. Fathers need to be included in research on sex and gender differences in child pain. With the exception of a few studies, fathers tend to be overlooked. In fact, 91% of child health psychology studies (including child pain), published from 1996 to 2003, involved only mothers or collapsed data from both parents (Phares et al., 2005). Particularly in research about sex and gender, the impact of parent gender on socialization cannot be ignored without compromising the meaningfulness of outcomes.

Conclusion

Although the study of sex differences in child pain is not as advanced as the adult pain literature, evidence for sex differences in child and adolescent pain has accumulated in the past decade. Studies of sex differences in children's responses to experimentally induced pain have largely focused on the cold pressor pain paradigm and have generally not uncovered sex differences. In contrast, epidemiological data indicate that girls are at an increased risk of a number of chronic pain conditions. Findings from child clinical pain studies are inconsistent, but generally suggest that boys and girls give comparable pain ratings. Findings from recent studies of needle pain are mixed but indicate that girls may give higher pain affect ratings. Postoperative pain findings are equivocal, with some studies indicating greater pain intensity in girls and others reporting no sex differences. Findings on sex differences in child pain coping strategies are remarkably similar to findings with adults. Girls appear to seek more social support for pain whereas boys are more likely to engage in distraction. Similar to the adult literature, some data also suggest that girls may be more likely than boys to catastrophize in response to pain. Although gender influences adult pain responses, the study of gender differences in child pain has not been extensive. Researchers have only just begun to delineate the impact of biological, family, and sociocultural factors on sex and gender differences in pain. Inconsistent findings highlight the need for further expansion of this field.

Acknowledgements

The authors acknowledge the assistance of Dr Paula Forgeron, University of Ottawa, in the preparation of the case examples.

References

Berkley, K. J. (1997). Sex differences in pain. *Behav Brain Sci,* 20, 371–380

Blankenburg, M., Boekens, H., Hechler, T., Maier, C., Krumova, E., Scherens, A., *et al.* (2010). Reference values for quantitative sensory testing in children and adolescents: developmental and gender differences of somatosensory perception. *Pain,* 149, 76–88.

Boldizar, J.P. (1991). Assessing sex typing and androgeny in children: the Children's Sex Role Inventory. *Dev Psychol,* 27, 505–515.

Brennan, T. J., Vendermeulen, E. P., and Gebhart, G. F. (1996). Characterization of a rat model of incisional pain. *Pain,* 64, 493–501.

Brun Sundblad, G. M., Saartok, T., and Engstrom, L.-M. T. (2007). Prevalence and co-occurence of self-rated pain and perceived health in school-children: age and gender differences. *Eur J Pain,* 11, 171–180.

Bush, F. M., Harkins, S. W., Harrington, W. G., and Price, D. D. (1993). Analysis of gender effects on pain perception and symptom presentation in temporomandibular pain. *Pain,* 53, 73–80.

Caes, L., Veroort, T., Eccleston, C., and Goubert, L. (2012). Parents who catastrophize about their child's pain prioritize attempts to control pain. *Pain,* 153, 1695–1701.

Caprilli, S., Anastasi, F., Grotto, R. P. L., Abeti, M. S., and Messeri, A. (2007). Interactive music as a treatment for pain and stress in children during venipuncture: a randomized prospective study. *J Dev Behav Pediatr,* 28, 399–403.

Chambers, C. T. (2003). The role of family factors in pediatric pain. In P. J. McGrath and G. A. Finley (eds) *Pediatric pain: biological and social context,* pp. 99–130. Seattle, WA: IASP Press.

Chambers, C. T., Craig, K. D., and Bennett, S. M. (2002). The impact of maternal behavior on children's pain experiences: an experimental analysis. *J Pediatr Psychol,* 27, 293–301.

Chambers, C. T., Giesbrecht, K., Craig, K. D., Bennett, S. M., and Huntsman, E. (1999). A comparison of faces scales for the measurement of pediatric pain: children's and parents' ratings. *Pain,* 83, 25–35.

Chambers, C. T., Hardial, J., Craig, K. D., Court, C., and Montgomery, C. (2005). Faces scales for the measurement of postoperative pain intensity in children following minor surgery. *Clin J Pain,* 21, 277–285.

Chang, L., Toner, B. B., Fukudo, S., Guthrie, E., Locke, G. R., Norton, N. J., *et al.* (2006). Gender, age, society, culture, and the patient's perspective in the functional gastrointestinal disorders. *Gastroenterology,* 130, 1435–1446.

Cohen, L. L., Blount, R. L., Cohen, R. J., and Johnson, V. C. (2004). Dimensions of pediatric procedural distress: children's anxiety and pain during immunizations. *J Clin Psychol Med S,* 11, 41–47.

Cohen, L. L., Manimala, R., and Blount, R. L. (2000). Easier said than done: what parents say they do and what they do during children's immunizations. *Child Health Care,* 29, 79–86.

Coldwell, S. E., Kaakko, T., Gartner-Makihara, A. B., Williams, T., Milgrom, P., Weinstein, P., *et al.* (2002). Temporal information reduces children's pain reports during a multiple-trial cold pressor procedure. *Behav Ther,* 33, 45–63.

Derbyshire, S. W., Nichols, T. E., Firestone, L., Townsend, D. W., and Jones, A. K. (2002). Gender differences in patterns of cerebral activation during equal experience of painful laser stimulation. *J Pain,* 3, 401–411.

Edwards, R. R., Haythornthwaite, J. A., Sullivan, M. J., and Fillingim, R. B. (2004). Catastrophizing as a mediator of sex differences in pain: differential effects for daily pain versus laboratory-induced pain. *Pain,* 111, 335–341.

Evans, S., Tsao, J. C. I., and Zeltzer, L. K. (2008). Relationship of child perceptions of maternal pain to children's laboratory and nonlaboratory pain. *Pain Res Manag,* 13, 211–218.

Fillingim, R. B. and Edwards, R. R. (2001). The association of hormone replacement therapy with experimental pain responses in postemenopausal women. *Pain,* 92, 229–234.

Fillingim, R. B., King, C. D., Ribeiro-Dasilva, M. C., Rahim-Williams, B., and Riley, J. L. (2009). Sex, gender, and pain: A review of recent clinical and experimental findings. *J Pain,* 10, 447–485.

Fordyce, W. (1976). *Behavioral methods for chronic pain and illness.* St. Louis, MO: Mosby.

Gibbs, T. S., Fleischer, A. B., Jr., Feldman, S. R., Sam, M. C., and O'Donovan, M. D. (2003). Health care utilization in patients with migraine: demographics and patterns of care in the ambulatory setting. *Headache,* 43, 330–335.

Gillies, M. L., Smith, L. N., and Parry-Jones, W. L. (1999). Postoperative pain assessment and management in adolescents. *Pain,* 79, 207–215.

Goodenough, B., Thomas, W., Champion, G. D., Perrott, D., Taplin, J. E., von Baeyer, C. L., *et al.* (1999b). Unravelling age effects and sex differences in needle pain: Ratings of sensory intensity and unpleasantness of venipuncture pain by children and their parents. *Pain,* 80, 179–190.

Goodenough, B., van Dongen, K., Brouwer, N., Abu-Saad, H. H., and Champion, G. D. (1999a). A comparison of the Faces Pain Scale and the Facial Affective Scale for children's estimates of the intensity and unpleasantness of needle pain during blood sampling. *Eur J Pain,* 3, 301–315.

Goodman, J. E. and McGrath, P. J. (2003). Mothers' modeling influences children's pain ratings during a cold pressor task. *Pain,* 104, 559–565.

Hatchette, J. E., McGrath, P. J., Murray, M., and Finley, G. A. (2008). The role of peer communication in the socialization of adolescents' pain experiences: a qualitative investigation. *BMC Pediatr,* 8. doi:10.1186/1471-2431-8-2. Available at: <http://www.biomedcentral.com/1471-2431/8/2>.

Hechler, T., Chalkiadis, G. A., Hasan, C., Kosfelder, J., Meyerhoff, U., Vocks, S., *et al.* (2009). Sex differences in pain intensity in adolescents suffering from cancer: differences in pain memories? *J Pain,* 10, 586–593.

Hechler, T., Vervoort, T., Hamann, M., Tietze, A. L., Vocks, S., Goubert, L., *et al.* (2011). Parental catastrophizing about their child's chronic pain: are mothers and fathers different? *Eur J Pain,* 15, 515.e1–515.e9

Hoffmann, D. E. and Tarzian, A. J. (2001). The girl who cried pain: a bias against women in the treatment of pain. *J Law Med Ethics,* 29, 13–27.

Huguet, A. and Miró, J. (2008). The severity of chronic pediatric pain: an epidemiological study. *J Pain,* 9, 226–236.

Hurley, R. W. and Adams, M. C. B. (2008). Sex, gender and pain: an overview of a complex field. *Anesth Analg,* 107, 309–317.

Jaaniste, T., Hayes, B., and von Baeyer, C. L. (2007). Effects of preparatory information and distraction on children's cold-pressor pain outcomes: a randomized controlled trial. *Behav Res Ther*, 45, 2789–2799.

Jensen, I., Nygren, A., Gamberale, F., Goldie, I., and Westerholm, P. (1994). Coping with long-term musculoskeletal pain and its consequences: is gender a factor? *Pain*, 57, 167–172.

Johnston, C. C., Campbell-Yeo, M., and Filion, F. (2011). Paternal vs. maternal kangaroo care for procedural pain in preterm neonates: a randomized crossover trial. *Arch Pediatr Adolesc Med*, 165, 792–796.

Kaczynski, K. J., Claar, R. L., and Logan, D. E. (2009). Testing gender as a moderator of associations between psychosocial variables and functional disability in children and adolescents with chronic pain. *J Pediatr Psychol*, 34, 738–748.

Kankkunen, P. M., Vehvilainen-Julkunen, K. M., Pietila, A. K., and Halonen, P. M. (2003). Parents' perceptions of their 1–6-year-old children's pain. *Eur J Pain*, 7, 203–211.

Keefe, F. J., Lefebvre, J. C., Egert, J. R., Affleck, G., Sullivan, M. J., and Caldwell, D. S. (2000). The relationship of gender to pain, pain behavior, and disability in osteoarthritis patients: The role of catastrophizing. *Pain*, 87, 325–334.

Keogh, E. and Eccleston, C. (2006). Sex differences in adolescent chronic pain and pain-related coping. *Pain*, 123, 275–284.

Kleiber, C., Schutte, D. L., McCarthy, A., Floria-Santos, M., Murray, J. C., and Hanrahan, K. (2007). Predictors of topical anesthetic effectiveness in children. *J Pain*, 8, 168–174.

Kotzer, A. M. (2000). Factors predicting postoperative pain in children and adolescents following spine fusion. *Issues Compr Pediatr Nurs*, 23, 83–102.

Kristjansdottir, G. (1996). Sociodemographic differences in the prevalence of self-reported stomach pain in school children. *Eur J Pediatr*, 155, 981–983.

Kroner-Herwig, B., Heinrich, M., and Morris, L. (2007). Headache in German children and adolescents: a population-based epidemiological study. *Cephalalgia*, 27, 519–527.

Lander, J., Fowler-Kerry, S., and Hill, A. (1990). Comparison of pain perceptions among males and females. *Can J Nurs Res*, 22, 39–49.

Larochette, A., Chambers, C. T., and Craig, K. D. (2006). Genuine, suppressed and faked facial expressions of pain in children. *Pain*, 126, 64–71.

Lash, S. J., Eisler, R. M., and Schulman, R. S. (1990). Cardiovascular reactivity to stress in men. *Behav Modif*, 14, 3–20.

LeResche, L. (1997). Epidemiology of temporomandibular disorder: Implications for the investigation of etiologic factors. *Crit Rev Oral Biol Med*, 8, 291–305.

Lu, Q., Zeltzer, L.K., Tsao, J.C.I., Kim, S.C., Turk, N. and Naliboff, B. D. (2005). Heart rate mediation of sex differences in pain tolerance in children. *Pain*, 118, 185–193.

Lu, Q., Tsao, J.C.I., Myers, C.D., Kim, S.C., and Zeltzer, L. K. (2007). Coping predictors of children's laboratory-induced pain tolerance, intensity, and unpleasantness. *J Pain*, 8, 708–717.

Lynch, A. M., Kashikar-Zuck, S., Goldschneider, K. R., and Jones, B. A. (2007). Sex and age differences in coping styles among children with chronic pain. *J Pain Symptom Manag*, 33, 208–216.

Martin, A. L., McGrath, P. A., Brown, S. C., and Katz, J. (2007). Children with chronic pain: Impact of sex and age on long-term outcomes. *Pain*, 128, 13–19.

Mechanic, D. (1964). The influence of mothers on their children's health attitudes and behavior. *Pediatrics*, 33, 444–453.

Meier, P. M., Berde, C. B., DiCanzio, J., Zurakowski, D., and Sethna, N. F. (2001). Quantitative assessment of cutaneous thermal and vibration sensation and thermal paindetection thresholds in healthy children and adolescents. *Muscle Nerve*, 24, 1339–1345.

Mikkelsson, M., Salminen, J. J., and Kautiainen, H. (1997). Non-specific musculoskeletal pain in preadolescents. Prevalence and 1-year persistence. *Pain*, 73, 29–35.

Moon, E. C. (2010). Parent and child behavior during child pain: the effects of sex and gender. Unpublished doctoral dissertation, Dalhousie University, Halifax, NS.

Moon, E. C., Chambers, C. T., Larochette, A.-C., Hayton, K., Craig, K. D., and McGrath, P. J. (2008). Sex differences in parent and child pain ratings during an experimental child pain task. *Pain Res Manag*, 13, 225–230.

Moon, E. C., Chambers, C. T., and McGrath, P. J. (2011). 'He says, she says': a comparison of fathers' and mothers' verbal behavior during child cold pressor pain. *J Pain*, 12, 1174–1181.

Moulton, E. A., Keaser, M. L., Gullapalli, R. P., Maitra, R., and Greenspan, J. D. (2006). Sex differences in cerebral BOLD signal response to painful heat stimuli. *Am J Physiol Regul Integr Comp Physiol*, 291, R257–267.

Myers, C. D., Riley, J. L., and Robinson, M. E. (2003). Psychosocial contributions to sex-correlated differences in pain. *Clin J Pain*, 19, 225–232.

Myers, C. D., Robinson, M. E., Riley, J. L., and Sheffield, D. (2001). Sex, gender and blood pressure: Contributions to experimental pain report. *Psychosomat Med*, 63, 545–550.

Myers, C. D., Tsao, J. C. I., Glover, D. A., Kim, S. C., Turk, N., and Zeltzer, L. K. (2006). Sex, gender, and age: contributions to laboratory pain responding in children and adolescents. *J Pain*, 7, 556–564.

Nayak, S., Shiflett, S. C., Eshun, S., and Levine, F. M. (2000). Culture and gender effects in pain beliefs and the prediction of pain tolerance. *Cross-Cult Res*, 34, 135–151.

Oh, M. C., Aw, M. M., Chan, Y. H., Tan, L. Z., and Quak, S. H. (2004). Epidemiology of recurrent abdominal pain among Singaporean adolescents. *Ann Acad Med, Singapore*, 33, S10–11.

Otto, M. W. and Dougher, M. J. (1985). Sex differences and personality factors in responsivity to pain. *Percept Mot Skills*, 61, 383–390.

Owen Blakemore, J. E., Berenbaum, S. A., and Liben, L. S. (2009). *Gender development*. New York: Psychology Press.

Paulson, P. E., Minoshima, S., Morrow, T. J., and Casey, K. L. (1998). Gender differences in pain perception and patterns of cerebral activation during noxious heat stimulation in humans. *Pain*, 76, 223–229.

Piira, T., Taplin, J. E., Goodenough, B., and von Baeyer, C. L. (2002). Cognitive-behavioural predictors of children's tolerance of laboratory-induced pain: Implications for clinical assessment and future directions. *Behav Res Ther*, 40, 571–584.

Piira, T., Hayes, B., Goodenough, B., and von Baeyer, C. L. (2006). Effects of attentional direction, age, and coping style on cold-pressor pain in children. *Behav Res Ther*, 44, 835–848.

Piira, T., Sugiura, T., Champion, G. D., Donnelly, N., and Cole, A. S. J. (2005). The role of parental presence in the context of children's medical procedures: a systematic review. *Child Care, Health Dev*, 31, 233–242.

Pepino, M. Y. and Mennella, J. A. (2005). Sucrose-induced analgesia is related to sweet preferences in children but not adults. *Pain*, 119, 210–218.

Phares, V., Lopez, E., Fields, S., Kamboukos, D., and Duhig, A. M. (2005). Are fathers involved in pediatric psychology research and treatment? *J Pediatr Psychol*, 30, 631–643.

Pool, G. J., Schwegler, A. F., Theodore, B. R., and Fuchs, P. N. (2007). Role of gender norms and group identification on hypothetical and experimental pain tolerance. *Pain*, 129, 122–129.

Ramchandani, P. G., Hotopf, M., Sandhu, B., Stein, A., and the Avon Longitudinal Study of Parents and Children Study Team (2005). The epidemiology of recurrent abdominal pain from 2 to 6 years of age: results of a large, population-based study. *Pediatrics*, 116, 46–50.

Reid, G. J., Gilbert, C. A., and McGrath, P. J. (1998). The Pain Coping Questionnaire: preliminary validation. *Pain*, 76, 83–96.

Riley, J. L., Robinson, M. E., Wise, E. A., Myers, C. D., and Fillingim, R. B. (1998). Sex differences in the perception of noxious experimental stimuli: A meta-analysis. *Pain*, 74, 181–187.

Riley, J. L., Robinson, M. E., Wise, E. A., and Price, D. D. (1999). A meta-analytic review of pain perception across the menstrual cycle. *Pain*, 81, 225–235.

Ring, C., Veldhuijzen van Zanten, J. J. C. S., and Kavussanu, M. (2009). Effects of sex, phase of the menstrual cycle and gonadal hormones on pain in healthy humans. *Biol Psychol*, 81, 189–191.

Robinson, M. E., Riley, J. L., Myers, C. D., Papas, R. K., Wise, E. A., Waxenberg, L. B., et al. (2001). Gender role expectations of pain: relationship to sex differences in pain. *J Pain*, 2, 251–257.

Robinson, M. E., Wise, E. A., Riley, J. L., and Atchison, J. W. (1998). Sex differences in clinical pain: a multisample study. *J Clin Psychol Med S*, 5, 413–423.

Rolke, R., Baron, R., Maier, C., Tölle, T. R., Treede, R. D., Beyer, A., et al. (2006). Quantitative sensory testing in the German Research Network on Neuropathic Pain (DFNS): standardized protocol and reference values. *Pain*, 123, 231–243.

Schechter, N. L., Bernstein, B. A., Beck, A., Hart, L., and Scherzer, L. (1991). Individual differences in children's response to pain: role of temperament and parental characteristics. *Pediatrics*, 87, 171–177.

Siegal, M. (1987). Are sons and daughters treated more differently by fathers than by mothers? *Dev Rev*, 7, 193–209.

Sparks, L. (2001). Taking the 'ouch' out of injections for children: using distraction to decrease pain. *MCN, Am J Matern Child Nurs*, 26, 72–78.

Stanford, E. A., Chambers, C. T., Biesanz, J. C., and Chen, E. (2008). The frequency, trajectories, and predictors of adolescent recurrent pain: a population-based approach. *Pain*, 138, 11–21.

Stewart, W. F., Linet, M. S., Celentano, D. D., Van Natta, M., and Ziegler, D. (1991). Age-and-sex-specific incidence rates of migraine with and without visual aura. *Am J Epidemiol*, 134, 1111–1120.

Stewart, W. F., Lipton, R. B., Celentano, D. D., and Reed, M. L. (1992). Prevalence of migraine headache in the United States: relation to age, income, race, and other sociodemographic factors. *JAMA*, 267, 64–69.

Thorn, B. E., Clements, K. L., Ward, L. C., Dixon, K. E., Kersh, B. C., Boothby, J. L., and Chaplin, W. F. (2004). Personality factors in the explanation of sex differences in pain catastrophizing and response to experimental pain. *Clin J Pain*, 20, 275–282.

Trapanotto, M., Pozziani, G., Perissinotto, E., Barbieri, S., Zacchello, F., and Benini, F. (2009). The cold pressor test for the pediatric population: refinement of procedures, development of norms, and study of psychological variables. *J Pediatr Psychol*, 34, 749–759.

Tsang, A., Von Korff, M., Lee, S., Alonso, J., Karam, E., Angermeyer, M. C., et al. (2008). Common chronic pain conditions in developed and developing countries: Gender and age differences and comorbidity with depression-anxiety disorders. *J Pain*, 9, 883–891.

Tsao, J. C. I., Lu, Q., Kim, S. C., and Zeltzer, L. K. (2006a). Relationships among anxious symptomatology, anxiety sensitivity and laboratory pain responsivity in children. *Cognitive Behavior Ther*, 35, 207–215.

Tsao, J. C. I., Lu, Q., Myers, C. D., Kim, S. C., Turk, N., and Zeltzer, L. K. (2006b). Parent and child anxiety sensitivity: relationship to children's experimental pain responsivity. *J Pain*, 7, 319–326.

Tsao, J. C. I., Myers, C. D., Craske, M. C., Bursch, B., Kim, S. C., and Zeltzer, L. K. (2004). Role of anticipatory anxiety and anxiety sensitivity in children's and adolescents' laboratory pain responses. *J Pediatr Psychol*, 29, 379–388.

Unruh, A. M. (1996). Gender variations in clinical pain experience. *Pain*, 65, 123–167.

Unruh, A. M. (1997). Why can't a woman be more like a man? *Behav Brain Sci*, 20, 467–468.

Unruh, A. M. and Campbell, M. (1999). Gender variation in children's pain experiences. In P. J. McGrath and G. A. Finley (eds) *Chronic and recurrent pain in children and adolescents*, pp. 199–241. Seattle, WA: IASP Press.

Unruh, A. M., Ritchie, J., and Merskey, H. (1999). Does gender affect appraisal of pain and pain coping strategies? *Clinical J Pain*, 15, 31–40.

von Baeyer, C. L., Spagrud, L. J., McCormick, J. C., Choo, E., Neville, K., and Connelly, M. A. (2009). Three new datasets supporting use of the Numerical Rating Scale (NRS) for children's self-reports of pain intensity. *Pain*, 143, 223–227.

Walker, L. S., Garber, J., and Van Slyke, D. A. (1995). Do parents excuse the misbehavior of children with physical or emotional symptoms? An investigation of the pediatric sick role. *J Pediatr Psychol*, 20, 329–345.

Walker, L. S., Williams, S. E., Smith, C. A., Garber, J., Van Slyke, D. A., and Lipani, T. A. (2006). Parent attention versus distraction: impact on symptom complaints by children with and without chronic functional abdominal pain. *Pain*, 122, 43–52.

Walker S.M., Franck L.S., Fitzgerald M., Myles J., Stocks J., and Marlow N. (2009). Long-term impact of neonatal intensive care and surgery on somatosensory perception in children born extremely preterm. *Pain*, 141, 79–87.

Wilson, R. and Cairns, E. (1988). Sex-role attributes, perceived competence, and the development of depression in adolescence. *J Child Psychol Psychiatry*, 29, 635–650.

Wilson, L., Dworkin, S. F., Whitney, C., and LeResche, L. (1994). Somatization and pain dispersion in chronic temporomandibular disorder pain. *Pain*, 57, 55–61.

World Health Organization. (n.d.). What do we mean by 'sex' and 'gender'? Available at: <http://www.who.int/gender/whatisgender/en/index.html>.

Zeman, J. and Garber, J. (1996). Display rules for anger, sadness, and pain: it depends on who is watching. *Child Dev*, 67, 957–973.

Zeman, J. and Shipman, K. (1996). Children's expression of negative affect: reasons and methods. *Dev Psychol*, 32, 842–849.

CHAPTER 15

Sleep and pain in children and adolescents

Bruce D. Dick, Penny Corkum, Manisha Witmans , and Christine T. Chambers

Summary

Ongoing pain is a problem that affects a large number of children and adolescents. It has been well documented that recurrent and chronic pain are associated with many difficulties related to both physical and psychological function. A major difficulty that many young people with chronic or recurrent pain experience is disrupted sleep. Sleep problems have been reported to exist in as many as 50% or more of children with chronic illnesses (Owens, 2007). In many cases, pain is reported by the sufferers to cause sleep fragmentation as well as significant difficulties with delayed sleep onset. As well, there is increasing evidence that disrupted sleep is associated with increased pain. Both pain and sleep disruption further complicate the patient's overall clinical picture by making it more difficult for children and teens to cope with health problems and associated difficulties. Further, there is evidence that childhood sleep problems can have important negative effects on adult sleep patterns and, thereby, influence health status later in life (Fricke-Oerkermann et al., 2007; Sivertsen et al., 2009). This chapter will address the prevalence, importance, and consequences of sleep problems in children and adolescents with pain. First, the prevalence and possible relationship between pain and sleep will be discussed. Next, we will highlight the assessment of sleep with a specific focus on assessment of sleep in paediatric pain populations. We will then review established and emerging medical and psychological treatment strategies used to effectively treat these important difficulties. Practical suggestions will also be provided as a general and basic guide for treatment of children and teens with pain and sleep problems.

Pain in children

For most children and adolescents, pain is a noxious experience that interrupts and negatively affects many aspects of function. As pain exists across a spectrum from acute and episodic to persistent and chronic, the disruptive effects of pain also range across a continuum from mild to disabling. Acute pain often plays an important protective role in alerting the sufferer to injury or illness and can therefore have a very disruptive effect on function, generally on a relatively short-term basis. Recurrent or persistent pain can have a useful function but often results in prolonged and more significant impairment. Chronic pain can become highly disruptive of function but generally tends not to have a useful or adaptive function, sometimes resulting in a complex web of negative outcomes that can have widespread effects on a young person's life.

Clinically, when pain becomes disruptive of function, it is frequently reported by child and adolescent sufferers to result in a range of negative outcomes. These negative effects include impairment of physical function and activity levels, decreased school attendance and academic performance, cognitive interruption, mood problems, particularly anxiety and depression, decreased social activity including negative effects on friendships, and poorer quality of life (Dick and Pillai Riddell, 2010; Forgeron et al. 2011). The nature and severity of the effects of these problems can interact with each other and can be associated with several negative vicious cycles.

Amidst all of these difficulties, sleep is a primary factor reported to be negatively affected by pain. In clinical settings, sleep is commonly reported to be one of the major complications caused by pain and a primary source of difficulty associated with mood problems, school attendance and performance, cognitive function, and quality of life (Owens, 2005). It is not uncommon for one or more of the major negative clinical features associated with pain to improve markedly when treatment results in improved sleep.

Sleep and pain

Sleep is of critical importance to the developing child. It has been found to be associated with physical health, growth, and function, development, learning, and cognitive function, several aspects of behaviour, mood, emotional regulation, and psychological health, coping, and family function (Durmer and Dinges, 2005; Forest and Godbout, 2000; Meltzer and Mindell, 2009 Mindell and Owens, 2003; Owens, 2005). Sleep problems are also associated with other health problems including cardiovascular disease, diabetes, obesity both in children and in adults (Cappuccio et al., 2008; Foley et al. 2004), and stress and other negative effects on parents of these children (Martin et al., 2007).

Table 15.1 Sleep-related symptoms in the context of pain in children (but not pain specific)

Daytime symptoms	Irritability, hyperactivity, daytime sleepiness, fatigue, increased pain, behavioural problems, anxiety, lower frustration tolerance
Bedtime symptoms	Delayed sleep onset, irritability, bedtime battles, anxiety, hyperactivity, increased pain
Sleep symptoms	Wakefulness after sleep onset, lower sleep efficiency, fragmented sleep (microarousals), nightmares, worse parasomnias resulting from sleep fragmentation, night-time arousals, irritability, sudden awakenings, inconsolability.

While sleep problems in children and teens in the general population are common, it has been recognized that children and adolescents with pain may be at particular risk for sleep problems (Owens, 2011). For example, adolescents with inflammatory bowel disease reported poorer quality sleep with increased disease severity. The parents of those adolescents also reported that their children experienced more nightmares and other sleep difficulties and that disease severity was associated with higher levels of daytime fatigue and an increase in the amount of time that their children spent sleeping during the day (Pirinen et al. 2010). In another study, Lewandowski and colleagues (2010) found that pain ratings were predicted by longer sleep duration and longer sleep onset delay. Given that pain can have such a dramatic effect on sleep quality, duration, and fragmentation, understanding the interaction between pain and sleep and how to effectively co-assess and treat these difficulties can have broader positive implications on child health and well-being in a variety of ways. It is remarkable how many common negative outcomes are uniquely associated with pain and/or sleep. Each problem can have a dramatic impact on function, mood, and cognition (Palermo, 2009; Sadeh, 2007). When pain and sleep problems coexist, the nature and extent of problems arising from the association can appear to be more complex and dynamic rather than simply additive. Chronic pain may also affect the child's sleep patterns over time and result in behavioural manifestations such as daytime irritability, moodiness, hyperactivity, and sleepiness. Unresolved sleep issues may make pain more difficult to manage. Table 15.1 provides common examples of behavioural manifestations in children struggling with sleep problems and pain.

Prevalence and impact of sleep problems

In recent years there has been tremendous advances in the study of the relationship between pain and sleep problems in children. Two prior reviews (Gagliese and Chambers, 2007; Lewin and Dahl, 1999) have highlighted the importance of sleep in the assessment and management of paediatric pain, and have summarized the prevalence of sleep problems among children with various painful conditions, such as headache, recurrent abdominal pain, sickle cell disease, musculoskeletal pain, and arthritis. There is a clear consensus that children with chronic pain are more likely to experience a variety of sleep difficulties than their healthy peers (Gagliese and Chambers, 2007). Estimates indicate that approximately 50% of children with chronic pain experience a significant sleep disturbance (Long et al., 2008; Palermo et al., 2007, 2011), in contrast to 10% to 20% in healthy peers. Sleep difficulties are also commonly experienced as a result of pain among children with intellectual and developmental disabilities (Breau and Camfield, 2011). Across studies and pain types, difficulties falling asleep (i.e. insomnia), night wakings, and daytime fatigue are the most common sleep disturbances in children with chronic pain (Gagliese and Chambers,

2007). Some conditions can be associated such as sleep disordered breathing has been reported to have a higher prevalence in children with sickle cell disease (Brooks et al., 1996; Fuggle et al., 1996). Not only are sleep problems more common in children with chronic pain, but the severity of sleep disturbances is generally related to pain intensity; children with more severe pain are likely to report a greater degree of sleep problems (Bloom et al., 2002; Miller et al., 2003).

Data evaluating the association between pain and sleep in children are emerging, most using self-report and subjective assessment tools. A small group of adolescent females with chronic musculoskeletal pain were found to have similar total sleep time compared to norms but significantly longer sleep onset latency, more night wakings, a later morning wake time, and more symptoms of daytime sleepiness using validated questionnaires (Meltzer et al., 2005). Some of these teens reported improvement in pain after a sleep period. Conversely, a study of children with polyarticular arthritis tracked pain severity and sleep quality over a period of 2 months and found that poorer sleep quality was associated with higher next-day ratings of pain (Butbul Aviel et al., 2011). These findings associating disturbed sleep and fatigue, with increased pain have been also found in other rheumatological conditions (Butbul Aviel et al., 2011) and result in lower quality of life (Gold et al., 2009; Long et al., 2008). There is currently adequate evidence to suggest that any programme involving treatment of pain should also address sleep parameters of the affected individuals.

A series of papers (Long et al., 2008; Tsai et al., 2008; Palermo and Owens, 2008; Valrie et al., 2008; Ward et al., 2008) published in a special issue of the *Journal of Pediatric Psychology* (2008, Volume 33, Issue 3) dedicated to sleep in children with medical conditions, have extended our current understanding of the importance of sleep in paediatric chronic pain. The results of these studies have confirmed that sleep problems are common in children with chronic pain, and highlight the importance of factors such as mood, stress, and daytime napping in helping to understand the relationship between pain and sleep in children with chronic pain. For example, Valrie and colleagues (2008) showed that, among children with sickle cell disease, a day with high pain was related to poor sleep quality that night, which was then related to higher pain the following day. The relationship between pain and sleep has been shown to be further exacerbated by high levels of stress (Valrie et al., 2007). Tsai and colleagues (2008) examined the important role of naps in children with chronic pain, finding that children with chronic pain were likely to engage in daytime naps to compensate for lost night time sleep, which may have a negative effect on night-time sleep.

Of concern, sleep problems in children and teens with chronic pain are associated with lower quality of life and a greater degree of functional disability (Chambers et al., 2008; Long et al., 2008; Palermo et al., 2007, 2008). Recent work examining behavioural and psychosocial factors associated with insomnia in adolescents with chronic pain has highlighted that, while sleep disruption may initially be a result of pain, sleep difficulties may evolve into a primary sleep disorder.

Relationships between sleep and pain

The interaction between pain, sleep, physical function, and emotional regulation is complex. Although the mechanisms of the interactions and pathogenesis of pain and sleep are poorly understood, it is probable that pain, sleep and emotion share common neurobiological pathways and neuronal mechanisms. The neurobiology of the specific pain condition based on its associated symptoms may have widespread effects that may be linked to sleep related cellular activity and neurotransmitter processing areas of the hypothalamus, amygdala, limbic region, and frontal cortical areas.

Recent studies involving neuroimaging and neurophysiology are shedding light on the altered functional and structural changes in chronic pain. For example, in fibromyalgia, the pain is thought to be neurogenic in origin and results from neurochemical imbalances that lead to amplification of pain perception and abnormal signal processing (Henry et al., 2011). This may be associated with changes in cellular activation or cortical sensory integration.

It has been suggested that other chronic pain syndromes also have similar dysfunction in pain processing within the brain, although the exact mechanisms have not been elucidated. Sleep deprivation or sleep fragmentation may further exacerbate the disruption in processing. It is then conceivable that the aberrant signal processing may not be related to pain alone, but potentially to other homeostatic mechanisms within the central nervous system, including the processes that govern sleep physiology and circadian rhythms. Whether poor sleep is the manifestation of underlying biological dysfunction or a result of such dysfunction remains to be determined. Of note, the same neurotransmitters that influence pain sensitivity such as dopamine, serotonin, and noradrenaline, are the same ones involved in sleep and emotional regulation (Saper et al., 2005).

Assessment of sleep in children with chronic pain

The assessment and evaluation of children with chronic pain and sleep issues is both challenging and complex because of the potential bidirectional relationship and mitigating factors that affect both sleep and pain. The assessment of a child with chronic pain condition should include a thorough history of sleep practices, routines, cultural beliefs and values related to sleep, sleep preferences, and screening for possible associated sleep disorders (such as sleep disordered breathing, restless legs syndrome, periodic limb movements, or disorders of excessive sleepiness). The evaluation should also include a typical comprehensive medical history, including details about psychiatric, developmental, social history and medication use. Further specific inquiry such as previous medication trials or complementary alternative therapy trials should also be included.

There are validated tools developed for children with chronic pain (Kashikar-Zuck et al., 2010, 2011; Palermo 2009). Validated questionnaires such as such as the Children's Sleep Habits Questionnaire (Owens et al., 2000), or the Pediatric Sleep Questionnaire (Chervin et al., 2007) have been used to identify sleep problems in various clinical and research populations but are not specifically designed for use with children or teens with chronic pain. Subjective, self-report measures for documenting sleep are available such as various

forms of sleep diaries which require recall of information about sleep quantity and timing (<http://www.sleepfoundation.org/; http://www.sleepforkids.org/pdf/SleepDiary.pdf>). An excellent detailed review of the strengths and limitations of subjective paediatric sleep measures is available (Lewandowski et al., 2011a).

Information on objective parameters of sleep and sleep quality in children with chronic pain are sparse and limited. An overnight polysomnogram, which involves monitoring multiple physiological signals related to sleep and breathing, is the gold standard of sleep assessment. Polysomnography has been widely used to document the presence or absence of sleep disordered breathing. The role of this test in populations with chronic pain is limited partially due to limited access to such testing in many geographic locations, a paucity of research related to its role in the care of these children, and the fact that, in many cases, monitoring only takes place over one night. Alternatively, actigraphy, a wrist-watch like device that uses accelerometers to monitor activity patterns, can provide ecologically valid objective information related to sleep. Actigraphs are extensively validated and widely used devices in sleep research with reasonable sensitivity and specificity. Moreover, in paediatric populations generally, actigraphs provide accurate estimates of total sleep time and sleep efficiency, but are generally poor at discerning wakefulness after sleep onset (Meltzer and Westin, 2011). Actigraphs have also been used in pain research in children to measure physical activity (Kashikar-Zuck et al., 2010; Long et al., 2008; Palermo et al., 2008).

As more ambulatory monitoring systems are developed, we can expect that such monitoring in the home environment will become more popular. What has been learned thus far is that polysomnography in children with juvenile fibromyalgia showed increased periodic limb movements in a subset of children but little is known about which children would benefit from having polysomnography testing (Tayag-Kier et al., 2000) without comorbid sleep complaints (Bromberg et al., 2011). Another study evaluating polysomnography in children with headache showed an association between migraine and sleep disordered breathing, and tension headache and bruxism (Vendrame et al., 2008) and less rapid eye movement sleep and slow wave sleep. Practically speaking, persistent sleep complaints or lack of improvement in symptoms with behavioural interventions would be reasonable indications for pursuing further detailed sleep evaluation, including polysomnography.

Another test to objectively measure sleepiness in children is the multiple sleep latency test. A patient is given nap opportunities at 2-hour intervals through the day, and the degree of sleepiness is documented objectively by determining how quickly the individual falls asleep using standardized testing parameters. However, the role of such testing in children with chronic pain is not known, especially in the context of medications that may be partially responsible for the daytime fatigue or sleepiness.

Optimizing sleep in children with chronic pain

Treatment of children with chronic pain who also have comorbid sleep problems requires a multidisciplinary, and often a multimodal approach. The multidisciplinary clinics often include an anaesthesiologist specialized in pain management, nurses, physiotherapists, occupational therapists, and child psychologists with interest and expertise in pain but often not the sleep medicine specialist. Either the addition of a sleep medicine specialist or involvement via consultation could help improve outcomes of both sleep and chronic pain. Despite the fact that pharmacological interventions are frequently used to treat insomnia in children and adults, the empirical evidence shows that psychological interventions are more effective in both children and adults, especially in the longer-term (Mindell et al., 2006a; Stiefel and Stagno, 2004).

There are emerging data about the use of behavioural and psychological treatments for children with chronic pain with positive results in improved pain intensity, functional impairment, and emotional functioning (Palermo, 2009). Cognitive-behavioural therapy (CBT) incorporates both cognitive strategies and behavioural techniques to improve sleep that have a well-established empiric basis in management of insomnia in adults. One randomized control trial provided CBT using Internet delivery of sleep-related advice during one session with promising results (Palermo et al., 2009). CBT does appear to be effective for functional disability in children with juvenile fibromyalgia but the role of sleep has not been specifically addressed (Kashikar-Zuck et al., 2010, 2012; Lewandowski et al., 2011b). Nevertheless, it is commonly accepted that sleep health counselling including healthy sleep habits (sleep hygiene) should be addressed as part of the treatment for chronic pain (Box 16.1). The added value of such interventions to an integrated pain programme warrants further evaluation (see Logan et al., Chapter 50, this volume).

Psychological treatments

Treatment studies can be used to tease apart the bi-directional relationship between sleep and pain, as well as provide clinicians with needed empirical support for selecting and implementing appropriate interventions. Of particular interest to the current review are studies that have treated sleep disturbances in individuals with chronic pain using psychological strategies. These studies examine how sleep problems in individuals with chronic pain respond to treatment. They also highlight the impact of improving sleep on pain and associated symptoms such as mood. In order to better understand the relationship between sleep and pain, and to highlight what we know about evidence-based psychological treatment of sleep problems in children with chronic pain, we will first review the empirical evidence for psychological treatment of sleep problems in otherwise healthy children. Due to the small amount of research on children in this area, adult studies are included.

Insomnia and sleep interventions

The most common sleep problem in both adults and children is insomnia. Approximately 30% of children and adults display some symptoms of insomnia and about 10% reach full diagnostic criteria for insomnia (Meltzer et al., 2010; Morin, 2010). This rate is even higher for individuals with chronic pain; up to 50% of children and 50% to 70% of adults with chronic pain report insomnia (Lewandowski et al., 2011b; Menefee et al., 2000). There are a number of treatment strategies that are effective in treating insomnia in adults. These strategies include sleep restriction (i.e. limiting total sleep time to number of hours currently sleeping and slowly increasing sleep time), stimulus control therapy (i.e. changing conditioned associations with bed and sleep, e.g., using the bed as a place for sleep only), relaxation exercises (such as progressive

muscle relaxation, guided imagery, deep breathing), and sleep hygiene (i.e. a range of strategies that lead to healthy sleep habits). These strategies, along with cognitive restructuring (i.e. identifying and challenging illogical and maladaptive thoughts related to sleep) have been combined into a multi-component treatment approach, labelled cognitive-behavioural therapy for insomnia (CBT-I). In adult populations, CBT-I has received strong research support, based on meta-analyses and systematic reviews, for the treatment of primary insomnia (i.e. insomnia without any other medical or psychological conditions; Morin 2010). Less is known about the use of this technique in children. Given that CBT requires cognitive skills that emerge as development progresses, using CBT-I methods would require matching the treatment task requirements to each child's individual needs.

Sleep interventions for children

Research examining the effectiveness of psychological treatments for insomnia in children has focused on testing the various treatment components in isolation or in combination, but has not specifically evaluated CBT-I. The vast majority of research has been conducted with infants and preschoolers and very little intervention research has been conducted with school-aged children and adolescents. Also, there have been very few randomized controlled trials (RCTs) conducted to document the efficacy of sleep interventions for children of any age. Mindell et al. (2006b) conducted a review of treatment randomized trials in young children and found that in the vast majority, children demonstrated improved sleep with the use of behavioural interventions. Not only did the children's sleep improve (80% of whom demonstrated clinically significant improvement), but also improvements in children's daytime functioning and parent well-being were noted (Mindell, et al., 2006b).

The primary goal of sleep interventions in children is to create positive associations with sleep, establish bedtime routines, and learn relaxation or self-soothing skills. The interventions that are considered well established by research are: extinction (i.e. parent not responding to child's attempt to re-engage parent to provide external soothing), graduated extinction (i.e. parent ignoring their child's attempt to re-engage for predetermined length of time), and parent education (i.e. teaching parents about children's sleep and appropriate sleep hygiene). Strategies considered to be probably efficacious include: scheduled awakenings (i.e. pre-emptive waking schedule for which parents wake their child 15 to 30 min prior to the time of typical night awakenings) and bedtime fading (i.e. putting the child to bed at a time that he/she is likely to fall asleep quickly and once successful backing up bedtime in 15-min increments).

Sleep interventions for children with chronic pain

Although there is strong support for some intervention techniques in certain age ranges, there is very little research testing the effectiveness of these interventions for children with physical or mental health diagnoses (Lewandowski et al., 2011b; Vriend and Corkum, 2011). There is even less research on children with chronic pain. Four studies have provided sleep intervention as part of a multicomponent treatment for pain (Bruni et al., 1999; Degotardi et al., 2006, Maynard et al., 2010, Palermo et al., 2009). Each of these studies is

Table 15.2 Intervention studies which included a sleep component for treating children with chronic pain

Author	Participants	Design	Treatment	Outcome
Child intervention studies				
Degotardi et al., 2006	N = 67 (59 females, 8 males); fibromyalgia; mean age: 13.9 years (SD = 2.8, range = 8–20)	Pre-post design; outcome was measured by questionnaires on physical (e.g. pain, sleep quality, fatigue) and psychological (e.g. anxiety, internalization, quality of life) symptoms completed by parents and children	8 weekly sessions which focused on psycho-education about pain and sleep, sleep improvement, pain management, and activities of daily living. Sleep treatment strategies included sleep hygiene, relaxation, self-reward, stimulus control, sleep restriction, and cognitive restructuring. Treatment was based on a CBT treatment manual developed by the authors	Improvements reported across all measures, including decreased pain, somatic symptoms, anxiety and fatigue as well as improved sleep quality. 24% of the children were reported to be pain free at the end of the intervention. Both self-reports and clinical observations showed dramatic improvements. Results were based on participants who completed the intervention (34% attrition rate)
Maynard et al., 2010	N = 41 (30 females, 11 males); pain-associated disability syndrome; mean age: 13.8 years (SD = 2.8, range = 8–21)	Retrospective chart review; outcome was measured by information in chart on school attendance, medication usage, sleep, functional disability, coping skills, and mobility	Treatment through an interdisciplinary inpatient rehabilitation programme including several components. Psychological treatment focused on CBT for pain and anxiety and the use of shaping to improve functional ability. Sleep intervention included relaxation strategies at bedtime	Improvement in functional ability, physical mobility, as well as school status, sleep, and medication use
Palermo et al., 2009	N = 48 (35 females, 13 males); chronic headache, abdominal, or musculoskeletal pain; mean age: 14.8 years (SD = 2.0, range = 11–17)	RCT; Internet-treatment group (n = 26), waitlist control group (n = 22); outcomes (e.g. recording pain and activity levels) were measured by daily diaries and questionnaires pre- and post-treatment	Internet-delivered CBT intervention which included 8 weeks of modules focused on treating pain through relaxation training, cognitive strategies, parent operant techniques, communication strategies, and sleep and activity interventions. Sleep intervention included information on sleep and good sleep hygiene practices	Improvements in pain intensity and activity levels at end of treatment and 3-month follow-up. No improvement in parental protectiveness or child mood symptoms
Bruni et al., 1999	N = 70 (32 females, 38 males); migraine sufferers with poor sleep hygiene; mean age: 9.7 years (SD = 1.5, range = 5–15 years)	RCT, assigned to treatment (n = 35), no treatment (n = 35); outcomes were assessed by tracking duration, frequency and severity of migraines	Treatment included application of sleep hygiene guidelines, but these were not specified in the paper	Improvement in frequency and duration of migraines for treatment group, but no change in severity

described in detail in Table 15.2. Results across these studies were generally positive, with improvements in both pain and sleep, as well as other associated areas (e.g. functional disability, fatigue). A series of randomized trials conducted among adults with chronic pain conditions (Currie et al., 2000; Edinger et al., 2005; Jungquist et al., 2010; Rybarczyk et al., 2005) has yielded similar positive results. More intervention research in this area is needed, with a focus on demonstrating that improvements in sleep does indeed result in improved pain outcomes.

Pharmacological treatments

Pharmacological therapy for chronic pain should take into consideration potential interactions with sleep. There are no approved medications for the treatment of insomnia in children or medications for chronic pain in children. Reviews about insomnia and treatment options in children are available (Owens and Moturi, 2009; Owens et al., 2005). Chronic pain in children is often managed with similar medications as in adults off label, but integration of behavioural strategies are often paramount, much like management

of childhood insomnia. Of note, many pain medications that are prescribed often have sleep-related effects. For example, tricyclic antidepressants and anticonvulsants often have sleepiness as a side effect which may help promote sleep. These same medications may also cause daytime sleepiness or fatigue which may further worsen functional adaptation in dealing with pain. In some instances, such as with the use of gabapentin for neuropathic pain, the medication may help reduce pain and possibly improve a comorbid sleep disorder such as restless legs syndrome. Selective serotonin reuptake inhibitors (e.g. paroxetine) may be used for treatment of comorbid psychological disorders rather than pain itself and the impact of these medications on sleep such as rapid eye movement suppression, or increased periodic limb movements (Vendrame et al., 2011) should not be overlooked. Similarly, opioid medications for chronic pain may worsen underlying sleep disordered breathing, or result in constipation and associated discomfort that impairs sleep. Controlled trials using medications for treating chronic pain in children and teens are lacking. Future research studies should add in components that address sleep specifically. (For more information on clinical use of opioids see Strassels, Chapter 45, and for drugs for neuropathic pain, see Rastogi and Campbell, Chapter 48, this volume.)

Key recommendations

Given the evidence to date, we recommend that children with pain and sleep problems be provided with a developmentally appropriate, evidence-based intervention for their sleep problems as one component of their pain management plan. A detailed description of these intervention strategies is beyond the scope of this review; however, Box 15.1 lists some healthy sleep habits for children and adolescents and Table 15.3 contains a list of resources. Some modifications or special considerations might be useful to consider when implementing sleep intervention for children with chronic pain (Smith et al., 2005). The clinician may have to explain to parents why treating sleep problems is important, as a study by Claar and Scharff (2007) found that parents did not see sleep interventions as likely to help with the treatment of pain in their children. It will also be important to develop sleep interventions that parents of children with chronic pain can readily access. For example, novel delivery methods, such as internet (Corkum and Davidson, 2011) or telehealth (Witmans et al., 2008) may help to reduce access barriers. Clinicians working with children with chronic pain may also want to consider the following when implementing sleep interventions:

- Managing pain will help the child be able to fall asleep and stay asleep. Also, making sure that medications taken by the child are not interfering with sleep.

- Many of the strategies used to help with pain management (e.g. proper diet and exercise) will also help with sleep. It is important that exercise does not occur close to bedtime and that foods that cause any intestinal distress not be eaten close to bedtime.

- Parents and children should be informed about the relationship between sleep and pain, so that they understand why it is important to treat sleep problems as part of the overall pain management plan. For example, it would be important to point out that poor sleep is associated with next-day pain as well as increased negative affect and decreased positive affect.

- Sleep hygiene is an important component for sleep treatment. For children with chronic pain, it is important that the bed/bedroom is not associated with any painful treatments (e.g. injections) and that the child's bed is as comfortable as possible in order to reduce any pain associated with sleeping.

- Given that children with pain may experience hyperarousal, it is important to include relaxation training as one of the sleep intervention strategies.

- Sleep restriction therapy should be used with caution given some evidence that sleep restriction can increase pain.

- Parents may require additional support when implementing sleep strategies. Many parents find implementing these strategies to be stressful and this may be more so for parents of children with chronic pain.

Conclusion

There is much more to learn about which sleep treatment components are most effective in this population, as well as how we might

---

Box 15.1 Healthy sleep habits for children and adolescents

- Ensure morning bright-light exposure
- Schedule daily physical activity (ideally earlier in the day)
- Avoid caffeine in the afternoon and evening
- Reduce (and avoid where possible) bright light in the evening and in the night
- Reduce stimulating activities before and at bedtime
- Set an age-appropriate bedtime
- Establish a regular, consistent bedtime routine
- Maintain a consistent schedule for weekdays and weekends
- Create an environment conducive to sleep: cool, dark, quiet, comfortable
- Remove electronics from the bedroom
- Use the bed only for sleep
- Monitor for side effects of medications that may affect sleep.

Table 15.3 Resources for sleep intervention in children

Journal articles	Hill, C. (2011). Practitioner review: effective treatment of behavioural insomnia in children. *J Child Psychol Psychiatry*, 52(7), 731–741. doi:10.1111/j.1469–7610.2011.02396.x
	Jan, J. E., Owens, J. A., Weiss, M. D., Johnson, K. P., Wasdell, M. B., Freeman, R. D., *et al.* (2008). Sleep hygiene for children with neurodevelopmental disabilities. *Pediatrics*, 122(6), 1343–1350. doi:10.1542/peds.2007–3308
	Meltzer, L. J. (2010). Clinical management of behavioral insomnia of childhood: treatment of bedtime problems and night wakings in young children. *Behav Sleep Med*, 8(3), 172–189. doi:10.1080/15402002.2010.487464
	Taylor, D. J., and Roane, B. M. (2010). Treatment of insomnia in adults and children: a practice-friendly review of research. *J Clin Psychol*, 66(11), 1137–1147. doi:10.1002/jclp.20733
	Vriend, J. and Corkum, P. (2011). Clinical management of behavioral insomnia of childhood. *Psychol Res Behav Manag*, 4, 69–79. doi: http://dx.doi.org/10.2147/PRBM.S14057
Books for professionals	Durand, V. M. (2008). *When children don't sleep well: parent workbook: interventions for pediatric sleep disorders (treatments that work)*. New York: Oxford University Press
	Mindell, J. A. and Owens, J.A. (2009). *A clinical guide to pediatric sleep: diagnosis and management of sleep problems* (2nd edn). Philadelphia, PA: Lippincott Williams & Wilkins
	Sheldon, S. S., Ferber, R. and Kryger, M. H. (2005). *Principles and practice of pediatric sleep medicine*. Philadelphia, PA: W.B. Saunders
	Stores, G. and Wiggs, L. (2001). *Sleep disturbance in children and adolescents with disorders of development: its significance and management*. London: MacKeith Press
Websites	Kidszzzsleep: <http://www.kidzzzsleep.org>
	National Sleep Foundation: <http://www.sleepfoundation.org>
	Sleep Net: <http://www.sleepnet.com/>
	Sleep for Kids: <http://www.sleepforkids.org/index.html>

have to modify existing sleep interventions to enhance effectiveness in children with chronic pain. However, at the current time, it would seem reasonable for clinicians working with children with chronic pain to assess and treat sleep problems. At a minimum, treating sleep problems will reduce the number of issues with which the child and parent is trying to cope, and could potentially improve pain while enhancing overall quality of life.

There is now a strong empirical base to conclude that sleep disturbances are indeed a significant problem for children with chronic pain. There remains much important work to do in this area. For example, more research is needed to examine the developmental trajectory of the relationship between sleep and pain problems across childhood and adolescence, the impact of the kinds and quantities of medication used by children with chronic pain and how these relate to sleep (Chambers et al., 2008). Future research is critically needed to develop and test the impact of interventions addressing sleep and pain among children and adolescents with chronic pain.

Case example: pain and sleep

Melissa is a 14-year-old girl with a 5-year history of recurrent abdominal pain, which had recently significantly worsened to the point that she was now unable to attend school. At the time of her pain clinic evaluation, Melissa was experiencing daily, severe stomach aches with no identifiable medical cause. When queried about sleep during her evaluation, Melissa noted that in addition to her pain she was experiencing significant difficulties falling asleep at night and would watch television in bed until late at night. Melissa was also having great difficulty getting out of bed at a reasonable time in the morning. Because she was not attending school, her parents tended to let Melissa sleep in to catch up on her sleep, and Melissa reported that she often napped in the afternoon while watching television and resting. Melissa reported feeling more irritable and fatigued during the day, and acknowledged that feeling this way was likely making it harder for her to deal with her pain. The pain management team recommended a comprehensive cognitive-behavioural intervention in order to help Melissa learn strategies to better cope with her pain as well as a graduated school re-entry plan. Melissa's sleep, in addition to her pain, was also identified as one of the primary treatment targets. The family was provided with basic information about sleep and sleep hygiene and links between pain and sleep problems. A session was scheduled to tailor those strategies to meet Melissa's needs and to help her parents coach and support her sleep changes. The importance of a regular sleep schedule, the removal of the television from the bedroom, and the negative impact of daytime naps on night sleep were discussed. As treatment progressed, Melissa noted significant improvements in her sleep and her ability to apply the pain coping strategies she was learning in clinic. At the end of treatment, Melissa was still experiencing mild stomach aches most days, but had returned to school, was sleeping much better, her mood had improved, and she reported feeling more energy and less irritability.

References

Bloom, B. J., Owens, J. A., McGuinn, M., Nobile, C., Schaeffer, L., and Alario, A. J. (2002). Sleep and its relationship to pain, dysfunction, and disease activity in juvenile rheumatoid arthritis. *J Rheumatol*, 29, 169–173.

Breau, L. M. and Camfield, C. S. (2011). Pain disrupts sleep in children and youth with intellectual and developmental disabilities. *Res Dev Disabil*, 32, 2829–2840.

Bromberg, M. H., Gil, K. M., and Schanberg, L. E. (2011). Daily sleep quality and mood as predictors of pain in children with juvenile polyarticular arthritis. *Health Psychol*, 31, 202–209.

Brooks, L. J., Koziol, S. M., Chiarucci, K. M., and Berman, B. W. (1996). Does sleep-disordered breathing contribute to the clinical severity of sickle cell anemia? *J Pediatr Hematol/Oncol*, 18, 135–139.

Bruni, O., Galli, F., and Guidetti, V. (1999). Sleep hygiene and migraine in children and adolescents. *Cephalalgia*, 19, 57–59.

Butbul Aviel, Y., Stremler, R., Benseler, S. M., Cameron, B., Laxer, R. M., Ota, S., *et al.* (2011). Sleep and fatigue and the relationship to pain, disease activity and quality of life in juvenile idiopathic arthritis and juvenile dermatomyositis. *Rheumatology*, 50, 2051–2060.

Cappuccio, F. P., Taggart, F. M., Kandala, N. B., Currie, A., Peile, E., Stranges, S., *et al.* (2008). Meta-analysis of short sleep duration and obesity in children and adults. *Sleep*, 31, 619–626.

Chambers, C. T., Corkum, P., and Rusak, B. (2008). Commentary: the importance of sleep in pediatric chronic pain—a wake-up call for pediatric psychologists. *J Pediatr Psychol*, 33, 333–334.

Claar, R. and Scharff, L. (2007). Parent and child perceptions of chronic pain treatments. *Child Health Care*, 36, 285–301.

Corkum, P. and Davidson, F. (2011). Sleep intervention for behavioural insomnia in children: impact on sleep and daytime functioning of typically developing children and children with ADHD. Presentation at the AACAP/CACAP Joint Annual Meeting, 18–23 October, Toronto, Ontario.

Currie, S. R., Wilson, K. G., Pontefract, A. J., and deLaplante, L. (2000). Cognitive–behavioral treatment of insomnia secondary to chronic pain. *J Consult Clin Psych*, 68, 407–416.

Degotardi, P. J., Klass, E. S., Rosenberg, B. S., Fox, D. G., Gallelli, K. A., and Gottlieb, B. S. (2006). Development and evaluation of a cognitive-behavioral intervention for juvenile fibromyalgia. *J Ped Psych*, 31, 714–723.

Dick, B. D. and Pillai Riddell, R. (2010). Cognitive and school functioning in children and adolescents with chronic pain: a critical review. *Pain Res Manag*, 15, 238–244.

Durmer, J. S. and Dinges, D. F. (2005). Neurocognitive consequences of sleep deprivation. *Semin Neurol*, 25, 117–129.

Edinger, J. D., Wohlgemuth, W. K., Krystal, A. D., and Rice, J. R. (2005). Behavioral insomnia therapy for fibromyalgia patients: a randomized clinical trial. *Arch Int Med*, 165, 2527–2535.

Foley, D., Ancoli-Israel, S., Britz, P., and Walsh, J. (2004). Sleep disturbances and chronic disease in older adults: results of the 2003 National Sleep Foundation Sleep in America Survey. *J Psychosom Res*, 56, 497–502.

Forest, G. and Godbout, R. (2000). Effects of sleep deprivation on performance and EEG spectral analysis in young adults. *Brain Cogn*, 43, 195–200

Forgeron, P. A., McGrath, P. J., Stevens, B., Evans, J., Dick, B. D., Finley, G. A., *et al.* (2011). Social information processing in adolescents with chronic pain: my friends don't really understand me. *Pain*, 152(12), 2773–2780.

Fricke-Oerkermann, L., Pluck, J., Schredl, M., Heinz, K., Mitschke, A., and Wiater, A. (2007). Prevalence and course of sleep problems in childhood. *Sleep*, 30, 1371–1377.

Fuggle, P., Shand, P. A. X., Gill, L. J., and Davies, S. C. (1996). Pain, quality of life and coping in sickle cell disease. *Arch Dis Child*, 75, 199–203.

Gagliese, L. and Chambers, C. T. (2007). Pediatric and geriatric pain in relation to sleep disturbances. In G. Lavigne, B. J. Sessle, M. Choiniere and P. J. Soja (eds) *Sleep and pain*, pp. 341–59. Seattle, WA: IASP Press.

Gold, J. I., Mahrer, N. E., Yee, J., and Palermo, T. M. (2009). Pain, fatigue, and health-related quality of life in children and adolescents with chronic pain. *Clin J Pain*, 25(5), 407–412.

Henry, D. E., Chiodo, A. E., and Yang, W. (2011). Central nervous system reorganization in a variety of chronic pain states: a review. *PM R*, 12, 1116–1125.

Jungquist, C. R., O'Brien, C., Matteson-Rusby, S., Smith, M. T., Pigeon, W. R., Xia, Y., and Perlis, M. L. (2010). The efficacy of cognitive-behavioral therapy for insomnia in patients with chronic pain. *Sleep Med*, 11, 302–309.

Kashikar-Zuck, S., Flowers S. R., Claar, R. L., Guite, J. W., Logan, D. E., Lynch-Jordan, A.M., *et al*. (2011). Clinical utility and validity of the functional disability inventory among a multicenter sample of youth with chronic pain. *Pain*, 152, 1600–1607.

Kashikar-Zuck, S., Flowers, S. R., Verkamp, E., Ting, T. V., Lynch-Jordan, A. M., Graham, T. B., *et al*. (2010). Actigraphy-based physical activity monitoring in adolescents with juvenile primary fibromyalgia syndrome. *J Pain*, 11, 885–93.

Kashikar-Zuck, S., Johnston, M., Ting, T. V., Graham, B. T., Lynch-Jordan, A. M., Verkamp, E., *et al*. (2010). Relationship between school absenteeism and depressive symptoms among adolescents with juvenile fibromyalgia. *J Pediatr Psychol*, 35, 996–1004.

Kashikar-Zuck, S., Ting, T. V., Arnold, L. M., Bean, J., Powers, S. W., Graham, T. B., *et al*. (2012). Cognitive behavioral therapy for the treatment of juvenile fibromyalgia: a multisite, single-blind, randomized, controlled clinical trial. *Arthritis Rheum*, 64, 297–305.

Kashikar-Zuck, S., Parkins, I. S., Ting, T. V., Verkamp, E., Lynch-Jordan, A., Passo, M., *et al*. (2010). Controlled follow-up study of physical and psychosocial functioning of adolescents with juvenile primary fibromyalgia syndrome. *Rheumatology*, 49, 2204–2209.

Lewandowski, A. S., Palermo, T. M., De la Motte, S., and Fu, R. (2010). Temporal daily associations between pain and sleep in adolescents with chronic pain versus healthy adolescents. *Pain*, 151(1), 220–225.

Lewandowski, A. S., Toliver-Sokol, M., and Palermo, T. M. (2011a). Evidence-based review of subjective pediatric sleep measures. *J Pediatr Psychol*, 36, 780–793.

Lewandowski, A. S., Ward, T. M. and Palermo, T. M. (2011b). Sleep problems in children and adolescents with common medical conditions. *Ped Clin N Am*, 58, 699–713.

Lewin, D. S. and Dahl, R. E. (1999). Importance of sleep in the management of pediatric pain. *J Dev Behav Pediatr*, 20, 244–252.

Long, A. C., Krishnamurthy, V., and Palermo, T. M. (2008). Sleep disturbances in school-age children with chronic pain. *J Pediatr Psychol*, 33, 258–268.

Long, A. C., Palermo, T. M., and Manees, A. M. (2008). Brief report: using actigraphy to compare physical activity levels in adolescents with chronic pain and healthy adolescents. *J Pediatr Psychol*, 33, 660–665.

Maynard, C. S., Amari, A., Wieczorek, B., Christensen, J. R., and Slifer, K. J. (2010). Interdisciplinary behavioral rehabilitation of pediatric pain-associated disability: retrospective review of an inpatient treatment protocol. *J Ped Psych*, 35, 128–137.

Martin, J., Hiscock, H., Hardy, P., Davey, B., and Wake, M. (2007). Adverse associations of infant and child sleep problems and parent health: an Australian population study. *Pediatrics*, 119(5), 946–955.

Meltzer, L. J., Johnson, C., Crosette, J., Ramos, M., and Mindell, J. A. (2010). Prevalence of diagnosed sleep disorders in pediatric primary care practices. *Pediatrics*, 125, e1410–e1418.

Meltzer, L. J., Logan, D. E., and Mindell, J. A. (2005). Sleep patterns in female adolescents with chronic musculoskeletal pain. *Behav Sleep Med*, 3, 193–208.

Meltzer, L. J. and Mindell, J. A. (2009). Pediatric sleep. In M. C. Roberts and R. G. Steele (eds) *Handbook of pediatric psychology* (4th edn), pp. 491–507. New York: The Guilford Press.

Meltzer, L. J. and Westin, A. M. (2011). A comparison of actigraphy scoring rules used in pediatric research. *Sleep Med*, 12, 793–796.

Menefee, L. A., Cohen, M. M., Anderson, W. R., Doghramji, K., Frank, E. D., and Lee, H. (2000). Sleep disturbance and nonmalignant chronic pain: a comprehensive review of the literature. *Pain Med*, 1, 156–172.

Miller, V. A., Palermo, T. M., Powers, S. W., Scher, M. S., and Hershey, A. D. (2003). Migraine headaches and sleep disturbances in children. *Headache*, 43, 362–368.

Mindell, J. A., Emslie, G., Blumer, J., Genel, M., Glaze, D., Ivanenko, A., and Banas, B. (2006a). Pharmacologic management of insomnia in children and adolescents: Consensus statement. *Pediatrics*, 117, e1223–e1232.

Mindell, J. A., Kuhn, B., Lewin, D. S., Meltzer, L. J., and Sadeh, A. (2006b). Behavioral treatment of bedtime problems and night wakings in infants and young children. *Sleep*, 29, 1263–1276.

Mindell, J. A. and Owens, J. A. (2003). Sleep problems in pediatric practice: clinical issues for the pediatric nurse practitioner. *J Pediatr Health Care*, 17(6), 324–331.

Morin, C. M. (2010). Chronic insomnia: recent advances and innovations in treatment developments and dissemination. *Can Psychol*, 51, 31–39.

Owens, J. A. (2005). Epidemiology of sleep disorders during childhood. In S. H. Sheldon, R. Ferber, and M. H. Kryger (eds) *Principles and practices of pediatric sleep medicine* (4th edn), pp. 27–33. Philadelphia, PA: Elsevier/Saunders.

Owens J. A. (2007). Classification and epidemiology of childhood sleep disorders. *Sleep Med Clin*, 2, 353–361.

Owens, J. A. (2011). Update in pediatric sleep medicine. *Curr Opin Pulm Med*, 17, 425–430.

Owens, J. A., Babcock, D., Blumer, J., Chervin, R., Ferber, R., Goetting, M., *et al*. (2005). The use of pharmacotherapy in the treatment of pediatric insomnia in primary care: rational approaches. A consensus meeting summary. *J Clin Sleep Med*, 15(1), 49–59.

Owens, J. A. and Moturi, S. (2009). Pharmacologic treatment of pediatric insomnia. *Child Adolesc Psychiatr Clin N Am*, 18, 1001–1016.

Owens, J. A., Spirito, A., and McGuinn, M. (2000). The Children's Sleep Habits Questionnaire (CSHQ): psychometric properties of a survey instrument for school-aged children. *Sleep*, 23(8), 1043–1051.

Palermo, T. M. (2009). Assessment of chronic pain in children: current status and emerging topics. *Pain Res Manag*, 14, 21–26.

Palermo, T. M., Fonareva, I., and Janosy, N. R. (2008). Sleep quality and efficiency in adolescents with chronic pain: relationship with activity limitations and health-related quality of life. *Behav Sleep Med*, 6, 234–250.

Palermo, T. M. and Owens, J. (2008). Introduction to the special issue: sleep in pediatric medical populations. *J Pediatr Psychol*, 33, 227–231.

Palermo, T. M., Toliver-Sokol, M., Fonareva, I., and Koh, J. L. (2007). Objective and subjective assessment of sleep in adolescents with chronic pain compared to healthy adolescents. *Clin J Pain*, 23, 812–820.

Palermo, T. M., Wilson, A. C., Lewandowski, A. S., Toliver-Sokol, M., and Murray, C. B. (2011). Behavioral and psychosocial factors associated with insomnia in adolescents with chronic pain. *Pain*, 152, 89–94.

Palermo, T. M., Wilson, A. C., Peters, M., Lewandowski, A., and Somhegyi, H. (2009). Randomized controlled trial of an internet-delivered family cognitive–behavioral therapy intervention for children and adolescents with chronic pain. *Pain*, 146, 205–213.

Pirinen, T., Kolho, K. L., Simola, P., Ashorn, M., and Aronen, E. T. (2010). Parent and self-report of sleep-problems and daytime tiredness among adolescents with inflammatory bowel disease and their population-based controls. *Sleep*, 33(11), 1487–1493.

Rybarczyk, B., Stepanski, E., Fogg, L., Lopez, M., Barry, P., and Davis, A. (2005). A placebo controlled test of cognitive-behavioral therapy for comorbid insomnia in older adults. *J Consult Clin Psychol*, 73, 1164–1174.

Sadeh, A. (2007). Consequences of sleep loss or sleep disruption in children. *Sleep Med Clinics*, 2, 513–520.

Saper, C. B., Cano, G., and Scammell, T. E. (2005). Homeostatic, circadian, and emotional regulation of sleep. *J Comp Neurol*, 493, 92–98.

Sivertsen, B., Hysing, M., Elgen, I., Stormark, K., and Lundervold, A. (2009). Chronicity of sleep problems in children with chronic illness: a longitudinal population-based study. *Child Adol Psychiat Ment Health*, 3, 1–7.

Smith, M. T., Huang, M. I., and Manber, R. (2005). Cognitive behavior therapy for chronic insomnia occurring within the context of medical and psychiatric disorders. *Clin Psychol Rev*, 25, 559–592.

Stiefel, F. and Stagno, D. (2004). Management of insomnia in patients with chronic pain conditions. *CNS Drugs*, 18, 285–296.

Tayag-Kier, C. E., Keenan, G. F., Scalzi, L. V., Schultz, B., Elliott, J., Zhao, R. H., *et al.* (2000). Sleep and periodic limb movement in sleep in juvenile fibromyalgia. *Pediatrics*, 106, E70.

Tsai, S. Y., Labyak, S. E., Richardson, L. P., Lentz, M. J., Brandt, P. A., Ward, T. M., *et al.* (2008). Actigraphic sleep and daytime naps in adolescent girls with chronic musculoskeletal pain. *J Pediatr Psychol*, 33, 307–311.

Valrie, C. R., Gil, K. M., Redding-Lallinger, R., and Daeschner, C. (2008). Brief report: daily mood as a mediator or moderator of the pain-sleep relationship in children with sickle cell disease. *J Pediatr Psychol*, 33, 317–322.

Valrie, C. R., Gil, K. M., Redding-Lallinger, R., and Daeschner, C. (2007). The influence of pain and stress on sleep in children with sickle cell disease. *Child Health Care*, 36, 335–53.

Vendrame, M., Kaleyias, J., Valencia, I., Legido, A., and Kothare, S.V. (2008). Polysomnographic findings in children with headaches. *Pediatr Neurol*, 39, 6–11.

Vendrame, M., Zarowski, M., Loddenkemper, T., Steinborn, B., and Kothare, S.V. (2011). Selective serotonin reuptake inhibitors and periodic limb movements of sleep. *Pediatr Neurol*, 45, 175–177.

Vriend, J. and Corkum, P. (2011). Clinical management of behavioral insomnia of childhood. *Psych Res Beh Man*, 4, 69–79.

Vriend, J. L., Davidson, F. D., Corkum, P. V., Rusak, B., McLaughlin, E. N., and Chambers, C. T. (2012). Sleep quantity and quality in relation to daytime functioning in children. *Child Health Care, 41(3), 204–222.*

Ward, T. M., Brandt, P., Archbold, K., Lentz, M., Ringold, S., Wallace, C. A., *et al.* (2008). Polysomnography and self-reported sleep, pain, fatigue, and anxiety in children with active and inactive juvenile rheumatoid arthritis. *J Pediatr Psychol*, 33, 232–241.

Witmans, M. B., Dick, B., Good, J., Schoepp, G., Dosman, C., Hawkins, M., and Witol, A. (2008). Delivery of pediatric sleep services via telehealth: the Alberta experience and lessons learned. *Behav Sleep Med*, 6, 207–219.

SECTION 4

Pain in specific populations and diseases

CHAPTER 16

Pain in children with intellectual or developmental disabilities

John L. Belew, Chantel C. Barney, Scott A. Schwantes, Dick Tibboel, Abraham J. Valkenburg , and Frank J. Symons

Summary

In this chapter, it is argued that it is time to bring the burgeoning work on pain together and develop a coherent clinically-informed research agenda addressing the problem of pain among children with intellectual or developmental disabilities (I/DD). The chapter starts with an introductory section providing a short overview of the problem of pain among children with I/DD including many definitional and historical issues. Subsequent sections include a review of the epidemiology and impact of pain in children with I/DD, followed by a review of pain assessment and then pain management in children with I/DD. The chapter ends with a summary and conclusions relevant for future research and practice.

Introduction

There is an enormous amount of scientific data about pain but comparatively little knowledge specific to children with intellectual or developmental disability. A PubMed search using the terms 'pain' and 'human' yielded over 100 000 publications for the 5-year period between 2005 and 2009 (the last full 5-year epoch) or, approximately 20 000 papers per year reporting on new discoveries, reviews, and theories regarding pain and the human condition. Only a fraction (3.7%) of those papers addressed paediatrics and pain (the topic of this volume). For that same 5-year period, there were a total of 30 scientific papers published specific to pain and children with I/DD—approximately 0.03% of the publication volume. Considering that approximately 1% to 7% of the world's population lives with an intellectual or related developmental disability (estimates vary widely between developed and developing countries; World Health Organization, 2001), the gap between what science has to tell us about pain in this population and what we probably need to know is striking (Figure 16.1). A contributing factor for this paucity of literature is most likely the routine exclusion of individuals with I/DD from research.

Pain—important and prevalent in children with I/DD

There is little doubt that pain is a universal phenomenon causing tremendous human suffering and compromising the quality of life for countless individuals. The US congress declared 2001 to 2010 as the Decade of Pain Control and Research, however we estimate a decade devoted to pain research yielded fewer than 80 papers about pain in children with I/DD. And yet, there is no good reason to believe that pain is any less frequent in a child with a developmental disability or intellectual impairment, or that such an individual would be insensitive or indifferent to pain. Numerous functional limitations as well as the underlying neurological condition itself frequently confound the presentation of pain. Regardless of the degree of the disability, however, pain is often a part of daily life for children with I/DD (Oberlander and Symons, 2006).

The majority of scientific activity devoted to pain and children with I/DD in the previous decade has been to 'build a better mousetrap'— improving behavioural assessment techniques to identify accurately the presence of pain and its source or type, when reliable self-report is not an option. The fruits of this labour are manifest in several rating scales and questionnaires designed to measure pain intensity/severity and its expression (these are reviewed in detail in later sections).

Although the terms *intellectual disability* and *developmental disability* are familiar ones, we encourage the reader to pay careful attention to the explanation of these terms. The term I/DD includes a population of children that is highly heterogeneous: children with conditions of diverse type and aetiology (e.g. Down syndrome, cerebral palsy (CP), Rett syndrome) are included along with children with neurodevelopmental disabilities of unknown origin. Therefore our attempt here is to portray common features related to pain experience and management that are found across this diverse group, and specifically within certain subpopulations. By the very nature of their underlying condition children with I/DD are particularly at risk for painful experiences disproportionate to their typically developing peers. Common vulnerabilities children with I/DD face

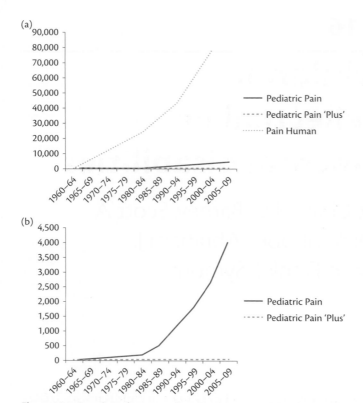

Figure 16.1 Cumulative frequency of paediatric pain research based on PubMed search results for full 5-year epochs using search terms 'pain', 'human', 'paediatric', and 'paediatric' *plus* 'intellectual disability', 'mental retardation', 'developmental disability (a) and results for 'pain', 'paediatric', and 'paediatric plus' only (b).

with respect to pain include increased prevalence of painful conditions, both acute and chronic, higher rate of exposure to painful procedures (diagnostic and therapeutic), and neurosensory concerns that heighten the pain experience as well as complicate pain assessment and management.

Pain concerns are usually first addressed in a medical context. An initial obstacle health care providers (HCPs) often face when providing care for children with I/DD is the inconsistency and lack of detail typically found in medical records regarding a child's neurodevelopmental disabilities. While school records may contain the results of extensive neurodiagnostic testing, medical records often lack key information regarding the child's specific cognitive, communication, and adaptive behaviour abilities. This can make it extremely difficult for the HCP to establish the specific neurodevelopmental status of a child with I/DD (Salvador-Carulla and Saxena, 2009). HCPs are left to guess or make assumptions based on 'clues' such as observed communication patterns and behaviour. Medical records frequently include non-specific use of terms like *autistic*, *mentally retarded*, or *developmentally delayed*. Used appropriately, the term *developmental delay* flags neurodevelopmental concerns in young children. However, this term is often included in the medical record of older children, even adults, when no more specific developmental descriptors have been established in the medical record.

Defining intellectual disability

Intellectual disability (ID; previously referred to as 'mental retardation' and referred to as 'learning disability' in the UK) is defined by the American Association on Intellectual and Developmental Disabilities (AAIDD) as a 'disability characterized by significant limitations both in intellectual functioning and in adaptive behaviour, which covers many everyday social and practical skills. This disability originates before the age of 18' (2012). Similarly, the International Association for the Scientific Study of Intellectual Disability (IASSID) considers ID as a 'significant intellectual deficit present from birth, or which originates at an early age or during the developmental period' (2012). There are key components to the definitions specific to the concept of 'intellectual functioning' and 'adaptive behaviour'. Intellectual functioning (i.e. intelligence) 'refers to general mental capacity, such as learning, reasoning, problem solving, and so on. One criterion to measure intellectual functioning is an IQ test. Generally, an IQ test score of around 70 or as high as 75 indicates a limitation in intellectual functioning' [i.e. greater than two standard deviations below average IQ] (AAIDD, <http://www.aaidd.org/content_100.cfm>). A similar approach is used to determine adaptive function. Specifically, standardized tests are used to determine limitations in adaptive behaviour, comprised of three specific skill types including conceptual skills (e.g. number concepts), social skills (e.g. social problem solving), and practical skills (e.g. activities of daily living). On the basis of a set of standardized measures designed to specifically assess and evaluate intelligence and adaptive behaviour it is determined whether a child has an ID (see Salvador-Carrulla et al. 2011 for an interesting discussion of ID in the medical context.)

Defining developmental disability

Developmental disability as defined in the US by the *Developmental Disabilities Assistance and Bill of Rights Act* (DD Act; PL. 98–527) refers to a 'severe, chronic disability' attributable to 'mental' and/or 'physical' impairments that are 'likely to continue indefinitely', resulting in substantial functional imitations in three or more 'major life activity areas: self-care, receptive or expressive language, learning, self-direction, capacity for independent living and economic self-sufficiency', are manifest by age 22 and require care, treatment or other services of lifelong extended duration. Some conditions may be included categorically, e.g. CP, spina bifida, autism. It is worth noting that unlike 'intellectual disability', classifying developmental disability does not benefit from a prescribed set of standardized assessment instruments, procedures, or professional training programmes. From a somewhat similar perspective, through the World Health Organization (WHO), The International Classification of Functioning, Disability and Health (referred to as ICF) also provides a classification system for health and health-related domains affected by disability. The domains are classified from body, individual and societal perspectives in two areas; (1) body functions and structure, and (2) activity and participation. The ICF is WHO's framework for measuring health and disability at both individual and population levels.

Issues for I/DD created by the definition of pain

Pain, as defined by the International Association for the Study of Pain (IASP), refers to 'an unpleasant sensory and emotional experience associated with actual or potential tissue damage, or described in terms of such damage' (Merskey and Bodguck, 1994). Because of problems created, in part, with the implicit requirement to self-report on the sensory or emotional experience, the definition was revised in 2002 with the clause 'the inability to communicate verbally does not negate the possibility that an individual is experiencing pain and is in need of appropriate pain-relieving treatment' (IASP, 2012). The overwhelming approach to considering pain, however, still relies extensively on self-report using language based on the spoken word (despite problems associated with almost exclusive reliance on self-report as a 'gold standard'; see Schiavenato and Craig, 2010). The obvious problem created by the original definition for children with I/DD is that different combinations and functional levels of language/communicative, motor, and cognitive impairments associated with I/DD make self-report of a complex experience such as pain difficult if not impossible for some children. There is a likelihood that pain among many of these children cannot be measured in conventional ways (or perhaps even detected), resulting in painful conditions that are untreated or undertreated.

Historical perspectives on pain and I/DD

Historically, there has been little recognizable sustained scientific investigation of pain among individuals with I/DD. At the same time, there is a long history of quasi-scientific perspectives regarding individuals with I/DD, including children, to be 'defective' in sensory function, particularly touch (including the ability to discriminate pain). So much so, as Sobsey (2006) points out, that the early tests for intellectual ability relied heavily on sensory discrimination tasks as well as notions of 'defects of vitality' and 'energy'. In his early account of autism, Bettelheim (1967) remarked that:

> Why these children are so unresponsive to physical pain is difficult to know. It is the more baffling because they seem to pay so little attention to the external world and to direct all their attention to themselves. Thus, ... they should be more sensitive to what comes from inside them, including pain, than are normal people. But actually, the opposite is true. (pp. 58–59)

The historical lack of scientific attention given to the issue of pain in children with I/DD may be, in part, due to longstanding cultural 'norms' and personal beliefs, held by some and reflected in Bettleheim's thinking, that people with I/DD do not feel pain (insensitive) or do not care about pain (indifferent) (Couston, 1954; Sobsey, 2006). From this perspective, it follows logically that pain thresholds among individuals with I/DD would be expected to be elevated. Further, this view would suggest that individuals with I/DD who experience noxious stimuli would have reduced pain sensation compared to comparable peers (age, gender) without disabilities experiencing the same degree of noxious stimulation. The problem with this view—which has persisted to the present in different forms (Malviya et al., 2005)—is that studies are rarely designed explicitly assessing the dimensions considered to be deficient (e.g. pain thresholds). As a consequence, there is a scientific vacuum concerning the state of our knowledge about sensory function in relation to pain experience among individuals with I/DD (see Defrin (2004) for an example of a threshold study specific to I/DD).

Considering the core definition of pain, the revision notwithstanding, there is a danger that the 'elevated thresholds' viewpoint (either pain insensitive and/or pain indifferent) as the only position regarding pain may persist for children with I/DD. This may be particularly true for those children with multiple impairments (intellectual, motor, communicative) resulting in severe or profound disability—because of the great difficulty in reliable access to a subjective state (Breau et al., 2003a; Symons et al., 2008). Caregivers and healthcare professionals often report that pain signs are ambiguous, paradoxical, altered, blunted, or that they confuse pain signs with stress or arousal (Oberlander and Symons, 2006). Although there is great heterogeneity within the population of children with I/DD and some individuals may experience altered pain sensation (similar to the general population), there is no current compelling reason to think that all children with I/DD would have such wholly affected nociceptive physiological systems. (We are aware of the fact that there are rare syndromes and conditions in which pain sensitivity is reduced or absent or that pain is sensed but the individual is indifferent to it (Nagasako et al., 2003).)

Epidemiology

Most children with I/DD have associated disabilities and chronic health conditions; the likelihood of these conditions increases with the severity of the disability, as does the frequency of painful procedures for diagnostic or therapeutic indications. There are several reasons that children with I/DD are at higher risk for experiencing recurrent pain than their peers without disability, including painful conditions associated with the underlying cause of the disability; higher rates of painful medical procedures; physical therapy regimens that might be painful; impaired cognitive or communication abilities, resulting in under-recognition or delay in recognition that the individual is experiencing pain; and nociceptive pain experienced for extended periods of time increasing the risk of developing neuropathic pain or other chronic pain states.

There is very limited scientific evidence describing the incidence or prevalence of pain among the general population of children with I/DD. In daily pain diaries recorded by parents of non-verbal children with severe cognitive impairments over 2 weeks (n = 34), 73% of the children had a painful experience on at least 1 day (Stallard et al., 2001) In a longitudinal study, children with moderate to profound ID (n = 94) were found to experience pain for an average of 9 h per week (Breau et al., 2003b). Most of the painful events were non-accidental and were not associated with medical procedures but were related to gastrointestinal or musculoskeletal problems. The limited available evidence supports a reasonable assumption that individuals with more significant impairments of cognition and communication are more vulnerable to experiencing painful events that are not recognized or adequately managed. For example, although a parent might recognize that the child is experiencing pain, the child might not be capable of providing key descriptive information regarding the location, type, or timing of the pain. Recurrent, pervasive pain experienced by these children can result in extensive suffering and limitation. For example, ongoing pain issues have been associated with sleep problems of both the child and the family (Breau and Camfield, 2011; Hemmingsson et al., 2009).

The population of children with I/DD is extremely heterogeneous with regard to underlying conditions, degree of disability, functional limitations, etc. It is not surprising, then, that the literature addressing pain prevalence among children with I/DD in recent years includes papers on specific disabilities. For example, in the single study exploring pain among children with spina bifida (n = 68), 49% reported experiencing pain weekly or more frequently (Clancy et al., 2005).

Down syndrome

From 40% to 60% of children with Down syndrome have congenital cardiac or intestinal anomalies requiring surgical intervention, and are therefore exposed to pain associated with major invasive procedures (Valkenburg et al., 2010). Later in life, children with Down syndrome are at risk for orthopaedic problems associated with pain. Quantitative sensory testing studies in adults with Down syndrome have shown that the response time to sensory stimuli is prolonged, localization is more difficult, and that adults with Down syndrome are possibly more sensitive to heat pain (Defrin et al., 2004; Hennequin et al., 2000).

Cerebral palsy

Recent population-based investigations place estimates of the prevalence of recurring pain among children with CP at between 50% and 75% (Doralp and Bartlett, 2010; Parkinson et al., 2010; Tüzün et al., 2010). The most common type of pain among children with CP is musculoskeletal pain. In addition, mobility limitations can result in secondary conditions that also cause significant pain, including pressure ulcers and constipation. The most common sites of pain include feet, legs, back, hips, hands, and arms (Engel et al., 2005). Children with CP often have low bone mineral density (attributable to limited weight-bearing, seizure medications, and other risk factors) which contributes to high fracture rates (Stevenson et al., 2006). It is important to note the heterogeneity of the population of children with CP, especially with regard to level of physical and cognitive limitations.

Although CP is often described in terms of motor impairments caused by anomalies in the brain, it is important to consider that the somatosensory system is also involved. The interplay between altered sensory functioning and pain experiences in individuals with CP has been increasingly recognized in a variety of conditions such as entrapment neuropathy (Frascarelli et al., 2005) or by applying sensory testing techniques (Riquelme and Montoya, 2010) or related approaches to investigating sensory issues (Riquelme et al., 2011). Although not all children with CP experience pain routinely, those who do are at risk for experiencing painful conditions through adulthood (Castle et al., 2007). With modern advances in medical management children with CP can be expected to live as long as their peers without disability (Strauss et al., 2007). The types of pain experienced in adulthood are likely to be associated with lifelong strain on muscles and joints (Turk, 2009).

Assessment

Reliably and validly assessing a complex construct like pain is fraught with challenges. There is no equivalent of a 'pain thermometer' and the difficulty of the task, already made difficult in a paediatric setting, is amplified in the presence of a cognitive, communicative, or motor impairment associated with I/DD. As such, the verbal and cognitive functioning relied on for self-report of pain is compromised. Part of the challenge is also in the varied nature of I/DD. There are multiple levels of cognitive functioning, verbal abilities, physical and motor impairments such that no one assessment approach fits for all children with I/DD. Further, there are often multiple people involved in the care of children with I/DD (e.g. parents, teachers, physicians, nurses, physical therapists, etc.) and so pain assessment and management may often be regarded as someone else's responsibility.

Self-report

Self-report is considered the 'gold standard' for pain assessment in other populations, however there is little evidence supporting its use with children with I/DD (Breau and Burkitt, 2009). For instance, Benini et al. (2004) taught children with I/DD on how to use self-report tools and then asked them to self-report on their own pain intensity and location following immunization. Despite having done well during training, only half of the children with I/DD were able to give consistent and accurate self-reports of their pain. Given the disparity between reporting pain during practice and during a real painful event, self-report is recommended to be used with great caution and in conjunction with other types of pain indicators (Breau and Burkitt, 2009; Breau et al., 2007).

Rating scales by proxy

To gain access to the pain condition when self-report has not proven reliable, observational methods have been used. Observational pain scales have been created based on measuring times when children are presumed to be in pain (e.g. during a needle stick, postoperative) versus times when children are not suspected to be in pain and examining behavioural cues that differ between the two conditions (Symons et al., 2008). A second approach has been to generate pain inventories or checklists based initially on interviews with caregivers that resulted in determining a list of pain cues. The initial lists are then reduced via item analysis and a rating scale is developed that in turn can be validated with different samples (Breau et al., 2002; Duivenvoorden et al., 2006; Hunt et al., 2004)

In multiple empirical studies there have been reports on the development of measurement tools that produce valid and reliable pain scores for children with I/DD (Breau et al., 2002; Hunt et al., 2004; Malviya et al., 2006). These measures focus on vocalizations, facial expression, physiological changes, and social changes. Each scale is unique (e.g. number of items, scoring method) but all share fundamentally similar pain descriptors. Three of the most promising paediatric pain measurement scales (NCCPC-R, PPP, r-FLACC) are reviewed in Table 16.1 (space precludes reviewing all relevant paediatric pain I/DD scales—see also Valkenburg et al. (2010) for a comprehensive scale review). It is important to acknowledge that it is sometimes difficult to distinguish pain from other responses such as fear, anxiety, sadness, or even contentment or excitement. Work continues with the emerging measurement tools to distinguish specific cues related to pain to provide a more clear understanding of when a child with I/DD may be experiencing pain. The scales have face validity, some empirical validity, and perhaps also clinical utility. All pain observation scales assess similar pain cues and all reviewed here have shown promising reliability and validity when used with children with I/DD (Breau et al., 2002; Hunt et al., 2004; Malviya et al., 2006). A different approach—used so far with adult samples with I/DD—developed by Bodfish et al. (2001; Phan et al., 2005) was to base the scoring of a scale on a standardized pain exam procedure. The most important choice particularly from a clinical perspective may not be *which* scale to use but rather to make a decision that pain *will be assessed* systematically and be aware that there are multiple measurement tools to choose from.

Treatment

Adequate pain management in children with I/DD is accomplished when one finds a balance between caring for the individual and seeing the broad picture of analgesic management and pain mechanisms. As already described, these children are more at risk to experience acute and chronic pain. Comorbidities can cause pain and their treatment can influence pain management. Caregivers in all disciplines should select the most appropriate and adequate pain management for the individual. Pain expression could be less apparent than in other children, but that is not necessarily a good reason to delay analgesia. Unfortunately, with the paucity of evidence on pain management in this heterogeneous population, the broad picture in terms of evidence-based practice is not yet very clear. The starting point should be treatment according to

Table 16.1 Sample paediatric pain assessment tools designed for intellectual and developmental disabilities

	Paediatric Pain Profile (PPP)	Non-Communicating Children's Pain Checklist-Revised (NCCPC-R)	Faces Legs Activity Cry Consolability Scale—Revised (r-FLACC)
Purpose	The purpose of the PPP is to provide an individualized measure for each child that is assessed. This scale is unique in that it asks caregivers to describe their child's good days and bad days	The purpose of the NCCPC-R is to provide one tool that is useful and accurate for all non-verbal children with IDD. The NCCPC-R quantifies pain responses observed by clinicians, parents, and caregivers regardless of how well they know the child. A postoperative version is available	The purpose of the r-FLACC is to provide a feasible method of quantifying an individual child's pain based on five domains and the specific criteria for scoring each of those domains. The original FLACC was revised to expand the descriptors for the subscales that were least reliable when used with children with IDD
Description of subscales and items	The PPP is a semi-individualized measure that allows caregivers to describe their child's behaviours related to pain. It also includes a 20-item questionnaires that is scored on a 0–3 scale	The NCCPC-R includes seven subscales (vocal, social, facial, activity, body and limbs, physiological, and eating/sleeping) each of which include multiple items that are scored from 0–3. There are a total of 30 items. The NCCPC postoperative version includes 27 of the same items but excludes the eating/sleeping subscale	The r-FLACC has five items (Face, Legs, Activity, Cry, Consolability) that are each scored from 0–2 based on the detailed descriptors specific to each item. The r-FLACC also provides caregivers the opportunity to write in other pain descriptors that may be unique to their child
Scale format	*Estimated time to complete:* 5–10 min *Scoring:* add item scores to determine a total score. The information written in by caregivers cannot be scored but provides valuable information specific to that child	*Estimated time to complete:* requires a 5–10-min observation period and <1 min to score. *Scoring:* item scores are added to determine the total score. A total score of 7 or greater indicates the child is in pain (accurate 77% of the time), and a score of 6 or less suggests the child does not have pain (accurate 84% of the time)	*Estimated time to complete:* 1–2 min *Scoring:* a total score of 0–3 is mild, 4–6 is moderate, and 7–10 is severe pain
Psychometric properties	*Sample used to test psychometric properties:* parents reported on 144 non-verbal children with various IDD (ages 1–18). The PPP is a valid, reliable, and sensitive measure for individual children; however, it does not provide generalizable measures across children because the information written in is unique to each child	*Sample used to test psychometric properties:* Caregivers of 71 non-verbal children with various IDD (ages 3–17). The NCCPC-R shows strong inter-rater reliability and internal consistency. This measure has also proved to have consistent scores over time. The NCCPC-R is sensitive and specific to pain and the scores are significantly related to parent pain rating	*Sample used to test psychometric properties:* 54 children ages 4–21 with various IDD pre and post surgery. The r-FLACC showed inter-rater reliability and test–retest reliability. The measure showed strong correlation between observer FLACC scores and a parent's global pain rating
Recommendations	The PPP is useful for distinguishing a child's good days from bad days and it is recommended for monitoring pain over time. Because the PPP provides the opportunity for parents to add detailed information about the child's unique pain expression, this scale may be especially beneficial for parents to complete and leave with healthcare professionals during a child's hospital stay	The NCCPC-R is recommended for use in research studies because it is a standardized scale that is consistent across children. The NCCPC-R has shown strong psychometric properties across multiple populations and settings and is consistently accurate. There is a required observation time that allows for more accurate assessment because observation is a key part of proxy assessment	The r-FLACC demonstrates clinical utility as it is fast and easy to use. It can be individualized for each child which is beneficial for children with unique pain signs. Because it is individualized it is more difficult to compare across children and to have a consistent pain score that serves to determine when a child is in pain or not
Where to obtain the scale	<http://www.ppprofile.org.uk>	<http://www.aboutkidshealth.ca/En/Documents/AKH_Breau_Everyday.pdf>	<http://deepblue.lib.umich.edu/bitstream/2027.42/72254/1/j.1460–9592.2005.01773.x.pdf>
References	Hunt et al. (2002)	Breau et al. (2002)	Malviya et al. (2006)

the WHO guidelines: by mouth, by the clock, and by the ladder (WHO, 1996, p. 36). For the perioperative setting, the American Society of Anesthesiologists published practice guidelines for acute pain management, with special recommendations for paediatric and cognitive impaired patients (2012).

Prospective randomized trials on analgesia in children with I/DD are scarce. Lower doses of intraoperative opioids have been observed (Koh et al. 2004; Long et al., 2009). Malviya et al. (2005) reported that 89% of the surveyed physicians had a tendency to prescribe subtherapeutic doses of analgesics in children with intellectual disability. However, less than 10% of surveyed anaesthetists report giving lower doses of intraoperative opioids in children with I/DD (Valkenburg et al., 2012b). From these observational studies it is clear that it can be challenging to provide adequate analgesia in this heterogeneous population, there are concerns about the risk of side effects and toxicity, and so far there is no proper evidence for dosing analgesia in these children.

On the positive side, the development of the pain assessment tools for children with I/DD (reviewed earlier) and the establishment of pharmacological research in children will make it feasible to start with pharmacokinetic and pharmacodynamic studies specific to children with I/DD that, in turn, will provide evidence for decision aids to manage their pain (Valkenburg et al., 2012a). Walker advocates that pain management is more than the measurement of pain intensity; it should include a global assessment of inter-related current conditions and general health, nature of the surgery (if relevant), prior pain experience, current response to analgesia in terms of efficacy, and side effects (Walker, 2012).

Pharmacokinetics

In general, children with I/DD are at greater risk to develop side effects (Reiss, 1997), but epidemiological data are missing. Case–control studies have shown that children and adults with Down syndrome are at increased risk to develop side effects and toxicity when treated with paracetamol (Griener et al., 1990) or methotrexate (Buitenkamp et al., 2010). After inhalational induction with sevoflurane, bradycardia and hypotension occurred in 57% of the children with Down syndrome versus in 12% of the children without Down syndrome (Kraemer et al., 2010). From observational clinical studies it is clear that there is variability in the dosing of analgesics and there is a high prevalence of comorbidities and treatment with psychotropic and anticonvulsant drugs in children with I/DD (Valkenburg et al., 2010).

For adequate pain management, it would be ideal to predict the pharmacokinetics (what the body does to a drug) and pharmacodynamics (what the drug does to the body) of the analgesics for the individual patient. It would mean that we have knowledge of the pharmacokinetic covariate effects (size, age, and organ function) as well as pharmacodynamic covariate effects (target organ perfusion, receptor sensitivity, efficacy, pharmacogenomic changes). As a group, children with I/DD are at risk for variability in both the pharmacokinetics and pharmacodynamics, due to, for example, the use of antiepileptic drugs, cerebral pathology, and genetic abnormalities such as trisomy 21. It will be a challenge to focus pharmacokinetic and pharmacodynamic studies on the drugs with the highest priority and the groups of children that are the most at risk for polypharmacy and side effects, but understanding of the factors that contribute to variability will help to individualize pain management.

Antiepileptic drugs

Epilepsy is common among children with I/DD; incidence rates from 14% to 79% have been reported (Beavis et al., 2007). The more severe and extensive the cerebral pathology, the greater is the risk for epilepsy. Different antiepileptic drugs have varying degrees of protein binding and (liver) enzyme induction (Kofke, 2010). Chronic treatment with antiepileptic drugs can affect also the pharmacokinetics of other drugs that are metabolized by the same (P450) enzymatic pathway. This could be an explanation for the finding that patients treated with antiepileptic drugs required higher doses of fentanyl during general anaesthesia (Tempelhof et al., 1990). A survey among Dutch anaesthesiologists revealed that around 75% adjust the dose of anaesthetic drugs in children treated with antiepileptic drugs (Valkenburg et al., 2012b). The interaction between antiepileptic drugs and analgesics as well as general anaesthetic drugs needs further attention.

Pain treatment in cerebral palsy

A key component of pain management in individuals with CP is the reduction of muscle spasticity that contributes to musculoskeletal pain. A variety of therapeutic modalities are used to relieve pain associated with muscle spasticity (Aisen et al., 2011; Roscigno, 2002). Oral antispasticity medications include baclofen, dantrolene, diazepam, and tizanidine. Baclofen can also be delivered intrathecally by an implanted pump. Botulinum toxin A is used through multiple injections made to targeted muscle groups, after local anaesthesia with EMLA® and procedural sedation or under general anaesthesia (depending on location of injection, number of muscle groups to be treated, age, comorbidities and previous experiences). The toxin's inhibition of the release of acetylcholine at the neuromuscular synapse results in relief of spasticity that lasts 3 to 4 months—and for some individuals there is corresponding pain reduction. Through neurosurgery selective dorsal rhizotomy involves the cutting of sensory nerves to reduce muscle spasms (Grunt et al., 2011). A randomized controlled trial in 27 children with CP showed that epidural analgesia can give better analgesia and less muscle spasms after selective dorsal rhizotomy than intravenous morphine infusions (Malviya et al., 1999). Non-pharmacological interventions including massage and other interventions are widely reported as effective in relieving pain and promoting comfort (Glew et al., 2010), though there has been little research-based evidence demonstrating these benefits.

Physical therapy

In addition to ID, many children with I/DD have a physical disability. CP causes motor disorders such as an altered muscle tone, impaired postural control, and muscle synergetic action (Martin et al., 2010). Motor development is often delayed in children with Down syndrome and they are at high risk for musculoskeletal disorders due to joint hypermobility and ligamentous laxity (Weijerman and de Winter, 2010). Physical therapy treatment goals are aimed at improving muscle strength, range of motion, gross motor function, endurance, and overall quality of life including pain reduction (Martin et al., 2010; Opheim et al., 2011). A survey among American physical therapists revealed that 80% of the respondents used pain assessment tools in children with I/DD. Distraction, procedural talk, and praise were the most used pain management techniques (Swiggum et al., 2010). Physical therapy will be used to treat and prevent pain from musculoskeletal disorders, but the therapy can be painful itself. Pain reduction should be evaluated over the course of physical therapy sessions and moderate to severe procedural pain should be treated.

Conclusion

Moving forward, the clinical and scientific agenda is clear—to continue to leverage discoveries from basic and clinical pain research and apply them to solve the problem of pain for children with I/DD.

The remarkable achievements in pain scale development in the last decade for communicatively and cognitively compromised individuals needs to be converted to demonstrations that pain is being more effectively and efficiently identified and managed in healthcare, rehabilitative, educational, and home environments.

Children with I/DD have been found to have a prevalence of chronic pain as high as 73%; this compares with recent estimates that approximately 33% of children in the general population experience chronic pain (Peterson et al., 2006; Roth-Isigkeit et al., 2004). Pain assessment is particularly challenging when encountering the array of individual cognitive and communication patterns found among children with I/DD. Early recognition and accurate assessment of pain is essential to prevent the development of pain syndromes resulting from untreated nociceptive pain. A broad array of instruments are available to support better pain management, and it is time for these instruments to be incorporated into randomized controlled trials and pharmacokinetic/pharmacodynamic studies in children with I/DD.

The notion of 'altered neural substrates' has only recently begun to be addressed (de Knegt and Scherder, 2011). At issue here is whether some point along the pain neuroaxis is compromised depending on the nature of the neural impairment leading to the intellectual or developmental disability. Although the specific brain pathophysiology underlying the myriad subgroups of I/DD is not often known, it may be reasonable to speculate on how known processing problems associated with some I/DDs and their neural correlates could affect pain (transduction, transmission, etc.). One reasonable framework could be to consider the three classic pain dimensions (sensory–discriminative, affective–motivational, cognitive–evaluative) as a way to organize imaging and neuropsychological assessment findings from different I/DD syndromes to consider whether specific features of pain processing are disrupted and whether the disruption co-varies with specific neurocognitive features of the I/DD. One pragmatic outcome of such an approach would be to broaden current approaches to pain assessment and management in the I/DD population beyond 'nociceptive' only pain (sensory-discriminative features) and push HCPs to consider relevant motivational, affective, and cognitive factors as well.

Clearly, there remains much work to be done. The weight of the (limited) evidence (provided, in part, by the scales developed during the last decade) suggests that children with I/DD have been subject to practices and procedures with little regard for their ability to experience or express pain. We need to continue to refine behavioural methods for the assessment of pain intensity, along with a measurement framework that can account for and predict the individual pain trajectory/course over time. More objective methods such as quantitative sensory testing (QST) might hold promise for the assessment of pain in children with I/DD, although modifications of these methods are needed to adapt to individuals not capable of cooperating with a standard QST protocol. In addition to cognitive and communication limitations, many other biopsychosocial factors are likely to contribute to inadequate pain management in this population, for example: atypical responses to treatment, polypharmacy, chronic pain conditions, repeated surgical intervention, genetic abnormalities, altered stress/arousal responses. Better specification of such variability will aid clinicians in developing pain management plans tailored to the needs of the individual child.

Research studies involving such a heterogeneous population must specify with as much detail as possible the specific features of study subjects with I/DD. When possible, evaluations of levels of cognitive and communicative functioning would be preferable to blanket characterizations (e.g. verbal versus non-verbal). Better specification of I/DD related features would permit more accurate determination of how these variables interact with the main phenomena—some aspect of pain—under investigation. Trials should be developed and designed in accordance with recent consensus statements from the IMMPACT group further bringing in line results from studies with children with I/DD with other paediatric pain trials (McGrath et al., 2008). The Initiative on Methods, Measurement, and Pain Assessment in Clinical Trials (IMMPACT—a recurring internationally-recognized consensus group of pain experts from academia, government agencies, the pharmaceutics industry, and self-help organizations) recommended a number of core pain outcome domains including: (1) pain intensity, (2) physical functioning, and (3) ratings of overall improvement. There is no reason that paediatric pain outcomes research focusing on children with I/DD cannot incorporate the same core outcome domains.

Case example: paediatric chronic pain I/DD case presentation

KL is a young girl (3 years, 6 months) with a past medical history significant for prenatal CMV (cytomegalovirus) exposure with resultant CP, spastic quadriparesis GMFCS (gross motor function classification system) class V, static encephalopathy, global developmental delay, intractable epilepsy, restrictive lung disease, disordered sleep, and cortical visual impairment who presents to clinic with a chief complaint of persistent distressing symptoms. The family has concerns that every 7 to 10 days, KL will have 2 to 3 days of increased crying, irritability, and discomfort. They state they have tried many medications including hydroxyzine, methadone, diazepam, oxycodone, ibuprofen, and acetaminophen. Of all the modalities the father states that ibuprofen and acetaminophen seem to be what gives the best relief; however, this is very transient. The day before some of these spells KL will usually be less engaged and they sense that she is 'winding up'. She will then have increasing amounts of 'whining' at which time they will administer ibuprofen or an extra dose of methadone. She will then enter an inconsolable crying spell where she will wake up and generally be crying all day and take a nap at 14.00. They can tell when KL is in pain as they have been using the TOPS scale and have been very adept at knowing when she is in distress. Additionally, the family states that when she is in one of these spells her heart rate is typically in the 170s and will stay there even when appearing calm. They state that there has been no major change in bowel or bladder function. They also do have concerns that she is hypertensive during these episodes. They feel as if some of these events can be precipitated by major temperature changes, which can cause her to 'lose it'. Additionally, they note an association with bowel or bladder discomfort that seems to 'set her off'.

Clinical decision-making

After reviewing the past medical history with the family, we worked with the notion that a significant amount of KL's distress was likely secondary to her underlying neurological insult with resultant autonomic dysfunction, exacerbated by pain, discomfort, temperature swings, and bowel and bladder dysfunction. The initial intervention included treatment of the underlying autonomic dysfunction with optimized doses of gabapentin and cyproheptadine. Additionally, KL was weaned off of her scheduled methadone. Finally, we offered the following 'rescue plan' protocol when KL was experiencing an exacerbation of her distressing symptoms:

a. Administer acetaminophen and ibuprofen in combination (180 mg and 120 mg respectively) via gastrostomy tube every 6 h as needed for pain or fever.

b. If no effect in 30 min may administer diphenhydramine 12.5 mg via gastrostomy tube every 6 h as needed for agitation.

c. If no effect in 30 min may administer diazepam 4 mg via gastrostomy tube every 6 h as needed for severe agitation.

d. If no effect within 30 min, may administer propranolol 3 mg via gastrostomy tube every 6 h as needed for autonomic storming.

Clinical outcomes

On 1-month follow-up, family had been able to enjoy positive changes in KL, including sleeping through the night. They stated that her irritability does continue, but it is intermittent, as opposed to constant, within the day. Most episodes during the day occur early in the evening, usually beginning at 18.00, and ending by 21.00. This was an improvement from the all-day 07.00 to 21.00 inconsolable crying. The family also notes that the 'rescue plan' has been working well at night-time; however, when tried during the day, it does not appear as effective. They state that overall they feel that KL appears more comfortable, she is more aware of her surroundings, and engaged at times when not irritable.

Based on this feedback, we further optimized her cyproheptadine and adjusted her protocol as follows:

a. Administer acetaminophen and ibuprofen in combination (180 mg and 120 mg, respectively) via gastrostomy tube every 6 h as needed for pain or fever.

b. If no effect in 30 min, may administer to give diazepam 4 mg via gastrostomy tube every 6 h as needed for severe agitation.

c. If no effect in 20 to 30 min, may administer diphenhydramine 12.5 mg via gastrostomy tube every 6 h as needed for agitation.

d. If no effect, may administer propranolol 3 mg via gastrostomy tube every 6 h as needed for autonomic storming.

e. If no effect, may administer oxycodone 1.5 mg via gastrostomy tube every 6 h as needed for severe pain.

The 3-month follow-up revealed significantly improved symptoms and KL and her family were able to enjoy many symptom-free days with flare-ups treated by employing the 'rescue plan' protocol.

Clinical issues

KL's distressing symptoms required both an extensive daily maintenance plan (cyproheptadine and gabapentin) as well as a 'rescue plan' protocol that could be administered by the family during flares. Educating and empowering the family while ensuring a plan that can be successful in the home was critical to the continued success in KL's comfort.

References

Aisen, M. L., Kerkovich, D., Mast, J., Mulroy, S., Wren, T. A. L., Kay, R. M., et al. (2011). Cerebral palsy: clinical care and neurological rehabilitation. *Lancet Neurol*, 10(9), 844–852.

American Association on Intellectual and Developmental Disabilities. (2012). American Association on Intellectual and Developmental Disabilities website. Available at: <http://www.aaidd.org> (accessed 15 February 2012).

American Society of Anesthesiologists. (2012). Practice guidelines for acute pain management in the perioperative setting: an updated report by the American Society of Anesthesiologists Task Force on Acute Pain Management. *Anesthesiology*, 116(2), 248–273.

Beavis, J., Kerr, M., and Marson, A. G. (2007). Pharmacological interventions for epilepsy in people with intellectual disabilities. *Cochrane Database Syst Rev*, 3, CD005399.

Benini, F., Trapanotto, M., Gobber, D., Agosto, C., Carli, G., Drigo, P., et al. (2004). Evaluating pain induced by venipuncture in pediatric patients with developmental delay. *Clin J Pain*, 20(3), 156–163.

Bettelheim, B. (1967). *The empty fortress: infantile autism and the birth of the self.* New York: Free Press.

Bodfish, J., Harper, V., Deacon, J., and Symons, F. (2001). *Identifying and measuring pain in persons with developmental disabilities: a manual for the Pain and Discomfort Scale (PADS).* Morganton, NC: Western Carolina Center Research Report.

Breau, L. M. and Burkitt, C. (2009). Assessing pain in children with intellectual disabilities. *Pain Res Manag*, 14(2), 116–120.

Breau, L. M. and Camfield, C. S. (2011). Pain disrupts sleep in children and youth with intellectual and developmental disabilities. *Res Dev Disabil*, 32(6), 2829–2840.

Breau, L. M., Camfield, C. S., McGrath, P. J. and Finley, G.A. (2007). Pain's impact on adaptive functioning. *J Intell Disabil Res*, 51(2), 125–134,

Breau, L. M., Camfield, C. S., McGrath, P. J., and Finley, G. A. (2003b). The incidence of pain in children with severe cognitive impairments. *Arch Pediatr Adolesc Med*, 157(12), 1219–1226.

Breau, L. M., Finley, G. A., McGrath, P. J., and Camfield, C. S. (2002). Validation of the Non-communicating Children's Pain Checklist-Postoperative Version. *Anesthesiology*, 96(3), 528–535.

Breau, L. M., MacLaren, J., McGrath, P. J., Camfield, C. S., and Finley, G. A. (2003a). Caregivers' beliefs regarding pain in children with cognitive impairment: relation between pain sensation and reaction increases with severity of impairment. *Clin J Pain*, 19(6), 335–344.

Buitenkamp, T. D., Mathôt, R. A., de Haas, V., Pieters, R., and Zwaan, C. M. (2010). Methotrexate-induced side effects are not due to differences in pharmacokinetics in children with Down syndrome and acute lymphoblastic leukemia. *Haematologica*, 95(7), 1106–1113.

Castle, K., Imms, C., and Howie, L. (2007). Being in pain: a phenomenological study of young people with cerebral palsy. *Dev Med Child Neurol*, 49(6), 445–449.

Clancy, C. A., McGrath, P. J., and Oddson, B. E. (2005). Pain in children and adolescents with spina bifida. *Dev Med Child Neurol*, 47(1), 27–34.

Couston, T. (1954). Indifference to pain in low-grade mental defectives. *Br Med J*, 1(4871), 1128–1129.

Defrin, R., Carmeli, E., and Pick, C. G. (2004). Behavioral indices of pain and pain threshold measurement in individuals with mental retardation. *Pain*, 110(3), 767–769.

Defrin, R., Pick, C. G., Peretz, C., and Carmeli, E. (2004). A quantitative somatosensory testing of pain threshold in individuals with mental retardation. *Pain*, 108(1–2), 58–66.

Doralp, S. and Bartlett, D. J. (2010). The prevalence, distribution, and effect of pain among adolescents with cerebral palsy. *Pediatr Phys Ther*, 22(1), 26–33.

Duivenvoorden, H. J., Tibboel, D., Koot, H. M., van Dijk, M., and Peters, J. W. 2006). Pain assessment in profound cognitive impaired children using the Checklist Pain Behavior; is item reduction valid? *Pain*, 126(1–3), 147–154.

Engel, J. M., Petrina, T. J., Dudgeon, B. J., and McKearnan, K. A. (2005). Cerebral palsy and chronic pain: a descriptive study of children and adolescents. *Phys Occup Ther Pediatr*, 25(4), 73–84.

Frascarelli, M., Frascarelli, F., Gentile, M. G., Serrao, M., De Santis, F., Pierelli, F., *et al.* (2005). Entrapment neuropathy in patients with spastic cerebral palsy. *Acta Neurol Scand*, 112(3), 178–182.

Glew, G. M., Fan, M. Y., Hagland, S., Bjornson, K., Beider, S., and McLaughlin, J. F. (2010). Survey of the use of massage for children with cerebral palsy. *Int J Ther Massage Bodywork*, 3(4), 10–15.

Griener, J., Msall, M., and Cooke, R. (1990). Noninvasive determination of acetaminophen disposition in Down's syndrome. *Clin Pharmacol Ther*, 48, 520–528.

Grunt, S., Becher, J. G., and Vermeulen, R. J. (2011). Long-term outcome and adverse effects of selective dorsal rhizotomy in children with cerebral palsy: a systematic review. *Dev Med Child Neurol*, 53(6), 490–498.

Hemmingsson, H., Stenhammar, A.M., and Paulsson, K. (2009). Sleep problems and the need for parental night-time attention in children with physical disabilities. *Child Care Health Dev*, 35(1), 89–95.

Hunt, A., Goldman, A., Seers, K., Crichton, N., Mastroyannopoulou, K., Moffat, V., *et al.* (2004). Clinical validation of the paediatric pain profile. *Dev Med Child Neurol*, 46(01), 9–18.

International Association for the Scientific Study of Intellectual Disability. (2012). *Frequently asked questions.* Available at: <https://www.iassid.org/about-iassid/frequently-asked-questions> (accessed 17 July 2012).

International Association for the Study of Pain. (2012). International Association for the Study of Pain website. Available at: <http://www.iasp-pain.org> (accessed 15 February 2012).

de Knegt N., and Scherder E. (2011). Pain in adults with intellectual disabilities. Pain, 152(5), 971–974.

Kofke, W. A. (2010). Anesthetic management of the patient with epilepsy or prior seizures. *Curr Opin Anaesthesiol*, 23(3), 391–399.

Koh, J. L., Fanurik, D., Dale Harrison, R., Schmitz, M. L., and Norvell, D. (2004). Analgesia following surgery in children with and without cognitive impairment. *Pain*, 111(3), 239–244.

Kraemer, F. W., Stricker, P. A., Gurnaney, H. G., McClung, H., Meador, M. R., Sussman, E., *et al.* (2010). Bradycardia during induction of anesthesia with sevoflurane in children with Down syndrome. *Anesth Analg*, 111(5), 1259–1263.

Long, L. S., Ved, S., and Koh, J. L. (2009). Intraoperative opioid dosing in children with and without cerebral palsy. *Pediatr Anesth*, 19(5), 513–520.

Malviya, S., Voepel-Lewis, T., Burke, C., Merkel, S., and Tait, A. R. (2006). The revised FLACC observational pain tool: improved reliability and validity for pain assessment in children with cognitive impairment. *Pediatr Anesth*, 16(3), 258–265.

Malviya, S., Voepel-Lewis, T., Merkel, S., and Tait, A. R. (2005). Difficult pain assessment and lack of clinician knowledge are ongoing barriers to effective pain management in children with cognitive impairment. *Acute Pain*, 7(1), 27–32.

Malviya, S., Pandit, U. A., Merkel, S., Voepel-Lewis, T., Zang, L., Siewert, M., *et al.* (1999). A comparison of continuous epidural infusion and intermittent intravenous bolus doses of morphine in children undergoing selective dorsal rhizotomy. *Region Anesth Pain Med*, 24(5), 438–443.

Martin, L., Baker, R., and Harvey, A. (2010). A systematic review of common physiotherapy interventions in school-aged children with cerebral palsy. *Phys Occup Ther Pediatr*, 30(4), 294–312.

McGrath, P. J., Walco, G. A., Turk, D. C., Dworkin, R. H., Brown, M. T., Davidson, K., *et al.* (2008). Core outcome domains and measures for pediatric acute and chronic/recurrent pain clinical trials: PedIMMPACT recommendations. *J Pain*, 9(9), 771–783.

Merskey, H. and Bogduk, N. (1994). *Classification of chronic pain, IASP Task Force on Taxonomy*. Seattle, WA: IASP Press.

Nagasako, E. M., Oaklander, A. L., and Dworkin, R. H. (2003). Congenital insensitivity to pain: an update. *Pain*, 101(3), 213–220.

Oberlander, T. F. and Symons, F. J. (2006). *Pain in children and adults with developmental disabilities*. Baltimore, MD: Paul H Brookes Publishing.

Opheim, A., Jahnsen, R., Olsson, E., and Stanghelle, J. K. (2011). Physical and mental components of health-related quality of life and musculoskeletal pain sites over seven years in adults with spastic cerebral palsy. *J Rehabil Med*, 43(5), 382–387.

Parkinson, K., Gibson, L., Dickinson, H., and Colver, A. (2010). Pain in children with cerebral palsy: a cross-sectional multicentre European study. *Acta Paediatr*, 99(3), 446–451.

Phan, A., Edwards, C. L., and Robinson, E. L. (2005). The assessment of pain and discomfort in individuals with mental retardation. *Res Dev Disabil*, 26(5), 433–439.

Reiss, S., and Aman, M. G. (1997). The international consensus process on psychopharmacology and intellectual disability. *J Intell Disab Res* 41(6), 448–455.

Roscigno, C. I. (2002). Addressing spasticity-related pain in children with spastic cerebral palsy. *J Neurosci Nurs*, 34(3), 123–133.

Roth-Isigkeit, A., Thyen, U., Raspe, H., Stöven, H., and Schmucker, P. (2004). Reports of pain among German children and adolescents: an epidemiological study. *Acta Paediatr*, 93(2), 258–263.

Salvador-Carulla L., Reed, G. M., Vaez-Azizi, L. M., Cooper, S. A., Martinez-Leal, R., Bertelli M., *et al.* (2011). Intellectual developmental disorders: towards a new name, definition and framework for 'mental retardation/intellectual disability' in ICD-11. *World Psychiatry*, 10(3), 175–80.

Salvador-Carulla, L. and Saxena, S. (2009. Intellectual disability: between disability and clinical nosology. *Lancet*, 374(9704), 1798–1799.

Schiavenato, M. and Craig, K. D. (2010). Pain assessment as a social transaction: beyond the 'gold standard'. *Clin J Pain*, 26(8), 667–676.

Sobsey, D. (2006). Pain and disability in an ethical and social context. In T. F. Oberlander and F. J. Symons (eds) *Pain in children and adults with developmental disabilities*, pp. 19–39. Baltimore, MD: Paul H Brookes Publishing.

Stallard, P., Williams, L., Lenton, S., and Velleman, R. (2001). Pain in cognitively impaired, non-communicating children. *Arch Dis Child*, 85(6), 460–462.

Stevenson, R., Conaway, M., Barrington, J., Cuthill, S., Worley, G., and Henderson, R. (2006). Fracture rate in children with cerebral palsy. *Pediatr Rehabil*, 9(4), 396–403.

Strauss, D., Shavelle, R., Reynolds, R., Rosenbloom, L., and Day, S. (2007). Survival in cerebral palsy in the last 20 years: signs of improvement? *Dev Med Child Neurol*, 49(2), 86.

Swiggum, M., Hamilton, M. L., Gleeson, P., and Roddey, T. (2010). Pain in children with cerebral palsy: implications for Pediatr Phys Ther, 22(1), 86–92.

Symons, F. J., Shinde, S. K., and Gilles, E. (2008). Perspectives on pain and intellectual disability. *J Intell Disab Res*, 52(Pt 4), 275–286.

Turk, M. A. (2009). Health, mortality, and wellness issues in adults with cerebral palsy. *Devel Med Child Neurol*, 51, 24–29.

Tüzün, E. H., Guven, D. K., and Eker, L. (2010). Pain prevalence and its impact on the quality of life in a sample of Turkish children with cerebral palsy. *Disabil Rehab*, 32(9), 723–728.

Valkenburg, A., van Dijk, M., de Leeuw, T., Meeussen, C., Knibbe, C., and Tibboel, D. (2012a). Anaesthesia and postoperative analgesia in surgical neonates with or without Down's syndrome: is it really different? *Br J Anaesth*, 108(2), 295–301.

Valkenburg, A. J., van der Kreeft, S. M., de Leeuw, T. G., Stolker, R. J., Tibboel, D., and van Dijk, M. (2012b). Pain management in intellectually disabled children: a survey of perceptions and current practices among Dutch anesthesiologists. *Pediatr Anesth*, 22(7), 682–689.

Valkenburg, A. J., van Dijk, M., de Klein, A., van den Anker, J. N., and Tibboel, D. (2010). Pain management in intellectually disabled children:

assessment, treatment, and translational research. *Dev Disabil Res Rev*, 16(3), 248–257.

Walker, S. M. (2012). Perioperative care of neonates with Down's syndrome: should it be different? *Br J Anaesth*, 108(2), 177–179.

Weijerman, M. E., and de Winter, J. P. (2010). Clinical practice: the care of children with Down syndrome. *Eur J Pediatr*, 169(12), 1445–1452.

World Health Organization. (1996) *Cancer pain relief: with a guide to opioid availability* (2nd edn). Geneva: World Health Organization.

World Health Organization. (2001). *International classification of functioning, disability, and health*. Geneva. World Health Organization.

CHAPTER 17

Paediatric cancer pain

Jennifer Hickman, Jaya Varadarajan, and Steven J. Weisman

Introduction

The publication of the World Health Organization (WHO)'s monograph *Cancer Pain Relief* in 1990 may be one of the groundbreaking events in the advancement of treatment for cancer pain (WHO, 1990). A result of this work was the first published guideline for the treatment of cancer pain in children (Berde et al., 1990; McGrath et al., 1990; Zeltzer et al., 1990). Since that time, several other guidelines and monographs have been published which provide very useful frameworks for the treatment of cancer pain (Anonymous, 1996; Benedetti et al., 2000; Miaskowski et al., 2004).

Although the incidence of childhood cancer has remained relatively stable over the last 35 years, the survival rate has increased dramatically. In 1975, approximately 14.7/100 000 children from 0 to 19 years were diagnosed with cancer (Howlader et al., 2012). Although the overall incidence did rise slightly to 17.0/100 000, mortality rate has decreased from 5.4/100 000 to 2.5/100 000 per year. In addition, the 5-year survival rates for paediatric cancer have improved from 61.7% to 83.1% between 1975 to 1977 and 2002 to 2008. Certain types of paediatric malignancy now have survival rates near or above 90% at 5 years (Hodgkin's lymphoma, 96.9%; Wilms' tumour 89.8%; and acute lymphoblastic leukaemia (ALL) 88.7%). These remarkable survival statistics have not come without a heavy burden and price. As described later in this chapter, these children have multiple challenges to overcome when exposed to aggressive treatments that include complex and repetitive surgeries, chemotherapeutic and radiation treatment regimens, and bone marrow transplantation.

As exemplified in the following case example, each patient seems to follow a unique trajectory and, for the pain clinician, will present unique challenges that require agility and flexibility to design satisfactory pain treatment protocols. Using a systematic approach that encompasses the notion that pain in paediatric cancer is usually the result of multiple intersecting causes will usually provide satisfactory results for the patients and their watchdog families supervising their care. For the continually decreasing numbers of children who cannot survive their disease, our palliative care colleagues can continue multimodal pain management in conjunction with their pain management resources to ensure a dignified and comfortable end of life.

Case example

A 9-year-old boy with high-functioning autism was hospitalized for a several-week history of low grade fevers, progressive fatigue, pharyngitis, night sweats, and diffuse lymphadenopathy. Workup revealed an elevated white cell count and led to a diagnosis of high-risk acute myelocytic leukaemia.

He received three courses of induction chemotherapy and was in remission after the first course. Given his poor prognosis he was slated for an unrelated bone marrow transplant (BMT). His post-transplant course was complicated by pseudomonas bacteraemia, G-tube site infection, steroid-induced hypertension, sinusitis, mucositis, neutropenia, and high fevers suggestive of graft-versus-host disease (GVHD), eventually resulting in non-engraftment and rejection. He required multiple visits to the operating room for maxillary sinus taps and irrigations. He was treated with methylprednisolone, and then received a second haploidentical bone marrow transplant from his mother. He developed serum sickness with anti-thymocyte globulin and GVHD of the skin, needing immune suppression. His prolonged hospital course was further complicated by streptococcal viridans bacteraemia, viraemia, haemorrhagic cystitis, respiratory syncytial virus upper respiratory infection requiring ribavirin therapy, *Clostridium difficile* enterocolitis, feeding issues requiring enteral and total parenteral nutrition, episodic premature atrial contractions, intermittent prolonged QT syndrome, constipation, pancreatitis, hyperglycaemia, seizures, and chronic pain. Many of these issues were complications of therapy for his primary illness, but some were related to medications used for pain, insomnia, and mood. He was discharged after 7 months in the hospital.

Almost 2 years after his initial diagnosis, the patient's condition seemed to stabilize and his physical symptoms began to improve. He remained in remission, continued to be transfusion-dependent, but with no further evidence of GVHD. He was taken off systemic immunosuppression 3 years after BMT. He was able to wean a number of his medications and returned to school in a special education programme. As part of his recovery, he enrolled in a therapeutic riding programme and won the Child Equestrian Award 2 years ago. He is still considered high risk for secondary malignancies and is screened yearly.

Aetiologies and characteristics of pain in cancer

Pain is one of the most prevalent symptoms in cancer (Collins et al., 2000; Ljungman et al., 1999; Miser et al., 1987a, 1987b). Pain in cancer can be a direct result of the disease, but it is largely due to cancer treatments or the combined long-term effects of both. The aetiologies of disease-related pain include bone pain from metastases or infiltration of tissues, somatic pain from solid tumours, visceral pain, and neuropathic pain (Box 17.1).

Treatment-related pain can be the result of chemotherapy, radiation therapy, acute and chronic postoperative pain, graft-versus-host disease, or procedure-related pain (Box 17.2).

Pain from bone marrow infiltration, primary malignant bone tumours, and metastases

About a third of childhood cancers are leukaemias, the most common being ALL. Along with cancers of the central nervous system (CNS) they make up more than half of childhood cancers (Howlader et al., 2012). The rapid growth of leukemic blast cells from leukemic infiltration in the bone marrow results in diffuse bone pain. Pain from primary or metastatic bone disease is somatic in nature. It is often described as being 'aching'

Box 17.1 Disease-related cancer pain

- Bone marrow infiltration (leukaemia, metastatic tumours)
- Visceral pain (invasion, obstruction, compression, bleeding)
- Somatic pain (rhabdomyosarcoma, osteosarcoma, Ewing's sarcoma, leukaemia)
- Neuropathic pain (neural compression/invasion, brain/spinal cord tumours).

Box 17.2 Treatment-related cancer pain

- Medical procedures
- Acute postoperative
- Chronic postoperative: phantom limb, radiculopathies
- Chemotherapy:
  - Mucositis
  - Neuropathic
  - Extravasation burns
- Radiation therapy:
  - Mucositis
  - Skin burns
  - Local tissue injury
- Graft-versus-host disease
- Infection.

---

or 'gnawing' in nature in children who are able to communicate. The clinical presentation varies depending on the age of the child and the bones affected. Very young children, who are unable to communicate their pain, may present with a limp or an inability to walk. Children who have recently started walking may actually demonstrate regression in motor function. An older child, who is able to communicate, might report diffuse pain all over the body that is difficult to localize. Adolescents may localize the pain to a specific long bone and might mistakenly attribute it to a sports-related injury, thus delaying diagnosis and treatment. Cortical thinning could result in a pathological fracture with localized pain at the site. Treatment then would involve treatment of both the primary illness and its sequelae.

Malignant bone tumours such as osteosarcoma and Ewing's sarcoma can cause significant pain in the paediatric cancer patient. Direct tumour invasion causes bone pain from destruction of the normal trabecular bone pattern while periosteal new bone formation causes soft tissue inflammation and, in turn, pain. The bone pain from these processes is often severe and requires multimodal therapy. Solid tumours such as neuroblastoma can metastasize to both bone marrow and long bones. Its bone pain can be similar to that in the leukaemias.

Treatment of the primary cancer is the most effective method for managing cancer pain. In younger patients with leukaemia, decrease in the leukaemic burden following chemotherapy results in dramatic improvement of bone pain. Adolescents may be more challenging to treat due to more resistant disease, and require consistent analgesia. Local radiation therapy can also cause a reduction in bony pain. This will often be employed for palliation in situations where primary treatment has failed. Pharmacological treatment involves administration of opioids, often as continuous infusions or using patient- (PCA) or parent/nurse-controlled analgesia (PNCA). Adjuvant analgesics are also often employed. It is important to consider that in patients with bone marrow infiltration, there is often concomitant bone marrow suppression with thrombocytopenia. Use of non-steroidal anti-inflammatory drugs (NSAIDs) can therefore place these patients at risk for bleeding from both quantitative and qualitative platelet defects.

Neuropathic pain

Neuropathic pain is the result of tumour compression or infiltration of peripheral nerves or the spinal cord. Direct injury to a nerve can also occur with soft tissue tumours in compartmental areas, such as with Ewing's sarcoma or rhabdomyosarcoma arising in the pelvis. Neuropathic pain can also occur as a result of inflammation of a nerve root from malignancy or infection. Reactivation of a herpes zoster infection can occur in the immune-compromised cancer patient causing neuropathic pain. Cancer treatment is a common cause of neuropathic pain. Vincristine is one of the chemotherapeutic agents known to cause neurotoxicity.

The pathognomonic feature of neuropathic pain is dysaesthesia, with or without a 'burning' quality to the pain. Patients may also complain of 'electrical' pain, paroxysmal, brief 'shooting' or 'stabbing' pain, or allodynia and hyperpathia. Neuropathic pain can be challenging to treat. Medications used include the adjuvant drugs such as tricyclic antidepressants, neuromodulators such as gabapentin, and local anaesthetics. Natural antidepressants such as St John's wort have also been used but with limited data on

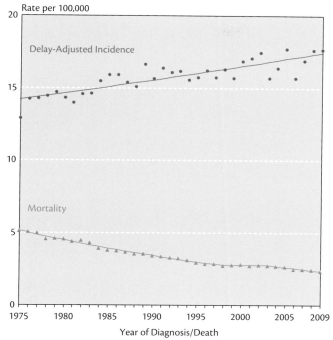

Figure 17.1 Cancer incidence and mortality in the United States 1975 to 2009. Reproduced from Howlader N et al. (eds), *SEER Cancer Statistics Review 1975–2009 (Vintage 2009 Populations), Section 28 Childhood Cancer by Site Incidence, Survival and Mortality*, Figure 28.1, National Cancer Institute, Bethesda, MD, USA, available from <http://seer.cancer.gov/csr/1975_2009_pops09/results_merged/sect_28_childhood_cancer.pdf>, based on November 2011 SEER data submission, posted to the SEER web site, April 2012.

effectiveness (Galeotti et al., 2010; Otto et al., 2007; Sindrup et al., 2001). Of the opioids, methadone is the one with the best data for being effective in neuropathic pain (Fisher et al., 2004; Lynch, 2005). Non-pharmacological approaches such as physical therapy, acupuncture, and cognitive-behavioural therapy (CBT) should always be considered.

Visceral pain

Visceral pain results from infiltration and distension of thoracic and abdominal viscera with capsular wall stretching, organ compression by primary or metastatic tumour, hollow organ obstruction from tumour, tumour regrowth within an organ, or peritoneal cavity bleeding. It is poorly localized pain and described as 'deep', 'squeezing', and 'pressure-like'. When acute, it could be associated with nausea, vomiting, and diaphoresis. Primary tumours of the liver, such as hepatoblastoma or hepatocellular carcinoma, and tumours that metastasize to the liver, such as neuroblastoma, result in visceral pain.

In the case of visceral pain due to organ invasion or tumour regrowth, reduction in tumour size is the primary modality for treatment of pain. In the setting of intestinal obstruction from tumour growth, treatment is determined by the nature of the tumour. For example when obstruction is from Burkitt's lymphoma, treatment consists of chemotherapy and/or radiation, as surgery is not effective (Delarue et al., 2008; England et al., 2012; Gupta et al., 2007; Meyer et al., 2012). A multimodal approach that includes surgery, chemotherapy, and/or radiotherapy is common in solid organ abdominal cancers, such as Wilms' tumour. Postoperative pain from

surgical resection needs early implementation of opioids. Regional techniques are also helpful if not contraindicated by the presence of coagulopathy due to thrombocytopenia, disseminated intravascular coagulation, or the presence of acquired factor inhibitors. Epidurals are effective in management of postoperative pain and they can be tunnelled for longer-term use. Coeliac plexus blocks can be useful for unresponsive tumours such as bladder rhabdomyosarcoma, neuroblastoma or pancreatic tumours, but have not gained widespread acceptance in the paediatric realm despite reports of their efficacy in terminal cancer pain in adults (Berde et al., 1990; Tanelian and Cousins, 1989). Newer radiographic techniques such as three-dimensional rotational angiography may facilitate correct placement of coeliac plexus blocks in children (Goldschneider et al., 2007).

Regardless of the aetiology of visceral pain, it is necessary to implement treatment early to prevent the later development of central pain syndromes and visceral hyperalgesia, which can be extremely challenging to treat. CBT must be included as part of the treatment protocol.

Pain with central nervous system tumours

CNS tumours are the most common solid tumours in childhood. The child often presents with symptoms suggestive of raised intracranial pressure from the mass effect of the tumour, such as headache or emesis. Surgical resection is undertaken for locally invasive tumours without metastatic potential such as astrocytomas (Sutton et al., 1995). Pain may persist from residual disease if complete surgical resection was not possible. In tumours that metastasize such as medulloblastoma, chemotherapy and/or radiation may be part of the treatment regimen either prior to or after surgical resection. Opioids are the mainstay of treatment in this population. Corticosteroids may be used to reduce cerebral oedema postoperatively. NSAIDs may be used if there is no contraindication due to the effects of chemotherapy or radiation therapy. The side effects of opioid treatment, such as nausea, emesis, and constipation, are best addressed pre-emptively, especially since the former symptoms can be confused with symptoms from the primary tumour. Adjuvant agents such as benzodiazepines may have a role in decreasing anxiety, facilitating sleep, and reducing muscle spasm postoperatively.

Acute pain due to cancer treatment

As cancer treatment protocols evolve, treatment-related pain has become more prevalent. Common treatment-related type pain includes, but is not limited to, mucositis, infection, antineoplastic therapy-related pain, and postoperative pain.

Mucositis is the painful inflammation of the mucous membranes lining the digestive tract in response to cancer treatments with chemotherapeutic agents and radiation. It can affect the entire digestive tract from mouth to anus and can be quite painful. Symptoms include swollen gums, ulcerations in the mouth, diarrhoea, abdominal cramping, or rectal ulcerations. Pain due to these symptoms often precludes talking, eating, and, on occasion, swallowing. Treatment for oral lesions involves using various mouthwash mixtures which can have agents such as saline, sodium bicarbonate, hydrogen peroxide, sucralfate, nystatin, or viscous lidocaine. In more severe cases, PCA may be necessary (Dunbar et al., 1995; Mackie et al., 1991).

Table 17.1 Adjuvant analgesics: major classes

Drug class	Examples
Multipurpose analgesics	
Antidepressants	
Tricyclic antidepressants	Amitriptyline (Elavil®) (tertiary amine) nortriptyline (Pamelor®), desipramine (Norpramin®); (secondary amines)
Selective serotonin reuptake inhibitors	Fluoxetine (Prozac®), paroxetine (Paxil®), sertraline (Zoloft®)citalopram (Celexa®), escitalopram (Lexapro®), fluvoxamine (Luvox®)
Noradrenaline/serotonin reuptake inhibitors	Venlafaxine (Effexor®), duloxetine (Cymbalta®), milnacipran (Savella®)
Others	Bupropion (Wellbutrin®)
Corticosteroids	Dexamethasone (Decadron®), prednisone(Deltasone®; Orasone®)
α2-adrenergic agonists	Clonidine (Catapres®), tizanidine(Zanaflex®)
Neuroleptics	Olanzapine (Zyprexa®)
For neuropathic pain	
Anticonvulsants	Gabapentin (Neurontin®), topiramate(Topamax®), lamotrigine(Lamictal®), carbamazepine(Carbatrol®; Tegretol®),levetiracetam (Keppra®),oxcarbazepine (Trileptal®),pregabalin (Lyrica®), tiagabine(Gabitril®), zonisamide(Zonegran®), phenytoin(Dilantin®), valproic acid(Depakene®)
Local anaesthetics	Lidocaine (Xylocaine®; Lidoderm®),mexiletine (Mexitil®)
N-methyl-D-aspartate receptor antagonists	Ketamine, dextromethorphan, memantine
	(Namenda®), amantadine (Symmetrel®)
Other	baclofen (Lioresal®)
	cannabinoids
	psychostimulant drugs: methylphenidate (Concerta®; Metadate CD®; Methylin®; Ritalin®), modafinil (Provigil®)
Topical drugs	Lidocaine/prilocaine (EMLA®), Lidocaine 4% (LMX4®), capsaicin
For bone pain	
Corticosteroids	Dexamethasone, prednisone
Calcitonin	(Miacalcin®)
Bisphosphonates	Pamidronate (Aredia®), zoledronic acid (Zometa®), risedronate (Actonel®), Alendronate (Fosamax®)
Radiopharmaceuticals	Strontium89, samarium153
For musculoskeletal pain	
Muscle relaxants	Cyclobenzaprine (Flexeril®), orphenadrine (Norflex®), carisoprodol (Soma®), metaxalone (Skelaxin®), methocarbamol (Robaxin®), Tizanidine (Zanaflex®) Baclofen (Lioresal®)
Benzodiazepines	Diazepam (Valium®), lorazepam (Ativan®), clonazepam (Klonopin®)
Adjuvants for pain from bowel obstruction	
Octreotide (Sandostatin®)	
Anticholinergics	Hyoscine (scopolamine), glycopyrrolate (Robinul®), hyoscyamine (Levsin®)
Corticosteroids	

Adapted with permission from David Lussier, Angela G. Huskey and Russell K. Portenoy, Adjuvant analgesics in cancer pain management, *The Oncologist*, Volume 9, Number 5, 571–591, Copyright © 2004 by AlphaMed Press.

Infection is common in children with cancer and can often be associated with pain. Common sites of pain include perioral, perirectal, abdominal, and skin infections. Severe abdominal pain can be due to typhlitis, infection of the cecum, in the immunocompromised, neutropenic patient (Hiruki et al., 1992). Treatment of the pain involves treatment of the infection. While being treated for the infection, analgesics such as opioids may need to be implemented on a short-term basis until the infection clears.

Injection of some chemotherapeutic agents may be associated with local pain at the time of injection. Thrombophlebitis

occasionally develops after injection of chemotherapy into a peripheral vein (Booth and Weiss, 1981). Intrathecal chemotherapy has been associated with arachnoiditis and meningeal irritation syndrome, which manifest as headache, nuchal rigidity, fever, nausea, and vomiting (D'Angio, 1983; Geiser et al., 1975).

Children with cancer undergo many surgical procedures such as port/line placements, tumour resections, peripheral and central biopsies, etc. These children have postoperative pain just as their non-cancerous counterparts do. Management of postoperative pain in the child with cancer is similar to the management of patients without malignancy. They will generally receive postoperative

Box 17.3 Using adjuvant analgesics in the management of cancer pain

1. Consider optimizing the opioid regimen before introducing an adjuvant analgesic.

2. Consider the burdens and potential benefits in comparison with other techniques used for pain that is poorly responsive to an opioid, including: (a) opioid rotation, (b) more aggressive side effect management, (c) a trial of spinal drug administration, and (d) trials of varied non-pharmacological approaches for pain control (e.g. nerve blocks, rehabilitative therapies, and psychological treatments).

3. Select the most appropriate adjuvant analgesic based on a comprehensive assessment of the patient, including inference about the predominating type of pain and associated factors (comorbidities) or symptoms.

4. Prescribe an adjuvant analgesic based on knowledge of its pharmacological characteristics, actions, approved indications, unapproved indications accepted in medical practice, likely side effects, potential serious adverse effects, and interactions with other drugs.

5. The adjuvant analgesics with the best risk:benefit ratios should be administered as first-line treatment.

6. Avoid initiating several adjuvant analgesics concurrently.

7. In most cases, initiate treatment with low doses and titrate gradually according to analgesic response and adverse effects.

8. Reassess the efficacy and tolerability of the therapeutic regimen on a regular basis, and taper or discontinue medications that do not provide additional pain relief.

9. Consider combination therapy with multiple adjuvant analgesics in selected patients.

Reprinted with permission from David Lussier, Angela G. Huskey and Russell K. Portenoy, Adjuvant analgesics in cancer pain management, *The Oncologist*, Volume 9, Number 5, 571–591, Copyright © 2004 by AlphaMed Press.

opioids, regional blocks, or neuraxial therapy to manage their pain. Patients who have been receiving preoperative opioids have usually developed some degree of opioid tolerance and should have their daily dose of opioids calculated into the postoperative treatment formula. This preoperative amount of opioid becomes their baseline to which additional opioids are added for the purpose of controlling new postoperative pain. If this principle is ignored, there will be dramatic under-dosing in the opioid-dependent oncology patient.

Procedure-related pain

Pain and suffering from painful procedures that take place for diagnosis, treatment, and surveillance of children with cancer are overall the greatest sources of distress. Angela Miser was the first to report the burden of procedure pain in paediatric oncology patients in 1987 (Miser et al., 1987). Further delineation of problem took place in a series of reports from Sweden in 1999 and 2000. Ljungman reported that over 40% of pain during cancer

treatment was attributed by the patients and families to procedures (Ljungman et al., 1999, 2000). In a follow-up study of paediatric oncology patients undergoing procedures including bone marrow aspiration and lumbar puncture, persistently high pain scores were reported, in spite of ostensibly therapeutic doses of analgesia (Weisman et al., 1998). Aggressive and widely available interventions for procedure pain management are an essential component of paediatric cancer treatment. Interventions range from simple cognitive-behavioural distraction techniques to formal training in biofeedback or hypnosis to active use of topical anaesthetics to mild or moderate pharmacologic sedation and, finally, to using general anaesthesia, when needed.

Oncology patients experience venepuncture, intravenous line placement, port access procedures, intramuscular and subcutaneous therapies, plus more invasive lumbar punctures and bone marrow aspirations or biopsies. Preparation by the staff or even staff specialized in cognitive-behavioural techniques can help prepare these patients for the complicated road they will traverse (Zeltzer et al., 1989, 1990). Topical analgesics can greatly reduce the discomfort of the painful cutaneous procedures mentioned (see Stevens and Zempsky, Chapter 2; Taddio, Chapter 19, this volume).

Many children will receive chemotherapy via a lumbar puncture. The drugs themselves may result in headache, but as many as 20% of teens are at risk for developing postdural tap headaches when standard 20- or 22-gauge needles are used for sampling and drug delivery (Burt et al., 1998; Scher et al., 1992; Wee et al., 2008). Pain is first managed with conservative bed rest, fluids, and analgesics. If symptoms persist for several days, an epidural blood patch, performed by an anaesthesiologist or pain specialist will usually result in resolution of the headache (Safa-Tisseront et al., 2001).

Bone marrow aspiration and biopsy are common procedures for children with leukaemia, certain sarcomas, and neuroblastoma. Cutaneous management, as discussed earlier, is essential. In addition, deeper tissue infiltration that includes the periosteum is critical to effective pain relief. Distress during these procedures is well described, over 30 years ago (Jay et al., 1983; Katz et al., 1980). These are often done in conjunction with lumbar puncture and hence it is widely accepted that these children will not only have some form of cutaneous anaesthesia, but they will also have procedural sedation, moderate, deep, or even general anaesthesia (see Cravero, Chapter 20, this volume).

Pain syndromes

Pain syndromes can occur as a consequence from the treatment of cancer. These syndromes can be a result of the surgical, chemotherapeutic, or radiation treatments undertaken while trying to cure the disease process. A variety of problems have been encountered in long-term survivors of childhood cancer that include, but are not limited to, chronic abdominal pain of uncertain aetiology, phantom limb pain, avascular necrosis of multiple joints, and neuropathic pain syndromes.

Amputation and limb-salvage procedures may be used as surgical approaches to achieve local control of a tumour that can lead to phantom limb pain. This pain is experienced when the patient continues to have pain appearing to come from where the affected amputated limb used to be. Krane and Heller (1995) found the prevalence of phantom pain in paediatric amputees to be 92%. The pain generally occurred within the first week after the loss of the limb.

The practitioner can use both pharmacological and non-pharmacological treatment modalities. The most important pharmacological treatment is effectively treating the pain preoperatively via the use of anaesthetic techniques such as an epidural. The use of epidurals prior to amputation can help prevent dorsal horn sensitization. After amputation, the focus becomes treating any neuropathic type symptoms. Chronic opioids are not usually effective in treating this type of neuropathic pain. A more successful approach usually involves the use of either gabapentin, pregabalin, or amitriptyline (or related tricyclic antidepressants). Non-pharmacological treatments or CAM treatments (complementary and alternative) can consist of hypnotherapy, massage, and acupuncture. An interesting approach to phantom limb treatment has emerged which uses mirror boxes (Chan et al., 2007; Ramachandran et al., 1996). This technique allows the amputee to place the remaining extremity into the mirror box. The projected image of the normal extremity appears to the patient to be the contralateral affected extremity. Repetitive therapeutic activity of the normal limb, viewed as the missing limb appears to 'retrain' and normalize neuronal pathways. Though phantom pain can be difficult to treat, in the paediatric population phantom pain tends to decrease over time regardless of the treatments.

Treatment regimens for cancer such as high-dose steroids and radiation treatments can have negative effects. These treatments can cause compromised blood supply to the bones which then leads to cell death in these areas resulting in avascular necrosis (AVN). The hip bone is the most common site, but knee, shoulder, and other bones can be affected. The incidence is 5% in childhood ALL and it usually develops during therapy although it has a latency period as long as 13 years after treatment is completed (Hanif et al., 2006; Mattano et al., 2000; Wei et al., 2000). Medical therapy for AVN is typically NSAIDs and physical therapy. However, if surgical intervention is needed it can include core decompression, bone grafting, osteotomies, or even joint replacement.

Chemotherapy-induced peripheral neuropathy (CIN) causes numerous debilitating symptoms and impairs functional capacity. Vincristine, vinblastine, cisplatin, oxaliplatin, and ifosfamide are most commonly implicated (Frisk et al., 2001; Gutiérrez-Gutiérrez et al., 2010; Le Deley et al., 2010; Lindeman et al., 1990; Reddy and Witek, 2003; Reinders-Messelink et al., 2000; Sandier et al., 1969). It can manifest with sensory symptoms, pain, motor symptoms, reflex loss, autonomic involvement, or a combination of these symptoms. Sensory symptoms tend to be most significantly manifested in the lower extremities. These manifest as itching, decreased or hyperactive responses to touch or vibration, and proprioception loss which can affect gait. Pain is an important side effect for many patients. It can occur early in treatment as painful paraesthesias or it can be a late and chronic consequence of treatment. Motor symptoms can be minor or more severe with athetoid movements and can progress to paralysis. There can be strength loss or symptomatic foot drop. Muscle cramping is also an underestimated motor manifestation. Reflexes can also be lost with the most common being the ankle reflex. Infrequently, patients develop symptoms of autonomic dysfunction. These can include orthostatic hypotension, constipation, or dysfunction of the urinary bladder (Windebank and Grisold, 2008). Prevention of CIN is the goal during treatment. There are agents that provide neuroprotection during therapy such as acetyl-L-carnitine, glutathione, vitamin E, or erythropoietin. These can be given to either prevent or even help treat developing

CIN. Supportive and symptomatic treatment is the mainstay of current CIN treatment. Management for CIN is similar to that of other neuropathic pain which entails analgesics, antidepressants, and antiepileptic drugs.

Management of pain in cancer

Recommendations for pain management in this population should encompass not only what we consider to be traditional pharmacological interventions, but must be founded in a truly interdisciplinary model that should include behavioural and psychological interventions and appropriate physical modalities. Psychological distress is invariably secondary to the pain of the disease or treatment. Obviously, children with underlying psychological diagnoses will require ongoing management of this during the course of their diagnosis and treatment for cancer. It is important for the pain specialist to understand the extent of the child's disease and oncological treatment plan, the role of anticancer therapy, duration of treatment, expected duration of side effects from anticancer treatments, the child's prior pain experiences and the expectations for pain management amongst the patient, guardians and oncology/surgery care team members.

Pharmacotherapy for management of cancer pain in children

The few analgesic studies that have been performed in children with cancer are limited by the paucity of subjects, and few are randomized controlled trials (Collins, 1998). Pharmacokinetic and pharmacodynamic properties of most opioids have been studied in children, but little information is available about oral bioavailability and potency ratios amongst the opioids (Collins and Weisman, 2003). There have been no controlled clinical trials of adjuvants drugs in paediatric cancer patients. The prescription of analgesics for children with cancer pain is based on various guidelines developed by content experts including the WHO guideline on cancer pain relief and palliative care in children (McGrath, 1996), the American Pain Society guideline for the management of cancer pain in adults and children (Miaskowski et al., 2004), the National Comprehensive Cancer Network practice guidelines for cancer pain (Benedetti et al., 2000), and *Supportive Care of Children with Cancer: Current Therapy and Guidelines from the Children's Oncology Group* (Altman and Children's Oncology Group, 2004). The original WHO ladder proposed that treatment of pain should begin with a non-opioid medication, progressing, as necessary, to a weak opioid and then to a more powerful opioid. It also included the possibility of adding adjuvants for neuropathic pain. Since its application into clinical practice in 1990 of the original guideline, the WHO stepladder has been quite useful for guiding the relief of pain from cancer (WHO, 1990). Its rationale and simplicity turned it into a very useful tool to unequivocally provide effective analgesia in malignant pain (American Pain Society, 2003). In recent years, several sources have proposed modifications to the original three-step ladder, recommending elimination of weaker opioids, use of stronger opioids as the first line in cancer pain treatment, using adjuvants early in the course of treatment, and incorporating neurolytic regional techniques in management when indicated (Jadad and Browman, 1995).

Non-opioid analgesics

Non-opioid analgesics include acetaminophen, traditional NSAIDs, selective cyclo-oxygenase (COX)-2 inhibitors, and tramadol (a unique analgesic described later in this section).

Acetaminophen is one of the most commonly used non-opioid analgesics used in children. It has analgesic and antipyretic effects. It inhibits prostaglandin synthesis primarily in the CNS. It does not have the side effects of gastritis and inhibition of platelet function that are concerns with aspirin and most of the NSAIDs (Lesko and Mitchell, 1999). Although it has the potential for hepatic and renal injury, this is usually not a concern in commonly used therapeutic doses (Sandler et al., 1989). It does not have an association with Reyes syndrome (Halpin et al., 1982; Hurwitz et al., 1985). The anti-pyretic action of acetaminophen may be contraindicated in neutropenic patients in whom monitoring of fever is critical.

The NSAIDS include the traditional non-selective COX inhibitors as well as the selective COX-2 inhibitors such as celecoxib and partially selective meloxicam. They are useful analgesics in children with adequate platelet number and function, both alone, and in combination with opioids or acetaminophen. They have anti-inflammatory, analgesic, and antipyretic potential. Chronic use increases the concern for analgesic nephropathy, gastritis, and haemostatic effects. The selective COX-2 inhibitors have a lower risk of gastrointestinal and minimal haemostatic adverse effects, but the risk of renal compromise appears no different (Brater, 1999). There are no data on the safety, efficacy, and tolerability of COX-2 inhibitors in children with cancer. The non-selective NSAID choline magnesium trisalicylate reportedly does not interfere with platelet aggregation, but its use should be avoided in children with platelet counts less than 20 000 or with active bleeding (Collins and Berde, 1997; Stuart and Pisko, 1981).

Tramadol is a synthetic, centrally acting analgesic that exerts its effects through the μ receptors, similar to opioids but not chemically related. It also stimulates the release of serotonin and inhibits reuptake of both serotonin and noradrenaline, thus simulating the properties of an antidepressant (Garrido et al., 2006). It is available in oral form alone in the US, but a parenteral form is being used in Europe and other countries. Long-acting forms are also available, allowing once-daily or twice-daily dosing. A concern with tramadol is that it lowers the seizure threshold, thus making its use challenging in cancer patients who could be on a multitude of other drugs with epileptogenic potential. It is currently a non-scheduled drug but concerns about its abuse potential have been raised (Grond et al., 1999).

Opioid analgesics

Opioids are now considered the first line of treatment in cancer (see Strassels, Chapter 45, this volume).

Morphine

Morphine is possibly the most widely used opioid for moderate to severe cancer pain in children. It can be administered by multiple routes including oral, sublingual, intravenous, subcutaneous, epidural, and intrathecal routes. An oral dose of 1 to 2 mg/kg/day is a reasonable starting point (Hunt et al., 1999). Oral morphine has a significant first-pass metabolism in the liver. A number of patients with cancer, however, require intravenous administration to address the severe pain associated with their disease and its sequelae. An oral to parenteral ratio of 3:1 is usually used for administration (Cherny and Foley, 1996; Cherny et al., 1995).

Some patients benefit from the convenience of a patient-controlled analgesic (PCA) pump. Typical initial morphine doses for intravenous PCA administration range from 0.01 to 0.02 mg/kg for both a basal infusion and demand dose. Sustained-release oral preparations of morphine are available and are usually administered once or twice daily. Dosing at 8 h intervals can also be used in cancer patients (Hunt et al., 1999). Sustained-release preparations are appropriate *only* in children who can swallow pills, as crushing produces immediate release of a large dose of morphine. Sustained-release capsules with time-released pellets (e.g. Kadian®) may be an option in the child unable to swallow pills, as they can be mixed with semisolids (Broomhead et al., 1997).

Hydromorphone

Hydromorphone is an alternative, when treatment is limited by the side effects of morphine. It is a safe drug to use in patients with impaired renal function, as its major metabolites are not active (Collins et al., 1996; Goodarzi, 1999). It is available for oral, intravenous, subcutaneous, epidural, and intrathecal administration and can also be used in a PCA pump, although dosing can be somewhat cumbersome in smaller patients. It has been reported to be an effective analgesic in several studies of patients with cancer (Babul et al., 1995; Broomhead et al., 1997; Dunbar et al., 1995, 1996; Weisman and Wishnie, 1996). It has been shown to be five to six times more potent than morphine in studies of children with cancer (Collins et al., 1996; Weisman and Wishnie, 1996). Little is known about its pharmacokinetics in infants and children (Babul et al., 1995; Murray and Hagen, 2005).

Oxycodone

Oxycodone is a semisynthetic opioid used for moderate to severe pain. It is available as a slow-release preparation and as an immediate-release preparation with or without acetaminophen. Oxycodone has a higher clearance value and a shorter elimination half-life in children than adults and appears to have a potency of about 1.5:1 with morphine (El-Tahtawy et al., 2006; Kokki et al., 2004, 2006; Poyhia et al., 1993). There are no controlled trials studying the use of oxycodone in children with cancer, but it is widely used with presumed efficacy (Collins, 2001).

Fentanyl

Fentanyl is a synthetic opioid approximately 50 to 100 times more potent than morphine with intravenous administration. It can be administered by intrathecal, epidural, transmucosal, and transdermal routes. It is an alternative for patients with dose-limiting side effects to morphine and hydromorphone (Cherny and Foley, 1996). It is commonly used in a transdermal form for patients requiring continuous opioids (Collins et al., 1999; Finkel et al., 2005). It has a proven track record for use in adult breakthrough cancer pain when administered by the transmucosal route (oral or nasal; Benitez-Rosario et al., 2005; Coluzzi et al., 2001; Payne et al., 2001; Zeppetella, 2000).

Methadone

Methadone is a synthetic opioid with a long and variable half-life (12–24 h). The oral to parenteral potency ratio is 2:1. Methadone provides equivalent but more prolonged analgesia than morphine (Berde et al., 1991; Davis and Walsh, 2001; Ripamonti et al., 1998). Its variable half-life predisposes to a risk of delayed sedation occurring several days after initiating treatment. Methadone does carry with it a cardiac risk with prolongation of QT intervals so serial electrocardiographic studies are advised in patients on long-term therapy (Kornick et al., 2003; Krantz et al., 2002, 2007). Methadone PCA has been reported as an effective delivery method in adults (Fitzgibbon and Ready, 1997; Shaiova et al., 2008).

In cancer patients, opioids should be administered at scheduled intervals to provide consistent pain relief. The dosing interval should be determined by the needs of the patient. Dose escalation may be required after treatment is initiated and periodically thereafter as tolerance to therapeutic effects is seen after a period of treatment (Portenoy, 1994b). Additional 'as needed' doses may be incorporated into the regimen for additional episodic breakthrough pain (Cleary, 1997). Oral and intravenous morphine and hydromorphone, and intranasal and oral transmucosal fentanyl are some of the options for breakthrough pain (Coluzzi et al., 2001; Zeppetella 2000).

Adjuvant analgesics

These are a heterogeneous group of medications that have a primary indication other than pain management, but are analgesic in some conditions (see also Rastogi and Campbell, Chapter 48, this volume). They are commonly prescribed in conjunction with primary analgesics (Portenoy, 1993). Their use is indicated when there is evidence of neuropathic pain, metastatic bone pain, anxiety, sleep disturbances, nausea and emesis, anorexia, poor appetite, cachexia, poor analgesic response to traditional analgesics, increased intracranial pressure, spinal cord compression, perineural oedema, and nerve compression (Lussier et al., 2004). They include drugs that come under the category of antidepressants, anticonvulsants, neuroleptics, psychostimulants, antihistamines, corticosteroids, and centrally acting skeletal muscle relaxants (George and Ahmedzai, 2000). Few adjuvants have been studied in the paediatric cancer population. To a large extent, drug selection, dosing, and monitoring approaches reflect extrapolation from the literature on non-malignant pain. Selection of an adjuvant is dictated by comorbid conditions and a comprehensive assessment of the patient. In some cases, the type of pain suggests the value of one category of adjuvant over another; in others, the existence of another symptom concurrent with pain favours the use of a specific drug.

Tricyclic antidepressants

These are often considered first-line treatment in the management of neuropathic pain of various aetiologies. They have been used for a variety of pain conditions including cancer pain (Magni, 1991; Magni et al., 1987a, 1987b). Although commonly used in practice, there is limited evidence from controlled trials evaluating their efficacy in cancer patients.

Since the antidepressants have established benefit in diverse types of neuropathic pain, the strongest indication for their use as an adjuvant in the cancer population occurs in the patient with neuropathic pain who has not derived much benefit from opioids. Early use of antidepressants is justified when pain is accompanied by depression. The sedating tricyclic antidepressants are often added when the patient complains of insomnia, while the anxiolytic selective serotonin reuptake inhibitors can be useful in anxious patients, and bupropion can be considered in sedated or fatigued patients.

Corticosteroids

These agents may have a role in managing bone pain due to metastatic bone disease, neuropathic pain from infiltration or compression of neural structures, headache due to increased intracranial pressure, metastatic spinal cord compression, arthralgia, pain due to obstruction of a hollow viscous, or organ capsule distension.

Dexamethasone is the most frequently used steroid on account of its high potency, duration of action, and minimal mineralocorticoid effect. Prednisone and methylprednisolone can also be used. Corticosteroids produce analgesia by a variety of mechanisms, including anti-inflammatory effects, reduction of tumour oedema, and potentially by a reduction of spontaneous discharges in injured nerves. They can improve appetite, nausea, malaise, and overall quality of life (Watanabe and Bruera, 1994).

Alpha 2 agonists

Clonidine, dexmedetomidine, and tizanidine may be used as adjuvants but side effects such as somnolence and hypotension can be limiting. Clonidine administered orally, transdermally, or intraspinally has been studied in non-malignant neuropathic pain. Intraspinal and epidural clonidine has been reported to be helpful in intractable cancer pain (Coombs et al., 1986; Eisenach et al., 1995). Limited experience with the use of dexmedetomidine as an adjuvant for refractory cancer pain has begun to appear in the literature (Roberts et al., 2011; Ugur et al., 2006). Hypotension occurs less commonly with tizanidine, which is an antispasticity/muscle relaxant agent. There is evidence for its use in myofascial pain syndrome and headaches, but not cancer (Chou et al., 2004).

Neuroleptic drugs

The neuroleptic drugs have been used for years in adults with cancer pain (Breitbart, 1998; Patt et al., 1994). There is little direct proof of their analgesic effect. These drugs do have profound sedating properties, which could explain the perception of co-analgesia (Richter and Burk, 1992). Methotrimeprazine appears to have analgesic properties in the setting of adult cancer pain (Beaver et al., 1966). However, this old neuroleptic drug is not being manufactured. Olanzapine (Zyprexa®) was reported to decrease pain intensity and opioid consumption, and improve cognitive function and anxiety, in cancer patients (Khojainova et al., 2002). Apart from these limited observations, evidence that commercially available neuroleptic drugs have analgesic properties is very meagre. The mechanism of analgesia and role as an adjuvant in paediatric cancer pain remains unclear. Given their potential for causing tardive dyskinesia and neuroleptic malignant syndrome, they are not routinely used as adjuvant analgesics unless delirium or agitation is present. The potential analgesic properties might allow a decrease in opioid consumption, which might in turn be helpful in resolving opioid-induced delirium. Neuroleptics tend to increase appetite, which may be desirable in some cancer patients.

Adjuvants for neuropathic pain

Anticonvulsants

Most view the anticonvulsants as the mainstays for managing neuropathic pain (Backonja 2000; Tremont-Lukats et al., 2000). Carbamazepine, phenytoin, and valproic acid have been the mainstay for years in treating neuropathic pain (Hardy et al., 2001; Harke et al., 2001; McCleane, 1999; Tanelian and Brose, 1991). Their use is limited by the potential haematological side effects, including neutropenia and thrombocytopenia. In recent years, gabapentin has been established in several types of non-malignant neuropathic pain, and it is now widely used to treat cancer-related neuropathic pain (Caraceni et al., 2004). Due to its proven analgesic effect in several types of neuropathic pain, its good tolerability, and low incidence of drug–drug interactions, gabapentin is now recommended as a first-line agent for the treatment of neuropathic pain of diverse aetiologies (Dworkin et al., 2007). The most common adverse effects are somnolence, dizziness, and unsteadiness. If titrated carefully, it is usually well tolerated.

Other newer anticonvulsants can be tried in patients who either have not responded satisfactorily to, have contraindications to, or have experienced adverse effects to gabapentin and other first-line adjuvants.

Local anaesthetics

Intravenous infusion of lidocaine has been shown to be effective in non-malignant neuropathic pain (Attal et al., 2000). Randomized clinical trials of lidocaine in neuropathic cancer pain have not been promising, but anecdotal reports of benefit may justify its use (Bruera et al., 1992; Buchanan and MacIvor, 2010; Ellemann et al., 1989). Relief is usually transient. If lidocaine is found to be effective, but pain recurs, long-term systemic local anaesthetic therapy can be initiated with an oral drug, mexiletine. For the rare patient that responds only to intravenous infusions, long-term subcutaneous infusion may be an option (Brose and Cousins, 1991). The predictive value of a lidocaine infusion for subsequent effectiveness of oral mexiletene has not been established. It is therefore reasonable to start therapy with the oral drug in patients that have not responded to antidepressants or anticonvulsants. There is a high rate of adverse effects and discontinuation due to toxicity, especially gastrointestinal distress.

N-methyl-D-aspartate (NMDA) receptor antagonists

These include the antitussive dextromethorphan, the dissociative anaesthetic ketamine, the antiviral amantadine, memantine, which is approved for Alzheimer's disease, and methadone. Ketamine has been shown to be effective in relieving cancer pain and reducing opioid requirements in children (Anghelescu and Oakes, 2005; Bell et al., 2003; Finkel et al., 2007). It is typically administered by the intravenous or subcutaneous routes, but oral therapy has also been used (Kannan et al., 2002, Lauretti et al., 1999). Dextromethorphan has been shown to improve analgesia and decrease analgesic requirements in patients undergoing surgery for cancer, but long-term results are mixed (Mercadante et al., 1998; Weinbroum et al., 2003). Amantadine is a non-competitive NMDA antagonist with conflicting data on its efficacy in cancer pain (Pud et al., 1998). Memantine also supposedly possesses analgesic properties (Grande et al., 2008). The role of these agents in cancer-related neuropathic pain is still unclear (Prommer, 2004). The d-isomer of the opioid methadone also blocks the NMDA receptor and might have a role in neuropathic cancer pain (Davis and Inturrisi 1999).

Miscellaneous

Oral dronabinol and Marinol® have been shown to be effective in cancer pain but more studies are needed (Campbell, 2001; Huskey, 2006). There is limited and conflicting evidence for analgesic effects from benzodiazepines, but a trial of clonazepam can be justified in refractory neuropathic pain, especially in the presence of anxiety.

Psychostimulants

There is evidence that psychostimulant drugs such as dextroamphetamine, methylphenidate, and caffeine have analgesic effects (Rozans et al., 2002). It appears, however, that their major use is in alleviating somnolence and sedation from opioids and other analgesics. The psychostimulants dextroamphetamine and methylphenidate have been used in children with cancer pain (Yee and Berde, 1994). Dextroamphetamine potentiates opioid analgesia and methylphenidate can reduce opioid-induced somnolence, improve cognition, treat depression, and alleviate fatigue. Potential side effects include anorexia, insomnia, and dysphoria. Modafinil, a newer psychostimulant, has been used to reduce opioid-induced somnolence in cancer patients (Webster et al., 2003). Although there are currently no scientific data supporting its use to reduce opioid-induced sedation, atomoxetine, a selective noradrenaline reuptake inhibitor, approved for the treatment of attention-deficit/hyperactivity disorder, has been used successfully in clinical practice.

Topicals

Options include EMLA® (eutectic mixture of prilocaine and lidocaine), topical lidocaine, liposomal lidocaine, and lidocaine 5% patches (Devers and Galer, 2000; Rowbotham et al., 1996). Topical capsaicin causes depletion of substance P and selective blockade of the TRPV1 receptor from the nerve terminals and decreased pain perception (Ellison et al., 1997). It has been helpful in postsurgical neuropathic pain in cancer patients and in HIV-neuropathy (Simpson et al., 2008).

Adjuvants for bone pain

An NSAID or steroid may be useful in multifocal bone pain. Calcitonin is useful in pain from bony metastases and neuropathic pain. It can be administered by the subcutaneous and intranasal routes for home care. There are also reports of epidural and intrathecal use in metastatic cancer (Blanchard et al., 1990). Monitoring of calcium and phosphorous is recommended. Bisphosphonates inhibit bone resorption. The analgesic efficacy of pamidronate and zoledronic acid has been well established in patients with metastases (Fulfaro et al., 1998; Rosen et al., 2001). These agents are also reported to decrease skeletal morbidity such as pathological fractures, need for radiation or surgery, spinal cord compression, and hypercalcaemia. Clodronate is an agent with good oral bio-availability (Ernst et al., 1992).

Radionuclide therapy

For painful osseous metastases the use of radionuclide therapy has been reported in the adult literature. They may be effective as monotherapy or as an adjunct to conventional radiation therapy

(Anderson, 2002; Silberstein 1993, 1994; Silberstein and Williams, 1985; Silberstein et al., 1992, 1998). Radionuclides are absorbed at areas of high bone turnover. They include strontium-89, phosphorus-32, iodine-131, tin-117m, and samarium-153. There are reports of their use in older children and adolescents. I[131] has been studied in children with painful metastatic bone disease from neuroblastoma (Cheung et al., 2001; Voute et al., 1988; Westlin et al., 1995). Given the potential for myelosuppression associated with their use, these drugs are considered when pain is refractory to other modalities.

Adjuvants for musculoskeletal pain

Cancer patients often have pain that originates in muscle or connective tissue. Muscle relaxants include drugs in a variety of classes including antihistamines (orphenadrine), tricyclics (cyclobenzaprine), and others such as carisoprodol, metazolone, and methocarbamol. Although the efficacy of these drugs in muscle spasm is fairly well established, their efficacy for musculoskeletal pain in the cancer population is unclear. Their risk:benefit ratio relative to the NSAIDs or opioids in also unknown. Sedation, which is a side effect with these drugs, can become an issue if it compounds the sedation caused by opioids and other centrally acting drugs in these patients. Caution is also advised when using these drugs in patients with a history of substance abuse. If muscle spasm is believed to be the primary cause for pain, drugs with established effects on skeletal muscle such as diazepam, other benzodiazepines, the α_2-agonist tizanidine, or baclofen should be used (Lussier et al., 2004). Botulinum toxin injections can be trialled for refractory musculoskeletal pain from spasms (Van Daele et al., 2002).

Adjuvants for pain caused by bowel obstruction

Management of malignant bowel obstruction is challenging, especially when surgery is not an option. There is the need to control pain and other symptoms such as nausea, vomiting, and distension. Opioid escalation may not be an option due to dose-limiting gastrointestinal side effects or sedation. Anecdotal reports suggest that anticholinergic drugs, the somatostatin analogue octreotide, and corticosteroids may be useful in this setting. Anticholinergic drugs reduce gut motility and secretions. Octreotide has similar effects but possibly causes them more rapidly (Mercadante et al., 2000; Yuan et al., 2000). Methylnaltrexone has recently been approved for the treatment of opioid-induced constipation and appears quite efficacious in adults (Thomas et al., 2008; Yuan and Foss, 2000). Steroids may also have a role in malignant bowel obstruction but the mode of action is unclear.

Complementary and alternative treatment options

There are multiple non-pharmacological therapies that can be employed for pain management in the paediatric cancer patient. These include the biobehavioural plus complementary and alternative medicine (CAM) therapies. CAM techniques are not often taught in medical schools, but can be powerful in the treatment of pain. These therapies are extensively discussed in Sections 7 and 8 and Chapters 59 (Weydert) and 60 (Zeltzer) in this volume. Specific issues related to malignancy are discussed in the rest of this section.

Physical

Radiotherapy, chemotherapy, and surgery can result in acute and long-term injury to the heart, lungs, and skeletal muscles. These impairments can affect the child's physical fitness, necessitating rehabilitation during and after treatment. *Physical therapy* should be an integral part of the treatment process in order to minimize systemic effects and improve pain control. There is growing evidence for the positive effects of physical training on organ system function, fatigue and physical well-being in children during and after treatment for cancer (Huang and Ness, 2011; Marchese et al., 2003).

Massage is one of the most commonly reported CAM therapies among children with cancer. It has positive effects on pain, stress, anxiety, and the immune system (Hughes et al., 2008; Post-White et al., 2009). However, specific massage guidelines, including type and duration for the incorporation of massage for children with cancer have yet to be developed. Also, in a study of children with ALL, a daily massage over a one month period was found to have an impact on the immune system (Field et al., 2001).

Acupuncture helps with pain, but it can also help with common symptoms experienced by child cancer patients such as headache, nausea, and vomiting. Acupuncture has not been widely disseminated into pain treatment regimens for the paediatric population due to the belief practitioners have that children will be afraid of the needles. On the contrary, it has been shown that for those children who have been referred to acupuncture for various chronic pain syndromes, over two-thirds report that it was a positive experience and an effective modality for treatment of their pain (Friedman et al., 1997; Pitetti et al., 2001).

Behavioural

There are many behavioural therapies that can be employed to assist with pain management.

Cognitive-behavioural therapy techniques are most commonly used to decrease distress and enhance a child's ability to cope with medical procedures (Chen et al., 1999; Liossi and Hatira, 2003; Zeltzer et al., 1991). These techniques have also been popularized as adjuvant therapy of the treatment of nausea and vomiting ding chemotherapy treatments (Rheingans, 2007). During non-painful procedures such as radiotherapy, children can be assisted by using hypnotic techniques.

References

Altman, A. J. and Children's Oncology Group. (2004). *Supportive care of children with cancer: current therapy and guidelines from the Children's Oncology Group* (3rd edn). Baltimore, MD: Johns Hopkins University Press.

American Pain Society. (2003). *Principles of analgesic use in the treatment of acute pain and cancer pain* (5th edn). Glenview, IL: American Pain Society.

Anderson, P. M. (2002). High-dose samarium-153 ethylene diamine tetramethylene phosphonate: low toxicity of skeletal irradiation in patients with osteosarcoma and bone metastases. *J Clin Oncol*, 20(1), 189–196.

Anghelescu, D. L. and Oakes, L. L. (2005). Ketamine use for reduction of opioid tolerance in a 5-year-old girl with end-stage abdominal neuroblastoma. *J Pain Symptom Manage*, 30(1), 1–3.

Anonymous. (1996). Practice guidelines for cancer pain management. A report by the American Society of Anesthesiologists Task Force on Pain Management, Cancer Pain Section. *Anesthesiology*, 84(5), 1243–1257.

Attal, N., Gaude, V., Brasseur, L., Dupuy, M., Guirimand, F., Parker, F., *et al.* (2000). Intravenous lidocaine in central pain: a double-blind, placebo-controlled, psychophysical study. *Neurology*, 54(3), 564–574.

Babul, N., Darke, A. C., and Hain, R. (1995). Hydromorphone and metabolite pharmacokinetics in children. *J Pain Symptom Manage*, 10(5), 335–337.

Backonja, M. M. (2000). Anticonvulsants (antineuropathics) for neuropathic pain syndromes. *Clin J Pain*, 16(2 Suppl), S67–72.

Beaver, W. T., Wallenstein, S. L., Houde, R. W., and Rogers, A. (1966). A comparison of the analgesic effects of methotrimeprazine and morphine in patients with cancer. *Clinical Pharmacology & Therapeutic*, 7(4), 436–446.

Bell, R., Eccleston, C., and Kalso, E. (2003). Ketamine as an adjuvant to opioids for cancer pain. *Cochrane Database Syst Rev*, 1, CD003351.

Benedetti, C., Brock, C., Cleeland, C., Coyle, N., Dube, J. E., Ferrell, B., *et al.* (2000). NCCN practice guidelines for cancer pain. *Oncology*, 14(11A), 135–150.

Benitez-Rosario, M. A., Martin, A. S., and Feria, M. (2005). Oral transmucosal fentanyl citrate in the management of dyspnea crises in cancer patients. *J Pain Symptom Manage*, 30(5), 395–397.

Berde, C., Ablin, A., Glazer, J., Miser, A., Shapiro, B., Weisman, S., *et al.* (1990). Report of the Subcommittee on Disease-Related Pain in Childhood Cancer. *Pediatrics*, 86(5), 818–825.

Berde, C. B., Beyer, J. E., Bournaki, M. C., Levin, C. R., and Sethna, N. F. (1991). Comparison of morphine and methadone for prevention of postoperative pain in 3- to 7-year-old children. *J Pediatr*, 119(1 (Pt 1)), 136–141.

Berde, C. B., Sethna, N. F., Fisher, D. E., Kahn, C. H., Chandler, P., and Grier, H. E. (1990). Celiac plexus blockade for a 3-year-old boy with hepatoblastoma and refractory pain. *Pediatrics*, 86(5), 779–781.

Blanchard, J., Menk, E., Ramamurthy, S., and Hoffman, J. (1990). Subarachnoid and epidural calcitonin in patients with pain due to metastatic cancer. *J Pain Symptom Manage*, 5(1), 42–45.

Booth, B. W., and Weiss, R. B. (1981). Venous thrombosis during adjuvant chemotherapy. *N Engl J Med*, 305(3), 170.

Brater, D. C. (1999). Effects of nonsteroidal anti-inflammatory drugs on renal function: focus on cyclooxygenase-2–selective inhibition. *Am J Med*, 107(6), 65–70.

Breitbart, W. (1998). Psychotropic adjuvant analgesics for pain in cancer and AIDS. *Psychooncology*, 7(4), 333–345.

Broomhead, A., Kerr, R., Tester, W., O'Meara, P., Maccarrone, C., Bowles, R., *et al.* (1997). Comparison of a once-a-day sustained-release morphine formulation with standard oral morphine treatment for cancer pain. *J Pain Symptom Manage*, 14(2), 63–73.

Brose, W. G. and Cousins, M. J. (1991). Subcutaneous lidocaine for treatment of neuropathic cancer pain. *Pain*, 45(2), 145–148.

Bruera, E., Ripamonti, C., Brenneis, C., Macmillan, K., and Hanson, J. (1992). A randomized double-blind crossover trial of intravenous lidocaine in the treatment of neuropathic cancer pain. *J Pain Symptom Manage*, 7(3), 138–140.

Buchanan, D. D., and J MacIvor, F. (2010). A role for intravenous lidocaine in severe cancer-related neuropathic pain at the end-of-life. *Support Care Cancer*, 18(7), 899–901.

Burt, N., Dorman, B. H., Reeves, S. T., Rust, P. F., Pinosky, M. L., Abboud, M. R., *et al.* (1998). Postdural puncture headache in paediatric oncology patients. *Can J Anaesth*, 45(8), 741–745.

Campbell, F. A. (2001). Are cannabinoids an effective and safe treatment option in the management of pain? A qualitative systematic review. *Br Med J*, 323(7303), 1–6.

Caraceni, A., Zecca, E., Bonezzi, C., Arcuri, E., Yaya Tur, R., Maltoni, M., *et al.* (2004). Gabapentin for neuropathic cancer pain: a randomized controlled trial from the Gabapentin Cancer Pain Study Group. *J Clin Oncol*, 22(14), 2909–2917.

Chan, B. L., Witt, R., Charrow, A. P., Magee, A., Howard, R., Pasquina, P. F., *et al.* (2007). Mirror therapy for phantom limb pain. *N Engl J Med*, 357(21), 2206–2207.

Chen, E., Zeltzer, L. K., Craske, M. G., and Katz, E. R. (1999). Alteration of memory in the reduction of children's distress during repeated aversive medical procedures. *J Consult Clin Psychol*, 67(4), 481–490.

Cherny, N. I. and Foley, K. M. (1996). Nonopioid and opioid analgesic pharmacotherapy of cancer pain. *Hematol Oncol Clin North Am*, 10(1), 79–102.

Cherny, N. J., Chang, V., Frager, G., Ingham, J. M., Tiseo, P. J., Popp, B., *et al.* (1995). Opioid pharmacotherapy in the management of cancer pain: a survey of strategies used by pain physicians for the selection of analgesic drugs and routes of administration. *Cancer*, 76(7), 1283–1293.

Cheung, N. K., Kushner, B. H., LaQuaglia, M., Kramer, K., Gollamudi, S., Heller, G., *et al.* (2001). N7: a novel multi-modality therapy of high risk neuroblastoma (NB) in children diagnosed over 1 year of age. *Med Pediatr Oncol*, 36(1), 227–230.

Chou, R., Peterson, K., and Helfand, M. (2004). Comparative efficacy and safety of skeletal muscle relaxants for spasticity and musculoskeletal conditions: a systematic review. *J Pain Symptom Manage*, 28(2), 140–175.

Cleary, J. F. (1997). Pharmacokinetic and pharmacodynamic issues in the treatment of breakthrough pain. *Semin Oncol*, 24(5 Suppl 16), S16–13–9.

Collins, J. J. (1998). Pharmacologic management of pediatric cancer pain. In R. K. Portenoy and E. Bruera (eds) *Topics in palliative care*, pp. 7–28. New York: Oxford University Press.

Collins, J. J. (2001). Cancer pain management in children. *Eur J Pain*, 5(SA), 37–41.

Collins, J. J., and Berde, C. B. (1997). Mangement of pain in children. In P. A. Pizzo and D. G. Poplack (eds) *Principles and practice of pediatric oncology* (3rd edn), pp. 1183–1199. Philadelphia, PA: Lippincott-Raven.

Collins, J. J., Byrnes, M. E., Dunkel, I. J., Lapin, J., Nadel, T., Thaler, H. T., *et al.* (2000). The measurement of symptoms in children with cancer. *J Pain Symptom Manage*, 19(5), 363–377.

Collins, J. J. and Weisman, S. J. (2003). Management of pain in childhood cancer. In N. L. Schechter, C. B. Berde, and M. Yaster (eds) *Pain in infants, children and adolescents* (2nd edn), pp. 517–538. Philadelphia, PA: Lippincott Williams & Wilkins.

Coombs, D. W., Saunders, R. L., Fratkin, J. D., Jensen, L. E., and Murphy, C. A. (1986). Continuous intrathecal hydromorphone and clonidine for intractable cancer pain. *J Neurosurg*, 64(6), 890–894.

D'Angio, G. J. (1983). Early and delayed complications of therapy. *Cancer*, 51(12 Suppl), 2515–2518.

Davis, A. M. and Inturrisi, C. E. (1999). D-methadone blocks morphine tolerance and N-methyl-D-aspartate-induced hyperalgesia. *J Pharmacol Exp Ther*, 289(2), 1048–1053.

Davis, M. P. and Walsh, D. (2001). Methadone for relief of cancer pain: a review of pharmacokinetics, pharmacodynamics, drug interactions and protocols of administration. *Support Care Cancer*, 9(2), 73–83.

Delarue, A., Bergeron, C., Mechinaud-Lacroix, F., Coze, C., Raphael, M., Patte, C., *et al.* (2008). Pediatric non-Hodgkin's lymphoma: primary surgical management of patients presenting with abdominal symptoms. Recommendations of the Lymphoma Committee of the French Society to Combat Pediatric Cancers (SFCE). *J Chir*, 145(5), 454–458.

Devers, A. and Galer, B. S. (2000). Topical lidocaine patch relieves a variety of neuropathic pain conditions: an open-label study. *Clin J Pain*, 16(3), 205–208.

Dunbar, P. J., Buckley, P., Gavrin, J. R., Sanders, J. E., and Chapman, C. R. (1995). Use of patient-controlled analgesia for pain control for children receiving bone marrow transplant. *J Pain Symptom Manage*, 10, 604–611.

Dunbar, P. J., Chapman, C. R., Buckley, F. P., and Gavrin, J. R. (1996). Clinical analgesic equivalence for morphine and hydromorphone with prolonged PCA. *Pain*, 68(2–3), 265–270.

Dworkin, R. H., O'Connor, A. B., Backonja, M., Farrar, J. T., Finnerup, N. B., Jensen, T. S., *et al.* (2007). Pharmacologic management of neuropathic pain: evidence-based recommendations. *Pain*, 132(3), 237–251.

Eisenach, J. C., DuPen, S., Dubois, M., Miguel, R., and Allin, D. (1995). Epidural clonidine analgesia for intractable cancer pain. The Epidural Clonidine Study Group. *Pain*, 61(3), 391–399.

Ellemann, K., Sjogren, P., Banning, A. M., Jensen, T. S., Smith, T., and Geertsen, P. (1989). Trial of intravenous lidocaine on painful neuropathy in cancer patients. *Clin J Pain*, 5(4), 291–294.

Ellison, N., Loprinzi, C. L., Kugler, J., Hatfield, A. K., Miser, A., Sloan, J. A., *et al.* (1997). Phase III placebo-controlled trial of capsaicin cream in the management of surgical neuropathic pain in cancer patients. *J Clin Oncol*, 15(8), 2974–2980.

El-Tahtawy, A., Kokki, H., and Reidenberg, B. E. (2006). Population pharmacokinetics of oxycodone in children 6 months to 7 years old. *J Clin Pharmacol*, 46(4), 433–442.

England, R. J., Pillay, K., Davidson, A., Numanoglu, A., and Millar, A. J. (2012). Intussusception as a presenting feature of Burkitt lymphoma: implications for management and outcome. *Pediatr Surg Int*, 28(3), 267–270.

Ernst, D. S., MacDonald, R. N., Paterson, A. H. G., Jensen, J., Brasher, P., and Bruera, E. (1992). A double-blind, crossover trial of intravenous clodronate in metastatic bone pain. *J Pain Symptom Manage*, 7(1), 4–11.

Field, T., Cullen, C., Diego, M., Hernandez-Reif, M., Sprinz, P., Beebe, K., *et al.* (2001). Leukemia immune changes following massage therapy. *J Bodywork Movement Ther*, 5(4), 271–274.

Finkel, J. C., Finley, A., Greco, C., Weisman, S. J., and Zeltzer, L. (2005). Transdermal fentanyl in the management of children with chronic severe pain: results from an international study. *Cancer*, 104(12), 2847–2857.

Finkel, J. C., Pestieau, S. R., and Quezado, Z. M. (2007). Ketamine as an adjuvant for treatment of cancer pain in children and adolescents. *J Pain*, 8(6), 515–521.

Fitzgibbon, D. R., and Ready, L .B. (1997). Intravenous high-dose methadone administered by patient controlled analgesia and continuous infusion for the treatment of cancer pain refractory to high-dose morphine. *Pain*, 73(2), 259–261.

Friedman, T., Slayton, W. B., Allen, L. S., Pollock, B. H., Dumont-Driscoll, M., Mehta, P., *et al.* (1997). Use of alternative therapies for children with cancer. *Pediatrics*, 100(6), e1.

Frisk, P., Stålberg, E., Strömberg, B., and Jakobson, Å. (2001). Painful peripheral neuropathy after treatment with high-dose ifosfamide. *Med Pediatr Oncol*, 37(4), 379–382.

Fulfaro, F., Casuccio, A., Ticozzi, C., and Ripamonti, C. (1998). The role of bisphosphonates in the treatment of painful metastatic bone disease: a review of phase III trials. *Pain*, 78(3), 157–169.

Galeotti, N., Vivoli, E., Bilia, A. R., Vincieri, F. F., and Ghelardini, C. (2010). St. John's Wort reduces neuropathic pain through a hypericin-mediated inhibition of the protein kinase Cgamma and epsilon activity. *Biochem Pharmacol*, 79(9), 1327–1336.

Garrido, M. J., Habre, W., Rombout, F., and Troconiz, I. F. (2006). Population pharmacokinetic/pharmacodynamic modelling of the analgesic effects of tramadol in pediatrics. *Pharmaceut Res*, 23(9), 2014–2023.

Geiser, C. F., Bishop, Y., Jaffe, N., Furman, L., Traggis, D., and Frei, E., 3rd. (1975). Adverse effects of intrathecal methotrexate in children with acute leukemia in remission. *Blood*, 45(2), 189–195.

George, R. M. and Ahmedzai, S. H. (2000). The management of neuropathic pain in cancer: clinical guidelines for the use of adjuvant analgesics. *Indian J Cancer*, 37(1), 4–9.

Goldschneider, K. R., Racadio, J. M., and Weidner, N. J. (2007). Celiac plexus blockade in children using a three-dimensional fluoroscopic reconstruction technique: case reports. *Reg Anesth Pain Med*, 32(6), 510–515.

Goodarzi, M. (1999). Comparison of epidural morphine, hydromorphone and fentanyl for postoperative pain control in children undergoing orthopaedic surgery. *Paediatr Anaesth*, 9(5), 419–422.

Grande, L. A., O'Donnell, B. R., Fitzgibbon, D. R., and Terman, G. W. (2008). Ultra-low dose ketamine and memantine treatment for pain in an opioid-tolerant oncology patient. *Anesth Analg*, 107(4), 1380–1383.

Grond, S., Radbruch, L., Meuser, T., Loick, G., Sabatowski, R., and Lehmann, K.A. (1999). High-dose tramadol in comparison to low-dose morphine for cancer pain relief. *J Pain Symptom Manage*, 18(3), 174–179.

Gupta, H., Davidoff, A. M., Pui, C. H., Shochat, S. J., and Sandlund, J. T. (2007). Clinical implications and surgical management of intussusception in pediatric patients with Burkitt lymphoma. *J Pediatric Surg*, 42(6), 998–1001; discussion 1001.

Gutiérrez-Gutiérrez, G., Sereno, M., Miralles, A., Casado-Sáenz, E., and Gutiérrez-Rivas, E. (2010). Chemotherapy-induced peripheral neuropathy: clinical features, diagnosis, prevention and treatment strategies. *Clin Transl Oncol*, 12(2), 81–91.

Halpin, T. J., Holtzhauer, F. J., Campbell, R. J., Hall, L. J., Correa-Villasenor, A., Lanese, R., *et al.* (1982). Reye's syndrome and medication use. *JAMA*, 248(6), 687–691.

Hanif, I., Mahmoud, H., and Pui, C. H. (2006). Avascular femoral head necrosis in pediatric cancer patients. *Med Pediatr Oncol*, 21(9), 655–660.

Hardy, J. R., Rees, E. A., Gwilliam, B., Ling, J., Broadley, K., and A'Hern, R. (2001). A phase II study to establish the efficacy and toxicity of sodium valproate in patients with cancer-related neuropathic pain. *J Pain Symptom Manage*, 21(3), 204–209.

Harke, H., Gretenkort, P., Ladleif, H. U., Rahman, S., and Harke, O. (2001). The response of neuropathic pain and pain in complex regional pain syndrome I to carbamazepine and sustained-release morphine in patients pretreated with spinal cord stimulation: a double-blinded randomized study. *Anesth Analg*, 92(2), 488–495.

Hiruki, T., Fernandes, B., Ramsay, J., and Rother, I. (1992). Acute typhlitis in an immunocompromised host. Report of an unusual case and review of the literature. *Dig Dis Sci*, 37(8), 1292–1296.

Howlader, N., Noone, A. M., Krapcho, M., Neyman, N., Aminou, R., Altekruse, S. F., *et al.* (2012). *SEER cancer statistics review, 1975–2009 (vintage 2009 populations), based on November 2011 SEER data submission*. Bethesda, MD: National Cancer Institute.

Huang, T. T. and Ness, K. K. (2011). Exercise interventions in children with cancer: a review. *Int J Pediatr*, 2011, 461512.

Hughes, D., Ladas, E., Rooney, D., and Kelly, K. (2008). Massage therapy as a supportive care intervention for children with cancer. *Oncol Nursing Forum*, 431–442.

Hunt, A., Joel, S., Dick, G., and Goldman, A. (1999). Population pharmacokinetics of oral morphine and its glucuronides in children receiving morphine as immediate-release liquid or sustained-release tablets for cancer pain. *J Pediatr*, 135(1), 47–55.

Hurwitz, E. S., Barrett, M. J., Bregman, D., Gunn, W. J., Schonberger, L. B., Fairweather, W. R., *et al.* (1985). Public Health Service study on Reye's syndrome and medications. Report of the pilot phase. *N Engl J Med*, 313(14), 849–857.

Huskey, A. (2006). Cannabinoids in cancer pain management. *J Pain Palliat Care Pharmacother*, 20(3), 43–46.

Jadad, A. R., and Browman, G. P. (1995). The WHO analgesic ladder for cancer pain management: stepping up the quality of its evaluation. *JAMA*, 274(23), 1870–1873.

Jay, S. M., Ozolins, M., Elliott, C. H., and Caldwell, S. (1983). Assessment of children's distress during painful medical procedures. *Health Psychol*, 2(2), 133–147.

Kannan, T. R., Saxena, A., Bhatnagar, S., and Barry, A. (2002). Oral ketamine as an adjuvant to oral morphine for neuropathic pain in cancer patients. *J Pain Symptom Manage*, 23(1), 60–65.

Katz, E. R., Kellerman, J., and Siegel, S. E. (1980). Behavioral distress in children with cancer undergoing medical procedures: developmental considerations. *J Consult Clin Psychol*, 48(3), 356–365.

Khojainova, N., Santiago-Palma, J., Kornick, C., Breitbart, W., and Gonzales, G. R. (2002). Olanzapine in the management of cancer pain. *J Pain Symptom Manage*, 23(4), 346–350.

Kokki, H., Rasanen, I., Lasalmi, M., Lehtola, S., Ranta, V.P., Vanamo, K., *et al.* (2006). Comparison of oxycodone pharmacokinetics after buccal and sublingual administration in children. *Clinical Pharmacokinet*, 45(7), 745–754.

Kokki, H., Rasanen, I., Reinikainen, M., Suhonen, P., Vanamo, K., and Ojanpera, I. (2004). Pharmacokinetics of oxycodone after intravenous, buccal, intramuscular and gastric administration in children. *Clin Pharmacokinet*, 43(9), 613–622.

Kornick, C. A., Kilborn, M. J., Santiago-Palma, J., Schulman, G., Thaler, H. T., Keefe, D. L., et al. (2003). QTc interval prolongation associated with intravenous methadone. *Pain*, 105(3), 499–506.

Krane, E. J. and Heller, L. B. (1995). The prevalence of phantom sensation and pain in pediatric amputees. *J Pain Symptom Manage*, 10(1), 21–29.

Krantz, M. J., Lewkowiez, L., Hays, H., Woodroffe, M. A., Robertson, A. D., and Mehler, P. S. (2002). Torsade de pointes associated with very-high-dose methadone. *Ann Internal Med*, 137(6), 501–504.

Krantz, M. J., Rowan, S. B., Schmittner, J., and Bucher Bartelson, B. (2007). Physician awareness of the cardiac effects of methadone: results of a national survey. *J Addict Dis*, 26(4), 79–85.

Lauretti, G. R., Lima, I. C., Reis, M. P., Prado, W. A., and Pereira, N. L. (1999). Oral ketamine and transdermal nitroglycerin as analgesic adjuvants to oral morphine therapy for cancer pain management. *Anesthiology*, 90(6), 1528–1533.

Le Deley, M. C., Rosolen, A., Williams, D. M., Horibe, K., Wrobel, G., Attarbaschi, A., et al. (2010). Vinblastine in children and adolescents with high-risk anaplastic large-cell lymphoma: results of the randomized ALCL99-vinblastine trial. *J Clin Oncol*, 28(25), 3987–3993.

Lesko, S. M. and Mitchell, A. A. (1999). The safety of acetaminophen and ibuprofen among children younger than two years old. *Pediatrics*, 104(4), e39.

Lindeman, G., Kefford, R., Stuart-Harris, R., Legha, S. S., and Mollman, J. E. (1990). Cisplatin neurotoxicity. *N Engl J Med*, 323(1), 64–65.

Liossi, C. and Hatira, P. 2003). Clinical hypnosis in the alleviation of procedure-related pain in pediatric oncology patients. *Int J Clin Exp Hypnosis*, 51(1), 4–28.

Ljungman, G., Gordh, T., Sorensen, S., and Kreuger, A. (1999). Pain in paediatric oncology: interviews with children, adolescents and their parents. *Acta Paediatr*, 88(6), 623–630.

Ljungman, G., Gordh, T., Sorensen, S., and Kreuger, A. (2000). Pain variations during cancer treatment in children: a descriptive survey. *Pediatr Hematol Oncol*, 17(3), 211–221.

Lussier, D., Huskey, A. G., and Portenoy, R. K. (2004). Adjuvant analgesics in cancer pain management. *Oncologist*, 9(5), 571–591.

Lynch, M. E. (2005). A review of the use of methadone for the treatment of chronic noncancer pain. *Pain Res Manag*, 10(3), 133–144.

Magni, G. (1991). The use of antidepressants in the treatment of chronic pain. A review of the current evidence. *Drugs*, 42(5), 730–748.

Magni, G., Arsie, D., and DeLeo, D. (1987a). Antidepressants in the treatment of cancer pain. A survey in Italy. *Pain*, 29(3), 347–353.

Magni, G., Conlon, P., and Arsie, D. (1987b). Tricyclic antidepressants in the treatment of cancer pain: a review. *Pharmacopsychiatry*, 20(4), 160–164.

Marchese, V. G., Chiarello, L. A., and Lange, B. J. (2003). Effects of physical therapy intervention for children with acute lymphoblastic leukemia. *Pediatr Blood Cancer*, 42(2), 127–133.

Mattano, L. A. Jr, Sather, H. N., Trigg, M. E., and Nachman, J. B. (2000). Osteonecrosis as a complication of treating acute lymphoblastic leukemia in children: a report from the Children's Cancer Group. *J Clin Oncol*, 18(18), 3262–3272.

McCleane, G. J. (1999). Intravenous infusion of phenytoin relieves neuropathic pain: a randomized, double-blinded, placebo-controlled, crossover study. *Anesth Analg*, 89(4), 985–988.

McGrath, P. A. (1996). Development of the World Health Organization guidelines on cancer pain relief and palliative care in children. *J Pain Symptom Manage*, 12(2), 87–92.

McGrath, P. J., Beyer, J., Cleeland, C., Eland, J., McGrath, P. A., and Portenoy, R. (1990). Report of the Subcommittee on Assessment and Methodologic Issues in the Management of Pain in Childhood Cancer. *Pediatrics*, 86(5 Pt 2), 814–817.

Mercadante, S., Ripamonti, C., Casuccio, A., Zecca, E., and Groff, L. (2000). Comparison of octreotide and hyoscine butylbromide in controlling gastrointestinal symptoms due to malignant inoperable bowel obstruction. *Support Care Cancer*, 8(3), 188–191.

Mercadante, S., Casuccio, A., and Genovese, G. (1998). Ineffectiveness of dextromethorphan in cancer pain. *J Pain Symptom Manage*, 16(5), 317–322.

Meyer, C. T., Wilsey, M. J., Hale, G. A., Monforte, H. L., and Danielson, P. D. (2012). Primary Burkitt's lymphoma of the colon—an uncommon cause of acute constipation and abdominal pain. *Fetal Pediatr Pathol*, 31(4), 254–259.

Miaskowski, C., Cleary, J., Burney, R., Coyne, P., Finley, R., Foster, R., et al. (2004). *Guideline for the management of cancer pain in adults and children, APS Clinical Practice Guidelines Series, No. 3*. Glenview, IL: American Pain Society.

Miser, A. W., Dothage, J. A., Wesley, R. A., and Miser, J. S. (1987a). The prevalence of pain in a pediatric and young adult cancer population. *Pain*, 29(1), 73–83.

Miser, A. W., McCalla, J., Dothage, J. A., Wesley, M., and Miser, J. S. (1987b). Pain as a presenting symptom in children and young adults with newly diagnosed malignancy. *Pain*, 29(1), 85–90.

Murray, A. and Hagen, N.A. (2005). Hydromorphone. *J Pain Symptom Manage*, 29(5), 57–66.

Otto, M., Bach, F. W., Jensen, T. S., and Sindrup, S. H. (2007). Health-related quality of life and its predictive role for analgesic effect in patients with painful polyneuropathy. *Eur J Pain*, 11(5), 572–578.

Patt, R. B., Proper, G., and Reddy, S. (1994). The neuroleptics as adjuvant analgesics. *J Pain Symptom Manage*, 9(7), 446–453.

Pitetti, R., Singh, S., Hornyak, D., Garcia, S.E., and Herr, S. (2001). Complementary and alternative medicine use in children. *Pediatr Emerg Care*, 17(3), 165–169.

Portenoy, R. K. (1994). Tolerance to opioid analgesics: clinical aspects. *Cancer Surv*, 21, 49–65.

Portenoy, R. K. (1993). Adjuvant analgesics in pain management. In D. Doyle, G. W. C. Hanks, and N. MacDonald (eds) *Oxford textbook of palliative medicine*, pp. 187–203. Oxford: Oxford University Press.

Post-White, J., Fitzgerald, M., Savik, K., Hooke, M.C., Hannahan, A. B., and Sencer, S. F. (2009). Massage therapy for children with cancer. *J Pediatr Oncol Nurs*, 26(1), 16–28.

Poyhia, R., Vainio, A., and Kalso, E. (1993). A review of oxycodone's clinical pharmacokinetics and pharmacodynamics. *J Pain Symptom Manage*, 8(2), 63–67.

Prommer, E. (2004). The other NMDA antagonists, amantadine, memantine, dextromethorphan: role in cancer therapeutics. *J Clin Oncol (Meeting Abstracts)*, 8223.

Pud, D., Eisenberg, E., Spitzer, A., Adler, R., Fried, G., and Yarnitsky, D. (1998). The NMDA receptor antagonist amantadine reduces surgical neuropathic pain in cancer patients: a double blind, randomized, placebo controlled trial. *Pain*, 75(2–3), 349–354.

Ramachandran, V. S. and Rogers-Ramachandran, D. (1996). Synaesthesia in phantom limbs induced with mirrors. *Proc Biol Sci*, 263(1369), 377–386.

Reddy, A. T., and Witek, K. (2003). Neurologic complications of chemotherapy for children with cancer. *Curr Neurol Neurosci Rep*, 3(2), 137–142.

Reinders-Messelink, H. A., Van Weerden, T. W., Fock, J. M., Gidding, C. E., Vingerhoets, H. M., Schoemaker, M. M., et al. (2000). Mild axonal neuropathy of children during treatment for acute lymphoblastic leukaemia. *Eur J Paediatr Neurol*, 4(5), 225–233.

Rheingans, J. I. (2007). A systematic review of nonpharmacologic adjunctive therapies for symptom management in children with cancer. *J Pediatr Oncol Nurs*, 24(2), 81–94.

Richter, P. A. and Burk, M. P. (1992). The potentiation of narcotic analgesics with phenothiazines. *J Foot Surg*, 31(4), 378–380.

Ripamonti, C., De Conno, F., Groff, L., Belzile, M., Pereira, J., Hanson, J., et al. (1998). Equianalgesic dose/ratio between methadone and other opioid agonists in cancer pain: comparison of two clinical experiences. *Ann Oncol*, 9(1), 79–83.

Roberts, S. B., Wozencraft, C. P., Coyne, P. J., and Smith, T. J. (2011). Dexmedetomidine as an adjuvant analgesic for intractable cancer pain. *J Palliat Med*, 14(3), 371–373.

Rosen, L. S., Gordon, D., Kaminski, M., Howell, A., Belch, A., Mackey, J., et al. (2001). Zoledronic acid versus pamidronate in the treatment of skeletal metastases in patients with breast cancer or osteolytic lesions of multiple myeloma: a phase III, double-blind, comparative trial. *Cancer J*, 7(5), 377–387.

Rowbotham, M. C., Davies, P. S., Verkempinck, C., and Galer, B. S. (1996). Lidocaine patch: double-blind controlled study of a new treatment method for post-herpetic neuralgia. *Pain*, 65(1), 39–44.

Rozans, M., Dreisbach, A., Lertora, J .J. L., and Kahn, M. J. (2002). Palliative uses of methylphenidate in patients with cancer: a review. *J Clin Oncol*, 20(1), 335–339.

Safa-Tisseront, V., Thormann, F., Malassine, P., Henry, M., Riou, B., Coriat, P., et al. (2001). Effectiveness of epidural blood patch in the management of post-dural puncture headache. *Anesthesiology*, 95(2), 334–339.

Sandier, S. G., Tobin, W., and Henderson, E. S. (1969). Vincristine-induced neuropathy A clinical study of fifty leukemic patients. *Neurology*, 19(4), 367–374.

Sandler, D. P., Smith, J. C., Weinberg, C. R., Buckalew, V. M. Jr., Dennis, V. W., Blythe, W. B., et al. (1989). Analgesic use and chronic renal disease. *N Engl J Med*, 320(19), 1238–1243.

Scher, C., Amar, D., Ginsburg, I., Reinsel, R., McDowall, R., and Barst, S. (1992). Post dural puncture headache in children with cancer. *Anesthesiology*, 77(3A), A1183.

Shaiova, L., Berger, A., Blinderman, C. D., Bruera, E., Davis, M. P., Derby, S., et al. (2008). Consensus guideline on parenteral methadone use in pain and palliative care. *Palliat Supp Care*, 6(02), 165–176.

Silberstein, E. B. (1993). The treatment of painful osseous metastases with phosphorus-32-labeled phosphates. *Semin Oncol*, 20(3 Suppl 2), 10–21.

Silberstein, E. B. (1994). The treatment of painful osteoblastic metastases: what can we expect from nuclear oncology? *J Nucl Med*, 35(12), 1994–1995.

Silberstein, E. B., Elgazzar, A. H., and Kapilivsky, A. (1992). Phosphorus-32 radiopharmaceuticals for the treatment of painful osseous metastases. *Semin Nucl Med*, 22(1), 17–27.

Silberstein, E. B. and Williams, C. (1985). Strontium-89 therapy for the pain of osseous metastases. *J Nucl Med*, 26(4), 345–348.

Simpson, D. M., Brown, S., and Tobias, J. (2008). Controlled trial of high-concentration capsaicin patch for treatment of painful HIV neuropathy. *Neurology*, 70(24), 2305–2313.

Sindrup, S. H., Madsen, C., Bach, F. W., Gram, L. F., and Jensen, T. S. (2001). St. John's wort has no effect on pain in polyneuropathy. *Pain*, 91(3), 361–365.

Srivastava, S. C., Atkins, H. L., Krishnamurthy, G. T., Zanzi, I., Silberstein, E. B., Meinken, G., et al. (1998). Treatment of metastatic bone pain with tin-117m Stannic diethylenetriaminepentaacetic acid: a phase I/II clinical study. *Clin Cancer Res*, 4(1), 61–68.

Stuart, J. J. and Pisko, E. J. (1981). Choline magnesium trisalicylate does not impair platelet aggregation. *Pharmatherapeutica*, 2(8), 547–551.

Sutton, L. N., Molloy, P. T., Sernyak, H., Goldwein, J., Phillips, P. L., Rorke, L. B., et al. (1995). Long-term outcome of hypothalamic/chiasmatic astrocytomas in children treated with conservative surgery. *J Neurosurg*, 83(4), 583–589.

Tanelian, D. L. and Brose, W. G. (1991). Neuropathic pain can be relieved by drugs that are use-dependent sodium channel blockers: lidocaine, carbamazepine, and mexiletine. *Anesthesiology*, 74(5), 949–951.

Tanelian, D. and Cousins, M. J. (1989). Celiac plexus block following high-dose opiates for chronic noncancer pain in a four-year-old child. *J Pain Symptom Manage*, 4(2), 82–85.

Thomas, J., Karver, S., Cooney, G. A., Chamberlain, B. H., Watt, C. K., Slatkin, N. E., et al. (2008). Methylnaltrexone for opioid-induced constipation in advanced illness. *N Engl J Med*, 358(22), 2332–2343.

Tremont-Lukats, I. W., Megeff, C., and Backonja, M. M. (2000). Anticonvulsants for neuropathic pain syndromes: mechanisms of action and place in therapy. *Drugs*, 60(5), 1029–1052.

Ugur, F., Gulcu, N., and Boyaci, A. (2006). Intrathecal infusion therapy with dexmedetomidine-supplemented morphine in cancer pain. *Acta Anaesthesiol Scand*, 51(3), 388–388.

Van Daele, D. J., Finnegan, E. M., Rodnitzky, R. L., Zhen, W., McCulloch, T. M., and Hoffman, H. T. (2002). Head and neck muscle spasm after radiotherapy: management with botulinum toxin A injection. *Arch Otolaryngol—Head Neck Surg*, 128(8), 956–959.

Voute, P. A., Hoefnagel, C. A., and de Kraker, J. (1988). 131I-meta-iodobenzylguanidine in diagnosis and treatment of neuroblastoma. *Bull Cancer*, 75(1), 107–111.

Watanabe, S. and Bruera, E. (1994). Corticosteroids as adjuvant analgesics. *J Pain Symptom Manage*, 9(7), 442–445.

Webster, L., Andrews, M., and Stoddard, G. (2003). Modafinil treatment of opioid-induced sedation. *Pain Med*, 4(2), 135–140.

Wee, L., Lam, F., and Cranston, A. (2008). The incidence of post dural puncture headache in children. *Anaesthesia*, 51(12), 1164–1166.

Wei, S. Y., Esmail, A. N., Bunin, N., and Dormans, J. P. (2000). Avascular necrosis in children with acute lymphoblastic leukemia. *J Pediatr Orthopaed*, 20(3), 331–335.

Weinbroum, A. A., Bender, B., Bickels, J., Nirkin, A., Marouani, N., Chazam, S., et al. (2003). Preoperative and postoperative dextromethorphan provides sustained reduction in postoperative pain and patient-controlled epidural analgesia requirement: a randomized, placebo-controlled, double-blind study in lower-body bone malignancy-operated patients. *Cancer*, 97(9), 2334–2340.

Weisman, S. J. and Wishnie, E. (1996). Postoperative hydromorphone epidural analgesia in children. Poster presentation at *8th World Congress on Pain, Vancouver, Canada*.

Westlin, J. E., Letocha, H., Jakobson, A., Strang, P., Martinsson, U., and Nilsson, S. (1995). Rapid, reproducible pain relief with [131I]iodine-meta-iodobenzylguanidine in a boy with disseminated neuroblastoma. *Pain*, 60(1), 111–114.

Windebank, A. J., and Grisold, W. (2008). Chemotherapy-induced neuropathy. *J Periph Nerv Syst*, 13(1), 27–46.

World Health Organization. (1990). *Cancer pain relief and palliative care. Report of a WHO expert committee.* Geneva: World Health Organization.

Yee, J. D. and Berde, C. B. (1994). Dextroamphetamine or methylphenidate as adjuvants to opioid analgesia for adolescents with cancer. *J Pain Symptom Manage*, 9(2), 122–125.

Yuan, C. S. and Foss, J. F. (2000). Oral methylnaltrexone for opioid-induced constipation. *JAMA*, 284(11), 1383–1384.

Yuan, C. S., Foss, J. F., O'Connor, M., Osinski, J., Karrison, T., Moss, J., et al. (2000). Methylnaltrexone for reversal of constipation due to chronic methadone use. *JAMA*, 283(3), 367–372.

Zeltzer, L. K., Altman, A., Cohen, D., LeBaron, S., Maunuksela, E. L., and Schechter, N. L. (1990). Report of the Subcommittee on the Management of Pain Associated with Procedures in Children with Cancer. *Pediatrics*, 86(Suppl.5), 826–831.

Zeltzer, L. K., Dolgin, M. J., LeBaron, S., and LeBaron, C. (1991). A randomized, controlled study of behavioral intervention for chemotherapy distress in children with cancer. *Pediatrics*, 88(1), 34–42.

Zeltzer, L. K., Jay, S. M., and Fisher, D. M. (1989). The management of pain associated with pediatric procedures. *Pediatr Clin North Am*, 36(4), 941–964.

Zeppetella, G. (2000). An assessment of the safety, efficacy, and acceptability of intranasal fentanyl citrate in the management of cancer-related breakthrough pain: a pilot study. *J Pain Symptom Manage*, 20(4), 253–258.

CHAPTER 18

Pain management in major paediatric trauma and burns

Greta M. Palmer and Franz E. Babl

Summary

Pain management in major paediatric trauma and burns is challenging. It involves many phases including pre-hospital and emergency department care, ward management frequently including intensive care, and multiple operative and procedural interventions (as inpatients and later outpatients). Distress, anxiety, post-traumatic stress disorder (from the primary event and the ensuing in-hospital and post-discharge course), itch, neuropathic pain (in addition to pain of nociceptive origin), and sleep disorders frequently affect major trauma and burns victims and can persist long term. An evidence-based discussion follows of the pharmacological and non-pharmacological interventions employed during these various phases to address pain and the associated issues in these patients.

Introduction

Paediatric patients with major trauma and burns represent significant pain management problems and present frequently to pre-hospital systems and emergency departments (EDs). Trauma and burn injury of moderate severity require ward and, when severe, intensive care unit (ICU) admission. Hospital stays may be prolonged. Surgery is commonly required, involving many surgical services. Pain, sedation, and anxiety management challenges occur throughout the patient's in-hospital stay and may persist during rehabilitation and post discharge.

Aims

This chapter details pain management of children with major trauma covering their overall trauma care and the patient journey from pre-hospital, through in-patient care to discharge highlighting:

◆ Acute pain management pre-hospital, in the ED and perioperatively.

◆ Procedural sedation provided in the ward setting.

◆ Weaning and step-down analgesic regimens.

This chapter addresses considerations specific to burn injuries. Evidence for practices, when available, will be included. Where possible, variations in international practice are presented.

Case example: trauma

A 14-year-old girl is inebriated and out with her teenage friends at midnight. They are 'train-surfing'—standing on top of a moving suburban train. Her two friends get off at a station but she decides to remain on and they see her balancing on top of the carriage, as the train moves away at speed. Shortly after leaving the station she is thrown from the roof of the train. Her friends see this and call emergency services with paramedics (ambulance officers) attending the scene within 10 min. She is crying in pain, confused, and smells of alcohol. She is tachypnoeic, tachycardic, and hypotensive. She has left chest wall tenderness and marked bruising over her upper abdomen; her right thigh is swollen, deformed, and tender.

Case example: burns

A 2-year-old boy is reported to have pulled a large saucepan of hot water from a stove top. The scalding water has led to burns of his face and anterior chest. His mother puts him under running water in the shower for 2 min and calls emergency services. The paramedics find a screaming toddler with extensive blistering, swelling, and redness extending from his face to below his rib cage. He has no hoarseness or stridor. The rest of his body is not affected.

Pre-hospital care

Care by paramedics occurs in a very different environment from hospital: resources are limited, backup is unavailable or only available remotely; initial assessment and care is often initiated in hostile environments, exposed to the elements with limited visibility; patients can be trapped requiring prolonged extrication; information can be limited and confusing; during transport assessment and procedures may be complicated by patient movement, crowding, and noise. Basic measures to assist with pain management include immobilisation and splinting of fractured limbs, the dressing of wounds, and covering of burns. Burns should be cooled under running tap water for 20 min, even if initial cooling is delayed (Allison and Porter, 2004; ANZBA, 2012) as supported by porcine data (Rajan et al., 2009). While decreasing ongoing heat-related tissue damage and providing pain relief, cooling of burn wounds in children can cause hypothermia. With larger burns and younger children, the wound should be cooled and the patient warmed (Allison and Porter, 2004). Temporary burns dressings should be applied in the pre-hospital setting to reduce pain caused by contact and draft and maintain wound sterility while allowing inspection of the underlying burn. They should not be applied circumferentially as the burnt and periburn tissue can swell with oedema and blistering, causing further pain and vascular compromise. Such temporary burns dressings include cellophane type kitchen wrap and clean/sterile sheets (Allison and Porter, 2004; ANZBA, 2012)

There is limited high-level data on pre-hospital pain care for traumatic injuries in children. In adults and children with obvious traumatic injury, pre-hospital analgesic administration occurs in a low percentage of patients (Rogovik and Goldman, 2007; Swor et al., 2005). The level of pain care provided in pre-hospital systems is largely determined by the type of staff, their level of training and competency, and the protocols guiding pre-hospital analgesic use. Protocols permit the early administration of analgesics by paramedical staff without requiring permission from a remote medical control physician. Earlier increased use of morphine (Pointer and Harlan, 2005; Porter, 2004) occurred when pre-hospital protocols were modified to improve analgesic care.

Morphine and *fentanyl* are extensively used in the pre-hospital setting including in air-transported paediatric trauma patients (DeVellis et al., 1998; Krauss et al., 2011). There may be advantages of fentanyl over morphine (see Sethna et al., Chapter 46, this volume). In a systematic review of pre-hospital adult analgesia with intravenous (IV) morphine and IV fentanyl (Park et al., 2010), no patients required ventilatory support and only one patient in each group required naloxone. More recently intranasal fentanyl (INF) has been used in pre-hospital systems and in EDs. INF has similar analgesic efficacy and time to onset compared to IV morphine. A recent review (Hansen et al., 2012) summarizes paediatric INF use as investigated in a number of randomized controlled trials (RCTs). Comparison of INF with established analgesic agents showed similar decreases in pain scores. No major adverse events occurred with paediatric analgesic INF use and Glasgow coma scale (GCS) and vital signs were unaffected (Hansen et al., 2012). Minor adverse events include nausea, vomiting, pruritis, drowsiness, and a bad taste in the mouth. INF as a sole agent has a low incidence of emesis. The hazards to staff of IV or intramuscular (IM) administration in a moving vehicle combined with difficulties of establishing IV access in children makes INF attractive (Bendall et al., 2011; Johnston et al., 2011). INF is administered by either a mucosal atomizer device (MAD®; attached to a syringe for metered dosing) or a drop-by-drop technique. Usual dosing is 1.5 mcg/kg, divided between each nostril. This administration route bypasses gastrointestinal and hepatic elimination (Hansen et al., 2012; Panagiotou and Mystakidou, 2010). A maximum volume limit of 0.15 ml was suggested to avoid pharyngeal run off (Dale et al., 2002; Hansen et al., 2012). In past studies high concentrations of usually 100 mcg/ml to 300 mcg/ml have been used (Borland et al., 2007; Hansen et al., 2012). However, two recent paediatric studies have demonstrated similar analgesic efficacy of INF using the standard IV

solution (50 mcg/ml; Borland et al., 2011; Crellin et al., 2010). The standard concentration solution has advantages of wide availability, lower cost, and potentially less error because it avoids stocking two concentrations of fentanyl.

Limited data are available on pre-hospital use of other opioids such as diamorphine, nalbuphine, and tramadol (Hyland-McGuire and Guly, 1998; Mackenzie, 2000; Roberts et al., 2003; Vergnion et al., 2001; Ward et al., 1997; Woollard et al., 2004). Successful pre-hospital use of femoral nerve blocks has also been reported (Barker et al., 2008; Lopez et al., 2003; Park et al., 2010). Data in children for these agents and techniques are scant.

Methoxyflurane is an inhaled volatile fluorinated hydrocarbon anaesthetic agent available in a portable, compact delivery system. In Australia and some other countries, it is administered as an analgesic by paramedics from a plastic tube inhaler. The dose lasts approximately 30 min. The total weekly dose must not exceed 15 ml because of the risk of cumulative dose-related irreversible nephrotoxicity (Medical Developments International, n.d.).

Case series indicate that it is an efficacious analgesic in children and adults (Bendall et al., 2011; Grindlay and Babl, 2009). In addition to nephrotoxicity, it has been implicated rarely in hepatotoxicity (Joshi and Conn, 1974). The previous manufacturer, Abbot, withdrew it from the US market in 2001, and the US Food and Drug Administration (FDA) has since removed it from the drug register because of the safety concerns (FDA, 2005).

The mechanism of methoxyflurane's nephrotoxicity is unknown. Methoxyflurane is contraindicated in renal impairment, diabetes, concurrent use of enzyme-inducing drugs or tetracycline, a history of liver damage secondary to anaesthesia, malignant hyperthermia or hypersensitivity to fluorinated anaesthetics (Medical Developments International, n.d.).

Nitrous oxide (N_2O) use on ambulances was described first in 1970 (Baskett, 1970). Recent reports indicate its continuing availability on ambulances in many pre-hospital systems (Bledsoe et al., 2005; Roberts et al., 2003; Siriwardena et al., 2010). It is usually administered in fixed concentration (50% N_2O and 50% oxygen) with a demand valve that limits its utility to children over 4 years of age, who can generate adequate negative pressure to open the valve. It is also problematic in cold environments (Borland et al., 2002). Trauma patients who have potential air trapping (e.g. suspected pneumothorax) may not receive N_2O.

Ketamine has also been used as an analgesic in the pre-hospital setting (Bredmose et al., 2009; Galinski et al., 2007; Jennings et al., 2012; Reid et al., 2011; Svenson and Abernathy, 2007). This includes use in paediatric trauma patients in parenteral and intranasal form (Bredmose et al., 2009; Reid et al., 2011; Svenson and Abernathy, 2007). In a physician-led air ambulance service, 164 children received IV or IM ketamine for analgesia for burns or for procedural sedation for fracture reduction (Bredmose et al., 2009). There were no adverse events or loss of airway, consistent with large scale ED data (Green et al., 2009a, 2009b). In an RCT of 135 adult trauma patients, IV morphine plus low-dose ketamine administered pre-hospital for moderate to severe pain provided superior analgesia to IV morphine alone but was associated with an increase in minor adverse events (Jennings et al., 2012).

Pre-hospital use of *non-pharmacological techniques* has also been described, including RCTs of acupressure in adults (Kober et al., 2002; Lang et al., 2007; McManus and Sallee, 2005).

Emergency department care of trauma

Definitions and classification of trauma

Trauma severity can be classified by injury extent, type, and severity. Injury extent centres around the number of body systems involved with multitrauma defined as involvement of two or more body areas. Injury type refers to penetrating versus blunt trauma. Injury severity groups trauma based on injury mechanism (such as a fall from a certain height) with findings during physical examination. High-risk trauma mechanisms have increased risk of clinical deterioration and require higher level care. A number of different paediatric trauma classification systems assist with patient triage, assess the severity of illness, and predict mortality (Marcin and Pollack, 2002).

Overall trauma management

Pain management in children with major traumatic injuries should be embedded in a standardized approach to trauma care such as the globally used and taught system of the American College of Surgeons' Advanced Trauma Life Support (ATLS®) Course (American College of Surgeons, 2008). ATLS® focuses on the recognition and management of life-threatening abnormalities of vital functions (primary survey and resuscitation) followed by a comprehensive systematic assessment of the trauma patient (secondary survey).

IV access is achieved to manage circulatory status, and is then available for IV analgesia. *Parenteral opioids* are the gold standard for analgesic management worldwide in the setting of moderate to severe trauma and burns management. If IV access is delayed in an unstable paediatric trauma patient, intraosseous access can be quickly established and permits fluid and drug administration including all analgesics (Von Hoff et al., 2008). If patients do not require IV access, such as in mild or isolated extremity trauma, INF provides an excellent alternative (Borland et al., 2007; Hansen et al., 2012) and its use can in itself reduce the need for IV access by 50% (Borland et al., 2008). Analgesic dosing is listed in Table 18.1.

Table 18.1 Analgesic doses used in for pre-hospital or emergency department setting

Analgesic categories and agents	Formulation	Initial or loading dose	Subsequent dosing	Maximum dose	Notes
Parenteral opioid					
IV morphine	10 mg/1ml	50–100 mcg/kg	10–50 mcg/kg	No ceiling but if 200 mcg/kg used consider adjuvant therapy	Gold standard; histamine release may cause hypotension
IV meperidine	100 mg/ml	–	–		Due to abuse and neurotoxic metabolite rarely used now
IV oxycodone	10 mg/1 ml	100–200 mcg/kg	25–50 mcg/kg		IV formulation recently available
IV hydromorphone	2 mg/ml	10–20 mcg/kg	2–10 mcg/kg		
IV fentanyl	100 mcg/2 ml	1–2 mcg/kg	0.25–0.5 mcg/kg		Shorter onset and shorter acting; bradycardia can occur (with hypotension)
Intranasal fentanyl	100 mcg/2 ml Or 300 mcg/2 ml	1.5 mcg/kg (50% in each nostril)		3 mcg/kg	Onset within 10 min with duration of c.60 min
IV remifentanil	1 mg, 2 mg ampoules	0.2–0.5 mcg/kg	Infusion 0.1–0.2 mcg/kg/min		Very potent; rapid onset and offset within 1–3 min; risk of respiratory depression/apnoea very high and so not used in pre-hospital setting
5HT/NA/opioid effects					
Tramadol IV Capsule/tablet Elixir	100 mg/2 ml 50 mg IR 10 mg/ml	1–3 mg/kg	1–2 mg/kg 6/24	100mg/dose 400mg/day	Lowers seizure threshold; avoid if serious head injury. Similar sedation, nausea and vomiting rates to opioids. M1 metabolite active at mu opioid receptors.
Non-opioid					
Acetaminophen IV oral tablet Syrup	500 mg/50 ml or 1000 mg/100 ml Typically 500 mg tablet And various mg/ml concentrations available	15 mg/kg if IV Some use loading doses of 20–30 mg/kg orally	15 mg/kg 4–6/24	1 g/dose 60 mg/kg/day	Some institutions use loading doses; no load and 6/24 prescribing introduced for uniformity across authors' institution Cost of IV 60–180x that of syrup-tablet dose

(Continued)

Table 18.1 (*Continued*)

Analgesic categories and agents	Formulation	Initial or loading dose	Subsequent dosing	Maximum dose	Notes
IV acetaminophen Neonates		10 mg/kg	10 mg/kg 6–12/24	Maximum depends on postmenstrual age	(Palmer et al., 2008)
NSAIDs					
Ibuprofen IV And oral Tablet, caplet Syrup	100 mg/1 ml 200 mg 100 and 200 mg/5 ml	5–10 mg/kg	10 mg/kg tds Give with meals if tolerating oral intake		Generally avoided in acute resuscitation phase as impair platelet adhesion (increasing bleeding risk) and glomerular filtration rate reversibly by 20% (Anderson, Chapter 43, this volume) and can precipitate renal failure in low output states
Diclofenac IV and rectal Tablet	25–100 mg suppositories 12–100 mg	1–2 mg/kg	1–1.5 mg/kg 8–12/24	50–100 mg/dose	Suggested ceiling effect; higher doses prescribed in practice
Indomethacin IV PO				100mg/dose	
IV Ketorolac	60 mg/ml 10 mg/ml	US 1 mg/kg Australia and New Zealand no load	0.5 mg/kg 6/24 0.2 mg/kg 6/24	Maximum 60 mg load then 30 mg per dose Maximum 10 mg/ dose	Not licensed for use in children <12years Costly
COX-2 inhibitors					
Rofecoxib oral	50 mg tablet		1 mg/kg	50 mg/day	Was licensed for use in acute pain. Withdrawn by FDA post cardiac events
Celecoxib Capsule	100 mg and 200 mg Suspension (not marketed; Donnelly et al., 2009)	–	2–4 mg/kg 12/24	400 mg/day	Not licensed for use in acute pain; can disperse capsule contents in water
IV Parecoxib	40 mg powder		1 mg/kg daily	40 mg/day	
NMDA antagonist					
IV Ketamine	200 mg/2 ml	Analgesia: 0.5 mg/kg Anaesthesia: 1–2 mg/kg	0.1–0.4 mg/kg boluses or infusion per hour	If infusion used, usual dose 0.2 mg/kg/h with maximum 0.4 mg/kg/h	Used in children older than 2 years as adjunct or sole agent
Benzodiazepines					
Midazolam	5 mg/ml OR 5 mg/5 ml	0.05–0.1 mg/kg IV 0.5 mg/kg PO 0.4 mg/kg rectal/nasal			Amnestic and muscle relaxant to treat spasm or assist reenlocation
Diazepam IV Tablet Syrup	10 mg/1 ml IV 1 mg/ml PO 5mg Suppositories	0.025–0.05 mg/kg IV 0.05–0.1 mg/kg PO/PR			To treat muscle spasm as an adjunct to opioids and regional, e.g. femoral nerve block
Inhalational					
Nitrous oxide	Entonox premix 50% adjustable system that delivers up to 70%	50–70% delivery for analgesia			Can cause nausea and vomiting; at higher concentrations can cause sedation. Avoid in closed pneumothorax, bowel obstruction
Methoxyflurane	Penthrox® whistle	0.1–0.3 MAC analgesic			

c = circa; FDA = Food and Drug Administration (US authority); IR = immediate release; IV = intravenous;NA = noradrenaline; NSAIDs = non-steroidal anti-inflammatory drugs; MAC = minimum alveolar concentration; NMDA = N-methyl D-aspartate; PO = oral; ® = registered trade mark; 5HT = serotonin

Burns assessment and management

The majority of paediatric burns are hot liquid scalds. Contact and flame burns are less frequent but cause deeper injury. Inhalation airway and lung burns are particularly problematic and in fires can be associated with carbon monoxide poisoning.

The majority of paediatric burn patients can be managed in EDs alone (Rawlins et al., 2007). Criteria for admission and transfer to specialized burn centres have been published (ANZBA, 2004).

Dressings for superficial and partial thickness burns have been Cochrane reviewed (Wasiak et al., 2008). Twenty-six RCTs were assessed and most were methodologically poor. The use of biosynthetic dressings is associated with a decrease in time to healing and reduction in pain during dressing changes. The use of the traditional silver sulphadiazine as comparator in some studies was considered problematic as it was associated with delay in wound healing and increased number of dressing changes. The existing evidence is of limited usefulness in aiding clinicians in choosing an optimal dressing.

Pain assessment

Pain assessment in the ED is often difficult, complicated by the urgency of critical medical issues with competing priorities, language barriers, patients affected by drugs or alcohol, and the difficulty of assessing patients with an immobilizing neck collar receiving oxygen or who are intubated, sedated, or medicated with muscle relaxants. In younger children, it is difficult to distinguish pain and distress. An inebriated, drug affected, or head-injured child or adolescent may be combative or uncooperative.

Pain is assessed using tools appropriate for the child's developmental stage, numeracy and literacy level, and intellectual capability (see chapters in Section 5 of this volume). Abnormal vital signs are sometimes used as proxies for pain, but in the trauma setting may reflect hypovolaemia and can be unreliable even in healthy subjects (Tousignant-Laflamme et al., 2005). The Critical Care Pain Observation Tool (CCPOT) has been developed to assess pain in critically ill ventilated adults. It has good inter-rater reliability (Gelinas and Johnston, 2007) with behavioural indicators providing more valid pain information than physiological indicators.

Case example: trauma (continued)

After placing a neck collar and providing oxygen by mask, the 14-year-old train-surfer was assessed for pain. A patient-reported pain scale could not be obtained due to poor cooperation. A paramedic assigned her a numerical pain scale of value 10/10. While on the train tracks she was offered methoxyflurane and coached in using it, decreasing the paramedic assessed pain score to 4/10. She had an IV placed and received fluid resuscitation. Her right leg was splinted. During the transport to the trauma centre, she received IV morphine (5 mg) due to ongoing pain. She was estimated to weigh 50 kg. On ED arrival, she was assessed by the trauma team. On her secondary survey she was found to have a left clavicle fracture, multiple left rib fractures with pulmonary contusion, abdominal tenderness, and a right mid-shaft femur fracture. She was treated with oxygen by face mask and a second fluid bolus for hypotension. Her pain was assessed as 7/10. Her

right leg was very tender. She had a femoral nerve block placed by the emergency physician under ultrasound guidance. She ceased complaints of leg pain and was log rolled to assess her back. Due to ongoing clavicle, chest, and abdominal pain of 5/10, she was given two further boluses of IV fentanyl followed by IV ketamine (5 mg = 0.1 mg/kg) which settled her pain. However, she became less responsive with a GCS score of 10. It was unclear if the decrease in consciousness was due to her alcohol ingestion, the opioid and ketamine used, or a concomitant head injury. An urgent computed tomography (CT) scan of the head showed bilateral cerebral contusions without midline shift, an abdominal CT showed a small liver laceration. On return from the CT scan her GCS score was 8 and she was intubated for airway protection by rapid sequence induction using thiopental and succinylcholine.

Case example: burns (continued)

The 2-year-old boy with scald burns was assessed to have 30-degree scald burns with large blisters developing over chest and upper abdomen. His burns were covered with a clean sheet by the paramedic services. He was screaming in pain. Paramedics administer INF at 1.5 mcg/kg. On arrival at the hospital, he had stopped crying. In the ED he was assessed to have no airway involvement and no circumferential burns were found. He had an IV placed and received hydration and IV morphine 0.1mg/kg. He was assessed by the burns team and his burns were covered with a silver containing dressing. Due to his burns' extent, he was admitted to a burns unit.

Emergency department analgesia options

Opioids—if the patient is still in pain, but is ventilating adequately and does not have a depressed conscious state, further IV opioids may be titrated (see Table 18.1 for dosing): if pain is mild, at 20% to 50% of loading doses; if pain is severe, repeat loading is appropriate, depending on the timing of the last opioid dose pre-hospital. If two loading doses have been given within the expected duration of the opioid's effect and pain is still severe, then adjunctive agents can be administered while reassessing the child. Compartment syndrome must be considered in the setting of limb fractures and circumferential burns when opioid requirements escalate or pain is uncontrolled. Monitoring and early referral for pressure testing, compartment release, or escharotomy is essential.

Tramadol (see Rastogi and Campbell, Chapter 48, this volume) is an alternative to opioids, also available in parenteral and oral forms. It is not licensed for use under 12 years of age and has not been studied in paediatric trauma or burns patients.

Non-opioid analgesics are used to spare opioid use, reducing opioid-related side effects.

Acetaminophen (paracetamol) is an effective analgesic (Anderson, Chapter 43, this volume). As it is available in IV form, it is a useful intervention in the acute trauma and burns setting (Babl et al., 2011) as patients are fasting and plasma levels are rapidly achieved (over the rectal or oral route). Patients admitted with trauma or burns typically receive acetaminophen for several days to weeks. Their liver function should be monitored and the daily maximum prescribed should take expected duration and probably ideal body weight into account.

Non-steroidal/non-selective anti-inflammatory drugs (NSAIDs; Anderson, Chapter 43, this volume) are *not used* in the acute moderate to severe trauma and burns setting due to their platelet inhibiting and renal effects. Platelet inhibition (although reversible with all except aspirin) may exacerbate bleeding propensity, particularly if coagulopathy is present. NSAIDs reduce renal arteriolar flow and reversibly reduce glomerular filtration, via cyclo-oxygenase (COX)-2 inhibition. If the patient is volume deplete, from blood or extracellular fluid loss (due to trauma and burns respectively), this NSAID effect may precipitate renal failure (Musu et al., 2011).

The *N-methyl-D-aspartate (NMDA) antagonist* ketamine (Cravero, Chapter 20, this volume) is used in the major trauma/burns ED setting usually as a second- or third-line agent to IV opioids and IV acetaminophen when pain is still problematic. It is generally given as intermittent boluses of analgesic doses of 0.1 to 0.2 mg/kg every 10 min (i.e. 10% of an anaesthetic dose). Morphine sparing efficacy of 0.2 mg/kg IV over placebo was found in adult trauma patients (n = 65; Galinski et al., 2007). Ketamine is not a respiratory depressant in its own right; however, it should be carefully titrated using a maximum single bolus of 0.5 mg/kg as opioid-induced respiratory depression can be precipitated once analgesia is achieved.

Benzodiazepines (BDZs), such as midazolam, diazepam, lorazepam, may be used in these patients' acute management for their muscle relaxant, anxiolytic, and sedative properties. They are used to supplement parenteral opioids or a regional block (e.g. fractured femur) to alleviate muscle spasm. They are used if the patient has escalating anxiety and/or distress (Kennedy, Chapter 34, this volume) not responding to analgesia and opioid titration. Midazolam has the additional benefit of antegrade amnesia and rapid onset (see Table 18.1).

Single-shot *nerve blocks* in trauma in the ED are useful (Barnett, 2009). Their application in trained hands is easily achieved, reducing or avoiding the need in multitrauma patients for opioids. In major trauma, a frequently used and useful block is the *femoral nerve block*. Paediatric femur fractures generally occur in the mid-shaft which is supplied by the femoral nerve (Barnett, 2009). Bupivacaine is usually used because of its longer duration of action. Following paediatric anaesthesiologists' practice (Flack and Anderson, 2012; Tsui and Suresh, 2010), the availability of ultrasound machines in EDs allows confirmation of the target nerve's position and avoids unwanted puncture and intravascular or intraneural injection (Frenkel et al., 2012; Reid et al., 2009). The alternative to a femoral nerve block is the fascia iliaca compartment block which has been successfully used in children in the ED. This block (performed without ultrasound; using ropivacaine) was compared to IV morphine for paediatric femoral fractures. It provided clinically superior pain management from 0.5 to 6 h (Wathen et al., 2007).

N2O can be used where short-acting sedation and analgesia is required for procedures associated with pain, discomfort or anxiety (see Cravero, Chapter 20, this volume). It can be used for minor trauma, instrumentation, and vascular access (Krauss and Green, 2006; Mace et al., 2008). N_2O should be combined with analgesia and topical, local, regional, or IV regional anaesthesia whenever possible to enhance the relatively weak analgesic properties of the agent for trauma-related procedures (Babl et al., 2008a). To achieve analgesia for painful procedures, N_2O can be combined with other techniques, such as INF (Seith et al., 2012), oral analgesia, and a haematoma block (Luhmann et al., 2006) or IV regional anaesthesia (Bier's block). N_2O reduces recall (Babl et al.,

2008a; Kanagasundaram et al., 2001). N_2O up to 70% for procedural sedation and analgesia is usually well tolerated by children with a low incidence of minor adverse events (5–8%: including vomiting, nausea, dizziness, and light-headedness) and rare serious or potentially serious adverse events (Babl et al., 2008b; Zier and Liu, 2011). Apnoea, aspiration, or the need for airway intervention has not been reported in large series after single-agent use of N_2O. In trauma patients N_2O should be avoided in patients with chest trauma and the possibility of an expanding pneumothorax or in head injured patients where there is a possibility of expanding intracranial air.

N_2O may also have adverse effects on staff or parents. Although there is no conclusive evidence for reproductive, genetic, haematological, genetic, or fetal effects (Axelsson et al., 1996; Rowland et al., 1992; Sanders et al., 2008), exposure should be minimized: using occupational health and safety approved sedation rooms, maintaining an adequate patient face-to-mask seal and using a suitable scavenging system. Exposure to N_2O should be avoided during pregnancy.

Ward management

Patient-controlled analgesia (PCA) delivery of opioids for alert, extubated patients over 7 years (McDonald and Cooper, 2001; Playfor et al., 2006) and *nurse-controlled analgesia* (NCA) (also described as continuous opioid infusions with nurse-initiated boluses) for younger patients, infants, and intubated patients (see Howard, Chapter 27, this volume) are universally used in the setting of major trauma/burns. These may be initiated in the ED and the patient continues to use this during their ward stay.

The most common opioid used is morphine but any opioid can be prescribed (Table 19.1). The usual prescription is for 1 to 2 ml boluses with a lockout of 5 to 7 min. Some institutions include a 1 or 4 h limit. In acute postoperative pain management, a background infusion on a PCA is generally avoided beyond 24 h (Howard, Chapter 27, this volume). In a trauma or a burn patient, a background is more often prescribed; when the continuous rate is higher than 2 ml/h, the bolus size is usually increased to match. An NCA involves the same concentration dilution infused at 0.5–4 ml/h with 1–2 ml boluses usually every 5 to 10 min.

Adjunctive *continuous ketamine infusion* (Howard, Chapter 27, this volume) is used frequently in these patients. Typical paediatric infusion prescriptions include ketamine 5 mg/kg in a total of 50 ml normal saline run at 0.1 to 0.3 mg/kg/h (1–3 ml per hour) (<http://www.rch.org.au/anaes/pain_management/Ketamine_Infusion/>). Higher infusion rates may be employed but hallucinations may occur (contributed to by polypharmacy, sepsis, and sleep deprivation). Our institution has infusion guidelines permitting additional ketamine bolus administration of 0.1 to 0.2 mg/kg every 30 min to be co-administered with opioid boluses or as an alternative if opioid side effects are prominent.

NSAIDs are particularly effective for pain of bony and muscular origin and may be used in the acute phase of analgesic management of musculoskeletal trauma and limb fractures, once volume resuscitation is complete, haemodynamic stability is achieved, and urine output is established (Anderson, Chapter 43, this volume). Parenteral forms are available. If NSAIDs are used when the patient is fasting or has an ileus, co-administration of a proton pump inhibitor is routine in moderate to severe burns or trauma patients to reduce the combined effects of stress and NSAIDs on the gastric mucosa. NSAIDs also impair osteoclast activity. This is desirable to reduce heterotropic bone formation but undesirable in the setting of extensive bone graft/fusion procedures. Reduced fusion has been reported in adult studies using high-dose ketorolac but not with normal-dose short-duration exposure (Li et al., 2011) and not in a retrospective review of teenagers (Sucato et al., 2008).

The newer *COX-2 inhibiting agents* (Anderson, Chapter 43, this volume) available are IV parecoxib (a prodrug of valdecoxib) and oral valdecoxib in its own right. Oral celecoxib is in capsule form which may be challenging to administer to children. A suspension is stable (Donnelly et al., 2009) but has not been marketed. These agents are used off licence in children during or post surgery where bleeding is a concern and reduction or avoidance of opioid use is desirable, e.g. in patients with respiratory or neurological compromise or obstructive sleep apnoea. COX-2s are without the platelet inhibition effect but still share the NSAIDs' renal effects and are thus used post-stabilization in acute trauma and burns. They are employed in skin graft surgery, to reduce opioid requirement particularly when pruritis with burns is prominent, or for bone grafting surgery when the clinicians wish to avoid NSAIDs.

Regional analgesia

Single-shot blocks performed in the ED can be repeated after ward admission and are employed perioperatively for these patients. Anaesthesiologists can offer *catheter techniques and local anaesthetic infusions* (see Zempsky, Chapter 47, this volume) (usually performed while anaesthetized) for internal fixation and limb reimplantation procedures of the upper (brachial plexus and interscalene techniques) and lower limbs (femoral and fascia iliaca), fractured ribs, flail segments, and thoracotomy (intercostal nerve blocks and paravertebral block/catheter) or for thoracic or abdominal surgery or lower limb fracture or graft surgery (epidural or caudal catheter/single shot). Other *perioperative single shot nerve blocks* employed are for free flaps and skin harvesting and/or grafting. These include lateral cutaneous nerve of thigh and transversus abdominis plane blocks and the aforementioned brachial plexus, femoral and fascia iliaca blocks (Sethna et al., Chapter 46, this volume).

ICU analgesia-sedation practices

These patients are typically on opioids for prolonged periods. The commonly administered agents in ICU for analgesia and sedation management are the opioids morphine and fentanyl and the benzodiazepines midazolam and lorazepam (Playfor et al., 2006; Stoddard et al., 2011b; Tobias, 2005; Twite et al., 2004). A consensus guideline has been created in the UK for critically ill children (Playfor et al., 2006). It suggests:

* Morphine infusions of 10 to 60 mcg/kg/h.
* Fentanyl infusions of 4 to 10 mcg/kg/h.
* Midazolam 2 to 10 mcg/kg/min.

Ketamine is not mentioned in the 2006 UK consensus. It is used in Australian and US ICUs (Twite et al., 2004). In our experience this patient group requires high infusion rates, e.g. greater than 5 to 7 mcg/kg/min or 300 to 400 mcg/kg/h, while a US review reports the use as sole agent at high sedative doses of 1 to 2 mg/kg/h (Tobias, 2005). We typically co-administer ketamine, opioid, and benzodiazepine infusions in these patients when in ICU for days to weeks.

One Canadian article reports ketamine use for 37 days in a child (White and Karsli, 2007).

There is no consensus on the indications for muscle paralysis (Playfor et al., 2007). Muscle relaxant administration is generally reserved for trauma-burn patients with head injury, facial–airway–pulmonary burns, smoke inhalation and primary or secondary respiratory disease, dyssynchrony with the ventilator, or use of the less physiological ventilation techniques such as high-frequency oscillation. Higher-dose analgesic administration has resulted with the move away from prolonged muscle relaxant administration during prolonged ventilation (Playfor et al., 2007; Twite et al., 2004). The patients frequently develop polytolerance (Playfor et al., 2006). As a result, achieving adequate sedation levels can be challenging and the patient may resist mechanical ventilation and require physical restraint despite receiving high doses of multiple agents. Delirium and emergence phenomena are experienced and complicate the clinical assessment of pain, distress, and septic episodes (Playfor et al., 2006).

These patients commonly receive supplementation with alternative sedative agents (Playfor et al., 2006; Tobias, 2005; Twite et al., 2004) including antihistamines, chloral hydrate (25–100 mg/kg, 4–6/24), psychoactive agents (haloperidol, chlorpromazine, and more recently olanzapine (Stoddard et al., 2006)), propofol infusions 1 to 3 mg/kg/h for limited periods (with the clinicians being aware of propofol infusion syndrome) and alpha-2 agonists clonidine (transdermal, intermittent IV bolus doses 2–5 mcg/kg three times daily or infusion 0.1–2 mcg/kg/h) and more recently dexmedetomidine by IV/subcutaneous (SC) infusion at (0.1–2 mcg/kg/h with or without loading dose of 0.5–1 mcg/kg) (Lin et al., 2011; Phan and Nahata, 2008; Tobias, 2007, 2008; Walker et al., 2006). ICU staff may involve an acute pain service early or prior to discharge to the standard ward.

Alpha-2 agonists

These agents have multiple desirable properties for use in burn or multitrauma patient management (Phan and Nahata, 2008). They are sedative, anxiolytic, reduce patient and distress, sympathetic outflow, and are adjunctive analgesics (Playfor et al., 2006). They are effective by reducing release of presynaptic catecholamines. The mechanism of analgesic effect is unclear with central (locus coeruleus) versus spinal (descending inhibition) versus peripheral effects (via substance P) proposed.

Clonidine causes a degree of bradycardia and hypotension which may be desirable in the polytolerant agitated patient but can be problematic during septic episodes. Interestingly in thermally injured rat studies, clonidine's vasoconstrictive effects were suggested to be detrimental by impairing healing (Cassuto et al., 2005b) and beneficial in terms of oedema reduction (Cassuto et al., 2005a). The bradycardic, hypotensive side effect also occurs with dexmedetomidine. Reports state it is well tolerated during sedation of the critically ill patient including paediatric cardiac or respiratory ICU patients (off-label use; Phan and Nahata, 2008; Tobias, 2007).

The doses for sedation are outlined in the 'ICU analgesia-sedation practices' section. Alpha-2 agonists are also useful premedicants prior to second-phase trauma or burns surgery: single-dose clonidine 2 to 5 mcg/kg orally or IV alone or combined with midazolam 0.5 mcg/kg oral or 0.1 mg/kg IV. Dexmedetomidine 2 mcg/kg has been used via the intranasal route and compared favourably to oral midazolam 0.5 mg/kg, as premedication prior to burns reconstructive surgery (Talon et al., 2009).

The 14-year-old train-surfer went to the operating room to have an intracranial pressure monitor placed and the right femoral fracture repaired with an internal fixation device. In the ICU she was sedated using morphine and midazolam infusions. After 24 h, sedation was stopped and she was extubated. She was neurologically normal but complained of severe left chest pain (rib fractures) and right thigh pain which was inadequately controlled with intermittent boluses of IV morphine. She was started on a PCA device with IV morphine and required this for 5 days. Her daily IV morphine consumption was 80 mg, 95 mg, 60 mg, 50 mg, and 40 mg respectively and so on day 6 she was converted to oxycodone CR and IR. She was still complaining of rib pain and disturbed sleep. She was prescribed OxyContin® 20 mg morning and 30mg at night and intermittent oxycodone IR 5 to 10 mg with amitriptyline 25 mg at night. She was discharged home on day 10 on OxyContin® 10 mg twice daily, oxycodone, ibuprofen, and amitriptyline 50 mg at night for review by her general practitioner.

The ongoing pain of the 2-year-old boy with scald burns was treated with oral acetaminophen and oral oxycodone. The burns were debrided in theatre on three occasions including grafting under a general anaesthetic. He required regular burns dressing changes which were conducted on the ward in the burns bath and later at the bedside under IV ketamine.

Step-down conversions from IV to oral opioids and tapering

The oral agent chosen and conversion plan in a burnt or multitrauma patient will depend on the:

◆ Rate/total dose and duration of treatment with opioids.

◆ Presence of tolerance.

◆ Presence of ongoing pain sources.

◆ Degree of background pain.

◆ Breakthrough pain associated with care (turns, dressing changes, physiotherapy, surgery).

◆ Prevention of opioid withdrawal syndrome when pain is absent or controlled.

◆ Routes available (oral versus gastric or jejunal feeding tube).

◆ Timing of further interventions.

When the patient is still experiencing pain but is tolerating oral intake, the parenteral opioid dose received in the preceding 24 to 48 h is calculated. If greater than 0.5 mg/kg/day of IV morphine equivalent was received, then approximately 50% to 80% of this is given as long-acting (depending on pain severity) with an immediate-release opioid prescribed as a rescue either as a single dose (usually at one-sixth of the patient's overall use) or with a range to allow for fluctuations, e.g. pre-emptive administration prior to aggressive

physical therapy. The long-acting component is weaned when the patient requires less than two rescues a day. The drop in dose is usually 'convenient' according to the available tablet size. Usually the morning dose is reduced first as the patient can request rescue medication while awake during the day. The night dose is maintained to facilitate comfort in sleep and weaned and ceased last.

A proscriptive opioid taper is prescribed when pain is minimal and tolerance is present with little data to support practices (Fisher, 2010). Previously slow tapers were performed similar in length to the duration of the opioid treatment. More recent practice is to taper by 10% to 20% daily, ceasing in 5 to 10 days. When an IV is no longer required, patients are switched to the SC route or enteric administration of either a longer acting formulation (Anand et al., 2010) or a different opioid at equivalent dosing. Withdrawal symptoms are ideally scored 8-hourly using the withdrawal assessment tool (WAT)-1 (Franck et al., 2012) or modified Finnegan score (Oschman et al., 2011). Morphine sulphate sustained-release granules or methadone elixir are convenient for enteric tube administration. Treatment can be guided according to withdrawal score tiers and either non-taper performed if moderate symptoms persist or rescue doses of immediate release opioids (or benzodiazepines or alpha-2 agonists) prescribed if symptoms are severe.

Fentanyl patches can be used if the enteric route is unavailable. A pilot study reports the use of patches in patients treated with high cumulative doses of IV fentanyl. This study (Johnson et al., 2010) inappropriately employed the practice of partly covering a fentanyl patch with Tegaderm®. Twelve-microgram patches are now available (but use in non-cancer pain is still off-licence).

Pruritis and neuropathic pain

Multitrauma patients experience neuropathic pain mechanistically related to their injury (e.g. compression or severance of peripheral nerves). They usually experience pruritis secondary to opioids. This is managed with antihistamines, optimization of non-opioid analgesics and opioid rotation, or small-dose naloxone (1 mcg/kg). Children and adult burns patients are frequently distressed by neurogenic pruritis (80–100% incidence). This is often severe, and persists for years after healing and successful grafting (Goutos et al., 2009, 2010). Neuropathic-like symptoms in the burn wound (hot sharp pain) are reported early from day 3 (Gray et al., 2011) and later (mean 4.3 months) post injury in adults (Schneider et al., 2006).

Agents used for pruritis in burns include antihistamines, topical doxepin or amitriptyline, massage therapy, topical treatments such as local anaesthetics, colloidal oatmeal, aloe vera and moisturizer, cool facewasher-icepack application, transcutaneous electrical nerve stimulation, compression garments, ondansetron and the gabapentinoids: gabapentin/pregabalin (Goutos et al., 2009). Five weeks of biweekly 15 min periburn massage sessions benefitted adolescents with burns with reduced pain, itching, and state anxiety versus controls (Parlak Gurol et al., 2010). Small open-label adult series of naltrexone (Jung et al., 2009; LaSalle et al., 2008) and IV lidocaine (Koppert et al., 2004) use have promise. More research is required to elucidate whether these agents or possibly clonidine could have beneficial roles if used early post injury.

The underlying mechanism of neurogenic itch and neuropathic pain-like symptoms probably has similar origin relating to C fibre in-growth, sprouting, increased spontaneous and high-frequency firing with stimuli, cross talk and descending inhibitory dysregulation supported in rat nerve (Radtke et al., 2010) and adult human punch biopsy study (Hamed et al., 2011). Gabapentinoids are consequently used in both neuropathic itch and neuropathic pain management.

A paediatric pilot study of gabapentin use for itch reported doses of 5 mg/kg morning, lunchtime, and 5 then 10 mg/kg nightly (Mendham, 2004). Itch reduced after 24 h of therapy and antihistamine use reduced or ceased. A stepwise approach was adopted in two groups of 50 patients (25% children). Itch was relieved better in the polytherapy groups: gabapentin (5 mg/kg (maximum 300 mg) three times a day), cetirizine, cyproheptadine group (95%) versus the chlorpheniramine, cetirizine, cyproheptadine group (84%) versus monotherapy with gabapentin (10%) or chlorpheniramine (44%) (Goutos et al., 2010). Another adult trial of 28 days of monotherapy reports all 40 gabapentin-treated patients achieving itch-free status compared to only three cetirizine treated (Ahuja et al., 2011).

Pregabalin (75–300 mg twice daily) has to date been studied in adults only. Neuropathic pain scale sharp, hot, and itch scores were impacted as were procedural pain scores (Gray et al., 2011). Statistical significance was achieved although the clinical impact was relatively small.

Antidepressants are increasingly prescribed in US ICUs (Stoddard et al., 2006, 2011b) and elsewhere for burn (and multitrauma) patients. Early psychopathology is common and anxiety and depression can persist for months (van Baar et al., 2011). Antidepressant drugs are used for their antineuropathic, sedative, psychomodulatory, antianxiety, and antidepressant effects (Stoddard et al., 2006). Antidepressant administration for paediatric neuropathic pain is sparsely studied with small sample sizes (see Rastogi and Campbell, Chapter 48, this volume). In a placebo-controlled crossover study, parents reported sertraline reduced post-traumatic stress symptoms without change in the children's report (Stoddard et al., 2011a). A placebo controlled trial in significantly burnt children suggests superiority of fluoxetine (72% response) versus imipramine (60%) and placebo (55%) (Robert et al., 2008). The same group published a chart review of the same agents (Tcheung et al., 2005) which was criticized for inadequate definition of acute stress disorder (Thombs et al., 2006)

The potential of antidepressant drug interactions must be carefully considered. Interactions can be both positive (e.g. adjuvant analgesia) and negative (CYP2D6 inhibition, serotonergic syndrome, e.g. with co-administration of tramadol).

Sleep disturbance

Most hospitalized patients have sleep disturbance which is more prominent in trauma and burns patients. Sleep deprivation results from multiple factors (Jaffe and Patterson, 2004):

- Physiological effects of trauma or burns with stress response, reduced growth hormone production, and fluid retention (exacerbation of obstructive sleep apnoea).

- Psychological effects—post-traumatic stress symptoms and disorder, anxiety and depression, distressing repeated procedures.

- Presence of prolonged periods of pain or pruritis.

- Treatment interventions such as frequent observation, sedative-analgesic administration that affect slow wave sleep (SWS) and rapid eye movement (REM) sleep, pharyngeal motility, and cause hypoventilation (opioids, benzodiazepines, barbiturates).

- Disrupted circadian rhythm, un-conducive environment (noise, light).

Non- pharmacological techniques are important and should be instituted as early as permissible in the unwell patient:

- Improve sleep hygiene (regular to bed and planned waking times), restrict napping, exercise during day.

- Light therapy: UV exposure, dawn simulation.

- Reduce stimuli: restrict visitors, reduce noise, stop TV/gaming.

- Nutritional: avoid caffeine and heavy evening meal.

- Relaxation training.

Pharmacological agents are introduced to restore the sleep wake cycle. They are commenced as early as feasible and include:

- Various benzodiazepines orally (PO)/IV or alternative BDZ receptor agonist (zolpidem: PO). These reduce sleep latency but negatively affect SWS/REM sleep and have rebound insomnia on cessation.

- Melatonin at doses of 0.5 escalating to 1.5 mg/kg PO. This agent should probably be first line in these patients as not only is it chronobiotic but it is a free radical scavenger, an antioxidant, reduces pro-inflammatory cytokines and adhesion molecules and may reduce thermal injury-related lymphocytopenia and oxidative damage (Maldonado et al., 2007). In rats at high dose (10 mg/kg), it reduces inflammatory marker elevation and coagulation disorder (Bekyarova et al., 2010) and gastric mucosal injury (Bekyarova et al., 2009).

- Haloperidol, particularly if delirium is present—0.1 mg/kg PO or 0.02 mg/kg IV.

- Sedative antihistamines—promethazine, chlorpromazine, etc. which may assist with pruritis but are simultaneously detrimental to sleep architecture.

- Clonidine 3 to 5 mcg/kg for sedative and anxiolytic properties.

- Antidepressants with sedative side effects: amitriptyline/nortriptyline 0.5 escalated to 1.5 to 2 mg/kg PO versus treatment of anxiety or depressive disorder with a morning SSRI, e.g. fluoxetine 5 to 20 mg.

- Gabapentinoids can be administered at higher evening versus morning doses and will assist pain, pruritis, anxiety, and cause sedation.

Procedural interventions

General anaesthesia, the performance of local anaesthetic blocks intraoperatively, and postoperative parenteral analgesic techniques are discussed elsewhere in this volume.

Procedures are often performed in the ward and later in the outpatient environment. During sedation-analgesia for a surgical intervention, opportunity can be taken for additional interventions such as IV or arterial line re-siting or dressing change, passive physical therapy, and naso-jejunal feeding tube insertion.

Techniques available to the patient during ward procedures include the following:

Propofol IV for light or deep sedation for ward procedures alone and in combination with opioids or ketamine. A study of paediatric burns dressing changes (n = 32) showed equal efficacy of IV propofol-fentanyl (1.2 mg: 1 mcg/kg) and propofol-ketamine (1.2 mg: 1 mg/kg) with less restlessness in the propofol-ketamine group (Tosun et al., 2008).

Ketamine is frequently used as a sole agent for burns dressing changes and burns baths. It can be given via various routes: intranasal, oral (0.5–2 mg/kg for analgesia and 5–7 mg/kg for sedation), and IV (0.5–2 mg/kg) in titrated boluses. Ketamine (and its active metabolite norketamine) pharmacokinetics have been studied in paediatric burns patients having general anaesthesia. Pharmacokinetic parameters were similar to those in paediatric ED fracture patients (Brunette et al., 2011). Simulation dosing data suggests 10 mg/kg orally followed by infusion of 1 mg/kg/h permits short-duration surgical dressing at 45 min. A large retrospective review reports protocolized IV ketamine administration (in conjunction with IV or oral midazolam) by nurse practitioners (Owens et al., 2006). Mean ketamine doses of 147 mg IV were given to children of mean weight 30 kg having 347 bedside procedures. Ten events (2.9%) required respiratory intervention: repositioning (2), oral airway insertion (1), supplemental oxygen via nasal prongs (1) and bag-mask ventilation (4) with none requiring intubation. Rectal S-ketamine 0.75 mg/kg in combination with midazolam 0.4 mg/kg is reported for 47 outpatient dressing changes in 30 young children with 5% to 15% burns. Sedation was good to excellent in the majority (Heinrich et al., 2004).

N2O alone is a popular inhaled analgesic management option during in and outpatient procedures (e.g. external fixateur adjustments) or dressing change. It can be used in conjunction with timely administration of IV, IN, and oral opioids and non-opioids or midazolam.

Single-dose benzodiazepine via various routes is useful for procedural sedation: midazolam providing amnesia and lorazepam and diazepam used for longer-duration anxiolysis-sedation.

Oral analgesic-sedative combinations for dressing changes include acetaminophen with a NSAID, opioid, and a benzodiazepine or clonidine and/or ketamine.

Non-pharmacological therapies include relaxation training, hypnosis, massage, and various forms of distraction therapy including music, play (including clown doctors), art, schooling, cartoon and favourite video/DVD viewing, hypnosis, massage, pet therapy, interactive videogames and virtual reality.

Interactive video games (IVGs) and virtual reality (VR)

IVGs have been studied in burns patients. Nintendo Wii® has been compared with Play station Eye Toy®. The latter was associated with higher demands and longer duration of active upper extremity motion indicating potential application in (post-burns) rehabilitation (Parry et al., 2012). *Immersive VR* involving a computer-generated virtual environment has been employed for painful physiotherapy. The patient wears head gear to exclude visual and aural input of their medical intervention (Sharar et al., 2007). In adult and paediatric burn patients, worst pain intensity, pain unpleasantness, and time spent thinking about pain are reduced (Sharar et al., 2007). Multiple use of immersive VR was assessed in children: pain scores were reduced and affect improved with patients experiencing fun although there was no difference in the maximum range of motion achieved (Schmitt et al., 2011).

For outpatient dressing changes, standard distraction (access to TV, video games, stories, toys, nursing staff soothing, and care giver support) was compared to multimodal distraction (MMD) involving a device that includes a procedural preparation video ('Bobby got a Burn') and includes games, 'touch and find' stories with multisensory feedback (visual, auditory, and vibratory). Parent and nursing pain scores were significantly less in the MMD group (reduced by 30% and 50% respectively; Miller et al., 2010). Virtual reality has been employed in a patient series (aged 9–40 years) having debridement in the hydrotank (burns bath; Hoffman et al., 2008).

Key recommendations

+ Pain management in trauma and burns patients should be embedded in a standardized approach to trauma care.

+ Opioid use is the mainstay of therapy and where possible opioid-sparing adjuvant agents should be introduced.

+ Intranasal fentanyl is a novel administration technique that has efficacy in the pre-hospital and ED setting for trauma patients. Its use is likely to extend to ward and outpatient settings for this patient group.

+ Local anaesthetic agents either topically, by infiltration, or as a nerve or regional block should be employed wherever possible to reduce the need for systemic agents (particularly opioids) and their subsequent systemic side effects.

+ Multimodal analgesia is essential in the effective management of pain in moderate to severe multitrauma or burn patients. Evidence supporting this practice in paediatrics is sparse.

+ Polypharmacy leads to polytolerance; withdrawal scoring should be a routine assessment performed in these patients during down-titration of opioids and sedatives.

+ Ketamine is useful as an analgesic and in anaesthetic doses for procedural sedation.

+ Alpha-2 agonists have multiple properties of therapeutic benefit in this patient group. The reported negative effects of clonidine in thermally injured rats need to be clarified as off-licence use of dexmedetomidine in this paediatric patient population is increasing. Both clonidine and dexmedetomidine offer advantages in sedation of these patients, and abstinence syndrome prevention and treatment.

+ Scientific understanding of the neurobiology of pain and the response to thermal injury at cellular, nerve fibre and tissue level is progressing.

+ Gabapentinoids offer benefits in neuropathic pain symptoms and pruritis. A multimodal approach is likely to be of benefit in these two conditions over mono-therapy alone.

+ Depression and anxiety symptoms are prominent several months to years post multitrauma or burn event. Antidepressant therapy should be considered early along with psychology/counselling to simultaneously address insomnia, neuropathic pain, pruritis, anxiety, depression, and post-traumatic and current stress.

+ Intervention to improve sleep should be employed as early as feasible. More study on the benefits of therapy with melatonin is required.

References

Ahuja, R. B., Gupta, R., Gupta, G., and Shrivastava, P. (2011). A comparative analysis of cetirizine, gabapentin and their combination in the relief of post-burn pruritus. *Burns*, 37, 203–207.

Allison, K. and Porter, K. (2004). Consensus on the pre-hospital approach to burns patient management. *Injury*, 35, 734–738.

American College of Surgeons. (2008). *ATLS®: Advanced Trauma Life Support for Doctors* (Student Course Manual). Chicago, IL: American College of Surgeons.

Anand, K. J. S., Willson, D. F., Berger, J., Harrison, R., Meert, K. L., Zimmerman, J., et al. (2010). Tolerance and withdrawal from prolonged opioid use in critically ill children. *Pediatrics*, 125, e1208–1225.

ANZBA. (2004). *Criteria for specialised burns treatment*. Australian and New Zealand Burn Association. Available at: <http://www.anzba.org.au/index.php?option=com_content&view=article&id=51&Itemid=58> (accessed September 2012).

ANZBA. (2012). *First aid in burns*. Australian and New Zealand Burn Association. Available at: <http://www.anzba.org.au/index.php?option=com_content&view=article&id=46&Itemid=103> (accessed September 2012).

Axelsson, G., Ahlborg, G. Jr., and Bodin, L. (1996). Shift work, nitrous oxide exposure, and spontaneous abortion among Swedish midwives. *Occup Environ Med*, 53, 374–378.

Babl, F. E., Oakley, E., Puspitadewi, A., and Sharwood, L. N. (2008a). Limited analgesic efficacy of nitrous oxide for painful procedures in children. *Emerg Med J*, 25, 717–721.

Babl, F. E., Oakley, E., Seaman, C., Barnett, P., and Sharwood, L. N. (2008b). High-concentration nitrous oxide for procedural sedation in children: adverse events and depth of sedation. *Pediatrics*, 121, e528–532.

Babl, F. E., Theophilos, T., and Palmer, G. M. (2011). Is there a role for intravenous acetaminophen in pediatric emergency departments? *Pediatr Emerg Care*, 27, 496–499.

Barker, R., Schiferer, A., Gore, C., Gorove, L., Lang, T., Steinlechner, B., et al. (2008). Femoral nerve blockade administered preclinically for pain relief in severe knee trauma is more feasible and effective than intravenous metamizole: a randomized controlled trial. *J Trauma Injury Infect Crit Care*, 64, 1535–1538.

Barnett, P. (2009). Alternatives to sedation for painful procedures. *Pediatr Emerg Care*, 25, 415–419.

Baskett, P. J. (1970). Use of Entonox in the ambulance service. *Br Med J*, 2, 41–43.

Bekyarova, G., Galunska, B., Ivanova, D., and Yankova, T. (2009). Effect of melatonin on burn-induced gastric mucosal injury in rats. *Burns*, 35, 863–868.

Bekyarova, G., Tancheva, S., and Hristova, M. (2010). The effects of melatonin on burn-induced inflammatory responses and coagulation disorders in rats. *Methods Find Exp Clin Pharmacol*, 32, 299–303.

Bendall, J. C., Simpson, P. M., and Middleton, P. M. (2011). Effectiveness of prehospital morphine, fentanyl, and methoxyflurane in pediatric patients. *Prehosp Emerg Care*, 15, 158–165.

Bledsoe, B., Braude, D., Dailey, M. W., Myers, J., Richards, M., and Wesley, K. (2005). Simplifying prehospital analgesia. Why certain medications should or should not be used for pain management in the field. *JEMS*, 30, 56–63.

Borland, M., Jacobs, I., King, B., and O'Brien, D. (2007). A randomized controlled trial comparing intranasal fentanyl to intravenous morphine for managing acute pain in children in the emergency department. *Ann Emerg Med*, 49, 335–340.

Borland, M., Milsom, S., and Esson, A. (2011). Equivalency of two concentrations of fentanyl administered by the intranasal route for acute analgesia in children in a paediatric emergency department: a randomized controlled trial. *Emerg Med Australas* 23, 202–208.

Borland, M. L., Clark, L. J., and Esson, A. (2008). Comparative review of the clinical use of intranasal fentanyl versus morphine in a paediatric emergency department. *Emerg Med Australas*, 20, 515–5120.

Borland, M. L., Jacobs, I., and Rogers, I. R. (2002). Options in prehospital analgesia. *Emerg Med*, 14, 77–84.

Bredmose, P. P., Grier, G., Davies, G. E., and Lockey, D. J. (2009). Pre-hospital use of ketamine in paediatric trauma. *Acta Anaesthesiol Scand*, 53, 543–545.

Brunette, K. E. J., Anderson, B. J., Thomas, J., Wiesner, L., Herd, D. W., and Schulein, S. (2011). Exploring the pharmacokinetics of oral ketamine in children undergoing burns procedures. *Paediatr Anaesth*, 21, 653–662.

Cassuto, J., Tarnow, P., Yregard, L., Lindblom, L., and Rantfors, J. (2005a). Adrenoceptor subtypes in the control of burn-induced plasma extravasation. *Burns*, 31, 123–129.

Cassuto, J., Tarnow, P., Yregard, L., Lindblom, L., and Rantfors, J. (2005b). Regulation of postburn ischemia by alpha- and beta-adrenoceptor subtypes. *Burns*, 31, 131–137.

Crellin, D., Ling, R. X., and Babl, F. E. (2010). Does the standard intravenous solution of fentanyl (50 microg/mL) administered intranasally have analgesic efficacy? *Emerg Med Australas*, 22, 62–67.

Dale, O., Hjortkjaer, R., and Kharasch, E. D. (2002). Nasal administration of opioids for pain management in adults. *Acta Anaesthesiol Scand*, 46, 759–770.

Devellis, P., Thomas, S. H., Wedel, S. K., Stein, J. P., and Vinci, R. J. (1998). Prehospital fentanyl analgesia in air-transported pediatric trauma patients. *Pediatr Emerg Care*, 14, 321–323.

Donnelly, R. F., Pascuet, E., Ma, C., and Vaillancourt, R. (2009). Stability of celecoxib oral suspension. *Can J Hosp Pharm*, 62, 464–468.

FDA (2005). Federal Drug Administration. Notice: human drugs: new drug applications- penthrane(methoxyflurane) inhalation liquid, 99.9. *Fed Regist*, 70(171), 53019.

Fisher, D. (2010). Opioid tapering in children: a review of the literature. *AACN Adv Crit Care*, 21, 139–145.

Flack, S. and Anderson, C. (2012). Ultrasound guided lower extremity blocks. *Paediatr Anaesth*, 22, 72–80.

Franck, L. S., Scoppettuolo, L. A., Wypij, D., and Curley, M. A. Q. (2012). Validity and generalizability of the Withdrawal Assessment Tool-1 (WAT-1) for monitoring iatrogenic withdrawal syndrome in pediatric patients. *Pain*, 153, 142–148.

Frenkel, O., Mansour, K., and Fischer, J. W. J. (2012). Ultrasound-guided femoral nerve block for pain control in an infant with a femur fracture due to nonaccidental trauma. *Pediatr Emerg Care*, 28, 183–184.

Galinski, M., Dolveck, F., Combes, X., Limoges, V., Smail, N., Pommier, V., et al. (2007). Management of severe acute pain in emergency settings: ketamine reduces morphine consumption. *Am J Emerg Med*, 25, 385–390.

Gelinas, C. and Johnston, C. (2007). Pain assessment in the critically ill ventilated adult: validation of the Critical-Care Pain Observation Tool and physiologic indicators. *Clin J Pain*, 23, 497–505.

Goutos, I., Dziewulski, P., and Richardson, P. M. (2009). Pruritus in burns: review article. *J Burn Care Res*, 30, 221–228.

Goutos, I., Eldardiri, M., Khan, A. A., Dziewulski, P., and Richardson, P. M. (2010). Comparative evaluation of antipruritic protocols in acute burns. The emerging value of gabapentin in the treatment of burns pruritus. *J Burn Care Res*, 31, 57–63.

Gray, P., Kirby, J., Smith, M. T., Cabot, P. J., Williams, B., Doecke, J., et al. (2011). Pregabalin in severe burn injury pain: a double-blind, randomised placebo-controlled trial. *Pain*, 152, 1279–1288.

Green, S. M., Roback, M. G., Krauss, B., Brown, L., McGlone, R. G., Agrawal, D., et al. (2009a). Predictors of airway and respiratory adverse events with ketamine sedation in the emergency department: an individual-patient data meta-analysis of 8,282 children. *Ann Emerg Med*, 54, 158–68.e1–4.

Green, S. M., Roback, M. G., Krauss, B., Brown, L., McGlone, R. G., Agrawal, D., et al. (2009b). Predictors of emesis and recovery agitation with emergency department ketamine sedation: an individual-patient data meta-analysis of 8,282 children. *Ann Emerg Med*, 54, 171–80.e1–4.

Grindlay, J. and Babl, F. E. (2009). Review article: efficacy and safety of methoxyflurane analgesia in the emergency department and prehospital setting. *Emerg Med Australas*, 21, 4–11.

Hamed, K., Giles, N., Anderson, J., Phillips, J. K., Dawson, L. F., Drummond, P., et al. (2011). Changes in cutaneous innervation in patients with chronic pain after burns. *Burns*, 37, 631–637.

Hansen, M. S., Mathiesen, O., Trautner, S., and Dahl, J. B. (2012). Intranasal fentanyl in the treatment of acute pain—a systematic review. *Acta Anaesthesiol Scand*, 56, 407–419.

Heinrich, M., Wetzstein, V., Muensterer, O. J., and Till, H. (2004). Conscious sedation: Off-label use of rectal S(+)-ketamine and midazolam for wound dressing changes in paediatric heat injuries. *Eur J Pediatr Surg*, 14, 235–239.

Hoffman, H. G., Patterson, D. R., Seibel, E., Soltani, M., Jewett-Leahy, L., and Sharar, S. R. (2008). Virtual reality pain control during burn wound debridement in the hydrotank. *Clin J Pain*, 24, 299–304.

Hyland-Mcguire, P., and Guly, H. R. (1998). Effects on patient care of introducing prehospital intravenous nalbuphine hydrochloride. *J Accid Emerg Med*, 15, 99–101.

Jaffe, S. E. and Patterson, D. R. (2004). Treating sleep problems in patients with burn injuries: practical considerations. *J Burn Care Rehabil*, 25, 294–305.

Jennings, P. A., Cameron, P., Bernard, S., Walker, T., Jolley, D., Fitzgerald, M., *et al.* (2012). Morphine and ketamine is superior to morphine alone for out-of-hospital trauma analgesia: a randomized controlled trial. *Ann Emerg Med*, 59, 497–503.

Johnson, P. N., Harrison, D., and Allen, C. (2010). Utility of transdermal fentanyl for prevention of iatrogenic opioid abstinence syndrome in children. *J Opioid Manage*, 6, 117–124.

Johnston, S., Wilkes, G. J., Thompson, J. A., Ziman, M., and Brightwell, R. (2011). Inhaled methoxyflurane and intranasal fentanyl for prehospital management of visceral pain in an Australian ambulance service. *Emerg Med J*, 28, 57–63.

Joshi, P. H., and Conn, H. O. (1974). The syndrome of methoxyflurane-associated hepatitis. *Ann Intern Med*, 80, 395–401.

Jung, S. I., Seo, C. H., Jang, K., Ham, B. J., Choi, I.-G., Kim, J.-H., *et al.* (2009). Efficacy of naltrexone in the treatment of chronic refractory itching in burn patients: preliminary report of an open trial. *J Burn Care Res*, 30, 257–260.

Kanagasundaram, S. A., Lane, L. J., Cavalletto, B. P., Keneally, J. P., and Cooper, M. G. (2001). Efficacy and safety of nitrous oxide in alleviating pain and anxiety during painful procedures. *Arch Dis Child*, 84, 492–495.

Kober, A., Scheck, T., Greher, M., Lieba, F., Fleischhackl, R., Fleischhackl, S., *et al.* (2002). Prehospital analgesia with acupressure in victims of minor trauma: a prospective, randomized, double-blinded trial. *Anesth Analg*, 95, 723–727.

Koppert, W., Weigand, M., Neumann, F., Sittl, R., Schuettler, J., Schmelz, M., *et al.* (2004). Perioperative intravenous lidocaine has preventive effects on postoperative pain and morphine consumption after major abdominal surgery. *Anesth Analg*, 98, 1050–1055.

Krauss, B. and Green, S. M. (2006). Procedural sedation and analgesia in children. *Lancet*, 367, 766–780.

Krauss, W. C., Shah, S., Shah, S., and Thomas, S. H. (2011). Fentanyl in the out-of-hospital setting: variables associated with hypotension and hypoxemia. *J Emerg Med*, 40, 182–187.

Lang, T., Hager, H., Funovits, V., Barker, R., Steinlechner, B., Hoerauf, K., *et al.* (2007). Prehospital analgesia with acupressure at the Baihui and Hegu points in patients with radial fractures: a prospective, randomized, double-blind trial. *Am J Emerg Med*, 25, 887–893.

Lasalle, L., Rachelska, G., and Nedelec, B. (2008). Naltrexone for the management of post-burn pruritus: a preliminary report. *Burns*, 34, 797–802.

Li, Q., Zhang, Z., and Cai, Z. (2011). High-dose ketorolac affects adult spinal fusion: a meta-analysis of the effect of perioperative nonsteroidal anti-inflammatory drugs on spinal fusion. *Spine*, 36, E461–468.

Lin, H., Faraklas, I., Sampson, C., Saffle, J. R., and Cochran, A. (2011). Use of dexmedetomidine for sedation in critically ill mechanically ventilated pediatric burn patients. *J Burn Care Res*, 32, 98–103.

Lopez, S., Gros, T., Bernard, N., Plasse, C., and Capdevila, X. (2003). Fascia iliaca compartment block for femoral bone fractures in prehospital care. *Reg Anesth Pain Med*, 28, 203–207.

Luhmann, J. D., Schootman, M., Luhmann, S. J., and Kennedy, R. M. (2006). A randomized comparison of nitrous oxide plus hematoma block versus ketamine plus midazolam for emergency department forearm fracture reduction in children. *Pediatrics*, 118, e1078–1086.

Mace, S. E., Brown, L. A., Francis, L., Godwin, S. A., Hahn, S. A., Howard, P. K., *et al.* (2008). Clinical policy: Critical issues in the sedation of

pediatric patients in the emergency department. *Ann Emerg Med*, 51, 378–99, 399.e1–57.

Mackenzie, R. (2000). Analgesia and sedation. *J Royal Army Med Corps*, 146, 117–127.

Maldonado, M.-D., Murillo-Cabezas, F., Calvo, J.-R., Lardone, P.-J., Tan, D.-X., Guerrero, J.-M., *et al.* (2007). Melatonin as pharmacologic support in burn patients: a proposed solution to thermal injury-related lymphocytopenia and oxidative damage. *Crit Care Med*, 35, 1177–1185.

Marcin, J. P. and Pollack, M. M. (2002). Triage scoring systems, severity of illness measures, and mortality prediction models in pediatric trauma. *Crit Care Med*, 30, S457–467.

McDonald, A. J. and Cooper, M. G. (2001). Patient-controlled analgesia: an appropriate method of pain control in children. *Paediatr Drugs*, 3, 273–284.

McManus, J. G. Jr. and Sallee, D. R., Jr. (2005). Pain management in the prehospital environment. *Emerg Med Clin N Am*, 23, 415–431.

Medical Developments International. (n.d.). Penthrox® (methoxyflurane) [Product information]. Available at: <http://www.medicaldev.com/clinical/penthrox-methoxyflurane/> (accessed September 2012).

Mendham, J. E. (2004). Gabapentin for the treatment of itching produced by burns and wound healing in children: a pilot study. *Burns*, 30, 851–853.

Miller, K., Rodger, S., Bucolo, S., Greer, R., and Kimble, R. M. (2010). Multi-modal distraction. Using technology to combat pain in young children with burn injuries. *Burns*, 36, 647–658.

Musu, M., Finco, G., Antonucci, R., Polati, E., Sanna, D., Evangelista, M., *et al.* (2011). Acute nephrotoxicity of NSAID from the foetus to the adult. *Eur Rev Med Pharmacol Sci*, 15, 1461–72.

Oschman, A., Mccabe, T., and Kuhn, R. J. (2011). Dexmedetomidine for opioid and benzodiazepine withdrawal in pediatric patients. *Am J Health Syst Pharm*, 68, 1233–8.

Owens, V. F., Palmieri, T. L., Comroe, C. M., Conroy, J. M., Scavone, J. A., and Greenhalgh, D. G. (2006). Ketamine: a safe and effective agent for painful procedures in the pediatric burn patient. *J Burn Care Res*, 27, 211–216.

Palmer, G. M., Atkins, M., Anderson, B. J., Smith, K. R., Culnane, T. J., McNally, C. M., *et al.* (2008). I.V. acetaminophen pharmacokinetics in neonates after multiple doses. *Br J Anaesth*, 101, 523–530.

Panagiotou, I. and Mystakidou, K. (2010). Intranasal fentanyl: from pharmacokinetics and bioavailability to current treatment applications. *Exp Rev Anticancer Ther*, 10, 1009–1021.

Park, C. L., Roberts, D. E., Aldington, D. J., and Moore, R. A. (2010). Prehospital analgesia: systematic review of evidence. *J R Army Med Corps*, 156, 295–300.

Parlak Gurol, A., Polat, S., and Akcay, M. N. (2010). Itching, pain, and anxiety levels are reduced with massage therapy in burned adolescents. *J Burn Care Res*, 31, 429–432.

Parry, I. S., Bagley, A., Kawada, J., Sen, S., Greenhalgh, D. G., and Palmieri, T. L. (2012). Commercially available interactive video games in burn rehabilitation: therapeutic potential. *Burns*, 38, 493–500.

Phan, H., and Nahata, M. C. (2008). Clinical uses of dexmedetomidine in pediatric patients. *Paediatr Drugs*, 10, 49–69.

Playfor, S., Jenkins, I., Boyles, C., Choonara, I., Davies, G., Haywood, T., *et al.* (2006). Consensus guidelines on sedation and analgesia in critically ill children. *Intensive Care Med*, 32, 1125–1136.

Playfor, S., Jenkins, I., Boyles, C., Choonara, I., Davies, G., Haywood, T., *et al.* (2007). Consensus guidelines for sustained neuromuscular blockade in critically ill children. *Paediatr Anaesth*, 17, 881–887.

Pointer, J. E. and Harlan, K. (2005). Impact of liberalization of protocols for the use of morphine sulfate in an urban emergency medical services system. *Prehosp Emerg Care*, 9, 377–381.

Porter, K. (2004). Ketamine in prehospital care. *Emerg Med J*, 21, 351–354.

Radtke, C., Vogt, P. M., Devor, M., and Kocsis, J. D. (2010). Keratinocytes acting on injured afferents induce extreme neuronal hyperexcitability and chronic pain. *Pain*, 148, 94–102.

Rajan, V., Bartlett, N., Harvey, J. G., Martin, H. C. O., La Hei, E. R., Arbuckle, S., *et al.* (2009). Delayed cooling of an acute scald contact burn injury in a porcine model: is it worthwhile? *J Burn Care Res*, 30, 729–734.

Rawlins, J. M., Khan, A. A., Shenton, A. F., and Sharpe, D. T. (2007). Epidemiology and outcome analysis of 208 children with burns attending an emergency department. *Pediatr Emerg Care*, 23, 289–293.

Reid, C., Hatton, R., and Middleton, P. (2011). Case report: prehospital use of intranasal ketamine for paediatric burn injury. *Emerg Med J*, 28, 328–329.

Reid, N., Stella, J., Ryan, M., and Ragg, M. (2009). Use of ultrasound to facilitate accurate femoral nerve block in the emergency department. *Emerg Med Australas*, 21, 124–130.

Robert, R., Tcheung, W. J., Rosenberg, L., Rosenberg, M., Mitchell, C., Villarreal, C., et al. (2008). Treating thermally injured children suffering symptoms of acute stress with imipramine and fluoxetine: a randomized, double-blind study. *Burns*, 34, 919–928.

Roberts, K., Allison, K. P., and Porter, K. M. (2003). A review of emergency equipment carried and procedures performed by UK front line paramedics. *Resuscitation*, 58, 153–158.

Rogovik, A. L., and Goldman, R. D. (2007). Prehospital use of analgesics at home or en route to the hospital in children with extremity injuries. *Am J Emerg Med*, 25, 400–405.

Rowland, A. S., Baird, D. D., Weinberg, C. R., Shore, D. L., Shy, C. M., and Wilcox, A. J. (1992). Reduced fertility among women employed as dental assistants exposed to high levels of nitrous oxide. *N Engl J Med*, 327, 993–997.

Sanders, R. D., Weimann, J., and Maze, M. (2008). Biologic effects of nitrous oxide: a mechanistic and toxicologic review. *Anesthesiology*, 109, 707–722.

Schmitt, Y. S., Hoffman, H. G., Blough, D. K., Patterson, D. R., Jensen, M. P., Soltani, M., et al. (2011). A randomized, controlled trial of immersive virtual reality analgesia, during physical therapy for pediatric burns. *Burns*, 37, 61–68.

Schneider, J. C., Harris, N. L., El Shami, A., Sheridan, R. L., Schulz, J. T., 3rd, Bilodeau, M.-L., et al. (2006). A descriptive review of neuropathic-like pain after burn injury. *J Burn Care Res*, 27, 524–528.

Seith, R. W., Theophilos, T., and Babl, F. E. (2012). Intranasal fentanyl and high-concentration inhaled nitrous oxide for procedural sedation: a prospective observational pilot study of adverse events and depth of sedation. [19(2), 238]. *Acad Emerg Med*, 19, 31–36.

Sharar, S. R., Carrougher, G. J., Nakamura, D., Hoffman, H. G., Blough, D. K., and Patterson, D. R. (2007). Factors influencing the efficacy of virtual reality distraction analgesia during postburn physical therapy: preliminary results from 3 ongoing studies. *Arch Phys Med Rehabil*, 88, S43–49.

Siriwardena, A. N., Shaw, D., and Bouliotis, G. (2010). Exploratory cross-sectional study of factors associated with pre-hospital management of pain. *J Eval Clin Pract*, 16, 1269–1275.

Stoddard, F. J., Jr., Luthra, R., Sorrentino, E. A., Saxe, G. N., Drake, J., Chang, Y., et al. (2011a). A randomized controlled trial of sertraline to prevent posttraumatic stress disorder in burned children. *J Child Adolesc Psychopharmacol*, 21, 469–477.

Stoddard, F. J., Jr., White, G. W., Kazis, L. E., Murphy, J. M., Sorrentino, E. A., Hinson, M., et al. (2011b). Patterns of medication administration from 2001 to 2009 in the treatment of children with acute burn injuries: a multicenter study. *J Burn Care Res*, 32, 519–528.

Stoddard, F. J., Usher, C. T., and Abrams, A. N. (2006). Psychopharmacology in pediatric critical care. *Child Adolesc Psychiatr Clin N Am*, 15, 611–655.

Sucato, D. J., Lovejoy, J. F., Agrawal, S., Elerson, E., Nelson, T., and McClung, A. (2008). Postoperative ketorolac does not predispose to pseudoarthrosis following posterior spinal fusion and instrumentation for adolescent idiopathic scoliosis. *Spine*, 33, 1119–1124.

Svenson, J. E., and Abernathy, M. K. (2007). Ketamine for prehospital use: new look at an old drug. *Am J Emerg Med*, 25, 977–980.

Swor, R., Mceachin, C. M., Seguin, D., and Grall, K. H. (2005). Prehospital pain management in children suffering traumatic injury. *Prehosp Emerg Care*, 9, 40–43.

Talon, M. D., Woodson, L. C., Sherwood, E. R., Aarsland, A., McRae, L., and Benham, T. (2009). Intranasal dexmedetomidine premedication is comparable with midazolam in burn children undergoing reconstructive surgery. *J Burn Care Res*, 30, 599–605.

Tcheung, W. J., Robert, R., Rosenberg, L., Rosenberg, M., Villarreal, C., Thomas, C., et al. (2005). Early treatment of acute stress disorder in children with major burn injury. *Pediatr Crit Care Med*, 6, 676–681.

Thombs, B. D., Bresnick, M. G., Magyar-Russell, G., and Kim, T. J. (2006). Early treatment of acute stress symptoms in pediatric burn patients with imipramine and fluoxetine. *Pediatr Crit Care Med*, 7, 498.

Tobias, J. D. (2005). Sedation and analgesia in the pediatric intensive care unit. *Pediatric Annals*, 34, 636–645.

Tobias, J. D. (2007). Dexmedetomidine: applications in pediatric critical care and pediatric anesthesiology. *Pediatr Crit Care Med*, 8, 115–131.

Tobias, J. D. (2008). Subcutaneous dexmedetomidine infusions to treat or prevent drug withdrawal in infants and children. *J Opioid Manage*, 4, 187–191.

Tosun, Z., Esmaoglu, A., and Coruh, A. (2008). Propofol-ketamine vs propofol-fentanyl combinations for deep sedation and analgesia in pediatric patients undergoing burn dressing changes. *Paediatr Anaesth*, 18, 43–47.

Tousignant-Laflamme, Y., Rainville, P., and Marchand, S. (2005). Establishing a link between heart rate and pain in healthy subjects: a gender effect. *J Pain*, 6, 341–347.

Tsui, B. and Suresh, S. (2010). Ultrasound imaging for regional anesthesia in infants, children, and adolescents: a review of current literature and its application in the practice of extremity and trunk blocks. *Anesthesiology*, 112, 473–492.

Twite, M. D., Rashid, A., Zuk, J., and Friesen, R. H. (2004). Sedation, analgesia, and neuromuscular blockade in the pediatric intensive care unit: survey of fellowship training programs. *Pediatr Crit Care Med*, 5, 521–532.

Van Baar, M. E., Polinder, S., Essink-Bot, M. L., Van Loey, N. E. E., Oen, I. M. M. H., Dokter, J., Box et al. (2011). Quality of life after burns in childhood (5–15 years): children experience substantial problems. *Burns*, 37, 930–938.

Vergnion, M., Degesves, S., Garcet, L., and Magotteaux, V. (2001). Tramadol, an alternative to morphine for treating posttraumatic pain in the prehospital situation. *Anesth Analg*, 92, 1543–1546.

Von Hoff, D. D., Kuhn, J. G., Burris, H. A. 3rd, and Miller, L. J. (2008). Does intraosseous equal intravenous? A pharmacokinetic study. *Am J Emerg Med*, 26, 31–38.

Walker, J., MacCallum, M., Fischer, C., Kopcha, R., Saylors, R., and McCall, J. (2006). Sedation using dexmedetomidine in pediatric burn patients. *J Burn Care Res*, 27, 206–210.

Ward, M. E., Radburn, J., and Morant, S. (1997). Evaluation of intravenous tramadol for use in the prehospital situation by ambulance paramedics. *Prehospital & Disaster Medicine*, 12, 158–162.

Wasiak, J., Cleland, H., and Campbell, F. (2008). Dressings for superficial and partial thickness burns. *Cochrane Database Syst Rev*, 4, CD002106.

Wathen, J. E., Gao, D., Merritt, G., Georgopoulos, G., and Battan, F. K. (2007). A randomized controlled trial comparing a fascia iliaca compartment nerve block to a traditional systemic analgesic for femur fractures in a pediatric emergency department. *Ann Emerg Med*, 50, 162–171, 171.e1.

White, M. C., and Karsli, C. (2007). Long-term use of an intravenous ketamine infusion in a child with significant burns. *Paediatr Anaesth*, 17, 1102–1104.

Woollard, M., Whitfield, R., Smith, K., Jones, T., Thomas, G., and Hinton, C. (2004). Less IS less: a randomised controlled trial comparing cautious and rapid nalbuphine dosing regimens. *Emerg Med J*, 21, 362–364.

Zier, J. L. and Liu, M. (2011). Safety of high-concentration nitrous oxide by nasal mask for pediatric procedural sedation: experience with 7802 cases. *Pediatr Emerg Care*, 27, 1107–1112.

CHAPTER 19

Needle procedures

Anna Taddio

Summary

All children undergo needle procedures as part of routine medical care. Numerous interventions are available for relieving pain from needle procedures. These interventions can be divided into four domains (4 Ps of pain management): procedural, pharmacological, psychological, and physical. Treating needle pain reduces pain and distress and improves satisfaction with medical care. Other potential benefits include a reduction in the development of needle fear and subsequent health care avoidance behaviour. Adoption of the 4Ps into routine clinical practice is feasible and should become a standard of care in the delivery of health care for children. This chapter is a narrative review of the current knowledge about: epidemiology, pain experience, practices and attitudes, and evidence-based interventions for pain management during common needle procedures.

Introduction

Despite their vital importance, needles are regarded as the negative symbol of health care (Schechter, 2006). This is because they cause anticipatory anxiety and pain. The needle is particularly concerning to children, who regard any procedure involving a needle as one of the most frightening and painful health-related events.

Epidemiology of needle procedures

Injections, venepunctures, and venous cannulations are among the most prevalent needle procedures undertaken in children and are the focus of this chapter. Injections consist primarily of intramuscular or subcutaneous administration of vaccines, and are experienced repeatedly throughout the lifespan. In the US, healthy children undergo over four dozen separate vaccine injections by the time they are adults (<http://www.immunize.org/catg.d/p4050.pdf>). Venepunctures and venous cannulations are the most common sources of needle pain for hospitalized children (Ellis et al., 2002; MacLean et al., 2007; Stevens et al., 2011; Zhu et al., 2012). In one study, venepuncture and venous cannulation accounted for almost two needle procedures per day among neonates in the first week of life (Stevens et al., 2003). In another study including hospitalized children of all ages, the mean frequency of all common needle procedures together was one every other day (Stevens et al., 2011).

Clinical impact of needle procedures

Although needle procedures are generally regarded as a source of 'mild' acute pain, there is substantial variability in the level of pain reported by different individuals. In general, children report needle procedures as being more painful than adults do (Goodenough et al., 2008; Schneider and LoBiondo-Wood, 1992) and regard any procedure involving a needle as one of the most frightening and painful health-related events (Cummings et al., 1996; Ellis et al., 2004; Humphrey, 1992). The majority of young children exhibit moderate-severe distress during needle procedures (wherein distress encompasses the combined effects of anxiety and pain). Since current methods of pain assessment do not allow pain to be differentiated from anxiety, pain responses in young children include anxiety responses as well. In one study of immunization injections, over 90% of children aged 15 to 18 months and 45% of those aged 4 to 6 years were seriously distressed (Jacobson et al., 2001). In two separate studies of venepuncture, 64% of 3 to 6-year-olds (Fradet et al., 1990) and 83% of 2½- to 6-year-olds (Humphrey et al., 1992) had high distress. The percentage with high distress decreased with increasing age: 51% and 28% for 7 to 12 years and 12 years and greater, respectively (Humphrey et al., 1992).

Needle procedures undertaken in infancy and childhood may impact on how pain is perceived in the future by altering the normal development of pain processing pathways (Fitzgerald and Walker, 2009) or by leading to the development of needle fears (Bijttebier and Vertommen, 1998; Chen et al., 2000; Jacobson et al., 2001; Rocha et al., 2003). Increased level of fearfulness, lower sense of control over health, and distrust of adults, particularly health providers, can occur after experience with repeated needle procedures in childhood as well (Rennick et al., 2002; Salmela et al., 2011) and such procedures may be perceived as more traumatic than the underlying disease (Hedstrom et al., 2003; Ljungman et al., 1999).

Recent studies demonstrate that about two-thirds of children have a fear of needles (Taddio et al., 2012c; <http://www.painfoundation.org/media/resources/pain-surveys.html>). Needle fears may be carried into adulthood whereby it is estimated that about one-quarter of adults are afraid (Taddio et al., 2012b) and one in ten have an outright phobia (Hamilton 1995). These fears place individuals at risk for adverse health and lifestyle consequences (Sokolowski et al., 2010). Individuals demonstrate health avoidance behaviours, including abstinence from: preventive health measures (e.g. immunizations, dental visits; Johnson et al., 2008; Sokolowski et al., 2010; Wright et al., 2009) and treatment interventions, even life-saving ones (e.g. diabetes management; Howe et al., 2011). Refusal of needle procedures can lead to social and legal consequences as well, including refused travel, education, employment, marriage, or pregnancy (Sokolowski et al., 2010). Reduced herd immunity from low immunization compliance rates may lead to outbreaks of vaccine-preventable diseases (Diekema, 2012; Omer et al., 2009).

Needle procedures carried out in children are also concerning for parents and clinicians. Alterations in physiological parameters (blood pressure, heart rate) and increased anxiety are documented for parents of children undergoing needle procedures (Smith et al., 2007). Both parents and clinicians report non-compliance with immunization in an effort to reduce pain in children (Harrington et al., 2000; Madlon-Kay and Harper, 1994; Woodin et al., 1995).

Pain management practices and attitudes

Historically, there has been under-utilization of pain-relieving interventions for needle procedures performed in children. Several audits conducted over the last decade reveal wide variations in practices (Carbajal et al., 2008; Ellis et al., 2002; Johnston et al., 2011; MacLean et al., 2007; Simons et al., 2003; Stevens et al., 2003; Chan et al, 2013; Zhu et al., 2012). Studies in hospitalized children, for instance, document pain-relieving interventions in 0% to 90% of needle procedures. Studies in neonates report higher utilization rates than those involving all ages of children. Intramuscular or subcutaneous injections are associated with higher utilization rates than venepuncture and venous cannulation. In one study comparing two time points, a lower number of procedures were documented in the more recent time period, suggesting a reduction in the burden of pain over time in hospitalized infants (Johnston et al., 2011). This finding contrasts with the outpatient setting, where the burden of pain has been steadily increasing over time due to the continual increase in the number of vaccines being introduced into routine clinical practice.

Taking care of a child's pain is important to parents (Ammentorp et al., 2005). Parents are prepared to wait longer and to pay to reduce their child's pain (Meyerhoff et al., 2001; Myrick and Barfield 2006; Walsh and Bartfield 2006; Wasserfallen et al., 2006). Clinicians regard pain management as the parents' responsibility. They focus on the technical aspects of a child's medical care, forgoing children's (and parents') experiences of that care, including associated pain. With respect to needle procedures, clinicians often hold a procedure-focused, rather than child-focused view, and dismiss concerns about pain by describing it as a self-limited process. Dismissive attitudes about pain in clinicians results in parental acceptance of pain as 'the necessary evil' that must be traded-off to obtain good health in their children (Parvez et al., 2010).

Since parents value pain management and pain management improves the quality of care that is delivered, it follows that the societal value of pain management is high. Pain management should thus be incorporated within the process of all needle procedures (Wasserfallen et al., 2006). Parents, health care providers, and institutions must partner together to address barriers to best practices. The model of family-centred care may serve as a theoretical framework for this partnership (Franck and Callery, 2004). Briefly, this model describes participation of the family in children's health care and in decision-making in order to achieve optimal health care delivery in children.

Evidence-based interventions for pain management

There are numerous effective, safe, and feasible interventions for managing pain from needle procedures. These interventions can be categorized into four domains: 'Procedural' techniques that operators can use when performing the procedure; and 'Pharmacological', 'Psychological', and 'Physical' techniques that parents, operators, and children can use to modify the experience of pain for children; herein referred to as the '4 Ps' of pain management. The remainder of this chapter reviews examples of interventions within these domains. Figure 19.1 illustrates the timeline for their use to mitigate pain from needle procedures undertaken in children. Systemic analgesics and adjuvant interventions are reviewed separately, in chapters in Section 6.

Procedural interventions

The best way to manage pain is to avoid it. Use of non-invasive technology is one way of avoiding pain—for instance, needle-free immunization (e.g. intranasal influenza vaccine) or non-invasive sampling devices (e.g. transcutaneous bilirubinometry; Yap et al., 2004). Children should undergo the minimum number of procedures possible. This is particularly important for hospitalized children, who frequently undergo unnecessary procedures due to lack of communication and coordination among hospital personnel. For children requiring ongoing or repeated intravenous access, long-term indwelling catheters can be inserted. With respect to injections, combination vaccines can be used rather than single-antigen ones to minimize the number of separate injections (Zareba, 2006).

Health care providers undertaking needle procedures can utilize a variety of approaches to mitigate pain, including selecting one particular procedure over another and using specific techniques to carry out a procedure. For example, blood sampling can be performed using venepuncture instead of heel lance (Shah and Ohlsson, 2011). For intramuscular immunization injections, injections can be carried out quickly without prior aspiration (Taddio et al., 2009a). When multiple injections are being given sequentially, pain can be reduced if the most painful one is administered last (Taddio et al., 2009a).

Since the physicochemical properties of the injectate can also influence pain, efforts should be made to administer the least painful formulation of a medication. In separate systematic reviews, pain from lidocaine infiltration (Cepeda et al., 2010) and measles–mumps–rubella vaccine injection (Taddio et al., 2009a) were reduced when a more physiological pH formulation was used. Such buffered lidocaine solutions, however, are not commercially available as they are not stable. They can be compounded prior to injection by adding 1 ml of sodium bicarbonate 8.4% to 9 ml of lidocaine 1% (Cepeda et al., 2010). Buffering is not recommended for vaccines as the effect on immunogenicity is not known.

The temperature of the injectate may also affect pain. Lidocaine solutions that are warmed to body temperature, for example, cause less pain during infiltration, even if the lidocaine is buffered (Hogan et al., 2011b). No benefit has been observed for warmed vaccines, and thus, is not recommended for vaccinations (Taddio et al., 2009a).

Pharmacological interventions

A variety of pharmacological interventions are available for reducing pain from needle procedures. The most common are local anaesthetics and sweet solutions.

Local anaesthetics

Local anaesthetics are the most studied class of pharmacological interventions for reducing pain from needle procedures in children.

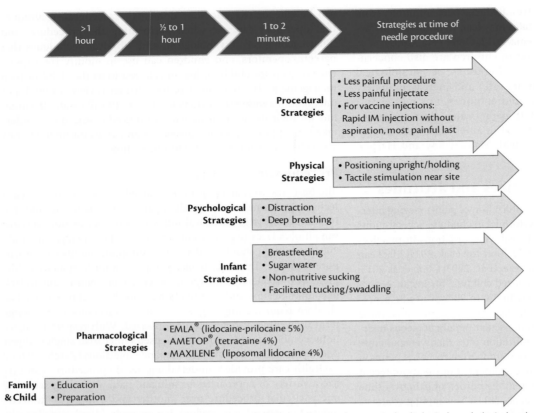

Figure 19.1 Timeline for pain relieving strategies prior to and during needle procedures: procedural, physical, psychological, and pharmacological strategies (plus infant and family/child). IM = intramuscular.

Local anaesthetics provide analgesia by blocking nociceptive transmission in nerve cells. They are administered to the site of the needle procedure using non-invasive (i.e. topical) and invasive (i.e. needle) methods.

Table 19.1 summarizes currently marketed products that are applied topically on intact skin and rely on passive diffusion to achieve dermal anaesthesia. Depending on the product, clinically reliable local anaesthesia is achieved after a contact time of 20 to 60 min. Commercial preparations available in a disc/patch formulation have the local anaesthetic embedded within the delivery system and are adhered to the skin. Other preparations require that the appropriate dosage (usually about 1 g) be applied to the skin in a mound, and then covered with an occlusive dressing. Occlusion facilitates absorption of the anaesthetic and prevents accidental removal and/or ingestion. It may be necessary to apply topical anaesthetics to more than one body region (or site) to account for multiple procedures. Care must be taken, however, to ensure that maximum recommended dosages are not exceeded in order to prevent systemic toxicity.

Needle procedures are usually undertaken right after the required contact time has been met and both the dressing and anaesthetic have been removed. If a procedure is not undertaken immediately, a non-toxic marker can be used to mark the site where the anaesthetic was applied—this prevents subsequent needle puncture in an unanaesthetized area. Attention should be given to the elapsed time following removal, as the anaesthetic effect will begin to fade thereafter. Elapsed times of more than 1 h are not generally recommended in order to minimize the risk of analgesic failure.

Table 19.1 Commercially available topical anaesthetics

Topical anaesthetic	Availability	Recommended application duration in minutes
Lidocaine 2.5%—prilocaine 2.5%	Cream, patch	60
Lidocaine 7%—tetracaine 7%	Heat delivery patch	20
Liposomal lidocaine 4%	Cream	30
Tetracaine 4%	Gel	40

Multiple systematic reviews and meta-analyses have concluded that local anaesthetics are effective and safe for reducing pain from common needle procedures (Fetzer, 2002; Lander et al., 2006; Shah et al., 2009) (see also Zemspky, Chapter 47, this volume). There is evidence that they may improve procedure success rate (e.g. insertion of indwelling cannula or procurement of blood sample is achieved on the first attempt) and reduce total procedure duration time as well, presumably due to reduced pain and movement during procedures (Taddio et al., 2005b). One meta-analysis found tetracaine to be superior to lidocaine-prilocaine for reducing pain from venepuncture (Lander et al., 2006), suggesting that not all preparations are equianalgesic. No differences, however, have been observed in procedural success rate among various preparations (Arendts et al., 2008).

Despite their demonstrated effectiveness, topical anaesthetics are under-utilized for needle procedures. This is due, at least in part, to perceptions about their effectiveness and feasibility. There is an expectation that topical anaesthetics will lead to painless needle procedures. However, this is not usually the case. Pain perception is complex, and a result of multiple interacting factors including anxiety and fear, which topical anaesthetics may not eliminate. In addition, anaesthetics do not block all sensation—sensations of pressure are still present, which may be interpreted by children and/or adults as pain. The depth of penetration is several millimetres, resulting in partial blockade of nociceptive input for most procedures. Finally, the presence of genetic polymorphisms may predispose some children to analgesic failure (Kleiber et al., 2007).

Another barrier to the use of topical anaesthetics relates to perceptions of feasibility. The requisite waiting time makes it impossible to use topical anaesthetics for emergency procedures. Most needle procedures, however, are not required on an urgent basis. Studies performed in a wide variety of clinical settings demonstrate that topical anaesthetics can be incorporated within usual waiting times for most needle procedures (Fein, 1999; MacLean et al., 2007; Robieux et al., 1990; Taddio et al., 2012a). The person applying the preparation must also know where to apply the topical anaesthetic. Concerns that parents are unable to apply topical anaesthetics to the appropriate site(s) are unsupported by primary research (Koh et al., 1999; Taddio et al., 1994).

Topical anaesthetics are well tolerated and considered safe in most children. When used for immunization, they do not appear to interfere with antibody response (Shah et al., 2009). Systemic toxicities have been reported rarely and have included seizures, dysrhythmias, and methaemoglobinaemia. Methaemoglobinaemia is a toxicity of lidocaine-prilocaine, owing to the oxidizing effects of metabolites of prilocaine. Neonates and young infants are more susceptible because of immature enzyme activity. For the most part systemic toxicities have only occurred after either excessive doses or durations of application were used. Careful attention to dose and duration of application are required to minimize significant absorption and systemic effects (Shachor-Meyouhas et al., 2008).

Transient local side effects are relatively common—they occur in one-quarter to one-half of individuals, and include transient skin colour changes (erythema, blanching), oedema, and itching. Allergic contact dermatitis is uncommon or rare, and may be more likely with ester-based topical anaesthetics (tetracaine; Shah et al., 2009).

To reduce the onset of action of topical anaesthetics and increase the depth of penetration of the active agent, alternative methods of administration have been used. Of these, injection of local anaesthetics is the oldest and most common method currently in use. Typically, small volumes (0.1–0.3 ml) of lidocaine 1% solution are injected intradermally or subcutaneously using a narrow-gauge (27 or 30) needle (Klein et al., 1995; Luhmann et al., 2004; Soliman et al., 1988). The onset of anaesthesia is approximately 1 to 3 min.

There is reluctance about using lidocaine injection in some clinical settings. This is not surprising, given its administration is associated with an additional needle puncture, and pain from the needle puncture and the lidocaine itself (which causes a burning/stinging sensation). It should be noted however, that the pain from lidocaine injection is less than that from the needle procedure for which it is being utilized; hence, there is an overall net benefit of less pain when lidocaine injection is used for needle procedures. Nevertheless, when lidocaine injection is utilized, it should be accompanied by strategies to reduce injection pain, including: buffering lidocaine with sodium bicarbonate (Cepeda et al., 2010) and warming the solution to body temperature (Hogan et al., 2011b).

More recently, novel technologies have been developed that allow for rapid administration of local anaesthetics without the need for needle puncture (Zempsky, 2008). For the most part, there is very limited experience with these technologies and they are not readily available in most clinical settings. These technologies offer alternative methods of administering local anaesthetics and may come to have an important role in the management of cutaneous pain in children in the future. They are discussed in further detail by Zempsky (Chapter 47, this volume).

With so many options available, the choice of which local anaesthetic administration method to use depends primarily on: urgency of procedure, procedure site, child factors, availability of equipment, and availability of experienced staff. If procedures are required urgently, only techniques with a short onset of action are suitable. For topical preparations, disc/patch dosage modalities may be more convenient to use provided that the contact surface area and geography of body region allow them to be suitably applied. The presence of specific child factors, such as age, distress levels, allergies, or child preferences lend themselves to the selection of certain preparations over others. Finally, the presence of requisite equipment and trained staff are needed to administer them.

Sweet solutions

Sweet solutions have analgesic effects in infants up to 12 months of age (Gaspardo et al., 2005; Harrison et al., 2010; Shah et al., 2009; Stevens et al., 2010). Their mechanism of action is unknown; however, it has been speculated to involve taste-induced release of endogenous opioids, calming through non-nutritive sucking, and/or distraction. There are a plethora of studies showing reduced pain behaviours in infants given sweet solutions while undergoing needle procedures (reviewed in detail by Harrison et al., Chapter 49, this volume). Of note, a recent study failed to demonstrate an effect on pain-specific brain activity (Slater et al., 2010), questioning whether sweet solutions are 'true analgesics'. However, at present, the clinical significance of that study is not known.

A variety of natural and artificial sweet compounds have been evaluated; the most widely used is sucrose (Taddio et al., 2009b). Sucrose solutions are administered on the infant's tongue with a pacifier, syringe, or cup. Administration with a pacifier stimulates non-nutritive sucking and may improve effectiveness (Buscemi et al., 2008; Stevens et al., 2010). The onset of action is fast (within 10 sec), with a peak effect at 2 min, and duration of action of up to 10 min (Buscemi et al., 2008). The usual single dose is 0.5 to 2 ml of 12% to 24% strength (weight/volume; Stevens et al., 2010). Multiple-dose regimens utilize lower single doses, particularly in preterm infants (Stevens et al., 2010) owing to concerns about potential adverse effects. It is not clear whether there is a dose–response effect (Harrison et al., 2010; Stevens et al., 1997).

Sucrose is well tolerated—adverse effects are rare and transient, including choking and oxygen desaturation (Stevens et al., 2010, Taddio et al., 2008). One multiple dose study in preterm infants, however, suggested worse neurobehavioural development and severity of illness scores at selected follow-up testing ages with increasing sucrose exposure (Johnston et al., 2002)—the significance of this finding is unknown (see Harrison et al., Chapter 49, this volume, for a more detailed review).

Psychological interventions

Psychological interventions include cognitive and behavioural techniques aimed at reducing child anxiety and pain. The proposed mechanism of action is hypothesized to involve the 'gate control theory' of pain, whereby descending nerve signals involving thoughts, beliefs, emotion, and attention modulate ascending pain signals (Cohen 2008; Schechter et al., 2007).

For the most part, psychological interventions do not require specialized equipment, and are devoid of toxicity. However, their effectiveness often hedges on the competence of individuals delivering them. Parents and clinicians may not be adequately trained, resulting in limited success.

Preparation of parents and children

Having parents present during needle procedures undertaken in children is consistent with parent and child preferences and hence, supports family-centred care (Gonzalez et al., 1989; Piira et al., 2005; Pruitt et al., 2008; Ross and Ross 1984; Stephens et al., 1999). Parental presence has the added benefit of promoting respect for the child's emotional welfare. Two separate studies correlated parental presence with enhanced use of pain strategies in hospitalized infants (Carbajal et al., 2008; Johnston et al., 2011), either because parents request pain-relieving interventions or their presence prompts clinicians to administer them (Carbajal et al., 2008; Johnston et al., 2011).

Parent behaviour significantly influences child distress and pain during needle procedures, both positively and negatively (Blount et al., 2001; Cohen et al., 2002; Frank et al., 1995; Gonzalez et al., 1993; Liossi et al., 2007; Rocha et al., 2003; Sweet and McGrath, 1998). Parents should therefore be targeted for education about strategies that reduce a child's distress and pain (Cohen, 2008). In general, children's distress responses are reduced when adults are calm and use *coping-promoting* strategies such as coaching children to cope and distracting children (diverting children's attention away from the procedure). Conversely, responses are increased when adults are anxious and use *distress-promoting* strategies such as apologizing, criticizing, reassuring, or empathizing. The latter may focus children's attention on the procedure by their nature and the manner in which they are communicated.

Children should be prepared for needle procedures ahead of time as prior preparation helps to reduce an individual's anxiety and pain perception (Jaaniste et al., 2007; Suls and Wan 1989). Preparation includes developmentally-appropriate explanations of procedural and sensory information, including: what will happen, how it will feel, what will be done to prevent discomfort, and what children can do to help (Schechter et al., 2007). It may also involve demonstrations and/or practice opportunities. Children should not be told 'it won't hurt'—this is an ineffective strategy and promotes distrust (Taddio et al., 2010a).

In general, preparation should not be performed too far in advance—this may cause children to become fixated on the event and become more anxious, or to forget procedure details (Cohen 2008). Children should have enough time to process the information and plan how they will cope. The information can be presented the day prior to or on the day of the procedure depending on the individual child (Cohen, 2008). Preparation may be suitable commencing at age greater than 2 years (Schechter et al., 2007); however, it may have greater benefit in children 7 years and older (Cohen, 2008).

Distraction

Distraction involves any technique that removes a child's attention from the needle procedure to something more pleasant. It is viewed as a key non-pharmacological intervention for essentially all ages of children. Multiple reviews and meta-analyses demonstrate the effectiveness of distraction for reducing pain during needle procedures (Chambers et al., 2009; DeMore and Cohen, 2005; Kleiber and Harper, 1999; Richardson et al., 2006; Uman et al., 2006) (see also Cohen et al., Chapter 53, this volume). Distraction is usually commenced before the procedure begins, and is continued during and afterwards—this helps reduce anticipatory anxiety and pain, and enhances recovery (Cohen, 2008).

Distraction interventions typically use a combination of cognitive and behavioural approaches. They can consist of relatively simple, cost-neutral or low-cost techniques, such as non-procedural talk, breathing exercises, bubble blowing, playing with toys/games, and watching movies. Alternatively, they can involve more complex and cognitively-based interventions such as hypnosis (Buscemi et al., 2008). The time required to teach an individual to use simple distractions is short (up to 15 min), making it feasible for most clinical settings (DeMore and Cohen, 2005). Cognitively-based interventions, however, usually require facilitation by a trained individual such as a child life specialist, hence, are not easily implemented. In addition, cognitive interventions can realistically only be used in children aged 3 years and older (Richardson et al., 2006).

The most effective distractors stimulate multiple sensory modalities (e.g. vision, hearing, touch), elicit positive affective states (e.g. laughing), or require overt behavioural responses (Cohen, 2008; DeMore and Cohen, 2005). The critical aspect for any distractor, however, is that a child is actively engaged in it—otherwise, it will be ineffective. To this end, it is important to select age-appropriate and engaging distractions (Schechter et al., 2007). Facilitation, either from a health provider or parent is also important, in order to ensure the child's attention is maintained on the distraction (Cohen, 2008; DeMore and Cohen, 2005).

For infants, the proposed primary methods of distraction include parental use of coping-promoting behaviours and physical interventions (Schechter, 2006) rather than the use of external items (e.g. toys, books). A recent systematic review and meta-analysis found insufficient evidence to recommend toy-mediated distraction in infants and young children (up to 3 years; Pillai Riddell et al., 2011). The same review, however, found sufficient evidence of effectiveness for video-mediated distraction in the same population (Pillai Riddell et al., 2011). Some of the observed inconsistencies in the overall effectiveness of distraction may be explained by who delivers the distraction (clinicians versus parents; Chambers et al., 2009). Parents may be less effective than clinicians because they are: (1) insufficiently trained or experienced to administer distraction, (2) unable to undertake other soothing behaviours while performing distraction, or (3) anxious and transmit their anxiety to children.

Physical interventions

Physical interventions target body position and physical activity. They are generally cost-neutral. Numerous physical interventions have been shown to reduce pain responses in infants and children undergoing needle procedures.

Breastfeeding for infants

Breastfeeding reduces pain responses in infants up to 1 year of age (Shah et al., 2007, 2009). Although categorized as a physical pain-relieving intervention, the analgesic effects of breast milk are hypothesized to be mediated by multiple mechanisms, including touch/maternal presence (skin-to-skin contact), non-nutritive sucking, sweet-taste and other potentially analgesic substances, and smell. Compared to other pain-relieving strategies such as sweet-tasting substances and local anaesthetics, breastfeeding offers a natural, cost-neutral, and convenient option. Breastfeeding is commenced before the needle puncture and continued throughout the procedure and afterward. Thus, an adequate latch must be established *prior to* the procedure commencing—this may take a few minutes.

Concerns have been raised about the potential for breastfeeding analgesia to cause infants to choke. To date, this adverse effect has not been documented. Another concern is that infants might learn to associate breastfeeding with pain, which will negatively impact on future breastfeeding. This adverse effect is also unlikely as needle procedures are sporadic; hence, breastfeeding would not be a reliable cue for an impending painful procedure (Shah et al., 2009).

Other physical interventions for infants and young children

A variety of physical interventions have been evaluated for their effectiveness in infants and young children undergoing painful medical procedures, including skin-to-skin contact (also called kangaroo care/kangaroo-mother care), non-nutritive sucking, rocking, and swaddling (Pillai Riddell et al., 2011; Taddio et al., 2009a; van Sleuwen et al., 2007).

Skin-to-skin contact involves holding infants clad only in a nappy against the bare skin of a parent. In a recent systematic review, there was sufficient evidence to support skin-to-skin contact as a pain relieving intervention in preterm infants but not full-term neonates (Pillai Riddell et al., 2011). At present, the optimal exposure time for skin-to-skin contact prior to needle procedures is unknown and an insufficient exposure time in full-term neonates may explain the inconsistent findings. Skin-to-skin contact is described further by Johnston and Campbell-Yeo (Chapter 58, this volume).

Non-nutritive sucking involves the placement of a pacifier in an infant's mouth to stimulate sucking. Sucking is postulated to release neurotransmitters that modify pain perception (Buscemi et al., 2008). Non-nutritive sucking has been shown to reduce pain responses in preterm infants, full-term neonates, and older infants (Pillai Riddell et al., 2011). Adults may be required to keep pacifiers in place. The combination of sweet solutions and non-nutritive sucking may improve the effectiveness of non-nutritive sucking (Buscemi et al., 2008; Stevens et al., 2010).

Facilitated tucking or swaddling involves containing the infant's limbs close to the infant's trunk in a flexed position. This physical intervention has been shown to reduce pain in preterm infants and neonates (Pillai Riddell et al., 2011). Care must be taken to avoid over-bundling which contributes to elevated body temperature (van Sleuwen et al., 2007).

Some aforementioned physical interventions require the presence of a parent. Involving parents supports their preferences to be included in their infant's care and promotes parent–infant bonding (Franck et al., 2005; Gale et al., 2004), however, this may not always be possible.

Upright positioning and holding

Upright position and parent holding are regarded as optimal ways to position children during needle procedures (Sparks et al., 2007; Taddio et al., 2009a). It is hypothesized that individuals feel less fear when positioned upright than when positioned supine (Lacey et al., 2008) and that parental holding adds support and comfort (Stephens et al., 1999). There are limited data, however, in young infants and one systematic review found conflicting evidence for a benefit of holding (and/or rocking; Pillai Riddell et al., 2011). Despite this result, upright positioning has been recommended beginning as soon as infants can hold themselves up (3–5 months; Stephens et al., 1999).

Several variations in positioning and holding have been suggested: the most popular involves seating children on a parent's lap, with the child facing the parent. Alternatively, children can sit on the examination table, with the parent holding the child around the trunk. Care must be taken to avoid restraining children as this can increase movement and distress (Stephens et al., 1999).

Upright positioning and parent holding is a simple, cost-free pain relieving intervention that can be employed in any clinical setting, provided that clinicians are comfortable with it. Some clinicians may be hesitant about this technique (Lacey et al., 2008; Sparks et al., 2007), due to perceptions that it is unsafe (i.e. children's extremities are insufficiently immobilized) and that it increases workload (i.e. requiring additional time or personnel). In addition, clinicians may have to modify their procedure technique to accommodate the child's position—this may cause some to feel insecure in their ability to carry out needle procedures successfully (Sparks et al., 2007). Methods to improve clinician experience and acceptability of this intervention are needed.

Tactile stimulation

Tactile stimulation is a physical intervention that involves touching the skin near the procedure site. It may be delivered using a variety of techniques including rhythmic rubbing, manual pressure, pressure devices (e.g. ShotBlocker™), and vibration devices (e.g. Buzzy™). Most of the studies evaluating this intervention have utilized either rubbing or manual pressure delivered by the operator performing the procedure—both techniques are ideally suited for use in any clinically setting as they do not require any equipment, advanced preparation, or additional cost (Taddio et al., 2009a). The proposed mechanism of action is hypothesized to involve the 'gate control theory' of pain, whereby nociceptive signal transmission to the brain is reduced by simultaneous competitive transmission of touch sensation. The end result is a lower pain signal reaching the brain.

Tactile stimulation is currently not recommended for use in children less than 4 years of age due to lack of data supporting its effectiveness. Limited research in the infant population (Beaver, 1987; Hogan et al., 2013; Jain et al., 2006) does not demonstrate a clear benefit. One possible explanation for the negative result observed in one trial (Hogan et al., 2013) is that tactile stimulation was delivered by a parent instead of the health care provider. It is possible that the intervention was not delivered appropriately or that it interfered with the parent's ability to soothe infants. Additional investigation of the effectiveness of clinician-led tactile stimulation is recommended in this population.

Cold

Skin refrigerants/vapocoolants

A variety of volatile chemicals are associated with an evaporation-induced cooling sensation after application to the skin. Based on the hypothesis that cooling reduces pain sensation in cutaneous sensory neurons, these agents have been investigated as potential analgesics for needle procedures (Zempsky, 2008). At present, there are two marketed preparations: Ethyl Chloride® and Pain Ease®. They are sprayed on the site continuously until blanching of the skin is observed (and for up to 10 sec). The cooling effect is short-lived, necessitating needle insertion within 1 min, or re-application. Some individuals experience discomfort with application of these cold solutions; otherwise side effects are limited with appropriate use.

Numerous studies conducted over the past two decades have not demonstrated a consistent analgesic effect of vapocoolants, irrespective of age of the individual (child or adult) or procedure (venous access or injection) (Hogan et al., 2011a). Possible reasons for inconsistent results include: increased or reduced pain perception arising from the cooling sensation, varied administration methods, or mild (equivocal) effects (Shah et al., 2009; Zempsky, 2008). Vapocoolant sprays are therefore not recommended for widespread use.

Ice

Based on the same mechanism of action as vapocoolant sprays, local cooling of the skin can be achieved via application of ice. Similar to studies of vapocoolant sprays, studies with ice do not demonstrate a consistent pattern of effectiveness (Movahedi et al., 2006; Taddio et al., 2009a). Hence, ice cannot be recommended as an analgesic for needle procedures.

Combining the 4 Ps of pain management for needle pain

Needle pain is an iatrogenic harm; hence, the goal of pain management is to prevent it (Chorney et al., 2010). No single pain-relieving intervention reliably achieves analgesia, thus interventions should be combined to improve effectiveness. Pain treatments that are consistently applied for all needle procedures experienced commencing from birth ensure the greatest likelihood that procedures are minimally painful, if not pain-free, and that the negative sequelae of unmitigated pain are averted. When children are sufficiently mature and/or have developed coping strategies and preferences, pain management can be tailored to their preferences (Cheng et al., 2003; Kortesluoma et al., 2008).

Pain and anxiety might not be completely eliminated by use of pain-relieving interventions. Children may still be anxious because of negative previous experiences, unfamiliar individuals and/or settings, or other reasons. These circumstances in no way negate the use of pain-relieving interventions; instead, they call for additional interventions.

Conclusion

Attending to pain from needle procedures undertaken in children supports children's health because it: (1) reduces acute suffering, which improves the experience of children undergoing needle procedures, their caregivers, and operators, and (2) reduces long-term harms, including non-compliance with future health care interventions as a result of minimizing the development of needle fears. Numerous evidence-based and feasible interventions are available, however, at present, they are underutilized. Knowledge translation initiatives that target the family, health providers, and institutions are recommended to improve current practices (Zhu et al, 2012; Chan et al, 2013; Schechter et al, 2010) (described in detail by Yamada and Hutchinson, Chapter 61, this volume).

References

Ammentorp, J., Mainz, J., and Sabroe, S. (2005). Parents' priorities and satisfaction with acute pediatric care. *Arch Pediatr Adolesc Med*, 159, 127–131.

Arendts, G., Stevens, M., and Fry, M. (2008). Topical anaesthesia and intravenous cannulation success in paediatric patients: a randomized double-blind trial. *Br J Anaesth*, 100, 521–524.

Beaver, P. K. (1987). Premature infants' response to touch and pain: can nurses make a difference? *Neonatal Netw*, 6, 13–17.

Bijttebier, P. and Vertommen, H. (1998). The impact of previous experience on children's reactions to venepunctures. *J Health Psychol*, 3, 39–46.

Blount, R. L., Bunke, V., Cohen, L. L., and Forbes, C. J. (2001). The Child-Adult Medical Procedure Interaction Scale-Short Form (CAMPIS-SF): validation of a rating scale for children's and adults' behaviors during painful medical procedures. *J Pain Symptom Manage*, 22, 591–599.

Buscemi, N., Vandermeer, B., and Curtis, S. (2008). The Cochrane Library and procedural pain in children: an overview of reviews. *Evid Based Child Health*, 3, 260–279.

Carbajal, R., Rousset, A., Danan, C., Coquery, S., Nolent, P., Ducrocq, S., *et al.* (2008). Epidemiology and treatment of painful procedures in neonates in intensive care units. *JAMA*, 300, 60–70.

Cepeda, M. S., Tzortzopoulou, A., Thackrey, M., Hudcova, J., Arora Gandhi, P. and Schumann, R. (2010). Adjusting the pH of lidocaine for reducing pain on injection. *Cochrane Database Syst Rev*, 8, CD006581.

Chan, S., Pielak, K., McIntyre, C., Deeter, B., and Taddio, A. (2013). Implementation of a new clinical practice guideline regarding pain management during childhood vaccine injections. *Paediatr Child Health*, 18: in press.

Chambers, C., Taddio, A., Uman, L.S., McMurtry, M., and HELPinKIDS. (2009). Psychological interventions for reducing pain and distress during routine childhood immunizations: a systematic review. *Clin Ther*, 31, S77–S103.

Chen, E., Zeltzer, L. K., Craske, M. G., and Katz, E. R. (2000). Children's memories for painful cancer treatment procedures: implications for distress. *Child Dev*, 71, 933–947.

Cheng, S. F., Foster, R. L., and Hester, N. O. (2003). A review of factors predicting children's pain experiences. *Issues Compr Pediatr Nurs*, 26, 203–216.

Cohen, L. L. (2008). Behavioral approaches to anxiety and pain management for pediatric venous access. *Pediatrics*, 122, S134–S139.

Cohen, L. L., Bernard, R. S., Greco, L. A., and McClellan, C. B. (2002). A child-focused intervention for coping with procedural pain: are parent and nurse coaches necessary? *J Pediatr Psychol*, 27, 749–757.

Cummings, E. A., Reid, G. J., Finley, G. A., McGrath, P. J., and Ritchie, J.A. (1996). Prevalence and source of pain in pediatric inpatients. *Pain*, 68, 25–31.

DeMore, M. and Cohen, L. L. (2005). Distraction for pediatric immunization pain: a critical review. *J Clin Psychol Med Sett*, 12, 281–291.

Diekema, D. S. (2012). Improving childhood vaccination rates. *N Engl J Med*, 366, 391–393.

Ellis, J. A., O'Connor, B. V., Cappelli, M., Goodman, J. T., Blouin, R., and Reid, C. W. (2002). Pain in hospitalized pediatric patients: how are we doing? *Clin J Pain*, 18, 262–269.

Ellis, J. A., Sharp, D., Newhook, K., and Cohen, J. (2004). Selling comfort: a survey of interventions for needle procedures in a pediatric hospital. *Pain Manage Nurs*, 5, 144–152.

Fein, J. A. (1999). Intravenous catheterization in the ED: is there a role for topical anesthesia? *Am J Emerg Med*, 17, 624–625.

Fetzer, S. J. (2002). Reducing venipuncture and intravenous insertion pain with eutectic mixture of local anesthetic: a meta-analysis. *Nurs Res*, 51, 119–124.

Fitzgerald, M. and Walker, S. M. (2009). Infant pain management: a developmental neurobiological approach. *Nature Clin Pract Neurol*, 5, 35–50.

Fradet, C., McGrath, P. J., Kay, J., Adams, S., and Luke, B. (1990). A prospective survey of reactions to blood tests by children and adolescents. *Pain*, 40, 53–60.

Franck, L. S., Allen, A., Cox, S., and Winter, I. (2005). Parents' views about infant pain in neonatal intensive care. *Clin J Pain*, 21, 133–139.

Franck, L. S. and Callery, P. (2004). Re-thinking family-centred care across the continuum of children's healthcare. *Child Care Health Dev*, 30, 265–277.

Frank, N. C., Blount, R. L., Smith, A. J., Manimala, M. R., and Martin, J. K. (1995). Parent and staff behavior, previous child medical experience, and maternal anxiety as they relate to child procedural distress and coping. *J Pediatr Psychol*, 20, 277–289.

Gale, G., Franck, L. S., Kools, S., and Lynch, M. (2004). Parents' perceptions of their infant's pain experience. *Int J Nurs Stud*, 41, 51–58.

Gaspardo, C. M., Linhares, M. B. M., and Martinez, F. E. (2005). The efficacy of sucrose for the relief of pain in neonates: a systematic review of the literature. *J Pediatr*, 81, 435–442.

Gonzalez, J. C., Routh, D. K., and Armstrong, F. D. (1993). Effects of maternal distraction versus reassurance on children's reactions to injections. *J Pediatr Psychol*, 18, 593–604.

Gonzalez, J. C., Routh, D. K., Saab, P., Armstrong, F. D., Shifman, L., Guerra, E., *et al.* (1989). Effects of parent presence on children's reactions to injections: behavioral, physiological, and subjective aspects. *J Pediatr Psychol*, 14, 449–462.

Goodenough, B., Perrott, D. A., van Dongen K., Brouwer, N., and Champion, G.D. (2008). Children's repose to vaccine fluid injection versus needle puncture pain during routine immunization. *Ambulat Child Health*, 6, 91–100.

Hamilton, J. G. (1995). Needle phobia: a neglected diagnosis. *J Family Pract*, 41, 169–175.

Harrington, P. M., Woodman, C., and Shannon, W. F. (2000). Low immunization uptake: is the process the problem? *J Epidemiol Comm Health*, 54, 394–400.

Harrison, D., Stevens, B., Bueno, M., Yamada, J., Adams-Webber, T., Beyene J., *et al.* (2010). Efficacy of sweet solutions for analgesia in infants between 1 and 12 months of age: a systematic review. *Arch Dis Child*, 95, 406–413.

Hedstrom, M., Haglund, K., Skolin, I., and von Essen, L. (2003). Distressing events for children and adolescents with cancer: child, parent, and nurse perceptions. *J Pediatr Oncol Nurs*, 20, 120–132.

Hogan, M. E., Kikuta, A., Shah, V., and Taddio, A. (2011a). Vapocoolants for pain reduction in children undergoing immunization, venipuncture, or venous cannulation. *Pediatric Academic Societies Meeting*, E-PAS20112904.58.

Hogan, M. E., Probst, J., Wong, K., Pillai Riddell, R., Katz, J., Taddio, A. (2013). A randomized controlled trial of parent-led tactile stimulation to reduce pain during infant immunization injections. *Clin J Pain, 9 May.* [Epub ahead of print.]

Hogan, M. E., Vandervaart, S., Perampaladas, K., Machado, M., Einarson, T. R., and Taddio, A. (2011b). Systematic review and meta-analysis of the effect of warming local anesthetics on injection pain. *Ann Emerg Med*, 58, 86–98.e1.

Howe, C. J., Ratcliffe, S. J., Tuttle, A., Dougherty, S., and Lipman, T. H. (2011). Needle anxiety in children with type 1 diabetes and their mothers. *MCN Am J Matern/Child Nurs*, 36, 25–31.

Humphrey, G. B., Boon, C. M., van Linden van den Heuvell, G. F., and van de Wiel, H. B. (1992). The occurrence of high levels of acute behavioral distress in children and adolescents undergoing routine veinpunctures. *Pediatrics*, 90, 87–91.

Jaaniste, T., Hayes, B., and von Baeyer, C. L. (2007). Providing children with information about forthcoming medical procedure: a review and synthesis. *Clin Psychol Sci Pract*, 14, 124–143.

Jacobson, R.M., Swan, A., Adegbenro, A., Ludington, S. L., Wollan, P. C., Poland, G. A., *et al.* (2001). Making vaccines more acceptable-methods to prevent and minimize pain and other common adverse events associated with vaccines. *Vaccine*, 19, 2418–2427.

Jain, S. and Kumar McMillan, D. D. (2006). Prior leg massage decreases pain responses to heel stick in preterm babies. *J Paediatr Child Health*, 42, 505–508.

Johnson, D. R., Nichol, K. L., and Lipczynski, K. (2008). Barriers to adult immunization. *Am J Med*, 121, S28–S35.

Johnston, C. C., Barrington, K. J., Taddio, A., Carbajal, R., and Filion, F. (2011). Pain in Canadian NICU's: have we improved over the past 12 years? *Clin J Pain*, 27, 225–232.

Johnston, C. C., Filion, F., Snider, L., Majnemer, A., Limperopoulos, C., Walker, C. D., *et al.* (2002). Routine sucrose analgesia during the first week of life in neonates younger than 31 weeks' postconceptional age. *Pediatrics*, 110, 523–528.

Kleiber, C. and Harper, D. C. (1999). Effects of distraction on children's pain and distress during medical procedures: a meta-analysis. *Nurs Res*, 48, 44–49.

Kleiber, C., Schutte, D. L., McCarthy, A. M., Floria-Santos, M., Murray, J. C., and Hanrahan, K. (2007). Predictors of topical anesthetic effectiveness in children. *J Pain*, 8, 168–174.

Klein, E. J., Shugerman, R. P., Leigh-Taylor, K., Schneider, C., Portscheller, D., and Koepsell, T. (1995). Buffered lidocaine: analgesia for intravenous line placement in children. *Pediatrics*, 95, 709–712.

Koh, J. L., Fanurik, D., Stoner, P. D., Schmitz, M. L., and VonLanthen, M. (1999). Efficacy of parental application of eutectic mixture of local anesthetics for intravenous insertion. *Pediatrics*, 103, e79.

Kortesluoma, R. L., Nikkonen, M., and Serlo, W. (2008). 'You just have to make the pain go away' – children's experiences of pain management. *Pain Manag Nurs*, 9, 143–149.

Lacey, C. M., Finkelstein, M., and Thygeson, M. V. (2008). The impact of positioning on fear during immunizations: supine versus sitting up. *J Pediatr Nurs*, 23, 195–200.

Lander, J. A., Weltman, B. J., and So, S. S. (2006). EMLA and amethocaine for reduction of children's pain associated with needle insertion. *Cochrane Database Syst Rev*, 19, CD004236.

Liossi, C., White, P., Franck, L., and Hatira, P. (2007). Parental pain expectancy as a mediator between child expected and experienced procedure-related pain intensity during painful medical procedures. *Clin J Pain*, 23, 392–399.

Ljungman, G., Gordh, T., Sorensen, S., and Kreuger, A. (1999). Pain in paediatric oncology: interviews with children, adolescents, and their parents. *Acta Paediatr*, 88, 623–630.

Luhmann, J., Hurt, S., Shootman, M., and Kennedy, R. (2004). A comparison of buffered lidocaine versus ELA-Max before peripheral intravenous catheter insertions in children. *Pediatrics*, 113, e217–e220.

Chorney, J. M., McGrath, P., and Finley, G. A. (2010). Pain as the neglected adverse event. *CMAJ*, 182, 732.

MacLean, S., Obispo, J., and Young, K.D. (2007). The gap between pediatric emergency department procedural pain management treatments available and actual practice. *Pediatr Emerg Care*, 23, 87–93.

Madlon-Kay, D. and Harper, P. (1994). Too many shots? parent, nurse, and physician attitudes toward multiple simultaneous childhood vaccinations. *Arch Family Med*, 3, 610–613.

Meyerhoff, A. S., Weniger, B. G., and Jacobs, R. J. (2001). Economic value to parents of reducing the pain and emotional distress of childhood vaccine injections. *Pediatr Infect Dis J*, 20, S57–S62.

Movahedi, A. F., Rostami, S., Salsali, M., Keikhaee, B., and Moradi, A. (2006). Effect of local refrigeration prior to venipuncture on pain related responses in school age children. *Aust J Adv Nurs*, 24, 51–55.

Myrick, B. and Barfield, J. M. (2006). Survey of parental willingness to pay and willingness to stay for 'painless' intravenous catheter placement. *Pediatr Emerg Care*, 22, 699–703.

Omer, S. B., Salmon, D. A., Orenstein, W. A., deHart, P., and Halsey, N. (2009). Vaccine refusal, mandatory immunization, and the risks of vaccine-preventable diseases. *N Engl J Med*, 360, 1981–1988.

Parvez, E., Stinson, J., Boon, H., Goldman, J., Shah, V., and Taddio, A. (2010). Mothers' beliefs about analgesia during childhood immunization. *Paediatr Child Health*, 15, 289–293.

Piira, T., Sugiura, T., Champion, G. D., Donnelly, N., and Cole, A. S. J. (2005). The role of parental presence in the context of children's medical procedures: a systematic review. *Child Care Health Dev*, 31, 233–243.

Pillai Riddell, R. R., Racine, N. M., Turcotte, K., Uman, L. S., Horton, R. E., Din Osmun, L., *et al.* (2011). Non-pharmacological management of infant and young child procedural pain. *Cochrane Database Syst Rev*, 5, CD006275.

Pruitt, L. M., Johnson, A., Elliott, J. C., and Polley, K. (2008). Parental presence during pediatric invasive procedures. *J Pediatr Health Care*, 22, 120–127.

Rennick, J. E., Johnston, C. C., Dougherty, G., Platt, R., and Ritchie, J. A. (2002). Children's psychological responses after critical illness and exposure to invasive technology. *J Dev Behav Pediatr*, 23, 133–144.

Richardson, J., Smith, J. E., McCall, G., and Pilkington, K. (2006). Hypnosis for procedure-related pain and distress in pediatric cancer patients: a systematic review of effectiveness and methodology related to hypnosis interventions. *J Pain Symptom Manage*, 31, 70–84.

Robieux, I. C., Kumar, R., Rhadakrishnan, S., and Koren, G. (1990). The feasibility of using EMLA cream in pediatric outpatient clinics. *Can J Hosp Pharm*, 43, 235–236, xxxii.

Rocha, E. M., Prkachin, K. M., Beaumont, S. L., Hardy, C. L., and Zumbo, B. D. (2003). Pain reactivity and somatization in kindergarten-age children. *J Pediatr Psychol*, 28, 47–57.

Ross, D. M. and Ross, S. A. (1984). Childhood pain: the school-aged child's viewpoint. *Pain*, 4, 179–191.

Salmela, M., Aronen, E. T., and Salantera, S. (2011). The experience of hospital-related fears of 4- to 6-year-old children. *Child Care Health Dev*, 37, 719–726.

Schechter, N. L. (2006). Treatment of acute and chronic pain in the outpatient setting. In G. A. Finley, P. J. McGrath, and C. T. Chambers (eds) *Bringing pain relief to children: treatment approaches*, pp. 31–58. Totwa, NJ: Humana Press.

Schechter, N. L., Zempsky, W. T., Cohen, L. L., McGrath, P. J., McMurtry, C. M., and Bright, N. S. (2007). Pain reduction during pediatric immunizations: evidence-based review and recommendations. *Pediatrics*, 119, e1184–e1198.

Schechter, N.L., Bernstein, B.A., Zempsky, W.T., Bright, N.S., and Willard, A.K. (2012). Educational outreach to reduce immunization pain in office settings. *Pediatrics*, 126, e1514–e1521.

Schneider, E. M. and LoBiondo-Wood, G. (1992). Perceptions of procedural pain: parents, nurses, and children. *Child Health Care*, 21, 157–162.

Shachor-Meyouhas, Y., Galbraith, R., and Shavit, I. (2008). Application of topical analgesia in triage: a potential for harm. *J Emerg Med*, 35, 39–41.

Shah, P. S., Aliwalas, L., and Shah, V. (2007). Breastfeeding or breastmilk to alleviate procedural pain in neonates: a systematic review. *Breastfeed Med*, 2, 74–82.

Shah, V. and Ohlsson, A. (2011). Venepuncture versus heel lance for blood sampling in term neonates. *Cochrane Database Syst Rev*, 5, CD001452.

Shah, V., Taddio, A., Rieder, M. J. and HELPinKIDS. (2009). Effectiveness and tolerability of pharmacologic and combined interventions for reducing injection pain during routine childhood immunizations: systematic review and meta-analysis. *Clin Ther*, 31, S104–S1051.

Simons, S.H., van Dijk, M. and Anand, K.S., Roofthooft, D., van Lingen, R. A., and Tibboel, D. (2003). Do we still hurt newborn babies? A prospective study of procedural pain and analgesia in neonates. *Arch Pediatr Adolesc Med*, 157, 1058–1064.

Slater, R., Cornelissen, L., Fabrizi, L., Patten, D., Yoxen, J., Worley, A., *et al.* (2010). Oral sucrose as an analgesic drug for procedural pain in newborn infants: a randomised controlled trial. *Lancet*, 376, 1225–1232.

Smith, R. W., Shah, V., Goldman, R. D., and Taddio, A. (2007). Caregivers' responses to pain in their children in the emergency department. *Arch Pediatr Adolesc Med*, 161, 578–582.

Sokolowski, C. J., Giovannitti, J. A. Jr., and Boynes, S. G. (2010). Needle phobia: etiology, adverse consequences, and patient management. *Dental Clin N Am*, 54, 731–744.

Soliman, I. E, Broadman, L. M., Hannallah, R. S., and McGill, W. A. (1988). Comparison of the analgesic effects of EMLA (eutectic mixture of local anesthetics) to intradermal lidocaine infiltration prior to venous cannulation in unpremedicated children. *Anesthesiology*, 68, 804–806.

Sparks, L. A., Setlik, J., and Luhman, J. (2007). Parental holding and positioning to decrease IV distress in young children: a randomized controlled trial. *J Pediatr Nurs*, 22, 440–447.

Stephens, B. K., Barkey, M. E., and Hall, H. R. (1999). Techniques to comfort children during stressful procedures. *Adv Mind-Body Med*, 15, 49–60.

Stevens, B., Abbott, L. K., Yamada, J., Harrison, D., Stinson, J., Taddio, A., *et al.* (2011). Epidemiology and management of painful procedures in children in Canadian hospitals. *CMAJ*, 19, E403–E410.

Stevens, B., McGrath, P., Gibbins, S., Beyene, J., Breau, L., Camfield, C., *et al.* (2003). Procedural pain in newborns at risk for neurologic impairment. *Pain*, 105, 27–35.

Stevens, B., Taddio, A., Ohlsson, A., and Einarson, T. (1997). The efficacy of sucrose for relieving procedural pain in neonates—a systematic review and meta-analysis. *Acta Paediatrica*, 86, 837–842.

Stevens, B., Yamada, J., and Ohlsson, A. (2010). Sucrose for analgesia in newborn infants undergoing painful procedures. *Cochrane Database Syst Rev*, 20, CD001069.

Suls, J. and Wan, C. K. (1989). Effects of sensory and procedural information on coping with stressful medical procedures and pain: a meta-analysis. *J Consult Clin Psychol*, 57, 372–379.

Sweet, S. D. and McGrath, P. J. (1998). Relative importance of mothers' versus medical staffs' behavior in the prediction of infant immunization pain behavior. *J Pediatr Psychol*, 23, 249–256.

Taddio, A., Appleton, M., Bortolussi, B., Chambers, C., Dubey, V., Halperin, S., *et al.* (2010a). Reducing the pain of childhood vaccination—an evidence-based clinical practice guideline. *CMAJ*, 182, E843–E855.

Taddio, A., Hogan, M. E., Gerges, S., Girgis, A., Moyer, P., Wang, L., *et al.* (2012a). Addressing parental concerns about pain during childhood vaccination: is there enough time to include pain management in the ambulatory setting? *Clin J Pain*, 28, 238–242.

Taddio, A., Ilersich, A. L., Ipp, M., Kikuta, A., Shah, V., and HELPinKIDS. (2009a). Physical interventions and injection techniques for reducing injection pain during routine childhood immunization: systematic review of randomized controlled trials and quasi-randomized controlled trials. *Clin Ther*, 31, S48–S76.

Taddio, A., Ipp, M., Thivakaran, S., Jamal, A., Parikh, C., Smart, S., *et al.* (2012b). Survey of the prevalence of immunization non-compliance due to needle fears in children and adults. *Vaccine*, 30, 4807–4812.

Taddio, A., Nulman, I., Goldbach, M., Ipp, M., and Koren, G. (1994). Use of lidocaine-prilocaine cream for vaccination pain in infants. *J Pediatr*, 124, 643–648.

Taddio, A., Shah, V., Hancock, R., Smith, R. W., Stephens, D., Atenafu, E, *et al.* (2008). Effectiveness of sucrose analgesia in newborns undergoing painful medical procedures. *CMAJ*, 179, 37–43.

Taddio, A., Soin, H., Schuh, S., Koren, G., and Scolnik, D. (2005b). A randomized controlled trial of liposomal lidocaine to improve procedural success rates and reduce procedural pain in children. *CMAJ*, 172, 1691–1695.

Taddio, A., Yiu, A., Smith, R., Katz, J., McNair, C., and Shah, V. (2009b). Variability in clinical practice guidelines for sweetening agents in newborn infants undergoing painful procedures. *Clin J Pain*, 25, 153–155.

Uman, L. S., Chambers, C. T., McGrath, P. J. and Kisely, S. (2006). Psychological interventions for needle-related procedural pain and distress in children and adolescents. *Cochrane Database Syst Rev*, 18, CD005179.

van Sleuwen, B. E., Engelberts, A. C., Boere-Boonekamp, M. M., Kuis, W., Schulpen, T. W. J. and L'Hoir, M. P. (2007). Swaddling: a systematic review. *Pediatrics*, 120, e1097–e1106.

Walsh, B. M. and Bartfield, J. M. (2006). Survey of parental willingness to pay and willingness to stay for 'painless' intravenous catheter placement. *Pediatr Emerg Care*, 22, 699–703.

Wasserfallen, J. B., Currat-Zweifel, C., Cheseaux, J. J., Hofer, M., and Fanconi, S. (2006). Parents' willingness to pay for diminishing children's pain during blood sampling. *Pediatr Anesth*, 16, 11–18.

Woodin, K. A., Rodewald, L. E., Humiston, S. G., Carges, M. S., Schaffer, S. J., and Szilagyi, P.G. (1995). Physician and parent opinions: are children becoming pincushions from immunizations? *Arch Pediatr Adolesc Med*, 149, 845–849.

Wright, S., Yelland, M., Heathcote, K. and Shu-Kay, N. (2009). Fear of needles: nature and prevalence in general practice. *Australian Family Physician*, 38, 172–176.

Yap, S. H., Mohammad, I., and Ryan, C. A. (2004). Avoiding painful blood sampling in neonates by transcutaneous bilirubinometry. *Ir J Med Sci*, 171, 188–190.

Zareba, G. (2006). A new combination vaccine for measles, mumps, rubella and varicella. *Drugs Today (Barc)*, 42, 321–329.

Zempsky, W. T. (2008). Pharmacologic approaches for reducing venous access pain in children. *Pediatrics*, 122, S140–S153.

Zhu, L., Stinson, J., Palozzi, L., Weingarten, K., Hogan, M. E., Duong, S., et al. (2012) Improvements in pain outcomes in a Canadian pediatric teaching hospital following implementation of a multifaceted knowledge translation initiative. *Pain Res Manag*, 17, 173–179.

CHAPTER 20

Procedural sedation

Joseph P. Cravero

Summary

Paediatric patients undergoing procedures often require sedation to provide the appropriate combination of anxiolysis, analgesia, and motionlessness. Due to the behavioural and developmental issues involved with this population, children actually require sedation to accomplish procedures much more often than adults. Paediatric sedation is a dynamic area of practice. Requests for this care continue to rise. The variety of providers involved in this care has also increased significantly. This chapter reviews the basic concepts involved in sedation delivery and then addresses the various considerations involved in sedation cases from the point of view of patient factors, procedure factors, and provider factors. Various drugs available for sedation are also reviewed with comments on appropriate strategies for a variety of common diagnostic and therapeutic procedures.

Introduction

Providing pain control for children requires recognition of the distinct nature of this population when compared to adults. Emotional and behavioural issues change with every developmental stage. Even if pain can be controlled, the presence of strangers and medical equipment will upset many children. The result can be unwanted physical and/or psychological trauma to the child and difficulty in accomplishing the procedure for the health care provider. As a result, sedation is sometimes required (in addition to analgesia) in order to provide optimal care.

Over the last 30 years the delivery of sedation for children has changed considerably. Procedural sedation was, and in many places still is, disseminated among a large group of providers with little organization or strategic planning and with wide variation in approach. The last 10 years has seen the formation of paediatric sedation services across North America and Europe staffed by a variety of specialists including anaesthesiologists, emergency medicine providers, intensivists, and hospital-based paediatricians (Cravero, 2009; Cravero et al., 2006, 2009; Rodrigo, 1991; Rodrigo et al., 1992; Weinbroum et al., 2001). These highly organized services have proven to be efficient, safe, and have decreased variation, as tracked by the Pediatric Sedation Research Consortium (Cravero et al., 2006). Training in sedation has become a fundamental component of paediatric emergency medicine and intensive care fellowships in the US, Europe, and Australia (Ilkhanipour et al., 1994; Mintegi et al., 2008). With these changes in care and training, the level of expectations for the delivery of safe, efficient, and highly effective procedural sedation has been raised significantly.

It is imperative that professionals who provide sedation clearly understand the concepts that are the keys to sedation practice including the nature of sedation depth, sedation monitoring, pharmacodynamics/pharmacokinetics of the sedative agents, core competencies for sedation management, and issues involving recovery of patients after sedation. It is only with a clear understanding of these concepts that the goal of safely eliminating pain and anxiety from the experience of hospital procedures and tests can be realized for children.

Background

Levels of sedation

Professional organizations have defined sedation in different ways. The American Academy of Pediatrics (AAP) and the American Academy of Pediatric Dentistry (AAPD) (Cote and Wilson, 2006), the American Society of Anesthesiologists (ASA; ASA Task Force on Sedation and Analgesia by Non-Anesthesiologists, 2002), and The Joint Commission (TJC; <http://www.TheJointCommision.com>) as well as the National Institute for Health and Clinical Excellence (NICE, 2010) in the UK have used the concept of levels of sedation ranging from minimally impaired consciousness to complete unconsciousness or general anaesthesia. On the other hand, the American College of Emergency Physicians prefers to refer to all sedation that is provided with the intent of accomplishing a test or procedure as 'procedural sedation' (Godwin, 2005) without emphasis on various depths of sedation.

Any provider who delivers sedation should recognize that different depths of sedation are possible and that risk for respiratory depression and cardiovascular changes are related to depth of sedation. Furthermore, a drug does not determine the depth of sedation that results from its administration. Any sedative drug, given a large enough dose, will produce complete unconsciousness and potentially dangerous outcomes (Cote et al., 2000b). The provider of sedation should be able to manage or rescue a patient from any level of sedation achieved.

The current levels of sedation defined by the AAP/AAPD, ASA, and NICE guidelines for management of patients during sedation include the following (Cote and Wilson, 2006):

Minimal sedation

A medically controlled state of depressed consciousness (formerly referred to as conscious sedation) which allows protective reflexes to be maintained; retains the patient's ability to maintain a patent airway independently and continuously; and permits appropriate response by the patient to physical stimulation or verbal commands such as 'open your eyes'. Although cognitive function and coordination may be impaired, ventilatory and cardiovascular functions are unaffected.

Moderate sedation/analgesia

A drug-induced depression of consciousness during which patients respond purposefully to verbal commands, either alone or accompanied by light tactile stimulation. No interventions are required to maintain a patent airway and spontaneous ventilation is adequate. Cardiovascular function is usually maintained.

Deep sedation

A medically controlled state of depressed consciousness or unconsciousness from which the patient is not easily aroused. It may be accompanied by a partial or complete loss of protective reflexes, and includes the inability to maintain a patent airway independently and respond purposefully to physical stimulation or verbal command. Patients may require assistance in maintaining a patent airway and spontaneous ventilation may be inadequate. Cardiovascular function is usually maintained.

General anaesthesia

General anaesthesia is a drug-induced loss of consciousness during which patients cannot be aroused, even by painful stimulation. The ability to independently maintain ventilatory function is often impaired. Patients often require assistance in maintaining a patent airway and positive pressure ventilation may be required because of depressed spontaneous ventilation or drug-induced depression of neuromuscular function. Cardiovascular function may be impaired.

The levels of sedation are *not* intended for use as a constant monitor of patient state. It is not practical to constantly stimulate patients to test their depth of sedation. Rather, these levels can be used to observe patient behaviour and codify patient risk based on response to stimuli that might occur during the course of a procedure.

Sedation depth monitoring

There are several monitors of depth of anaesthesia/sedation. The most commonly employed monitor is the Bispectral Index (BIS) monitor. This instrument uses a proprietary algorithm to process selected electroencephalographic (EEG) output into a number (from 0 to 100) that reflects the depth of sedation. While some investigators have validated its use during sedation of children (McDermott et al., 2003), it has not been found to be particularly useful during procedural sedation. Studies have found the BIS reading does not match well with clinical assessment of the depth of sedation, particularly when ketamine or combinations of sedation medications are utilized (Shields et al., 2005).

Several sedation monitoring scales are available for use during sedation activity. Unfortunately most have been designed for sedation depth monitoring in the intensive care unit (ICU) environment and, in order to test the depth of sedation, most of them require stimulation and documentation of response. The University of Michigan Sedation Score (UMSS) (Box 20.1) has been widely used and has undergone testing for validity. It is simple to use (repeatedly) during the course of a sedation activity (Malviya et al., 2002; Mason et al., 2004) Other sedation scores include the

---

Box 20.1 University of Michigan Sedation Score

Level state:

0 = Awake/alert.

1 = Minimally sedated: tired/sleepy, appropriate response to verbal conversation and/or sounds.

2 = Moderately sedated: somnolent/sleeping, easily aroused with light tactile stimulation.

3 = Deeply sedated: deep sleep, arousable only with significant physical stimulation.

4 = Unarousable

Copyright © The Regents of the University of Michigan. Reprinted with permission from Malviya S et al., Depth of sedation in children undergoing computed tomography: validity and reliability of the University of Michigan Sedation Scale (UMSS), *British Journal of Anaesthesia*, Volume 88, Issue 2, pp. 241–25, 2002.

Observer's Assessment of Alertness/Sedation Scale (Chernik et al., 1990), Comfort Score, Modified Ramsey Sedation Score, and the Children's Hospital of Wisconsin Sedation Scale (Ista et al., 2005). All of these scales measure levels of consciousness and agitation while the Comfort Scale and the Modified Ramsey Scale also include an assessment of pain and ventilation. While the scales have been compared to one another in various studies over the years, no specific scale has been shown to improve patient outcome or sedation provision over the others (De Jonghe et al., 2000).

Planning for sedation

There are many factors that impact the manner in which sedation should be provided. Every child should undergo a pre-sedation health assessment. This assessment should include age, weight, past medical history, vital signs, physical examination, and ASA status (Cote and Wilson, 2006).

While the pre-sedation examination of the patient is undoubtedly important in planning sedation for a procedure or test, this assessment is only one of a larger number of factors that must be considered including those related to the patient, the procedure, and the provider.

Factors relating to the patient

Past experience

As part of a detailed sedation history prior to the procedure the previous experiences of the patient should be elicited. For example, a patient who became combative with a dose of oral midazolam would not be well served by repeating that drug for another procedure. The sedation provider should also consider the anxiety level of the patient and family. The severely anxious patient will often need significantly more pharmacological sedation where a relaxed patient may only need support or distraction (Mintegi et al., 2008). Child life or play therapists can play an integral role in determining the optimal strategy for managing each patient's emotional and psychological needs (Brewer et al., 2006, Stevenson et al., 2005).

Allergies and adverse reactions

It is imperative that a drug allergy and adverse reaction history be elicited prior to providing sedation. Reports of an allergy to a given medication should be followed up with a history of the nature of the reaction. Drugs that were associated with truly allergic symptomatology (such as rash or wheezing) should be avoided. Families commonly interpret nausea or odd behaviour after sedation as an allergy. In fact these issues are often commonly known reactions to a medication or procedure. Nausea and vomiting are always possible after sedation—particularly with medications such as ketamine (Langston et al., 2008). Anticipatory treatment with 5HT3 inhibitors or steroids may decrease nausea and vomiting effects (Gan et al., 2007). Approximately 2% of patients will have paradoxical reactions to sedative medications such as midazolam or chloral hydrate (Sakurai et al. 2010). In these cases crying and combative behaviour is elicited shortly after administration rather than the desired sedation. Observational studies suggest the use of the benzodiazepine reversal agent romazicon can be useful in truncating the behaviour (Rodrigo, 1991; Weinbroum et al., 2001). Emergence agitation has been described during the recovery phase after sedation (Karaaslan et al., 2006). In these cases, patients may be delirious and combative for a period of 10 to 30 min (rarely longer) on awakening from sedation.

NPO status and assessment of aspiration risk

The ASA and AAP (ASA Task Force on Preoperative Fasting, 1999, Cote and Wilson, 2006) guidelines have historically taken the approach that anyone receiving moderate sedation or deep sedation should be treated similarly to those receiving anaesthesia regarding the timing of oral intake to prevent aspiration (Table 20.1) The authors argue that since sedation depth is variable it is possible that patients will enter a state where they will have impaired airway protective reflexes even when moderated sedation is targeted.

In the UK, NICE guidelines recommend nothing by mouth (NPO) intervals of 2 h for clear liquids, 4 h for breast milk, and 6 h for solids (NICE, 2010) Fasting is not recommended for individuals who will receive minimal sedation or moderate sedation where verbal contact will be monitored and maintained throughout.

Recently, two retrospective reviews have questioned the application of these guidelines to the field of paediatric sedation. These studies reviewed the charts of over 2400 emergency department paediatric sedation encounters and found no relationship between NPO duration prior to sedation and adverse outcomes (Agrawal et al., 2003; Roback et al., 2004). In light of this data, the American College of Emergency Physicians has developed its own set of fasting guidelines that differs significantly from the ASA (Green et al., 2007).

In addition to the history of oral intake, the ASA Practice Guidelines for Perioperative Fasting recommend that a history of gastro-oesophageal reflux disease should be considered a risk factor for pulmonary aspiration during sedation or anaesthesia (ASA Committee on Standards and Practice Parameters, 2011).

General health

The general health status for each patient who presents for sedation should be assessed. A general physical examination with focus on the airway, cardiovascular, and respiratory systems is critical.

The ASA status classification system categorizes individuals based on a general health (ASA Committee on Standards and Practice Parameters, 2011) (Table 20.2). Rather than focus on any specific disease entity, the ASA status is intended to group patients together based on their health status in order to better assess the risk of anaesthesia or sedation. Several studies have documented that the risk for any complication during sedation (desaturation episodes, airway obstruction, hypotension) rises by four- to fivefold with increasing ASA status (Cravero et al., 2009; Krauss and Green, 2008).

Airway issues

As part of the pre-sedation evaluation, specific abnormalities of the airway should be noted. These issues can be divided into two general categories: (1) the difficult functional airway, and (2) the difficult anatomical airway (Sims and von Ungern-Sternberg, 2012).

The difficult functional airway refers to those patients who are expected to have difficulty exchanging air through their natural airway when sedated. Children in this category would include those with severe sleep apnoea, obesity, recurrent croup, markedly enlarged tonsils, or those with congenital anomalies that make sleeping supine difficult or impossible (Donnelly et al., 2000). When children in this category are sedated to the point of unconsciousness, airway obstruction would be much more common than in healthy children (Adewale, 2009).

Table 20.1 ASA fasting guidelines for sedation or anaesthesia

Food	Hours of fasting required
Clear liquids	2
Breast milk	4
Formula or light meal (no fat)	6
Full meal	8

Reprinted with permission from Practice Guidelines for Preoperative Fasting and the Use of Pharmacologic Agents to Reduce the Risk of Pulmonary Aspiration: Application to Healthy Patients Undergoing Elective Procedures: An Updated Report by the American Society of Anesthesiologists Committee on Standards and Practice Parameters, *Anesthesiology*, Volume 114, Issue 3, pp. 495–511, Copyright © 2011 of the American Society of Anesthesiologists. A copy of the full text can be obtained from ASA, 520 N. Northwest Highway, Park Ridge, Illinois 60068–2573.

Table 20.2 Outline of the ASA physical status criteria

ASA class	Description
1	A normal, healthy patient, without organic, physiological, or psychiatric disturbance
2	A patient with controlled medical conditions without significant systemic effects
3	A patient having medical conditions with significant systemic effects intermittently associated with significant functional compromise
4	A patient with a medical condition that is poorly controlled, associated with significant dysfunction and is a potential threat to life
5	A patient with a critical medical condition that is associated with little chance of survival with or without the surgical procedure
6	A patient who is brain dead and undergoing anaesthesia care for the purposes of organ donation
E	This modifier is added to any of the above classes to signify a procedure that is being performed as an emergency and may be associated with a suboptimal opportunity for risk modification

Reprinted with permission of the American Society of Anesthesiology, Copyright © 2013 of the American Society of Anesthesiologists. A copy of the full text can be obtained from ASA, 520 N. Northwest Highway, Park Ridge, Illinois 60068–2573.

The difficult anatomical airway subgroup includes patients in whom the visualization of the airway with a standard direct laryngoscopy is expected to be difficult. The sedation provider must note this issue even if intubation is not planned. Since definitive airway management with an endotracheal tube is the ultimate rescue manoeuvre for children who are severely compromised during sedation, it is critical to anticipate if this is going to be a difficult intervention. A small or malformed mandible or a large tongue is often associated with difficult visualization of the glottis (Sims and von Ungern-Sternberg, 2012). Teeth that are protruding or particularly loose should be noted as they may hinder airway visualization or be knocked free during manipulation. Furthermore any patient who has limited neck mobility (such as trauma or burn patients) may be difficult to position in a manner that makes laryngoscopy possible. Finally any syndrome that results in an unusual facial appearance should be carefully noted as they may also be associated with an airway that is difficult to visualize (Candido et al., 2000; Sarvet and Brewer, 2011).

Developmental issues

The neurodevelopmental status of the child should be noted prior to planning sedation. Requirements for sedation will change greatly for any child who is severely delayed and/or autistic (Pasternak, 2002). Furthermore induction of sedation can be very difficult in large patients who cannot, or will not, cooperate with starting an intravenous (IV) line or taking oral medications (Rodrigo, 1995). Input from the family, primary care givers, and/or Child Life Specialists can be critical in determining the best strategies for accomplishing sedation and the amount of intervention that will be required for a given procedure (Mintegi et al., 2008).

Cardiac and respiratory systems

As already mentioned, the cardiac and pulmonary systems must be assessed prior to beginning sedation. In particular, patients with pulmonary hypertension may have significantly adverse reactions to hypoventilation and increased carbon dioxide (CO_2), or hypoxia, which can easily occur with sedation (Carmosino et al., 2007). In children with complex anatomical defects, the degree of left-to-right or right-to-left shunting may be changed by pulmonary or systemic vasodilation which can be a side effect of sedation medications. Patients with complex congenital heart disease should be sedated by practitioners who understand their physiology completely and also understand the physiological implications of sedation.

Respiratory illness

Although little data exists concerning the risk of sedation for patients with asthma, data from anaesthesia literature indicate that an asthmatic should be in the patient's best possible condition prior to beginning the procedure (Dones et al., 2012). Management should include administration of all currently prescribed inhalers prior to the sedation and assuring that the child is not actively wheezing at the time of sedation (Doherty et al., 2005).

There is little data to indicate the impact of an upper respiratory tract infection (URTI) on the success or safety of procedural sedation. URTIs are extremely common during the winter months with as many as 20% to 30% of the paediatric population having symptoms of an upper respiratory infection (Zaman et al., 1997). While it is simply not practical to cancel all procedures in this patient group, several studies have found an increase in airway and respiratory complications when they have surgery while experiencing a URTI (Homer et al., 2007). These problems include oxygen desaturation, increased secretions, laryngospasm, and coughing. The risk period exists not only during the time the child has the URI, but for approximately 2 weeks after the child is symptomatically improved (von Ungern-Sternberg et al., 2010). Fortunately, the frequency of severe complications (such as cardiac arrest, unexpected admissions, neurological injury, or death) have not been determined to be increased for this population (Tait and Malviya, 2005). It is prudent for sedation providers to consider the presence of a URTI when evaluating a child for sedation. If the procedure is going to be extended and/or if absolute movement control is required, it may be wise to reschedule an elective intervention even if symptoms are limited to the upper airway. If sedation is provided for those with a limited URTI the post-procedural observation may need to be extended (Homer et al., 2007). Elective sedation should be postponed in children who have a fever, or those with a significant cough and sputum production, rales, or wheezing.

Factors relating to the procedure

When choosing a sedation medication or technique, the provider should consider the time that the procedure will require to be accomplished. For drugs that are given as a single dose orally or nasally it is appropriate to match the duration of the procedure with the duration of the sedative. For short acting sedatives that are given as infusions—such as propofol, short or long duration procedures are equally easily accommodated. (Cravero et al., 2009; Wheeler et al., 2003)

An essential aspect of sedation that must be considered is the presence or absence of pain with any given procedure. Many of the sedatives that are commonly used for sedation—such as chloral hydrate, benzodiazepines, and even propofol—have no analgesic component (Jayabose et al., 2001; White and Romero, 2006). Options such as fentanyl, ketamine, and/or local anaesthesia should be considered to complement the effects of the purely sedative medications in these cases (Singh et al., 2010). It should be noted however, that the addition of opiates to other sedatives will significantly potentiate the probability of apnoea or airway obstruction (Taylor et al., 1986).

The provider must consider the position that the patient will be in during the procedure. Position can affect access to the airway during the procedure. Most children will maintain an open airway in the supine position when deeply sedated as long as the neck can be slightly extended and jaw lifted slightly forward (Shorten et al., 1995). If there is no access to the head, or if the head must be flexed during a procedure or a scan, obstruction of the airway will be much more likely (Isono et al., 2004). Care should be taken to avoid deep sedation unless the provider is ready to provide positive pressure ventilation. Airway resistance is actually decreased when a child is placed in the lateral decubitus or prone position (Vialet and Nau, 2009). While definitive management of the airway may be more complicated in these positions, spontaneous ventilation is often improved when compared to supine position if all other factors are unchanged.

Sedation should be considered for procedures that are particularly emotionally stressful even if not necessarily painful, but where a brief period of unconsciousness will allow the patient to avoid an emotionally harmful experience. Often these procedures involve invasion or examination of the genitalia (such as sexual abuse evaluations) or voiding cystourethrograms (Harari and Netzer, 1994).

Factors related to the sedation provider

When moderate or deep sedation is induced at least one person, in addition to the clinician performing the procedure, should be present to help care for the patient (Cote and Wilson, 2006). This person's responsibility is to monitor parameters such as pulse oximetry, heart rate, ventilation, and blood pressure and to assist in any supportive or resuscitation measures, as required. It is strongly encouraged that this individual at a minimum be trained in paediatric basic life support. Current knowledge of the emergency cart access/inventory as well as knowledge of how to activate back-up systems is critical (ASA Task Force on Sedation and Analgesia by Non-Anesthesiologists, 2002; Cote et al., 2006).

Sedation systems and sedation providers must recognize that the skill and training of providers of sedation varies greatly. The provider should be readily able to rescue that patient from the potential side effects of unexpected deepening sedation—which includes loss of airway integrity and spontaneous ventilation. Those who provide deep sedation for children should be able to rescue a child from the possible effects of general anaesthesia including definitive management of the airway and cardiovascular depression.

Studies of sedation related critical events have shown that severe adverse outcomes are most common in venues where a good backup or rescue system is not available (Cote et al., 2000a, 2000b, 2000c). Furthermore, sedation rescue has been shown to vary greatly between sedation providers and sedation settings (Blike et al., 2001). Given this evidence, it is logical that a protocol for accessing the backup help for sedation critical events (hospital resuscitation team or emergency medical systems) should be clearly laid out and tested.

Equipment needs for sedation

The following equipment is necessary for sedation. A bag and mask for positive pressure ventilation, masks of appropriate size for any patient, a second backup source of oxygen, a variety of sizes of oral and nasal suction equipment.

Vital signs, including oxygen saturation via pulse oximetry and heart rate, should be documented at least every 5 min in a time-based record. While the pulse oximeter measures oxygenation it does not directly measure ventilation. Depending on the amount of oxygen that the patient is breathing, there can be significant lag time between the onset of apnoea and oxygen desaturation (Langhan et al., 2012; Lightdale et al., 2006). In addition, a patient may experience significant hypoventilation but have acceptable oxygen saturation if receiving high-flow oxygen.

There are several methods for monitoring ventilation. The most basic is direct observation of the patient—noting coordinated chest wall/abdominal wall motion. When observation is not possible, other methods such as a precordial stethoscope or capnography should be used.

Capnography measures and displays CO_2 levels sampled from the breathing interface of the patient. For patients who are not intubated, a side stream detection technique is most often employed in which a small amount of gas (50–100 cc/min) is continuously sampled from the nasal cannula or inside of the mask on the patient. Apnoea is detected as soon as it occurs since it would result in an immediate loss of the expired CO_2 waveform (Figure 20.1).

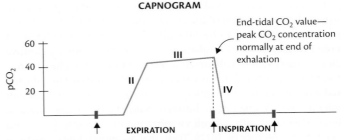

Figure 20.1 Key aspects of the capnogram.

Components of the normal capnogram:

I—(near zero baseline). Exhalation of CO_2 free gas contained in dead space.

II—(rapid sharp rise). Exhalation of mixed dead space and alveolar gas.

III—(alveolar plateau). Exhalation of mostly alveolar gas.

IV—(rapid sharp downstroke). Inhalation.

Sedation drugs

Hypnotic medications (sedatives)

Chloral hydrate

Chloral hydrate is a halogenated hydrocarbon that has been used as a sedative for 90 years. The common doses used vary between 20 to 75 mg/kg orally. Most practitioners limit the dose to 100 mg/kg or a total dose of 2 g (Greenberg et al., 1991). The pharmacokinetics of chloral hydrate are somewhat prolonged. The peak effect may not be seen for 60 min and the plasma half-life is 4 to 9 h. The drug can result in prolonged sedation, particularly in infants, with peak effect occurring well after the intended time of desired sedation (Cote, 1994, Malviya et al., 2000). On the other hand, the drug rarely results in respiratory depression (Sanborn et al., 2005). The potential for respiratory compromise does exist however, and is most marked when combined with opioids or other sedatives. Deaths have been reported with doses of chloral hydrate in the recommended range.

This drug is of limited use for painful procedures since it lacks analgesic effect. In addition, the prolonged onset time and duration do not match well with many paediatric procedures. Emergence can be marked by behavioural disturbances and agitation. It may still have a niche for use during radiology procedures such as magnetic resonance imaging (MRI) scans or for electroencephalograms. The drug is most effective in infants and toddlers.

In the spring of 2012 the only manufacturer of chloral hydrate in the US ceased production. It is still available in most areas outside of the US including Canada, Europe, and Asia (FDA, 2012).

Midazolam

Midazolam is a short-acting benzodiazepine that is widely used for anxiolysis and sedation. It has become particularly popular because of its short duration, predictable onset, and lack of active metabolites. Prominent effects include skeletal muscle relaxation, amnesia, and anxiolysis (Kain et al., 2000).

Although originally formulated for IV use, the same medication used orally has proven very successful in producing minimal to moderate sedation and amnesia (Malinovsky et al., 1995;

McMillan et al., 1992). The recommended oral dose is 0.5 to 0.75 mg/kg, with onset of sedation in approximately 15 min. Offset occurs approximately 30 min after the peak effect is noted. Oral midazolam is excellent for minor invasive procedures such as IV catheter placement or minor laceration repair when combined with local anaesthesia.

Midazolam may be given by the intranasal route at doses of 0.2 to 0.4 mg/kg (Harcke et al., 1995). Onset time is intermediate between the oral and IV routes of administration (10–15 min). The effectiveness of this route of administration is well established as a premedication for anaesthesia and sedation for minor procedures but its use is limited by significant discomfort on administration. Recent studies have noted that discomfort may be minimized through the use of a mucosal atomizer device for administration and pretreatment with lidocaine on the nasal mucosa (Chiaretti et al., 2011).

IV midazolam is titrated to effect with fractionated doses of 0.05 to 0.10 mg/kg that may be repeated at intervals of 3 to 4 min to a total dose of 0.5 to 0.7 mg/kg. IV midazolam reaches peak effect in 2 to 3 min. Slow IV administration is recommended with close observation for respiratory depression. When combined with IV opioids for painful procedures, midazolam has much more potent sedative and respiratory depressant effects when compared to its use as a single agent.

Respiratory depression is rare with administration of midazolam in recommended doses regardless of the route of administration. Patients are generally relaxed and drowsy after administration. One of the most desirable side effects is the anterograde amnesia. The extent of this effect will vary with the age of the patient and the dose employed.

Certain underlying conditions or medications may prolong the effects of midazolam. Heparin decreases protein binding and increases the free fraction. Hepatic metabolism is inhibited by cimetidine which prolongs the elimination half-life. Patients in renal failure may have three times the free fraction of the drug secondary to decreased protein binding.

Pentobarbital

Pentobarbital has potent sedative hypnotic properties, but it has no analgesic properties. Onset of action after IV administration is rapid, resulting in moderate–deep sedation within 3 to 5 min. The effective dose ranges from 3 to 6 mg/kg for over 98% of patients (Greenberg et al., 2000). Highest success rates are reported when the drug is used for patients under 12 years old and under 50 kg. The incidence of respiratory depression is less than 1% when pentobarbital is used as a sole agent at the recommended dosages (Sanborn et al., 2005). Failure to achieve sedation rates have been reported in 1.2% of patients when confined to this population. Paradoxical reactions leading to agitation occur in approximately 1% of patients. Pentobarbital is used in 14% of all sedations from an international collaboration of over 30 institutions (Cravero et al., 2006). Given the collected data on this drug reviewed above, pentobarbital is a reasonable choice for patients undergoing painless radiological procedures.

Intravenous propofol

Propofol is a 2, 6-diisopropylphenol compound that has potent sedative and hypnotic properties. The highly lipophilic nature of the drug requires that it be delivered in a lipid emulsion. It can only be delivered by the IV route. Onset of action is extremely rapid and induction of deep sedation/anaesthesia may be achieved with 2 to 3 mg/kg in 95% of patients within 60 to 90 sec. Sleep may be induced with as little as 1.5 mg/kg and maintenance of sedation is usually accomplished through the use of an IV infusion at 50 to 200 mcg/kg/minute. Recovery from the drug is faster than with any other IV sedative (2–3 min redistribution time) and the incidence of prolonged sedation or vomiting is extremely low. A dose-related decrease in blood pressure is noted that is similar to that found with other anaesthetics (Hertzog et al., 1999).

To reduce pain associated with injection a small dose of lidocaine (1 mg/kg) can be given through the IV catheter prior to administration or propofol can be given through a fast-flowing IV line into a large vein.

Some hospitals limit propofol use to anaesthesia personnel however studies have described the role of this drug in the ICU and emergency department (Barbi et al., 2003; Bassett et al., 2003; Guenther et al., 2003). A recent report found excellent effectiveness with a low rate of adverse events among sedation services using propofol for procedural sedation in children (Cravero et al., 2009). Airway interventions (intubation, bag-mask ventilation, or oral/nasal airway insertions) were required in approximately one out of 65 sedated patients in this cohort. The authors of these and other studies emphasize that safe use of propofol for sedation requires proven competencies in airway management.

Intravenous dexmedetomidine

Dexmedetomidine (DEX) has become increasingly popular as a sedative for radiological tests and procedures. This drug produces a sedated state with a small component of analgesia and little decrease in respiratory drive. DEX is an α2 agonist with a short half-life that is generally given in a bolus (0.5–1 mcg/kg over 10 min) followed by constant infusion (0.5–2 mcg/kg/h; Tobias and Berkenbosch, 2002; Tobias et al., 2003). In order to maximize effectiveness, doses two to three times this amount have been reported in patients aged 1 to 8 years (Mason et al., 2008b).

DEX has been reported for sedation of children on ventilators in the paediatric intensive care unit and as a sedative for procedures (Berkenbosch et al., 2005; Tobias and Berkenbosch, 2002). In one series of over 700 patients given 2 to 3 mcg/kg as a loading dose followed by infusions of 1.5 to 2.0 mcg/kg/h, no respiratory adverse events were reported (Mason et al., 2008c). Caution is warranted as hypertension, hypotension, and bradycardia have been reported side effects with DEX (Mason et al., 2008a, 2008b).

Analgesic medications

Fentanyl

Fentanyl is a synthetic opioid which is 100 times more potent than morphine. It has a very high degree of fat solubility that allows for very rapid penetration of the blood–brain barrier (Cote, 1994). The sedation effects are relatively brief as the offset of the drug is dependent on redistribution rather than elimination.

The IV dose recommendation for fentanyl is 0.5 to 1 mcg/kg/dose for procedures associated with significant pain such as lumbar punctures, bone marrow biopsies, bronchoscopies, minor surgical procedures, and central venous catheter placement (Chiaretti et al., 2011). Fentanyl as a sole agent offers excellent pain relief with mild sedation at these doses. Maximal effect occurs within 5 min when administered intravenously. Opioid effects last for 30 to 40 min. More often fentanyl is combined with sedatives to provide an analgesic component to sedation. There are reports of its use in combination with benzodiazepines or propofol for endoscopy (Langhan et al., 2012), haematology/oncology procedures (Langhan, 2011; Langhan et al., 2012), and invasive line placement (Chiaretti et al., 2011).

Chest wall rigidity may occur with IV fentanyl dosing and is particularly problematic when the drug is rapidly administered (Scamman, 1983). Respiratory depression is markedly increased when the drug is combined with midazolam or other sedative (Kennedy et al., 1998). Naloxone should be readily available when Fentanyl is administered.

Ketamine

Ketamine is a phencyclidine derivative. It blocks N-methyl-D-aspartate receptors to produce intense analgesic and sedative qualities. Its use has been described for over 40 years as a sedative for painful procedures in children (Green et al., 1990, 2001). A functional dissociation is created between the cortical and limbic systems of the brain. Spontaneous respirations and airway reflexes are maintained. Patients may exhibit random tonic movements of the extremities that make this drug inappropriate for procedures where the patient must lie perfectly still (i.e. computed tomography and MRI scans). Ketamine generally causes an increase in heart rate, blood pressure, cardiac output, and intracranial pressure. Oral secretions may be mildly increased although a recent meta-analysis of ketamine data suggests an increase in complications when combined with anticholinergics (Green et al., 2009). Ketamine has bronchodilator qualities making it ideal for use in children with issues relating to bronchospasm.

Ketamine can be given orally at a dose of 5 to 6 mg/kg. Onset of sedation occurs in 15 to 30 min and effects may be prolonged with this route—lasting 3 to 4 h (Rowland et al., 1995; Srinivasan et al., 2012). Intramuscular (IM) ketamine reaches peak blood levels and clinical effect in 5 min after a 3 to 5 mg/kg IM injection. Recovery from dissociation occurs within 15 to 30 min with coherence and purposeful neuromuscular activity returning in 30 to 120 min (Sanderson, 1997). There are two formulations for ketamine—10 mg/ml and 100 mg/ml. The more concentrated formulation of ketamine is preferred for IM administration. IM ketamine has been widely reported in the paediatric emergency medicine literature for sedation during painful procedures such as facial laceration repair, fracture reduction, abscess incision and drainage, and foreign body removal (Bloomfield et al., 1993; Sanderson, 1997). Ketamine can also be given intramuscularly to uncooperative patients in whom IV or oral administration of ketamine or other sedatives is not possible (Pershad et al., 2007).

Ketamine may be given in small IV doses of 0.5 to 1 mg/kg to produce rapid and profound sedation with analgesia. Peak concentrations occur within 1 min and allow almost immediate induction of clinical effects and lasts 15 min if no additional doses are given (Clements and Nimmo, 1981). Painful procedures are tolerated well following administration of ketamine because of its profound analgesic properties. IV ketamine is ideal for painful procedures such as burn debridement, foreign body removal, abscess incision, and orthopaedic procedures with a success rate over 98% (Baculard et al., 2007; Kienstra et al., 2004).

Adverse events under ketamine sedation are similar regardless of the route of administration. Nausea and vomiting has been described in 5% to 13% of children receiving ketamine (Bloomfield et al., 1993) while agitation on emergence is noted in 12% to 22% (Kienstra et al., 2004). Respiratory drive is not inhibited by ketamine and airway reflexes are largely left intact. A pooled analysis of ketamine sedation in over 8000 patients found an airway adverse event rate of less than 4% with the majority of events consisting of oxygen desaturation responsive to minimal intervention (Green et al., 2009).

Nitrous oxide

Nitrous oxide (N_2O) was described for use as an analgesic/anaesthetic over 100 years ago. It is a colourless, odourless gas that has analgesic, anxiolytic, and weak sedative effects. The drug may be delivered alone at concentrations of 30% to 70% for moderately painful procedures (Zier et al., 2008) or in combination with a mild sedative at lower concentrations for similar effect (Litman et al., 1998a). Onset of sedation and analgesia occurs in minutes and is terminated rapidly when the gas is discontinued. N_2O has minimal cardiovascular and respiratory effects when *not* combined with a potent sedative or opioid. It appears to cause a synergistic increase in sedation when used with other sedative or analgesic medications. (Litman et al., 1998b)

Current systems for administering N_2O include continuous flow systems that deliver anywhere from 0% to 70% N_2O and older 'demand valve' systems that use a premixed 50% mixture of N_2O in oxygen. Demand valve systems require the patient to initiate negative pressure to open the inspiratory valve of the system (Farrell et al., 2008). This can be difficult for some toddlers and thus the continuous flow systems are preferable for the youngest patients. Scavenging systems should be available for N_2O at any location that it is being delivered (Rowland et al., 1995). Recent studies have shown excellent safety outcomes (no apnoea or airway interventions in over 5000 patient encounters) for 70% N_2O administered by continuous flow to paediatric patients (Farrell et al., 2008; Zier and Liu, 2011).

Reversal agents

Reversal agents should be available when performing sedation with a benzodiazepine or opioid. Flumazenil can be used to reverse the effects of benzodiazepines and should be immediately available when using benzodiazepines for sedation. A dose of 0.01 mg/kg should be administered initially. Although rare, re-sedation may occur and additional doses of flumazenil may be required.

Naloxone (Narcan®) is an opioid antagonist and can be given intravenously, intramuscularly, or subcutaneously. The drug should be given in a slowly titrated manner when possible. The standard preparation contains 0.4 mg/cc of naloxone. The dose for children is 0.1 mg/kg for children under 20 kg. The dose for children over 20 kg is 2 mg (Table 20.3).

Discharge

The criteria for discharge from a sedated procedure should include stable vital signs; pain under control; a return to the level of consciousness that is similar to the baseline for that patient; adequate head control and muscle strength to maintain a patent airway; nausea and/or vomiting should be controlled; and the patient should be adequately hydrated.

Table 20.3 Sedation regimens

Propofol	50–200 mcg/kg/min IV	Non-painful procedures
Pentobarbital	3–6 mg/kg IV or PO	Radiology imaging
Midazolam	0.5–0.75 mg/kg PO 0.025–0.5 mg/kg IV 0.2 mg/kg intranasal	Anxiolysis, premedication, procedural sedation along with a topical anaesthetic or opioid
Chloral hydrate	50–100 mg/kg PO	Imaging, EEG, not commercially available in the US. Prolonged sedation
Dexmedetomidine	0.5–2.0 mcg/kg bolus (over 10 min) followed by 1–2 mcg/kg/h infusion.	For procedural sedation
Propofol with fentanyl	Fentanyl 1–2 mcg/kg IV with Propofol.5–1mg/kg boluses	Painful procedures
Midazolam with fentanyl	Midazolam 0.020mg/kg IV Fentanyl 1–2mcg/kg IV	Painful procedures
Ketamine	3–4 mg/kg IM 1–2 mg/kg IV	Painful procedures

Even when these criteria are used children have been found to be discharged with residual sedation effects (Malviya et al., 2004). In particular, children who have received a large dose of long-acting sedation medications (such as chloral hydrate) are very prone to re-sedation after vigorous efforts are made to rouse them. These patients should not be discharged until they have demonstrated that they can maintain wakefulness for 15 min or more.

Case example

Presentation: an 8-year-old, 35-kg girl with acute lymphoblastic leukaemia presents for a lumbar puncture with intrathecal chemotherapy administration.

Management: the child is held in mother's arms (as is her preference) while an IV infusion begun. She is given 0.5 mcg/kg of fentanyl followed by 1 mg/kg of propofol as a slow IV push. As she starts to become sleepy she is placed in a left lateral decubitus position with nasal cannula oxygen equipped with end-tidal CO_2 monitoring. A pulse oximeter and blood pressure cuff are also placed. After 3 min she is deeply sedated as evidenced by no response to voice and minimal movement when 2 mg of 2% lidocaine is infiltrated subcutaneously in the L3 to L4 interspace. She receives no further sedation and does not move during the lumbar puncture procedure. Heart rate is steady at 90 and her pulse oximeter remains at 98%. Breathing is partially obstructed and is easily improved with minimal jaw thrust—not required after about 2 min. She wakes up 9 min after procedure is completed and eats an ice lolly at that point.

Comment: this case is an example of a painful procedure where an analgesic (fentanyl) is used in conjunction with the sedative (propofol). The combination results in deep sedation which can (and does in this case) result in partial loss of airway tone requiring some airway manipulation. The sedation is very effective and results in movement control that would likely not be possible if analgesic were not added to the propofol. Of note, the providers allowed the child to choose how she would approach induction. This is particularly important for children such as this who will undergo a large number of procedures and tend to focus on the process over time.

Conclusions: procedures result in fear and anxiety and may involve pain as well in children. Sedation is not always required, but may help eliminate unwanted long-term behavioural and psychological outcomes from invasive procedures. The need for pharmacological intervention should be determined by the developmental status, the level of anxiety, and context of the procedure. The formation of expert teams of providers is critical to optimal outcomes.

References

Adewale, L. (2009). Anatomy and assessment of the pediatric airway. *Paediatr Anaesth*, 19(Suppl.1), 1–8.

Agrawal, D., Manzi, S. F., Gupta, R., and Krauss, B. (2003). Preprocedural fasting state and adverse events in children undergoing procedural sedation and analgesia in a pediatric emergency department. *Ann Emerg Med*, 42, 636–646.

ASA Committee on Standards and Practice Parameters. (2011). Practice guidelines for preoperative fasting and the use of pharmacologic agents to reduce the risk of pulmonary aspiration: application to healthy patients undergoing elective procedures. *Anesthesiology*, 114, 495–511

ASA Task Force on Preoperative Fasting. (1999). Practice guidelines for preoperative fasting and the use of pharmacologic agents to reduce the risk of pulmonary aspiration: application to healthy patients undergoing elective procedures. *Anesthesiology*, 90, 896–905.

ASA Task Force on Sedation and Analgesia by Non-Anesthesiologists. (2002). Practice guidelines for sedation and analgesia by non-anesthesiologists. *Anesthesiology*, 96, 1004–1017.

Baculard, F., Rieutord, A., Eslami, A., Cousin, J., Van Den Abbeele, T., and Francois, M. (2007). [Rectal pentobarbital sedation for children undergoing auditory brainstem response testing]. *Ann Otolaryngol Chir Cervicofac*, 124, 61–65.

Barbi, E. G. T., Marchetti, F., Neri, E., Verucci, E., Bruno, I., Martelossi, S., et al. (2003). Deep sedation with propofol by non-anesthesiologists: a prospective pediatric experience. *Arch Pediatr Adolesc Med*, 157, 1097–1103.

Bassett, K. E., Anderson, J. L., Pribble, C. G., and Guenther, E. (2003). Propofol for procedural sedation in children in the emergency department. *Ann Emerg Med*, 42, 773–782.

Berkenbosch, J., Wankum, P., and Tobias, J. (2005). Prospective evaluation of dexmedetomidine for noninvasive procedural sedation in children. *Pediatr Crit Care Med*, 6, 435–9.

Blike, G., Cravero, J., and Nelson, E. (2001). Same patients, same critical events – different systems of care, different outcomes: description of a human factors approach aimed at improving the efficacy and safety of sedation/analgesia care. *Qual Manag Health Care*, 10, 17–36.

Bloomfield, E. L., Masaryk, T. J., Caplin, A., Obuchowski, N. A., Schubert, A., Hayden, J., Ebrahim, Z. Y., et al. (1993). Intravenous sedation for MR imaging of the brain and spine in children: pentobarbital versus propofol. *Radiology*, 186, 93–97.

Brewer, S., Gleditsch, S. L., Syblik, D., Tietjens, M. E., and Vacik, H. W. 2006. Pediatric anxiety: child life intervention in day surgery. *J Pediatr Nurs*, 21, 13–22.

Candido, K. D., Saatee, S., Appavu, S. K., and Khorasani, A. (2000). Revisiting the ASA guidelines for management of a difficult airway. *Anesthesiology*, 93, 295–298.

Carmosino, M. J., Friesen, R. H., Doran, A., and Ivy, D. D. (2007). Perioperative complications in children with pulmonary hypertension undergoing noncardiac surgery or cardiac catheterization. *Anesth Analg*, 104, 521–527.

Chernik, D. A., Gillings, D., Laine, H., Hendler, J., Silver, J. M., Davidson, A. B., et al. (1990). Validity and reliability of the Observer's Assessment of Alertness/Sedation Scale: study with intravenous midazolam. *J Clin Psychopharmacol*, 10, 244–251.

Chiaretti, A., Barone, G., Rigante, D., Ruggiero, A., Pierri, F., Barbi, E., et al. (2011). Intranasal lidocaine and midazolam for procedural sedation in children. *Arch Dis Child*, 96, 160–163.

Clements, J., and Nimmo, W. (1981). Pharmacokinetics and analgesic effect of ketamine in man. *Fr J Anaeth* 53, 27.

Cote, C., Notterman, D., Karl, H., Weinberg, J., and McCloskey, C. (2000a). Adverse sedation events in pediatrics: a critical incident analysis of contributing factors. *Pediatrics*, 105, 805–814.

Cote, C. J. (1994). Sedation for the pediatric patient. A review. *Pediatr Clin N Am*, 41, 31–58.

Cote, C. J., Karl, H. W., Notterman, D. A., Weinberg, J. A., and McCloskey, C. (2000b). Adverse sedation events in pediatrics: analysis of medications used for sedation. *Pediatrics*, 106, 633–644.

Cote, C. J., Karl, H. W., Notterman, D. A., Weinberg, J. A., and McCloskey, C. (2000c). Adverse sedation events in pediatrics: analysis of medications used for sedation. *Pediatrics*, 106, 633–644.

Cote, C. J. and Wilson, S. (2006). Guidelines for monitoring and management of pediatric patients during and after sedation for diagnostic and therapeutic procedures: an update. *Pediatrics*, 118, 2507–2602.

Cravero, J. P. (2009). Risk and safety of pediatric sedation/anesthesia for procedures outside the operating room. *Curr Opin Anaesthesiol*, 22, 509–513.

Cravero, J. P., Beach, M. L., Blike, G. T., Gallagher, S. M., and Hertzog, J. H. (2009). The incidence and nature of adverse events during pediatric sedation/anesthesia with propofol for procedures outside the operating room: a report from the Pediatric Sedation Research Consortium. *Anesth Analg*, 108, 795–804.

Cravero, J. P., Blike, G. T., Beach, M., Gallagher, S. M., Hertzog, J. H., Havidich, et al. (2006). Incidence and nature of adverse events during pediatric sedation/anesthesia for procedures outside the operating room: report from the Pediatric Sedation Research Consortium. *Pediatrics*, 118, 1087–1096.

De Jonghe, B., Cook, D., Appere-De-Vecchi, C., Guyatt, G., Meade, M., and Outin, H. (2000). Using and understanding sedation scoring systems: a systematic review. *Intensive Care Med*, 26, 275–285.

Doherty, G. M., Chisakuta, A., Crean, P., and Shields, M. D. (2005). Anesthesia and the child with asthma. *Paediatr Anaesth*, 15, 446–454.

Dones, F., Foresta, G., and Russotto, V. (2012). Update on perioperative management of the child with asthma. *Pediatr Rep*, 4, e19.

Donnelly, L. F., Strife, J. L., and Myer, C. M., 3rd. (2000). Glossoptosis (posterior displacement of the tongue) during sleep: a frequent cause of sleep apnea in pediatric patients referred for dynamic sleep fluoroscopy. *AJR Am J Roentgenol*, 175, 1557–1560.

Farrell, M. K., Drake, G. J., Rucker, D., Finkelstein, M., and Zier, J. L. (2008). Creation of a registered nurse-administered nitrous oxide sedation program for radiology and beyond. *Pediatr Nurs*, 34, 29–35.

Federal Drug Administration. (2012). *Drugs to be discontinued*. Available at: <http://www.fda.gov/Drugs/DrugSafety/DrugShortages/ucm050794.htm>.

Gan, T. J., Meyer, T. A., Apfel, C. C., Chung, F., Davis, P. J., Habib, A. S., et al. (2007). Society for Ambulatory Anesthesia guidelines for the management of postoperative nausea and vomiting. *Anesth Analg*, 105, 1615–1628.

Godwin, S. A., Caro, D. A., Wolf, S. J., Jagoda, A. S., Charles, R., Marett, B. E., et al. (2005). Clinical policy: procedural sedation and analgesia in the emergency department. *Ann Emerg Med*, 45(2), 177–196.

Green, S. M., Denmark, T. K., Cline, J., Roghair, C., Abd Allah, S., and Rothrock, S. G. (2001). Ketamine sedation for pediatric critical care procedures. *Pediatr Emerg Care*, 17, 244–248.

Green, S. M., Nakamura, R., and Johnson, N. E. (1990). Ketamine sedation for pediatric procedures: Part 1, A prospective series. *Ann Emerg Med*, 19, 1024–1032.

Green, S. M., Roback, M. G., Krauss, B., Brown, L., McGlone, R. G., Agrawal, D., et al. (2009). Predictors of airway and respiratory adverse events with ketamine sedation in the emergency department: an individual-patient data meta-analysis of 8,282 children. *Ann Emerg Med*, 54, 158–68.e1–4.

Green, S. M., Roback, M. G., Miner, J. R., Burton, J. H., and Krauss, B. (2007). Fasting and emergency department procedural sedation and analgesia: a consensus-based clinical practice advisory. *Ann Emerg Med*, 49, 454–461.

Greenberg, S., Adams, R., and Aspinall, C. (2000). Initial experience with intravenous pentobarbital sedation for children undergoing MRI at a tertiary care pediatric hospital: the learning curve. *Pediatr Radiol*, 30, 689–691.

Greenberg, S., Faerber, E., and Aspinall, C. (1991). High dose chloral hydrate sedation for children undergoing CT. *J Comp Assist Tomogr*, 15, 467–469.

Guenther, E., Pribble, C. G., Junkins, E. P., Jr., Kadish, H. A., Bassett, K. E., and Nelson, D. S. (2003). Propofol sedation by emergency physicians for elective pediatric outpatient procedures. *Ann Emerg Med*, 42, 783–791.

Harari, M. D., and Netzer, D. 1994. Genital examination under ketamine sedation in cases of suspected sexual abuse. *Arch Dis Child*, 70, 197–8.

Harcke, H., Grissom, L., and Meister, M. (1995). Sedation in pediatric imaging using intranasal midazolam. *Pediatr Radiol*, 25, 341–343.

Hertzog, J. H., Campbell, J. K., Dalton, H. J., and Hauser, G. J. (1999). Propofol anesthesia for invasive procedures in ambulatory and hospitalized children: experience in the pediatric intensive care unit. *Pediatrics*, 103, E30.

Ilkhanipour, K., Juels, C. R., and Langdorf, M. I. (1994). Pediatric pain control and conscious sedation: a survey of emergency medicine residencies. *Acad Emerg Med*, 1, 368–372.

Isono, S., Tanaka, A., Tagaito, Y., Ishikawa, T., and Nishino, T. (2004). Influences of head positions and bite opening on collapsibility of the passive pharynx. *J Appl Physiol*, 97, 339–346.

Ista, E., VAN Dijk, M., Tibboel, D., and De Hoog, M. (2005). Assessment of sedation levels in pediatric intensive care patients can be improved by using the COMFORT 'behavior' scale. *Pediatr Crit Care Med*, 6, 58–63.

Jayabose, S., Levendoglu-Tugal, O., Giamelli, J., Grodin, W., Cohn, M., Sandoval, C., et al. (2001). Intravenous anesthesia with propofol for painful procedures in children with cancer. *J Pediatr Hematol Oncol*, 23, 290–3.

Kain, Z., Hofstadtr, M., Mayes, L., Krivutza, D., Alexander, G., Wang, S., et al. (2000). Midazolam: effects on amnesia and anxiety in children. *Anesthesiology*, 93, 676–84.

Karaaslan, D., Peker, T. T., Alaca, A., Ozmen, S., Kirdemir, P., Yorgancigil, H., et al. (2006). Comparison of buccal and intramuscular dexmedetomidine premedication for arthroscopic knee surgery. *J Clin Anesth*, 18, 589–593.

Kennedy, R. M, Porter, F. L., Miller, J. P., and Jaffe, D. M. (1998). Comparison of fentanyl/midazolam with ketamine/midazolam for pediatric orthopedic emergencies. *Pediatrics*, 102, 956–963.

Kienstra, A. J., Ward, M. A., Sasan, F., Hunter, J., Morriss, M. C., and Macias, C. G. (2004). Etomidate versus pentobarbital for sedation of children for head and neck CT imaging. *Pediatr Emerg Care*, 20, 499–506.

Krauss, B. and Green, S. M. (2008). Training and credentialing in procedural sedation and analgesia in children: lessons from the United States model. *Paediatr Anaesth*, 18, 30–35.

Langhan, M. (2011). Availability and clinical utilization of capnography in the prehospital setting. *Conn Med*, 75, 197–201.

Langhan, M. L., Auerbach, M., Smith, A. N., and Chen, L. (2012). Improving detection by pediatric residents of endotracheal tube dislodgement with capnography: a randomized controlled trial. *J Pediatr*, 160, 1009–14 .e1.

Langston, W. T., Wathen, J. E., Roback, M. G., and Bajaj, L. (2008). Effect of ondansetron on the incidence of vomiting associated with ketamine sedation in children: a double-blind, randomized, placebo-controlled trial. *Ann Emerg Med*, 52, 30–34.

Lightdale, J. R., Goldmann, D. A., Feldman, H. A., Newburg, A. R., Dinardo, J. A., and Fox, V. L. (2006). Microstream capnography improves patient monitoring during moderate sedation: a randomized, controlled trial. *Pediatrics*, 117, e1170–1178.

Litman, R., Kottra, J., Verga, K., Berkowitz, R., and Ward, D. (1998a). Chloral hydrate sedation: the additive sedative and respiratory depressant effects of nitrous oxide. *Anesth Analg*, 86, 724–728.

Litman, R. S., Kottra, J. A., Berkowitz, R. J., and Ward, D. S. (1998b). Upper airway obstruction during midazolam/nitrous oxide sedation in children with enlarged tonsils. *Pediatr Dent*, 20, 318–320.

Malinovsky, J.-M., Populaire, C., and Cozian, A. (1995). Premedication with midazolam in children. Effect of intranasal, rectal, and oral routes on plasma midazolam concentrations. *Anaesth*, 50, 351.

Malviya, S., Voepel-Lewis, T., Ludomirsky, A., Marshall, J., and Tait, A. (2004). Can we improve the assessment of discharge readiness? A comparative study of observational and objective measures of depth of sedation in children. *Anesthesiology*, 100, 218–224.

Malviya, S., Voepel-Lewis, T., Prochaska, G., and Tait, A. R. (2000). Prolonged recovery and delayed side effects of sedation for diagnostic imaging studies in children. *Pediatrics*, 105, E42.

Malviya, S., Voepel-Lewis, T., Tait, A. R., Merkel, S., Tremper, K., and Naughton, N. (2002). Depth of sedation in children undergoing computed tomography: validity and reliability of the University of Michigan Sedation Scale (UMSS). *Br J Anaesth*, 88, 241–235.

Mason, K. P., Sanborn, P., Zurakowski, D., Karian, V. E., Connor, L., Fontaine, P. J., *et al.* (2004). Superiority of pentobarbital versus chloral hydrate for sedation in infants during imaging. *Radiology*, 230, 537–542.

Mason, K. P., Zgleszewski, S. E., Prescilla, R., Fontaine, P. J., and Zurakowski, D. (2008a). Hemodynamic effects of dexmedetomidine sedation for CT imaging studies. *Paediatr Anaesth*, 18, 393–402.

Mason, K. P., Zurakowski, D., Zgleszewski, S., Prescilla, R., Fontaine, P. J., and Dinardo, J. A. (2008b). Incidence and predictors of hypertension during high-dose dexmedetomidine sedation for pediatric MRI. *Paediatr Anaesth*, 20, 516–523.

Mason, K. P., Zurakowski, D., Zgleszewski, S. E., Robson, C. D., Carrier, M., Hickey, P. R., *et al.* (2008c). High dose dexmedetomidine as the sole sedative for pediatric MRI. *Paediatr Anaesth*, 18, 403–411.

McDermott, N. B., Vansickle, T., Motas, D., and Friesen, R. H. (2003). Validation of the bispectral index monitor during conscious and deep sedation in children. *Anesth Analg*, 97, 39–43.

McMillan, C., Spahr-Schopfer, I., and Sikech, N. (1992). Premedication of children with oral midazolam. *Can J Anaesth*, 39, 545.

Mintegi, S., Shavit, I., and Benito, J. (2008). Pediatric emergency care in Europe: a descriptive survey of 53 tertiary medical centers. *Pediatr Emerg Care*, 24, 359–363.

National Institute for Health and Clinical Excellence (NICE). (2010). *Sedation in children and young people: sedation for diagnostic and therapeutic procedures in children and young people.* Available at: <http://www.nice.org.uk/nicemedia/live/13296/52132/52132.pdf>.

Pasternak, L. R. (2002). ASA practice guidelines for preanesthetic assessment. *Int Anesthesiol Clin*, 40, 31–46.

Pershad, J., Wan, J., and Anghelescu, D. L. (2007). Comparison of propofol with pentobarbital/midazolam/fentanyl sedation for magnetic resonance imaging of the brain in children. *Pediatrics*, 120, e629–636.

Rachel, H. J., Elwood, T., Peterson, D., and Rampersad, S. (2007). Risk factors for adverse events in children with colds emerging from anesthesia: a logistic regression. *Paediatr Anaesth*, 17, 154–161.

Roback, M. G., Bajaj, L., Wathen, J. E., and Bothner, J. (2004). Preprocedural fasting and adverse events in procedural sedation and analgesia in a pediatric emergency department: are they related? *Ann Emerg Med*, 44(5), 454–459.

Rodrigo, C. (1995). Flumazenil in dentistry. *Anesth Prog*, 42, 121–125.

Rodrigo, C. R. (1991). Flumazenil reverses paradoxical reaction with midazolam. *Anesth Prog*, 38, 65–68.

Rodrigo, M. R., Chan, L., and Hui, E. (1992). Flumazenil reversal of conscious sedation for minor oral surgery. *Anaesth Intensive Care*, 20, 174–176.

Rowland, A. S., Baird, D. D., Shore, D. L., Weinberg, C. R., Savitz, D. A., and Wilcox, A. J. (1995). Nitrous oxide and spontaneous abortion in female dental assistants. *Am J Epidemiol*, 141, 531–538.

Sakurai, Y., Obata, T., Odaka, A., Terui, K., Tamura, M., and Miyao, H. (2010). Buccal administration of dexmedetomidine as a preanesthetic in children. *J Anesth*, 24(1), 49–53

Sanborn, P., Michna, E., Zurakowski, D., Burrows, P., Fontaine, P., Connor, L., and Mason, K. (2005). Adverse cardiovascular and respiratory events during sedation of pediatric patients for imaging examinations. *Radiology*, 237, 288–294.

Sanderson, P. M. (1997). A survey of pentobarbital sedation for children undergoing abdominal CT scans after oral contrast medium. *Paediatr Anaesth*, 7, 309–315.

Sarvet, B. and Brewer, S. (2011). Anxiety disorders in pediatric primary care. *Pediatr Ann*, 40, 499–505.

Scamman, F. (1983). Fentanyl-O2-N2O rigidity and pulmonary compliance. *Anesth Analg* 62, 332–334.

Shields, C. H., Styadi-Park, G., McCown, M. Y., and Creamer, K. M. (2005). Clinical utility of the bispectral index score when compared to the University of Michigan Sedation Scale in assessing the depth of outpatient pediatric sedation. *Clin Pediatr*, 44, 229–236.

Shorten, G. D., Armstrong, D. C., Roy, W. I., and Brown, L. (1995). Assessment of the effect of head and neck position on upper airway anatomy in sedated paediatric patients using magnetic resonance imaging. *Paediatr Anaesth*, 5, 243–248.

Sims, C., and Von Ungern-Sternberg, B. S. (2012). The normal and the challenging pediatric airway. *Paediatr Anaesth*, 22, 521–526.

Singh, R., Batra, Y. K., Bharti, N., and Panda, N. B. (2010). Comparison of propofol versus propofol-ketamine combination for sedation during spinal anesthesia in children: randomized clinical trial of efficacy and safety. *Paediatr Anaesth*, 20, 439–444.

Srinivasan, M., Turmelle, M., Depalma, L. M., Mao, J., and Carlson, D. W. (2012). Procedural sedation for diagnostic imaging in children by pediatric hospitalists using propofol: analysis of the nature, frequency, and predictors of adverse events and interventions. *J Pediatr*, 160, 801–806.e1.

Stevenson, M. D., Bivins, C. M., O'Brien, K., and Gonzalez Del Rey, J. A. (2005). Child life intervention during angiocatheter insertion in the pediatric emergency department. *Pediatr Emerg Care*, 21, 712–718.

Tait, A. R. and Malviya, S. (2005). Anesthesia for the child with an upper respiratory tract infection: still a dilemma? *Anesth Analg*, 100, 59–65.

Taylor, M. B., Grounds, R. M., Mulrooney, P. D., and Morgan, M. (1986). Ventilatory effects of propofol during induction of anaesthesia. Comparison with thiopentone. *Anaesthesia*, 41, 816–820.

Tobias, J. and Berkenbosch, J. (2002). Initial experience with dexmedetomidine in paediatric-aged patients. *Paediatric Anaesthesia*, 12, 171–175.

Tobias, J. D., Berkenbosch, J. W., and Russo, P. (2003). Additional experience with dexmedetomidine in pediatric patients. *South Med J*, 96, 871–875.

Vialet, R., and Nau, A. (2009). Effect of head posture on pediatric oropharyngeal structures: implications for airway management in infants and children. *Curr Opin Anaesthesiol*, 22, 396–399.

Von Ungern-Sternberg, B. S., Boda, K., Chambers, N. A., Rebmann, C., Johnson, C., Sly, P. D., *et al.* (2010). Risk assessment for respiratory complications in paediatric anaesthesia: a prospective cohort study. *Lancet*, 376, 773–783.

Weinbroum, A. A., Szold, O., Ogorek, D., and Flaishon, R. (2001). The midazolam-induced paradox phenomenon is reversible by flumazenil. Epidemiology, patient characteristics and review of the literature. *Eur J Anaesthesiol*, 18, 789–797.

Wheeler, D. S., Vaux, K. K., Ponaman, M. L., and Poss, B. W. (2003). The safe and effective use of propofol sedation in children undergoing diagnostic and therapeutic procedures: experience in a pediatric ICU and a review of the literature. *Pediatr Emerg Care*, 19, 385–392.

White, P. and Romero, G. (2006). *Nonopioid intravenous anesthesia*. Philadelphia, PA: Lippincott Williams & Wilkins.

Zaman, K., Baqui, A. H., Yunus, M., Sack, R. B., Bateman, O. M., Chowdhury, H. R., *et al.* (1997). Acute respiratory infections in children: a community-based longitudinal study in rural Bangladesh. *J Trop Pediatr*, 43, 133–137.

Zier, J. L. and Liu, M. (2011). Safety of high-concentration nitrous oxide by nasal mask for pediatric procedural sedation: experience with 7802 cases. *Pediatr Emerg Care*, 27, 1107–1112.

Zier, J. L., Rivard, P. F., Krach, L. E., and Wendorf, H. R. (2008). Effectiveness of sedation using nitrous oxide compared with enteral midazolam for botulinum toxin A injections in children. *Dev Med Child Neurol*, 50, 854–858.

CHAPTER 21

Neuropathic pain in children

Suellen M. Walker

Summary

Lesions or disease of the somatosensory nervous system can produce neuropathic pain (NP). Typical features include spontaneous or paroxysmal pain, often described as burning, shooting, like electric shocks, or pins and needles. NP does occur in childhood, but age at the time of injury may influence the risk of NP following traumatic nerve injuries. While conditions commonly associated with NP in adults may be less common in childhood (e.g. trigeminal neuralgia) other conditions (e.g. Fabry's disease and erythromelalgia), may present with pain in childhood and present a diagnostic challenge for paediatric practitioners.

Introduction

Neuropathic pain (NP) has been defined as pain caused by a lesion or disease of the somatosensory nervous system (Jensen et al., 2011). Chronic pain is reported by up to 6% of children and adolescents (van Dijk et al., 2006), but the proportion with NP is not clear. However, children with neuropathic pain or complex regional pain syndrome (CRPS) comprise a significant proportion of cases referred to paediatric chronic pain clinics (Howard, 2011; Martin et al., 2010). Epidemiological studies suggest a prevalence of chronic pain with neuropathic features of 3.3% to 8.2% in the adult population (Haanpaa et al., 2011; Smith and Torrance, 2012); but conditions associated with NP in children differ from those commonly reported in adults (Borsook, 2012):

- Many conditions associated with NP in adults are rare or not associated with significant pain in children (e.g. Parkinson's disease, Alzheimer's disease, post-stroke pain).

- The incidence of post-herpetic neuralgia and trigeminal neuralgia is much lower in children (Hall et al., 2006).

- Painful diabetic neuropathy is a feature of more prolonged disease and is rarely reported before 14 years of age (Hall et al., 2006), but sensory changes have been detected in children prior to onset of pain (Blankenburg et al., 2012).

- Some NP conditions are increasingly recognized in children (e.g. CRPS, phantom limb pain, or NP following trauma or surgery; Walco et al., 2010).

- NP may be the presenting symptom during childhood of specific genetic conditions (e.g. Fabry's disease or erythromelalgia; Fischer and Waxman, 2010; Ramaswami, 2008).

- Children may have increased susceptibility to certain types of painful neurological injury (e.g. toxicity following mercury exposure; Celebi et al., 2008).

NP may be considered as a clinical entity in its own right with a common pattern of symptoms and signs, often with similar management irrespective of the underlying cause (Table 21.1). In later sections of this chapter, NP associated with specific conditions in children will be outlined. The classification of CRPS as a neuropathic pain condition is debated, but in this volume is included in Chapter 24 by Clinch. Pharmacological management of NP is often extrapolated from adult data (Attal et al., 2010; Dworkin et al., 2010; see Rastogi and Campbell, Chapter 48, this volume). Laboratory data regarding mechanisms and effects of nerve injury in early life are discussed by Vega-Avelaria and Beggs (Chapter 7, this volume).

Assessment and diagnostic features

Current guidelines for the assessment and diagnosis of NP are designed for adults (Haanpaa et al., 2011), but are often extrapolated to older children or adolescents features include:

- Screening questionnaires to identify neuropathic pain include: LANSS, Leeds Assessment of Neuropathic Symptoms and Signs (Bennett, 2001); DN4, Douleur Neuropathique en 4 questions (Bouhassira et al., 2005); NPQ, Neuropathic Pain Questionnaire (Krause and Backonja, 2003); painDETECT (Freynhagen et al., 2006); and ID-Pain, identify Pain (Portenoy, 2006). The sensitivity (66–91%) and specificity (74–94%) of these tools fall within reasonable ranges in adults (Bennett et al., 2007; Haanpaa et al., 2009) but they have not yet been validated in children.

- Pain history including: evaluation of intensity (assessed by numerical rating scale or visual analogue scale), quality (sensory descriptors), temporal aspects of pain (frequency, spontaneous/paroxysmal or continuous, aggravating/relieving factors), and response to treatment. History remains the mainstay of diagnosis, and many children use descriptors that are considered 'typical' of NP, such as burning, shooting, radiating, burning, electricity-like, pain on contact, stabbing, pricking, tingling, pins and needles, and pinching (Krane and Heller, 1995; Wilkins et al., 1998, 2004). However, young children may be unable to clearly describe their pain in these terms.

- Sensory examination to verify the lesion of the somatosensory system (sensory, motor, and autonomic signs; allodynia and

Table 21.1 Neuropathic pain conditions in children

Classification	Examples
Trauma	◆ Post surgery ◆ Phantom limb pain ◆ Brachial plexus injury ◆ Peripheral nerve injury ◆ Spinal cord injury
Complex regional pain syndrome	◆ Following trauma/fracture ◆ No precipitating cause
Neurological and neuromuscular disease	◆ Guillain–Barré disease ◆ Trigeminal neuralgia ◆ Multiple sclerosis
Metabolic disease	◆ Fabry's disease
Neuropathy following infection	◆ HIV/AIDS ◆ Post-herpetic neuralgia
Tumour	◆ Nervous system tumour (neurofibromatosis) ◆ Invasion/compression by tumour ◆ Effect of treatment (e.g. post surgery, chemotherapy)
Genetic	◆ Erythromelalgia ◆ Paroxysmal extreme pain disorder

hyperalgesia; hypoaesthesia and hypoalgesia). Sensory abnormalities on clinical examination are more difficult to elicit in infants and young children. Quantitative sensory testing evaluates patterns of change in association with NP in adults (Maier et al., 2010), but paediatric use of this technique is often limited to research studies (Lebel et al., 2008;Sethna et al., 2007; see also Hermann, Chapter 40, this volume).

◆ Assessment of disability, quality of life, sleep, and mood. In adults, NP is associated with a greater disease burden than other forms of chronic pain, with effects on quality of life, impaired sleep, higher anxiety/depression scores, and increased use of health care and specialist services (Attal et al., 2011; Smith and Torrance, 2012). The impact of chronic pain on quality of life, mood, and disability is covered in many chapters throughout this text, but relatively few paediatric series have evaluated the impact of NP per se on quality of life (Jan and Wilson, 2004).

◆ Additional tests may be indicated, although many are limited to research settings or specific cases (e.g. electroneuromyography, microneurography, functional brain imaging, skin biopsy). Investigations may be required to confirm a specific underlying diagnosis (e.g. Fabry's disease) or to exclude other causes.

Neuropathic pain following trauma and surgery

Laboratory models of traumatic peripheral nerve injury have demonstrated a reduced susceptibility to neuropathic pain if the injury is performed at a younger age (first 3 postnatal weeks in the rodent; see Vega-Avelaria and Beggs, Chapter 7; Walker, Chapter 3, this volume). Clinical studies are also suggestive of an increased likelihood of neuropathic pain following trauma or surgery at older ages.

Post-surgical neuropathic pain

Neuropathic pain can occur acutely or as a feature of persistent post-surgical pain in adults (Kehlet et al., 2006; Macintyre et al., 2010). There has been limited prospective evaluation of postoperative NP in children, and most data comes from retrospective questionnaires.

The largest study (response rate 63%, n = 651) surveyed 18- to 19-year-olds who had undergone inguinal hernia repair before 5 years of age (Aasvang and Kehlet, 2007). Pain from the operated groin was reported by 13.5% of respondents; 5.2% had pain at rest with an average intensity of 2.5 (range 1–9 on 0–10 visual analogue scale, VAS); and in 2% pain was frequent and moderate or severe (VAS 6.3, range 4–9). Neuropathic descriptors were reported by 53% and sensory descriptors by 72%, including tender, annoying, and shooting. There was no difference in incidence if surgery was performed before 3 months of age. Pain was frequently precipitated by exercise and activity, and this led the authors to conclude that a significant component of the pain may arise from muscle and/or ligamentous sources rather than being predominantly neuropathic pain.

Eighty-eight of 91 patients who underwent thoracotomy for repair of coarctation of the aorta between 1965 and 1985 at ages between 0 and 25 years were assessed at an average time of 39.3±7.7 years following surgery (Kristensen et al., 2010). An increased proportion reported pain for greater than 3 months following their surgery if it was performed at a later age: 1/31 at 0 to 6 years; 7/36 at 7 to 12 years, and 6/21 at 13 to 25 years. Three patients, who had initial surgery between 7 and 25 years, still reported pain with neuropathic descriptors at the surgery site. As the authors noted, this retrospective study is subject to significant recall bias, particularly for those who had surgery before 6 years of age.

Neuropathic pain was reported in six children (within a group of approximately 40) with cerebral palsy undergoing multilevel surgery to reduce contractures (tendon release/lengthening/transfer) and/or improve sitting position or gait. Pain with neuropathic descriptors commenced 4 to 9 days after surgery, was associated with allodynia in five of six patients, and required referral and ongoing management in a chronic pain clinic (Lauder and White, 2005).

Early-onset localized pain in surgical scars was reported in three cases following surgery at 14 to 17 years. Symptom onset was delayed for 6 to 12 months in a further two cases following surgery at 8 and 10 years respectively (Nayak and Cunliffe, 2008).

Ulna nerve injury with sensory and/or motor signs occurred in 6% of children (average age 6.5 years) having pins inserted for supracondylar fractures of the humerus. Recovery occurred after a mean of 9.3 (range 6–36) weeks, but the presence or absence of associated NP was not specifically reported (Eberl et al., 2011).

In summary, neuropathic pain can occur following surgery in children, but additional larger studies are required to evaluate the prevalence and duration of symptoms, and also determine if susceptibility is related to age at time of surgery.

Phantom limb pain

Altered sensory function following limb amputation is generally classified as non-painful phantom sensations or phantom limb pain. The majority of current literature is based on retrospective case series with differing methodology and variable response rates (Table 21.2).

Characteristics of phantom pain

Pain that is experienced in the region of the missing limb following amputation (i.e. phantom limb pain) has been described by

Table 21.2 Studies on phantom pain in children

Study	Pain incidence overall + subgroups	Sensation incidence	Identified patients	Number	Age
Krane and Heller, 1995	Overall: 83%; 1/2 congenital deformity; 9/10 cancer; 10/12 trauma/infection	100%	Medical records 2 hospitals; amputations between 1980 and 1990; children <19 years age	n = 24; (54 mailed; 12 undelivered) 24/42 = 57% RR	Current age: 5–19 yrs; Age at operation 2–16 yrs Time since op. 1 mth–7 yrs
Wilkins et al., 1998	Overall: 29%; 1/27 congenital deficiency 16/33 surgery (≤6 yrs 9/19; >6 yrs 14/14)	42% 2/27 congenital deficiency 23/33 surgery	Recruit from Canadian Child Amputee Program (CHAMP)	n = 60 (247 letters sent; 74 responded; 60 agreed) 60/247 = 24% RR	Current age: congenital 12.4±2.6 yrs; surgery 12.7±2.4 yrs (time since op. 6.6±4.3 yrs
Thomas et al., 2003	Overall: 38%; major burn injury 20% (3/15) flame 53% (10/19) electrical		Retrospective medical record review; single hospital ~1972–2002	n = 34 (39 cases, 4 died, one major neurological injury)	Age at amputation: median 11 yrs (3–22 yrs)
Melzack et al., 1997	4% (3/75) congenital deficient; 22% (11/49) amputation <6 yrs	20% (15/76) congenital deficient; 50% (26/49) amputation <6 yrs	Recruit from Canadian Child Amputee Program (CHAMP) and single hospital	n = 125 (184/329 questionnaires returned; 46 interviewed at hospital; 125 met inclusion criteria)	Age at assessment: 14.7 yrs
Burgoyne et al., 2012	Overall: 76%; 26 cancer (20/26 primary bone tumours)		Retrospective medical record review; single hospital 2000–2007	n = 26 (2 excluded based on age 5/12 and 2 yrs old)	Age at assessment: 6 to 27 yrs; (median 15 yrs; 9/26 >18 yrs)
Smith and Thompson, 1995	Overall: 44%; 48% (32/67) cancer; 12% (1/8) trauma		Retrospective medical record review; single hospital 1983–1993	n = 75 (293 records reviewed, 75 met inclusion criteria)	5–17 years

children as sharp, tingling, stabbing, pins and needles, throbbing, piercing, squeezing, tight and uncomfortable (Krane and Heller, 1995; Wilkins et al., 1998, 2004).

Phantom pain is frequently of moderate or severe intensity, with reported mean ratings of 5.29±2.4 (Wilkins et al., 1998) and 6.4±1.8 out of 10 (Wilkins et al., 2004). Typically, pain is episodic, lasts for seconds or minutes, with a frequency varying from daily to monthly, and only a small proportion of children have reported constant pain (Wilkins et al., 2004).

Exercise, objects approaching the stump, cold weather, and 'feeling nervous' have been reported to trigger episodes of phantom pain (Wilkins et al., 1998). Psychosocial triggers were more common in girls, whereas pain was triggered by physical stimuli in a higher proportion of boys (Wilkins et al., 2004).

Phantom pain has been reported to produce minimal interference with daily activity (Wilkins et al., 1998). In a series of 88 children, five of 24 following lower limb amputation and one of 64 with congenital lower limb deficiency reported phantom pain, but 89% were able to use their prosthesis for the whole day; 95% were able to walk; and 93% of those over 4 years were able to cycle (Boonstra et al., 2000). It is not clear from this series if phantom pain influenced the ability to tolerate the prosthesis, but it has been reported that phantom limb sensations were less apparent while wearing a prosthesis (Melzack et al., 1997).

Associated phenomena

Non-painful sensations experienced in the region of the missing limb (i.e. phantom sensations) are reported by 50% to 100% of children following surgical amputation and in 7% to 20% of children with congenitally deficient limbs (Table 22.2). These have been described as tingling, pins and needles, tickling, 'feels asleep',

numb, itching, and prickling (Krane and Heller, 1995; McGrath and Hillier, 1992; Wilkins et al., 1998, 2004). Despite reported mean intensities of 4 to 5 (0 = no sensation, 10 = strongest imaginable sensation), phantom sensations had minimal impact on daily activities (Wilkins et al., 1998, 2004).

Stump pain often coexists with phantom limb pain but may also occur in isolation. A higher incidence has been reported following surgery than in children with a congenitally absent limb (Wilkins et al., 1998, 2004).

Incidence of phantom limb pain

It is now well established that NP can follow amputation in children, but it is difficult to accurately estimate the incidence. Much of the data comes from retrospective questionnaires with response rates below 50% or from medical case notes that may not accurately record all symptoms. Samples are often small, may be derived from the community or clinics, and the duration between surgery and assessment is often variable.

Reported incidences of phantom limb pain are summarized in Table 21.2. Factors that have been associated with an increased incidence in children include:

◆ Surgical amputation (49–76%) versus congenitally deficient limbs (3–4%).

◆ Older age at time of amputation. A negative correlation has been reported between age at disruption and onset of a phantom limb (i.e. amputation at older age, shorter time to phantom onset) but it is not clear if this relationship holds for phantom pain as well as phantom sensations (Melzack et al., 1997)

◆ Cancer and chemotherapy. Phantom pain following amputations for cancer has been reported in 48–90% of children (Burgoyne et al., 2012; Krane and Heller, 1995), and in one small series the rate was higher than following amputations for trauma (32/67 versus 1/8; Smith and Thompson, 1995). Chemotherapy may also increase the risk of phantom pain as the incidence ranged from 74% in children exposed to chemotherapy before or at the time of amputation, to 44% if chemotherapy was only administered after the amputation, and was lowest (12%) in those who did not require chemotherapy (Smith and Thompson, 1995). Other causes of cancer-related neuropathic pain are discussed later in the chapter.

♦ Major burns due to electrical (10/19) versus flame (3/15) injury (Thomas et al., 2003).

♦ Preoperative pain. The presence of pain prior to amputation was reported in 35% to 75% of patients who developed phantom pain (Krane and Heller, 1995; Wilkins et al., 1998). The impact of preoperative pain on the incidence or degree of phantom pain has not been assessed in children, although in one series both patients with the most persistent pain had also experienced pain prior to amputation (Burgoyne et al., 2012)

Time course

Onset of pain in the early postoperative period was reported in 85% (Krane and Heller, 1995) and 53% (Wilkins et al., 1998) of children with phantom pain, within weeks or months in 20% or 30%, and in one patient from both series the onset of pain was delayed for more than a year. An earlier onset of phantom pain (mean 6 days versus 12.3 days) was noted in children receiving perioperative chemotherapy (Smith and Thompson, 1995). The mean time to onset of phantom limb sensations was 2.3 years in children with surgical amputation before 6 years, and 9 years in those with a congenitally absent limb (Melzack et al., 1997).

There is a perception that phantom limb pain resolves more rapidly in children than in adults, but there is limited supporting evidence. Phantom pain is often poorly documented in medical case notes (Krane and Heller, 1995), and there has been little prospective follow-up, although in a single case a progressive reduction in the duration, frequency and intensity of phantom pain episodes was noted over the first 28 postoperative days (McGrath and Hillier, 1992). In 20 children requiring amputation for cancer, trauma or infection, pain reduced in intensity and frequency in 13 (with resolution after months in two and years in four), but was unchanged in seven (Krane and Heller, 1995). Phantom limb pain was documented in the charts of 19 of 25 patients (age 6 to 27 years) after cancer-related amputation, and only two patients (both of whom were older than 18 years and had pain prior to the amputation) still had pain at 1 year (Burgoyne et al., 2012).

Obstetric brachial plexus injury (OBPI)

The brachial plexus innervates the upper limb and is formed from the lower cervical (C5,6,7,8) and the first thoracic (T1) nerve roots. Obstetric complications, such as shoulder dystocia or breech delivery can be associated with traction injuries of the brachial plexus injury in the newborn. The associated nerve lesions range in degree from neuropraxia to complete root avulsion, and can affect part or all of the plexus. Surgical exploration and repair, where possible, is often performed if there is no spontaneous recovery or elbow flexion by 3 to 6 months (Malessy and Pondaag, 2011). Associations between OBPI and pain in later life have been assessed in a number of series, which vary in the outcomes measured and the time since injury.

In addition, it is difficult to differentiate neuropathic pain associated with the initial injury from pain related to: re-innervation following early microsurgical repair and nerve grafts; subsequent surgical procedures (e.g. tendon transfers or rotational osteotomies) that may be required throughout childhood to improve function; trophic injuries associated with reduced sensory function; and musculoskeletal pain. These issues are highlighted by the following case series.

♦ Twenty-four patients with OBPI (20 operated and four non-operated) were assessed at intervals ranging from 3 to 23 years. Neither patients nor parents reported symptoms suggestive of neuropathic pain in the affected limb. Pain in a scar associated with surgery at 4 years was reported in one case. Restoration of sensory function and accurate stimulus localization was documented in 16/20 following microsurgical repair (Anand and Birch, 2002).

♦ A retrospective chart review of OBPI cases between 1990 and 2002 noted self-mutilating behaviour in 3.9% (11/280) of infants (McCann et al., 2004), which may be a response to sensory loss, and/or painful dysaesthesias in a hypoaesthetic or reinnervated area. The incidence was influenced both by the occurrence and the type of prior surgery; increasing from 1.4% (2/147) in the non-surgical group, to 6.8% (9/133) in those who had surgery prior to developing self-mutilating behaviour. Within the surgical group, the rate was much higher in association with microsurgery involving the plexus (29.1%; 7/24) than following bone or tendon surgery (1.8%, 2/109). The median onset 8 months after surgery and resolution of behaviour 4 to 7 months later also suggest a time course related to re-innervation dysaesthesia in at least some patients.

♦ A survey of 53 7- to 8-year-old children with OBPI (61% response rate) reported pain in the shoulder, upper arm and neck, particularly during writing, in 45% of children. The authors attributed pain to musculoskeletal causes (Spaargaren et al., 2011).

♦ Pain in the affected upper limb was reported by 31% of 112 patients, on average 13.5 (range 5.6–31.5) years after OBPI. In nine patients, local pain was associated with non-union of the clavicle (divided to improve access during initial surgery). It is not clear if patients had features suggestive of neuropathic pain, related either to the initial or to subsequent injuries which were relatively common (11% burns, 15% other injuries; Kirjavainen et al., 2008). Persistent neuropathic pain was reported in one of 70 patients with OBPI, now aged 7 to 20 years. 'Most participants' reported discomfort in the arm, usually in the shoulder or elbow after exercise. Quantitative sensory testing demonstrated reduced thermal sensitivity in 16% of patients, but as seen in other studies, there was better recovery of sensory than motor function (Strombeck et al., 2007).

Trauma during childhood

Brachial plexus injury during childhood

Trauma during childhood can result in brachial plexus injury (BPI), but the number of reports and details of associated pain are limited. Ten children aged 3 to 16 years had BPI and fractures following motor vehicle accidents. Reconstructive surgery was performed 1 to 8 months later, and there were no reports of deafferentation pain (El-Gammal et al., 2003). In a further 25 cases of traumatic BPI (2/12 to 14 years) related to motor vehicle accidents, 16 required plexus exploration and several subsequent orthopaedic procedures. Two teenagers with root avulsions complained of moderate pain, but there are no further details of the nature or time course of symptoms (Dumontier and Gilbert, 1990). By contrast, BPI in association with proximal humerus fracture in four patients (10–14 years), was associated with neurological recovery by 5 to 9 months, but all had NP (often described as burning) for at least 6 months (Hwang et al., 2008).

Peripheral nerve injury

A series of 49 children with distal upper limb nerve injury were followed for an average 2 years and 3 months (Atherton et al., 2008). As seen following amputation, an increased proportion of older children developed neuropathic symptoms. No children under 5 years (0/15) had pain or allodynia, whereas the five children with spontaneous pain were all aged over 12 years at the time of injury. A further eight children aged older than 5 years had increased sensitivity to thermal or pinprick stimuli (Atherton et al., 2008).

Spinal cord injury (SCI)

Pain after SCI in adults is classified as nociceptive (musculoskeletal, visceral, other) or neuropathic (Bryce et al., 2012), with the latter categorized as:

+ 'At level SCI pain' occurring in a segmental pattern within three dermatomes of the neurological level of the injury, and likely due to injury to the nerve roots and/or cord.

+ 'Below level SCI pain' occurring more than three dermatomes below the neurological level of injury, which is a result of damage to the spinal cord, and can occur following either complete (no motor function preserved below the level) or incomplete injuries.

+ Other coexistent causes of NP not related to the spinal lesion (e.g. trigeminal neuralgia).

Only 3% to 5% of new cases of SCI are in children, but SCI can occur in neonates as a complication of delivery, and tends to have a better recovery than seen at older ages (Pape, 2012). Complete cord lesions are more common in younger age groups, and there is a male predominance at all ages. Follow-up an average of 15 years following SCI (mean age at injury 14 years, n = 216) reported an overall incidence of pain at any site of 69%, with younger age at injury associated with orthopaedic complications such as scoliosis and hip subluxation, and older age at injury associated with ankle pain and spasticity (Vogel et al., 2002). NP has been reported to be less common if injury occurs at a younger age: 26% (24/91) before 20 years of age versus 45% (139/311) at older ages (Werhagen et al., 2004). In a series of 31 participants, aged between 5 months and 18 years at the time of SCI, 65% reported chronic pain, and this had neuropathic features in 19%, but was associated with less interference in daily activities than in adults (Jan and Wilson, 2004).

Cancer-related neuropathic pain

Neuropathic pain occurs in 20% to 40% of adult patients with cancer (Bennett et al., 2012). The overall rate of cancer-related neuropathic pain is likely to be lower in children, but as noted earlier phantom limb pain is more common in children who require amputations for cancer and perioperative chemotherapy. Significant pain may occur in specific populations:

+ *Primary tumours* within the nervous system. Neurofibromatosis type 1 (NF1) and type 2 (NF2) are neurocutaneous disorders associated with tumours affecting the central and peripheral nervous systems (Ardern-Holmes and North, 2011; Jett and Friedman, 2010). Pain is experienced by up to 46% of children with plexiform neurofibromas (Serletis et al., 2007), and increasing pain and rapid growth of the tumour may indicate development of a malignant nerve sheath tumour (Ardern-Holmes and North, 2011). Pain can also have significant impact on health-related quality of life in children with NF (Krab et al., 2009) and this condition is also discussed by Mherekumombe and Collins (Chapter 32, this volume).

+ *Tumour invasion or compression* of neural structures (spinal cord, spinal nerve roots, nerve plexus, peripheral nerves). As the incidence of solid tumours is lower in children, tumour invasion/compression is less common in children than in adults, but can result in severe pain with high analgesic requirements. Pain may be difficult to control with opioids alone, and in some cases requires regional blockade with local anaesthetic (Butkovic et al., 2006; Collins et al., 1995; Cooper et al., 1994).

Cancer treatment-related neuropathic pain

Treatment-related NP may occur following surgery (e.g. post-amputation pain; see 'Phantom limb pain' section) or chemotherapy. Perioperative chemotherapy has also been associated with an increased incidence and earlier onset of post-amputation pain (Smith and Thompson, 1995).

Peripheral neuropathy occurs in 50% to 90% of those treated with platinum compounds (cisplatin) and almost half with vinca alkaloids (vincristine; Vondracek et al., 2009). In 21 children with solid tumours and nine with leukaemia aged between 10 and 17 years, neuropathic pain symptoms (paraesthesia, numbness and burning pain in the fingers and toes, hyperalgesia and tactile allodynia) commenced within days of beginning chemotherapy. In addition, pain was severe (mean baseline VAS >75/100) (Vondracek et al., 2009). In a retrospective review, 174/498 patients developed peripheral neurotoxicity with vincristine treatment for acute lymphoblastic leukaemia (Anghelescu et al., 2011). Associated NP occurred in 35%, with recurrent episodes in 16% to 30.6%. Age at diagnosis ranged from 1 to 19 years, but had minimal influence on the rate of NP, which varied from 31% in the 1- to 5-year-group, to 40% in those aged 16 to 20 years. Pain was described as aching, burning, cramping, tingling, numbness, sharp, or stinging; and was most common in the lower limbs, back and jaw (Anghelescu et al., 2011).

Treatment of high-risk neuroblastoma with a monoclonal antibody directed against the tumour-associated disialoganglioside GD2 can result in severe acute pain in children (Wallace et al., 1997; Yu et al., 2010). Laboratory studies have confirmed mechanical allodynia as a result of C-fibre activation (Xiao et al., 1997) and complement activation (Sorkin et al., 2010), which is reduced by gabapentin (Gillin and Sorkin, 1998). Current clinical treatment protocols incorporate NP management strategies, such as oral gabapentin, and addition of intravenous ketamine or lidocaine if pain is inadequately controlled by intravenous opioid (Wallace et al., 1997; see also Rastogi and Campbell, Chapter 48, this volume).

Metabolic disorders

Fabry's disease

Clinical features

Pain is a common presenting symptom in Fabry's disease, and often has an onset during childhood (Hoffmann et al., 2007;

Pintos-Morell and Beck, 2009; Ries et al., 2005). As pain may be the only feature for some years, Fabry's disease should be considered in the differential diagnosis of pain clinic referrals (Pagnini et al., 2011). Episodic burning pain and 'pins and needles' may initially be restricted to the hands and feet, but pain becomes more persistent and generalized with time (Hoffmann et al., 2007) and can be triggered by changes in environmental or body temperature, exercise, or emotional stress (Ries et al., 2005). Pain is not only present in over 70%, with a higher incidence in males (80% versus 65%; Hoffmann et al., 2007), but it has a significant impact on quality of life (Ramaswami et al., 2006; Ries et al., 2005). Other features of Fabry's disease include hypo- or hyperhidrosis, gastrointestinal disturbances and abdominal pain, angiokeratomas, and ophthalmological abnormalities (cornea verticillata) (Mehta et al., 2010; Ramaswami, 2008).

Pathophysiology

Fabry's disease is an X-linked recessive disorder, and females typically have less severe symptoms that develop at a later age. Mutations in the *GLA* gene that encodes the lysosomal enzyme alpha-galactosidase A result in failure to catabolize lipids containing alpha-D-galactosyl moieties. Accumulation of glycolipids, including globotriaosylceramide (Gb3) in cells and tissues results in dysfunction of multiple organ systems including heart, kidney, gastrointestinal tract, and nervous system (Hoffmann et al., 2007). Small fibre loss in peripheral tissues and glycolipid accumulation in the dorsal root ganglia or nerves may underlie the neuropathic pain symptoms (Borsook, 2012).

Age

Reported ages at diagnosis range from 5 to 77 years (Pagnini et al., 2011). However, pain has been reported from 3 years of age in boys and 6 years in girls, with neuropathic features at a mean age of 7.8±3.2 years (Ries et al., 2005). Similarly, neuropathic pain was reported in 59% of boys (median 7 years) and 41% of girls (median 9 years) (Hopkin et al., 2008).

Diagnosis and management

The diagnosis is based on measurement of plasma alpha-galactosidase A activity (although levels may be normal in carrier females), and of plasma or urinary Gb3 or lyso-Gb3; and is confirmed by genetic analysis of *GLA* gene (Mehta et al., 2010).

Enzyme replacement therapy with alpha-galactosidase A reduces glycolipid storage in tissues, but effects on pain take time. Improvement in all dimensions of pain perception after 24 months has been reported (Hoffmann et al., 2007), with reductions in neuropathic 'pain at its worst' scores in both boys and girls (2.8 to 1.5) and 'average pain' from 2.2 to 0.9, and a reduced requirement for neuropathic treatment with anti-convulsants (Pintos-Morell and Beck, 2009). In others, the overall prevalence of pain was not altered by enzyme replacement therapy, but those with pain at the onset of therapy did show a decrease in severity (Ramaswami et al., 2011).

Neurological disorders

Neuropathic pain is a feature of several neurological conditions. Pain associated with neurofibromatosis, Guillain–Barré syndrome, neuromuscular disorders and pain associated with HIV are covered by Mherekumombe and Collins (Chapter 32, this volume).

Multiple sclerosis

Multiple sclerosis (MS) is a chronic inflammatory disease producing demyelination and axonal damage in the brain and spinal cord (Mariotti et al., 2010). Pain is common in adults with a prevalence from 57% to 65%, and 43% to 54% have pain at the time of diagnosis. Patients with MS may experience multiple types of pain (including tonic spasms, back pain, and headache) but additionally may experience central neuropathic pains.

- Dysaesthetic extremity pain occurs in up to 23% of patients. Pain is burning, typically bilateral, often in the legs and feet, worse at night, and is exacerbated by exercise.

- Trigeminal neuralgia is more common than in the general population with a higher rate of bilateral symptoms.

- Brief electric shock sensations in the back of the neck, lower back, or other parts of body, are brought on by neck flexion (Lhermitte's sign).

An estimated 2% to 5% of patients experience their first symptoms of MS before 16 years of age, with onset usually between 8 and 14 years, and a higher incidence in females (ranging from 1.3 to 3 times). Cohorts of paediatric MS patients report sensory symptoms in 13% to 69%, but there is little information about the proportion with neuropathic pain (Ness et al., 2007). Headache is more frequent in paediatric than in adult patients with MS (Mariotti et al., 2010). The course of the disease may be slower in children, but can have a significant impact on schooling and psychosocial function (Ness et al., 2007); further reductions in quality of life have been associated with increasing age and duration of illness. The impact of disease-modifying therapies, such as interferon, on pain symptoms are not clear (O'Connor et al., 2008).

Postherpetic neuralgia

Reactivation of varicella zoster virus infection, which has been dormant within sensory neurons, results in painful eruptions along the distribution of the nerve (also known as shingles), and approximately 14% of adults develop persistent neuropathic pain (i.e. postherpetic neuralgia, PHN; Delaney et al., 2009). Overall, zoster infection and PHN are less common in children (Hall et al., 2006), but children who are immunocompromised, particularly in association with cancer treatment, are at higher risk. In a series of 226 children with acute lymphoblastic leukaemia, zoster eruptions occurred 90 times, with recurrent episodes in 14 children. All experienced pain with the acute eruption and were treated with acyclovir, and five developed postherpetic neuralgia, which persisted for greater than 2 months in two patients (Sorensen et al., 2011).

Trigeminal neuralgia

Clinical features

Clinical features of trigeminal neuralgia include (Bender et al., 2011; Solth et al., 2008; Yue, 2004):

- Unilateral pain in the distribution of the trigeminal nerve. The trigeminal innervation is divided into three zones: V1 ophthalmic (scalp, forehead, upper eyelid, eye), V2 maxillary (lower eyelid, cheek, nose, upper teeth and gums), and V3 mandibular (lower teeth and gums, jaw, parts of external ear). Pain may be experienced in one or more zones—most commonly V2 followed by V2/3 combined.

* Pain is described as sharp, lancinating or shooting, electric-shock like, and occasionally burning.

* Pain is intermittent and paroxysmal.

* Intermittent paroxysms of pain can be triggered by light touch in the trigeminal region (cutaneous trigger zones), chewing, brushing the teeth, cold wind, or exercise.

Pain may also be associated with spasm of the facial muscles, or *tic douloureux*.

Incidence

The incidence of trigeminal neuralgia is much lower in children (Hall et al., 2006), and less than 1.5% of patients with trigeminal neuralgia report an onset of symptoms before 18 years of age (Bender et al., 2011). Case series report trigeminal neuralgia in children aged from 3 to 18 years, with median ages of 11 to 13 years (Bender et al., 2011; Resnick et al., 1998; Yue, 2004).

Pathophysiology

Trigeminal neuralgia may be classified as idiopathic or result from compression within the intracranial course of the nerve either by vasculature (Bender et al., 2011; Resnick et al., 1998; Solth et al., 2008) or by tumour (da Silva et al., 2006). As idiopathic trigeminal neuralgia and glossopharyngeal neuralgia (pain in the posterior tongue, pharynx, beneath angle of lower jaw and/or in ear) are rare in children, appropriate imaging and investigations are required to exclude underlying causes (Arruda et al., 2011). A 1-year-old child who presented with episodic crying and raising the hand towards the left ear, had marked allodynia over the ear, and was found to have a schwannoma in the trigeminal nerve (da Silva et al., 2006).

Neuropathic pain and genetic disorders

Erythromelalgia

Clinical features

Erythromelalgia (EM) is characterized by severe episodic pain and redness affecting the hands and feet (Waxman and Dib-Hajj, 2005). Bilateral pain and redness of the ears may also represent a variant of EM (Brill et al., 2009; Vivas et al., 2011). Pain is aggravated by warmth, prolonged standing and exercise, and relieved by cooling and submersion in iced water, but is often poorly responsive to analgesia.

Pathophysiology

The pathophysiology of EM has been attributed to vascular, inflammatory and neuropathic causes (Waxman and Dib-Hajj, 2005). Both microvascular ischaemic (vasoconstrictive) and reactive-hyperaemic (vasodilatory) subtypes have been postulated, resulting in treatment with a wide range of vasoactive drugs (Cohen, 2000). EM has also been reported in association with myeloproliferative or auto-immune disorders, and in such cases may be termed secondary EM (Novella et al., 2007).

Primary EM has recently been associated with a genetic mutation, which may occur spontaneously, or in association with a positive family history. Nine subtypes of voltage gated sodium channels have been identified ($Na_V1.1$ to $Na_V1.9$). $Na_V1.7$ is of particular importance for pain as it is selectively expressed within nociceptive dorsal root ganglion and sympathetic ganglion neurons (Dib-Hajj et al., 2009; Drenth and Waxman, 2007; Fischer and Waxman, 2010). Mutations in the *SCN9A* gene, which encodes the $Na_V1.7$ channel, can result in either:

(1) Loss of function and congenital insensitivity to pain (Cox et al., 2006; Staud et al., 2011), or

(2) Gain of function and increased pain (Cummins et al., 2007; Dib-Hajj et al., 2005; Waxman and Dib-Hajj, 2005). Point mutations at different sites result in two distinct phenotypes: paroxysmal extreme pain disorder (PEPD) or primary EM (Cheng et al., 2010; Fertleman et al., 2006; Estacion et al., 2008). Mutations associated with EM alter channel activation, reduce threshold and increase firing frequency, and increase excitability.

Age-dependent effects

The degree of change in channel kinetics varies with the site of the mutation, and larger depolarizing shifts have been associated with onset of symptoms at younger ages (Ahn et al., 2010; Han et al., 2009). However, variable expression of neonatal and adult isoforms of the channel may also influence the age at which symptoms first appear (Choi et al., 2010).

Management

Diverse views of the pathophysiology of EM have resulted in a range of treatments directed at vascular (vasoactive drugs such as topical GTN, sodium nitroprusside infusion, clonidine; Cohen, 2000), anti-inflammatory, and neuropathic aetiologies (amitriptyline, gabapentin; Natkunarajah et al., 2009). With awareness of the potential involvement of $Na_V1.7$ in EM, there has been increased use of drugs with sodium channel blocking activity. Different EM-related mutations may be more responsive to either mexiletine (Choi et al., 2009; Iqbal et al., 2009; Nathan et al., 2005) or carbamazepine (Fischer et al., 2009).

Paroxysmal extreme pain disorder

PEPD can present soon after birth with episodic pain in association with redness over the buttocks, legs and feet. Through infancy and childhood, the condition progresses to include episodes of (Fertleman et al., 2006):

* Rectal pain, often induced by a bowel movement, and burning pain and redness in the lower limbs.

* Brief episodes of intense burning ocular pain associated with redness around the eyes and runny nose and eyes.

* Bilateral mandibular pain and redness, which may be triggered by cold, eating or emotional state.

Mutations at different points in the *SCN9A* gene result in altered channel kinetics (impaired inactivation, prolonged action potential, and repetitive firing) and a phenotype that differs from EM (Estacion et al., 2008). PEPD has been reported to be differentially sensitive to carbamazepine (Fertleman et al., 2006).

Conclusion

Neuropathic pain is a frequent reason for referral to a paediatric chronic pain clinic, and diagnosis is predominantly based on the pain history and descriptors. NP following trauma is more common when the initial injury occurs later in childhood (e.g. following amputation at greater than 6 years). However, NP can occur at younger ages, particularly in higher-risk populations (e.g. cancer, chemotherapy and immunosuppression) or in association with specific conditions (e.g. Fabry's disease). Pharmacological management of NP is largely extrapolated from adult studies (see Rastogi and Campbell, Chapter 48, this volume). However, pain is often severe and only partially responsive to pharmacological interventions, and multidisciplinary care is required. As discussed in other chapters throughout this text, assessment and management of chronic pain (including NP) must also encompass non-pharmacological and psychological interventions, include family or caregivers, and address issues related to poor sleep and school attendance.

Case example

A 10-year-old boy with severe vascular malformations of the lower leg has had multiple episodes of infection and of bleeding requiring transfusion and now presents for a below-knee amputation. Preoperative preparation has included discussions with rehabilitation specialists and psychologists, and his perioperative pain management has been planned in coordination with the anaesthetist, pain service, and surgical team. As there are no contraindications, consent is gained for epidural catheter insertion and an infusion of local anaesthetic and opioid is commenced immediately prior to surgery and continued for the first 3 postoperative days, with good control of pain. Following cessation of the epidural he develops a sensation of a larger than normal lower leg which is pointing down through the bed at an unusual angle. In addition, he has paroxysms of shooting pain extending below the stump, which are not relieved by oral opioids, and which are significantly disrupting his sleep. He is commenced on oral amitriptyline at night and oral gabapentin. The episodes of pain become less frequent, but remain severe, and gradually improve with escalation of the gabapentin dose over the next 7 days. He is subsequently discharged for rehabilitation at a different centre, where he receives ongoing multidisciplinary care (that includes psychological and family support and input from the pain service) regarding management of his amputation, phantom limb pain, fitting of a prosthesis, and a gradual return to school is planned. Three months later he returns to the chronic pain clinic for review. He has occasional episodes of pain during the day, ongoing non-painful phantom sensations (although the size of the phantom has significantly reduced), and is sleeping well at night but feels a little drowsy in the morning. The amitriptyline is weaned without any increase in pain, and he continues to be reviewed with a plan to gradually wean the gabapentin as tolerated.

References

Aasvang, E. K., and Kehlet, H. (2007). Chronic pain after childhood groin hernia repair. *J Pediatr Surg*, 42, 1403–1408.

Ahn, H. S., Dib-Hajj, S. D., Cox, J. J., Tyrrell, L., Elmslie, F. V., Clarke, A. A., et al. (2010). A new Nav1.7 sodium channel mutation I234T in a child with severe pain. *Eur J Pain*, 14, 944–950.

Anand, P. and Birch, R. (2002). Restoration of sensory function and lack of long-term chronic pain syndromes after brachial plexus injury in human neonates. *Brain*, 125, 113–122.

Anghelescu, D. L., Faughnan, L. G., Jeha, S., Relling, M. V., Hinds, P. S., Sandlund, J.T., et al. (2011). Neuropathic pain during treatment for childhood acute lymphoblastic leukemia. *Pediatr Blood Cancer*, 57, 1147–1153.

Ardern-Holmes, S. L., and North, K. N. (2011). Therapeutics for childhood neurofibromatosis type 1 and type 2. *Curr Treat Options Neurol*, 13, 529–543.

Arruda, M. A., Albuquerque, R. C., and Bigal, M. E. (2011). Uncommon headache syndromes in the pediatric population. *Curr Pain Headache Rep*, 15, 280–288.

Atherton, D. D., Taherzadeh, O., Elliot, D., and Anand, P. (2008). Age-dependent development of chronic neuropathic pain, allodynia and sensory recovery after upper limb nerve injury in children. *J Hand Surg Eur Vol*, 33, 186–191.

Attal, N., Lanteri-Minet, M., Laurent, B., Fermanian, J., and Bouhassira, D. (2011). The specific disease burden of neuropathic pain: results of a French nationwide survey. *Pain*, 152, 2836–2843.

Attal, N., Cruccu, G., Baron, R., Haanpaa, M., Hansson, P., Jensen, T. S., et al. (2010). EFNS guidelines on the pharmacological treatment of neuropathic pain: 2009 revision. *Eur J Neurol*, 17(9), 1113–e88.

Bender, M. T., Pradilla, G., James, C., Raza, S., Lim, M., and Carson, B. S. (2011). Surgical treatment of pediatric trigeminal neuralgia: case series and review of the literature. *Childs Nerv Syst*, 27, 2123–2129.

Bennett, M. (2001). The LANSS Pain Scale: the Leeds assessment of neuropathic symptoms and signs. *Pain*, 92, 147–157.

Bennett, M. I., Attal, N., Backonja, M. M., Baron, R., Bouhassira, D., Freynhagen, R., et al. (2007). Using screening tools to identify neuropathic pain. *Pain*, 127, 199–203.

Bennett, M. I., Rayment, C., Hjermstad, M., Aass, N., Caraceni, A., and Kaasa, S. (2012). Prevalence and aetiology of neuropathic pain in cancer patients: a systematic review. *Pain*, 153, 359–365.

Blankenburg, M., Kraemer, N., Hirschfeld, G., Krumova, E. K., Maier, C., Hechler, T., et al. (2012). Childhood diabetic neuropathy: functional impairment and non-invasive screening assessment. *Diabet Med*, 29(11), 1425–1432.

Boonstra, A. M., Rijnders, L. J., Groothoff, J. W., and Eisma, W. H. (2000). Children with congenital deficiencies or acquired amputations of the lower limbs: functional aspects. *Prosthet Orthot Int*, 24, 19–27.

Borsook, D. (2012). Neurological diseases and pain. *Brain*, 135, 320–344.

Bouhassira, D., Attal, N., Alchaar, H., Boureau, F., Brochet, B., Bruxelle, J., et al. (2005). Comparison of pain syndromes associated with nervous or somatic lesions and development of a new neuropathic pain diagnostic questionnaire (DN4). *Pain*, 114, 29–36.

Brill, T. J., Funk, B., Thaci, D., and Kaufmann, R. (2009). Red ear syndrome and auricular erythromelalgia: the same condition? *Clin Exp Dermatol*, 34, e626–628.

Bryce, T. N., Biering-Sorensen, F., Finnerup, N. B., Cardenas, D. D., Defrin, R., Lundeberg, T., et al. (2012). International spinal cord injury pain classification: part I. Background and description. *Spinal Cord*, 50, 413–417.

Burgoyne, L. L., Billups, C. A., Jiron, J. L. Jr., Kaddoum, R. N., Wright, B. B., Bikhazi, G. B., et al. (2012). Phantom limb pain in young cancer-related amputees: recent experience at St Jude's research hospital. *Clin J Pain*, 28, 222–225.

Butkovic, D., Toljan, S., and Mihovilovic-Novak, B. (2006). Experience with gabapentin for neuropathic pain in adolescents: report of five cases. *Paediatr Anaesth*, 16, 325–329.

Celebi, N., Canbay, O., Aycan, I. O., Sahin, A., and Aypar, U. (2008). Mercury intoxication and neuropathic pain. *Paediatr Anaesth*, 18, 440–442.

Cheng, X., Dib-Hajj, S. D., Tyrrell, L., Wright, D. A., Fischer, T. Z., and Waxman, S. G. (2010). Mutations at opposite ends of the DIII/S4-S5 linker of sodium channel Na V 1.7 produce distinct pain disorders. *Mol Pain*, 6, 24.

Choi, J. S., Cheng, X., Foster, E., Leffler, A., Tyrrell, L., Te Morsche, R. H., et al. (2010). Alternative splicing may contribute to time-dependent manifestation of inherited erythromelalgia. *Brain*, 133, 1823–1835.

Choi, J. S., Zhang, L., Dib-Hajj, S. D., Han, C., Tyrrell, L., Lin, Z., et al. (2009). Mexiletine-responsive erythromelalgia due to a new Na(v)1.7 mutation showing use-dependent current fall-off. *Exp Neurol*, 216, 383–389.

Cohen, J. S. (2000). Erythromelalgia: new theories and new therapies. *J Am Acad Dermatol*, 43, 841–847.

Collins, J. J., Grier, H. E., Kinney, H. C., and Berde, C. B. (1995). Control of severe pain in children with terminal malignancy. *J Pediatr*, 126, 653–657.

Cooper, M. G., Keneally, J. P., and Kinchington, D. (1994). Continuous brachial plexus neural blockade in a child with intractable cancer pain. *J Pain Symptom Manage*, 9, 277–281.

Cox, J. J., Reimann, F., Nicholas, A. K., Thornton, G., Roberts, E., Springell, K., *et al.* (2006). An SCN9A channelopathy causes congenital inability to experience pain. *Nature*, 444, 894–898.

Cummins, T. R., Sheets, P. L., and Waxman, S. G. (2007). The roles of sodium channels in nociception: Implications for mechanisms of pain. *Pain*, 131, 243–257.

da Silva, H. M., Boullosa, J. L., and Arruda, M. A. (2006). Secondary intermedius neuralgia-like pain in a young child. *Cephalalgia*, 26, 1483–1484.

Delaney, A., Colvin, L. A., Fallon, M. T., Dalziel, R. G., Mitchell, R., and Fleetwood-Walker, S. M. (2009). Postherpetic neuralgia: from preclinical models to the clinic. *Neurotherapeutics*, 6, 630–637.

Dib-Hajj, S. D., Binshtok, A. M., Cummins, T. R., Jarvis, M. F., Samad, T., and Zimmermann, K. (2009). Voltage-gated sodium channels in pain states: Role in pathophysiology and targets for treatment. *Brain Res Rev*, 60, 65–83.

Dib-Hajj, S. D., Rush, A. M., Cummins, T. R., Hisama, F. M., Novella, S., Tyrrell, L., *et al.* (2005). Gain-of-function mutation in Nav1.7 in familial erythromelalgia induces bursting of sensory neurons. *Brain*, 128, 1847–1854.

Drenth, J. P., and Waxman, S. G. (2007). Mutations in sodium-channel gene SCN9A cause a spectrum of human genetic pain disorders. *J Clin Invest*, 117, 3603–3609.

Dumontier, C. and Gilbert, A. (1990). Traumatic brachial plexus palsy in children. *Ann Chir Main Memb Super*, 9, 351–357.

Dworkin, R. H., O'Connor, A. B., Audette, J., Baron, R., Gourlay, G. K., Haanpää, M. L., *et al.* (2010). Recommendations for the pharmacological management of neuropathic pain: an overview and literature update. *Mayo Clin Proc*, 85, S3–14.

Eberl, R., Eder, C., Smolle, E., Weinberg, A. M., Hoellwarth, M. E., and Singer, G. (2011). Iatrogenic ulnar nerve injury after pin fixation and after antegrade nailing of supracondylar humeral fractures in children. *Acta Orthop*, 82, 606–609.

El-Gammal, T. A., El-Sayed, A., and Kotb, M. M. (2003). Surgical treatment of brachial plexus traction injuries in children, excluding obstetric palsy. *Microsurgery*, 23, 14–17.

Estacion, M., Dib-Hajj, S. D., Benke, P. J., Te Morsche, R. H., Eastman, E. M., Macala, L. J., *et al.* (2008). NaV1.7 gain-of-function mutations as a continuum: A1632E displays physiological changes associated with erythromelalgia and paroxysmal extreme pain disorder mutations and produces symptoms of both disorders. *J Neurosci*, 28, 11079–11088.

Fertleman, C. R., Baker, M. D., Parker, K. A., Moffatt, S., Elmslie, F. V., Abrahamsen, B., *et al.* (2006). SCN9A mutations in paroxysmal extreme pain disorder: allelic variants underlie distinct channel defects and phenotypes. *Neuron*, 52, 767–774.

Fischer, T. Z., Gilmore, E. S., Estacion, M., Eastman, E., Taylor, S., Melanson, M., *et al.* (2009). A novel Nav1.7 mutation producing carbamazepine-responsive erythromelalgia. *Ann Neurol*, 65, 733–741.

Fischer, T. Z., and Waxman, S. G. (2010). Familial pain syndromes from mutations of the NaV1.7 sodium channel. *Ann N Y Acad Sci*, 1184, 196–207.

Freynhagen, R., Baron, R., Gockel, U., and Tolle, T. R. (2006). painDETECT: a new screening questionnaire to identify neuropathic components in patients with back pain. *Curr Med Res Opin*, 22, 1911–1920.

Gillin, S. and Sorkin, L. S. (1998). Gabapentin reverses the allodynia produced by the administration of anti-GD2 ganglioside, an immunotherapeutic drug. *Anesth Analg*, 86, 111–116.

Haanpaa, M., Attal, N., Backonja, M., Baron, R., Bennett, M., Bouhassira, D., *et al.* (2011). NeuPSIG guidelines on neuropathic pain assessment. *Pain*, 152, 14–27.

Haanpaa, M. L., Backonja, M. M., Bennett, M. I., Bouhassira, D., Cruccu, G., Hansson, P. T., *et al.* (2009). Assessment of neuropathic pain in primary care. *Am J Med*, 122, S13–21.

Hall, G. C., Carroll, D., Parry, D., and McQuay, H. J. (2006). Epidemiology and treatment of neuropathic pain: the UK primary care perspective. *Pain*, 122, 156–162.

Han, C., Dib-Hajj, S. D., Lin, Z., Li, Y., Eastman, E. M., Tyrrell, L., *et al.* (2009). Early- and late-onset inherited erythromelalgia: genotype-phenotype correlation. *Brain*, 132, 1711–1722.

Hoffmann, B., Beck, M., Sunder-Plassmann, G., Borsini, W., Ricci, R., and Mehta, A. (2007). Nature and prevalence of pain in Fabry disease and its response to enzyme replacement therapy—a retrospective analysis from the Fabry Outcome Survey. *Clin J Pain*, 23, 535–542.

Hopkin, R. J., Bissler, J., Banikazemi, M., Clarke, L., Eng, C. M., Germain, D. P., *et al.* (2008). Characterization of Fabry disease in 352 pediatric patients in the Fabry Registry. *Pediatr Res*, 64, 550–555.

Howard, R. F. (2011). Chronic pain problems in children and young people. *Contin Educ Anaesth Crit Care Pain*, 11, 219–223.

Hwang, R. W., Bae, D. S., and Waters, P. M. (2008). Brachial plexus palsy following proximal humerus fracture in patients who are skeletally immature. *J Orthop Trauma*, 22, 286–290.

Iqbal, J., Bhat, M. I., Charoo, B. A., Syed, W. A., Sheikh, M. A., and Bhat, I. N. (2009). Experience with oral mexiletine in primary erythromelalgia in children. *Ann Saudi Med*, 29, 316–318.

Jan, F. K., and Wilson, P. E. (2004). A survey of chronic pain in the pediatric spinal cord injury population. *J Spinal Cord Med*, 27 Suppl 1, S50–53.

Jensen, T. S., Baron, R., Haanpaa, M., Kalso, E., Loeser, J. D., Rice, A. S., *et al.* (2011). A new definition of neuropathic pain. *Pain*, 152, 2204–2205.

Jett, K. and Friedman, J. M. (2010). Clinical and genetic aspects of neurofibromatosis 1. *Genet Med*, 12, 1–11.

Kehlet, H., Jensen, T. S., and Woolf, C. J. (2006). Persistent postsurgical pain: risk factors and prevention. *Lancet*, 367, 1618–1625.

Kirjavainen, M., Remes, V., Peltonen, J., Rautakorpi, S., Helenius, I., and Nietosvaara, Y. (2008). The function of the hand after operations for obstetric injuries to the brachial plexus. *J Bone Joint Surg Br*, 90, 349–355.

Krab, L. C., Oostenbrink, R., de Goede-Bolder, A., Aarsen, F. K., Elgersma, Y., and Moll, H. A. (2009). Health-related quality of life in children with neurofibromatosis type 1: contribution of demographic factors, disease-related factors, and behavior. *J Pediatr*, 154, 420–425, 425 e421.

Krane, E. J., and Heller, L. B. (1995). The prevalence of phantom sensation and pain in pediatric amputees. *J Pain Symptom Manage*, 10, 21–29.

Krause, S. J., and Backonja, M. M. (2003). Development of a neuropathic pain questionnaire. *Clin J Pain*, 19, 306–314.

Kristensen, A. D., Pedersen, T. A., Hjortdal, V. E., Jensen, T. S., and Nikolajsen, L. (2010). Chronic pain in adults after thoracotomy in childhood or youth. *Br J Anaesth*, 104, 75–79.

Lauder, G. R., and White, M. C. (2005). Neuropathic pain following multilevel surgery in children with cerebral palsy: a case series and review. *Paediatr Anaesth*, 15, 412–420.

Lebel, A., Becerra, L., Wallin, D., Moulton, E. A., Morris, S., Pendse, G., *et al.* (2008). fMRI reveals distinct CNS processing during symptomatic and recovered complex regional pain syndrome in children. *Brain*, 131, 1854–1879.

Macintyre, P. E., Schug, S. A., Scott, D. A., Visser, E. J., and Walker, S. M. (2010). *APM:SE Working Group of the Australian and New Zealand College of Anaesthetists and Faculty of Pain Medicine. Acute pain management: scientific evidence. Third edition.* Melbourne: ANZCA & FPM.

Maier, C., Baron, R., Tölle, T. R., Binder, A., Birbaumer, N., Birklein, F., *et al.* (2010). Quantitative sensory testing in the German Research Network on Neuropathic Pain (DFNS): somatosensory abnormalities in 1236 patients with different neuropathic pain syndromes. *Pain*, 150, 439–450.

Malessy, M. J., and Pondaag, W. (2011). Nerve surgery for neonatal brachial plexus palsy. *J Pediatr Rehabil Med*, 4, 141–148.

Mariotti, P., Nociti, V., Cianfoni, A., Stefanini, C., De Rose, P., Martinelli, D., *et al.* (2010). Migraine-like headache and status migrainosus as attacks of multiple sclerosis in a child. *Pediatrics*, 126, e459–464.

Martin, J., Osterman, M. J. K., and Sutton, P. D. (2010). Are preterm births on the decline in the United States? Recent data from the National Vital Statistics System. *NCHS Data Brief*, May(39), 1–8.

McCann, M. E., Waters, P., Goumnerova, L. C., and Berde, C. (2004). Self-mutilation in young children following brachial plexus birth injury. *Pain*, 110, 123–129.

McGrath, P. A., and Hillier, L. M. (1992). Phantom limb sensations in adolescents: a case study to illustrate the utility of sensation and pain logs in pediatric clinical practice. *J Pain Symptom Manage*, 7, 46–53.

Mehta, A., Beck, M., Eyskens, F., Feliciani, C., Kantola, I., Ramaswami, U., et al. (2010). Fabry disease: a review of current management strategies. *QJM*, 103, 641–659.

Melzack, R., Israel, R., Lacroix, R., and Schultz, G. (1997). Phantom limbs in people with congenital limb deficiency or amputation in early childhood. *Brain*, 120 (Pt 9), 1603–1620.

Nathan, A., Rose, J. B., Guite, J. W., Hehir, D., and Milovcich, K. (2005). Primary erythromelalgia in a child responding to intravenous lidocaine and oral mexiletine treatment. *Pediatrics*, 115, e504–507.

Natkunarajah, J., Atherton, D., Elmslie, F., Mansour, S., and Mortimer, P. (2009). Treatment with carbamazepine and gabapentin of a patient with primary erythermalgia (erythromelalgia). Identified to have a mutation in the SCN9A gene, encoding a voltage-gated sodium channel. *Clin Exp Dermatol*, 34, e640–642.

Nayak, S. and Cunliffe, M. (2008). Lidocaine 5% patch for localized chronic neuropathic pain in adolescents: report of five cases. *Paediatr Anaesth*, 18, 554–558.

Ness, J. M., Chabas, D., Sadovnick, A. D., Pohl, D., Banwell, B., and Weinstock-Guttman, B. (2007). Clinical features of children and adolescents with multiple sclerosis. *Neurology*, 68, S37–45.

Novella, S. P., Hisama, F. M., Dib-Hajj, S. D., and Waxman, S.G. (2007). A case of inherited erythromelalgia. *Nat Clin Pract Neurol*, 3, 229–234.

O'Connor, A. B., Schwid, S. R., Herrmann, D. N., Markman, J. D., and Dworkin, R. H. (2008). Pain associated with multiple sclerosis: systematic review and proposed classification. *Pain*, 137, 96–111.

Pagnini, I., Borsini, W., Cecchi, F., Sgalambro, A., Olivotto, I., Frullini, A., et al. (2011). Distal extremity pain as a presenting feature of Fabry's disease. *Arthritis Care Res (Hoboken)*, 63, 390–395.

Pape, K. E. (2012). Developmental and maladaptive plasticity in neonatal SCI. *Clin Neurol Neurosurg*, 114(5), 475–482.

Pintos-Morell, G. and Beck, M. (2009). Fabry disease in children and the effects of enzyme replacement treatment. *Eur J Pediatr*, 168, 1355–1363.

Portenoy, R. (2006). Development and testing of a neuropathic pain screening questionnaire: ID Pain. *Curr Med Res Opin*, 22, 1555–1565.

Ramaswami, U. (2008). Fabry disease during childhood: clinical manifestations and treatment with agalsidase alfa. *Acta Paediatr Suppl*, 97, 38–40.

Ramaswami, U., Parini, R., Pintos-Morell, G., Kalkum, G., Kampmann, C., and Beck, M. (2011). Fabry disease in children and response to enzyme replacement therapy: results from the Fabry Outcome Survey. *Clin Genet*, 81(5), 485–490.

Ramaswami, U., Whybra, C., Parini, R., Pintos-Morell, G., Mehta, A., Sunder-Plassmann, G., Widmer, U., et al. (2006). Clinical manifestations of Fabry disease in children: data from the Fabry Outcome Survey. *Acta Paediatr*, 95, 86–92.

Resnick, D. K., Levy, E. I., and Jannetta, P. J. (1998). Microvascular decompression for pediatric onset trigeminal neuralgia. *Neurosurgery*, 43, 804–807; discussion 807–808.

Ries, M., Gupta, S., Moore, D. F., Sachdev, V., Quirk, J. M., Murray, G. J., et al. (2005). Pediatric Fabry disease. *Pediatrics*, 115, e344–355.

Serletis, D., Parkin, P., Bouffet, E., Shroff, M., Drake, J. M., and Rutka, J. T. (2007). Massive plexiform neurofibromas in childhood: natural history and management issues. *J Neurosurg*, 106, 363–367.

Sethna, N. F., Meier, P. M., Zurakowski, D., and Berde, C. B. (2007). Cutaneous sensory abnormalities in children and adolescents with complex regional pain syndromes. *Pain*, 131, 153–161.

Smith, B. H., and Torrance, N. (2012). Epidemiology of neuropathic pain and its impact on quality of life. *Curr Pain Headache Rep*, 16(3), 191–8.

Smith, J. and Thompson, J. M. (1995). Phantom limb pain and chemotherapy in pediatric amputees. *Mayo Clin Proc*, 70, 357–364.

Solth, A., Veelken, N., Gottschalk, J., Goebell, E., Pothmann, R., and Kremer, P. (2008). Successful vascular decompression in an 11-year-old patient with trigeminal neuralgia. *Childs Nerv Syst*, 24, 763–766.

Sorensen, G. V., Rosthoj, S., Wurtz, M., Danielsen, T. K., and Schroder, H. (2011). The epidemiology of herpes zoster in 226 children with acute lymphoblastic leukemia. *Pediatr Blood Cancer*, 57, 993–997.

Sorkin, L. S., Otto, M., Baldwin, W. M. 3rd, Vail, E., Gillies, S. D., Handgretinger, R., et al. (2010). Anti-GD(2) with an FC point mutation reduces complement fixation and decreases antibody-induced allodynia. *Pain*, 149, 135–142.

Spaargaren, E., Ahmed, J., van Ouwerkerk, W. J., de Groot, V., and Beckerman, H. (2011). Aspects of activities and participation of 7–8 year-old children with an obstetric brachial plexus injury. *Eur J Paediatr Neurol*, 15, 345–352.

Staud, R., Price, D. D., Janicke, D., Andrade, E., Hadjipanayis, A. G., Eaton, W. T., et al. (2011). Two novel mutations of SCN9A (Nav1.7) are associated with partial congenital insensitivity to pain. *Eur J Pain*, 15, 223–230.

Strombeck, C., Remahl, S., Krumlinde-Sundholm, L., and Sejersen, T. (2007). Long-term follow-up of children with obstetric brachial plexus palsy II: neurophysiological aspects. *Dev Med Child Neurol*, 49, 204–209.

Thomas, C. R., Brazeal, B. A., Rosenberg, L., Robert, R. S., Blakeney, P. E., and Meyer, W. J. (2003). Phantom limb pain in pediatric burn survivors. *Burns*, 29, 139–142.

van Dijk, A., McGrath, P. A., Pickett, W., and VanDenKerkhof, E. G. (2006). Pain prevalence in nine- to 13-year-old schoolchildren. *Pain Res Manag*, 11, 234–240.

Vivas, A. C., Escandon, J., and Kirsner, R. S. (2011). Refractory erythromelalgia of the ears: response to mexiletine. *Am J Otolaryngol*, 32, 168–170.

Vogel, L. C., Krajci, K. A., and Anderson, C. J. (2002). Adults with pediatric-onset spinal cord injuries: part 3: impact of medical complications. *J Spinal Cord Med*, 25, 297–305.

Vondracek, P., Oslejskova, H., Kepak, T., Mazanek, P., Sterba, J., Rysava, M., et al. (2009). Efficacy of pregabalin in neuropathic pain in paediatric oncological patients. *Eur J Paediatr Neurol*, 13, 332–336.

Walco, G. A., Dworkin, R. H., Krane, E. J., LeBel, A. A., and Treede, R. D. (2010). Neuropathic pain in children: Special considerations. *Mayo Clin Proc*, 85, S33–41.

Wallace, M. S., Lee, J., Sorkin, L., Dunn, J. S., Yaksh, T., and Yu, A. (1997). Intravenous lidocaine: effects on controlling pain after anti-GD2 antibody therapy in children with neuroblastoma—a report of a series. *Anesth Analg*, 85, 794–796.

Waxman, S. G., and Dib-Hajj, S. (2005). Erythermalgia: molecular basis for an inherited pain syndrome. *Trends Mol Med*, 11, 555–562.

Werhagen, L., Budh, C. N., Hultling, C., and Molander, C. (2004). Neuropathic pain after traumatic spinal cord injury—relations to gender, spinal level, completeness, and age at the time of injury. *Spinal Cord*, 42, 665–673.

Wilkins, K. L., McGrath, P. J., Finley, G. A., and Katz, J. (1998). Phantom limb sensations and phantom limb pain in child and adolescent amputees. *Pain*, 78, 7–12.

Wilkins, K. L., McGrath, P. J., Finley, G. A., and Katz, J. (2004). Prospective diary study of nonpainful and painful phantom sensations in a preselected sample of child and adolescent amputees reporting phantom limbs. *Clin J Pain*, 20, 293–301.

Xiao, W. H., Yu, A. L., and Sorkin, L. S. (1997). Electrophysiological characteristics of primary afferent fibers after systemic administration of anti-GD2 ganglioside antibody. *Pain*, 69, 145–151.

Yu, A. L., Gilman, A. L., Ozkaynak, M. F., London, W. B., Kreissman, S. G., Chen, H. X., et al. (2010). Anti-GD2 antibody with GM-CSF, interleukin-2, and isotretinoin for neuroblastoma. *N Engl J Med*, 363, 1324–1334.

Yue, W. L. (2004). Peripheral glycerol injection for the relief of facial neuralgia in children. *Int J Pediatr Otorhinolaryngol*, 68, 37–41.

CHAPTER 22

Inflammatory arthritis and arthropathy

Peter Chira and Laura E. Schanberg

Summary

Musculoskeletal pain is a common symptom in inflammatory arthritides such as juvenile idiopathic arthritis; however, identifying the underlying pathological process is often challenging for health care providers due to the extensive differential diagnoses. In children with inflammatory arthritides, physical examination abnormalities including swelling and/or pain on movement and joint limitation accompany the pain at initial presentation. Control of disease activity through anti-inflammatories and other disease-modifying agents can limit disease progression and joint damage; however, pain may persist in spite of these measures. Optimal treatment of pain in juvenile idiopathic arthritis and related conditions is based on a biopsychosocial model, which addresses biological, environmental, and cognitive-behavioural factors. Analgesics such as opioids and neuropathic pain medications, in conjunction with other modalities such as pain coping skills training, aerobic exercise, and improved sleep hygiene may be appropriate in certain circumstances. Further research is needed to prospectively identify patients and families early in the course of disease who would benefit from additional support to optimize pain management and limit distress. In addition, future clinical trials should assess the impact of study interventions on pain as a primary endpoint, assessed independently from other response variables.

Introduction

The evaluation of children with musculoskeletal pain is often challenging for health care providers due to the extensive differential diagnoses. Identifying any underlying pathological process in a thoughtful, expeditious manner is extremely important in order to minimize distress of patients and families and prevent long-term disability. Many practitioners lack comfort and familiarity in determining if musculoskeletal symptoms and pain complaints are related to an inflammatory process such as juvenile idiopathic arthritis (JIA) or other inflammatory disorders. Prompt recognition and diagnosis of an underlying rheumatic disorder allow for early treatment to reduce pain and other symptoms. Ideally, through treatment, long-term damage to joint or muscle is prevented, limiting physical disability and/or emotional distress. Additionally, control of inflammation may decrease pain signalling and prevent long-term alteration of

pain processing. However, aggressive medical therapy alone is not sufficient to optimally treat pain in children with rheumatic conditions. Other important concomitant factors besides disease activity impact pain perception and management. A biopsychosocial model of pain more completely addresses all factors contributing to the pain symptoms of a child with an underlying rheumatic disease, serving as an effective framework for treatment (Figure 22.1).

Mechanisms of arthritis pain

Much of what is understood about the biology of joint pain comes from the study of neural pathways in mice models of experimental inflammatory arthritis (McDougall, 2006; McDougall and Larson, 2006). Schaible's extensive work on the basis of pain resulting from inflammatory arthritides such as rheumatoid arthritis (RA) and JIA (Schaible et al., 2002, 2005, 2009) have described two primary mechanisms: peripheral sensitization (increased sensitivity of nociceptive primary afferent neurons) and central sensitization (hyperexcitability of nociceptive neurons in the central nervous system). Degenerative processes within joints, along with inflammation, can trigger and exacerbate sensitization of pain pathways, resulting in the development and perpetuation of chronic pain. Current mechanistic theories behind the development of pain associated with inflammation and arthritis in children with rheumatic disease have been reviewed (Kimura and Walco, 2007).

Primary afferent neurons have three main functions in nociception: detection of noxious or damaging stimuli (transduction), conveyance of sensory input from the periphery to the spinal cord (conduction), and synaptic transfer of input to neurons within specific laminae of the dorsal horn of the spinal cord (transmission) (Kidd and Urban, 2001). C-fibre nociceptors are activated by thermal, mechanical, and chemical stimuli, and can also be sensitized by mediators of the inflammatory response (e.g. prostaglandin E2 and bradykinin; see Walker and Baccei, Chapter 6, this volume). Once sensitization occurs, low-level previously non-noxious stimulation elicits neural activity (Giordano, 2006), and pain can be precipitated by routine movement in the presence of inflammation or joint damage from trauma or tissue injury. In inflammatory arthritis, a complex interplay of mechanical factors and chemical mediators such as release of bradykinins, prostaglandins, neuropeptides, cytokines, and ion channels is triggered, resulting in a decrease in

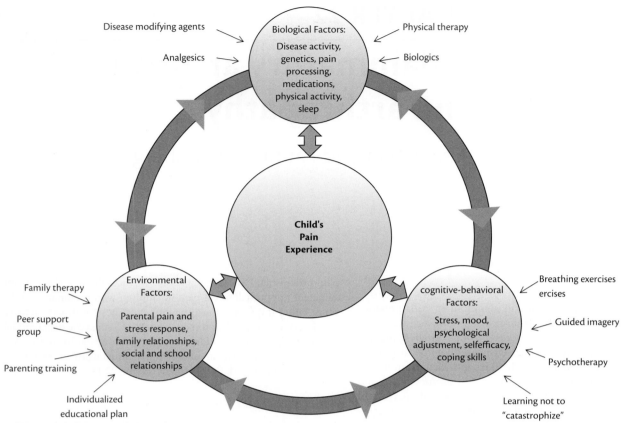

Figure 22.1 Biopsychosocial model of pain. Arthritis pain has multiple factors (biological, environmental, and cognitive-behavioural) that can contribute to a child's perception of pain. Treatment strategies should address the various components that can include pharmacological and non-pharmacological therapies.

the normal pain threshold within a joint and causing hyperalgesia and allodynia in local tissues. Inflammatory cytokines such as tumour necrosis factor alpha (TNF-α), interleukin 1, and interleukin 6 can directly activate nociceptors and contribute to effects of inflammation itself (via swelling affecting mechanical nociception), which helps to initiate and perpetuate the pain signal (Kidd and Urban, 2001; Oen et al., 2005). Thus, newer biological agents to control inflammatory arthritis using anticytokine therapies may impact arthritis pain directly, as well by decreasing disease activity.

Joint inflammation also produces central sensitization occurs when various neurotransmitters (e.g. L-glutamate) and neuropeptides (e.g. substance P, neurokinin A) activate and/or modulate synapses within the dorsal horn in the spinal cord, leading to enhancement of the pain signal and potential expansion of pain receptive fields via postsynaptic receptor activation (Schaible et al., 2009). Pain can be modulated by: reducing central sensitization via antagonism of postsynaptic receptors (e.g. N-methyl-D-aspartate (NMDA); Schaible et al., 2006); local inhibitory and excitatory interneuron circuits within the dorsal horn; as well as descending pathways (e.g. from the rostral medulla) that can facilitate or inhibit spinal nociceptive processing (Schaible et al., 2005). Imaging studies in adults have also shown that cortical processes have a major role in the mediation of pain processing that includes elements of cognition, arousal state, attention, and expectation (Seifert and Maihofner, 2009; see also Fitzgerald, Chapter 8; Hermann, Chapter 40, this volume).

Increasingly recognized as an important factor in the establishment of chronic pain is the role of accessory glial cells in the

perpetuation of pain signals (Milligan and Watkins, 2009; see also Vega-Avelaira and Beggs, Chapter 7, this volume). In inflammatory arthritides such as JIA, the role of glial cells in perpetuating pain is unclear but growing evidence suggests that cytokines released as part of the inflammatory cascade can affect and alter glial mediated central pain processing, resulting in dysfunctional pain signalling (Milligan and Watkins, 2009).

Chronic pain in children with rheumatic disease is the result of an integration of biological processes (e.g. glial cell activation, peripheral and central sensitization), psychological factors (e.g. anxiety, poor coping), and sociocultural contexts (e.g. parental emotional distress, peer relationships) within a developmental framework (Zeltzer et al., 1997). Disease activity and day to day life experiences, including emotional state, sleep quality, and family and peer relationships, all impact the severity, characteristics, and regularity of pain with time. Ongoing pain can result in sensitization of the peripheral and central nervous systems, producing neurophysiological, neurochemical, and neuroanatomical changes (Woolf and Salter, 2000), which may continue despite low disease activity or the absence of tissue damage. In addition, the extent of disability associated with a specific chronic pain level varies from person to person based on genetics as well as many of the biopsychosocial factors that impact pain perception. In summary, pain perception is multifactorial and best understood using a biopsychosocial framework including developmental status, coping ability, mood, stress levels, as well as environmental and family factors, in addition to disease status and severity (Rapoff and Lindsley, 2000).

Clinical presentation

Children and adolescents presenting with rheumatic disease may not have musculoskeletal pain as their sole, primary presenting complaint. However, for children with chronic inflammatory arthritis, joint pain can be a major presenting symptom. Interestingly, McGee looked at all patients presenting to a paediatric rheumatology clinic, and of 111 patients with an initial chief complaint of isolated musculoskeletal pain, only one had arthritis or other rheumatic disease (McGhee et al., 2002). These findings confirmed earlier data, which showed that the majority of patients referred to paediatric rheumatology clinics across the US do not have primary rheumatic disease but rather non-specific musculoskeletal complaints or abnormal laboratory studies (such as a positive antinuclear antibody; Bowyer and Roettcher, 1996). Both studies highlight the need for health care professionals to distinguish those with non-specific musculoskeletal pain from those with inflammatory conditions.

When joint pain is the primary complaint for a patient presenting with inflammatory arthritis such as JIA, it is accompanied by overt abnormalities on examination such as swelling and/or pain on movement with limitation of motion, or tenderness noted at the joint line along with limitation. The pain of arthritis is typically described as mild to moderate, dull or achy discomfort, with joint stiffness that worsens with inactivity (sleeping or sitting for prolonged periods) and improves with movement. Pain at rest is unusual. Pain commonly varies from day to day; however, the physical examination abnormalities are constantly present. Often, the stiffness is described as a 'gel phenomenon' in which inactivity causes a sensation within the affected joint(s) similar to gelatin setting or glue drying, although the exact pathophysiology of why this occurs is not understood. Arthritis pain rarely causes night awakening; therefore, other causes of joint or bone pain must be ruled out including malignancy, infection, or bone tumours (osteoid osteoma) if night pain is the primary complaint. Other signs of chronic inflammatory arthritis include gait abnormality such as limp, warmth of the joint (not necessarily associated with erythema), and muscle atrophy of proximally or distally affected areas. If there is erythema and/or exquisite tenderness with palpation of joints or bones, infection (such as osteomyelitis or septic arthritis), reactive processes (such as rheumatic fever or Henoch–Schönlein purpura), malignancy (such as leukaemia, lymphoma, or neuroblastoma), or trauma should be considered before making the diagnosis of JIA or other rheumatic disease. Table 22.1 lists the differential diagnoses to consider when children present with musculoskeletal pain.

Pain variables in arthritis

The intensity of pain reported by children and adolescents with JIA is quite variable. Early studies of pain in children with JIA erroneously suggested the condition was less painful than RA (Laaksonen and Laine, 1961). More recent studies in the 1990s, incorporating more developmentally appropriate measures, showed disease-related pain is often underestimated in children with JIA and other rheumatic disorders. In fact, using daily diary methodology, Schanberg and colleagues reported that children with JIA report pain on 70% of days (Schanberg et al., 2003). Most children reported mild to moderate pain, but 25% of children reported pain in the severe range. Interestingly, disease activity predicts less than half of reported pain variance, and day-to-day variations of pain are influenced by factors such as mood, stress, parental and child coping, and parental pain and health beliefs (Schanberg et al., 2003, 2005).

Although a relationship between increased disease activity and increased pain exists (Malleson et al., 2004; Vandvik and Eckblad, 1990; Varni et al., 1987), research consistently has demonstrated limited predictive value for disease status variables. Across studies, disease status variables typically predict only a small to medium proportion of the variance in children's pain ratings (8–28%; Malleson et al., 2004; Schanberg et al., 1997; Thompson et al., 1987; Vandvik and Eckblad, 1990). Therefore, it is important to delineate other influential factors in the pain experience of children with JIA.

The most highly predictive models of pain variance conceptualize pain report as influenced by multiple factors, including disease variables, demographic variables, psychological variables (such as coping and mood), and environmental factors. In a sample of 56 children with chronic arthritis, Ross and colleagues reported that increased child anxiety, increased maternal distress, and increased family harmony were associated with higher child pain ratings averaged over a 1-month time period (Ross et al., 1993). The authors hypothesized that increased family harmony might lend itself to increased responsiveness to children's pain behaviour, serving to reinforce pain behaviour and pain reporting in children.

Demographic variables such as age may influence JIA-related pain, but findings in cross-sectional studies have not been reproducible. Hagglund and Malleson both identified older age as a predictor of pain in their respective cohorts (Hagglund et al., 1995; Malleson et al., 2004), but other investigators have not found this relationship (Ross et al., 1993; Vandvik and Eckblad, 1990).

The role of psychosocial variables such as emotional distress, mood, stress, and pain-coping strategies in children's pain reporting has been studied in many settings. Schanberg and co-workers investigated interrelationships of daily stress, daily mood, and disease expression. Results of multilevel random effects models indicated that day-to-day fluctuations in mood and stressful events were related to daily symptoms in children with polyarticular forms of juvenile chronic arthritis (Schanberg et al., 2000, 2005). Specifically, worse mood and more stressful events predicted increased daily pain, fatigue, and stiffness. These results confirm other studies which indicate that increased psychological distress (e.g. stress, depression, and anxiety) is related to increased pain reporting and poorer functional outcomes, such as decreased participation in school and social activities (Hoff et al., 2006; Margetic et al., 2005; Ross et al., 1993). Hoff and colleagues found that depressive symptoms reported by children with JIA at a baseline evaluation were predictive of reports of pain and functional disability 6 and 12 months later (Hoff et al., 2006).

Children's coping with pain is another influential factor. The use of catastrophizing (i.e. engaging in overly negative thinking about pain) and decreased pain-coping efficacy predict higher pain intensity across several pain measures and more painful body locations, even after controlling for demographic variables and medical status variables (Schanberg et al., 1997). In a laboratory setting, catastrophizing also predicted higher pain intensity, decreased pain tolerance, and increased pain-related discomfort in children with JIA undergoing experimental cold pressor pain (Thastum et al., 1997, 2001). Recent studies by Thastum and colleagues underscore the

Table 22.1 Differential diagnoses for musculoskeletal pains in children

Category	Diagnosis	Hallmarks
Anatomic or mechanical issues	Avascular necrosis	Pain with weight bearing
	Osteochondroses (e.g. Legg–Calf–Perthes)	Hip pain and limp
	Apophysitis (e.g. Osgood–Schlatter)	Tibial tuberosity pain
	Ligamentous laxity (e.g. patellar dislocation)	Mobile patella with pain
	Benign hypermobility syndrome	Multi-joint hyperextensibility
Trauma	Fracture	Multiple fractures in young children suggest child abuse; growth plate fractures not seen on X-ray
	Sprain, muscular strain	Physically active teens, unusual <4 years of age
	Haemarthrosis (e.g. haemophilia)	Warm, pain with motion, grossly bloody arthrocentesis
Infections	Reactive arthritis	Post-diarrhoeal or genitourinary infections
	Rheumatic fever	Exquisitely tender migratory polyarthritis of large joints
	Lyme disease	Oligo- or polyarthritis is a manifestation of late Lyme infection
	Viral arthritis (e.g. Epstein–Barr virus, cytomegalovirus, parvo B19)	Often with rash and fever
	Infectious osteomyelitis (bacterial, fungal, tuberculosis)	May be associated with sympathetic effusion of adjacent joint
	Septic arthritis	Typically is associated with redness, warmth, pain with motion, elevated inflammatory markers
Malignancy or other tumours	Leukaemia	Severe night pain can be associated with bony point tenderness and complete blood count abnormalities
	Lymphoma	Matted lymph nodes
	Osteoid osteoma	Night-time pain, often alleviated by NSAIDs
	Neuroblastoma	Abdominal mass
Rheumatic diseases	Juvenile idiopathic arthritis	Multiple subgroups based on clinical characteristics
	Systemic lupus erythematosus	Non-erosive polyarthritis
	Henoch–Schönlein purpura	Purpuric rash on legs, buttocks; arthritis of lower extremities
	Dermatomyositis	Bilateral proximal muscle weakness and rash on face, eyelids, and extensor surfaces of joints
	Sarcoidosis	Joints boggy and painless, associated with rash and inflammatory eye disease
Other inflammatory conditions	Arthropathy related to inflammatory bowel disease	Peripheral arthritis reflects gastrointestinal (GI) disease activity versus axial skeletal arthritis which is independent of GI disease
	Auto-inflammatory disorders	Periodic fever syndromes, C1AS mutations
	Chronic recurrent multifocal osteomyelitis (non-infectious)	Multi-focal affecting long bones as well as mandible, spine, and clavicles; bone biopsy needed for diagnosis
	Arthritis from immunodeficiency	Combined variable immunodeficiency
Pain amplification disorders	Complex regional pain syndrome	Type 1 associated with trauma and with diffuse swelling and discoloration of affected limb
	Fibromyalgia	Sleep disturbance, fatigue and tender points
	Benign limb pains of childhood (e.g. growing pains)	Night awakenings with extremity pain relieved by massage or warm packs
Metabolic and endocrinological	Rickets	Flaring at bony metaphyses on X-ray
	Mucopolysaccharidoses	Gaucher or Hurler

impact of cognitive health beliefs on pain in children with JIA (Thastum and Herlin, 2011; Thastum et al., 2005). Results suggested beliefs about control over pain and the ability to function despite the presence of pain influence the development of effective pain-coping strategies, while dysfunctional health beliefs persist over time in patients with high pain.

Finally, parent and family environmental variables are related to pain report of children with JIA. These variables include the nature of family relationships (family harmony or conflict), increased parent psychological distress, parental responses to child pain, and parent and family pain history (Connelly et al., 2010; Iobst et al., 2007; Reid et al., 2005). For example, in a sample of school-aged children with chronic arthritis, Schanberg and colleagues found that a more extensive parent and family history of pain was related to increased child self-reported pain intensity (Schanberg et al., 2001). Moreover, within the context of hierarchical regression analyses, child catastrophizing mediated the relationship. In other words, parent and family pain variables influenced a child's use of catastrophizing as a coping strategy, which in turn influenced child reporting of pain.

Diagnosis

The diagnosis of chronic inflammatory arthritis is based on clinical examination and history. No laboratory or radiographic studies make the diagnosis of JIA. Duration of symptoms is extremely important as diagnostic criteria for all the chronic arthritides require the presence of objective joint abnormalities on physical examination (either swelling or pain/tenderness with limitation) in the same joint for at least 6 weeks' time. Acute presentations of joint pain and/or swelling caused by infections, injury, or reactive processes are more common than JIA, and often are self-limited, resolving before 6 weeks. The paediatric Gait, Arms, Legs screen (pGALs) is an excellent screening tool for use by non-rheumatologists that includes a focused joint examination for affected areas which incorporates inspection, palpation, and range of motion (Foster et al., 2006).

Classification

The nomenclature for childhood onset arthritis has evolved through the years. The current classification system was developed by the International League Against Rheumatism (ILAR; Fink, 1995; Petty et al., 1998, 2004) and uses the term juvenile idiopathic arthritis (JIA) instead of juvenile rheumatoid arthritis (American College of Rheumatology classification; Brewer et al., 1972, 1977) or juvenile chronic arthritis (European League Against Rheumatism classification; Wood, 1978). While the different classification systems have similarities, they are not interchangeable. Within the ILAR classification of JIA, there are seven categories corresponding to different onset subtypes based on the first 6 months of presentation, which include: oligoarticular, polyarticular-rheumatoid factor negative, polyarticular-rheumatoid factor positive, psoriatic, enthesitis-related, systemic, and unclassified arthritis. The ILAR criteria were developed to help provide prognostic information for various subtypes of JIA, as well as provide a framework for research; however, the classification scheme is cumbersome and often misused even by paediatric rheumatologists. In addition, large numbers of patients fall into the unclassified category (Berntson et al., 2001; Kunjir et al., 2010; Merino et al., 2001; Petty, 2001; Ravelli et al., 2011).

Diagnostic studies

Although inflammatory arthritis is typically a clinical diagnosis, laboratory and/or radiographic evaluations can be helpful in classifying the subtype of JIA or determining if arthritis is part of a systemic disorder. A complete blood count with manual differential, erythrocyte sedimentation rate (ESR) and/or C-reactive protein are often performed to assess for generalized inflammation. A comprehensive metabolic panel, including uric acid and lactate dehydrogenase to look for possible increased cellular turnover noted in malignancies, and urinalysis are useful to assess organ damage or involvement. If pain is not localized at a joint but more diffuse, muscle enzymes such as creatine kinase or aldolase as well as vitamin D and thyroid function levels may be helpful. Often, these ancillary studies are useful in identifying other aetiologies of joint or bony pain such as metabolic diseases and malignancies.

The utility of screening autoantibodies varies depending on the context of ordering the test. If joint or musculoskeletal pain is the only complaint without obvious joint pathology such as swelling or pain on movement/tenderness with limitation (arthralgias), then screening tests have little value and cause undue consternation if abnormal (Wong et al., 2012). In the presence of true arthritis, screening for anti-nuclear antibody, rheumatoid factor (especially for polyarticular presentation), anti-citrullinated cyclic peptide, and HLA-B27 is helpful to determine prognosis and risk of eye disease (Anonymous, 1993; Heiligenhaus et al., 2007).

Radiographic studies assess bony abnormalities or joint destruction such as erosions, but often in JIA these diagnostic studies are negative, especially early in the disease course. MRI and ultrasound are newer modalities used in assisting the diagnosis of arthritis by demonstrating effusions, synovial proliferation, early erosions, increased blood flow, and bone marrow oedema from inflammation, but there are issues with regard to normal standards in the growing skeleton. Therefore, imaging studies are best evaluated by an experienced paediatric musculoskeletal radiologist in conjunction with a paediatric rheumatologist.

Other rheumatic conditions

Systemic lupus erythematosus, juvenile dermatomyositis, and vasculitis can all present with arthritis as a primary manifestation. Joint or muscle pain can be the presenting symptom for these patients. Typically, other signs and symptoms including rash and constitutional symptoms such as malaise, fever, fatigue, or anorexia guide further evaluation. Screening for organ system damage by looking at renal, cardiopulmonary, and neuropsychiatric function can be helpful in making diagnoses of other rheumatic conditions.

Treatment/management of pain in children with JIA

The biopsychosocial model of pain provides a useful framework from which to approach managing pain in JIA. In addition to aggressively treating the biological basis of disease, a combination of pharmacological and non-pharmacological modalities can be used to manage pain. Reducing disease activity is associated with improved radiographic outcomes, functional capability and reduced symptoms including pain; however, disease control is not sufficient to eliminate pain and other symptoms. Further goals of treatment in children and adolescents are to alleviate pain, improve or preserve function, and restore normal growth. Unfortunately, no clinical trials in JIA have addressed pain management as a primary endpoint. Even the original studies of non-steroidal anti-inflammatories (NSAIDs) in children with JIA used disease activity outcomes that included pain, rather than pain alone, to prove efficacy (Giannini et al., 1990; Laxer et al., 1988; Nicholls et al., 1982; Steans et al., 1990).

Initial treatment of pain related to inflammatory arthritides is NSAIDS, adding acetaminophen for acutely painful events. Therapy may be escalated based on disease severity, symptom intensity, functional disability or lack of efficacy, to include: corticosteroids (systemic or intra-articular injections); disease modifying antirheumatic drugs (DMARDs) such as methotrexate, sulfasalazine, hydroxychloroquine, or leflunomide; and biological therapies such as TNFα blockers (etanercept, infliximab, adalimumab, golimumab, certolizumab), interleukin-1 blockade (anakinra, rilonacept, canakinumab), B-cell depletion (rituximab), interleukin-6 inhibition (tocilizumab) and T-cell costimulation blockade (abatacept). Recently, studies of early aggressive treatment (Tynjälä et al., 2011; Wallace et al., 2012) have led to development of algorithms and treatment protocols for various subtypes of JIA (Beukelman et al., 2011; DeWitt et al., 2012; Tynjälä et al., 2011; Wallace et al., 2012). Table 22.2 shows the dosing of agents commonly used to treat pain in JIA.

Intra-articular injection of long-acting corticosteroids can be a highly effective means of immediately reducing joint inflammation and pain, especially for monoarticular or oligoarticular JIA, as well as persistently symptomatic joints in polyarticular disease (Wallen and Gillies, 2006). Because of wide ranging and distressing side effects, as well as concerns about obscuring a diagnosis of cancer, the routine use of systemic corticosteroids to reduce pain is discouraged, except in cases of severe systemic JIA following a bone marrow biopsy to rule out cancer, when arthritis is so severe the child will otherwise become bedridden or wheelchair-bound, or for short-term use while starting a new agent or intervention with delayed effect (Connelly and Schanberg, 2006).

As one of the oldest and most potent anti-inflammatory medication available, systemic corticosteroids have historically been used by practitioners to reduce pain in rheumatic disease even without overt evidence of active inflammation. While corticosteroids immediately reduce inflammation and may secondarily decrease pain with substantial symptom relief, corticosteroids unfortunately do not change the long-term course of arthritis and are not remittive agents so the actual benefit is limited. Corticosteroids can also mask the presence of malignancy or other rheumatic disease and should not be used in the absence of a clear diagnosis or without consultation with a paediatric rheumatologist. In addition, chronic use of systemic corticosteroids has many undesired side effects (e.g. growth retardation, osteoporosis, avascular necrosis, cataracts, and immunosuppression), which are especially devastating for children. Nevertheless, 27% of paediatric rheumatologists surveyed about pain treatment in JIA preferentially prescribed systemic corticosteroids over analgesics to treat residual pain in children with arthritis because of discomfort and lack of training in the use of opioid pain medications (Kimura et al., 2006).

Specific medications

NSAIDs are the mainstay of pain treatment in paediatric patients with rheumatic diseases (Table 22.2) providing rapid and effective analgesia in a variety of well-tolerated oral preparations (liquid, chewable tablets, tablets, capsules). NSAIDs work peripherally inhibiting cyclo-oxygenase (COX), which reduces prostaglandin production and subsequently pain (see also Anderson, Chapter 43, this volume). Analgesia from NSAIDs may be additive to that of opioids and other adjuvant medications. NSAIDs have a ceiling effect (i.e. increased doses have no further benefit). COX-2 selective inhibitors (meloxicam and celecoxib) are approved by the US Federal Drug Administration (FDA) for use in JIA and are effective and safe (Foeldvari et al., 2009; Ruperto et al., 2005), although there is little information regarding long-term cardiovascular risks in children taking either selective or non-selective NSAIDs.

Significant potential adverse effects from NSAIDs and COX-2 inhibitors include gastrointestinal toxicity (dyspepsia, gastritis, ulcers, constipation and diarrhoea), renal toxicity (interstitial nephritis, papillary necrosis, decreased blood flow, hypertension), hepatotoxicity (hepatocellular injury, cholestasis); cardiovascular toxicity has thus far been reported only in adults. Platelet inhibition occurs with most NSAIDs and needs to be considered in patients with a coexisting bleeding diathesis or prior to a surgical procedure. NSAIDs (especially naproxen) have also been associated with pseudoporphyria, which can cause significant scarring (Lang and Finlayson, 1994). Typically, fair-skinned children are at greatest risk for pseudoporphyria with sun exposure. The skin lesions present as small linear scratches in sun-exposed areas such as the face or arms. Sunscreen use is encouraged while on NSAIDs.

Acetaminophen is an appropriate analgesic for mild to moderate pain and can be used in combination with NSAIDs. Patients must be cautioned not to take more than the recommended dosage (10–15 mg/kg/dose every 4–6 h, maximum of 4 g in 24 h). Larger doses, especially taken chronically, can cause significant hepatotoxicity and are an important cause of liver failure. It is important to remember that many analgesics contain acetaminophen as well as the principal analgesic (e.g. Percocet® contains acetaminophen in addition to oxycodone) in order to avoid overdosing patients with acetaminophen.

Opioids (see also Strassels, Chapter 45, this volume) which act as agonists blocking principally μ and less commonly κ receptors in the central nervous system, are gaining acceptance to treat chronic, non-malignant pain in adults and children (Kalso et al., 2004; Slater et al., 2010). However, a recent Cochrane systematic review did not find strong evidence for long-term use in adult RA (Whittle et al., 2011). Opioids may be better tolerated, have more rapid onset of action, and are potentially less toxic than aggressive immunosuppression. Tramadol is a weak opioid that provides fairly effective relief of mild to moderate pain when NSAIDs and acetaminophen have failed. While there is fair evidence of its efficacy in osteoarthritis (Manchikanti et al., 2011), it has not been studied specifically in children with arthritis. Additional choices for acute pain include various oxycodone preparations, and for long-term pain management methadone (which also acts as an antagonist of NMDA receptors) may be useful. Methadone is not well studied in children but several studies suggest dosing only two to three times per day may be effective (Berde et al., 1991; Brown et al., 2004; Shir et al., 1998).

Table 22.2 Medications used to treat pain in rheumatic diseases

Name	Dosage	Max. dose/day	How supplied
NSAIDs			
Aspirin	60–100 mg/kg/day	20–30 mg/dl level	Chewable tablet, tablet
	Divided 3 times/day		
Ibuprofen	30–40 mg/kg/day	2400 mg	Liquid, chewable tablets, tablets
	Divided 3 times/day		
Naproxen	10–20 mg/kg/day	1000 mg	Liquid, tablet
	Divided 2 times/day		
Indomethacin	2–4 mg/kg/day	200 mg	Liquid, capsule, tablet
	Divided 2–3 times/day		
Meloxicam	0.125–0.25 mg/kg	7.5 mg	Liquid, tablet
	Once daily		
Celecoxib	50 mg/dose (12–25 kg) 100 mg/dose (>25 kg) 200 mg/dose (>50 kg) } 2 times/day	400 mg	Capsule
Tolectin	40 mg/kg/day	1600 mg	Tablet
	Divided 3 times/day		
Etodolac SR	20–30 mg/day (by age)	1000 mg	Tablet
	Once daily		
Nabumetone	30 mg/kg/day	2000 mg	Tablet
	Divided 1–2 times/day		
Analgesics, including opioids			
Acetaminophen	10–15 mg/kg/dose	2–4 g	Liquid, chewable tablet, tablet
	Every 4–6 h		
Hydrocodone	0.15 mg/kg	Limited by side effects	Liquid, tablet
	Every 3–6 h		
Oxycodone	0.005–0.2 mg/kg	Limited by side effects	Liquid, capsule, tablet
	Every 3–6 h		
Tramadol	25–100 mg	300 mg	Tablet
	Every 6–8 h		
Methadone	0.2–0.4 mg/kg	Limited by side effects	Liquid, tablet
	Every 6–12 h		
Hydromorphone	0.03–0.08 mg/kg/dose	Limited by side effects	Liquid, tablet
	Every 4 h		
Other agents			
Gabapentin	8–35 mg/kg/day	3600 mg	Tablet
	Divided 3 times/day		
Amitriptyline	10–30 mg/day	75 mg	Tablet
	At bedtime		
Pregabalin[a]	150–300 mg/day	450 mg	Tablet
	Divided 2 times/day[b]		
Duloxetine[a]	30–60 mg/day	60 mg	Tablet
	Once daily[c]		

[a]Not FDA approved in children <18 years.

[b]Trials in children 12–17 have starting dose of 25 mg with slow titration until effect achieved.

[c]Trials in children from 13–17, starting dose of 30 mg.

Despite potential benefits, paediatric rheumatologists rarely use opioids to treat JIA-related pain with nearly 60% expressing refusal to use opioids for chronic pain management in a recent survey even though more than 75% of respondents reported caring for patients with significant arthritis-related pain despite adequate medical treatment (Kimura et al., 2006). Side effect concerns such as drowsiness, fatigue, and constipation as well as respiratory depression strongly influenced paediatric rheumatologists' attitudes toward opioid use, but those opposed to opioid use were most concerned about addiction and dependence (χ^2 5.51, p = 0.019). Most side effects, including sedation, nausea, and pruritis are reversible and short term. Additional complications such as respiratory distress can be avoided by starting at low dose and titrating to effect. A pre-emptive bowel regimen, including a stool softener and stimulant, can prevent constipation (Connelly and Schanberg, 2006).

Adjuvant medications often are useful for managing chronic pain in children with JIA. The most commonly used medication of this type is amitriptyline, a tricyclic antidepressant used in low doses at night for generalized chronic pain associated with sleep disturbance. However, in an N of 1 Bayesian trial in six children with JIA, Huber found low-dose amitriptyline did not improve pain scores (Huber et al., 2007). Selective serotonin re-uptake inhibitors (SSRIs) may be used to treat comorbid mood disorders in children and adolescents with JIA. Given FDA-mandated black box labelling for SSRIs, these medications should only be used with close follow-up and extensive parent education about the increased risk of suicidality. Adding medications that address neuropathic pain has been advocated in adult arthritis (e.g. gabapentin, pregabalin, duloxetine), but there are no published studies looking specifically at their usage to treat chronic pain in JIA or other childhood-onset rheumatic diseases.

Surgical interventions

The role of surgery in treating pain and disability in children with chronic arthritis is not straight forward; although several studies suggest children experience marked pain reduction after surgery (Dell'Era et al., 2008; Iesaka et al., 2006; Parvizi et al., 2003). Surgical interventions including synovectomy, soft-tissue release, and arthroplasty are generally limited to children with marked functional impairment, severe disabling pain, or deformity. Whenever possible, the age and skeletal maturity of the child should be considered, and surgery should be delayed until growth plate closure. Surgical interventions should be performed in specialized clinics at tertiary centres with awareness of the presence of arthritis in the cervical spine and temporomandibular joints, if intubation is planned. Pharmacological advances in treating children with chronic arthritis have brought into question the role of surgical interventions and likely will be an increasingly rare occurrence in the future.

Non-pharmacological interventions

The growing acceptance of the biopsychosocial model of pain has prompted the development and study of non-pharmacological interventions for JIA-related pain. Research on non-pharmacological interventions has included programmes for improving physical conditioning and sleep hygiene, massage therapy, and, perhaps most importantly, cognitive behavioural therapy.

Cognitive-behavioural therapy (CBT) aims to manage pain by improving self-reliance and facilitating normal activities through the use of coping skills, decreasing cognitive responses to pain, and using behavioural strategies including progressive muscle relaxation, distraction, and guided imagery (see also Logan et al., Chapter 50, this volume). Addressing coping strategies through CBT is integral to pain management in JIA, as pain coping accounts for a large amount of the variance in self-reported pain intensity over and above the effect of disease activity (Sawyer et al., 2004; Schanberg et al., 1997; Thastum et al., 2005).Two published studies demonstrated improvement in self-reported pain ratings of children with chronic arthritis after CBT both immediately after treatment and at 6-month follow-up (Lavigne et al., 1992; Walco et al., 1992). The studies are limited by small sample size, abbreviated scope of the CBT intervention, and the lack of functional outcome variables. Although future studies of CBT are necessary to understand fully its role in treatment of children with JIA, a systematic review of controlled trials of psychological therapy for chronic pain concluded that there is evidence to support the use of CBT to treat headaches and other types of recurrent and chronic pain in children and adolescents (Palermo et al., 2010). The lack of side effects and the generalizability of the skills make CBT an attractive adjunctive intervention.

Physical therapy and exercise programmes can help reduce pain in children with arthritis, who tend to be less physically active and more deconditioned than their peers (Takken et al., 2008). Decreased physical activity as a result of disease symptoms leads to decreased aerobic capacity and endurance, decreased exercise time, and decreased peak workload as compared with healthy controls (Giannini and Protas, 1991; Klepper and Giannini, 1994). Klepper et al. studied the effect of an exercise regimen in 25 children with arthritis, showing that improved aerobic conditioning was achieved and was associated with decreased pain, without disease exacerbation (Klepper 1999, 2008). Several other studies have demonstrated decreases in active joint count and disease severity with initiation of a therapeutic exercise programme, as well as decreased pain and improved cardiovascular fitness, but noted difficulty in motivating patients to continue achieving aerobic goals (Singh-Grewal et al., 2006, 2007; Takken et al., 2008). Future studies are necessary to delineate the most appropriate exercise for children with arthritis.

Improving *sleep quality* often is overlooked in the treatment of pain. One study described frequent night waking, parasomnias, sleep anxiety, sleep-disordered breathing, and daytime fatigue in children with arthritis compared with controls and disturbed sleep was associated with increased pain (Bloom et al., 2002). Bromberg and colleagues found that self-reported nightly sleep quality was highly predictive of pain the following day, with better mood attenuating the effect (Bromberg et al., 2012). Thus, even simple measures to improve sleep, including use of a supportive but soft mattress and sleeping in warm pyjamas (e.g. sweat clothes), should be recommended to children with JIA. Physical therapists also can suggest sleep positions that maximize level of comfort depending on the unique combination of active joints. Relaxation techniques, such as progressive muscle relaxation or guided imagery taught within the context of cognitive behavioural therapy, also can be useful in improving sleep hygiene.

Other interventions, including integrative approaches (see Zeltzer, Chapter 60, this volume) to improve pain in children with JIA have not been well studied; however, limited research includes studies of the use of massage and orthotics in children with JIA and several interventions in adult RA. Field and colleagues evaluated the effectiveness of massage in decreasing pain in a sample of 20 children with mild to moderate arthritis (Field et al., 1997). Children were randomly assigned to either a massage therapy or relaxation techniques control group. Immediately after treatment, children who received massage had lower levels of anxiety and decreased salivary cortisol levels. They also reported less present pain, less pain during the past week, and fewer painful locations than children in the control condition. A controlled trial of 40 children investigating the effectiveness of custom orthotics showed significant improvements in pain, ambulation speed, and self-related functionality and activity, when compared to children using over-the-counter inserts and supportive athletic shoes (Powell et al., 2005).

An evidence based review of non-pharmacological treatments for adults with rheumatoid arthritis found that aerobic physical exercise, sports, and muscle-strengthening exercises demonstrated positive benefit in pain and health related quality of life; however, there was little evidence that dietary measures, nutritional supplements and elimination diets were effective (Gossec et al., 2006).Further controlled studies on these and other non-pharmacological interventions are required before reaching conclusions relating to the effectiveness of these approaches in children with JIA-related pain.

Outcomes

More comprehensive assessment and tracking of pain in children with rheumatic conditions are needed upon which to base future treatment considerations. Currently, there is no generally accepted, standardized method of assessing pain for children with rheumatic conditions and pain improvement is not considered independently in either pharmaceutical or investigator-initiated medication efficacy trials, despite a call from the international paediatric pain community to perform more comprehensive pain assessments in children participating in clinical trials (McGrath et al., 2008). A Childhood Arthritis and Rheumatology Research Alliance (CARRA) initiative has sought to formalize pain assessment as part of the routine evaluation of children and adolescents presenting to paediatric rheumatology clinics (Stinson et al., 2012). Additionally, more in depth understanding of the context of pain in JIA is needed to guide development of more effective interventions. Symptom tracking using electronic diaries or other mobile technologies can reveal the ecological momentary impact of pain in JIA, demonstrating hourly as well as daily variability not apparent in cross sectional pain assessments during routine clinic visits (Connelly et al., 2007; Schanberg et al., 2003; Stinson et al., 2006, 2008).

Extremely important in any assessment of pain is gathering information directly from children themselves as studies show a lack of concordance between provider, parent, and patient perceptions of pain, especially as children get older and depression or other psychological distress is more common (Garcia-Munitis et al., 2006;

Lal et al., 2011; Palermo et al., 2004). Tong and colleagues' recent systematic review of qualitative studies about the experiences of children with JIA identified six major themes: aversion to being different, striving for normality, stigma and understanding, suspension in uncertainty, managing treatment, and desire for knowledge (Tong et al., 2012). Of note, pain from JIA, its impact and management were pervasive within all themes and the author's conclusions reinforce the concepts and framework of the biopsychosocial pain model.

Chronic recurrent pain in children, which likely includes those with JIA, is known to have negative short-term impact including poorer social and peer relationships, missed school and decreased functionality, and emotional and psychological distress (Connelly et al., 2012; Eccleston and Crombez, 2007; Haverman et al., 2012; Palermo, 2000; Roth-Isigkeit et al., 2005). Without properly addressing pain as a standard part of JIA treatment, long-term disability and increased medical expenditures may result (Arkela-Kautiainen et al., 2006; Foster et al., 2003). Understanding relationships between pain, school attendance, sleep, stress, emotion regulation, and mood will guide development of interventions designed to enhance the functionality and productive coping of children and adolescents with JIA.

To improve routine care of children with JIA, pain assessment and control are included in proposed standards for health care delivery quality measurements (Lovell et al., 2011). Consensus assessment and treatment plans addressing pain in children with JIA are being developed through CARRA and will provide recommendations regarding use of various treatment modalities to manage the multifactorial nature of pain in rheumatic conditions. Additionally, validation and standardization of outcome measurements for the assessment of paediatric rheumatic conditions, which includes pain intensity assessment, are being addressed through worldwide efforts through organizations such as Paediatric Rheumatology INternational Trials Organisation (PRINTO) and Pediatric Rheumatology Collaborative Study Group (PRCSG). With the advent of newer agents introduced earlier in the disease course to quickly limit inflammation, new studies are needed to investigate if shifts in the treatment paradigm result in fewer pain complaints and less pain related functional limitation. Consensus derived algorithms will standardize assessment and treatment of JIA-related pain in clinical settings. Through comparative effectiveness research studies using the CARRA network, we can evaluate the best modalities to approach pain.

Conclusion

Pain is common in children with inflammatory arthritis despite aggressive treatment of JIA with contemporary medications. Pain is an important, but often neglected, aspect of care for children with arthritis, negatively impacting well-being and function. Further research is needed to prospectively identify patients and families early in the course of disease who would benefit from additional support to optimize pain management and limit distress. In addition, future clinical trials should assess the impact of study interventions on pain as a primary endpoint, assessed independently from other response variables.

Case example

A 15-year-old adolescent female presents for evaluation of diffuse musculoskeletal pain, which has been ongoing for 2 years. In the past, she was able to cope with the pain and keep playing basketball, her favourite sport. Over the past 6 months, she stopped playing basketball due to swollen knees and lower back pain. Every morning she is stiff for 2 h. Physical exam shows arthritis of both knees, but also exquisite tenderness at bilateral sacroiliac joints with poor flexion of the lumbar spine. She also has enthesitis (tenderness at the bony insertion points of tendons and ligaments) at bilateral Achilles tendons, greater trochanteric heads, tibial tuberosities, and anterior superior iliac crests (see Figure 22.2). Laboratory evaluation includes normal blood counts with elevated ESR of 50. HLA B27 is positive but antinuclear antibody, rheumatoid factor, and anti-citrullinated cyclic peptide are negative. MRI and plain films reveal erosions at her sacroiliac joints. Her primary care provider has started ibuprofen 600 mg three times daily. Since starting the medication, she is moving better with morning stiffness lasting only an hour. Her knee swelling is unchanged.

Given the clinical picture, she was diagnosed with enthesitis-related juvenile idiopathic arthritis, also known as a seronegative spondyloarthropathy, by a paediatric rheumatologist. Because of the severity of joint findings on imaging, she immediately was started on a TNF-α blocker and underwent intra-articular joint injections for her knees. With initiation of treatment, her inflammatory lab markers normalized, her knee swelling fully resolved and she resumed most normal daily activities. Unfortunately in follow-up, she still complained of back pain, which she now characterized as extending up her entire back into her neck, shoulder blades and including her lower back. She is worried that the newly diagnosed arthritis is worsening since her pain has changed, and is now sharper, more stabbing in nature and seems to affect more body parts including hips, knees, shoulders and elbows. She also is fatigued, often missing school. A short course of oral prednisone does not provide relief or improvement in her symptoms.

On further history, she endorses non-restorative sleep and multiple psychosocial and emotional stressors, including recently breaking up with her boyfriend. Previously, she was physically active but has not engaged in aerobic activity since onset of the knee arthritis. She expresses desperation to get to back to feeling normal. Re-examination shows no obvious joint abnormalities but she has diffuse musculoskeletal tenderness at her gluteal insertions and other tender points. To address the current concerns, she was started on low-dose amitriptyline to help with sleep and provided a regimented physical therapy programme including range of motion and core strengthening exercises, as well as a conditioning programme to work on aerobic capacity for eventual resumption of her previous physical activities. Additionally, she is referred to a therapist for counselling regarding pain coping strategies.

In the setting of enthesitis-related JIA (also known as juvenile spondyloarthropathy), fibromyalgia overlay can occur, especially in females, making the diagnosis and assessment of current health status especially challenging (Aloush et al., 2007; Fitzcharles and Boulos, 2003). Characteristically, this form of JIA is more frequent in males than females and is not associated with autoantibodies such as rheumatoid factor or antinuclear antibodies. Because arthritis may be limited to the axial skeleton, overt joint abnormalities may not be present. Entheseal tenderness can overlap or be in similar locations as fibromyalgia tender points (Figure 22.3), for example, as noted in the gluteal region and hip girdle (Fitzcharles and Esdaile, 1997). TNF-α blockade (such as etanercept, infliximab, golimumab, or adalimumab) treats the inflammatory component of this form of JIA extremely well, even helping heal destructive changes noted in the axial skeleton.

Secondary fibromyalgia is common in adult patients with rheumatic conditions, but also occurs in children and adolescents. Treatment of pain should incorporate a biopsychosocial model addressing all elements that may be contributing to her current health status: anti-inflammatories and immune modulators for inflammation, physical exercise for fatigue and functional limitations, and counselling to improve pain coping and address psychological and emotional confounders. For this teen, initiation of amitriptyline to improve sleep quality, graduated aerobic exercise in addition to adjunctive treatment with a TENS unit or massage therapy, as well as cognitive behavioural therapy will help manage residual pain. Escalation of arthritis treatment such as using courses of oral or parenteral corticosteroids do not treat the central pain processing changes underlying diffuse persistent pain or impact factors moderating pain in the case of this teen.

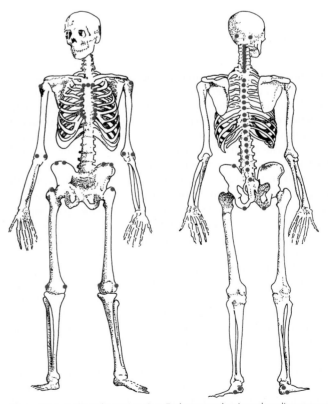

Figure 22.2 Entheseal insertion sites. Entheses are the sites where ligaments and tendons insert into bone. Reproduced from *Annals of the Rheumatic Diseases*, M. Mander et al., Studies with an enthesis index as a method of clinical assessment in ankylosing spondylitis, Volume 46, Issue 3, p. 198, Copyright © 1987, with permission from BMJ Publishing Group Ltd, http://ard.bmj.com/.

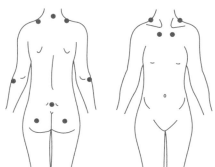

- Tenderness of
  skin overlaying trapezius
- Low cervical spine
- Midpoint of trapezius
- Supraspinatus
- Pectoralis, maximal lateral
  to the second
  costochondral junction
- Lateral epicondyle of
  the elbow
- Upper gluteal area
  Low lumbar spine
- Medial fat pad of the knee

Figure 22.3 Fibromyalgia tender points. Tender points are a hallmark of the generalized musculoskeletal pain of patients with fibromyalgia. Adapted from Hakim, A., Clunie, G., and Haq, I. (eds), *Oxford Handbook of Rheumatology*, 3rd Edition, Oxford University Press, Oxford, UK, pp. 179, Copyright © 2011, by permission of Oxford University Press.

References

Aloush, V., Ablin, J. N., Reitblat, T., Caspi, D., and Elkayam, O. (2007). Fibromyalgia in women with ankylosing spondylitis. *Rheumatol Int*, 27(9), 865–868.

Anonymous. (1993). American academy of pediatrics section on rheumatology and section on ophthalmology: guidelines for ophthalmologic examinations in children with juvenile rheumatoid arthritis. *Pediatrics*, 92(2), 295–296.

Arkela-Kautiainen, M., J. Haapasaari, J., Kautiainen, H., Leppänen, L., Vilkkumaa, I., Mälkiä, E., *et al.* (2006). Functioning and preferences for improvement of health among patients with juvenile idiopathic arthritis in early adulthood using the WHO ICF model. *J Rheumatol*, 33(7), 1369–1376.

Berde, C. B., Beyer, J. E., Bournaki, M. C., Levin, C. R., and Sethna, N. F. (1991). Comparison of morphine and methadone for prevention of postoperative pain in 3- to 7-year-old children. *J Pediatr*, 119(1 Pt 1), 136–141.

Berntson, L., Fasth, A., Andersson-Gäre, B., Kristinsson, J., Lahdenne, P., Marhaug, G. *et al.* (2001). Construct validity of ILAR and EULAR criteria in juvenile idiopathic arthritis: a population based incidence study from the Nordic countries. International League of Associations for Rheumatology. European League Against Rheumatism. *J Rheumatol*, 28(12), 2737–2743.

Beukelman, T., Patkar, N. M., Saag, K. G., Tolleson-Rinehart, S., Cron, R. Q., DeWitt, E. M., *et al.* (2011). 2011 American College of Rheumatology recommendations for the treatment of juvenile idiopathic arthritis: initiation and safety monitoring of therapeutic agents for the treatment of arthritis and systemic features. *Arthritis Care Res*, 63(4), 465–482.

Bloom, B. J., Owens, J. A., McGuinn, M., Nobile, C., Schaeffer, L., and Alario, A. J. (2002). Sleep and its relationship to pain, dysfunction, and disease activity in juvenile rheumatoid arthritis. *J Rheumatol*, 29(1), 169–173.

Bowyer, S. and Roettcher, P. (1996). Pediatric rheumatology clinic populations in the United States: results of a 3 year survey. Pediatric Rheumatology Database Research Group. *J Rheumatol*, 23(11), 1968–1974.

Brewer, E. J.Jr., Bass, J., Baum, J., Cassidy, J. T., Fink, C., Jacobs, J., *et al.* (1977). Current proposed revision of JRA Criteria. JRA Criteria Subcommittee of the Diagnostic and Therapeutic Criteria Committee of the American Rheumatism Section of The Arthritis Foundation. *Arthritis Rheum*, 20(2 Suppl), 195–199.

Brewer, E. J.Jr., Bass, J., and Caassidy, T. J. (1972). Criteria for the classification of juvenile rheumatoid arthritis. *Bull Rheum Dis*, 23(5), 712–719.

Bromberg, M. H., Gil, K. M., and Schanberg, L. E. (2012). Daily sleep quality and mood as predictors of pain in children with juvenile polyarticular arthritis. *Health Psychol*, 31(2), 202–209.

Brown, R., Kraus, C., Fleming, M., and Reddy, S. (2004). Methadone: applied pharmacology and use as adjunctive treatment in chronic pain. *Postgrad Med J*, 80(949), 654–659.

Connelly, M., Anthony, K. K., Sarniak, R., Bromberg, M. H., Gil, K. M., and Schanberg, L. E. (2010). Parent pain responses as predictors of daily activities and mood in children with juvenile idiopathic arthritis: the utility of electronic diaries. *J Pain Symptom Manage*, 39(3), 579–590.

Connelly, M., Bromberg, M. H., Anthony, K. K., Gil, K. M., Franks, L., and Schanberg, L. E. (2012). Emotion regulation predicts pain and functioning in children with juvenile idiopathic arthritis: an electronic diary study. *J Pediatr Psychol*, 37(1), 43–52.

Connelly, M., Keefe, F. J., Affleck, G., Lumley, M. A., Anderson, T., and Waters, S. (2007). Effects of day-to-day affect regulation on the pain experience of patients with rheumatoid arthritis. *Pain*, 131(1–2), 162–170.

Connelly, M. and Schanberg, L. (2006). Opioid therapy for the treatment of refractory pain in children with juvenile rheumatoid arthritis. *Nat Clin Pract Rheumatol*, 2(12), 636–637.

Dell'Era, L., Facchini, R., and Corona, F. (2008). Knee synovectomy in children with juvenile idiopathic arthritis. *J Pediatr Orthop*, B17(3), 128–130.

DeWitt, E. M., Kimura, Y., Beukelman, T., Nigrovic, P. A., Onel, K., Prahalad, S., et al. (2012). Consensus treatment plans for new-onset systemic juvenile idiopathic arthritis. *Arthritis Care Res (Hoboken)*, 64(7), 1001–1010.

Eccleston, C. and Crombez, G. (2007). Worry and chronic pain: a misdirected problem solving model. *Pain*, 132(3), 233–236.

Field, T., Hernandez-Reif, M., Seligman, S., Krasnegor, J., Sunshine, W., Rivas-Chacon, R., *et al.* (1997). Juvenile rheumatoid arthritis: benefits from massage therapy. *J Pediatr Psychol*, 22(5), 607–617.

Fink, C. W. (1995). Proposal for the development of classification criteria for idiopathic arthritides of childhood. *J Rheumatol*, 22(8), 1566–1569.

Fitzcharles, M. A., and Boulos, P. (2003). Inaccuracy in the diagnosis of fibromyalgia syndrome: analysis of referrals. *Rheumatology*, 42(2), 263–267.

Fitzcharles, M.-A., and Esdaile, J. M. (1997). The overdiagnosis of fibromyalgia syndrome. *Am J Med*, 103(1), 44–50.

Foeldvari, I., Szer, I. S., Zemel, L. S., Lovell, D. J., Giannini, E. H., Robbins, J. L., *et al.* (2009). A prospective study comparing celecoxib with naproxen in children with juvenile rheumatoid arthritis. *J Rheumatol*, 36(1), 174–182.

Foster, H. E., Kay, L. J., Friswell, M., Coady, D., and Myers, A. (2006). Musculoskeletal screening examination (pGALS) for school-age children based on the adult GALS screen. *Arthritis Rheum* 55(5), 709–716.

Foster, H. E., Marshall, N., Myers, A., Dunkley, P., and Griffiths, I. D. (2003). Outcome in adults with juvenile idiopathic arthritis: a quality of life study. *Arthritis Rheum*, 48(3), 767–775.

Garcia-Munitis, P., Bandeira, M., Pistorio, A., Magni-Manzoni, S., Ruperto, N., Schivo, A., *et al.* (2006). Level of agreement between children, parents, and physicians in rating pain intensity in juvenile idiopathic arthritis. *Arthritis Rheum*, 55(2), 177–183.

Giannini, E. H., Brewer, E. J., Miller, M. L., Gibbas, D., Passo, M. H., Hoyeraal, H. M., *et al.* (1990). Ibuprofen suspension in the treatment of juvenile rheumatoid arthritis. Pediatric Rheumatology Collaborative Study Group. *J Pediatr*, 117(4), 645–652.

Giannini, M. J., and Protas, E. J. (1991). Aerobic capacity in juvenile rheumatoid arthritis patients and healthy children. *Arthritis Care Res*, 4(3), 131–135.

Giordano, J. (2006). The neuroscience of pain and analgesia. In M. Boswell, B. E. Cole, and R. S. Weiner, (eds) *Weiner's pain management: a guide for clinicians*, pp. 15–34. Boca Raton, FL: CRC Taylor & Francis.

Gossec, L., Pavy, S., Pham, T., Constantin, A., Poiraudeau, S., Combe, B., *et al.* (2006). Nonpharmacological treatments in early rheumatoid arthritis: clinical practice guidelines based on published evidence and expert opinion. *Joint Bone Spine*, 73(4), 396–402.

Hagglund, K. J., Schopp, L. M., Alberts, K. R., Cassidy, J. T., and Frank, R. G. (1995). Predicting pain among children with juvenile rheumatoid arthritis. *Arthritis Care Res*, 8(1), 36–42.

Haverman, L., Verhoof, E. J., Maurice-Stam, H., Heymans, H. S., Gerlag, D. M., van Rossum, M. A., *et al.* (2012). Health-related quality of life and psychosocial developmental trajectory in young female beneficiaries with JIA. *Rheumatology*, 51(2), 368–374.

Heiligenhaus, A., Niewerth, M., Ganser, G., Heinz, C., and Minden, K. (2007). Prevalence and complications of uveitis in juvenile idiopathic arthritis in a population-based nation-wide study in Germany: suggested modification of the current screening guidelines. *Rheumatology*, 46(6), 1015–1019.

Hoff, A. L., Palermo, T. M., Schluchter, M., Zebracki, K., and Drotar, D. (2006). Longitudinal relationships of depressive symptoms to pain intensity and functional disability among children with disease-related pain. *J Pediatr Psychol*, 31(10), 1046–1056.

Huber, A. M., Tomlinson, G. A., Koren, G., and Feldman, B. M. (2007). Amitriptyline to relieve pain in juvenile idiopathic arthritis: a pilot study using Bayesian metaanalysis of multiple N-of-1 clinical trials. *J Rheumatol*, 34(5), 1125–1132.

Iesaka, K., Kubiak, E. N., Bong, M. R., Su, E. T., and Di Cesare, P. E. (2006). Orthopedic surgical management of hip and knee involvement in patients with juvenile rheumatoid arthritis. *Am J Orthop (Belle Mead NJ)*, 35(2), 67–73.

Iobst, E., Nabors, L., Brunner, H. I., and Precht, B. (2007). Pain, fatigue, family functioning, and attitude toward illness in children with juvenile rheumatic diseases. *J Dev Phys Disabil*, 19(2), 135–144.

Kalso, E., Edwards, J. E., Brunner, H. I., and Precht, B. (2004). Opioids in chronic non-cancer pain: systematic review of efficacy and safety. *Pain*, 112(3), 372–380.

Kidd, B. L., and Urban, L. A. (2001). Mechanisms of inflammatory pain. *Br J Anaesth*, 87(1), 3–11.

Kimura, Y. and Walco, G. A. (2007). Treatment of chronic pain in pediatric rheumatic disease. *Nat Clin Pract Rheumatol*, 3(4), 210–218.

Kimura, Y., Walco, G. A., Sugarman, E., Conte, P. M., and Schanberg, L. E. (2006). Treatment of pain in juvenile idiopathic arthritis: a survey of pediatric rheumatologists. *Arthritis Rheum*, 55(1), 81–85.

Klepper, S. E. (1999). Effects of an eight-week physical conditioning program on disease signs and symptoms in children with chronic arthritis. *Arthritis Care Res*, 12(1), 52–60.

Klepper, S. E. (2008). Exercise in pediatric rheumatic diseases. *Curr Opin Rheumatol*, 20(5), 619–624.

Klepper, S. E., and Giannini, M. J. (1994). Physical conditioning in children with arthritis: assessment and guidelines for exercise prescription. *Arthritis Care Res*, 7(4), 226–236.

Kunjir, V., Venugopalan, A., and Chopra, A. (2010). Profile of Indian patients with juvenile onset chronic inflammatory joint disease using the ILAR classification criteria for JIA: a community-based cohort study. *J Rheumatol*, 37(8), 1756–1762.

Laaksonen, A. L., and Laine, V. (1961). A comparative study of joint pain in adult and juvenile rheumatoid arthritis. *Ann Rheum Dis*, 20, 386–387.

Lal, S. D., McDonagh, J., Baildam, E., Wedderburn, L. R., Gardner-Medwin, J., Foster, H. E., *et al.* (2011). Agreement between proxy and adolescent assessment of disability, pain, and well-being in juvenile idiopathic arthritis. *J Pediatr*, 158(2), 307–312.

Lang, B. A., and Finlayson, L. A. (1994). Naproxen-induced pseudoporphyria in patients with juvenile rheumatoid arthritis. *J Pediatr*, 124(4), 639–642.

Lavigne, J. V., Ross, C. K., Berry, S. L., Hayford, J. R., and Pachman, L. M. (1992). Evaluation of a psychological treatment package for treating pain in juvenile rheumatoid arthritis. *Arthritis Care Res*, 5(2), 101–110.

Laxer, R. M., Silverman, E. D., St-Cyr, C., Tran, M. T., and Lingam, G. (1988). A six-month open safety assessment of a naproxen suspension formulation in the therapy of juvenile rheumatoid arthritis. *Clin Ther*, 10(4), 381–387.

Lovell, D. J., Passo, M. H., Beukelman, T., Bowyer, S. L., Gottlieb, B. S., Henrickson, M., *et al.* (2011). Measuring process of arthritis care: a proposed set of quality measures for the process of care in juvenile idiopathic arthritis. *Arthritis Care Res*, 63(1), 10–16.

Malleson, P. N., Oen, K., Cabral, D. A., Petty, R. E., Rosenberg, A. M., and Cheang, M. (2004). Predictors of pain in children with established juvenile rheumatoid arthritis. *Arthritis Rheum*, 51(2), 222–227.

Manchikanti, L., Ailinani, H., Koyyalagunta, D., Datta, S., Singh, V., Eriator, I. *et al.* (2011). A systematic review of randomized trials of long-term opioid management for chronic non-cancer pain. *Pain Physician*, 14(2), 91–121.

Margetic, B., Aukst-Margetic, B., Bilić, E., Jelusić, M., and Tambić Bukovac, L. (2005). Depression, anxiety and pain in children with juvenile idiopathic arthritis (JIA). *Eur Psychiatry*, 20(3), 274–276.

McDougall, J. J. (2006). Arthritis and pain. Neurogenic origin of joint pain. *Arthritis Res Ther*, 8(6), 220.

McDougall, J. J., and Larson, S. E. (2006). Nociceptin/orphanin FQ evokes knee joint pain in rats via a mast cell independent mechanism. *Neurosci Lett*, 398(1–2), 135–138.

McGhee, J. L., Burks, F. N., Sheckels, J. L., and Jarvis, J. N. (2002). Identifying children with chronic arthritis based on chief complaints: absence of predictive value for musculoskeletal pain as an indicator of rheumatic disease in children. *Pediatrics*, 110(2 Pt 1), 354–359.

McGrath, P. J., Walco, G. A., Turk, D. C., Dworkin, R. H., Brown, M. T., Davidson, K., *et al.* (2008). Core outcome domains and measures for pediatric acute and chronic/recurrent pain clinical trials: PedIMMPACT recommendations. *J Pain*, 9(9), 771–783.

Merino, R., De Inocencio, J., and García-Consuegra, J. (2001). Evaluation of ILAR classification criteria for juvenile idiopathic arthritis in Spanish children. *J Rheumatol*, 28(12), 2731–2736.

Milligan, E. D., and Watkins, L. R. (2009). Pathological and protective roles of glia in chronic pain. *Nat Rev Neurosci*, 10(1), 23–36.

Nicholls, A., Hazleman, B., Todd, R. M., Murray-Leslie, C., Kühnen, H., and Cain, A. R. (1982). Long-term evaluation of naproxen suspension in juvenile chronic arthritis. *Curr Med Res Opin*, 8(3), 204–207.

Oen, K., Malleson, P. N., Cabral, D. A., Rosenberg, A. M., Petty, R. E., Nickerson, P., *et al.* (2005). Cytokine genotypes correlate with pain and radiologically defined joint damage in patients with juvenile rheumatoid arthritis. *Rheumatology*, 44(9), 1115–1121.

Palermo, T. M. (2000). Impact of recurrent and chronic pain on child and family daily functioning: a critical review of the literature. *J Dev Behav Pediatr*, 21(1), 58–69.

Palermo, T. M., Eccleston, C., Lewandowski, A. S., Williams, A. C., and Morley, S. (2010). Randomized controlled trials of psychological therapies for management of chronic pain in children and adolescents: an updated meta-analytic review. *Pain*, 148(3), 387–397.

Palermo, T. M., Zebracki, K., Cox, S., Newman, A. J., and Singer, N. G. (2004). Juvenile idiopathic arthritis: parent-child discrepancy on reports of pain and disability. *J Rheumatol*, 31(9), 1840–1846.

Parvizi, J., Lajam, C. M., Trousdale, R. T., Shaughnessy, W. J., and Cabanela, M. E. (2003). Total knee arthroplasty in young patients with juvenile rheumatoid arthritis. *J Bone Joint Surg Am*, 85-A(6), 1090–1094.

Petty, R. E. (2001). Growing pains: the ILAR classification of juvenile idiopathic arthritis. *J Rheumatol*, 28(5), 927–928.

Petty, R. E., Southwood, T. R., Baum, J., Bhettay, E., Glass, D. N., Manners, P., *et al.* (1998). Revision of the proposed classification criteria for juvenile idiopathic arthritis: Durban, 1997. *J Rheumatol*, 25(10), 1991–1994.

Petty, R. E., Southwood, T. R., Baum, J., Bhettay, E., Glass, D. N., Manners, P., *et al.* (2004). International League of Associations for Rheumatology classification of juvenile idiopathic arthritis: second revision, Edmonton, 2001. *J Rheumatol*, 31(2), 390–392.

Powell, M., Seid, M., and Szer, I. S. (2005). Efficacy of custom foot orthotics in improving pain and functional status in children with juvenile idiopathic arthritis: a randomized trial. *J Rheumatol*, 32(5), 943–950.

Rapoff, M. A., and Lindsley, C. B. (2000). The pain puzzle: a visual and conceptual metaphor for understanding and treating pain in pediatric rheumatic disease. *J Rheumatol Suppl*, 58: 29–33.

Ravelli, A., Varnier, G. C., Oliveira, S., Castell, E., Arguedas, O., and Magnani, A. (2011). Antinuclear antibody-positive patients should be grouped as a separate category in the classification of juvenile idiopathic arthritis. *Arthritis Rheum*, 63(1), 267–275.

Reid, G. J., McGrath, P. J., and Lang. B. A. (2005). Parent-child interactions among children with juvenile fibromyalgia, arthritis, and healthy controls. *Pain*, 113(1–2), 201–210.

Ross, C. K., Lavigne, J. V., Hayford, J. R., Berry, S. L., Sinacore, J. M., and Pachman, L. M. (1993). Psychological factors affecting reported pain in juvenile rheumatoid arthritis. *J Pediatr Psychol*, 18(5), 561–573.

Roth-Isigkeit, A., Thyen, U., Stöven, H., Schwarzenberger, J., and Schmucker, P. (2005). Pain among children and adolescents: restrictions in daily living and triggering factors. *Pediatrics*, 115(2), e152–e162.

Ruperto, N., Nikishina, I., Pachanov, E. D., Shachbazian, Y., Prieur, A. M., Mouy, R., *et al.* (2005). A randomized, double-blind clinical trial of two doses of meloxicam compared with naproxen in children with juvenile idiopathic arthritis: short- and long-term efficacy and safety results. *Arthritis Rheum*, 52(2), 563–572.

Sawyer, M. G., Whitham, J. N., Roberton, D. M., Taplin, J. E., Varni, J. W., and Baghurst, P. A. (2004). The relationship between health-related quality of life, pain and coping strategies in juvenile idiopathic arthritis. *Rheumatology*, 43(3), 325–330.

Schaible, H. G., Del Rosso, A., and Matucci-Cerinic, M. (2005). Neurogenic aspects of inflammation. *Rheum Dis Clin North Am*, 31(1), 77–101, ix.

Schaible, H. G., Ebersberger, A., Von Banchet, G. S. (2002). Mechanisms of pain in arthritis. *Ann N Y Acad Sci*, 966: 343–354.

Schaible, H. G., Richter, F., Ebersberger, A., Boettger, M. K., Vanegas, H., Natura, G., *et al.* (2009). Joint pain. *Exp Brain Res*, 196(1), 153–162.

Schaible, H. G., Schmelz, M., and Tedeger, I. (2006). Pathophysiology and treatment of pain in joint disease. *Adv Drug Deliv Rev*, 58(2), 323–342.

Schanberg, L. E., Anthony, K. K., Gil, K. M., Lefebvre, J. C., Kredich, D. W., and Macharoni, L. M. (2001). Family pain history predicts child health status in children with chronic rheumatic disease. *Pediatrics*, 108(3), E47.

Schanberg, L. E., Anthony, K. K., Gil, K. M., and Maurin, E. C. (2003). Daily pain and symptoms in children with polyarticular arthritis. *Arthritis Rheum*, 48(5), 1390–1397.

Schanberg, L. E., Gil, K. M., Anthony, K. K., Yow, E., and Rochon, J. (2005). Pain, stiffness, and fatigue in juvenile polyarticular arthritis: contemporaneous stressful events and mood as predictors. *Arthritis Rheum*, 52(4), 1196–1204.

Schanberg, L. E., Lefebvre, J. C., Keefe, F. J., Kredich, D. W., and Gil, K. M. (1997). Pain coping and the pain experience in children with juvenile chronic arthritis. *Pain*, 73(2), 181–189.

Schanberg, L. E., Sandstrom, M. J., Starr, K., Gil, K. M., Lefebvre, J. C., Keefe, F. J., *et al.* (2000). The relationship of daily mood and stressful events to symptoms in juvenile rheumatic disease. *Arthritis Care Res*, 13(1), 33–41.

Seifert, F., and Maihofner, C. (2009). Central mechanisms of experimental and chronic neuropathic pain: findings from functional imaging studies. *Cell Mol Life Sci*, 66(3), 375–390.

Shir, Y., Shenkman, Z., Shavelson, V., Davidson, E. M., and Rosen, G. (1998). Oral methadone for the treatment of severe pain in hospitalized children: a report of five cases. *Clin J Pain*, 14(4), 350–353.

Singh-Grewal, D., Schneiderman-Walker, J., Wright, V., Bar-Or, O., Beyene, J., Selvadurai, H., *et al.* (2007). The effects of vigorous exercise training on physical function in children with arthritis: a randomized, controlled, single-blinded trial. *Arthritis Rheum*, 57(7), 1202–1210.

Singh-Grewal, D., Wright, V., Bar-Or, O., and Feldman, B. M. (2006). Pilot study of fitness training and exercise testing in polyarticular childhood arthritis. *Arthritis Rheum*, 55(3), 364–372.

Slater, M.-E., De Lima, J., Campbell, K., Lane, L., and Collins, J. (2010). Opioids for the management of severe chronic nonmalignant pain in children: a retrospective 1-year practice survey in a children's hospital. *Pain Med*, 11(2), 207–214.

Steans, A., Manners, P. J., and Robinson, I. G. (1990). A multicentre, long-term evaluation of the safety and efficacy of ibuprofen syrup in children with juvenile chronic arthritis. *Br J Clin Pract*, 44(5), 172–175.

Stinson, J. N., Connelly, M., Jibb, L. A., Schanberg, L. E., Walco, G., Spiegel, L. R., *et al.* (2012). Developing a standardized approach to the assessment of pain in children and youth presenting to pediatric rheumatology providers: a Delphi survey and consensus conference process followed by feasibility testing. *Pediatr Rheumatol Online J*, 10(1), 7.

Stinson, J. N., Petroz, G. C., Tait, G., Feldman, B. M., Streiner, D., McGrath, P. J., *et al.* (2006). e-Ouch: usability testing of an electronic chronic pain diary for adolescents with arthritis. *Clin J Pain*, 22(3), 295–305.

Stinson, J. N., Stevens, B. J., Feldman, B. M., Streiner, D., McGrath, P. J., Dupuis, A., *et al.* (2008). Construct validity of a multidimensional electronic pain diary for adolescents with arthritis. *Pain*, 136(3), 281–292.

Takken, T., Van Brussel, M., Engelbert, R. H., Van Der Net, J., Kuis, W., and Helders, P. J. (2008). Exercise therapy in juvenile idiopathic arthritis: a Cochrane Review. *Eur J Phys Rehabil Med*, 44(3), 287–297.

Thastum, M. and Herlin, T. (2011). Pain-specific beliefs and pain experience in children with juvenile idiopathic arthritis: a longitudinal study. *J Rheumatol*, 38(1), 155–160.

Thastum, M., Herlin, T., and Zachariae R. (2005). Relationship of pain-coping strategies and pain-specific beliefs to pain experience in children with juvenile idiopathic arthritis. *Arthritis Rheum*, 53(2), 178–184.

Thastum, M., Zachariae, R., and Herlin, T. (2001). Pain experience and pain coping strategies in children with juvenile idiopathic arthritis. *J Rheumatol*, 28(5), 1091–1098.

Thastum, M., Zachariae, R., Schøler, M., Bjerring, P., and Herlin, T. (1997). Cold pressor pain: comparing responses of juvenile arthritis patients and their parents. *Scand J Rheumatol*, 26(4), 272–279.

Thompson, K. L., Varni, J. W., and Hanson, V. (1987). Comprehensive assessment of pain in juvenile rheumatoid arthritis: an empirical model. *J Pediatr Psychol*, 12(2), 241–255.

Tong, A., Jones, J., Craig, J. C., and Singh-Grewal, D. (2012). Children's experiences of living with juvenile idiopathic arthritis: thematic synthesis of qualitative studies. *Arthritis Care Res*, 64(9), 1392–1404.

Tynjälä, P., Vähäsalo, P., Tarkiainen, M., Kröger, L., Aalto, K., Malin, M., *et al.* (2011). Aggressive combination drug therapy in very early polyarticular juvenile idiopathic arthritis (ACUTE–JIA), a multicentre randomised open-label clinical trial. *Ann Rheum Dis*, 70(9), 1605–1612.

Vandvik, I. H., and Eckblad, G. (1990). Relationship between pain, disease severity and psychosocial function in patients with juvenile chronic arthritis (JCA). *Scand J Rheumatol*, 19(4), 295–302.

Varni, J. W., Thompson, K. L., and Hanson, V. (1987). The Varni/Thompson Pediatric Pain Questionnaire. I. Chronic musculoskeletal pain in juvenile rheumatoid arthritis. *Pain*, 28(1), 27–38.

Walco, G. A., Varni, J. W., and Ilowite, N. T. (1992). Cognitive-behavioral pain management in children with juvenile rheumatoid arthritis. *Pediatrics*, 89(6 Pt 1), 1075–1079.

Wallace, C. A., Giannini, E. H., Spalding, S. J., Hashkes, P. J., O'Neil, K. M., Zeft, A. S., *et al.* (2012). Trial of early aggressive therapy in polyarticular juvenile idiopathic arthritis. *Arthritis Rheum*, 64(6), 2012–2021.

Wallen, M. and Gillies, D. (2006). Intra-articular steroids and splints/rest for children with juvenile idiopathic arthritis and adults with rheumatoid arthritis. *Cochrane Database Syst Rev*, 1, CD002824.

Whittle, S. L., Richards, B. L., Husni, E., and Buchbinder, R. (2011). Opioid therapy for treating rheumatoid arthritis pain. *Cochrane Database Syst Rev*, 11, CD003113.

Wong, K. O., Bond, K., Homik, J., Ellsworth, J. E., Karkhaneh, M., Ha, C., *et al.* (2012). *Antinuclear antibody, rheumatoid factor, and cyclic-citrullinated peptide tests for evaluating musculoskeletal complaints in children*. AHRQ Comparative Effectiveness Reviews. Rockville, MD: Agency for Healthcare Research and Quality (US).

Wood, P. (1978). Special meeting on: nomenclature and classification of arthritis in children. In E. Munthe, (ed.) *The Care of Rheumatic Children*, pp. 47–50. Basel: EULAR.

Woolf, C. J., and Salter, M. W. (2000). Neuronal plasticity: increasing the gain in pain. *Science*, 288(5472), 1765–1769.

Zeltzer, L., Bursch, B., and Walco, G. (1997). Pain responsiveness and chronic pain: a psychobiological perspective. *J Dev Behav Pediatr*, 18(6), 413–422.

CHAPTER 23

Chronic pain syndromes in childhood: one trunk, many branches

Neil L. Schechter

Summary

Although this volume is replete with detailed discussions about specific pain problems, the focus of this chapter is on a discussion of the commonalities in aetiology, associated symptoms, and treatment of many of the frequent chronic pain problems. We will explore in brief the data that demonstrates the co-occurrence of many of the common chronic pain problems in children and the epidemiological similarities that exist between affected individuals. Then we will review the concept of central sensitization and the physiological evidence that supports its presence in many of the functional pain problems. We will briefly review some of the symptoms associated with these entities (orthostatic intolerance, sleep disturbance, depression, anxiety, hypermobility, family distress). Finally, we will discuss briefly a general approach to these problems emphasizing the collection of specific information in the history and physical examination, the critically important presentation of the formulation to the family, and the treatment modalities that appear to be effective for many of these conditions. In-depth discussion of each of these pain problems is available in chapters specifically designated to review them in detail.

Introduction

In this chapter, we will highlight relevant issues around the frequent co-occurrence of common chronic pains. This overlap may easily escape the notice of busy specialists who tend to focus on the specific symptoms most relevant to their discipline. For example, it would not be unusual for a child who is being evaluated for persistent abdominal pain by a gastroenterologist to simultaneously be experiencing headache or widespread musculoskeletal pain. Because these symptoms are not the focus or expertise of the gastroenterologist, he or she may ignore these additional symptoms assuming that they will be addressed by others. As a result, the frequency with which these pains co-occur and the similarities in their aetiology and treatment may not be fully appreciated. By the end of this chapter, we hope that the reader will appreciate the importance of recognizing the common elements that bind these entities together and the importance of their simultaneous evaluation and treatment. Such an approach will hopefully reduce the burden of unnecessary investigation and treatment in these children who are often already overwhelmed by the collective efforts of the medical community.

Epidemiology of chronic pain in children

There has been long-standing recognition that children and adolescents experience chronic pain and that it is a relatively common experience for them. In a large community sample, Perquin et al. (2000) reported an incidence of chronic pain (defined as recurrent or continuous pain for more than 3 months) of 25% with headache, abdominal pain, and limb pain the most common presentations. There have been multiple other large-scale surveys which report a similar incidence.

Additionally, the co-occurrence of chronic pain problems has been recognized for many years in the adult literature. Table 23.1 presents selected data adapted from a comprehensive review of this subject by Yunus (2007a). He summarizes the data which demonstrates the likelihood of having a second chronic pain syndrome in individuals who have at least one. For example, he reports that the prevalence of irritable bowel syndrome is 45% in individuals with fibromyalgia (with a range of 32–70% depending on the study). Yunus identified the co-occurrence of fibromyalgia, chronic fatigue syndrome, irritable bowel syndrome, tension and migraine headaches, temporomandibular disorders, primary dysmenorrhoeal pain, post-traumatic stress disorder, and multiple chemical sensitivities. As is evident from this chart of studies on adults, there is frequent overlap among these entities which Yunus calls central sensitivity syndromes based on his hypothesis of their aetiology.

The overlap of these syndromes in the paediatric population is a more recent discovery. Although Zuckerman et al. (1987) noted the frequent coexistence (22%) of headache and stomach aches in preschool children in England when surveying the community for the incidence of these pain problems, the significance of this overlap in children was not a focus of research in the paediatric literature until 1997, when Krstjansdottir (1997) studied this phenomenon

Table 23.1 Associations among central sensitivity syndromes (CSS)

Condition	Mean prevalence (%) of another CSS in patients with this condition (range of %)	Total no. of studies	Total no. patients
FMS	CFS 39 (22–74)	6	214
	IBS 45 (32–70)	17	1776
	Migraine 38 (22–49)	3	183
	UHA 50 (35–56)	5	558
	TTH 42 (22–60)	5	889
CFS	FMS 48 (16–80)	2	57
	IBS 36	1	25
IBS	FMS 36 (28–65)	5	179
	CFS 14	1	200
	UHA 42 (31–50)	3	297
Migraine	CFS 51	1	63

FMS = fibromyalgia syndrome; IBS = irritable bowel syndrome; TTH = tension headache; UHA= unspecified headache.

Adapted from *Seminars in Arthritis and Rheumatism*, Volume 36, Issue 6, Muhammad B. Yunus, Fibromyalgia and overlapping disorders: the unifying concept of central sensitivity syndromes, pp. 339–356, Copyright © 2007, with permission from Elsevier, http://www.sciencedirect.com/science/journal/00490172.

directly. She reported that over a 3-month period, 21% of children who had one pain had at least one other. Subsequently, other investigators found a co-occurrence rate that ranged from a low of 5% (Larsson and Sund, 2007) to a high of 50% (Kroner-Herwig et al., 2011) depending on definitions of chronic pain. Fichtel and Larsson (2002) found that almost 15% of their Scandinavian sample of children with chronic pain had four or more pain sites.

Shared biological and clinical features

The recognition that multiple pain sites are common in individuals who have chronic pain has prompted a more in-depth look for similarities between these entities. The fact of their frequent co-occurrence has significant research implications as it requires an explanatory model that is broader than focus on a specific end organ (stomach, back, head, etc.). It is not only the frequency of overlap of these entities that is noteworthy, however, but also the co-occurrence of many other associated features. These include female predominance, association with psychological disorders, school and sleep disruption, frequent fatigue and loss of mental clarity. Additionally, many of the same centrally acting non-specific treatments (exercise, stress reduction, acupuncture, neuromodulating drugs such as antidepressants and anticonvulsants) are effective for these all of these syndromes. These shared characteristics provide further support for the linkage of these entities and add to the critical importance of a multidisciplinary approach which allows the insights of researchers who had been narrowly exploring one type of pain to influence the thinking of those exploring other pain problems. In this section, we will review the evidence that supports the existence of the numerous commonalities among these entities. Because much of the work stems from adult research, we will use the schema devised by Mayer and Bushnell (2009) in the final section of their seminal volume on functional pain syndromes where they attempt to synthesize what we have learned about the inter-relationship of these common problems in adults and add paediatric data where it is available.

Evidence for shared biological mechanisms

Although the data is still emerging, it appears from multiple streams of evidence that many of the functional pain syndromes are associated with abnormalities of nociceptive processing which may account for the fact that individuals with these conditions often experience severe pain without evidence of structural pathology or other physiological derangement. This may result from, depending on the condition and situation, enhanced neurotransmission stemming from hyperarousal of central neurons (central sensitization) (Geisser et al., 2008; Giesecke et al., 2004; Woolff, 2001), autonomic nervous system dysfunction (Janig, 2009), hypothalamic–pituitary–adrenal axis dysfunction (Chang et al., 2009), and/or from dysfunction of descending pain modulatory abilities (Johannesson et al., 2007; Lautenbacher and Rollman, 1997). Even though the mechanistic details require more research and may vary from individual to individual, there is a robust literature which suggests that individuals with functional pain syndromes often have an altered response to clinical and experimental pain exemplified by increased spontaneous firing, decreased threshold, increased response amplitude, expanded receptive field. This is evident on both oral reports of increased pain in clinical situations and on laboratory induced pain as well as on functional magnetic resonance imaging evaluations which suggest an altered pain response in individuals with chronic pain as compared to controls.

This recognition has led a number of investigators to conclude that at their core, many of these entities have a similar aetiology—a hypersensitivity to noxious and non-noxious stimuli typically known as central sensitization (Woolf, 2011) which is multifactorial in origin. In fact, Yunus (2007a, 2008) has recently clustered a number of these entities together under the rubric of 'central sensitivity disorders' implying the centrality of central sensitization in their aetiology. He identified research that demonstrated an altered response to pressure, heat, cold, and auditory sensations in adults with migraine, fibromyalgia, and irritable bowel syndrome. Similarly, Von Baeyer and Champion (2011) conclude that these problems are all manifestations of an underlying pain vulnerability which stems from multiple sources but yields similar outcomes.

The origins for this increased susceptibility to pain are quite complex and not fully understood and likely vary from individual to individual. Mayer and Bushnell (2009) and Yunus (2007b) have suggested that this alteration may emerge from multiple mechanisms, both biological and social. These may include genetic predisposition, anxiety or depression, increased psychosocial stressors, early life adversity, infections, and/or inflammation. Microtrauma such as that stemming from hypermobility or overuse may also play a role. These factors may impact on the central nervous system and cause the hyperexcitability that is called central sensitization which they feel is the core biological link and final common pathway to the creation of functional pain disorders. Other models suggest while acknowledging the centrality of central sensitization that psychological factors exert their influence independently and not necessarily through a hyperexcited central neurons.

As should be evident from the preceding discussion, if one assumes that functional pain disorders emerge from a composite of biological vulnerabilities and psychosocial factors which jointly create abnormalities of pain processing or the misperception of those signals, then the notion that pain can be categorized as strictly physical or psychological is highly outdated and in fact destructive. Unfortunately, however, many families may become frustrated by the traditional approach to unexplained pain—extensive laboratory investigation and imaging which if negative results in referral to a mental health professional. It is essential that the child and family understand that declaring the pain syndrome to be functional does not at all imply psychogenesis. The pain itself is the disease.

Shared clinical features

Besides abnormalities of nociceptive processing, there are a number of other clinical and epidemiological characteristics of functional pain syndromes that link them together—they occur predominantly in females, there is often a family history of pain problems, there is an association with early life trauma, and they frequently occur in individuals with specific personality types and mental health disorders. Additionally, they often co-occur with other clinical conditions in which there is autonomic dysregulation such as postural orthostatic tachycardia syndrome. Finally, they all seem to respond, at least somewhat, to centrally acting interventions such as anticonvulsants and antidepressants, exercise, acupuncture, stress management, and cognitive-behavioural therapy.

Greater prevalence in girls and women

For reasons that are not entirely clear at this time, adolescent girls and women are much more likely to experience chronic pain than boys and men. In community-based studies, girls are twice as likely as boys to report chronic pain (Perquin et al., 2001). A similar finding is reported in analyses of paediatric chronic pain attendees where in one study, 73% were female (Vetter, 2008). The numbers vary depending on the study but the incidence of abdominal pain, fibromyalgia, and migraine headache is much higher in girls than in boys. Although there is much speculation as to the origin of these differences, the finding that girls report more chronic pain than boys is robust and consistent. There is certainly precedent for sex differences in neurological phenomena. For example, the incidence of attention deficit-hyperactivity disorder, enuresis, and learning disabilities is much higher in boys than girls.

Family history

There is strong evidence that chronic pain problems tend to run in families. This is most likely due to a number of factors including the genetics of nociception, genetic inheritance of painful conditions, and parental modelling of pain behaviour.

Studies have attempted to evaluate the relative contributions of genetics to variations in pain sensitivity, in both animals and humans (Foulkes and Wood, 2008). For example, Mogil and colleagues compared the pain thresholds within and between 11 inbred laboratory mouse strains using multiple laboratory-induced pain modalities and identified significant genetic contributions to nociception and a variety of candidate genes (Mogil et al., 1999).

In addition to experimentally induced pain, several studies have investigated the genetic contribution to differences in severity of and susceptibility to certain chronic pain conditions. A recent study by Kato and colleagues which included 15,950 pairs of twins, found a genetic contribution of about 50% to the likelihood of developing fibromyalgia (Kato et al., 2006). The inheritance of other chronic pain problems has been studied. Migraines (with and without aura) all have a substantial risk of familial recurrence. Concordance rates for migraine are consistently higher among monozygotic than dizygotic twins (Montagna, 2008). Thirty-three per cent of individuals with irritable bowel syndrome have a family history (Whorwell et al., 1986). There is similar data for other central sensitivity syndromes.

Additionally, a number of environmental characteristics may play an important role. Parental modelling of pain behaviour has been demonstrated to increase pain behaviour in their children. Parents with pain are more likely to have children with pain and children are more likely to have pain sites that are similar to their parents (Evans et al., 2007). Parents' interactions with their children may have a role in influencing the likelihood that the pain will affect the child's functioning (Goodman and McGrath, 2003). The relative contribution of genetics, modelling, and parental response to the pain experience probably varies from child to child but it is clear that chronic pain aggregates in families. Schanberg and colleagues (2001) reviewed the family history of 100 patients seen in a paediatric rheumatology clinic and found that 90% of parents reported at least one chronic pain condition, typically lower back pain, shoulder/neck pain, and migraine headache. On average, parents reported a history of 3.5 chronic pain conditions. Ninety-three per cent of parents reported at least one relative with chronic pain in their immediate family. It is critical therefore that a detailed family history be obtained to further our understanding of the factors contributing to the child's chronic pain.

History of adverse life events

There is an emerging literature on the impact of early life events on the development of nociceptive pathways and on the development of chronic pain subsequently. The strongest work in this field comes from the animal literature in which rodents are subjected to a variety of noxious experiences and the impact of those on subsequent pain responsiveness is assessed. Rat pups subjected to daily foot shocks during their equivalent developmental phase to the human neonatal period demonstrated long-term effects on sensitivity to pain and on their response to morphine subsequently (Shimada et al., 1990). Likewise, rat pups subjected to inflammatory pain, skin wounding, and visceral stimulation such as colorectal distension demonstrated increased visceral sensitivity and other changes in sensory pathways long after the stimulation had ceased (Al-Chaer et al., 2000).

More subtle adverse experiences in animals have also been shown to impact pain sensitivity and pain thresholds as well. In a series of studies, rat pups subjected to maternal separation experienced both a dampening of their stress response as evidenced by decreased stress hormone output and a heightened sensitivity, depending on the timing of the separation. Interestingly, in one study, pregnant rats were subjected to inescapable stress during the last week of pregnancy. Stress appeared to cause cognitive delays, anxiety, and hypersensitivity of the adrenal stress response in their offspring. Together, this work suggests that noxious events early on, both subtle and pronounced, can impact on the subsequent pain experience of rodents (Al-Chaer and Weaver, 2009).

The literature in humans on the relationship of early adverse life events and pain is more tenuous although suggestive of a similar relationship to that found in animals. For example, Hermann and colleagues (2006) compared the responses on quantitative nerve testing between a group of 9- to 14-year-old children who had prolonged time in the neonatal intensive care unit with those who did not. They found that consistent with animal findings, pain experiences in the neonatal period were associated with alterations in thermal pain responsivity in school-aged children who had been born preterm suggesting that those experiences created measurable differences in nociception many years after they had occurred.

Additional literature to support the long term impact of early life events on pain emerges from the abuse literature. Chartier et al. (2007) identified the fact that individuals who had been abused as children had statistically more physical complaints than those who were not abused. In a community sample of women, individuals with chronic pain were far more likely to have an abuse history than those who did not have chronic pain (Walsh et al., 2007). Together, this animal and human research strongly suggests that early life circumstances can alter nociception.

Temperament/personality

A number of studies have investigated the relationship of temperament, generally assumed to be the innate biological underpinning of personality, in children and response to painful procedures. Schechter et al. (1991) in a prospective study identified that children with a 'difficult temperament cluster' were more reactive to immunization than children other children. Chen et al. (2000) constructed a pain-sensitive temperament cluster and found that children with acute lymphocytic leukaemia who rated more highly on that scale were more likely to report a higher level of distress during lumbar punctures than those who did not.

The literature on the relation of personality and chronic pain is a bit more complex and far beyond the scope of this chapter but it is likely that personality may have a role in the development of chronic pain and certainly on one's ability to cope with it.

Comorbidity with disorders of mood and affect

Research on comorbid psychiatric disorders in chronic pain reveals that patients with mental health disorders are significantly overrepresented in chronic pain clinics (Bair et al., 2008; Lynch et al., 2006; Varni et al., 1996; White and Farrell, 2006). The relationship between psychological factors and both acute and chronic pain is extensively explored throughout this volume. There is clearly the need for population-based prospective studies to examine this issue but few could disagree with the frequent co-occurrence of mental

health concerns and pain. Regardless, whether anxiety and depression stem from having chronic pain and/or are precursors to it is less relevant to this discussion than the fact that these disorders require treatment as part of a comprehensive approach to pain.

Response to centrally acting, non-specific therapies

Another intriguing overlap between these disorders is their response to centrally acting and often non-specific treatments. It is clear, for example, that centrally acting drugs such as selective serotonin re-uptake inhibitors and serotonin–noradrenaline reuptake inhibitors, tricyclic antidepressants such as amitriptyline or nortriptyline, and anticonvulsants such as gabapentin or pregabalin seem to decrease chronic pain symptoms in most functional pain syndromes. Additionally, other non-pharmacological approaches such as exercise, stress reduction, cognitive-behavioural strategies, and acupuncture all have demonstrated efficacy in diminishing pain in individuals with many of these pain disorders.

There are numerous studies that support the efficacy of non-specific treatments in chronic pain. For example, amitriptyline appears effective at reducing pain in functional abdominal pain, tension and migraine headaches, and in fibromyalgia (Goldenberg et al., 1996; Hershey et al., 2000; Rajagopalani et al., 1998). Likewise, there is evidence that both exercise and acupuncture is also effective for all three of these entities (Drossman, 1999; Köseoglu et al., 2003; Martin et al., 2006; Meiworm et al., 2000; Melchart et al., 1999; Takahash, 2006). Finally, studies have identified that cognitive-behavioural therapies and stress reduction techniques diminish pain in chronic pain syndromes as well (Drossman, 1993; Nelson, 2006; Thorn et al., 2007). The fact that similar interventions are effective for many different types of chronic pain in children adds further credence to the notion that they are fundamentally linked at some level.

Orthostatic intolerance

It has become increasingly clear that chronic pain is often associated with autonomic dysregulation. This is often manifested through orthostatic intolerance, the prime example which is postural orthostatic tachycardia syndrome (POTS) which is often present in individuals with chronic pain. POTS typically occurs following illness or injury. Ohja et al. (2011) identified the fact that in patients with POTS, 75% had gastrointestinal pain, 40% had headache, and 98% had a sleep disorder. Kitzberger et al. (2011) examined the relationship between chronic pain, autonomic function, physical disability, and psychological function and found that heart rate changes of greater than 30 beats per minute associated with positional change (the traditional adult POTS criteria) in patients with chronic pain were associated with higher levels of disability, depression, and anxiety. Although there is some debate as to whether a 30-beat increase is an appropriate threshold for children (Singer et al., 2012), evaluating the child for orthostatic intolerance should be part of the physical examination of any child with chronic pain.

Hypermobility

There are a number of studies which suggest that joint hypermobility is associated with chronic fatigue and fibromyalgia (Castori et al., 2011; Voermans et al., 2010). Rozen et al. (2006) has suggested that cervical hypermobility is more frequent in individuals with headache disorders than in the general population. Sacheti et al. (1997) reported on the high incidence of abdominal pain in individuals with Ehlers–Danlos, hypermobile type. The mechanism may stem from central sensitization due to a continuous afferent stimulation from frequent microtrauma due to subluxations or dislocations or from other factors, but hypermobility is often identified in individuals with chronic pain.

Sleep dysfunction

Roth-Isigkeit et al. (2005) reported that the incidence of sleep disturbance in a cadre of children with various chronic pains was 53%. Most clinicians who work with children with all types of persistent pain would agree that issues around sleep are a common occurrence in their patients. Clearly, pain and sleep are inversely related—the more pain, the less sleep; the less sleep, the more pain. It appears that poor sleep increases pain perception and reduces one's ability to cope with pain thus increasing pain and further decreasing sleep. Sleep difficulties may present as delays in sleep initiation, multiple night awakenings, non-restorative sleep, or early morning awakening. Palermo and Fonareva (2006) have reviewed this topic and suggest that although the adult literature is replete with studies which identify a relationship between chronic pain and poor sleep, there is a paucity of such studies in children. The few studies that have attempted to use theoretically objective measures to assess sleep (polysomnography and actigraphy) have yielded somewhat inconclusive results although the preponderance of evidence suggests that like in adults, sleep is often impaired in individuals with chronic pain and it should be addressed as part of comprehensive approach.

Impact on school and family life

In addition to their similar biological and clinical features, these syndromes have a similar impact on children and their families. All chronic pain problems interfere with the child's schooling and enjoyment of daily life. They have a direct impact on the family as well, causing both financial and emotional distress.

Impact on school

It is intuitive that chronic pain would have an impact on school performance and numerous studies validate this assumption. The frequency of school absence has been formally studied in many of the functional pain disorders and is clearly increased compared to the non-pain population (Sato et al., 2007). In fact, rates of school absence for children with chronic pain often exceed those with other chronic health conditions (Palmero, 2000). For a small group of children, that impact is so pronounced that they formally withdraw from school. Vetter found that 12% of children with a variety of chronic pain problems are home schooled and that those who are not miss on average 3 days of school per month (Vetter, 2008). Logan and colleagues (2008) reviewed the school performance of over 200 children attending a chronic pain clinic. They examined data on the school performance using a variety of sources including child and parent reports and school records and found surprising concordance among informants. They found that many adolescents with chronic pain miss a significant amount of school, experience a decline in grades, and perceive pain to interfere with their school success. Why do some children with chronic pain attend school and others with similar conditions do not? Obviously the answer is complex and a number of factors are probably at play. Breuner et al. (2004) studied almost 300 children with headache and found that children with high absences (greater than 2 days in the last

6 months for pain) differed from the low absence group (less than 2 days) primarily on two variables. The high-absence group was more likely to have depressed mood and a lower academic performance than the low-absence group. School avoidance may be a significant contributory factor in a subgroup of these children.

It is clear, therefore, that school absence is a critical issue in the rehabilitation of children with chronic pain. The more school one misses, the greater the anxiety that surrounds school re-entry which may potentiate the pain experience which will promote further school absence. This cycle must be addressed as part of a comprehensive approach to chronic pain.

Family distress

The persistence of pain in a child, regardless of its aetiology, often takes a significant toll on the family at multiple levels. Watching your child suffer with pain that you cannot ameliorate is agonizing for many parents and frequently leads to emotional distress. In a study by Eccleston et al. (2004), 40% of parents of children with chronic pain had depressive symptoms and 60% had a high level of general anxiety; 66% of parents had high scores on parenting stress indices. Feelings of guilt and inadequacy are frequent and parental conflict commonly increases.

Adding to family distress are the financial burdens typically associated with paediatric chronic pain. Sleed et al. (2005) examined the economic impact of chronic pain in an adolescent rheumatology clinic in the UK. She found that the cost of adolescent chronic pain averaged about £8000 —approximately £14 000 for those with non-rheumatological disorders and £4500 for those with rheumatic disease. In addition to the direct costs of medical care (diagnostic testing, medical visits, hospitalizations, medications), the burden of which will vary depending on the specific health care system, there are many indirect costs to families. She found that in the 52 families of children who had chronic pain that she evaluated, family members missed on average 78 work days per year (20% of the working year). In addition to time off from work, there were expenses associated with lost productivity, transportation, additional childcare expenses, non-prescription medications, special foods, plus a number of other out of pocket expenses which all add to the financial pressures on families. Coupled with the emotional stressors, these create a great weight on families who must grapple with these complexities.

Treatment implications

As should be clear from the previous discussion, the purpose of this chapter is to highlight the commonalities that exist among functional pain problems which may not be evident if one focuses solely on individual pain sites. Importantly, many of the similarities in aetiology and impact between these entities have treatment implications. In fact, a number of the interventions that may be recommended to address the abdominal pain in Constance, the young woman in the case example presented in this chapter may be equally efficacious for her headache and musculoskeletal pain as well.

The first goal of treatment is to evaluate the patient for red flags that would imply traditional organic disease. Even if these are identified, however, symptom treatment is still critical as merely treating the disease does not necessarily immediately eliminate distressing symptoms. The following discussion, however, assumes that organic disease is not present or has been well controlled yet pain persists.

Feedback to families

Goals of the feedback session

The feedback session in which the nature of the functional pain problem that the child is experiencing is explained is critical to the successful rehabilitation of it. The discussion is remarkably similar regardless of the specific site of the pain or the number of sites involved. At its conclusion, the family should be reassured that the doctor understands the child's problem, that he or she does not believe it is solely in their child's head, and that all are comfortable with a functional diagnosis with minimal subsequent testing necessary. Lindley identified the factors associated with limited improvement after one year in children with functional abdominal pain and reported that acceptance of the diagnosis by the child and family was essential to recovery (Lindley et al., 2005). The feedback session should also emphasize that improvement will be gradual, and that both parent and child participation in the process are essential.

Setting the stage

It is not uncommon for children with functional pain syndromes, especially those who have multiple pain sites, to have seen a number of clinicians and to have had extensive imaging and laboratory investigation. Because functional problems often have no confirmatory tests, if no traditional organic explanation is uncovered at the end of the investigative journey, families will sometimes urge clinicians to order additional tests in the hope that the answer lies in the results of the next investigation. It is therefore important to present a functional pain diagnosis not as one of exclusion but in a positive way. Merely stating what the diagnosis is not and what has been ruled out (not cancer, not arthritis, etc.), is far less satisfying to parents than stating that this pattern (the location, the family history, the time course, the quality of the pain, the negative physical examination, the lack of red flags for organic disease) supports a functional pain diagnosis. Obviously, the clinician cannot be completely certain that there is not an organic diagnosis that has been missed and the question of how much testing is enough always arises. This is especially difficult when parents produce case reports from the internet or the neighbourhood in which a rare entity with similar symptoms has been missed by clinicians for years. If after a reasonable investigation, the clinician states that a functional diagnosis is most likely but he or she will continue carefully monitoring the child ('watchful waiting'; Herzog and Harper, 1981) and will pursue new symptoms if they emerge, most parents will be satisfied. Additionally, it is important that the physician not imply that the lack of a clear organic diagnosis suggests a psychological explanation. Although psychological factors should not be dismissed, except in rare cases, the symptoms are the result of a complex interplay of a variety of factors and triggers; therefore, implying solely psychological origin not only distances the clinician from the family, but is in fact incorrect. If families feel that their child's suffering is being trivialized or dismissed, even if that is not the intent of the clinician, many families will then continue their search for an organic explanation subjecting the child to additional often unnecessary testing and adding to their own and the health care system's financial burden.

Specific content

The nature of the discussion with the family about functional pain problems should be individualized based on the educational, social, and cultural characteristics of the family. Regardless, the complex nature of pain and the biopsychosocial dimensions should be emphasized. The key element is that a number of factors (inflammation, infection, genetic predisposition, stress, depression, injury) may have altered the transmission of pain information in the child and that sensation is now the problem, making the child pain vulnerable. Use of key phrases ('the pain is hurting but not harming you'; 'the pain you are experiencing is not protective') as well as the use of analogies is often helpful. There are a number of analogies that are often used (Coakley and Schechter, 2013). The hardware/software discussion (the pain represents a software problem (the pain message) and not a hardware problem (the bowel, head, muscles, etc.)) is helpful in computer-savvy families. Another frequently used analogy is the false alarm analogy—the continuous pain is like a false car alarm—annoying but not representing a genuine problem. Most clinicians develop their own analogies and explanatory models to help families understand this complex concept that does not follow the traditional medical model.

Typical treatment recommendations

Specific treatment recommendations are available throughout this volume in the sections that address each of the functional pain problems individually. In general, however, regardless of the site of the functional pain problem, a number of elements should be addressed as part of the treatment.

School reintegration

As mentioned earlier, school absence is a frequent phenomenon in children with chronic pain. For children with frequent absences, the return to school may be highly stressful. Children may assert that they are not worried about returning to school after a prolonged absence, yet concern about missed work and academic performance and promotion, difficulties with concentration due to pain, worries about discussion with peers regarding the reasons for the absence and about being jostled in the hallway, fears of not being believed by other students and teachers along with a host of other considerations create an inevitable anxiety in the returning student who must deal with these issues while not feeling that well.

It is imperative therefore that school reintegration be carefully orchestrated and often gradual. Depending on the country, there may be legal protections available to the student (a 504 plan in the US, for example) which may ease the return. Regardless of how the school re-entry plan is configured, it should be followed religiously. Decisions about school attendance should not be made in the morning when the child reports he or she is not feeling well enough to return to school. School attendance is expected unless the child has a fever or a contagious process. Accommodations can be made regarding the length of the school day and in the workload but the expectation must be that the child attends school every day.

Sleep

Addressing issues of sleep is imperative. As mentioned earlier, inadequate and often non-restorative sleep is extremely common in chronic pain. A detailed sleep history should be obtained and identified issues should be addressed. Issues of sleep hygiene (getting into bed when tired, no television in the room, etc.) should be discussed. Relaxation strategies are also often helpful and can be taught by the clinician or by a colleague with experience in these techniques. If sleep remains an issue despite the introduction of psychological strategies, a number of pharmacological agents may be considered. In particular, some of the agents typically administered for pain or spasm often have a side effect of sedation which can be an added benefit of their use if they are taken at bedtime.

Physical activity

It is not uncommon when one is in pain to limit physical activity. This may occur because of associated pain, anxiety about pain which may occur as a result, depression, or diminished interest in social activities but regardless, it often leads to deconditioning which increases pain and disability. Decreased exercise and weight bearing can also promote osteopenia.

It is often valuable to have a skilled physical therapist evaluate the child's musculoskeletal system to determine whether formal physical therapy may be needed or whether a home exercise programme will suffice. The therapist can also evaluate the need for desensitization and can emphasize the importance of pacing and stretching. He or she can identify particularly tight or weak areas and if the child is hypermobile, can help with strengthening specific muscles to compensate for ligamentous laxity and promote joint stability. If only core strengthening and building endurance are felt to be necessary, then physical therapy may not be necessary and a graduated exercise programme may be substituted. Either way, increasing movement will promote a sense of well-being and an inevitable reduction of pain.

Addressing anxiety and depression

As mentioned repeatedly, anxiety and depression are often fellow travellers with chronic pain and may have a role in initiating it, maintaining it, or both. Clinicians should address this with families in the context of the numerous factors involved with chronic pain, as opposed to the organic versus psychological paradigm. There is an extensive literature on psychological strategies reducing the arousal in pain sensitive individuals and response to these strategies does not imply psychological causation (Eccleston et al., 2009). The psychologist can teach relaxation strategies, can address catastrophization, and explore the thoughts that might be promoting incapacitation from a nociceptive stimulus. Most paediatric pain programmes employ or are connected to paediatric psychologists and their evaluation should be a critical part of the assessment and treatment of pain in children. Many families may be resistant to this part of the evaluation and they often fear that they will be blamed for their child's pain. As a result, they may state (sometimes quite strongly) that that component of the evaluation is unnecessary as their child's pain is real. It is important to dispel the notion that the purpose of psychological evaluation and treatment in chronic pain is to unearth subtle psychological causation and blame parents for the child's problem. It is to identify every trigger that may promote and maintain pain and to teach techniques to help ameliorate it. Occasionally, psychopharmacological intervention may be necessary as well.

Attending to other symptoms

Other symptoms may amplify the incapacitation associated with chronic pain, regardless of site. Dizziness, nausea, and fatigue may result from pain but may also potentiate it. If at all possible, these symptoms should be addressed. Often POTS may be associated with these symptoms or with a general sensation of feeling unwell but it is often not considered and orthostatic vital signs are not obtained. Because the treatment of POTS is often relatively straightforward and its amelioration can dramatically help the child's pain and mood, obtaining blood pressure and heart rate measurements both lying down and then standing up should be a routine part of the evaluation of any type of chronic pain.

Provider communication

Because children with multiple pain problems typically see multiple specialists (neurology for headache, rheumatology for joint and musculoskeletal pain, gastroenterology for abdominal pain, orthopaedics for back pain, cardiologists for POTS) in addition to their primary care providers, it is imperative that a mechanism for communication among providers be developed. Specialists may not address or even ask about other pain sites which they perceive are out of their realm of expertise and assume those will be addressed by others. They may offer suggestions that they perceive are helpful for the specific problem that they are asked to address but may in fact be detrimental to the whole child. Additionally, there is also often significant variability of opinion among providers as to the aetiology, evaluation and treatment of chronic pain problems. Konenjiberg et al. (2004) gave 135 paediatricians a series of case scenarios involving chronic pain and asked how clinicians would address them. There was limited consensus on aetiology, on specific diagnostic testing, and on treatment. A similar situation likely occurs in clinical practice as these problems are often quite confusing and subject to multiple diagnostic opinions. As a result, families may feel confused by the lack of clarity among their physicians and continue a futile search for the right answer. Tests may often be unnecessarily repeated and agents prescribed that may interact negatively. It is imperative therefore in situations in which multiple pains exist that the clinical team be in communication and speak, as much as possible, in one voice.

Conclusion

This chapter has attempted to review the commonalities and overlaps between the common pain problems that children experience, most of which are functional in nature. This area has had limited attention in the past, most likely due to the fact that pain problems are typically evaluated by experts in the specific organ system from which the pain seems to stem and they may not have expertise in pain that stems from other areas. When one looks at these problems from a distance however, there are remarkable similarities in their theoretical aetiologies, in their impact on the child and family, in associated symptoms, and in their treatment. The adequate care of these problems demands an appreciation of the biopsychosocial model which looks at the child as a whole and on a multidisciplinary approach which allows for multiple streams of information to impact on the child's care.

Case example

Constance Payne is a 15-year-old young woman who was referred to the gastroenterology programme by her primary care provider for longstanding abdominal pain which had recently escalated in intensity. Constance has had periumbilical pain since the age of 12 but recently since high school entry her discomfort had increased. In the past, Constance had missed 1 to 2 days of school a month for her abdominal pain, but in the fall of ninth grade began missing at least one day per week.

The gastroenterologist who evaluated her identified no pattern to her symptoms and no obvious triggers for it. Her physical examination and subsequent laboratory investigation did not offer a specific pathological explanation for her pain nor did the endoscopy that was performed subsequently. A number of medications were prescribed for Constance including hyoscyamine and omeprazole which were both ineffective.

During the course of this evaluation, she reported that recently, she had developed an almost continuous headache and she often felt dizzy. Additionally, she described her vision as 'blurry'. She was subsequently referred to a neurologist who ordered a magnetic resonance imaging scan of her head and sent her to an ophthalmologist. None of these investigations yielded an explanation for her pain. Constance began taking ibuprofen to dampen her headache but stated that this medication aggravated her stomach pain. Concern was raised about her dizziness and she was referred to a cardiologist who identified a significant disparity between her heart rate when she changed position from lying to standing. He suggested a trial of salt and increased fluids.

Because of these multiple complaints, Constance became increasingly inactive. This inactivity was aggravated by additional reports of achiness in her neck, knees, and back. She became increasingly incapacitated and was referred to an orthopaedic surgeon and rheumatologist, neither of whom could explain her pain and deterioration. Her sleep became increasingly disordered and she began napping during the day and having difficulty falling asleep at night and awakening in the morning. She complained of crushing fatigue.

Constance and her mother began appearing frequently in the emergency department because, according to her mother, 'something has to be done'. Two of these visits ended in hospitalization for observation and pain control. Constance began losing interest in friends and in activities that had previously brought her pleasure.

With all of these complaints and no explanation, Mrs Payne began to express her worry that her cadre of doctors was missing something essential that would explain this unique constellation of findings. She herself had a cousin who had similar symptoms and was eventually found to have a serious underlying disease. She stated that in September she had a healthy daughter who did well in school and was an excellent athlete. Now, Constance can barely care for herself. Even though she herself has fibromyalgia, Mrs Payne feels she has to stay home and care for Constance. She reports as well the fact that although Constance sees many doctors, her physicians never seem to talk to each other and she feels the overwhelming burden of coordinating her daughter's care due to her fear that something will be missed if she is not perpetually vigilant.

References

Al-Chaer, E. D., Kawasaki, M., and Pasricha, P. J. (2000). A new model of chronic visceral hypersensitivity in adult rats by colon irritation during postnatal development. *Gastroenterology*, 119, 1277–1285.

Al-Chaer, E. D., and Weaver, S. (2009). Early life trauma and chronic pain. In E. A. Mayer and M. C. Bushnell (eds) *Functional pain syndromes: presentation and pathophysiology*, pp. 423–452. Seattle, WA: IASP Press,

Bair, M. J., Wu, J., Damush, T. M., Sutherland, J. M., and Kroenke, K. (2008). Association of depression and anxiety alone and in combination with chronic musculoskeletal pain in primary care. *Psychosom Med*, 70, 890–897.

Breuner, C. C., Smith, M. S., and Womack, W. M. (2004). Factors related to school absenteeism in adolescents with recurrent headache. *Headache*, 44, 217–222.

Castori, M., Celletti, C., Camerota, F., and Grammatico, P. (2011). Chronic fatigue syndrome is commonly diagnosed in patients with Ehlers-Danlos syndrome hypermobility type/joint hypermobility syndrome. *Clin Exp Rheumatol*, 29, 597–598.

Chang, L., Sundaresh, S., Elliott, J., Anton, P. A., Baldi, P., Licudine, A., et al. (2009). Dysregulation of the HPA axis in irritable bowel syndrome. *Neurogastroenterol Motil*, 21, 149–159.

Chartier, M. J., Walker, J. R., and Naimark, B. (2007). Childhood abuse, adult health, and health care utilization: results from a representative community sample. *Am J Epidemiol*, 165, 1031–1038.

Coakley, R. and Schechter, N. L. (2013). Chronic pain is like… :the use of analogy and metaphor in the treatment of chronic pain in children. *Pediatr Pain Lett*, 15(1), 1–8.

Chen, E., Craske, M. G., Katz, E. R., Schwartz, E., and Zeltzer, L. K. (2000). Pain-sensitive temperament: does it predict procedural distress and response to psychological treatment among children with cancer? *J Pediatr Psychol*, 25, 269–278.

Drossman, D. A. (1999). An integrated approach to the irritable bowel syndrome. *Aliment Pharmacol Ther*, 13(Supplement s2), 3–14.

Eccleston, C., Crombez, G., Scotford, A., Clinch, J., and Connell, H. (2004). Adolescent chronic pain: patterns and predictors of emotional distress in adolescents with chronic pain and their parents. *Pain*, 108, 221–229

Eccleston, C., Palermo, T. M., deWilliams, A. C., Lewandowski, A., and Morley, S. (2009). Psychological therapies for the management of chronic and recurrent pain in children and adolescents. *Cochrane Database Syst Rev*, 2, CD003968.

Evans, S., Keenan, T. R., and Shipton, E. A. (2007). Psychosocial adjustment and physical health of children living with maternal chronic pain. *J Paediatr Child Health*, 43, 262–270.

Fichtel, A. and Larsson, B. (2002). Psychosocial impact of headache and comorbidity with other pains among Swedish school adolescents. *Headache*, 42, 766–7758.

Foulkes, T. and Wood, J. N. (2008). Pain genes. *PLoS Genet*, 4, e1000086. doi: 10.1371/journal.pgen.1000086.

Geisser, M. E., Glass, J. M., Rajcevska, L. D., Clauw, D. J., Williams, D. A., Kileny, P. R., et al. (2008). A psychophysical study of auditory and pressure sensitivity in patients with fibromyalgia and healthy controls. *J Pain*, 9, 417–422.

Giesecke, T., Gracely, R.H., Grant, M. A., Nachemson, A., Petzke, F., Williams, D. A., et al. (2004). Evidence of augmented central pain processing in idiopathic chronic low back pain. *Arthritis Rheum*, 50, 613–623.

Goldenberg, D., Mayskiy, M., Mossey, C., Ruthazer, R., and Schmid, C. (1996). A randomized, double-blind crossover trial of fluoxetine and amitriptyline in the treatment of fibromyalgia. *Arthritis Rheum*, 39, 1852–1859.

Goodman, J. E., and McGrath, P. J. (2003). Mothers' modeling influences children's pain during a cold pressor task. *Pain*, 104, 559–565.

Hermann, C., Hohmeister, J., Demirkca, S., Zohsel, K., and Flor, H. (2006). Long term alteration of pain sensitivity in school aged children with early pain experiences. *Pain*, 125, 278–285.

Hershey, A. D., Powers, S. W., Bentti, A. L., and Degrauw, T. J. (2000). Effectiveness of amitriptyline in the prophylactic management of childhood headaches. *Headache*, 40, 539–549.

Herzog, D. B., and Harper, G. B. (1981). Diagnostic dilemmas and principles of management. *Clin Pediatr*, 20(12), 761–767

Janig, W. (2009). Autonomic nervous system dysfunction. In E. A. Mayer, and M. C. Bushnell (eds) *Functional pain syndromes*, pp. 265–300. Seattle, WA: IASP Press.

Johannesson, U., de Boussard, C. N., Brodda, J. G., and Bohm-Starke, N. (2007). Evidence of diffuse noxious inhibitory controls (DNIC) elicited by cold noxious stimulation in patients with provoked vestibulodynia. *Pain*, 130, 31–39.

Kato, K., Sullivan, P. F., Evengard, B., and Pedersen, N. L. (2006). Importance of genetic influences on chronic widespread pain. *Arthritis Rheum*, 54, 1682–1686.

Konijnenberg, A. Y., DeGraeff-Meeder, E. R., Kimpen, J. L. L., van der Hoeven, J., Buitelaar, J. K., Uiterwaal, C. S., et al. (2004). Children with unexplained chronic pain: do pediatricians agree regarding the diagnostic approach and presumed primary cause. *Pediatrics*, 114, 1220–1226.

Köseoglu, E., Akboyraz, A., and Ersoy, A. O. (2003). Aerobic exercise and plasma beta endorphin levels in patients with migrainous headache without aura. *Cephalalgia*, 23, 972–976.

Kritzberger, C. J., Antiel, R. M., Wallace, D. P., Zacharias, J. D., Brands, C. K., Fischer, P. R., *et al.* (2011). Functional disability in adolescents with orthostatic intolerance and chronic pain. *J Child Neurol*, 26, 593–598.

Kroner-Herwig, B., Gassmann, J., van Gessel, H., and Vath, N. (2011). Multiple pains in children and adolescents: a risk factor analysis in a longitudinal study. *J Pediatr Psychol*, 36, 420–427.

Krstjansdottir, G. (1997). Prevalence of pain combinations and overall pain: a study of headache, stomach pain, and back pain among schoolchildren. *Scand J Soc Med*, 25, 58–63.

Larsson, B. and Sund, A. M. (2007). Emotional, behavioral, social correlates and one year predictors of frequent pains among early adolescents. *Eur J Pain*, 11, 57–65

Lautenbacher, S. and Rollman, G. B. (1997). Possible deficiencies of pain modulation in fibromyalgia. *Clin J Pain*, 13, 189–96.

Lindley, K. J., Glaser, D., and Milla, P. J. (2005). Consumerism in healthcare can be detrimental to child health: lessons from children with functional abdominal pain. *Arch Dis Child*, 90, 35–37.

Logan, D. E., Simons, L. E., Stein, M. J., and Chastain, L. (2008). School impairment in adolescents with chronic pain. *J Pain*, 9, 407–416.

Lynch, A. M., Kashikar-Zuck, S., Goldschneider, K. R., and Jones, B. A. (2006). Psychosocial risks for disability in children with chronic back pain. *J Pain*, 7, 244–251.

Martin, D. P., Sletten, D., Williams, B. A., and Berger, I. H. (2006). Improvement in fibromyalgia symptoms with acupuncture: results of a randomized controlled trial. *Mayo Clinic Proc*, 81, 749–757.

Mayer, E. A., and Bushnell, M. C. (2009). Functional pain disorders: time for a paradigm shift. In E. A. Mayer, and M. C. Bushnell (eds) *Functional pain syndromes: presentation and pathophysiology*, pp. 531–565. Seattle, WA: IASP Press.

Meiworm, L., Jakob, E., and Walker, U. A. (2000). Patients with fibromyalgia benefit from aerobic exercise. *Clin Rheumatol*, 19, 253–257.

Melchart, D., Linde, K., Fischer, P., White, A., Allais, G., Vickers, A., *et al.* (1999). Acupuncture for recurrent headaches: a systematic review of randomized controlled trials. *Cephalgia*, 19, 779–786.

Mogil, J. S., Wilson, S. G., Bon, K., Lee, S. E., Chung, K., Raber, P., *et al.* (1999). Heritability of nociception 1: responses of 11 inbred mouse strains on 12 measures of nociception. *Pain*, 80, 67–82.

Montagna, P. (2008). The primary headaches: genetics, epigenetics and a behavioural genetic model. *J Headache Pain*, 9, 57–69

Nelson, B. R. (2006). Cognitive behavioral therapy for fibromyalgia. *Nat Clin Pract Rheum*, 8, 416–424.

Ohja, A., Chelminsky, T. C., and Chelminsky, G. (2011). Comorbidities in pediatric patients with postural orthostatic tachycardia syndrome. *J Pediatr*, 158, 20–23.

Palermo, T. M. (2000). Impact of recurrent and chronic pain on child and family daily functioning: a critical review of the literature. *J Dev Behav Pediatr*, 21, 58–69.

Palermo, T. M., and Fonareva, I. (2006). Sleep in children and adolescents with chronic pain. *Pediatr Pain Lett*, 8, 11–15

Perquin, C. W., Hazebroek-Kampschreur, A. A., Hunfeld, J. A., Bohnen, A. M., van Suijlekom-Smit, L. W., Passchier, J., *et al.* (2000). Pain in children and adolescents: a common experience. *Pain*, 87, 51–58

Perquin, C. W., Hunfeld, J. A. M., Hazebroek-Kampschreur, A. A., van Suijlekom-Smit, L. W., Passchier, J., Koes, B. W., *et al.* (2001). Insights in the use of health care services in chronic benign pain childhood and adolescents. *Pain*, 94, 205–213

Rajagopalani, M., Kurian, G., and Jacob, J. (1998). Symptom relief with amitriptyline in the Irritable Bowel syndrome. *J Gastroenterol Hepatol*, 13, 738–741.

Roth-Isigkeit, A., Thyen, U., Stoven, H., Schwarzenberger, J., and Schmucker, P. (2005). Pain among children and adolescents: restrictions in daily living and triggering factors. *Pediatrics*, 115, 152–162.

Rozen, T. D., Roth, J. M., and Denenberg, N. (2006). Cervical spine joint hypermobility: a possible predisposing factor for new daily persistent headache. *Cephalalgia*, 26, 1182

Sacheti, A., Szemere, J., Bernstein, B., Tafas, T., Schechter, N., and Tsipouras, P. (1997). Chronic pain is a manifestation of the Ehlers-Danlos syndrome. *J Pain Symptom Manage*, 14, 88–93

Sato, A., Hainsworth, K. R., Khan, K. A., Ladwig, R. J., Weismand, S. J., Davies, W. H. *et al.* (2007). School absenteeism in pediatric chronic pain: identifying lessons learned from the general school absenteeism literature. *Child Health Care*, 36, L355–372

Schanberg, L. F., Anthony, K. K., Gil, K. M., Lefebvre, J. C., Kredich, D. W., and Macharoni, L. M. (2001). Family pain history predicts child health status in children with chronic rheumatic disease. *Pediatrics*, 108, E47.

Schechter, N. L., Bernstein, B., Beck, A., Hart, L., and Scherzer, L. (1991). Individual differences in children's response to pain: role of temperament and parental characteristics. *Pediatrics*, 87, 171–177.

Shimada, C., Kurumiya, S., Noguchi, Y., and Umemoto, M. (1990). The effect of neonatal exposure to chronic footshock on pain responsiveness and sensitivity to morphine after maturation in the ratr. *Behav Brain Res*, 36, 105–111.

Singer, W., Sletten, D. M., Opfer-Gehrking, T. L., Brands, C. K., Fischer, P. R., and Low, P. A. (2012). Postural tachycardia in children and adolescents: what is abnormal? *J Pediatr*, 160, 222–226.

Sleed, M., Eccleston, C., Beecham, J., Knapp, M., and Jordan, A. (2005). The economic impact of chronic pain in adolescence: methodological considerations and a preliminary costs of illness study. *Pain*, 119, 183–190.

Takahashi, T. (2006). Acupuncture for functional gastrointestinal disorders. *J Gastroenterol*, 41, 408–417.

Thorn, B. E., Pence, L. B., Ward, L. C., Kilgo, G., Clements, K. L, Cross, T. H., *et al.* (2007). A randomized clinical trial of targeted cognitive behavioral treatment to reduce catastrophizing in chronic headache sufferers. *J Pain*, 8, 938–949.

Varni, J. W., Rapoff, M. A., Waldron, S. A., Gragg, R. A., Bernstein, B. H., and Lindsley, C. B. (1996). Chronic pain and emotional distress in childrena and adolescents. *J Dev Behav Pediatr*, 17, 154–161.

Vetter, T. R. (2008). A clinical profile of a cohort of patients referred to an anesthesiology based pediatric chronic pain medicine program. *Anesth Analg*, 106, 786–793.

Voermans, N. C., Knoop, H., van de Kamp, N., Hamel, B. C., Bleijenberg, G., and van Engelen, B. G. (2010). Fatigue is a frequent and clinically relevant problem in Ehlers-Danlos syndrome. *Semin Arthritis Rheum*, 40, 267–274.

Von Baeyer, C. L. and Champion, G. D. (2011). Commentary: multiple pains as functional pain syndromes. *J Pediatr Psychol*, 36, 433–437.

Walsh, C. A., Jamieson, E., MacMillan, H., and Boyle, M. (2007). Child abuse and chronic pain in a community survey of women. *J Interpers Violence*, 22, 1536–1554.

White, K. S. and Farrell, A. D. Anxiety and psychosocial stress as predictors of headache and abdominal pain in urban early adolescents. *J Pediatr Psychol*, 31, 582–596

Whorwell, P. J., McCallum, M., and Creed, F. H. (1986). Non-colonic features of IBS. *Gut*, 27, 37–40.

Woolf, C. J. (2011). Central sensitization: implications for the diagnosis and treatment of pain. *Pain*, 152(Suppl. 3), S2–15.

Yunus, M. B. (2007a). Fibromyalgia and overlapping disorders: the unifying concept of central sensitivity syndromes. *Semin Arthritis Rheum*, 36, 339–356.

Yunus, M. B. (2007b). Role of central sensitization in symptoms beyond muscle pain and the evaluation of a patient with widespread pain. *Best Practice and Research in Clinical Rheumatol*, 21, 481–497.

Yunus, M. B. (2008). Central sensitivity syndromes: a new paradigm and group nosology for fibromyalgia and overlapping conditions, and the related issue of disease versus illness. *Semin Arthritis Rheum*, 37, 339–352.

Zuckerman, B., Stevenson, J., and Bailey, V. (1987). Stomachaches and headaches in a community sample of preschool children. *Pediatrics*, 79, 677–682.

CHAPTER 24

Non-inflammatory musculoskeletal pain

Jacqui Clinch

Summary

Non-inflammatory musculoskeletal pain is common in children and adolescents, and when persistent or widespread, can have a negative impact on physical and psychological well-being. Diagnostic labels and criteria are not uniform in the current literature, but musculoskeletal pain may present as widespread pain or juvenile fibromyalgia, complex regional pain syndrome, or in association with joint hypermobility. Chronic musculoskeletal pain, irrespective of its trigger, can bring persistent and recurrent distress, disability, and widespread family disruption. Once serious medical causes have been excluded by history, examination, and relevant investigations, the focus should be on rehabilitation. Multidisciplinary team management to facilitate cohesive working and the introduction of psychological and physical therapies can improve outcome. Further research is required to define the role of pharmacological interventions.

Introduction

The most common chronic musculoskeletal pain conditions reviewed in paediatric rheumatology settings include diffuse idiopathic musculoskeletal pain (DIP; also called juvenile fibromyalgia or chronic widespread pain), chronic pain related to childhood joint hypermobility, complex regional pain syndrome (CRPS), chronic back pain, and persistent joint pain following previous or controlled inflammation (e.g. juvenile idiopathic arthritis (JIA)) (Malleson and Clinch, 2003; O'Sullivan et al., 2011).

For many young people presenting to clinic, regardless of whether the cause of their pain is known, the chronic experience of pain has often had a large and wholly negative impact on their physical and psychological well-being, and their family (Malleson and Clinch, 2003). Children who suffer persistent musculoskeletal pain and other symptoms also have a significant chance of developing chronic widespread pain and pain-associated disability in adult life (Jones et al., 2007).

This chapter will review: (1) the epidemiology of musculoskeletal pain in childhood, (2) evaluation of the impact of chronic pain, (3) the clinical features of common pain presentations and their relevance to diagnosis and treatment planning, and (4) rehabilitation interventions aimed at the management of chronic musculoskeletal pain.

Epidemiology

There is limited data on the prevalence and incidence of musculoskeletal pain in youth, and on the prevalence of pain-associated suffering or disability. However, pain is a common experience during childhood. One study showed that 83% of school-aged children had experienced an episode of pain during the preceding 3 months (Roth-Isigkeit et al., 2005). Pain is a normal sensation but becomes disabling when it persists and is associated with suffering. In this same study, 30.8% of the children and adolescents stated that the pains had been present for over 6 months. Musculoskeletal pains accounted for 64% of all the pains that were reported (Roth-Isigkeit et al., 2005). Other studies support this finding (Brattberg, 2004; Perquin et al., 2000).

♦ The epidemiology of DIP (also referred to as juvenile fibromyalgia or chronic widespread pain) is difficult to accurately assess. There are no universally agreed diagnostic criteria, although some authors have suggested using the term juvenile fibromyalgia and proposed diagnostic criteria akin to the adult fibromyalgia criteria (Kashikar-Zuck et al., 2006). The HUNT study (Hoftun et al., 2008) showed 8.5% of a population of 7373 adolescents in Norway fulfilled the criteria for DIP; whereas a UK study showed the prevalence of chronic widespread pain in 17-year-old school children to be 4.3% (Deere et al., submitted).

♦ Hypermobility, as currently defined, is present in 19.8% of the normal UK adolescent population (Clinch et al., 2011). There is a relationship between localized pain and significant hypermobility (Beighton score 6 or above); this is discussed later in the chapter (Tobias et al., 2013).

♦ Low-back pain (LBP) is commonly reported. A UK observational cohort study reported the prevalence of LBP as 16.3% in 17-year-old adolescents (Deere et al., submitted). A cross-sectional study of school-age children showed prevalence of LBP that lasted for at least 1 month was 24% (Watson et al., 2002), the HUNT study showed this to be 16.7% for girls and 11% for boys (1 day a week for at least 3 months; Hoftun et al., 2011).

♦ The prevalence of CRPS in adults is 26 per 100 000 person years (De Mos et al., 2007). In children the epidemiology has not been robustly evaluated but recent studies have demonstrated that approximately 90% of the cases reported are females in a range of 8 to 16 years (Sherry et al., 1999). There tends to be a delay in recognizing the diagnosis (Stanton Hicks, 2010). A complicating factor is the lack of clear diagnostic criteria for children.

♦ In JIA it is clear that persistent pain is a significant problem for many children (Anthony et al., 2007). Approximately 40% describe pain 5 years after diagnosis (Lovell and Walco, 1989). A significant minority progress to develop localized or diffuse musculoskeletal pain that is not directly related to the control of their inflammatory condition (Haverman et al., 2012).

Looking generally across studies a number of features are clear:

♦ Girls experience more musculoskeletal pain than boys (Groholt, 1994; Hoftun et al., 2011).

♦ Children living in low-educated, low-income families have a 1.4-fold increase in the odds of having back pain (Groholt et al., 1994).

♦ The incidence of chronic widespread musculoskeletal pain peaks in older adolescence (Hoftun et al., 2011).

♦ Multiple common symptoms (including joint pain, headaches, abdominal pain) in childhood are associated with a moderately increased risk of chronic widespread pain in adulthood (Jones et al., 2007).

Clinical features of chronic musculoskeletal pain

As many features of musculoskeletal pain conditions are shared by most children, it is appropriate to describe the general presentations at this stage, and then concentrate on specific pain-related conditions in their own right.

General features

It is not unusual for musculoskeletal pain to start in a localized area of the body (Buskila and Neumann, 2000). The pain can intensify and radiate to other areas. It is associated often with a reluctance to mobilize, and avoidance of movement. In adults, avoidance and fear of pain and movement can reduce fitness and further increase in pain (Elbaz et al., 2009), but in children this occurs on the background of a musculoskeletal system that is still developing. Discomfort and pain intensity increase and become constant. As discrete pains multiply and continue, the young person may avoid contact with, or use of, an area of the body affected, and this can then lead to muscular spasms, and abnormalities of posture and gait. As gait alters, the resultant asymmetry can lead to other vulnerable sites (including lower lumbar, anterior knee, and lateral aspect of pelvis) taking an altered load and causing further discomfort. Over time, affected limbs may adopt flexed positions, and tendons tighten, further exaggerating imbalance and pain.

Associated symptoms and signs

♦ Hypervigilance and pain sensitivity that is greater than expected from a given physical trigger. Children often report a heightened awareness of pain and pain associated cues (American Pain Society, 2012; Malleson and Clinch, 2003; O'Sullivan et al., 20011). It is unclear whether this is caused by fear of pain, or increased sensitivity of pain signalling. Clinically, this presents as young people describing unbearable pain on minimal skin contact, and heightened fear of being touched, for example, on examination.

♦ Perceived thermodysregulation—this is observed more commonly in adolescent girls. Limbs are particularly cool and mottled. Occasionally there will be areas that are very red and hot to touch on a background of the mottled skin. There may also be an abnormal perception of temperature, but an increase in thermal pain sensitivity has only been documented in adults (Geisser et al., 2003).

♦ Autonomic dysfunction—pain is a powerful stressor. Continuous pain signals, immobility, and fatigue act directly on the autonomic system (Cohen et al., 2001). In an environment of physical and emotional anxiety, the sympathetic system is more active. This leads to tachycardia, hyperventilation (compounded with panic attacks), cold sweats, blurred vision, abdominal pain and extreme pallor. Girls particularly complain of nausea, dizziness, and episodes of feeling faint. Children look unwell during these episodes of increased pain. It is not unusual for attending paediatricians to investigate cardiovascular, neurological, and gastrointestinal systems in an attempt to elicit pathology.

♦ Musculoskeletal disequilibrium—these young people are still growing, often in their peripubertal growth spurt, and musculoskeletal pain can have lasting effects on the final positioning (Lightman et al., 1987). Proprioceptive signals from the joints are reduced and the limb held in a rigid, fixed position (Sherry et al., 1999; Walco et al., 2010). Legs may 'give way'. Knees and hips are held flexed, feet are inverted, and hands are clenched with flexed wrists. These positions are often described as the most comfortable. Muscles and tendons quickly tighten and this complicates the pain and disability. The adaptive positioning of a young person with leg or abdominal pains particularly affects the gait and resting positions and thus alters the loads on the spine and pelvis.

There are a number of influences on physical behaviour, including psychosocial factors. What can first appear as a structural anomaly or physical constraint may be better explained by fear of pain on movement, or postural compensation due to overprotection of a painful body part. Although an important area, there is very little research of the effects of a chronic stressor such as pain during critical periods of physical development, or in the measurement of movement constrained by pain.

Specific childhood musculoskeletal pain conditions

Diffuse idiopathic pain syndromes (juvenile fibromyalgia/chronic widespread pain)

This describes widespread pain, often located over muscles and joints, and with significant pain associated disability (Malleson et al., 2001). The term juvenile fibromyalgia has been used, with diagnostic criteria similar to those used in adults (Hoftun et al., 2011), including a history of widespread pain for at least 3 months, and the presence of 11 of 18 bilateral tender points (occiput, low cervical, trapezius, supraspinatus, second rib, lateral epicondyle, gluteal, greater trochanter, and knees). It should be noted that these American College of Rheumatology criteria have recently been revised and now do not include tender points as it is recognized that widespread pain and related symptoms are good markers for adult fibromyalgia (Wolfe et al., 2010).

The onset of pain in DIP/juvenile fibromyalgia is often gradual. There may have been an initial insult or trauma but often there is no obvious trigger and only vague recollections of the time of onset. The pain is generalized. There may be areas of allodynia (profound hypersensitivity to light touch) and subjective hyperalgesia but there is often an absence of the autonomic changes (including reduced cutaneous perfusion, localized swelling, shiny stretched appearance) seen in more localized pain conditions (O'Sullivan et al., 2011).

What is striking in the young people with diffuse pain is the associated fatigue, poor sleep pattern, and extremely low mood. It is widely believed, however, that low mood in adolescents are reactive (to the pain-associated disability) rather than a primary depression. This is in contrast to adults with fibromyalgia where primary depression is frequently seen (Buskila et al., 1995). Menstrual cycling has been shown to affect fibromyalgia-related symptoms in nearly 50% of adult patients (Pamuk and Cakir, 2005), and this may be relevant in the adolescent female population.

Complex regional pain syndrome

Although it is almost 20 years since this condition first received attention in children, the diagnosis and treatment of CRPS continues to be poorly understood. Many children receive investigations and rehabilitation for other presumed conditions, resulting in a long journey before CRPS is recognized, and often a worsening of the symptoms and associated disability (Berde and Lebel, 2005; Connelly and Schanberg, 2006). The diagnosis of CRPS remains a clinical one, and in adults is based on the Budapest Criteria (Box 24.1) (Harden et al., 2010). Although there is frequently a precipitating trauma, this is not present in around 10% of cases, and pain is usually out of proportion to the inciting event and accompanied by allodynia (Stanton Hicks, 2010). Children most often describe the pain as burning, with sensations akin to dysaesthesia. CRPS in paediatric patients is clinically distinct from the adult condition (Connelly and Schanberg, 2006; Stanton Hicks, 2010):

- The lower limb is more commonly involved than the upper limb.

- There is a marked female predominance.

- The peak incidence is in early adolescence (median 13 years).

- Dystrophic changes and long-term disability are less common than in adults.

Signs and symptoms may completely resolve within several months to a few years, but relapses may also occur (Connelly and Schanberg, 2006; Stanton Hicks, 2010). Occasionally more than one limb may be affected at presentation (Stanton Hicks, 2010) or symptoms may progress or migrate to a hand or other leg. This may be due in part to an increase in mechanical load through the arms through the use of crutches and subsequent mechanical pain. Autonomic changes include swelling, reduced cutaneous perfusion, and thermodynamic instability. The affected limb develops a purplish hue with other colour changes that can cause concern to the child and family (Figure 24.1). The skin takes on a shiny, stretched appearance, with coarse hairs developing in patches (Harden et al., 2010). In rare cases, severe trophic changes develop with ulceration and marked wasting. Figure 24.2 shows the marked changes on thermography (reduction in cutaneous blood flow represented

---

Box 24.1 Budapest clinical diagnostic criteria for complex regional pain syndrome

1. Continuing pain, which is disproportionate to any inciting event.

2. Must report at least one symptom in *three of the four* following categories:
   a. *Sensory:* reports of hyperesthesia and/or allodynia.
   b. *Vasomotor:* reports of temperature asymmetry and/or skin colour changes and/or skin colour asymmetry.
   c. *Sudomotor/oedema:* reports of oedema and/or sweating changes and/or sweating asymmetry
   d. *Motor/trophic:* reports of decreased range of motion and/or motor dysfunction (weakness, tremor, dystonia) and/or trophic changes (hair, nail, skin).

3. Must display at least one sign at time of evaluation in *two or more* of the following categories:
   a. *Sensory:* evidence of hyperalgesia (to pinprick) and/or allodynia (to light touch and/or deep somatic pressure and/or joint movement).
   b. *Vasomotor:* evidence of temperature asymmetry and/or skin colour changes and/or asymmetry.
   c. *Sudomotor/oedema:* evidence of oedema and/or sweating changes and/or sweating asymmetry.
   d. *Motor/trophic:* evidence of decreased range of motion and/or motor dysfunction (weakness, tremor, dystonia) and/or trophic changes (hair, nail, skin).

4. There is no other diagnosis that better explains the signs and symptoms.

Reproduced from Harden, R. N. et al., Validation of proposed diagnostic criteria (the 'Budapest Criteria') for complex regional pain syndrome, *Pain®*, Volume 150, Issue 2, August 2010, pp. 268–274 with permission of the International Association for the Study of Pain® (IASP). The figure may NOT be reproduced for any other purpose without permission.

---

by lack of heat detected) of the wasted, flexed, ulcerated foot that is shown in Figure 24.3. Magnetic resonance imaging (MRI) changes early in the condition can show bone oedema that may be confused with other musculoskeletal conditions. Later radiology may show osteopenia secondary to disuse (Berde and Lebel, 2005). Limbs can become distorted and feet/hands held in seemingly fixed and often flexed positions.

While the pathophysiology of CRPS is poorly understood, a number of aetiologies have been proposed: a peripheral small fibre neuropathy, autonomic dysfunction, and exaggerated regional inflammation (Stanton Hicks, 2010). However, inflammatory aspects differ from those seen in other conditions involving tissue inflammation. The suggestion that CRPS in children is a different clinical entity than that seen in the adult, is probably incorrect, as recent evidence would suggest that the pathophysiology is most likely to involve similar endocrine, behavioural, developmental, and environmental factors (Stanton Hicks, 2010). Many features, particularly the neurological abnormalities, suggest both peripheral

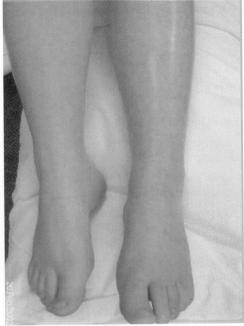

Figure 24.1 Early CRPS changes, left leg.
Reproduced from Richard Watts, Philip Conaghan, Chris Denton, Helen Foster, John Issacs, and Ulf Müller-Ladner (eds) *Oxford Textbook of Rheumatology*, Fourth Edition, Oxford University Press, Oxford, UK, Copyright © 2014, by permission of Oxford University Press.

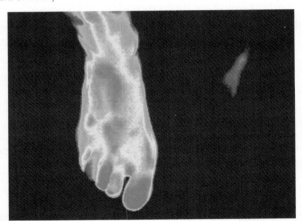

Figure 24.2 Loss of cutaneous capillary blood flow in left foot on thermography.
Reproduced from Richard Watts, Philip Conaghan, Chris Denton, Helen Foster, John Issacs, and Ulf Müller-Ladner (eds) *Oxford Textbook of Rheumatology*, Fourth Edition, Oxford University Press, Oxford, UK, Copyright © 2014, by permission of Oxford University Press.

and central nervous system (CNS) involvement, and considerable CNS circuitry changes have recently been shown with functional MRI in young people with a diagnosis of CRPS (Lebel et al., 2008).

Back pain

Recent research has shown that the prevalence of LBP has increased among children and adolescents ranging from 16.4% to 36% (Deere et al., submitted; Kjaer et al., 2011). Mid-back pain and neck pain are also frequently seen (9.4% and 8.9% respectively of adolescent population; Deere et al., submitted) but the literature evaluating these areas is less robust.

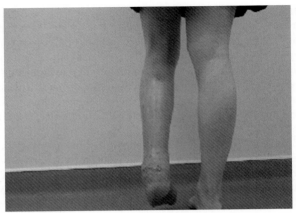

Figure 24.3 Wasted, ulcerated left leg in advanced CRPS.
Reproduced from Richard Watts, Philip Conaghan, Chris Denton, Helen Foster, John Issacs, and Ulf Müller-Ladner (eds) *Oxford Textbook of Rheumatology*, Fourth Edition, Oxford University Press, Oxford, UK, Copyright © 2014, by permission of Oxford University Press.

Factors related to LBP in children and adolescents include:

♦ LBP is more common among girls and increases with age (Kjaer et al., 2011; Watson et al., 2002).

♦ Risk factors are poor physical condition, reduced strength in muscles that support the back (Diepenmaat et al., 2006), intensive sports (Lundin et al., 2006), and reduced hamstring length (Sjolie, 2004).

♦ A prospective study of adolescents showed a strong correlation between LBP, emotional and behavioural problems, as well as other physical problems such as headaches, stomach aches, sore throat, and fatigue (Watson et al., 2002).

The vast majority of children with LBP who come to paediatric rheumatology clinics improve with physiotherapy; however, a minority proceed to develop increasing pain-related disability (Ahlqwist et al., 2008). Chronic pain among adults may, in part, be rooted in untreated painful experiences in childhood and young people who have suffered from LBP are more likely to suffer from these problems as adults (Kjaer et al., 2011).

Few treatment studies on children and adolescents with LBP have been published. One study of children and adolescents shows that individual assessment and follow-up, including an active treatment intervention by an experienced physiotherapist, improves self-perceived health and function and reduces pain, while increasing mobility and strength (Ahlqwist et al., 2008). Another study shows that an exercise programme tailored for children and adolescents with recurrent non-specific LBP has beneficial effects, including reduced pain intensity (Jones et al., 2007).

Red flags for pathology include nocturnal pain, presentation in young children, or neurological symptoms indicating nerve compression/damage. These cases should be fully investigated to exclude:

♦ Malignancies (e.g. sarcoma, neuroblastoma, metastases).

♦ Vertebral damage (trauma—accidental and non-accidental).

♦ Infection (osteomyelitis, abscess) and inflammation (arthritis, disciitis).

♦ Rare conditions such as chronic recurrent osteomyelitis, Langerhans' histiocytosis, and collapse secondary to iatrogenic or idiopathic osteoporosis.

Juvenile idiopathic arthritis and pain

Despite significant advances in medical treatments for children with JIA, persistent pain is a common complaint (Anthony and Schanberg, 2007; see also Chira and Schanberg, Chapter 22, this volume). Pain has been shown to be a primary determinant of the physical, emotional, and social functioning in these children (Anthony and Schanberg, 2007). The degree of disabling pain does not always mirror inflammatory joint activity, and a growing body of research highlights the importance of environmental and cognitive behavioural influences in the pain experience of children, in addition to the contribution of disease activity (Connelly et al., 2010; Vuorimaa et al., 2009).

Idiopathic chronic limb pains

There are many presentations of musculoskeletal pain in children that do not meet the criteria for DIP/juvenile fibromyalgia or CRPS. These include the poorly understood 'growing pains', described as recurrent, bilateral, non-articular pain in the lower extremities that occur late in the evening or at night. They have been observed to coexist with vascular pain problems including migraines, leading to speculation that there may be a vascular component to the bone pain experienced. A recent small study challenged this theory (Hashkes et al., 2005). Others describe growing pains as a form of overuse injury (Friedland et al., 2005). The jury remains out.

Joint hypermobility and pain

Joint hypermobility results from ligamentous laxity and may occur in individuals with a primary genetic disorder affecting connective tissue matrix proteins (e.g. osteogenesis imperfecta or Marfan's syndrome) or other syndromes (e.g. trisomy 21, bony dysplasias, or velocardiofacial syndrome). In the majority of cases, hypermobility exists as an isolated finding (referred to as 'generalized joint laxity'), but it may also be associated with musculoskeletal symptoms such as pain and 'clicking joints' in the absence of known genetic causes, in which case it is referred to as 'hypermobility syndrome' (Clinch et al., 2011).

A method of examining and scoring for hypermobility (Figure 24.4) was developed by Beighton in 1973 (Beighton et al., 1973). The Beighton score was devised in South Africa and based on 1083 Tswana Africans and has subsequently been used internationally to define generalized joint laxity in all populations and all age groups. It has not been validated in children.

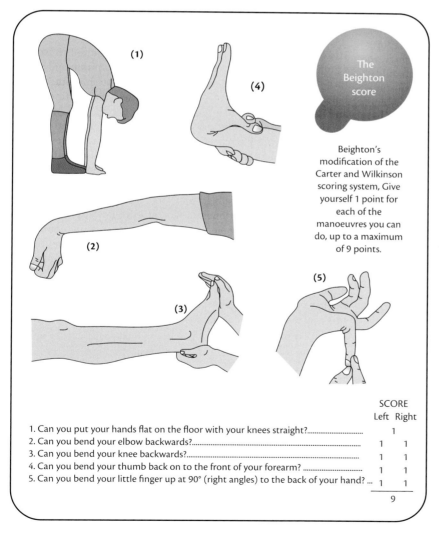

The Beighton score

Beighton's modification of the Carter and Wilkinson scoring system, Give yourself 1 point for each of the manoeuvres you can do, up to a maximum of 9 points.

	SCORE	
	Left	Right
1. Can you put your hands flat on the floor with your knees straight?	1	
2. Can you bend your elbow backwards?	1	1
3. Can you bend your knee backwards?	1	1
4. Can you bend your thumb back on to the front of your forearm?	1	1
5. Can you bend your little finger up at 90° (right angles) to the back of your hand?	1	1
	9	

Figure 24.4 Calculation of the Beighton score. Reproduced with kind permission from Arthritis Research <http://www.arthritisresearchuk.org/>.

It is widely believed that children are more flexible than adolescents, but there is very little supporting literature. For example, one rigorous population-based study from Sweden (Jansson et al., 2004) investigated 1845 children aged 9, 12, or 15 years from 48 geographically randomly selected schools and showed that at all ages, girls had a higher degree of generalized joint laxity as assessed by the modified Beighton criteria. Girls had the highest degree of general joint laxity at the age of 15 years, whereas joint laxity in boys decreased with increasing age. Similarly, a study of high school basketball players (Quatman et al., 2008) showed that after the onset of puberty, girls exhibited greater joint laxity than boys. A recent robust UK population-based cohort study showed that the prevalence of generalized joint laxity in girls and boys (mean age 13.8 years) was 27.5% and 10.6%, respectively, when the commonly used cut-off of four hypermobile joints from the modified Beighton 9-point scoring system was used (total of 1156/6022 children; Clinch et al., 2011). This is arguably within the normal variance of the adolescent population, and suggests that a higher cut-off (such as ≥6/9) or a new, more meaningful measure is needed.

The extent to which generalized joint laxity is associated with significant clinical sequelae, including joint pain, is unclear. A proportion of children noted to be hypermobile can present with recurrent lower-limb arthralgia, anterior knee pain syndromes, and back pain. The prevalence of pain among children with generalized joint laxity has been reported to range from 30% (El-Garf et al., 1998) to 55% (Qvindesland and Jonsson, 1999). However, reports linking hypermobility with joint pain in school children suffer from problems with sample size, methods of assessing hypermobility, and methods of assessing pain. By contrast, a cross-sectional study of schoolchildren showed no association between joint laxity and pain (Leone et al., 2009). A recent evaluation of over 4000 17-year-old adolescents using a higher cut-off for the Beighton score (≥6 joints) showed that there is a relationship at this age between hypermobility and pain in the knees and shoulders. There was no relationship between hypermobility and chronic widespread pain/fibromyalgia or back pain (Tobias et al., 2013). A large cohort study has also shown a positive association between generalized joint laxity (Beighton score ≥6) and habitual levels of physical activity, body mass index, and maternal education in girls (Deere et al., submitted).

What seems clear is that the majority of hypermobile individuals will not have significant pain or have any risk for specific musculoskeletal disorders (including osteoarthritis) in later life. Screening tools such as the Beighton score are likely to be inadequate in children as they are generally more mobile than adults (Deere et al., submitted). The challenge remains to interpret symptoms correctly as being related to the joint hypermobility and to predict why some children become symptomatic. The answer is likely to involve physiological and psychosocial factors.

The impact of chronic musculoskeletal pain on the child and family

Chronic musculoskeletal pain, irrespective of its trigger, can be associated with persistent and recurrent distress, disability, adult attention, and widespread family disruption (Perquin et al., 2000). Pain-related anxiety in JIA is a significant problem for many children and independently affects their social development (Gauntlett-Gilbert et al., 2013a). Most families have relatively successful mechanisms for dealing with short-lived demands or disruption. However, a young person with significant musculoskeletal chronic pain typically demands sustained physical, emotional, and financial resources (Roth-Isigkeit et al., 2005). Young people with musculoskeletal chronic pain report sleep disturbance, disordered mood, appetite disruption, low feelings (depression is often masked in this population), social isolation, and unwelcome dependency on parents. These are experienced chronically and can serve to maintain pain and disability. They are also difficult to manage in isolation from other symptoms. Adolescence is by definition a time of change and experimentation; adolescents with chronic pain report that they are less socially developed on virtually every metric than their peers (Eccleston et al., 2008).

Parents also report significant distress from living with a child in persistent pain. Levels of parental stress are clinically significant (Eccleston et al., 2004) and parents experience severe distress and conflict in parenting their child. Typically, they report struggling with the desire to cure their child's pain, and comfort their child, recognizing that the desire to protect may be counterproductive (Jordan et al., 2007).

Managing chronic musculoskeletal pain in childhood/adolescence

Assessment

History, examination, and investigations are required to exclude significant underlying disease. Although it is common and necessary to be clinically conservative and investigate multiple potential causes, if prolonged this can also lead to a diagnostic vacuum in treatment planning that allows for fear, disability, and depression to grow. With serious medical causes excluded one can then safely move on to rehabilitation. In paediatric practice this may be more difficult as there can be a tendency to catastrophize about persistent pain by the family, and sometimes by the physician. The need to find a cause for the pain can be overwhelming and, in this way, the child may be subject to a large number of medical investigations and interventions that are, at best, not appropriate and cause anxiety. For example, adolescents commonly present to paediatric rheumatology clinics with back pain; it is important to rule out pathology including malignancy and inflammation but to then move forward swiftly with reassurance and rehabilitation. All too often children are moved between different specialities and have further investigations over a long time period; in many instances this causes delay in rehabilitation and increased disability (Clinch and Eccleston, 2009)

History

For the physician, the goals of history taking are to exclude serious possible causes, identify key problems, build a trusting relationship with the patient (and family), and, if possible, identify a treatment plan. The main differential diagnoses in musculoskeletal pain are trauma, inflammation, infection and malignancy (Box 24.2). Many children with persistent musculoskeletal pain not only have a chronic experience of pain and distress, but a chronic experience of medical settings, feelings of being doubted, having the validity of their pain contested, and often a history of failed and pain exacerbating interventions. Three key psychological features of this setting are worth keeping in mind:

Box 24.2 Key pathology to exclude in musculoskeletal history

1. Inflammation:

   a. JIA: pain centred around joint but may be poorly localized (particularly in younger children). Usually more severe in morning and accompanied by stiffness. Reports of joint swelling in peripheral joints. Inflammatory backpain (including sacroiliitis) worse in morning and can wake child up at night.

   b. Discitis: inflammation of vertebral discs. More common in young children. Severe back pain, worse on movement and can wake at night.

   c. Myositis: inflammation of muscle groups. Muscle pain and fatigue. May follow infection or a presenting feature of rare conditions such as juvenile dermatomyositis (rash will accompany this).

   d. Chronic recurrent osteomyelitis: rare inflammatory condition affecting discrete portions of bone. Severe bone pain, may wake at night. Bone swelling seen if severe (particularly on clavicle).

   e. Osteoid osteoma: benign painful lesions in bones. Pain at any time. May wake at night. Localized.

2. Infection:

   a. Septic arthritis: usually acute presentation but can persist. Hot, swollen, painful joint. Child may be systemically unwell.

   b. Infective osteomyelitis: again usually acute but can develop Brodie's abscess and persistent bone pain if not identified early.

   c. Tuberculosis: TB can seed in the spine (Potts disease) or joint and cause persistent pain/swelling. A history of travel or contact is important.

3. Trauma:

   a. Accidental: enquire about any accidents, sporting injury. This can be missed.

   b. Non-accidental injury: it is extremely important that unusual musculoskeletal pain patterns or inconsistent history of events is investigated.

   c. Osteogenesis imperfecta: these children may have a history of bone pain with no or very little trauma. They suffer multiple fractures.

4. Malignancy:

   a. Haematological malignancy: bone pain (night and day) and effusions can be the presenting features of leukaemia.

   b. Osteosarcoma, Ewing's sarcoma: localized persistent pain (day and night).

   c. Neuroblastoma: often in younger children. Localized joint pain with or without history of swelling.

Note: a full medical history is important to exclude other diseases associated with joint pain (including inflammatory bowel disease, cystic fibrosis).

♦ Both child and family are likely to be fearful, hoping for a cure, desperate to be helpful, but often 'on their best behaviour', so may not immediately appear to be distressed, and may have flat or neutral affect.

♦ Because of their history, any attempt to shift the treatment goal from one of cure to management or symptom control may be heard to be patient and carer(s) blaming, and so should be done only after building trust.

♦ What matters is not necessarily what information has been given to the patient and carers, but what they believe to be true. Typically both patient and family will have heard a variety of stories about what may be happening to them (Clinch and Eccleston, 2009). For example, a family who have a child with many painful joints and associated disability may have family members or friends who have a history of bone pain related to other pathology (arthritis, cancer, infection, etc.). Despite reassurance this fear often remains. Inconsistent messages from health professionals and repeat investigations serve to reinforce the anxiety.

Physical examination

Time spent on full physical examination at the beginning may prevent repetition and unnecessary, distressing investigations at a later date (Anthony and Schanberg, 2007; Clinch and Eccleston, 2009). If there is concern regarding the diagnosis, then this is the time to order all investigations and ensure that these are followed up. Undue delay leads to fear and often a worsening of pain symptoms and associated disability. On assessment a full musculoskeletal examination would show evidence of, and target investigations to rule out:

♦ Inflammation (including JIA, myositis, myopathy, connective tissue disease, chronic recurrent mulitfocal osteomyelitis).

♦ Infection (including septic arthritis, infective osteomyelitis).

♦ Malignancy (including osteosarcoma, Ewing's sarcoma, leukaemia, neuroblastoma).

♦ Trauma (including non-accidental injury).

Paediatric GALS screening (child version of the Gait, Arms, Legs, and Spine adult examination) is a musculoskeletal examination that can be completed within a short time period on children of all ages (Foster et al., 2006; <http://www.arthritisresearchuk.org/health-professionals-and-students/video-resources/pgals>).

Psychometric instruments

Musculoskeletal pain intensity in children has long been measured using simple severity measurement tools, such as the visual analogue scale (VAS; Carlsson, 1983; see von Baeyer, Chapter 36, this volume). These give a subjective measure of the pain intensity according to the adolescent and/or pain perceived by their carer. While useful measures, they give no indication of the impact of pain on the young person's life (see Tham et al., Chapter 41, this volume). Two recently developed multidisciplinary tools that have been validated in JIA-related chronic pain and the more general paediatric pain population include:

♦ Bath Adolescent Pain Questionnaire (Eccleston et al., 2005) for measuring the impact of pain on adolescents with chronic pain (now used in many tertiary paediatric rheumatology settings).

♦ Bath Adolescent Pain Questionnaire for Parents (Jordan et al., 2008) for measuring the impact of adolescent chronic pain on parents.

Physiological measures of pain-related indices

There are little data on the role or utility of measuring physiological processes in the context of childhood chronic musculoskeletal pain. The role of thermography and bone scintigraphy in CRPS has been studied (Goldsmith et al., 1989; Lightman et al., 1987) in the early and late stages of this pain condition, but opinion is divided on their usefulness. Functional MRI has recently been shown to be a useful tool in evaluating CNS changes in childhood CRPS (Lebel et al., 2008). Quantitative sensory testing (QST) is a valuable tool for assessing sensory perception (including pain) in children (Blankenburg et al., 2010; see also Hermann, Chapter 40, this volume).

Rehabilitation and self-management

The primary treatment approach to the young person with chronic musculoskeletal pain is one of symptom management and psychosocial rehabilitation. Although it may be tempting to focus solely on the amelioration of the suffering of the child, one of the most important aspects of rehabilitation is 'inclusion'. A dedicated team that works consistently with the adolescent and family will facilitate communication, ensure effective delivery of therapy, reduce iatrogenic influences and enable goals to be reached earlier (Christie and Wilson, 2005;Walco et al., 2010; see also Birnie et al., Chapter 12, this volume). Most approaches to rehabilitation share common features that include education, symptom control, behavioural science and physical therapy. How these strands are delivered is debated. Certainly early recognition and intervention in an outpatient or inpatient setting is key and, in most cases, leads to a more favourable outcome (Anthony and Schanberg, 2007).

There is no current evidence favouring a dedicated outpatient over inpatient service for musculoskeletal pain; however anecdotally it is reported that treating children away from busy acute settings and keeping them in their local area, if possible, is beneficial (Clinch and Eccleston, 2009; Eccleston et al., 2003).

Dedicated pain residential units are able to provide physical and psychological intense treatment for children with significant pain associated disability. Musculoskeletal pain comprises approximately 60% of the presenting conditions in these units and over 80% of the children have related limb/back pain. Outcomes from these units show that pain does not significantly change but function (including back to school), anxiety and coping is measurably improved (Eccleston et al., 2003). Recently the role of parents in pain behaviour has been evaluated (McCracken and Gauntlett-Gilbert, 2011), and parents are key in rehabilitation plans. Specific parent programmes in residential pain centres have been developed and show that changing parent behaviour and responses to their child's pain, assists the child moving on to more optimal outcomes (Gauntlett-Gilbert, 2013a; McCracken and Gauntlett-Gilbert, 2011).

Education

Although the evidence for education alone as a treatment for behaviour change is lacking, the provision of a rationale for what are often counter-intuitive instructions in self-management is essential. Additionally, one should never underestimate that the average understanding of musculoskeletal anatomy and physiology is often limited. A critical first step in rehabilitation is to offer, reoffer, and reinforce an understanding of how one's body may be working to maintain pain.

Education about pain may be difficult to grasp because there is a dominant cultural view of pain in joints and muscles as a warning sign that a disease process or abnormality is present, and there is often a need for the young person and family to identify a cause. Education can play a valuable role as a fear reduction strategy, providing information to counter beliefs that that they have a unique medical complication, or that their symptoms are related to an underlying mysterious disease (Clinch and Eccleston, 2009). Children and their parents often have inflexible or rigid ideas not only about the cause of pain, but also of pain as an important signal of damage or disease. Back pain is extremely common but rarely related to malignancy or arthritis. It can be helpful to show and reinforce to the family the fact that many childhood pains have no function, or have outlived their usefulness. Rhetorical devices (metaphors, stories, examples, pictures) that counter this rigid thinking can be helpful. Explaining the fascinating case of phantom limb experiences can also be helpful, to introduce flexibility to the idea that brain signals must signify peripheral damage.

Pharmacotherapy

Many analgesics and different interventions have been used for children with chronic musculoskeletal pain, but are not supported by well-controlled therapeutic trials. It is becoming widely accepted, however, that any analgesic intervention should only be used alongside multidisciplinary therapy (Eccleston et al., 2003, 2009).

Psychological therapies

A Cochrane systematic review reported that psychological therapies are effective for headache and may improve pain control in children with musculoskeletal pain (Eccleston et al., 2009). Small studies using cognitive-behavioural therapy (CBT) in juvenile fibromyalgia (chronic widespread pain) show significant improvement in the child's confidence with managing the pain, but disappointing effect on functional disability and depressive symptoms (Kashikar-Zuck, 2006; see also Logan et al., Chapter 50, this volume). For children who have significant pain-associated disability (school absence, limited mobility, lost independence, extremely low mood, disturbed sleep) there are no randomized controlled trials of multidisciplinary multicomponent CBT; however, there is evidence that an interdisciplinary programme has a positive impact for adolescents disabled with chronic pain (Eccleston et al., 2003). The role of the physician is often as an educator, to oversee analgesic withdrawal and to support the overall message that it is safe to increase activity despite pain and reduce reliance on medical support (Clinch and Eccleston, 2009).

Physical therapies

In conditions such as CRPS, early intensive physiotherapy (including desensitization) with behavioural support can provide dramatic reversal of the presenting signs and symptoms for some patients (Littlejohn, 2004). The aim is accelerated mobilization (Lee et al., 2002), but this is hindered if the diagnosis is delayed and access to appropriate physical and psychological rehabilitation is limited (Littlejohn, 2004). Many cases of diffuse pain will require a gentle, paced approach. In all cases, the increase of activity should be consistent despite the pain. With musculoskeletal pains the more active the musculoskeletal system becomes the more likely the muscle spasms and tightening are to reduce.

Proprioception improves (Lee et al., 2002; Low et al., 2007) and autonomic changes subside. Where possible the young person should work to devise his or her own 'fitness plan'. Using a local gym rather than a hospital physiotherapy gym allows them to start to return to a more normal environment (Eccleston et al., 2003). Working in this consistent and paced manner can be extremely hard for the young person and their parents. The pain invariably continues at the beginning (if not throughout) and motivation is poor. Parental anxiety is high (Lee et al., 2002) and there is a fear that damage will be done. Psychological support during this time is important. The young person will need help setting goals, learning how to communicate pain to peers and family, maintaining motivation on 'bad days', managing low mood, dealing with anger and frustration, and overcoming fears. Often they have not been at school for a long period of time and need help in preparing again for this difficult environment. In some cases, there may be other mental health needs that can be identified and appropriately treated. See also Holsti et al. (Chapter 57, this volume) and Tupper et al. (Chapter 56, this volume) for further details.

There are ongoing studies that show promise with visual counter-stimulation, specifically in patients with CRPS. Mirror therapy, focusing on the hypothesis that incongruence between motor output and sensory input produces CRPS, is being evaluated in adults (McCabe et al., 2003) but there is no data for children.

It is common for young people with musculoskeletal pain to have contact with complementary medicines (often sourced by their parents). While the evidence supporting many of these therapies in children and adolescents is poor (Tsao and Zeltzer, 2005), some children report benefit with topical treatments that are massaged into the painful area (e.g. back pain) (see also Weydert, Chapter 59; Zeltzer, Chapter 60, this volume).

Natural history and long-term outcomes

The natural history of chronic musculoskeletal pain in children shows that, in many cases, functional and psychosocial outcomes are improved when compared with adults (Bursch et al., 1998; Gedalia et al., 2000). Early multidisciplinary input (including CBT) has been associated with improved outcomes (Eccleston et al., 2003). CRPS in children generally has a favourable prognosis if early physiotherapy is initiated (with psychological support; Sherry et al., 1999; Stanton Hicks, 2010). This is improved if the parents are involved in the rehabilitation process (Gauntlett-Gilbert et al., 2013b). However, a prolonged time to treatment and the presence of marked autonomic changes are poor prognostic indicators in this condition.

Summary points

- Untreated complex paediatric pain is personally, socially, and financially burdensome for individuals, families, and societies.

- Ensure an early, thorough history and physical musculoskeletal examination to rule out new or suboptimally treated pathology in children with chronic musculoskeletal pain.

- Evaluate the impact of the pain on the child and family (not just the level of pain) so that rehabilitation can be tailored

- Involve a multidisciplinary team early (ideally in joint clinics) to facilitate cohesive working and the introduction of psychological and physical therapies.

- Evidence shows that early dedicated therapy can significantly improve the outcome of childhood chronic musculoskeletal pain.

- Key areas for further research include evaluating the physiology of childhood musculoskeletal pain, the role of parents, and evaluating the efficacy of pharmacological interventions.

Case example

Anna is a 12-year-old previously well girl, who develops pain in her left ankle following a fall during her gymnastics class. She attends the Accident and Emergency (A&E) department, no fracture is seen on X-ray, and her ankle is bandaged. She is advised to rest, take paracetamol and ibuprofen for the pain, avoid weight bearing and use crutches until the pain settles. One week later, she returns to A&E as she still has severe pain. Repeat X-ray is normal, but her ankle is immobilized in a below-knee cast and she is referred for an orthopaedic opinion at her local hospital. Four weeks later the cast is removed, her lower leg is noted to be swollen, red, warm, and slightly sweaty, and she is still unable to weight bear due to pain. She is given codeine for analgesia, an MRI confirms swelling but there is no localized infection or bony injury. Anna is referred for physiotherapy, but is unable to perform most of the suggested exercises, as her leg is too painful. Over the next 2 months, the pain extends to involve her whole lower limb, her leg is now cold and mottled, and she can no longer wear shoes and socks as the skin is sensitive to touch. Anna can now only walk for short distances with crutches, is using a wheelchair to mobilize, cannot manage at school, and is sleeping poorly.

Both Anna and her parents are concerned that an important diagnosis has been missed, and request referral to another specialist. A bone scan is performed which shows a generalized decrease uptake, and she is commenced on gabapentin for her pain. Despite increasing doses of gabapentin, and continued use of codeine and ibuprofen, Anna's pain does not improve. She is referred to a multidisciplinary clinic. Anna reports continuing pain, she is unable to tolerate trousers on her left leg, and her leg feels weak. On examination, she is sitting in a wheel chair and is reluctant to stand, her lower leg appears swollen, light touch is painful but her left foot feels colder than the right, and she has reduced range of movement in both the ankle and knee. CRPS is diagnosed, and the nature of the condition and management are discussed with Anna and her parents. Her investigations are reviewed and reassurance given that other diagnoses have been excluded and no further investigations are required. Anna is referred for an intensive rehabilitation programme which includes physiotherapy, psychological interventions, and education. Her parents are still concerned, and angry that it has taken so long for the diagnosis to be made, but agree to attend family sessions during the programme. Despite initial reluctance to do physiotherapy exercises which exacerbated her pain, Anna is given a graded programme, and her mobility gradually improves. Three weeks later, she still has residual pain, but she is able to walk without aids, is weaning off her medications, and her sleep and mood have improved. Prior to discharge, Anna is given instructions about continuing management at home, including the need to deal with potential flare-ups. On review 3 months later, Anna has returned to full-time school and although she had a relapse of pain and swelling in her leg 4 weeks previously, she was able to manage this with increasing exercises and maintained weight bearing.

References

Ahlqwist, A., Hagman, M., Kjellby-Wendt, G., and Beckung, E. (2008). Physical therapy treatment of back complaints on children and adolescents. *Spine*, 33(20), E721–727.

American Pain Society. (2012). *Assessment and management of children with chronic pain*. The American Pain Society: Position statement. Available at: <https://www.ampainsoc.org/advocacy/downloads/aps12-pcp.pdf>.

Anthony, K. K., and Schanberg, L. E. (2007). Assessment and management of pain syndromes and arthritis pain in children and adolescents. *Rheum Dis Clin North Am*, 33, 625–660.

Brattberg, G. (1994). The incidence of back pain and headache among Swedish school children. *Qual Life Res*, 3(Suppl.1), S27–31.

Beighton, P., Solomon, L., and Soskolne, C. L. (1973). Articular mobility in an African population. *Ann Rheum Dis*, 32, 413–418.

Berde, C. B., and Lebel, A. (2005). Complex regional pain syndrome in children and adolescents. *Anesthesiology*, 102(2), 252–255.

Blankenburg, M., Boekens, H., Hechler, T., Maier, C., Krumova, E., Scherens, A., *et al.* (2010). Reference values for quantitative sensory testing in children and adolescents: developmental and gender differences of somatosensory perception. *Pain*, 149(1), 76–88.

Brattberg, G. (2004). Do pain problems in young school children persist into early adulthood? A 13-year follow-up. *Eur J Pain*, 8, 187–199.

Bursch, B., Walco, G. A., and Zeltzer, L. (1998). Clinical assessment and management of chronic pain and pain-associated disability syndrome. *Dev Behav Pediatr*, 1, 45–53.

Buskila, D., Neumann, L., Herschman, E., Gedalia, A., Press, J., and Sukenik, S. (1995). Fibromyalgia syndrome in children-an outcome study. *J Rheumatol*, 22, 525–528.

Buskila, D. and Neumann, L. (2000). Musculoskeletal injury as a trigger for fibromyalgia/posttraumatic fibromyalgia. *Curr Rheumatol Rep*, 2, 104–108.

Carlsson, A. M. (1983). Assessment of chronic pain. I. Aspects of the reliability and validity of the visual analogue scale. *Pain*, 16, 87–101.

Christie, D. and Wilson, C. (2005). CBT in paediatric and adolescent health settings: a review of practice-based evidence. *Pediatr Rehabil*, 8, 241–247.

Clinch, J., Deere, K., Sayers, A., Palmer, S., Palmer, S., Riddoch, C., *et al.* (2011). Epidemiology of generalized joint laxity (hypermobility) in fourteen-year-old children from the UK. *Arthritis Rheum*, 63, 2819–2827.

Clinch, J. and Eccleston, C. (2009). Chronic musculoskeletal pain in children: assessment and management. *Rheumatology*, 48, 466–474.

Cohen, H., Neumann, L., Kotler, K., and Buskila, D. (2001). Autonomic nervous system derangement in fibromyalgia syndrome and related disorders. *Isr Med Assoc J*, 3, 755–760.

Connelly, M., Anthony, K. K., Sarniak, R., Bromberg, M. H., Gil, K. M., and Schanberg, L. E. (2010). Parent pain responses as predictors of daily activities and mood in children with juvenile idiopathic arthritis: the utility of electronic diaries. *J Pain Symptom Manage*, 39(3), 579–90.

Connelly, M. and Schanberg, L. (2006). Latest developments in the assessment and management of chronic musculoskeletal pain syndromes in children. *Curr Opin Rheumatol*, 18, 496–502.

De Mos, M., de Bruijn, A. G., Huygen, F. J., Dieleman, J. P., Stricker, B. H., and Sturkenboom, M. C. (2007). The incidence of complex regional pain syndrome: a population based study. *Pain*, 129, 12–20.

Deere, K., Clinch, J., Sayers, A., Palmer, S., Clarke, E. M., and Tobias, J. (submitted). Female sex and obesity are risk factors for non-specific musculoskeletal pain in adolescents: findings from a population based cohort.

Diepenmaat, A. C., van der Wal, M. F., de Vet, H. C., and Hirasing, R. A. (2006). Neck/shoulder, low back, and arm pain in relation to computer use, physical activity, stress, and depression among Dutch adolescents. *Pediatrics*, 117, 412–416.

Eccleston, C., Crombez, G., Scotford, A., Clinch, J., and Connell, H. (2004). Adolescent chronic pain:patterns and predictors of emotional distress in adolescents with chronic pain and their parents. *Pain*, 108, 221–229.

Eccleston, C., Jordan, A., McCracken, L. M., Connell, H., and Clinch, J. (2005). The Bath Adolescent Pain Questionnaire (BAPQ): development and preliminary psychometric evaluation of an instrument to assess the impact of chronic pain on adolescents. *Pain*, 118, 263–270.

Eccleston, C., Malleson, P. M., Clinch, J., Connell, H., and Sourbut, C. (2003). Chronic pain in adolescents: evaluation of a programme of interdisciplinary cognitive behaviour therapy. *Arch Dis Child*, 88, 881–858.

Eccleston, C., Palermo, T. M., Williams, A. C., Lewandowski, A., and Morley, S. (2009). Psychological therapies for the management of chronic and recurrent pain in children and adolescents. *Cochrane Database Syst Rev*, 2, CD003968.

Eccleston, C., Wastell, S., Crombez, G., and Jordan, A. (2008). Adolescent social development and chronic pain. *Eur J Pain*, 12(6), 765–774.

Elbaz, A., Mirovsky, Y., Mor, A., Enosh, S., Debbi, E., Segal, G., *et al.* (2009). A novel biomechanical device improves gait pattern in patient with chronic nonspecific low back pain. *Spine*, 34(15), E507–512.

El-Garf, A. K., Mahmoud, G. A., and Mahgoub, E. H. (1998). Hypermobility among Egyptian children: prevalence and features. *J Rheumatol*, 25, 1003–1005.

Foster, H. E., Kay, L. J., Friswell, M., Coady, D., and Myers, A. (2006). Musculoskeletal screening examination (pGALS) for school-age children based on the adult GALS screen. *Arthritis Rheum*, 55(5), 709–716.

Friedland, O., Hashkes, P. J., Jaber, L., Cohen, H. A., Eliakim, A., Wolach, B., *et al.* (2005). Decreased bone speed of sound in children with growing pains measured by quantitative ultrasound. *J Rheumatol*, 32, 1354–1357.

Gauntlett-Gilbert, J., Kavirayani, A., and Clinch, J. (2013a). Physical and social functioning in adolescents with rheumatological conditions. *Acta Pediatr*, 102(3), e131–136.

Gauntlett-Gilbert, J., Connell, H., Clinch, J., Eccleston, C., and McCracken, L. (2013b). Acceptance and values based treatment of adolescents with chronic pain: outcomes and process. *J Ped Psych*, 38(1), 72–81.

Gedalia, A., Garcia, C. O., Molina, J. F., Bradford, N. J., and Espinoza, L. R. (2000). Fibromyalgia syndrome: experience in a pediatric rheumatology clinic. *Clin Exp Rheumatol*, 18, 415–419.

Geisser, M. E., Casey, K. L., Brucksch, C. B., Ribbens, C. M., Appleton, B. B., and Crofford, L. J. (2003). Perception of noxious and innocuous heat stimulation among healthy women and women with fibromyalgia: association with mood, somatic focus, and catastrophizing. *Pain*, 102, 243–250.

Goldsmith, D. P., Vivino, F. B., Heyman, S., Athreya, B. H., and Heyman, S. (1989). Nuclear imaging and clinical features of childhood reflex neurovascular dystrophy: comparison with adults. *Arthritis Rheum*, 32, 480–485.

Groholt, E. K. (2003). Recurrent pain in children, socio-economic factors and accumulation in families. *Eur J Epidemiol*, 18, 965–975.

Harden, R. N., Bruehl, S., Perez, R. S., Birklein, F., Marinus, J., Maihofner, C., *et al.* (2010). Validation of proposed diagnostic criteria (the 'Budapest Criteria') for Complex Regional Pain Syndrome. *Pain*, 150(2), 268–274.

Hashkes, P. J., Gorenberg, M., Oren, V., Friedland, O., and Uziel, Y. (2005). 'Growing pains' in children are not associated with changes in vascular perfusion patterns in painful regions. *Clin Rheumatol*, 24, 342–345.

Haverman, L., Grootenhuis, M. A., van den Berg, J. M., van Veenendaal, M., Dolman, K. M., Swart, J. F., *et al.* (2012). Predictors of health-related quality of life in children and adolescents with juvenile idiopathic arthritis: results from a web-based survey. *Arthritis Care Res*, 64(5), 694–703.

Hoftun, G. B., Romundstad, P. R., Zwart, J. A., and Rygg, M. (2011). Chronic idiopathic pain in adolescence—high prevalence and disability: The young HUNT study 2008. *Pain*, 152, 2259–2266.

Jansson, A., Saartok, T., Werner, S., and Renstrom, P. (2004). General joint laxity in 1845 Swedish school children of different ages: age- andgender-specific distributions. *Acta Paediatr*, 93, 1202–1206.

Jones, G. T., Silman, A. J., Power, C., and Macfarlane, G. J. (2007). Are common symptoms in childhood associated with chronic widespread body pain in adulthood? Results from the 1958 British Birth Cohort Study. *Arthritis Rheum*, 56, 1669–1675.

Jones, M., Stratton, G., Reilly, T., and Unnithan, V. (2007). The efficacy of exercise as an intervention to treat recurrent nonspecific low back pain in adolescents. *Pediatr Exerc Sci*, 19(3), 349–359.

Jordan, A., Eccleston, C., McCracken, L. M., Connell, H., and Clinch, J. (2008). The Bath Adolescent Pain—Parental Impact Questionnaire (BAP-PIQ): development and preliminary psychometric evaluation of an instrument to assess the impact of parenting an adolescent with chronic pain. *Pain*, 137, 478–487.

Jordan, A. L., Eccleston, C., and Osborn, C. (2007). Being a parent of the adolescent with complex chronic pain. *Eur J Pain*, 11, 49–56.

Kashikar-Zuck, S. (2006). Treatment of children with unexplained chronic pain. *Lancet*, 367, 380–382.

Kjaer, P., Wedderkopp, N., Korsholm, L., and Leboeuf-Yde, C. (2011). Prevalence and tracking of back pain from childhood to adolescence. *BMC Musculoskelet Disord*, 12, 98.

Lebel, A., Becerra, L., Wallin, D., Moulton, E. A., Morris, S., Pendse, G., et al. (2008). fMRI reveals distinct CNS processing during symptomatic and recovered complex regional pain syndrome in children. *Brain*, 131(Pt 7), 1854–1879.

Lee, B. H., Schariff, L., Sethna, N. F., McCarthey, C. F., Scott-Sutherland, J., Shea, A. M., et al. (2002). Physical therapy and cognitive behavioural treatment for complex regional pain syndromes. *J Pediatr*, 141, 135–140.

Leone, V., Tornese, G., Zerial, M., Locatelli, C., Ciambra, R., Bensa, M., et al. (2009). Joint hypermobility and its relationship to musculoskeletal pain in schoolchildren: a cross-sectional study. *Arch Dis Child*, 94, 627–632.

Lightman, H. I., Pochaczevsky, R., Aprin, H., and Ilowite, N. (1987). Thermography in childhood reflex sympathetic dystrophy. *J Pediatr*, 111, 551–555.

Littlejohn, G. O. (2004). Reflex sympathetic dystrophy in adolescents: lessons for adults. *Arthritis Rheum*, 51, 151–153.

Lovell, D. J., and Walco, G. A. (1989). Pain associated with juvenile rheumatoid arthritis. *Pediatr Clin North Am*, 36(4), 1015–1027.

Low, A. K., Ward, K., and Wines, A. P. (2007). Pediatric complex regional pain syndrome. *J Pediat Orthop*, 27(5), 567–572.

Lundin, O., Hellström, M., Nilsson, I., and Swärd, L. (2001). Back pain and radiological changes in the thoraco-lumbar spine of athletes. A long-term follow-up. *Scand J Med Sci Sports*, 11(2), 103–109.

Malleson, P. and Clinch, J. (2003). Pain syndromes in children. *Curr Opin Rheumatol*, 15, 572–580.

Malleson, P. N., Connell, H., Bennett, S. M., and Eccelston, C. (2001). Chronic musculoskeletal and other idiopathic pain syndromes. *Arch Dis Child*, 84, 189–192.

McCabe, C. S., Haigh, R. C., Ring, E. F., Halligan, P. W., Wall, P. D., and Blake, D. R. (2003). A controlled pilot study of the utility of mirror visual feedback in the treatment of complex regional pain syndrome (type 1). *Rheumatology*, 42, 97–101.

McCracken, L. M., and Gauntlett-Gilbert, J. (2011). Role of psychological flexibility in parents of adolescents with chronic pain: development of a measure and preliminary correlation analyses. *Pain*, 152(4), 780–785.

O'Sullivan, P., Beales, D., Jensen, L., Murray, K., and Myers, T. (2011). Characteristics of chronic non- specific musculoskeletal pain in children and adolescents attending a rheumatology outpatients clinic: a cross-sectional study. *Pediatric Rheumatol*, 9, 3.

Pamuk, O. N., and Cakir, N. (2005). The variation in chronic widespread pain and other symptoms in fibromyalgia patients. The effects of menses and menopause. *Clin Exp Rheumatol*, 23(6), 778–782.

Perquin, C. W., Hazebroek-Kampschreur, A. A., and Hunfield, J. A. (2000). Pain in children and adolescents: a common experience. *Pain*, 87, 51–58.

Quatman, C. E., Ford, K. R., Myer, G. D., Paterno, M. V., and Hewett, T. E. (2008). The effects of gender and pubertal status on generalized joint laxity in young athletes. *J Sci Med Sport*, 11, 257–263.

Qvindesland, A. and Jonsson, H. (1999). Articular hypermobility in Icelandic 12-year olds. *Rhematology*, 38, 1014–1016

Roth-Isigkeit, A. (2005). Pain among children and adolescents: restrictions in daily living and triggering factors. *Pediatrics*, 115, 152–162.

Sherry, D. D., Wallace, C. A., Kelley, C., Kidder, M., and Sapp, L. (1999). Short- and long-term outcomes of children with complex regional pain syndrome type I treated with exercise therapy. *Clin J Pain*, 15(3), 218–223.

Sjolie, A. N. (2004). Persistence and change in nonspecific low back pain among adolescents: a 3-year prospective study. *Spine*, 29(21), 2452–2457

Stanton Hicks, M. (2010). Plasticity of complex regional pain syndrome (CRPS) in children *Pain Med*, 11(8), 1216–1223.

Tobias, J., Deere, K., and Clinch, J. (2013). Hypermobility and mechanical pain. *Arthritis Rheum*, 65(4), 1107–1115.

Tsao, J. C., and Zeltzer, L. K. (2005). Complementary and alternative medicine approaches for pediatric pain: a review of the state-of-the-science. *Evid Based Complement Altern Med*, 2, 149–159.

Vuorimaa, H., Tamm, K., Honkanen, V., Komulainen, E., Konttinen, Y. T., and Santavirta, N. (2009). Parents and children as agents of disease management in JIA. *Child Care Health Dev*, 35(4), 578–585.

Walco, G. A., Dworkin, R. H., Krane, E. J., LeBel, A. A., and Treede, R. D. (2010). Neuropathic pain in children: special considerations. *Mayo Clin Proc*, 85(3 Suppl), S33–41.

Watson, K. D., Papageorgiou, A. C., Jones, G. T., Taylor, S., Symmons, D. P., Silman, A. J., and Macfarlane, G. J. (2002). Low back pain in schoolchildren: occurrence and characteristics. *Pain*, 97(1–2), 87–92.

Wolfe, F., Clauw, D. J., Fitzcharles, M. A., Goldenberg, D. L., Katz, R. S., Mease, P., et al. (2010). The American College of Rheumatology preliminary diagnostic criteria for fibromyalgia and measurement of symptom severity. *Arthritis Care Res*, 62(5), 600–610.

CHAPTER 25

Pain in sickle cell disease

Carlton Dampier and Lamia Barakat

Summary

Sickle cell disease (SCD) presents a complex pain disorder to clinicians. Pain from vaso-occlusion of sickle erythrocytes can occur in multiple musculoskeletal locations, several internal viscera such as the spleen, as well as the penis. Such pain is typically intermittent in childhood, shares features of acute pain with other pain disorders, and often responds to non-steroidal anti-inflammatory drugs (NSAIDs) and opioid analgesics. Adolescents with SCD often experience more frequent pain, and those with bone disease in spine, hips, or shoulders may experience chronic pain. Like other chronic pain disorders, this pain often responds poorly to opioids, but there is limited current clinical or research data to support alternative medications. Many cognitive-behavioural strategies are helpful as part of multidisciplinary pain management, particularly in adolescents, who may also benefit from psychological support to treat coexistent mood disorders, to increase coping skills, and to support appropriate school and family functioning. Future advances in pharmacological and psychological therapies are needed to ameliorate the substantial burden of pain in children and adolescents with SCD.

Introduction

Sickle cell disease (SCD) is a complex autosomal recessive disorder of haemoglobin structure characterized by variable degrees of haemolytic anaemia and intermittent episodes of vaso-occlusion that cause or contribute to a variety of acute and chronic complications, and ultimately leads to the development of chronic organ damage. These cumulative disease effects cause significant morbidity, reduced quality of life, and shortened life expectancy. Studies from the former Comprehensive Sickle Cell Centers suggest that it is the occurrence of vaso-occlusive pain that has the strongest negative effect on child or adult-reported health-related quality of life compared to any other acute or chronic SCD-related complications (Dampier et al., 2010a, 2010b). Healthcare utilization for pain management and their associated costs are substantial in this disorder. Yearly estimates of hospitalization frequency in the US range from 70 000 to 90 000, and over 200 000 to 230 000 for emergency department (ED) visits based on data from the Nationwide Emergency Department Sample, most of which (>80%) are for adults, with pain as the major indication (Lanzkron et al., 2010). This ED utilization is three times higher than for congestive heart failure, HIV, or asthma. Lifetime costs for SCD care have been estimated at over $US450 000 per individual including home care, and annual charges have been estimated at $US350 million for ED visits and $US1 to $US2 billion for hospitalizations, depending on study methodology (Kauf et al., 2009).

SCD pathophysiology

The pathophysiology of vaso-occlusion in SCD is quite complex and involves mechanisms beyond sickle polymer formation. One such mechanism demonstrated in *in vitro* systems (Walmet et al., 2003) and in animal models (Embury et al., 2004) is the adhesion of sickle erythrocytes, and perhaps other cellular elements including leucocytes and platelets (Turhan et al., 2002), to vascular endothelium. Their potential importance in vaso-occlusive pain in children has been demonstrated in biomarker studies (Dampier et al., 2004b), and specific anti-adhesive therapies are now being tested in preliminary efficacy studies in both paediatric and adult populations. Cellular adhesion is further enhanced by the release of cytokines from ischaemic tissue injury resulting from vaso-occlusion, which act both by upregulating the surface expression of receptors (interleukin (IL)-1, IL-6, tumour necrosis factor (TNF)), or by increasing integrin avidity (IL-8) (Pathare et al., 2003).

The tissue damage from ischaemia caused by sickle vaso-occlusion is an obvious source of an inflammatory response, and anti-inflammatory agents such as steroids and NSAIDs have clinical efficacy in the treatment of pain in SCD patients The molecules involved in the inflammatory response likely cause alterations in the properties of peripheral nerves leading to increased spontaneous firing known as 'peripheral sensitization', and the enhanced excitability of nociceptors leads to the development of primary hyperalgesia (see Walker and Baccei, Chapter 6, this volume, for additional details). These consequences of the pro-inflammatory component of vaso-occlusion likely contribute to the challenge in treating pain associated with SCD.

Epidemiology of pain in SCD

Pain is the most common symptom of SCD, but remains poorly characterized, and can begin early in the first year of life as levels of fetal haemoglobin decline in susceptible individuals. In a prospective longitudinal study of 103 infants with SCD from birth to 7 years of age (Dampier et al., 2010a), the total frequency of days that children had pain was 1.6%. This represented distinct episodes of pain typically lasting several days (3±2.9 days, range 1–23 days), of which only 14% required hospitalizations. Over 80% of the children reported to have pain in the 0- to 12-month age interval had pain locations (hands/feet) and signs/symptoms (swelling or tenderness) consistent with dactylitis, which became progressively less prevalent in older age intervals reaching a level of about 10% by age 48 to 60 months. The prevalence of sickle pain occurrence is consistently higher and its duration longer in the children with the typically more severe type of SCD, SS or SB0 thalassaemia, compared to those with the milder SCD type, SC or SB+ thalassaemia, at all age groups. The time to first reported occurrence of pain is also influenced by sickle genotype, and is significantly shorter in children with SS with a mean of 18.5±2.5 months, compared to 39.0±4.9 months for those with SC, 24.4±3.8 months in SB+ thalassaemia, and 37.9±11.7 months in SB0 thalassaemia (p = 0.003, log rank test). Similar genotype differences are noted for time to the second reported pain event (SS 21.3±2.3 months, SC 43.5±4.3 months, SB+ thalassaemia 30.3±3.9 months, also p = 0.003). Longitudinal modelling of pain trajectories over this early childhood period suggests about 70% of SCD infants and young children remain relatively asymptomatic while about 10% to 15% have relatively frequent pain over this period and a similar number develop frequent pain after age 2 to 3 years of age.

Almost all children with SCD experience increasing pain as they progress through childhood into adolescence and young adulthood, but studies suggest that the large majority of these painful episodes continue to be managed at home (Dampier et al., 2002a, 2002b). However, a small minority of children transition, often in their early adolescent years, from sporadic episodic acute pain to frequent recurrent acute pain, and these individuals represent the majority of paediatric patients hospitalized for acute pain (Platt et al., 1991).

There are no studies in paediatric SCD describing the prevalence of chronic pain, but daily opioid usage has been suggested as a surrogate for chronic pain. Data on the self-reported usage of daily oral opioids was obtained from the patient registry (Dampier et al., 2010b) of the 10 SCD programmes of former Comprehensive Sickle Cell Centers Clinical Trial Consortium. Usage was relatively infrequent prior to adolescence, particularly in the SC/SB+ cohort, and widespread throughout the adult age range. The incidence of new onset daily opioid usage was 3% per year, and once initiated was not often discontinued in the subsequent 2 years (<30%).

Pain is a more complex experience in adults with SCD, with features of both acute recurrent and chronic pain. A study of a cohort of adults using daily pain diaries documented that pain was reported on 56% of days and exacerbations of pain (crises) on 13% of days, with almost 30% of patients reporting pain in greater than 95% of diary days (Smith et al., 2008).

Beyond vaso-occlusion: other pain syndromes in SCD

Other pain syndromes distinct from vaso-occlusive episodes are also common (Table 25.1). Young children with acute splenic sequestration, an often life-threatening trapping of sickled erythrocytes in the spleen, can experience acute left upper quadrant visceral pain from rapid enlargement of the splenic capsule. Older children can similarly experience episodic right upper quadrant colicky abdominal pain and jaundice from cholelithiasis, as chronic haemolysis results in bilirubin accumulation in the gall bladder. Bone infarction leading to avascular necrosis in the vertebral column, shoulder, or hips,

Table 25.1 Other pain syndromes in sickle cell disease

Syndrome	Body site	Characteristics
Acute bone infarction	Ribs, long bones	Acute necrosis of bone marrow
Acute cholelithiasis	Gall bladder	Acute visceral pain from pigment gallstone irritation or common bile duct obstruction
Acute splenic sequestration	Spleen	Acute visceral pain related to stretch of splenic capsule from rapid splenic enlargement
Avascular necrosis	Hips, shoulders, vertebrae	Progressive collapse of bone cortex related to persistent vascular compromise of cortex and marrow
Headache	Head	Headache pain with or without migrainous characteristics
Leg ulcers	Ankles, feet	Acute and chronic pain from ischaemic damage to skin and underlying soft tissue
Osteomyelitis	Any bone	Bacterial infection of bone cortex or marrow, often related to chronic ischaemia
Splenic infarction	Spleen	Acute visceral pain from splenic infarction involving splenic tissue extending to splenic capsule

can be a source of acute pain as well as chronic pain in adolescent and young adult patients. Physical therapy is often helpful for initial symptom management of hip pain, but some patients will have progressive collapse, particularly in the head of the femur, that will ultimately require joint replacement for relief of chronic pain or to improve physical functioning. While uncommon in the paediatric age group, leg ulcers, typically over the medial malleolus of either or both ankles, can be a source of considerable pain and disability (Minniti et al., 2010). Headaches, as an isolated pain syndrome, or as part of a vaso-occlusive event, are relatively common, but not well characterized (Niebanck et al., 2007). Some have features characteristic of migraine headaches, others may be more typical of tension-type headaches, while a small number of individuals satisfy current diagnostic criteria for chronic daily headache. Headaches may be somewhat more frequent in children with a history of sickle cell-related cerebrovascular events.

Assessment

Multidimensional assessment of chronic and acute sickle cell and other pain across settings (home, school, and hospital) is the foundation of effective pain management. Age-appropriate pain intensity measures used for other acute pain disorders or for post-operative pain (McGrath et al., 2008) also have been validated in SCD. Inclusion of measures with body diagrams is particularly useful given that multiple sites of pain are often present (Walco and Dampier, 1990). Measures of pain interference with physical functioning, such as the Child Activity Limitation Interview, CALI (Palermo et al., 2004), or the Pediatric PROMIS (Patient Reported Outcome Measurement Information System) pain interference scale (Varni et al., 2010), also may provide additional important information useful in assessing treatment responses.

The importance of including child report of pain is highlighted in sickle cell disease (Graumlich et al., 2001). Limited concordance between child and caregiver sickle pain reports has been noted, similar to other disorders. Parents and children's report of child SCD pain are only moderately consistent and are particularly divergent for interference with activities and pain descriptors (Barakat et al., 2008b). Objective evaluations of sleep (Law et al., 2012) or physical activity with actigraphy (Wilson and Palermo, 2012) may help clarify discrepant reports. Moreover, emerging technologies have provided opportunities to facilitate daily patient report on pain. Electronic assessment was found to feasible for children and adolescents with SCD to monitor skills practice and daily pain using an electronic handheld device (McClellan et al., 2009). Data were complete when devices were accessed for daily pain diary data entry, and devices were accessed on 76% of pain diary days. Moreover, children, adolescents, and parents were highly satisfied with accessing device to provide information on pain. Similar electronic monitoring to guide analgesic medication usage has been recently described using cell phone technology, and appear particularly promising (Jacob et al., 2012) given the ubiquitous use of cell phones in the adolescent and young adult populations.

Psychological therapies

Cognitive-behavioural approaches, specifically deep breathing and progressive muscle relaxation, guided imagery, and calming self-talk, have been the most promising psychological therapies to address sickle cell-related and other pain among children and adolescents with SCD (Anie and Green, 2012; Chen et al., 2004). Chen and colleagues (2004), in their review of 22 interventional studies targeting pain and adherence, reported that cognitive-behavioural approaches were superior to educational interventions and probably efficacious in addressing both pain and health care contracts. In contrast, behavioural and educational approaches alone are not sufficient to modify adherence or pain. Findings regarding psychological interventions for SCD are consistent with the broader literature on efficacious interventions for paediatric chronic pain in which a recent meta-analysis indicated the superiority of cognitive-behavioural interventions (multicomponent, relaxation, and biofeedback approaches) to address pain across paediatric chronic pain conditions including SCD (Palermo et al., 2010).

Initial efforts to identify psychological interventions for children with SCD have been promising. Hypnosis delivered in group format and including caregivers over an 18-month period reduced sickle cell-related and other pain for children, adolescents, and adults with SCD (Dinges et al., 1997). In an effort to develop brief pain interventions, Gil and colleagues (Gil et al., 1997, 2001) reported on the results of an intervention for children and adolescents with SCD that was initiated during a clinic visit, and supported through phone calls and taped instructions. The intervention comprised deep breathing relaxation, pleasant imagery, and calming self-talk. Reduced laboratory task-based pain and less negative thinking were reported at the end of treatment. However, at follow-up, the treatment group endorsed more pain but also more active coping. When the children had pain and practised coping strategies, they had fewer health care contacts and missed fewer days of school. Also, the treatment group had less negative thinking on days with low levels of pain.

More recent psychological intervention trials have been guided by reported associations of environmental factors with pain and functional disability (e.g. socioeconomic status; Barakat et al., 2007; Palermo et al., 2008) and parenting stress as mediator of pain's association with reduced quality of life (Barakat et al., 2008a), which underscores the need to develop family-focused interventions to support communication around and management of SCD complications, in particular pain, to minimize caregiver's distress in response to SCD-related events. Targets of these interventions are more broadly defined in terms of sickle cell knowledge, pain coping and adherence, family functioning, and quality of life. A six-session family psychoeducational intervention (Kaslow et al., 2000) produced improvements in knowledge of sickle cell disease that were maintained at a 6-month follow-up but had no effect on psychological adjustment, family functioning, and social functioning and support. Similarly, four-session, family-based, cognitive-behavioural intervention for adolescents with SCD showed promise in terms of percentage of pain days, disease knowledge, and family cohesion (Barakat et al., 2010); however, both groups reported improved psychosocial functioning, including a decrease in percentage of days with interference with daily activities at both time points, and decrease in pain-related hindrance of goals.

More research is needed to evaluate components that may support maintenance of effects past the immediate post-intervention period and generalization of effects beyond pain to health care contacts, functional ability, and quality of life. In addition, evaluation of format for delivery of the intervention (i.e. therapist-delivered versus self-administered, individual versus group format) and inclusion of family members or other supports is important. Psychological interventions described in the literature were developed for and implemented with children and/or adolescents with SCD; however, no studies of psychological interventions for young children with SCD were identified. Given that parents experience uncertainty about their ability to manage pain at home (Ievers-Landis et al., 2001), interventions that support development of parenting skills that address but do not reinforce pain are essential. Finally, there is a need to evaluate whether tailoring of pain interventions to better match African American values and systems, such as through inclusion of extended family and integration of culturally sensitive content and components, improves the efficacy of psychological interventions for SCD pain (Schwartz et al., 2007). Importantly, related to accessibility of interventions, preliminary data from an Internet-delivered intervention (Palermo et al., 2009) with children and adolescents with chronic pain using a family cognitive-behavioural therapy approach showed significant effects in terms of reduced pain and increased activities maintained through a 3-month follow-up compared to a treatment as usual control group. This interactive, self-paced intervention involved eight online sessions and targeted improved knowledge, skills to address sleep, activity, and pain (relaxation, distraction, cognitive coping skills), parenting skills, and pain communication skills.

A new approach to pain management, that may be effective for children and adolescents with SCD, is acceptance and commitment therapy (ACT). ACT emphasizes the promotion of daily functioning and quality of life while teaching a willingness to experience difficult and possibly unavoidable private events (e.g. pain, discomfort, fatigue, anxiety) without defence when doing so serves valued ends. A recently published case study of a 16-year-old with SCD indicated improvements in pain, functional ability, and quality of life at a 3-month follow-up assessment (Masuda et al., 2011). Further larger studies are in progress.

Physical therapies

Physical therapies, especially heat therapy, are commonly used to provide symptomatic relief at home (Dampier et al., 2004a), but few such therapies have been subjected to rigorous evaluations. Massage therapy implemented for 20 min per day for 30 days by caregivers resulted in less pain, improved functional status, and lower levels of depression and anxiety during intervention and at immediate post-intervention follow-up for children and adolescents with SCD compared to an attention placebo control group (Lemanek et al., 2009). Unfortunately, caregivers in the massage therapy group had higher depression, suggesting that the demands of the intervention contributed to care provider stress. Transcutaneous electrical nerve stimulation (TENS) has also been studied in a small clinical trial (Wang et al., 1988), and showed some modest clinical benefit during vaso-occlusive pain.

Pharmacological therapies

Pharmacology of opioid analgesics in SCD

A unique feature of SCD pain treatment is the impact of chronic anaemia on analgesic pharmacokinetics. One of the normal compensatory mechanisms to chronic anaemia is increased cardiac output with resultant increase in hepatic blood flow, as well as increased renal blood flow and glomerular filtration rate. Many analgesics, such as morphine, that have a component of their metabolic pathway dependent on hepatic or renal clearance will have accelerated plasma clearance in individuals with SCD. Plasma morphine clearances in paediatric subjects aged 6 to 19 years ranged from 6.2 to 59.1 ml/min/kg (mean, 35.5±12.4) during steady-state infusions compared to 20 to 25 ml/min/kg in children with cancer or postoperative pain (Dampier et al., 1995). Over the age range studied clearance values were negatively correlated with age. Pharmacokinetic modelling suggested a two-compartment model with a short initial distribution phase (mean half-life = 4.5 min) and a rapid terminal elimination half-life (77.6±19.2 min). Similarly, in a study of 20 adult SCD patients in steady state (Darbari et al., 2011), a mean morphine clearance of 68 ml/min/kg (4.1±1.1 L/h/kg) was observed, which is also over twice that typical in adult individuals without SCD. The pharmacokinetics of other analgesics or analgesic adjuvants have not been determined in patients with SCD, but those dependent exclusively or renal clearance, such as gabapentin or pregabalin (Bockbrader et al., 2010) will likely be cleared more quickly so conventional drug dosing recommendations may result in subtherapeutic drug levels in many SCD individuals. These considerations underscore the need to conduct formal pharmacokinetic studies of commonly used analgesic medications and novel investigational agents in this population.

Home management

Most families prefer to manage their child's vaso-occlusive pain at home, as the home setting is likely to be more comfortable for children and less disruptive to the family. Many families have also experienced negative attitudes towards patients with sickle cell disease by health care providers in the ED setting, often based on a profound fear of catering to opioid addiction, that can compromise analgesic therapy (Zempsky, 2009). Successful home management optimally requires the presence of a caregiver relatively skilled in pain assessment with access to appropriate analgesic medication,

and some extended family support as these episodes may last for several days and usually require around-the-clock medication for adequate management. Home management and appropriate emergency department utilization is also facilitated by access to trusted medical health professionals with experience in sickle cell disease and pain management who can help optimize analgesic therapy. Families need to be reminded to provide these medications on an appropriate time-contingent basis as most studies and anecdotal experience suggest that families administer these medications less frequently than recommended (Dampier et al., 2002b). Since complete pain relief is unlikely, families also need to be counselled on appropriate home therapy goals of maximizing comfort and function while minimizing troublesome analgesic side effects.

Low-potency analgesics, such as acetaminophen or ibuprofen, are typically chosen as initial therapy by most families and are often adequate for less intense pain, particularly in younger children. These analgesics are often chosen out of concern for the adverse consequences of opioid analgesics and have the advantage of little sedation and subsequent disruption of age-appropriate distracting activities.

A substantial variety of oral opioid analgesics of varying potency are available in liquid and tablet formulations for management of more intense pain in children with SCD. However, comparative efficacy or potency data is not available in the SCD population so opioid selection is generally individualized based on patient-specific efficacy and side effect profiles. While labelled dosing and frequency are usually recommended, the enhanced hepatic and renal clearance of morphine in this population (Dampier et al., 1995), the potential impact of prevalent genotypes impacting morphine metabolism (Joly et al., 2012), and the potential occurrence of opioid tolerance suggests that dose and frequency of oral opioids may need to be individualized. There is little published literature or clinical trial experience with the use of newer buccal or intranasal opioid preparations in the SCD population, but these medications may have a more potential useful role for rapid pain relief in the ED setting rather than at home.

There have been few comparative studies of adjunctive non-opioid analgesic medications in this population. The combination of potent opioids and ibuprofen likely provides the most pain relief in the home setting compared to weaker opioid combinations, particularly for older children with more intense pain (Dampier et al., 2002b). An observational study using pharmacy claims data suggested that pharmacological treatments for sickle pain consisted mainly of NSAIDs and weak opioids (Jerrell et al., 2011). Significantly more SCD patients with more than three yearly inpatient or ER visits for pain management were prescribed stronger opioids, antidepressants, and anticonvulsants. Prescriptions of both stronger opioids and antidepressants or anticonvulsants were significantly associated with lower cumulative rates of acute sickle pain visits over time in this cohort. Further clinical trial data is needed to support these clinical findings and establish comparative efficacy and safety data for various analgesic and anticonvulsant or antidepressant combinations, particularly as many of these classes of medications are not currently labelled for use in paediatric age groups.

Families naturally use both medical and psychological interventions to address symptomatic treatment of pain. Several studies of caregivers of children with SCD have found that a large percentage of families use complementary approaches of prayer, spiritual healing, massage, and relaxation in addition to medication to manage their child's pain at home (Dampier et al., 2004a; Yoon and Black, 2006). In both studies, complementary approaches were used more frequently with higher levels of pain or medication use.

Management of chronic/persistent pain

In contrast to acute pain management in SCD, the management of chronic pain has not been described, particularly in adolescents and young adults, and management strategies are often extrapolated from adult literature. Currently, such management in SCD has largely relied on use of long-acting opioid preparations, either in oral or transdermal formulations, but there is an increasing realization in the general US adult population that such daily opioid usage is more frequent in individuals with comorbid psychological and psychiatric disorders (Edlund et al., 2010), and has substantial long-term adverse effects, especially in large doses, including a risk for opioid-induced hyperalgesia, addiction, tolerance, constipation, nausea, somnolence, and immune suppression (Hutchinson et al., 2011; Kalso et al., 2004). Studies are needed in paediatric SCD to further characterize appropriate patient selection and dosing for chronic daily opioids, the role of alternative non-opioid analgesics, antidepressants, anticonvulsants, and their long-term health outcomes. Adolescents and young adults with SCD started on daily opioids should also receive concurrent psychosocial and psychiatric support given the role that emotional, social, and psychiatric issues negatively contribute to the pain experience (Sullivan and Ballantyne, 2012).

In-patient/ED pain management

Authoritative guidelines are available for the management of severe SCD pain in the acute care setting (Benjamin, 1999; Rees et al., 2003), but are somewhat outdated. However, more contemporary single site pain management practices from a number of paediatric hospitals have been published (Morrissey et al., 2009; Zempsky et al., 2008). A recent 'snapshot' of clinical analgesic practice, across a large number of paediatric hospitals participating in an observational study of the development of acute chest syndrome after hospitalization for sickle pain management, suggested the use of opioid-based patient-controlled analgesia (PCA) was the most common analgesic practice (Miller et al., 2012). Opioid doses varied widely, but appeared to be somewhat higher for those individuals receiving PCA compared to time-contingent opioids, and for those receiving hydromorphone compared to morphine. The relationship between opioid dosing and prior daily opioid usage was not described in this cohort, but adult chronic pain patients with chronic opioid use have been shown to report higher postoperative pain scores after surgery and have a slower rate of pain resolution (Chapman et al., 2011), and a similar pattern is likely in sickle cell disease.

Nausea, pruritus, and constipation are common opioid-related adverse effects during such treatment (Dampier et al., 2011b), and require symptomatic management. The use of concurrent low-dose opioid antagonist (naloxone) has been shown in several small cohorts (Koch et al., 2008; Monitto et al., 2011) to ameliorate many CNS opioid-related symptoms without compromising analgesia, and may have particular benefit in SCD where respiratory depression may enhance the risk for pulmonary complications such as acute chest syndrome. Common GI-related opioid adverse effects may be significantly ameliorated by peripherally acting opioid antagonists, such as methylnaltrexone (Gatti and Sabato, 2012) and similar agents, but they have not been studied in SCD, and are not yet labelled for paediatric patients.

The concurrent use parenteral NSAIDs, usually ketorolac, is a widespread clinical practice in the ED and in-patient setting as an additional analgesic, and may have additional benefit as an anti-inflammatory agent given the increase evidence for the role of inflammation in sickle cell disease pathophysiology (Dworkis et al., 2011), but large scale efficacy studies are lacking and caution advised in those children with SCD and impaired renal function. Evidence of efficacy of other adjuvant analgesics for acute sickle pain, as have been proposed for postoperative pain (Wu and Raja, 2011) have not been subjected to clinical trials. Benefit from concurrent low-dose ketamine has been described in a small case series (Zempsky et al., 2010), and there is anecdotal experience with the use of oral or transdermal clonidine, an α2-adrenergic agonist, to enhance analgesia and to reduce symptoms of opioid withdrawal following prolonged periods of opioid PCA.

Emerging and future directions in sickle pain

Prevention of sickle pain

Fundamentally the best way to prevent pain in sickle cell disease is to prevent vaso-occlusion. Current therapy with hydroxyurea is often not able to produce a high enough fetal haemoglobin response to prevent sickling and subsequent vaso-occlusion in some patients, particularly those with relatively low baseline fetal haemoglobin levels. Alternative fetal haemoglobin inducers are being developed based on other mechanisms of action including histone deacetylase inhibitors, and novel thalidomide analogues (Akinsheye et al., 2011; Sankaran, 2011), both of which have entered clinical trials. Rather than reducing sickle polymer formation by decreasing the intracellular sickle haemoglobin content, other approaches to prevent sickling attempt to directly modify the properties of the sickle haemoglobin molecule. A naturally occurring aromatic aldehyde, 5-hydroxymethyl-2-furfural (5HMF) has been shown to form a high-affinity Schiff-base adduct with sickle haemoglobin and inhibits red cell sickling by allosterically shifting oxygen equilibrium curves towards the left (Abdulmalik et al., 2005). This compound has begun phase I/II clinical trials.

An improved understanding of the pathogenesis of vaso-occlusion has led to the targeting of several pathways contributing to vaso-occlusion. Hypoxia from ischaemia leads to alterations in many factors and metabolites which may contribute to the pathogenesis of pain and enhance further vaso-occlusion. Drug discovery approaches have identified that increased adenosine levels promoted sickling, haemolysis and damage to multiple tissues in SCD transgenic mice and promoted sickling of human erythrocytes mediated through adenosine A(2B) receptor (A(2B)R)-mediated induction of 2,3-diphosphoglycerate, an erythrocyte-specific metabolite that decreases the oxygen binding affinity of haemoglobin (Zhang et al., 2011). Antagonists of the adenosine A(2B) receptor are being developed and tested in early phase clinical trials for amelioration of sickle pain.

Similarly, a number of cell surface receptors on sickle erythrocytes or endothelial cells participate in promoting the adherence of blood cells during vaso-occlusion (Kaul et al., 2009). Polymorphonuclear neutrophils (PMNs) also can capture circulating sickle red blood cells in inflamed venules, leading to critical reduction in blood flow and vaso-occlusion suggesting a role for the selectin family of cell adhesion molecules. P-selectin-specific inhibitors (aptamers; Gutsaeva et al., 2011) and pan-selectin inhibitors (Chang et al., 2010) have shown efficacy in animal models of vaso-occlusion, and are also in early phase clinical trials for sickle cell crises.

Sickle pain pathophysiology

Several studies in mouse models of SCD have described sensory changes consistent with altered nociceptor function. Paw withdrawal threshold and withdrawal latency (to mechanical and thermal stimuli, respectively) and grip force were lower in homozygous and hemizygous Berkley mice, which express only human sickle haemoglobin, compared with control mice expressing human haemoglobin A consistent with deep/musculoskeletal and cutaneous hyperalgesia (Kohli et al., 2010). This mechanical hypersensitivity is further exacerbated when hypoxia is used to induce acute sickling (Hillery et al., 2011). Several research groups are working with these and similar mouse models to define unique molecular mechanisms of pain and identify potential therapeutic targets.

Preliminary human studies suggest similar sensory changes consistent with hyperalgesia in children and adults with SCD. Early studies suggested reduced pressure pain thresholds in school-age and adolescent SCD children compared to age-matched children with juvenile idiopathic arthritis, or compared to control children with asthma (Walco et al., 1990). In a recent cross-sectional study using quantitative sensory testing to thermal and mechanical stimuli in SCD paediatric patients in baseline health (n = 55) and race-matched controls (n = 57), SCD patients when compared to controls had significantly lower cold pain thresholds and heat pain thresholds, but not mechanical pain thresholds (Brandow et al., 2011). Older age was associated with lower cold pain thresholds, lower heat pain thresholds, and lower mechanical pain thresholds. Further studies will be necessary to characterize the risk factors and time course for these changes in processing of nociceptive signalling in both children and young adults with SCD, and to determine their implications for analgesic management.

Conclusion

SCD is a complex pain disorder that remains poorly understood with limited evidence base for analgesic therapies. Pain from vaso-occlusion of sickle erythrocytes can occur in multiple musculoskeletal locations, several internal viscera such as the spleen, as well as the penis. Such pain is typically intermittent in childhood, and often responds to NSAIDs and opioid analgesics similarly to acute pain in many other pain disorders. Adolescents with SCD often experience more frequent pain, and those with bone disease in spine, hips, or shoulders may experience chronic pain, which may show limited responses to opioids as in other chronic pain disorder. Many cognitive-behavioural strategies are helpful as part of multidisciplinary pain management, particularly in adolescents, who may also benefit from psychological support for coexistent mood disorders, to increase coping skills, and to support appropriate school and family functioning. Future advances are needed to further the evidence base for efficacious pharmacological and psychological therapies to ameliorate the substantial burden of pain in children and adolescents with SCD. Ultimately preventive therapies for vaso-occlusion, inflammatory and ischaemic tissue damage, and development of hyperalgesia will finally change the face of this common genetic disorder (Figure 25.1).

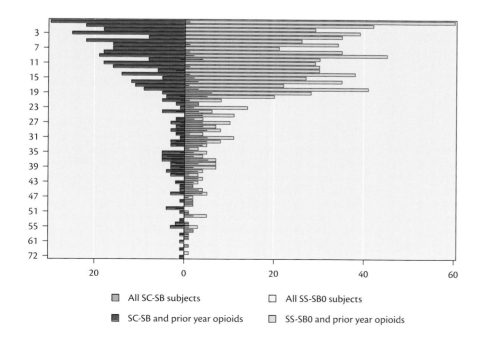

Figure 25.1 Age distribution of opioid usage in the year prior to registry enrolment. Bars represent the number of individuals in each year of age, with bars on the left representing SC or SB + thal subjects, while bars on the right represent the number of subjects with SS or SB0thal. Dark bars within each group represent the number of subjects reporting chronic daily opioid usage.

Case example

JK is a 18-year-female with homozygous sickle cell disease (SS) diagnosed at birth through the local state newborn hae-moglobinopathy screening programme. Her mother noticed prominent swelling of the dorsum of left hand and fingers of her daughter associated with reduced voluntary movement and discomfort with palpation at age 18 months preceded by a mild upper respiratory infection that responded to oral ibuprofen. Several subsequent episodes involving one or both hands and feet or sometimes her lower legs occurred over the next several years and were managed at home with oral ibuprofen and oral acetaminophen/codeine. Her family would often apply warm compresses and massage her limbs to help relieve swelling and pain. At age 5 she was admitted for several days with more severe pain managed with intravenous fluids, NSAIDs, and intravenous opioids (morphine). By age 12, similar admissions began to occur once to twice per year, which were interspersed with less severe episodes once or twice a month lasting several days. She began to miss considerable amounts of school and became somewhat withdrawn and spent less time with her friends. Oral hydroxyu-rea was started but had little impact on her pain complaints, in part because of poor adherence. More potent intermittent oral opioids were started, and provided some initial improvement in pain relief, but subsequently poorly controlled pain necessitated a switch to daily oral methadone. A variety of adjuvant medica-tions were tried but were found to be too sedating or had other significant side effects. A TENS unit was provided, which she found to be useful for mild to moderate pain. At age 13, her phys-ical activity was further compromised by persistent right-sided hip pain; hip X-rays and MRI demonstrated significant avascular necrosis of her right femoral head with partial collapse.

When she was 15 years of age, her family, who were increas-ingly concerned with her isolation, depression, and poor school performance, requested a multidisciplinary case conference with members of the sickle cell team, physical therapy, the hospital-based school teacher, child psychology, and a representative from the local hospital-based pain team. A comprehensive man-agement plan was developed with the concurrence of JK and her family that included a 12- to 18-month period of chronic transfusions in an attempt to ameliorate her underlying SCD, intensive physical therapy to improve conditioning and to assist with physical mobility of her hips, and individual and family psy-chology sessions to teach more effective communication styles and more successful active coping skills. A variety of relaxation techniques were to be taught to assist with stress management and to improve sleep hygiene. Under careful medical and psychologi-cal supervision, off-label use of duloxetine was started to improve pain control based on data from other pain disorders, and provide some antidepressant action. She was encouraged to become more active in her local church youth group, and was referred to a local African American college sorority programme that provided high school academic tutoring and role-modelling. Her frequency of hospitalization gradually decreased on this intensive supportive care programme, and she was able to be weaned to a small dose of daily opioids with further improvements in her pain charac-teristics, suggestive of some previous degree of opioid-induced hyperalgesia. She restarted oral hydroxyurea with an improved clinical response. With the assistance of her volunteer tutors, she was able to graduate from high school with her class, and will be starting a reduced schedule of community college classes in preparation for a healthcare-related degree programme.

References

Abdulmalik, O., Safo, M. K., Chen, Q., Yang, J., Brugnara, C., Ohene-Frempong, K., *et al.* (2005). 5-hydroxymethyl-2-furfural modifies intracellular sickle haemoglobin and inhibits sickling of red blood cells. *Br J Haematol*, 128, 552–561.

Akinsheye, I., Alsultan, A., Solovieff, N., Ngo, D., Baldwin, C. T., Sebastiani, P., *et al.* (2011). Fetal hemoglobin in sickle cell anemia. *Blood*, 118, 19–27.

Anie, K. A., and Green, J. (2012). Psychological therapies for sickle cell disease and pain. *Cochrane Database Syst Rev*, 2, CD001916.

Barakat, L. P., Patterson, C. A., Daniel, L. C., and Dampier, C. (2008a). Quality of life among adolescents with sickle cell disease: mediation of pain by internalizing symptoms and parenting stress. *Health Qual Life Outcomes*, 6, 60.

Barakat, L. P., Schwartz, L. A., Salamon, K. S., and Radcliffe, J. (2010). A family-based randomized controlled trial of pain intervention for adolescents with sickle cell disease. *J Pediatr Hematol/Oncol*, 32, 540–547.

Barakat, L. P., Schwartz, L. A., Simon, K., and Radcliffe, J. (2007). Negative thinking as a coping strategy mediator of pain and internalizing symptoms in adolescents with sickle cell disease. *J Behav Med*, 30, 199–208.

Barakat, L. P., Simon, K., Schwartz, L. A., and Radcliffe, J. (2008b). Correlates of pain-rating concordance for adolescents with sickle cell disease and their caregivers. *Clin J Pain*, 24, 438–446.

Benjamin, L. J., Dampier, C. D., Jacox, A., Odesina, V., Phoenix, D., Shapiro, B., *et al.* (1999). *Guideline for the management of acute and chronic pain in sickle-cell disease.* Glenview, IL: American Pain Society.

Bockbrader, H. N., Wesche, D., Miller, R., Chapel, S., Janiczek, N., and Burger, P. (2010). A comparison of the pharmacokinetics and pharmacodynamics of pregabalin and gabapentin. *Clin Pharmacokinet*, 49, 661–669.

Brandow, A. M., Kattappuram, R., Stucky, C. L., Hillery, C. A., and Panepinto, J. A. (2011). Patients with sickle cell disease have increased sensitivity to cold and heat stimuli, 2. *ASH Annual Meeting Abstracts*, 118, 2116.

Chang, J., Patton, J. T., Sarkar, A., Ernst, B., Magnani, J. L., and Frenette, P. S. (2010). GMI-1070, a novel pan-selectin antagonist, reverses acute vascular occlusions in sickle cell mice. *Blood*, 116, 1779–1786.

Chapman, C. R., Davis, J., Donaldson, G. W., Naylor, J., and Winchester, D. (2011). Postoperative pain trajectories in chronic pain patients undergoing surgery: the effects of chronic opioid pharmacotherapy on acute pain. *J Pain*, 12, 1240–1246.

Chen, E., Cole, S. W., and Kato, P. M. (2004). A review of empirically supported psychosocial interventions for pain and adherence outcomes in sickle cell disease. *J Pediatr Psychol*, 29, 197–209.

Dampier, C., Ely, E., Aertker, L., Brodecki, D., Kesler, K., and Stuart, M. (2010a). Pain in infants and young children with sickle cell disease-a prospective longitudinal analysis. *Blood*, 116, 366.

Dampier, C., Ely, B., Brodecki, D., and O'Neal, P. (2002a). Characteristics of pain managed at home in children and adolescents with sickle cell disease by using diary self-reports. *J Pain*, 3, 461–470.

Dampier, C., Ely, E., Brodecki, D., and O'Neal, P. (2002b). Home management of pain in sickle cell disease: a daily diary study in children and adolescents. *J Pediatr Hematol Oncol*, 24, 643–647.

Dampier, C., Ely, E., Eggleston, B., Brodecki, D., and O'Neal, P. (2004a). Physical and cognitive-behavioral activities used in the home management of sickle pain: a daily diary study in children and adolescents. *Pediatr Blood Cancer*, 43, 674–678.

Dampier, C., Lebeau, P., Rhee, S., Lieff, S., Kesler, K., Ballas, S., *et al.* (2011a). Health-related quality of life in adults with sickle cell disease (SCD):

a report from the Comprehensive Sickle Cell Centers Clinical Trial Consortium. *Am J Hematol*, 86, 203–205.

Dampier, C., Lieff, S., Lebeau, P., Rhee, S., McMurray, M., Rogers, Z., et al. (2010b). Health-related quality of life in children with sickle cell disease: a report from the Comprehensive Sickle Cell Centers Clinical Trial Consortium. *Pediatr Blood Cancer*, 55, 485–494.

Dampier, C., Setty, B.N., Eggleston, B., Brodecki, D., O'Neal, P., and Stuart, M. (2004b). Vaso-occlusion in children with sickle cell disease: clinical characteristics and biologic correlates. *J Pediatr Hematol Oncol*, 26, 785–790.

Dampier, C.D., Setty, B.N., Logan, J., Ioli, J.G., and Dean, R. (1995). Intravenous morphine pharmacokinetics in pediatric patients with sickle cell disease. *J Pediatr*, 126, 461–467.

Dampier, C.D., Smith, W.R., Kim, H.Y., Wager, C.G., Bell, M.C., Minniti, C.P., et al. (2011b). Opioid patient controlled analgesia use during the initial experience with the IMPROVE PCA trial: A phase III analgesic trial for hospitalized sickle cell patients with painful episodes. *Am J Hematol*, 86(12), E70–73.

Darbari, D.S., Neely, M., Van Den Anker, J., and Rana, S. (2011). Increased clearance of morphine in sickle cell disease: implications for pain management. *J Pain*, 12, 531–538.

Dinges, D.F., Whitehouse, W.G., Orne, E.C., Bloom, P.B., Carlin, M.M., Bauer, N.K., et al. (1997). Self-hypnosis training as an adjunctive treatment in the management of pain associated with sickle cell disease. *Int J Clin Exp Hypn*, 45, 417–432.

Dworkis, D.A., Klings, E.S., Solovieff, N., Li, G., Milton, J.N., Hartley, S.W., et al. (2011). Severe sickle cell anemia is associated with increased plasma levels of TNF-R1 and VCAM-1. *Am J Hematol*, 86, 220–223.

Edlund, M.J., Martin, B.C., Devries, A., Fan, M.Y., Braden, J.B., and Sullivan, M.D. (2010). Trends in use of opioids for chronic noncancer pain among individuals with mental health and substance use disorders: the TROUP study. *Clin J Pain*, 26, 1–8.

Embury, S.H., Matsui, N.M., Ramanujam, S., Mayadas, T.N., Noguchi, C.T., Diwan, B.A., et al. (2004). The contribution of endothelial cell P-selectin to the microvascular flow of mouse sickle erythrocytes in vivo. *Blood*, 104, 3378–3385.

Gatti, A. and Sabato, A.F. (2012). Management of opioid-induced constipation in cancer patients: focus on methylnaltrexone. *Clin Drug Investig*, 32, 293–301.

Gil, K.M., Anthony, K.K., Carson, J.W., Redding-Lallinger, R., Daeschner, C.W., and Ware, R.E. (2001). Daily coping practice predicts treatment effects in children with sickle cell disease. *J Pediatr Psychol*, 26, 163–173.

Gil, K.M., Wilson, J.J., Edens, J.L., Workman, E., Ready, J., Sedway, J., et al. (1997). Cognitive coping skills training in children with sickle cell disease pain. *Int J Behav Med*, 4, 364–377.

Graumlich, S.E., Powers, S.W., Byars, K.C., Schwarber, L.A., Mitchell, M.J., and Kalinyak, K.A. (2001). Multidimensional assessment of pain in pediatric sickle cell disease. *J Pediatr Psychol*, 26, 203–214.

Gutsaeva, D.R., Parkerson, J.B., Yerigenahally, S.D., Kurz, J.C., Schaub, R.G., Ikuta, T., et al. (2011). Inhibition of cell adhesion by anti-P-selectin aptamer: a new potential therapeutic agent for sickle cell disease. *Blood*, 117, 727–735.

Hillery, C.A., Kerstein, P.C., Vilceanu, D., Barabas, M.E., Retherford, D., Brandow, A.M., et al. (2011). Transient receptor potential vanilloid 1 mediates pain in mice with severe sickle cell disease. *Blood*, 118, 3376–3388.

Hutchinson, M.R., Shavit, Y., Grace, P.M., Rice, K.C., Maier, S.F., and Watkins, L.R. (2011). Exploring the neuroimmunopharmacology of opioids: an integrative review of mechanisms of central immune signaling and their implications for opioid analgesia. *Pharmacol Rev*, 63, 772–810.

Ievers-Landis, C.E., Brown, R.T., Drotar, D., Bunke, V., Lambert, R.G., and Walker, A.A. (2001). Situational analysis of parenting problems for caregivers of children with sickle cell syndromes. *J Dev Behav Pediatr*, 22, 169–178.

Jacob, E., Stinson, J., Duran, J., Gupta, A., Gerla, M., Ann Lewis, M., et al. (2012). Usability testing of a smartphone for accessing a web-based e-diary for self-monitoring of pain and symptoms in sickle cell disease. *J Pediatr Hematol Oncol*, 34(5), 326–335.

Jerrell, J.M., Tripathi, A., and Stallworth, J.R. (2011). Pain management in children and adolescents with sickle cell disease. *American J Hematol*, 86, 82–84.

Joly, P., Gagnieu, M.C., Bardel, C., Francina, A., Pondarre, C., and Martin, C. (2012). Genotypic screening of the main opiate-related polymorphisms in a cohort of 139 sickle cell disease patients. *Am J Hematol*, 87, 534–536.

Kalso, E., Edwards, J.E., Moore, R.A., and Mcquay, H.J. (2004). Opioids in chronic non-cancer pain: systematic review of efficacy and safety. *Pain*, 112, 372–380.

Kaslow, N.J., Collins, M.H., Rashid, F.L., Baskin, M.L., Griffith, J.R., Hollins, L. et al. (2000). The efficacy of a pilot family psychoeducational intervention for pediatric sickle cell disease (SCD). *Families Syst Health*, 18, 381–404.

Kauf, T.L., Coates, T.D., Huazhi, L., Mody-Patel, N., and Hartzema, A.G. (2009). The cost of health care for children and adults with sickle cell disease. *Am J Hematol*, 84, 323–327.

Kaul, D.K., Finnegan, E., and Barabino, G.A. (2009). Sickle red cell-endothelium interactions. *Microcirculation*, 16, 97–111.

Koch, J., Manworren, R., Clark, L., Quinn, C.T., Buchanan, G.R., and Rogers, Z.R. (2008). Pilot study of continuous co-infusion of morphine and naloxone in children with sickle cell pain crisis. *Am J Hematol*, 83, 728–731.

Kohli, D.R., Li, Y., Khasabov, S.G., Gupta, P., Kehl, L.J., Ericson, M.E., et al. (2010). Pain related behaviors and neurochemical alterations in mice expressing sickle hemoglobin: modulation by cannabinoids. *Blood*, 116(3), 456–465.

Lanzkron, S., Carroll, C.P., and Haywood, C., Jr. (2010). The burden of emergency department use for sickle-cell disease: an analysis of the national emergency department sample database. *Am J Hematol*, 85, 797–799.

Law, E.F., Dufton, L., and Palermo, T.M. (2012). Daytime and nighttime sleep patterns in adolescents with and without chronic pain. *Health Psychol*, 31(6), 830–833.

Lemanek, K.L., Ranalli, M., and Lukens, C. (2009). A randomized controlled trial of massage therapy in children with sickle cell disease. *J Pediatr Psychol*, 34, 1091–1096.

Masuda, A., Cohen, L.L., Wicksell, R.K., Kemani, M.K., and Johnson, A. (2011). A case study: acceptance and commitment therapy for pediatric sickle cell disease. *J Pediatr Psychol*, 36, 398–408.

McClellan, C.B., Schatz, J.C., Puffer, E., Sanchez, C.E., Stancil, M.T., and Roberts, C.W. (2009). Use of handheld wireless technology for a home-based sickle cell pain management protocol. *J Pediatr Psychol*, 34, 564–573.

McGrath, P.J., Walco, G.A., Turk, D.C., Dworkin, R.H., Brown, M.T., Davidson, K., et al. (2008). Core outcome domains and measures for pediatric acute and chronic/recurrent pain clinical trials: PedIMMPACT recommendations. *J Pain*, 9, 771–783.

Miller, S.T., Kim, H.Y., Weiner, D., Wager, C.G., Gallagher, D., Styles, L., et al. (2012). Inpatient management of sickle cell pain: a 'snapshot' of current practice. *Am J Hematol*, 87, 333–336.

Minniti, C.P., Eckman, J., Sebastiani, P., Steinberg, M.H., and Ballas, S.K. (2010). Leg ulcers in sickle cell disease. *Am J Hematol*, 85, 831–833.

Monitto, C.L., Kost-Byerly, S., White, E., Lee, C.K., Rudek, M.A., Thompson, C., et al. (2011). The optimal dose of prophylactic intravenous naloxone in ameliorating opioid-induced side effects in children receiving intravenous patient-controlled analgesia morphine for moderate to severe pain: a dose finding study. *Anesthesia and analgesia*, 113, 834–842.

Morrissey, L.K., Shea, J.O., Kalish, L.A., Weiner, D.L., Branowicki, P., and Heeney, M.M. (2009). Clinical practice guideline improves the treatment of sickle cell disease vasoocclusive pain. *Pediatr Blood Cancer*, 52, 369–372.

Niebanck, A.E., Pollock, A.N., Smith-Whitley, K., Raffini, L.J., Zimmerman, R.A., Ohene-Frempong, K., et al. (2007). Headache in children with sickle cell disease: prevalence and associated factors. *J Pediatr*, 151, 67–72, 72.e1.

Palermo, T. M., Eccleston, C., Lewandowski, A. S., Williams, A. C., and Morley, S. (2010). Randomized controlled trials of psychological therapies for management of chronic pain in children and adolescents: an updated meta-analytic review. *Pain*, 148, 387–397.

Palermo, T. M., Riley, C. A., and Mitchell, B. A. (2008). Daily functioning and quality of life in children with sickle cell disease pain: relationship with family and neighborhood socioeconomic distress. *J Pain*, 9, 833–840.

Palermo, T. M., Wilson, A. C., Peters, M., Lewandowski, A., and Somhegyi, H. (2009). Randomized controlled trial of an Internet-delivered family cognitive-behavioral therapy intervention for children and adolescents with chronic pain. *Pain*, 146, 205–213.

Palermo, T. M., Witherspoon, D., Valenzuela, D., and Drotar, D. D. (2004). Development and validation of the Child Activity Limitations Interview: a measure of pain-related functional impairment in school-age children and adolescents. *Pain*, 109, 461–470.

Pathare, A., Kindi, S. A., Daar, S., and Dennison, D. (2003). Cytokines in sickle cell disease. *Hematology*, 8, 329–337.

Platt, O. S., Thorington, B. D., Brambilla, D. J., Milner, P. F., Rosse, W. F., Vichinsky, E., *et al.* (1991). Pain in sickle cell disease. Rates and risk factors. *N Engl J Med*, 325, 11–16.

Rees, D. C., Olujohungbe, A. D., Parker, N. E., Stephens, A. D., Telfer, P., and Wright, J. (2003). Guidelines for the management of the acute painful crisis in sickle cell disease. *Br J Haematol*, 120, 744–752.

Sankaran, V. G. (2011). Targeted therapeutic strategies for fetal hemoglobin induction. *Hematol Am Soc Hematol Educ Program*, 2011, 459–465.

Schwartz, L. A., Radcliffe, J., and Barakat, L. P. (2007). The development of a culturally sensitive pediatric pain management intervention for African American adolescents with sickle cell disease. *Child Health Care*, 36, 267–283.

Smith, W. R., Penberthy, L. T., Bovbjerg, V. E., McClish, D. K., Roberts, J. D., Dahman, B., *et al.* (2008). Daily assessment of pain in adults with sickle cell disease. *Ann Intern Med*, 148, 94–101.

Sullivan, M. D., and Ballantyne, J. C. (2012). What are we treating with long-term opioid therapy? *Arch Intern Med*, 172, 433–434.

Turhan, A., Weiss, L. A., Mohandas, N., Coller, B. S., and Frenette, P. S. (2002). Primary role for adherent leukocytes in sickle cell vascular occlusion: a new paradigm. *Proc Natl Acad Sci U S A*, 99, 3047–3051.

Varni, J. W., Stucky, B. D., Thissen, D., Dewitt, E. M., Irwin, D. E., Lai, J. S., *et al.* (2010). PROMIS Pediatric Pain Interference Scale: an item response theory analysis of the pediatric pain item bank. *J Pain*, 11, 1109–1119.

Walco, G. A., and Dampier, C. D. (1990). Pain in children and adolescents with sickle cell disease: a descriptive study. *J Pediatr Psychol*, 15, 643–658.

Walco, G. A., Dampier, C. D., Hartstein, G., Djordjevic, D., and Miller, L. (1990). The relationship between recurrent clinical pain and pain threshold in children. *Adv Pain Res Ther*, 15, 333–340.

Walmet, P. S., Eckman, J. R., and Wick, T. M. (2003). Inflammatory mediators promote strong sickle cell adherence to endothelium under venular flow conditions. *Am J Hematol*, 73, 215–224.

Wang, W. C., George, S. L., and Wilimas, J. A. (1988). Transcutaneous electrical nerve stimulation treatment of sickle cell pain crises. *Acta Haematol*, 80, 99–102.

Wilson, A. C., and Palermo, T. M. (2012). Physical activity and function in adolescents with chronic pain: a controlled study using actigraphy. *J Pain*, 13, 121–130.

Wu, C. L., and Raja, S. N. (2011). Treatment of acute postoperative pain. *Lancet*, 377, 2215–2225.

Yoon, S. L., and Black, S. (2006). Comprehensive, integrative management of pain for patients with sickle-cell disease. *J Altern Complement Med*, 12, 995–1001.

Zempsky, W. T. (2009). Treatment of sickle cell pain: fostering trust and justice. *JAMA*, 302, 2479–2480.

Zempsky, W. T., Loiselle, K. A., Corsi, J. M., and Hagstrom, J. N. (2010). Use of low-dose ketamine infusion for pediatric patients with sickle cell disease-related pain: a case series. *Clin J Pain*, 26, 163–167.

Zempsky, W. T., Loiselle, K. A., McKay, K., Blake, G. L., Hagstrom, J. N., Schechter, N. L., *et al.* (2008). Retrospective evaluation of pain assessment and treatment for acute vasoocclusive episodes in children with sickle cell disease. *Pediatr Blood Cancer*, 51, 265–268.

Zhang, Y., Dai, Y., Wen, J., Zhang, W., Grenz, A., Sun, H., *et al.* (2011). Detrimental effects of adenosine signaling in sickle cell disease. *Nature Med*, 17, 79–86.

CHAPTER 26

Pain and gastroenterological diseases

Akshay Batra, Amanda Bevan and R. Mark Beattie

Summary

Pain is a common complaint in children with gastrointestinal tract pathology and it has significant consequences for patients' quality of life. A thorough evaluation should be performed to determine the cause and severity. Understanding the pathophysiology of pain in various conditions is key to effective management. This chapter outlines the aetiology and general principles of the management of pain in gastrointestinal disease. The specific management of common gastrointestinal conditions associated with pain, e.g. inflammatory bowel disease, gastro-oesophageal reflux disease, pancreatitis, and gut dysmotility disorders are discussed.

Introduction

Pain is an important and common symptom of gastrointestinal disease. It can be the first indication of a new pathology, or it can signify a change in a known condition. The recognition of the pain pattern and its significance is crucial to the early diagnosis and treatment. The relief of pain is frequently of diagnostic importance and is often the best indicator of successful treatment. This chapter will focus on the various gastrointestinal disorders causing pain and their management with special emphasis on conditions causing acute debilitating pain. Recurrent abdominal pain is reviewed by Schurman et al. (Chapter 29, this volume).

Innervation of the gastrointestinal tract

The lining of the gastrointestinal tract is the largest vulnerable surface that faces the external environment. Pain perception in the gastrointestinal tract is mediated via a complex pathway of enteric, autonomic, and central nervous system (CNS) structures (Knowles and Aziz, 2009).

Enteric nervous system

The enteric nervous system provides the intrinsic innervation to the gut. It is composed of Auerbach's and Meissner's plexuses. Auerbach's plexus is a myenteric plexus which lies between the longitudinal and circular muscle layers. Its role is mainly to control the contractions of the smooth muscle in the bowel. The submucosal Meissner's plexus lies below the mucosal layer and performs a predominantly sensory function in obtaining information about the luminal contents.

Three broad classes of primary afferent neurons associated with the gut are:

- Intrinsic primary afferent neurons (IPANs), with cell bodies and connections in the gut wall, either in the myenteric plexus or in the submucus plexus, and processes extending to muscularis mucosa. They are the primary sensors and regulators of the enteric nervous system (Gershon et al., 2005).

- Extrinsic primary afferent neurons, with cell bodies in vagal and dorsal root (spinal) ganglia, carry information about the state of the gastrointestinal tract to the CNS. They appear to monitor all aspects of gut function, and also carry nociceptive information via thinly myelinated $A\delta$ and unmyelinated C fibres (Sengupta, 1994; Sikander and Dickenson, 2012). Both the submucosal and muscular nerve plexus respond to multiple stimuli and transmit pain to the CNS.

- Intestinofugal neurons, with cell bodies in the gut and projections to neurons outside the gut wall.

Visceral sensory nerves follow three main anatomical pathways from the gastrointestinal tract to the CNS: the vagal, splanchnic, and pelvic nerves (Kirkup et al., 2001; Sikandar and Dickenson, 2012) (Figure 26.1). The splanchnic afferent neurons transmit pain sensation, whereas the parasympathetic afferent fibres transmit physiological information and non-noxious sensation (Goyal et al., 1996). The cell bodies of primary visceral afferent neurons are contained in the nodose ganglia (vagal afferents) and dorsal root ganglia (spinal afferents). The central terminals of vagal sensory neurons are in the brainstem, whereas the central terminals of spinal visceral afferent neurons are organized diffusely over several spinal segments. The vagal afferents do not directly participate in pain signalling but can indirectly modify spinal pain processing.

The autonomic nervous system, by way of the sympathetic and parasympathetic systems, also controls the secretory and muscular functions of the gut. Parasympathetic efferent fibres run in the vagus and sacral nerves, and exert an excitatory effect on the enteric neurons. The sympathetic efferent fibres inhibit gastrointestinal activity. The enteric nervous system though functioning independently interacts with the CNS allowing bidirectional communication. As a result the brain can integrate information from the gastrointestinal tract and respond appropriately. This is especially true for stimuli

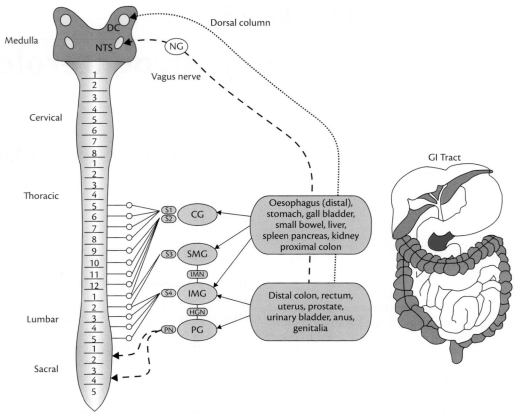

Figure 26.1 Schematic of gastrointestinal tract innervation. Visceral afferents innervating organs in thoracic and abdominal cavities travel either along the vagus nerve with cell bodies in the nodose ganglion (NG) and central terminals in the nucleus tractus solitarii (NTS), or along the dorsal column pathway (dotted line) with cell bodies in dorsal column nuclei (DC) in the brainstem. Other afferents innervating the same organs have terminals in the spinal cord, before passing through pre- and/ or paravertebral ganglia en route with cell bodies in dorsal root ganglia (not illustrated). Straight lined pathways indicate sympathetic innervation and hyphenated pathways indicate parasympathetic innervation. Prevertebral ganglia, CG: coeliac ganglion; SMG: superior mesenteric ganglion; IMG: inferior mesenteric ganglion; PG: pelvic ganglion. Nerves, S1, S2, S3, S4: greater, less, least, and lumbar splanchnic nerves, respectively; IMN: intermesenteric nerve; HGN: hypogastric nerve; PN: pelvic nerve. Republished from Sikandar, Shafaq and Dickenson, Anthony H, Visceral pain: the ins and outs, the ups and downs, *Current Opinion in Supportive and Palliative Care*, Volume 6, Issue 1, pp. 17–26, Copyright © 2012 Lippincott Williams & Wilkins, Inc., http://journals.lww.com/co-supportiveandpalliativecare/pages/default.aspx.

like hunger, satiety, and defecation (Blackshaw and Gebhart, 2002) thus providing a degree of conscious control over these functions; however, we are normally unaware of the complex signalling events which continuously occur within our internal organs.

Various neurotransmitters within the enteric nervous system take part in relaying this information. The excitatory neurotransmitters include acetylcholine, and substance P and inhibitory transmitters include adenosine triphosphate, vasoactive intestinal peptide, and nitric oxide. Serotonin, a monoamine neurotransmitter, plays a key role in the initiation of peristaltic and secretory reflexes, and in modulation of visceral sensations.

Neural pathways for pain

Peripheral visceral mechanisms

Sensory nerve endings (i.e. visceral nociceptors), in the mucosal or muscular layer are activated by a range of stimuli, such as mucosal and serosal inflammation, traction on the mesentery, rapid luminal distention, ischaemia, and forceful smooth muscle contraction. *Mucosal* afferents appear as bare endings in the lamina propria of intestinal villi and respond to luminal and local chemical stimulation of the mucosal surface. This may involve (Berthoud et al. 1995; Gebhart, 2000):

- Direct activation or mucosal damage due to excess hydrogen ions in conditions such as oesophagitis.

- Activation by pro-inflammatory neurotransmitters (e.g. histamine and substance P) that increase excitability of the receptors (i.e. peripheral sensitization) in inflammatory bowel disease.

- Direct involvement of the nerve in the inflammatory process (i.e. neuritis) as is seen in transmural inflammation with Crohn's disease.

Muscular afferents respond to mechanical stimuli, especially distention, and consist of specialized terminals which surround myenteric ganglia termed intraganglionic laminar endings (ILEs; Lynn et al., 2003). Pain can result from pathological conditions in which distention is beyond the tolerance threshold of the organ (e.g. acute intestinal obstruction); or be associated with a lower tolerance to distention, which is a proposed mechanism in functional abdominal pain. In conditions like chronic pseudo-obstruction there is a combination of the two factors: perception of distention is altered secondary to neuropathy, and there is also excessive distention secondary to myopathic changes (Gebhart, 2000). In addition, a subgroup of visceral afferent fibres are mechanically insensitive, so-called mechanically insensitive afferents (MIAs) or 'silent' nociceptors, but which acquire spontaneous activity and mechanosensitivity after tissue insults such as inflammation or mechanical trauma (Feng et al., 2012).

As the density of visceral sensory innervation is relatively sparse and there is marked divergence of visceral input into the spinal cord, visceral pain tends to be diffuse and poorly localized (Sikandar and Dickenson, 2012).

Peritoneal pain

Pain may also be produced by chemical stimulation, ischaemia, inflammation, or stretching of the parietal peritoneum, which is innervated by branches from somatic efferent and afferent nerves that also supply the muscles and skin of the overlying body wall. The parietal peritoneum lining the anterior abdominal wall is supplied by lower six thoracic and first lumbar nerves; and in the pelvis is mainly supplied by the obturator nerve, which is a branch of the lumbar plexus. Parietal pain is sharp, severe, and very well localized, and experienced in conditions such as peritonitis, appendicitis, and pancreatitis.

Central processing of visceral pain

In the spinal cord, visceral afferent input converges with somatic afferent input, resulting in referred visceral pain. In addition, ongoing activity due to sensitization of peripheral afferents, recruitment of MIAs, and interactions with intestinal immune cells (mast cells, macrophages, and lymphocytes) can result in sensitization of central nociceptive processing. Visceral pain sensitivity can also be modulated by descending pathways, particularly from the rostro-ventral medulla, and this may contribute to associations between of anxiety, stress, and functional abdominal pain (Feng et al., 2012; Sikander and Dickenson, 2012).

Postnatal development of visceral pain mechanisms

Age-related changes in the distribution or function of gastrointestinal afferents have not been directly evaluated throughout postnatal development (Christianson et al. 2009). However, it is clear that visceral mechanisms are functional in neonates and infants, as referred visceral hyperalgesia can be measured by changes in abdominal skin reflexes (Andrews et al., 2002), and repeated noxious stimuli in early life may contribute to persistent hyperalgesia (Anand et al., 2004).

Assessment

Assessment of a child with abdominal pain requires a careful and detailed history and examination. The main aim is to locate the cause of the pain, where possible (Table 26.1), and determine its severity and resulting disability. The history should focus on the site and radiation, type and duration of pain, aggravating and relieving factors, and its intensity. Pain needs to be interpreted in the context of any known pathology, potential new pathology, and the impact of pain on functioning. Examination includes overall impression (e.g. ill/well, malnourished, pale) and assessment of the systemic impact of pain with regard to changes in heart rate and blood pressure. Abdominal examination may help identify the site of pain by associated features including tenderness, guarding, and rebound, and identify any other associated factors such as organomegaly or palpable masses.

Pain assessment

Pain assessment is discussed elsewhere in this text, but examples of use in children with abdominal pain include:

Table 26.1 Classification of conditions presenting with abdominal pain

Gastrointestinal conditions presenting with abdominal pain

Diseases affecting the mucosal lining	Esophagitis: ◆ Reflux esophagitis ◆ Eosinophillic esophagitis ◆ Infections of oesophagus
	Gastritis
	Peptic ulcer disease
	Duodenal ulcers
	Inflammatory bowel disease
	Crohn's disease
	Ulcerative colitis
	Indeterminate colitis
	Eosinophillic gastroenteritis
	Infective enterocolitis
Diseases affecting the smooth muscles	Acute intestinal obstruction
	Chronic intestinal pseudo-obstruction
	Functional recurrent abdominal painv
	Distal intestinal obstruction syndrome (DIOS)
	Constipation
Diseases involving the parietal peritoneum	Pancreatitis
	Appendicitis
	Peritonitis

Non-gastrointestinal causes of abdominal pain

Lower respiratory tract infection
Urinary tract infection
Cholecystitis
Henoch–Schönlein purpura
Sickle cell crisis
Testicular torsion
Pelvic inflammatory disease
Pyelonephritis
Diabetic ketoacidosis
Haemolytic uremic syndrome

◆ Self-report tools have been used to quantify pain intensity with good agreement between the Wong–Baker Faces Scale and visual analogue scale in children (8–17 years) presenting to the emergency department with acute pain, of whom 19% had abdominal pain (Garra et al. 2010).

◆ Multidimensional Measure for Recurrent Abdominal Pain (MM-RAP) also quantifies non-pain symptoms associated with bowel disease (nausea or vomiting, heartburn, diarrhoea, constipation, flatulence, loss of appetite, bloating, sour taste, bad breath, sleep problems, and problems with ingestion of milk) and disability. It is best used in an outpatient setting for children with long standing recurrent abdominal pain (Malaty et al., 2005; see also Schurman et al., Chapter 29, this volume).

Inflammatory bowel disease

Inflammatory bowel disease (IBD) is a chronic relapsing illness affecting the gastrointestinal system that includes:

+ Crohn's disease (CD) is a chronic, idiopathic transmural inflammation which can affect one or several segments anywhere in the digestive tract. CD is also characterized by the type of disease into inflammatory, fistulating, and structuring disease.

+ Ulcerative colitis (UC) is a chronic idiopathic mucosal inflammation limited to the colon. It extends from the rectum continuously over a variable length of the colon from the distal to the proximal end.

+ Indeterminate colitis (IC) is reserved for cases of colitis in which findings are not sufficient to allow differentiation between CD and UC. The disease is characterized based on its severity ranging from mild to severe and its distribution in the gastrointestinal tract.

The aetiologies of both UC and CD remain unknown, but a response to environmental triggers like infection, drugs, or chemical agents in genetically susceptible individuals is the current consensus. Approximately 20% to 30% of patients with IBD present before the age of 18 years (Heyman et al., 2005; Sawczenko et al., 2001; Vind et al., 2006).

Clinical presentation

The common presenting features are abdominal pain, diarrhoea, and weight loss. Other features can include rectal bleeding, lethargy, anaemia, anal fissures or abscesses, mouth ulcers, or arthritis. Abdominal pain is a presenting feature in up to 72% of children with IBD (Sawczenko and Sandhu, 2003), and is the most debilitating symptom. Evaluation of pain is an important part of assessing disease severity and is a component of several disease activity indices. Pain may be due to ongoing intestinal inflammation or secondary to complications such as strictures, subacute bowel obstruction and abscesses seen in CD, or toxic megacolon in UC. Other conditions causing pain in IBD include gall stones, renal calculi, and chronic pancreatitis, and management principally involves treating the underlying pathology. Perianal disease can result in localized severe and difficult to control pain.

About 20% to 30% of adults with IBD continue to have pain without evidence of active inflammation, obstruction, or other biologically defined abnormalities (Bielefeldt et al., 2009; Colombel et al., 2010). Similarly, ongoing pain in children with IBD could be due to persistent sensitization in the gastrointestinal tract following inflammation and high rates of irritable bowel syndrome. Psychological and cognitive factors may also influence pain experience (Docherty et al., 2011).

Management

In patients with active inflammation, analgesics alone are generally less effective until the underlying cause is resolved. Inflammation or stricture formation requiring more intense medical or even surgical therapy likely explain why significant pain requiring analgesic therapy is a negative prognostic indicator (Lichtenstein et al., 2006).

Inflammation can be controlled by the following (Sandhu et al., 2010):

+ *Exclusive enteral nutrition* is an effective treatment for children with Crohn's disease and induces remission in 60% to 80% of the cases (Fell et al., 2000). Polymeric or elemental diets are equally effective. Duration of exclusive enteral nutrition is usually 6 weeks, and depending on patient symptoms, food may be cautiously reintroduced whilst weaning the enteral feed over 1 to 3 weeks.

+ *Corticosteroids* are potent anti-inflammatory agents for moderate to severe relapses of both UC and CD. They act through inhibition of several inflammatory pathways—suppressing interleukin transcription, induction of IκB that stabilizes the NFκB complex, suppression of arachidonic acid metabolism, and stimulation of apoptosis of lymphocytes within the lamina propria of the gut (Steinhart et al., 2001). Commonly used steroids are prednisolone in the dose of 2 mg/kg/day (max 40mg/day). Side effects include acne, moon face, sleep and mood disturbance, dyspepsia, or glucose intolerance. Effects associated with prolonged use include osteoporosis, osteonecrosis of the femoral head, myopathy, impaired growth, and susceptibility to infection.

+ *Monoclonal antibody therapy* such as infliximab, a chimeric antitumour necrosis factor monoclonal antibody with potent anti-inflammatory effects. It was initially developed for use in patients with moderate to severe luminal or fistulizing CD who are refractory to standard medical therapy, but is now being used more widely. Although used predominantly to treat CD, recent data suggest that infliximab also may have a role in the management of UC (Lawson et al., 2006).

Surgery, such as abscess drainage or fistulotomy, may be required for complications (Sandhu, 2010).

Pain management in inflammatory bowel disease

Non-steroidal anti-inflammatory drugs (NSAIDs) act by inhibiting the production of prostaglandins by cyclo-oxygenase (COX) enzymes (see Anderson, Chapter 43, this volume). The effect is mediated through inhibition of both the inducible form of the enzyme, COX-2, and the constitutively produced COX-1 enzyme, resulting in reduced prostaglandin production, which may also result in gastrointestinal side effects. NSAIDs have been linked in some reports to a higher likelihood of disease exacerbation. A 20% to 30% increase in risk of flare-ups was seen with use of NSAIDs in IBD, and all NSAID-treated patients experiencing a flare were able to re-attain remission simply by stopping the NSAID (Takeuchi et al., 2006). Even though controlled trials using NSAIDs in IBD are lacking, a large study including 500 adults failed to find any association between disease relapse and use of NSAIDs (Bernstein et al., 2010). NSAIDs can probably be safely used in children with IBD, particularly in the short term, but should be withdrawn if gastrointestinal side effects are seen or the disease flares and the NSAIDs are felt to be a factor. NSAID-induced enterocolitis is seen rarely (Geramizadeh et al., 2009).

Hyoscine butylbromide blocks the effects of acetylcholine at muscarinic receptors in the periphery, and has no central effects (unlike hyoscine hydrobromide) as it does not cross the blood–brain barrier. Hyoscine butylbromide has an inhibitory effect on smooth muscle and reduces gastrointestinal motility. As only 2% to 8% of an oral dose is absorbed, effects are mainly related to topical actions in the proximal gut, with no effect on the jejunum. Intravenous administration inhibits motility throughout the bowel (Dollery, 1998).

Opioids are mainly used for the management of acute pain in IBD, and have a well-defined role in the management of postoperative pain in children with IBD requiring surgery. The use in acute cases of disease flare-up is controversial, as opioids can induce significant adverse effects on gastrointestinal function and gut motility. Even at low doses, morphine decreases gastric motility, and may prolong gastric emptying time by up to 12 h as the tone of the antral portion of the stomach and the first part of the duodenum is increased. Propulsive contractions are reduced in the duodenum and colon, and colonic muscle tone is increased (the ileum is less affected), leading to constipation which can be severe (Brunton et al., 2011). Opioids also exert complex effects on the immune system via centrally mediated and direct cellular effects; and immunomodulatory effects are an area of active research in inflammatory bowel disease (Mani and Moore, 2009; Philippe et al., 2006; Zagon and McLaughlin, 2011).

In children presenting with an acute flare of IBD, opioids should be used with extreme caution and close monitoring for signs of toxic megacolon (e.g. tachycardia, fall in blood pressure, and increasing abdominal distension). The N-methyl-D-aspartate antagonist ketamine has been shown to reduce acute visceral hyperalgesia in adult volunteers (Willert et al., 2004), but efficacy and potential long-term side-effects have not been evaluated in children with gastro-enterological disease.

Long-term opioid use in children with IBD is discouraged, and has been associated with poorer outcomes in adults (Cross et al., 2005). The TREAT registry prospectively followed over 6000 patients with Crohn's disease, half of whom received infliximab. Chronic narcotic analgesics use was associated with an increased risk of infection (odds ratio, 2.38; 95% confidence interval 1.56–3.63; Lichtenstein et al., 2006). However, the increased complications associated with opioid use may be an indicator of more severe IBD, as adults treated with opiates were more likely to have increased disease activity, and were almost twice as likely to require surgical intervention (Cross et al., 2005).

Gastro-oesophageal reflux disease

Gastro-oesophageal reflux results in passage of the gastric juices and acid into the oesophagus. It is a normal physiological process occurring several times a day, particularly in the post-prandial period. Frequent episodes of transient relaxation of the lower oesophageal sphincter in response to gastric distention and vagal stimulation normally last for 10 to 30 sec, allowing retrograde flow of the stomach contents. Infants develop symptoms, such as vomiting, irritability and coughing after feeds if there are prolonged or excessively frequent relaxations of the sphincter (Box 26.1). Symptoms resolve by 6 months of age in 60% of children with reflux, and by 1 year in approximately 90% of infants (Martin et al., 2002).

A higher frequency of transient lower oesophageal sphincter relaxation and prolonged duration of oesophageal acid exposure may result in pathological gastro-oesophageal reflux disease (GORD), with associated complications such as erosive oesophagitis, respiratory complications, or weight loss. When symptoms

---

Box 26.1 Symptoms and signs of gastro-oesophageal reflux disease (GORD)

Symptoms

- Recurrent regurgitation with/without vomiting
- Weight loss or poor weight gain
- Irritability
- Ruminative behaviour
- Heartburn or chest pain
- Dysphagia, odynophagia
- Wheezing
- Stridor
- Cough
- Feeding refusal.

Signs

- Esophagitis
- Oesophageal stricture
- Barrett oesophagus
- Laryngeal/pharyngeal inflammation
- Recurrent pneumonia
- Anaemia
- Dental erosion
- Dystonic neck posturing (Sandifer syndrome)
- Apnoea spells.

---

persist beyond 18 months of age, there is higher likelihood of a pathological cause (Gold, 2004). Alterations in several protective mechanisms allow physiological reflux to become GORD: delay in gastric emptying, poor clearance of refluxed gastric juices from the oesophagus, or abnormal position of the lower oesophageal sphincter in the thoracic cavity (Cosgrove and Dodge, 1998).

Diagnosis

The diagnosis of GORD is predominantly based on history and examination or on response to treatment. It is important to differentiate this condition from foregut dysmotility, in which infants present with symptoms of vomiting and discomfort after feeds, but the typical features of arching, excess salivation, and feed refusal are absent. Infants with dysmotility have associated intermittent abdominal distension and altered bowel habits. A pH study can quantify oesophageal acid exposure by the number and duration of reflux episodes (pH <4.0) and the percentage of the entire record that oesophageal pH is less than 4.0. Although this test has established normal ranges, it is likely that a continuum between physiological GORD and pathological GORD exists, and the severity of pathologic acid reflux does not consistently correlate with symptom severity or demonstrable complications. Oesophageal pH monitoring can also help determine if a temporal association exists between episodes of reflux and atypical symptoms (chronic cough, stridor, wheezing, apnoea, irritability, or opisthotonic posturing) and evaluate the efficacy of antisecretory therapy (Colletti et al., 1995).

Management

Management of GORD in children is based on its severity, the degree of functional impairment, and presence or absence of complications. The goals for treatment are to relieve symptoms, heal oesophagitis if present, maintain remission of symptoms, and manage or prevent complications. Treatment options include:

* *Dietary management* by modifying infant feeding techniques and changing formula composition with addition of thickening agents. In one study, this improved vomiting and irritability in approximately one-quarter of infants with GORD symptoms (Shalaby et al., 2003). As symptoms of milk protein allergy can overlap those of GORD, a 2-week trial of hypoallergenic formula can be considered (Rudolph et al., 2001).

* *Pharmacological therapy* suppresses gastric acid production by histamine H_2 receptor blockers such as ranitidine, or proton pump inhibitors (PPIs) such as omeprazole, which have been shown to be more effective in reducing gastric acidity (van der Pol et al., 2011). Omeprazole given for 12 weeks resolved moderate-to-severe GORD symptoms in all but 7% of paediatric patients aged 1 to 16 years (Hassal et al., 2000). There is some conflicting data on whether histological findings as well as symptoms are improved (van der Pol et al., 2011). PPIs are safe and well tolerated in children of all ages (Faure et al., 2001; Hassal et al., 2000), with adverse events (headache, constipation, diarrhoea, and abdominal pain) in less than 5% of patients.

* *Surgery* may be indicated for failed medical therapy or symptom recurrence. Fundoplication is performed with consideration of a pyloroplasty if there is delayed gastric emptying, and/or a gastrostomy if there are feeding problems (Granderath et al., 2002). Postoperative analgesic requirements did not differ in a randomized trial of laparoscopic versus open fundoplication (McHoney et al., 2011), and a meta-analysis reported reduced postoperative complications, faster recovery, but an increased risk of reoperation following laparoscopic versus open surgery (Peters et al., 2009).

Pancreatitis

Pancreatitis is an inflammatory process associated with autodigestion of the gland by its enzymes, and can be acute or chronic. Although relatively rare in children, it is associated with high morbidity, but mortality rates are lower than in adult populations (Mekitarian et al., 2012). In a series of 279 paediatric cases, causes of pancreatitis in children included trauma (36%), systemic disease (22%), metabolic (6%), biliary (5%), drugs (3%), and viral illness (2%); but 25% were deemed idiopathic (Nydegger et al., 2007) (Box 26.2).

Pathophysiology

Mechanisms of pain associated with chronic pancreatitis may include (Tsiotou 2000):

* Increased pressure and tension within the gland due to blockage of the ducts. This hypothesis prompted development of techniques to endoscopically decompress the gland.

* Mechanical blockage of surrounding structures such as the duodenum secondary to enlargement of the gland, resulting in partial obstruction and pain.

* Local nerve injury and neuropathic pain.

Box 26.2 Aetiology of acute and chronic pancreatitis in children

Acute pancreatitis

* Infectious:
  * Coxsackie B virus
  * Epstein–Barr Virus
  * Hepatitis
  * Measles
  * Rubella
  * Malaria
  * Mumps
  * Mycoplasma
  * Influenza A & B.

* Hereditary pancreatitis.

* Drugs and toxins:
  * Alcohol
  * Azathioprine/6-mercaptopurine
  * Corticosteroids
  * Valproic acid
  * Sulfonamides
  * Erythromycin
  * Enalapril
  * L-aspariginase
  * Vincristine.

* Trauma.

* Obstructive:
  * Pancreatic duct abnormality
  * Biliary tract malformations
  * Sphincter of oddi dysfunction
  * Pancreas divisum
  * Choledocal cyst
  * Duplication cyst
  * Complication of endoscopic retrograde cholangio-pancreatography (ERCP)
  * Tumours.

* Systemic disease:
  * Alpha 1 antitrypsin deficiency
  * Cystic fibrosis
  * Haemochromatosis
  * Haemolytic uraemic syndrome
  * Malnutrition
  * Hyperparathyroidism
  * Vasculitis syndromes

Box 26.2 (Continued)

- ◆ Hypercalcaemia
- ◆ Hyperlipidaemia
- ◆ Sepsis/shock.

Chronic pancreatitis

- ◆ Hereditary pancreatitis
- ◆ Idiopathic fibrosing pancreatitis
- ◆ Cystic fibrosis
- ◆ Hyperlipidaemia/hypercalcaemia
- ◆ Trauma
- ◆ Congenital anomalies
- ◆ Wilson's disease.

The innervation of the pancreas is complex, involving both somatic–visceral and autonomic nerves. Painful stimuli, such as pressure, acid or chemicals released by cellular necrosis activate receptors on somatic–visceral nociceptive neurons in the pancreatic bed. The signal passes cephalad along both unmyelinated C-fibres and small myelinated Aδ fibres, through the celiac plexus via the left and right greater splanchnic nerves, and through the sympathetic trunk ganglia to the cell body in the dorsal root ganglia, to synapse in the spinal cord at levels T5 to T9. Sensory neurons from the back and epigastric rectus abdominus muscles are also found at this level, resulting in pain of pancreatitis being referred to the back and/or epigastric region.

Clinical presentation

Acute pancreatitis presents with vomiting and abdominal pain, which is characteristically a sharp, steady pain of sudden onset, aggravated by eating and improved by drawing the knees up to the chest. The pain is generally epigastric, but may be experienced in the middle or even lower abdomen, or referred to the back. Physical signs include fever and tachycardia. White cell count and inflammatory markers may be increased. Serum amylase is usually elevated and starts to subside by 3 to 5 days, but the degree of elevation does not correlate directly with severity of disease severity, and normal levels do not rule out the diagnosis (Lautz et al., 2011). Serum lipase may also remain elevated for 1 to 2 weeks. Ultrasound imaging can demonstrate an enlarged, oedematous pancreas, a dilated main pancreatic duct indicates obstruction, and calcifications are often seen in older children with recurrent pancreatitis.

Most episodes of acute pancreatitis in children are isolated and self-limited, but patients with recurrent episodes may progress to chronicity. Recurrent acute pancreatitis is commonly associated with congenital malformations of pancreatico-biliary tract, gall-stones, cystic fibrosis, and familial pancreatitis (Nydegger et al., 2006). Familial pancreatitis has been associated with mutations in: cationic trypsinogen gene (e.g. *PRSS1*) which enhances trypsin activation; *SPINK1* (serine protease inhibitor Kazal type 1) gene resulting in an abnormal pancreatic secretory trypsin inhibitor; and the *CFTR* (cystic fibrosis transmembrane conductance regulator) gene, which reduces the pancreatic fluid secretion capacity (Nydegger et al., 2006).

Management

Management of children with pancreatitis requires analgesia, fluid replacement, nutritional support, and treatment of any initiating cause (Table 26.2) or associated complications (Mekitarian et al., 2012):

- ◆ *Analgesia*: providing adequate analgesia is an important part of management of acute pancreatitis, and opioids are commonly used. There is no definitive human study to support the widespread belief that morphine exacerbates pancreatitis by stimulating the sphincter of Oddi to contract (Toouli et al., 2002), and no studies suggest that use of morphine is contraindicated in acute pancreatitis (Thompson 2001). Other drugs which may be beneficial include acetaminophen and non-steroidal anti-inflammatory agents. Drugs for neuropathic pain may be considered in chronic cases (see Rastogi and Campbell, Chapter 48, this volume). Pregabalin reduces acute acid-induced hyperalgesia in adult volunteers (Chua et al., 2012), but there is currently no data to confirm efficacy or inform appropriate patient selection in children who may have visceral hyperalgesia.

- ◆ *Pancreatic rest*: in acute cases, preventing oral intake 'rests' the pancreas and provides symptomatic relief (Lordan et al., 2009). Without any food being presented to the gut, secretions from the gastric glands are reduced, and reduced enzyme release by the pancreas decreases both autodigestion and pancreatic distension. Nutrition is critically important in patients with pancreatitis and an early positive nitrogen balance improves survival rates in adults (Meier et al., 2006). In adult studies, placement of a nasojejunal tube for feeding has been shown to as effective as parenteral nutrition, with reduced infectious complications (Kalfarentzos et al., 1997), and both assist in controlling pain (Raimondo et al., 2005). In patients with chronic pancreatitis there is limited research on the benefit of restricted diets, and it would be prudent to provide a well-balanced nutritionally complete diet (Shea et al., 2000; Toouli et al., 2002).

- ◆ *Somatostatin analogues*: octreotide has been used in adults for management of acute pain in pancreatitis as it suppresses cholecystokinin and pancreatic secretions (Uhl et al., 1999), and some but not all data suggests improved outcome (Beechey Newman 1993; Heikenen et al., 2002). Paediatric data is limited to case reports, and octreotide is not routinely used in children with acute pancreatitis, although some benefit has been shown for the

Table 26.2 Groups of medication used in management of constipation

Class of drug	Example	Mechanism of action
Osmotic laxatives	Lactulose, macrogols, magnesium sulphate, phosphate enema	Draws and retain water in large bowel by osmosis
Stimulant laxatives	Anthraquinones, e.g. senna Bisacodyl, picosulphate	Increase intestinal motility
Lubricants/softeners	Arachis oil, liquid paraffin, docusate	Softens impacted stool
Bulking agents	Fibre, bran, isphagula, methylcellulose	Increase faecal mass and improves peristalsis
Prokinetics	Erythromycin	Improves transit by increasing peristalsis

management of complications, such as ascites and pseudocysts. (Bosman-Vermeeren et al., 1996; Rushforth et al., 1993).

♦ Administration of oral pancreatic enzymes may reduce pain via negative feedback inhibition to the pancreas, with some benefit shown in adults (Layer et al., 1990), but data in children is lacking.

♦ Antioxidant therapy has been suggested for chronic pancreatitis in adults (Bhardwaj et al., 2004), but there is conflicting data about efficacy, and further research is needed (Gachago et al., 2008).

♦ Antibiotics may prevent secondary bacterial infections, limit complications, and improve outcome; however, they are best reserved for severe cases, especially where pancreatic necrosis is present (Sainio et al., 1995).

♦ Surgical intervention is rarely required in management of pancreatitis except in cases of congenital malformations or management of complications such as drainage of pseudocysts.

Constipation

Constipation is a very common (5–30%) cause of abdominal pain in children (van den berg et al., 2006). Most children do not have an underlying cause and the ROME III criteria for diagnosis of functional constipation include presence of two or more of the following for more than 1 month (Rasquin et al., 2006):

♦ Two or fewer defecations per week.

♦ At least one episode/week of incontinence after the acquisition of toileting skills.

♦ History of excessive stool retention.

♦ History of painful or hard bowel movements.

♦ Presence of a large faecal mass in the rectum.

♦ History of large-diameter stools which may obstruct the toilet.

History and clinical examination aim to assess the severity of symptoms and resulting functional impairment. Symptoms and signs that are suggestive of underlying pathology (Box 26.3) should be sought to ensure diagnosis or exclusion of organic conditions.

Management

The UK National Institute for Health and Clinical Excellence (NICE) produced a clinical guideline '*CG99 Constipation in children and young people: Diagnosis and management of idiopathic childhood constipation in primary and secondary care*' in May 2010 (<http://www.nice.org.uk/cg99>). The management of chronic functional constipation often requires a multidisciplinary approach, based on the following principles:

♦ Explanation of normal bowel function aids the family's understanding and improves compliance. Parents and children should be reassured that constipation is common and responds well to treatment.

♦ High-fibre diet is recommended along with adequate fluid intake because it adds bulk to the stool.

♦ Regular exercise promotes peristalsis and helps bowel transit.

♦ Regular toileting is a crucial part of the management to encourage regular emptying of the rectum.

♦ Behavioural advice and reward schemes (star charts) are helpful to gain child's trust in the management. Rewards can be given

---

Box 26.3 Symptoms and signs suggestive of underlying pathology in children with constipation

♦ Constipation reported from birth or first few weeks of life.

♦ Failure to pass meconium/delay (more than 48 h) in a term baby.

♦ Infrequent/very large (ribbon) stools.

♦ Faltering growth.

♦ Previously known or undiagnosed weakness in legs/locomotor delay.

♦ Abdominal distension with vomiting.

♦ Perianal inspection—abnormal appearance/patency/position of anus, anteriorly placed anus or absent anal wink, fissures, fistulae, bruising, tight or patulous anus.

♦ Gross abdominal distension, palpable faecal mass (in at least half of these patients).

♦ Spine and gluteal examination—asymmetry of gluteal muscles, scoliosis, evidence of sacral agenesis, overlying skin over sacral region with discoloration, naevi, sinus, hairy patch, lipoma or central pit.

♦ Deformity in lower limbs such as talipes.

♦ Abnormal neuromuscular signs unexplained by any existing condition, such as cerebral palsy.

♦ Abnormal tendon reflexes.

---

for compliance (sitting on the toilet) at first and then for success (opening bowel in the toilet).

♦ Drug treatment: laxatives are used in the management of acute as well as chronic constipation. As abdominal pain in these children is principally due to faecal impaction it is poorly responsive to analgesics.

♦ Disimpaction of stools can reduce pain (Poenaru et al., 1997). Senna or polyethylene glycol can be used as sole agents in high doses. In severe cases, sodium picosulphate (liquid or sachets) may be required. Rectal medications (suppositories, enemas) are used if all oral medications have failed. Manual evacuation of the bowel under anaesthesia is rarely considered, and only if oral and rectal treatments fail.

♦ Laxatives are often needed for prolonged maintenance therapy, but need to be closely monitored, weaned only after a sustained period of normal bowel actions with no soiling, and used in conjunction with other supportive strategies. Polyethylene glycol (Movicol®) is widely used. Senokot® given in the evening, at reasonable doses, is effective. The choice of agent depends on local preference as well as individual patient circumstances (Table 26.2). Young children should remain on laxatives until toilet training is well established.

Neuromuscular motility disorders

Motility disorders present with features of gastrointestinal obstruction in the absence of a mechanical cause. The spectrum of motility disorders ranges from relatively benign conditions such as gastro-oesophageal reflux and functional constipation, to life-threatening illnesses such as chronic intestinal pseudo-obstruction. It can result from any process that interferes with coordinated patterns of propulsive movement of intestinal musculature. Chronic disorders of motility account for 15% of patients with intestinal failure necessitating the use of parenteral nutrition (Connor et al., 2006) and irreversible cases may require intestinal transplant (Gupte et al., 2007)

Intestinal pseudo-obstruction can be divided into acute or chronic. Chronic pseudo obstruction can be primary or secondary to systemic illness. Primary pseudo-obstruction is a result of disorders of intestinal smooth muscle (myopathic) or myentric plexus (neuropathic), and can involve either the whole of or a localized segment of the bowel (Box 26.4). Neuropathic disorders are more common and may be primary or secondary (e.g. *in utero* insults such as fetal alcohol syndrome or postnatal injuries such as ischaemic events or viral infections; Rudolph et al., 1997). Antroduodenal manometry measures the intraluminal pressure of the antrum and duodenum and is useful to distinguish myopathy (contraction amplitude is reduced but spatial and temporal organisation is preserved), from neuropathy (contractions have normal amplitude but are uncoordinated and lack normal physiologic patterns) (Hyman et al., 1993).

Mitochondrial disorders such as mitochondrial neurogastrointestinal encephalopathy (MNGIE; an autosomal recessive multisystem disorder caused by thymidine phosphorylase deficiency) may also be complicated by pseudo-obstruction, with gastrointestinal symptoms (diarrhoea, dysphagia, and failure to thrive) often preceding the neurological dysfunction (leucoencephalopathy, external ophthalmoparesis and demyelinating peripheral neuropathy) (Shoffner et al., 2010). Recently, abnormalities of the gastrointestinal pacemaker cells, the interstitial cells of Cajal, have been described in patients with motility disorders. In most paediatric

---

Box 26.4 Neuromuscular motility disorders associated with primary chronic pseudo-obstruction

- Aganglionosis:
  - Hirschsprung's disease.
- Primary visceral myopathies:
  - Familial myopathy with megaduodenum
  - Megacystis microcolon
  - Hollow visceral myopathy
  - Myotonic dystrophy
  - Duchenne muscular dystrophy
  - Autoimmune myositis.
- Primary neuropathies:
  - Familial visceral neuropathies
  - Ganglioneuromatosis with MEN type IIb
  - Disorders of interstitial cells of Cajal
  - Autoimmune ganglionitis
  - Chagas disease
  - Kawasaki disease.

---

cases, symptoms are present from birth or early infancy. Pain is usually a prominent feature and is a result of uncoordinated contraction of bowel musculature (Takahashi, 2005).

Management

Management requires a multidisciplinary team that includes a gastroenterologist, surgeon, dietician, and psychologist. Chronic abdominal pain or the fear of pain is a common problem in children with chronic intestinal pseudo-obstruction. Luminal dilatation, repeated invasive procedures, and mucosal inflammation may all contribute to the development of visceral hyperalgesia with sensitization of peripheral and central pain pathways (Anand et al., 2004; Christianson et al., 2009; Feng et al., 2012). The stress of chronic disease can also influence pain report and altered family dynamics (see also Birnie et al., Chapter 12; Fogeron and King, Chapter 13, this volume).

Analgesics may have limited efficacy, and use of morphine can worsen symptoms due to further slowing of gut (Brunton et al., 2011). Controlling bowel dilatation and inflammation can reduce pain. Prokinetics used to improve gastric emptying and gut motility include erythromycin (Ng et al., 2012), domperidone, and neostigmine in severe cases (Gmora et al., 2002). Octreotide is being increasingly studied as a prokinetic to increase small intestinal motility, inhibit gastric emptying, and gallbladder contractility, but benefit has only been reported in adults (Soudah et al., 1991).

Stimulant laxatives have shown to be beneficial in relieving constipation as well as increasing motility (Connor et al., 2006). Reduced motility is also associated with bacterial overgrowth which causes further mucosal inflammation and damage, and worsens the gastrointestinal motility. Oral antibiotics help reduce inflammation and reduce distension by limiting gas-forming bacteria. Probiotics along with antibiotics have also been used in cases of overgrowth though their superiority above a placebo is yet to be proven (Shanahan, 2003). A dilated non-motile segment of the gut can be surgically removed or gastrostomy, jejunostomy, or loop enterostomy may be required to shorten the gut and facilitate transit of intraluminal contents, and can improve enteral feed tolerance in some cases (Shibata et al., 2003). Small intestinal transplantation is indicated in total parenteral nutrition (TPN)-dependent pseudo-obstruction patients with life-threatening complications of PN or with dwindling venous access (Mittal et al., 2003).

Conclusion

Pain is an important and common symptom of gastrointestinal disease. Pain may be the presenting feature, or an indicator of acute complications, that requires symptomatic treatment until the underlying gastrointestinal disorder is controlled by specific treatments. Pain needs to be interpreted in the context of any known pathology, potential new pathology, and the impact of pain on functioning, and persistent or chronic pain associated with gastrointestinal disease requires coordinated interdisciplinary management.

References

Anand, K. J., Runeson, B., and Jacobson, B. (2004). Gastric suction at birth associated with long-term risk for functional intestinal disorders in later life. *J Pediatr*, 144, 449–454.

Andrews, K. A., Desai, D., Dhillon, H. K., Wilcox, D. T., and Fitzgerald, M. (2002). Abdominal sensitivity in the first year of life: comparison of infants with and without prenatally diagnosed unilateral hydronephrosis. *Pain*, 100, 35–46.

Beechey-Newman, N. (1993). Controlled trial of high-dose octreotide in treatment of acute pancreatitis. Evidence of improvement in disease severity. *Dig Dis Sci*, 38, 644–647.

Berthoud, H. R., Kressel, M., Raybould, H. E., and Neuhuber, W. L. (1995). Vagal sensors in the rat duodenal mucosa: distribution and structure as revealed by in vivo DiI-tracing. *Anat Embryol (Berl)*, 191, 203–212.

Bernstein, C. N., Singh, S., Graff, L. A., Walker, J. R., Miller, N., and Cheang, M. (2010). A prospective population-based study of triggers of symptomatic flares in IBD. *Am J Gastroenterol*, 105, 1994–2002.

Bhardwaj, P., Thareja, S., Prakash, S., and Saraya, A. (2004). Micronutrient antioxidant intake in patients with chronic pancreatitis. *Trop Gastroenterol*, 25, 69–72.

Bielefeldt, K., Davis, B., and Binion, D. G. (2009). Pain and inflammatory bowel disease. *Inflamm Bowel Dis*, 15(5), 778–788.

Blackshaw, L. A., and Gebhart, G. F. (2002). The pharmacology of gastrointestinal nociceptive pathways. *Curr Opin Pharmacol*, 2, 642–649.

Brunton, L., Chabner, B.A., and Knollman, B. (eds) (2011). *Goodman and Gilman's: the pharmacological basis of therapeutics* (12th edn). New York: McGraw-Hill Medical.

Bosman-Vermeeren, J. M., Veereman-Wauters, G., Broos, P., and Eggermont, E. (1996). Somatostatin in the treatment of a pancreatic pseudocyst in a child. *J Pediatr Gastroenterol Nutr*, 23, 422–425.

Christianson, J. A., Bielefeldt, K., Altier, C., Cenac, N., Davis, B.M., Gebhart, G. F., *et al.* (2009). Development, plasticity and modulation of visceral afferents. *Brain Res Rev*, 60, 171–186.

Chua, Y. C., Ng, K. S., Sharma, A., Jafari, J., Surguy, S., Yazaki, E., *et al.* (2012). Randomised clinical trial: pregabalin attenuates the development of acid-induced oesophageal hypersensitivity in healthy volunteers—a placebo-controlled study. *Aliment Pharmacol Ther*, 35(3), 319–326.

Connor, F. L., and Di Lorenzo, C. (2006). Chronic intestinal pseudo-obstruction: assessment and management. *Gastroenterology*, 130(2 Suppl 1), S29–36.

Colletti, R. D., Christie, D. L., and Orenstein, S. R. (1995). Statement of the North American Society for Pediatric Gastroenterology and Nutrition (NASPGN). (1995). Indications for pediatric esophageal pH monitoring. *J Pediatr Gastroenterol Nutr*, 21, 253–262.

Colombel, J. F., Sandborn, W. J., Reinisch, W., Mantzaris, G. J., Kornbluth, A., Rachmilewitz, D., *et al.* (2010). Infliximab, azathioprine, or combination therapy for Crohn's disease. *N Engl J Med*, 362, 1383–1395.

Connor, F. L., and Di Lorenzo, C. (2006). Chronic intestinal pseudo-obstruction: assessment and management. *Gastroenterology*, 130(2 Suppl 1), S29–36.

Cosgrove, M. and Dodge, J. (1998). Gastro-oesophageal reflux in children. *Eur J Gastroenterol Hepatol*, 7 (10), 547–548.

Cross, R. K., Wilson, K. T., and Binion, D. G. (2005). Narcotic use in patients with Crohn's disease. *Am J Gastroenterol*, 100(10), 2225–2229.

Docherty, M. J., Jones, R. C. W., and Wallace, M. S. (2011). Managing pain in inflammatory bowel disease. *Gastroenterol Hepatol*, 7, 592–601.

Dollery, C. (1998). *Therapeutic drugs*. London: Churchill Livingstone.

Faure, C., Michaud, L., Shaghaghi, E. K., Popon, M., Laurence, M., Mougenot, J. F., *et al.* (2001). Lansoprazole in children: pharmacokinetics and efficacy in reflux oesophagitis. *Aliment Pharmacol Ther*, 15, 1397–1402.

Fell, J. M., Paintin, M., Arnaud-Battandier, F., Beattie, R. M., Hollis, A., Kitching, P., *et al.* (2000). Mucosal healing and a fall in mucosal pro-inflammatory cytokine mRNA induced by a specific oral polymeric diet in paediatric Crohn's disease. *Aliment Pharmacol Ther*, 14, 281–289.

Feng, B., La, J. H., Schwartz, E. S., and Gebhart, G. F. (2012). Neural and neuro-immune mechanisms of visceral hypersensitivity in irritable bowel syndrome. *Am J Physiol Gastrointest Liver Physiol*, 302(10), G1085–1098.

Gachago, C. and Draganov, P. (2008). Pain management in chronic pancreatitis. *World J Gastroenterol*, 14(20), 3137–3148.

Garra, G., Singer, A. J., Tiaras, B. R., Chohan, J., Cardoz, H., Chisena, E., *et al.* (2010). Validation of the Wong-Baker FACES Pain Rating Scale in pediatric emergency department patients. *Acad Emerg Med*, 17(1), 50–54.

Gebhart, G.F. (2000). Visceral afferent contributions to the pathobiology of visceral pain. *Am J Physiol Gastrointest Liver Physiol* 278, G834–G838.

Geramizadeh, B., Taghavi, A., and Banan, B. (2009). Clinical, endoscopic and pathologic spectrum of non-steroidal anti-inflammatory drug-induced colitis. *Indian J Gastroenterol*, 28(4), 150–153.

Gershon, M. D. (2005). Nerves, reflexes, and the enteric nervous system. *J Clin Gastroenterol*, 39, S184–193.

Gmora, S., Poenaru, D., and Tsai, E. (2002). Neostigmine for the treatment of pediatric acute colonic pseudo-obstruction. *J Pediatr Surg*, 37(10), E28.

Gold, B. D. (2004). Gastro oesophageal reflux disease: could intervention in childhood reduce the risk of later complications? *Am J Med*, 117(Suppl 5A), 23S–29S.

Goyal, R. K., and Hirano, I. (1996). Mechanisms of disease: the enteric nervous system. *N Engl J Med*, 334, 1106–1115.

Gupte, G. L., Beath, S. V., Protheroe, S., Murphy, M. S., Davies, P., Sharif, K., *et al.* (2007). Improved outcome of referrals for intestinal transplantation in the UK. *Arch Dis Child*, 92, 147–152.

Granderath, F. A., Kamolz, T., Schweiger, U. M., Pasiut, M., Haas, C. F., Whkypiel, H., *et al.* (2002). Long-term results of laparoscopic antireflux surgery. *Surg Endosc*, 16, 753–757.

Heikenen, J., Pohl, J., Werlin, S., and Bucuvalas, J. (2002). Octreotide in pediatric patients. *J Pediatr Gastroenterol Nutr*, 35(5), 600–609.

Heyman, M. B., Kirschner, B. S., Gold, B. D., Ferry, G., Baldassano, R., Cohen, S. A., *et al.* (2005). Children with early-onset inflammatory bowel disease (IBD): analysis of a pediatric IBD consortium registry. *J Pediatr*, 146, 35–40.

Hyman, P. E., Di Lorenzo, C., McAdams, L., and Garvey, T. Q. 3rd. (1993). Predicting the clinical response to cisapride in children with chronic intestinal pseudo-obstruction. *Am J Gastroenterol*, 88, 832–836.

Kalfarentzos, F., Kehagias, J., Mead, N., Kokkinis, K., and Gogos, C. A. (1997). Enteral nutrition is superior to parenteral nutrition in severe acute pancreatitis: results of a randomized prospective trial. *Br J Surg*, 84, 166–169.

Kirkup, A. J., Brunsden, A. M., and Grundy, D. (2001). Receptors and transmission in the brain-gut axis: potential for novel therapies. I. Receptors on visceral afferents. *Am J Physiol Gastrointest Liver Physiol*, 280, G787–794.

Knowles, C. H., and Aziz, Q. (2009). Basic and clinical aspects of gastrointestinal pain. *Pain*, 141(3), 191–209.

Lautz, T. B., Chin, A. C., and Radhakrishnan, J. (2011). Acute pancreatitis in children: spectrum of disease and predictors of severity. *J Pediatr Surg*, 46(6), 1144–1149.

Lawson, M. M., Thomas, A. G., and Akobeng, A. K. (2006). Tumour necrosis factor alpha blocking agents for induction of remission in ulcerative colitis. *Cochrane Database Syst Rev*, 3, CD005112.

Layer, P., Jansen, J. B., Cherian, L., Lamers, C. B., and Goebell, H. (1990). Feedback regulation of human pancreatic secretion. Effects of protease inhibition on duodenal delivery and small intestinal transit of pancreatic enzymes. *Gastroenterology*, 98, 1311–1319.

Lichtenstein, G. R., Feagan, B. G., Cohen, R. D., Salzberg, B. A., Diamond, R. H., Chen, D. M., *et al.* (2006). Serious infections and mortality in association with therapies for Crohn's disease: TREAT registry. *Clin Gastroenterol Hepatol*, 4(5), 621–630.

Lordan, J. T., Phillips, M., Chun, J. Y., Worthington, T. R., Menezes, N. N., Lightwood, R., *et al.* (2009). A safe, effective, and cheap method of achieving pancreatic rest in patients with chronic pancreatitis with refractory symptoms and malnutrition. *Pancreas*, 38(6), 689–692.

Lynn, P. A., Olsson, C., Zagorodnyuk, V., Costa, M., and Brookes, S. J. (2003). Rectal intraganglionic laminar endings are transduction sites of extrinsic mechanoreceptors in the guinea pig rectum. *Gastroenterology*, 125, 786–794.

Martin, A. J., Pratt, N., Kennedy, J. D., Ryan, P., Ruffin, R. E., Miles, H., *et al.* (2002). Natural history and familial relationships of infant spilling to 9 years of age. *Pediatrics*, 109, 1061–1067.

Malaty, H. M., Abudayyeh, S., O'Malley, K. J., Wilsey, M. J., Fraley, K., Gilger, M. A., *et al.* (2005). Development of a multidimensional measure for recurrent abdominal pain in children: population-based studies in three settings. *Pediatrics*, 115(2), e210–215.

Mani, A. R., and Moore, K. P. (2009) New insights into the role of endogenous opioids in the pathogenesis of gastrointestinal and liver disease. *Gut*, 58, 893–895.

McHoney, M., Wade, A. M., Eaton, S., Howard, R. F., Kiely, E. M., Drake, D.P., *et al.* (2011). Clinical outcome of a randomized controlled blinded trial of open versus laparoscopic Nissen fundoplication in infants and children. *Ann Surg*, 254(2), 209–216.

Meier, R. F., and Beglinger, C. (2006). Nutrition in pancreatic diseases. *Best Pract Res Clin Gastroenterol*, 20, 507–529.

Mekitarian Filho, E., Carvalho, W. B., and Silva, F. D. (2012). Acute pancreatitis in pediatrics: a systematic review of the literature. *J Pediatr (Rio J)*, 88(2), 101–114.

Mittal, N. K., Tzakis, A. G., Kato, T., and Thompson, J. F. (2003). Current status of small bowel transplantation in children: update 2003. *Pediatr Clin North Am*, 50, ix, 1419–1433.

National Institute for Health and Clinical Excellence (NICE). (2010). *Constipation in children and young people* (Clinical Guideline 99). Available at: <http://publications.nice.org.uk/constipation-in-children-and-young-people-cg99>.

Ng, Y. Y., Su, P. H., Chen, J. Y., Quek, Y. W., Hu, J. M., Lee, I. C., *et al.* (2012). Efficacy of intermediate-dose oral erythromycin on very low birth weight infants with feeding intolerance. *Pediatr Neonatol*, 53(1), 34–40.

Nydegger, A., Couper, R., and Oliver, M. R. (2006). Childhood pancreatitis. *J Gastroenterol Hepatol*, 21, 499–509.

Nydegger, A., Heine, R. G., Ranuh, R., Gegati-Levy, R., Crameri, J., and Oliver, M. R. (2007). Changing incidence of acute pancreatitis: 10-year experience at the Royal Children's Hospital, Melbourne. *J Gastroenterol Hepatol*, 22(8), 1313–1316.

Peters, M. J., Mukhtar, A., Yunus, R. M., Khan, S., Pappalardo, J., Memon, B., *et al.* (2009). Meta-analysis of randomized clinical trials comparing open and laparoscopic anti-reflux surgery. *Am J Gastroenterol*, 6, 1548–1561.

Poenaru, D., Roblin, N., Bird, M., Duce, S., Groll, A., Pietak, D., *et al.* (1997). The Pediatric Bowel Management Clinic: initial results of a multidisciplinary approach to functional constipation in children. *J Pediatr Surg*, 32(6), 843–848.

Philippe, D., Chakass, D., Thuru, X., Zerbib, P., Tsicopoulos, A., Geboes, K., *et al.* (2006). Mu opioid receptor expression is increased in inflammatory bowel disease: implications for homeostatic intestinal inflammation. *Gut*, 55, 815–823.

Rasquin, A., Di Lorenzo, C., Forbes, D., Guiralde, E., Hyams, J. S., Staiano, A., *et al.* (2006). Childhood functional gastrointestinal disorders: child/adolescent. *Gastroenterology*, 130, 1527–1537.

Raimondo, M. and Scolapio, J. S. (2005). What route to feed patients with severe acute pancreatitis: vein, jejunum, or stomach? *Am J Gastroenterol*, 100, 440–441.

Rudolph, C. D., Hyman, P. E., Altschuler, S. M., Christensen, J., Colletti, R. B., Cucchiara, S., *et al.* (1997). Diagnosis and treatment of chronic intestinal pseudo-obstruction in children: report of consensus workshop. *J Pediatr Gastroenterol Nutr*, 24, 102–112.

Rudolph, C. D., Mazur, L. J., Liptak, G. S., Baker, R. D., Boyle, J. T., Colletti, R. B., *et al.* (2001). Guidelines for evaluation and treatment of gastroesophageal reflux in infants and children: recommendations of the North American Society for Pediatric Gastroenterology and Nutrition. *J Pediatr Gastroenterol Nutr*, 32(Suppl), S1–S31.

Rushforth, J. A., Beck, J. M., McMahon, M., and Puntis, J. W. (1993). Resolution of pancreatic ascites with octreotide. *Arch Dis Child*, 68, 135–136.

Sainio, V., Kemppainen, E., Puolakkainen, P., Taavit-sainen, M., Kivisaari, L., Valtonen, V., *et al.* (1995). Early antibiotic treatment in acute necrotising pancreatitis. *Lancet*, 346, 663–667.

Sandhu, B. K., Fell, J. M., Beattie, R. M., Mitton, S. G., Wilson, D. C., Jenkins, H.; on behalf of the IBD Working Group of the British Society of Paediatric Gastroenterology, Hepatology, and Nutrition. (2010). Guidelines for the management of inflammatory bowel disease in children in the United Kingdom. *J Pediatr Gastroenterol Nutr*, 50, S1–S13.

Sawczenko, A. and Sandhu, B. (2003). Presenting features of inflammatory bowel disease in Great Britain and Ireland. *Arch Dis Child*, 88, 995–1000.

Sawczenko, A., Sandhu, B. K., Logan, R. F., Jenkins, H., Taylor, C. J., Mian, S., *et al.* (2001). Prospective survey of childhood inflammatory bowel disease in the British Isles. *Lancet*, 357, 1093–1094.

Sengupta, J. N., and Gebhart, G. F. (1994). Gastrointestinal afferent fibers and sensation. In L. R. Johnson, (ed.) *Physiology of the gastrointestinal tract* (3rd edn), pp. 483–519. New York: Raven Press.

Shanahan, F. (2003). Probiotics: a perspective on problems and pitfalls. *Scand J Gastroenterol*, 38(Suppl), 34–36.

Shalaby, T. M., and Orenstein, S. R. (2003). Efficacy of telephone teaching of conservative therapy for infants with symptomatic gastroesophageal reflux referred by pediatricians to pediatric gastroenterologists. *J Pediatr*, 142, 57–61.

Shea, J. C., Hopper, I. K., Blanco, P. G., and Freedman, S. D. (2000). Advances in nutritional management of chronic pancreatitis. *Curr Gastroenterol Rep*, 2, 323–326.

Shibata, C., Naito, H., Funayama, Y., Fukushima, K., and Sasaki, I. (2003). Surgical treatment of chronic intestinal pseudo-obstruction: report of three cases. *Surg Today*, 33, 58–61.

Shoffner, J. M. (2010). Mitochondrial neurogastrointestinal encephalopathy disease. 22 April 2005 (updated 11 May 2010). In R. A. Pagon, T. D. Bird, C. R. Dolan, K. Stephens, and M. P. Adam (eds) *GeneReviews™* [Internet]. Seattle, WA: University of Washington, 1993–2005. Available at: <http://www.ncbi.nlm.nih.gov/books/NBK1179/>.

Sikandar, S. and Dickenson, A. H. (2012). Visceral pain: the ins and outs, the ups and downs. *Curr Opin Support Palliat Care*, 6(1), 17–26.

Soudah, H. C., Hasler, W. L., and Owyang, C. (1991). Effect of octreotide on intes- tinal motility and bacterial overgrowth in scleroderma. *N Engl J Med*, 325, 1461–1467.

Steinhart, A. H., Ewe, K., Griffiths, A. M., Modigliani, R., and Thomsen, O. O. (2001). Corticosteroids for maintaining remission of Crohn's disease. *Cochrane Database Syst Rev*, 3, CD000301.

Takahashi, A. (2005). The role of interstitial cells of cajal on gastrointestinal motility and pathological conditions of gastrointestinal disease. *Jpn J Pediatr Surg*, 37(4), 473–478.

Takeuchi, K., Smale, S., Premchand, P., Maiden, L., Sherwood, R., Thjodleifsson, B., *et al.* (2006). Prevalence and mechanism of nonsteroidal anti-inflammatory drug-induced clinical relapse in patients with inflammatory bowel disease. *Clin Gastroenterol Hepatol*, 4(2), 196–202.

Thompson, D. R. (2001). Narcotic analgesic effects on the sphincter of Oddi: a review of the data and therapeutic implications in treating pancreatitis. *Am J Gastroenterol*, 96(4), 1266–1272.

Toouli, J., Brook-Smith, M., Bassi, C., Carr-Locke, D., Telford, J., Freeny, P., *et al.* (2002). Guidelines for the management of acute pancreatitis. *J Gastroenterol Hepatol*, 17(Suppl.), S15–39.

Tsiotou, A. G., and Sakorafas, G. H. (2000). Pathophysiology of pain in chronic pancreatitis: clinical implications from a surgical perspective. *Int Surg*, 85(4), 291–296.

Uhl, W., Anghelacopoulos, S. E., Friess, H., Büchler, M. W. The role of octreotide and somatostatin in acute and chronic pancreatitis. *Digestion*, 60(Suppl.2), 23–31.

van der Pol, R. J., Smits, M. J., van Wijk, M. P., Omari, T. I., Tabbers, M. M., and Benninga, M. A. (2011). Efficacy of proton-pump inhibitors in children with gastroesophageal reflux disease: a systematic review. *Pediatrics*, 127, 925–935.

Van Den Berg, M., Benninga, M. A., and Di Lorenzo, C. (2006). Epidemiology of childhood constipation: a systematic review. *Am J Gastroenterol*, 101(10), 2401–2409.

Vind, I., Riis, L., Jess, T., Knudsen, E., Pedersen, N., Elkjaer, M., *et al.* (2006). Increasing incidences of inflammatory bowel disease and decreasing surgery rates in Copenhagen City and County, 2003–2005: a population-based study from the Danish Crohn colitis database. *Am J Gastroenterol*, 101, 1274–1282.

Willert, R. P., Woolf, C. J., Hobson, A. R., Delaney, C., Thompson, D. G., and Aziz, Q. (2004). The development and maintenance of human visceral pain hypersensitivity is dependent on the N-methyl-D-aspartate receptor. *Gastroenterology*, 126(3), 683–692.

Zagon, S. and McLaughlin, P. J. (2011). Targeting opioid signalling in Crohn's disease: new therapeutic pathways. *Expert Rev Gastroenterol Hepatol*, 5, 55–58.

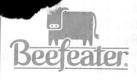

Total
PIN VERI.
AUTHORISED
012799
Ref: 1261
Merchant: 540436504447731
CHECK:28562
Receipt: 1431686836287

Date: 15/05/15 Time: 11:47
Please Keep This Receipt For
Your Records

CHAPTER 27

Postoperative pain management

Richard F. Howard

Introduction

Postoperative pain management begins prior to surgery and includes not only the prevention and pharmacological treatment of pain, but also a holistic and well-coordinated strategy that allays fears and anxieties, and allows children and their carers to participate in the selection and implementation of safe and suitable analgesia. Admission to hospital for surgery is a significant and potentially traumatic event. Coping with a strange and unknown environment, fear of separation, anticipation of painful procedures, and postoperative pain or adverse effects such as nausea are all prominent causes of anxiety and stress that can increase the perception of pain and impact on the quality of perioperative care. Therefore, a successful postoperative pain management programme will include: ongoing training of hospital staff, adequate preparation of children and families that provides timely verbal and written information, and the development and implementation of audited institutional analgesic protocols that ensure the safety and efficacy of pain management strategies in a child-friendly and secure environment.

Aims

- Understand basic principles of postoperative analgesia.

- Ability to select an age-appropriate postoperative pain assessment tool.

- Understand the pharmacology, advantages and disadvantages of the principal analgesics, and analgesic techniques.

- Ability to describe suitable analgesic regimens for frequently encountered surgical procedures and in special situations.

General principles

Postoperative pain is predictable, but pain intensity and the response to analgesia are subject to many different patient-determined variables that are not fully predictable. Therefore, postoperative pain should be anticipated and its intensity assessed frequently during the postoperative period so that appropriate analgesia can be administered promptly, and the response to treatment assessed. Analgesia should be planned according to the expected intensity and duration of pain, but must always be titrated against clinical response, as treatment must be flexible enough to adapt to inter-individual variation and unexpected circumstances or events. Side effects, such as PONV (postoperative nausea and vomiting), over-sedation, or depression of respiration should also be anticipated, monitored, and managed.

Pain after surgery can vary in intensity and duration, but is virtually always greatest in the early perioperative period. Pain intensity decreases in the succeeding days or weeks depending not only on the type and extent of surgery but also on less predictable inter-individual factors, but can normally be expected to resolve spontaneously over time. In practical terms this implies that in the first postoperative hours and days analgesia should be given regularly, by the clock, until requirements start to fall. Analgesia can then be given 'when required' at times when pain is reported or measured, or pain is anticipated, e.g. prior to mobilization. A number of professional organizations have produced detailed and helpful guidelines on the analgesic management of postoperative pain in children. 'Good Practice in Postoperative and Procedural Pain' from the Association of Paediatric Anaesthetists of Great Britain and Ireland are comprehensive, systematically developed, evidence-based guidelines on procedure-specific analgesic strategies for postoperative pain in neonates and children (Howard et al., 2012). 'Acute Pain Management: Scientific Evidence' from the Australian and New Zealand College of Anaesthetists (Macintyre et al., 2010), and 'Practice Guidelines for Acute Pain Management in the Perioperative Setting' from the American Society of Anesthesiologists also include advice on the management of postoperative pain in children (American Society of Anesthesiologists, 2012). The paediatric anaesthesiologist is responsible for the selection and initiation of an appropriate perioperative analgesic regimen. In many institutions ongoing care is devolved to a multidisciplinary postoperative pain management service, but all providers of postoperative pain treatment should be familiar with the methods, indications, doses, and side effects of the most commonly used analgesics and analgesic techniques.

Negative effects of postoperative pain

Aside from its unpleasant and distressing qualities, poorly managed pain has negative physiological, psychological, and behavioural consequences. Changes in cardiorespiratory, gastrointestinal, endocrine, and immune function that can be prevented by effective analgesia are known to occur (see *Acute Pain Management: Scientific Evidence* (3rd edition) for an up-to-date account; Macintyre et al., 2010). Postoperative pain can delay re-mobilization and recovery from surgery and can lead to undesirable long-term effects.

Pain and injury during infancy and childhood can adversely influence pain processing mechanisms in later life, including the response to subsequent pain and injury many years later (see Walker, Chapter 3, this volume). In addition, a small proportion of children may experience persistent postsurgical pain for months or years. Predisposing factors include poorly controlled postoperative pain, extensive or repeated surgery involving nerve damage, and psychological vulnerability (Kehlet et al., 2006; Macintyre et al., 2010; Macrae, 2008). Poorly managed postoperative pain also contributes to adverse and problematic changes in children's behaviour and sleep pattern, which may be observed for prolonged periods after surgery, and cause considerable distress and disruption to family life (Karling et al., 2007; Kotiniemi et al., 1997a; Power et al., 2012).

Postoperative pain management services

Anaesthesiology-led acute pain management services were developed to improve the quality and consistency of care following surgery. Their responsibilities include: provision of education programmes for staff, provision and maintenance of specialized equipment (such as patient-controlled analgesia (PCA) pumps), and overall supervision of pain management and recognition/management of side effects or complications (Box 27.1).

Multidisciplinary institutional Pain Management Services have been established in many hospitals to fulfil this role, several models have been described; they are an essential resource to ensure the quality and consistency of care (Lloyd-Thomas and Howard, 1994; Shapiro et al., 1991; Stomberg et al., 2003). Such services have facilitated the introduction of complex and innovative infusion techniques for pain management in children including PCA, nurse-controlled analgesia (NCA), and continuous regional local anaesthesia (LA), e.g. epidural and paravertebral blocks.

Pain assessment and measurement

Effective pain assessment is central to the prevention and relief of postoperative pain (Finley et al., 2005; Howard, 2003; Taylor et al., 2008; Walter-Nicolet et al., 2010). Postoperative pain should be assessed frequently, its intensity documented, and appropriate remedial action taken when indicated. The outcome and effectiveness of pain management strategies should then be confirmed by

---

Box 27.1 Role of postoperative Pain Management Services

- ◆ Education and training
- ◆ Development and implementation of pain management protocols
- ◆ Provision of written information for children, parents, and carers
- ◆ Supervision of pain assessment practice
- ◆ Oversee safe delivery of appropriate analgesia
- ◆ Monitoring for side effects
- ◆ Quality control and audit of outcomes.

---

re-assessment; thereby establishing a cycle of evaluation and treatment that should continue throughout the postoperative period (Howard, 1997). This requires training of health care professionals in the principles of acute pain assessment and the selection and use of structured pain measurement tools that are suitable for the developmental age of the child and the context in which they are to be used. As postoperative pain management must often continue at home following discharge from hospital, parents and carers may also require guidance and instruction on the assessment of pain.

Basic principles of measurement

For pain to be measured as accurately as possible, the principles underpinning assessment at different developmental ages and in different settings must be understood. Standardized pain measurement tools use various different methods of self-report or observations to quantify pain intensity. Older children are able to use self-report scales such as the visual analogue scale (VAS) or numerical rating scale (NRS) but these methods are not accurate in children who are too young to understand such concepts and cannot be used in infants and pre-verbal or non-verbal children. In order to overcome these obstacles a variety of scales have been devised using three basic methods of measurement:

1. Self-report (e.g. using diagrams or pictures).

2. Observations of behaviour.

3. Observations of physiological parameters.

As some of these methods are relatively indirect, and not appropriate for all ages and all settings, a pain measurement tool should be scientifically 'validated' prior to its adoption for clinical use. An important consequence of this is that pain measurement tools should not generally be adapted or changed from their original validated form, as even minor adaptations can change the psychometric properties of the tool and alter its accuracy (Howard et al., 2012). Validation of pain assessment and measurement tools and detailed description of tools suitable for different ages and settings are covered in more detail elsewhere (see Brummelte et al., Chapter 38; Chorney and McMurty, Chapter 37; Lee and Stevens, Chapter 35; von Baeyer, Chapter 36, this volume).

Children's self-report of pain is the preferred approach whenever possible, and is usually feasible in children older than 5 years (Stinson et al., 2006). An observational measure should be used in conjunction with self-report with 3- to 5-year-olds because the evidence for the reliability and validity of self-report measures of pain intensity alone in this age group is quite limited, and a number of potential problems and biases have been identified when children do not fully understand the scale or the concepts underpinning it (Howard et al., 2012; von Baeyer et al., 2009a). Physiological measures, such as changes in cardiovascular or respiratory parameters are unreliable indicators of pain as they are very non-specific and therefore prone to error. Their use in clinical practice is unproven and therefore they are not recommended as a sole modality, however physiological measures are sometimes used in combination with observations of behaviour in some 'composite' pain assessment tools (Buttner and Fincke, 2000; van Dijk et al., 2001).

Measurement tools for postoperative pain

A considerable number of acute pain measurement tools exist, but despite the availability of tools they are not always used consistently or well (Broome et al., 1996; Franck and Bruce, 2009; Karling et al., 2002). An evidence-based guideline 'The Recognition and Assessment of Acute Pain in Children' that provides an evaluation of many currently available tools and advice on selecting appropriate tools has been recently revised by the UK Royal College of Nursing (RCN, 2009).

The suitability of a pain assessment tool depends on the age, cognitive level, language, ethnic/cultural background of the child, the setting for which it is to be used and the tool's psychometric properties i.e. validity, reliability, etc. (Breau and Burkitt, 2009; Mathew and Mathew, 2003; Merkel et al., 2002; Stinson et al., 2006; von Baeyer, 2006; von Baeyer and Spagrud, 2007). All such factors should be taken into consideration when making choices about which acute pain measurement tool to use.

Self-report scales suitable for postoperative pain include the linear VAS, NRS, and diagrammatic scales such as the Faces Pain Scale Revised (FPS-R; Hicks et al., 2001; von Baeyer et al., 2009b) and the Wong–Baker Faces scale (Wong and Baker, 1988). Observational scales include the Face, Legs, Activity, Cry, Consolability (FLACC) scale and the COMFORT scale (Merkel et al., 2002; van Dijk et al., 2005). For children with neurocognitive deficits or developmental delay, a small number of special pain measurement tools have been devised. Examples are the Non-communicating Children's Pain Checklist-Postoperative Version (NCCPC-PV) that is valid for 3- to 19-year-olds, and the Paediatric Pain Profile (PPP) valid for 1 to 18 years (Breau et al., 2002; Hunt et al., 2004). The FLACC scale, one of the most widely used tools in clinical practice, has also been adapted (revised FLACC) and validated for use with cognitively impaired children (Malviya et al., 2006). The Postoperative Pain Measure for Parents has been specially devised and validated for parents to assess their child's pain (Chambers et al., 1996). For postoperative pain assessment in children of normal cognitive ability, Table 27.1 shows some of the most suitable and widely used tools.

Analgesia

Analgesics and analgesic techniques are selected according to the expected intensity and duration of postoperative pain. Analgesic

Table 27.1 Measures for postoperative pain by age

Child's age[a]	Measure/tool[b]
Newborn-3 years old	COMFORT or FLACC
4 years old	FPS-R + COMFORT or FLACC
5–7 years old	FPS-R
8 years and older	VAS or NRS or FPS-R

[a]Assuming normal cognitive development.

[b]See text for explanation of tools and abbreviations.

Adapted with permission from Howard, R. F. et al., Special Issue: Good Practice in Postoperative and Procedural Pain Management, 2nd Edition, *Pediatric Anesthesia*, Volume 22, Issue Supplement s1, pp. 1–79, Copyright © 2012 Blackwell Publishing Ltd, http://onlinelibrary.wiley.com/journal/10.1111/%28ISSN%291460-9592.

requirements fall with time as pain intensity decreases, and the 'reverse pain ladder' concept is often used to provide a simple guide to treatment (Figure 27.1). Local anaesthesia combined with two or more systemic analgesics such as paracetamol, non-steroidal anti-inflammatory drug (NSAID), and an opioid are often used as part of a multimodal analgesic strategy (see later in chapter). Physical and psychological techniques, including reassurance, distraction, and hypnosis, have proven effectiveness for brief procedural pain (see Taddio, Chapter 19, this volume). Non-pharmacological techniques also have a role as a supplement to analgesic drugs in the perioperative period, by helping to allay fear and anxiety during potentially painful care such as blood sampling, placing, changing or removing nasogastric tubes, bladder catheters, chest drains, or sutures and during postoperative mobilization.

Routes of drug administration

The route of administration of a drug is an important determinant of its effectiveness. However, in the postoperative setting the number of routes may be limited (e.g. during fasting and nil oral periods), and choice of route is an important issue that requires discussion with children and their families (Seth et al., 2000). It is well known that children dislike needles, but children are sometimes

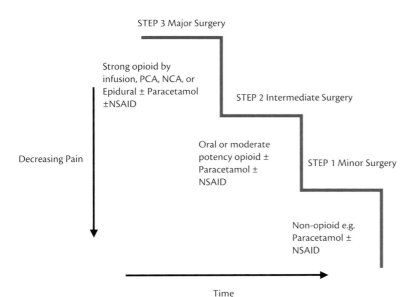

STEP 3 Major Surgery

Strong opioid by infusion, PCA, NCA, or Epidural ± Paracetamol ±NSAID

STEP 2 Intermediate Surgery

Decreasing Pain

Oral or moderate potency opioid ± Paracetamol ± NSAID

STEP 1 Minor Surgery

Non-opioid e.g. Paracetamol ± NSAID

Time

Figure 27.1 Reverse pain ladder.
Adapted with permission from the World Health Organization, original available from <http://www.who.int/cancer/palliative/painladder/en/>.

reluctant to take oral medications if they find their taste or consistency unpalatable, rectal administration may be unacceptable to some families, and children may, or may not, be willing or able to use a self-administration technique such as PCA. It is important that children's views are taken into consideration whenever possible and that their wishes and those of their families are respected when decisions are made regarding the route and method of pain relief. When available, the oral route is usually preferred above all others for its safety, simplicity, and convenience, although acceptable formulations or combinations of drugs with favourite drinks or food may be necessary for them to be tolerated. In the immediate perioperative period, and sometimes for many days later depending on the type of surgery, the oral route cannot be used and so drugs are most commonly given by the intravenous (IV) route.

An advantage of LA techniques is that they may reduce the need for analgesia during the early postoperative period when the oral route is not available. 'Single-shot' nerve blocks (see 'Multimodal analgesia' section), performed under general anaesthesia typically provide analgesia of several hours' duration, which is often sufficient for resumption of oral intake. Other options when analgesics cannot be given orally include subcutaneous, sublingual, and buccal routes. Subcutaneous opioid infusions are particularly useful when IV access is difficult or limited and must be preserved for other drugs or treatments such as chemotherapy or parenteral nutrition. In the future, novel technologies such as transcutaneous drug administration may become a viable choice in the perioperative period, but at present the available formulations are generally unsuitable.

Multimodal analgesia

Since the approach of multimodal analgesia was first suggested (Kehlet, 1997), the efficacy of combinations of analgesics and analgesic strategies have been shown in numerous studies of postoperative pain in children. However, there have been few studies with sufficient sensitivity to demonstrate the individual contribution of a single analgesic. In theory, the use of multiple analgesics that are effective on different mechanisms of nociception will increase efficacy whilst minimizing the dose, and therefore potential for adverse effects, of each drug. For example, avoiding side effects such as sedation, PONV, or respiratory depression from higher doses of opioid analgesics is clearly an important potential advantage. A recent meta-analysis of studies involving the use of NSAIDs has shown that as part of a multimodal technique they can also reduce opioid consumption and the incidence of PONV (Michelet et al., 2012). Adjuvant analgesics such as ketamine are sometimes

co-administered with opioids to improve postoperative analgesia and reduce opioid dose but supporting evidence is weak and optimum doses are not known (Dahmani et al., 2011; Elshammaa et al., 2011). Similarly, there has been recent interest in the use of preoperative gabapentin prior to potentially nerve-damaging major surgery; postoperative opioid requirements may be reduced in children but again few data are available (Rusy et al., 2010). LA blocks, such as wound infiltration and simple nerve blocks such as ilio-inguinal or penile dorsal nerve block, are relatively easy to perform and analgesia extends into the early postoperative phase following a single injection, thereby reducing the need for other analgesics. These techniques, or 'single-shot' caudal epidural block, can also be combined with non-opioid analgesics after a range of 'intermediate' surgeries at and below the inguinal region, e.g. inguinal hernia repair, orchidopexy or circumcision. For guidance on which combinations are effective for individual procedures, see evidence-based guidelines (Howard et al., 2012; Macintyre et al., 2010).

Selection of an appropriate analgesic requires specific knowledge of its developmental pharmacology; a summary for some of the most important analgesics used for postoperative pain is given here, for more detailed information see chapters where indicated.

Paracetamol and NSAIDs

Paracetamol and NSAIDs can be used singly or combined for minor surgery and at home following day surgery (see Anderson, Chapter 43, this volume, for detailed pharmacology of paracetamol and NSAIDs). As part of a multimodal analgesic regimen they are used throughout the postoperative period to supplement other techniques (see Figure 27.1).

Paracetamol (acetaminophen)

Paracetamol has been studied extensively in children, its developmental pharmacokinetic characteristics are relatively well understood, and it can be used safely in the neonatal period provided dosage guidelines are followed (Anderson and Palmer, 2006). Paracetamol is available for oral administration in syrup, tablet, and dispersible forms, can be given per rectum (but there is very wide variation in the bioavailability of rectal paracetamol) and an IV preparation of paracetamol is also available. Dosage regimens depend on the age of the child, the route of administration and the duration of treatment (Tables 27.2 and 27.3). Clearance in neonates is reduced, and the volume of distribution is increased, therefore the dose and dose interval are modified for neonates. The maximum

Table 27.2 Paracetamol dosing guide—oral and rectal administration

Age	Route	Loading dose	Maintenance dose	Interval	Maximum daily dose	Duration at maximum dose
28–32 weeks PCA	Oral	20 mg/kg	10–15 mg/kg	8–12 h	30 mg/kg	48 h
	Rectal	20 mg/kg	15 mg/kg	12 h		
32–52 weeks PCA	Oral	20 mg/kg	10–15 mg/kg	6–8 h	60 mg/kg	48 h
	Rectal	30 mg/kg	20 mg/kg	8 h		
>3 months	Oral	20 mg/kg	15 mg/kg	4 h	90 mg/kg	48 h
	Rectal	40 mg/kg	20 mg/kg	6 h		

PCA = post-conceptional age.

Table 27.3 Paracetamol dosing guide—intravenous administration

Weight (kg)	Dose	Interval	Maximum daily dose
<5 (term neonate)	7.5 mg/kg	4–6 h	30 mg/kg
5–10	10 mg/kg	4–6 h	40 mg/kg
10–50	15 mg/kg	4–6 h	60 mg/kg
>50	1 g	4–6 h	4 g

daily dose of paracetamol is limited by the potential for hepatotoxicity which can occur following overdose (single or repeated doses exceeding 150 mg/kg in total). Multiple therapeutic doses may also lead to accumulation and toxicity in children who are malnourished or dehydrated.

NSAIDs

NSAIDs are effective for the treatment of postoperative pain, used alone or in combination as part of a multimodal strategy, as they reduce opioid requirements and the combination of NSAIDs and paracetamol produces better analgesia than either drug alone (Michelet et al., 2012). A number of different NSAIDs and formulations are available and suitable for postoperative use, e.g. ibuprofen tablets and syrup, a sublingual dispersible tablet, diclofenac tablets (dispersible and enteric coated), suppositories, and parenteral formulations (Table 27.4). NSAIDs are widely available and generally considered to be safe; nevertheless it is important to understand how their mode of action can make them a potentially undesirable choice of analgesic in certain situations.

The mechanism of action of NSAIDs is via inhibition of cyclo-oxygenase (COX) activity, thereby blocking the synthesis of prostaglandins and thromboxane. Because COX is ubiquitous and responsible for many physiological regulatory activities NSAIDs have the potential to cause adverse effects, sometimes at therapeutic plasma levels:

- As NSAIDs reduce platelet aggregation and prolong bleeding time, they are contraindicated in children with coagulation disorders or in those who are receiving anticoagulant therapy and relatively contraindicated when there is a high risk of postoperative bleeding.

- NSAIDs can cause gastric irritation and gastrointestinal bleeding, and therefore are relatively contraindicated in children with a history of peptic ulcer disease. The risk of adverse gastrointestinal effects is low when NSAID use is limited to 1 to 3 days, e.g. in the postoperative period, and may be further reduced by co-prescription of proton pump inhibitors such as omeprazole, or histamine (H_2) receptor antagonists in patients at higher risk. NSAIDs can inhibit prostaglandin mediated renal function and this effect is greater in the presence of renal disease and dehydration.

- Renal toxicity is very low in healthy children, but NSAIDs should not be administered concurrently with other agents known to cause nephrotoxicity.

- NSAIDs have the potential to exacerbate asthma in a predisposed subset of NSAID-sensitive asthmatics who show cross-sensitivity with aspirin. It is estimated that 2% of asthmatic children are susceptible to aspirin induced bronchospasm, and 5% of this subgroup are likely to be cross sensitive to other NSAIDs. A history of previous uneventful NSAID exposure should be established in

Table 27.4 Dosage of NSAIDs

NSAID	Dose	Interval	Maximum daily dose
Ibuprofen	5–10 mg/kg	6–8 h	30 mg/kg
Diclofenac	1 mg/kg	8 h	3 mg/kg
Ketorolac	0.5 mg/kg	6 h	2 mg/kg
Naproxen	7.5 mg/kg	12 h	15 mg/kg
Piroxicam	0.5 mg/kg	24 h	0.5 mg/kg
Ketoprofen	1 mg/kg	6 h	4 mg/kg

asthmatic children whenever possible but there is reassuring data regarding the safety of short-term use of ibuprofen and diclofenac in asthmatic children (Lesko et al., 2002; Short et al., 2000). Nevertheless, they should be avoided in children with severe acute asthma, and are contraindicated in status asthmaticus.

- Studies in animals using high doses of ketorolac found that bone fusion was delayed: This has led to concern that the use of NSAIDs in children may delay bone healing following fracture or bony surgery. This has not been supported by human studies and the analgesic benefits of short-term NSAID use often outweigh the hypothetical risk of delayed bone healing (Howard et al., 2012).

The risks of side effects are often considered to outweigh the analgesic benefits in infants and neonates and so these drugs are rarely prescribed for pain for age less than 3 months. Attempts to reduce the undesirable effects of NSAIDs have led to the development of compounds that specifically inhibit COX-2, the COX enzyme responsible for the generation of pain and inflammation. However, these compounds have been shown to cause cardiovascular side effects in adults and have been little studied, and are little used, for postoperative pain in children (Turner and Ford, 2004).

Opioids

Opioids remain the most potent and efficacious group of systemic analgesics for postoperative pain. They can be given by many routes and are safe for all ages, provided accepted dosing regimens are used and appropriate monitoring and education of staff are in place. Morphine is the prototype opioid; diamorphine, hydromorphone, oxycodone, and tramadol, are frequent alternatives to morphine in the postoperative period, and Table 27.5 shows the relative potency to morphine. The synthetic family of opioids (fentanyl, sufentanil, alfentanil, and remifentanil) have a role after major surgery and in

Table 27.5 Relative potency of opioids

Drug	Potency relative to morphine	Single dose (oral)	Continuous infusion (IV)
Tramadol	0.1	1–2 mg/kg	100–400 mcg/kg/h
Codeine[a]/dihydrocodeine	0.1–0.12	0.5–1 mg/kg	N/A
Morphine	1	200–400 mcg/kg	10–40 mcg/kg/h
Hydromorphone	5	40–80 mcg/kg	2–8 mcg/kg/h

[a]Relative potency of codeine depends on metabolizer status—see chapter text.

intensive care practice, and can be used intraoperatively to provide analgesia reduce the stress response to surgery. The so-called moderate potency opioids, codeine and dihydrocodeine, are sometimes used for short-term treatment of postoperative pain of low intensity or in non-hospital settings. Codeine is usually not recommended for postoperative pain because it is a pro-drug, and the production of the active metabolite morphine is very variable and unpredictable, and can result in either ineffective analgesia in poor metabolizers (Williams et al., 2001) or relative overdose and toxicity in ultrarapid metabolizers (Kelly et al., 2012; see also Chau and Koren, Chapter 42, this volume). The synthetic opioid pethidine (meperidine) is not recommended for children, due to the adverse effects of its main metabolite norpethidine.

Opioids can cause a wide range of adverse effects but substantial clinical experience in their use in children means that they can be given safely for postoperative pain, provided dosage guidelines and some relatively straightforward management principles are followed. Side effects of opioids such as nausea and vomiting, sedation, and depression of respiration are usually dose related. However, their occurrence is not uniform between different opioids or even between patients taking the same drug. The incidence and severity of side effects in an individual patient are influenced by both the specific opioid, dose, route of administration, genetic, and developmental factors (see also Hathway, Chapter 44; Strassels, Chapter 45, this volume). Appropriate monitoring and adverse effect management should always be included when potent opioids are prescribed, i.e. frequent monitoring of respiratory rate and level of sedation, and prophylaxis and treatment of PONV.

Intravenous opioid analgesia, PCA, and NCA

For moderate to severe postoperative pain, especially after major surgery, continuous IV analgesia using opioids is usually indicated, with the addition of intermittent 'extra' analgesia when required for breakthrough or incident pain (Howard et al., 2012). In recent years, the techniques of PCA and NCA have also become popular, which allow for bolus administration with a lock-out period, with or without a background infusion. Some institutions have even introduced the concept of PCA-by-proxy (Anghelescu et al., 2005; Howard, 2003; Howard et al., 2010; Lloyd-Thomas and Howard, 1994; Nelson et al., 2010). Opioid infusions, including PCA and NCA, have utilized a range of opioids (e.g. morphine, fentanyl, oxycodone, tramadol) and can provide adequate titration of analgesia with an acceptable level of side effects (Morton and Errera, 2010). Some typical doses and infusion rates for PCA and NCA are given in Tables 27.6 and 27.7.

PCA has been extensively used in children as young as 5 years of age who can understand the necessary concepts, and compares favourably with continuous morphine infusion but with the added benefits of autonomy and ease of titration for patients. PCA infusion programming variables are bolus size (mg/kg), continuous infusion rate (mg/kg/h), and bolus lock-out interval (min). An important difference between PCA in young children and PCA in adults, is that it is not unusual to run a small background infusion for young patients. This is regarded as improving analgesia without compromising safety, provided there is adequate monitoring for sedation and depression of respiration (Morton and Errera, 2010).

NCA is an analgesic infusion where a nurse activates the button to provide on-demand analgesia within pre-established guidelines. NCA can provide safe and flexible analgesia for children who are too young or unable to use PCA; it has been used safely in large numbers of children (Howard et al., 2010; Lloyd-Thomas and Howard, 1994). NCA can also been used in the neonatal period but some dosing modifications have been recommended (see later section related to neonatal analgesia).

Regional analgesia

Local anaesthetics and techniques

LA is popular in the perioperative setting because it allows profound and specific analgesia at the site of surgery, often without systemic side effects. The amide LAs bupivacaine, levobupivacaine, and ropivacaine are most often used for perioperative pain, either as a single dose with a duration of action of 2 to 4 h, or by continuous infusion. The principal drawback of LA techniques is the relatively limited duration of action with single-shot intraoperative blocks, and the potential for serious side effects if recommended doses are exceeded (Table 27.8). Strategies designed to prolong the action of LA include the use of infusion catheters near peripheral nerves, into the epidural space, or elsewhere. Vasoconstrictors may be added to reduce the systemic absorption of local anaesthetic

Table 27.6 Patient-controlled analgesia doses and infusion rates

Opioid	Loading dose (mcg/kg)	Bolus (mcg/kg)	Lock-out (min)	Background (mcg/kg/h)
Morphine	50–100	10–20 (max 1mg)	5–10	0–4
Fentanyl	0.5–1.0	0. 25–0.5 (max 50 mcg.)	5–10	0–0.1
Oxycodone	50–100	10–20 (max 1mg)	5–10	0–4

Table 27.7 Nurse-controlled analgesia doses and infusion rates (not neonates)

Opioid	Loading dose (mcg/kg)	Bolus (mcg/kg)	Lock-out (min)	Background (mcg/kg/h)
Morphine	50–100	10–20 (max 1 mg)	20–30	4–10
Fentanyl	0.5–1.0	0. 25–0.5 (max 50 mcg.)	0–30	0–0.1
Oxycodone	50–100	10–20 (max 1 mg)	20–30	0–4

Table 27.8 Suggested maximum dose of bupivacaine, levobupivacaine, and ropivacaine

Single bolus injection	Maximum dosage
Neonates	2 mg/kg
Children	2.5 mg/kg

Continuous postoperative infusion	Maximum infusion rate
Neonates	0.2 mg/kg/h
Children	0.4 mg/kg/h

Table 27.9 Dose and side effects of epidural neuraxial analgesics

Drug	Single dose	Infusion	Side effects
Clonidine	1–2 mcg/kg	0.08–0.2 mcg/kg/h	Sedation; dose related hypotension and bradycardia (5 mcg/kg); delayed respiratory depression and bradycardia in neonates
Morphine	15–50 mcg/kg	0.2–0.4 mcg/kg/h	Nausea and vomiting; urinary retention; pruritis; delayed respiratory depression
Fentanyl	0.5–1 mcg/kg	0.3–0.8 mcg/kg/h	Nausea and vomiting
Tramadol	0.5–2 mg/kg		Nausea and vomiting

and to prolong their effects, and neuraxial analgesics may be been co-administered with the LA to prolong the effect of central nerve blocks (Walker and Yaksh, 2012).

LA techniques include:

- Wound infiltration (often performed intraoperatively by the surgeon).
- Peripheral nerve blocks, e.g. penile dorsal nerve block, ilio-inguinal-iliohypogastric nerve block.
- Field block such as the transversus abdominis plane (TAP) block.
- Plexus blocks, e.g. axillary brachial plexus block.
- Central neuraxial blocks such as caudal epidural block, lumbar or thoracic epidural block, and intrathecal spinal block.

Ultrasound guidance for regional blocks has become popular as it potentially allows greater accuracy in placement of LA and therefore improved safety and effectiveness (Ivani and Mossetti, 2010; Tsui and Suresh, 2010).

Continuous lumbar and thoracic epidural blocks are complex techniques whose potential complications include epidural infection or haematoma that could lead to significant permanent neurological deficit. The safety of these techniques is likely to depend on many factors including training standards and technical proficiency, the use of screening tests for coagulopathy and effective aseptic technique, and the monitoring and management of neurological signs and symptoms. Recent audits of large numbers of continuous epidural blocks have found that the overall risk of permanent neurological harm in children is less than 1:10 000 (Ecoffey et al., 2010; Llewellyn and Moriarty, 2007; Walker and Yaksh, 2012), a figure that is broadly similar to the risk of serious complications following continuous opioid infusions (Howard et al., 2010; Morton and Errera, 2010).

Neuraxial and adjuvant analgesics

Drugs that produce a specific spinally mediated analgesic effect following epidural or intrathecal administration are referred to as neuraxial analgesic drugs. Clonidine, ketamine, and opioids have been used for neuraxial analgesia (see Table 27.9 for typical doses and side effects). In combination with LA neuraxial analgesics can increase the duration of analgesia but the use of some neuraxial analgesics has declined in recent years; due to side effects in the case of opioids, and because of potential neurotoxicity for ketamine (Engelman and Marsala, 2012; Schnabel et al., 2011; Walker and Yaksh, 2012; Walker et al., 2010).

Clonidine is an α2-adrenergic agonist and has sedative, anxiolytic, and analgesic properties that can be given orally, transdermally, intravenously, or epidurally. It has an established role as a neuraxial analgesic in paediatric practice as clonidine via the intrathecal or caudal/epidural route has a greater effect than the same dose intravenously (Akin et al., 2010; Disma et al., 2011). Sensitivity to side effects of clonidine (apnoea, oxygen desaturation, and bradycardia) is greater in neonates, and cardiovascular and sedative side effects have been reported following doses of 5 mcg/kg caudal clonidine in children (Schnabel et al., 2011). Epidural clonidine 0.08 to 0.12 mcg/kg/h produces dose-dependent analgesia when added to LA infusion (De Negri et al., 2001), and higher doses of clonidine alone (0.2 mcg/kg/h preceded by bolus of 2 mcg/kg) provide analgesia at rest following abdominal surgery (Klamt et al., 2003).

Special situations

Day surgery

Most surgery in children is done on a day-stay basis. Day surgery has social advantages for children and their families, and for health care providers there are significant economic benefits. A long-recognized disadvantage is that potentially large numbers of children suffer unnecessary pain and other symptoms at home after day surgery that can last for several weeks (Kotiniemi et al., 1997b; Power et al., 2012; Wolf, 1999). Ensuring that effective pain management continues at home after day surgery is an important priority. Initiatives designed to improve the quality of care after day surgery include better information for parents about the use of analgesics and non-pharmacological pain management strategies, training in pain assessment, 'take home packs' of medication and rapid access telephone or online support systems. The quality of analgesia at home and the incidence and management of symptoms should always be closely monitored and audited.

Neonates

Neonates are a particularly vulnerable group who are also susceptible to higher rates of serious complications due to surgery and medications, including analgesics. For example, severe complications following paediatric regional analgesic techniques are rare, but the incidence is higher in neonates and infants: 0.4% versus 0.1% for all regional blocks or 1.1% versus 0.49% for epidural blocks (Walker and Yaksh, 2012). Similarly, the incidence of serious adverse events during NCA morphine analgesia, at 2.5%, was almost ten times higher in neonates (<1 month of age) compared with 0.27% in those older than 1 month (Howard et al., 2010). In addition, there may be long-term consequences to the developing nervous system as injury, pain, and analgesia have been associated with long-term changes in sensory processing systems in laboratory surgery models and in children following neonatal surgery (Fitzgerald and Walker, 2009; Peters et al., 2005; Schmelzle-Lubiecki et al., 2007; Walker et al., 2009). Drugs such as general anaesthetics and some analgesics with N-methyl-D-aspartate antagonist and/or γ-aminobutyric acid agonist activity are known to increase neuronal apoptosis (spontaneous neuronal cell death) in the developing brain in rodents and primates (Stratmann, 2011). Clearly, immaturity of organ systems renders them vulnerable to dysregulation and even permanent damage necessitating modification of analgesic drug choice and dosage regimens together with increased vigilance for adverse effects by staff with specialist training and skills.

Analgesic doses must be modified in the neonatal period as rapid and profound changes in body composition and organ function occur in the first few weeks of life. Changes in body water, fat distribution and composition, and plasma protein binding capacity alter the volume of drug distribution and other pharmacokinetic variables in neonates. Immaturity of hepatic metabolizing systems and slower renal elimination prolong the elimination time of many drugs such that doses and dose intervals must be modified. Larger inter-individual variations in the response to analgesics and their adverse effects add further unpredictability (Walker and Howard, 2004; see also Chau and Koren, Chapter 42, this volume).

Paracetamol

The pharmacokinetics of paracetamol in neonates has been relatively well studied (Allegaert et al., 2011; see also Anderson et al., 2002, Chapter 43, this volume), with recommendations for doses adjusted for age (see Tables 27.3 and 27.4). Although paracetamol is used extensively in the neonatal period the potential for overdose due to drug accumulation with repeated dosing, prescription or administration error are always present.

NSAIDs

Although this group of drugs is used for pharmacological closure of patent ductus arteriosus in premature neonates they are not generally a suitable choice for postoperative pain until after 3 months of age. Prostaglandins, inhibited by NSAIDs, have multiple regulatory roles and are especially important in early development. Increased risk of pulmonary hypertension, changes in cerebral blood flow, decreased renal function- ibuprofen has been shown to reduce glomerular filtration rate in neonates by 20%, deficient thermoregulation, and disrupted sleep cycle are just some of the increased risks anticipated with the use of these drugs in the neonatal period.

Opioids

Plasma clearance of opioids is reduced in neonates, and correlates with weight and post-conceptual age (Bouwmeester et al., 2004; Kart et al., 1997; Lynn et al., 2000). Although the plasma concentration of morphine associated with analgesia is not known, both pharmacokinetic and pharmacodynamic factors contribute to reduced dose requirements in neonates (see also Hathway, Chapter 44; and

Strassels, Chapter 45, this volume). Opioids are indicated postoperatively and are safe in neonates, provided dosage guidelines are followed with individual titration against response. The risk of respiratory depression is higher in neonates receiving postoperative NCA, particularly those with intercurrent illness or prematurity (Howard et al., 2010; Morton and Errera, 2010). Adequate training of staff and monitoring for side effects is essential, and in some centres may warrant nursing in high-dependency or intensive care settings. NCA regimens for neonates frequently utilize bolus-only administration without background infusions (Howard, 2010; Howard et al., 2010).

Local anaesthesia

LA techniques are an appealing option for the immediate perioperative period as the need for general anaesthesia and potent systemic analgesics is reduced. Nevertheless, the toxicity of LAs is also greater in neonates and so maximum recommended doses are lower, and must not be exceeded (Berde, 1993). Bupivacaine is highly protein-bound to α1-acid glycoprotein and albumin. The concentration and affinity of α1-acid glycoprotein for bupivacaine is reduced in neonates, thus increasing the proportion of free unbound drug, but during epidural infusion techniques reduced hepatic clearance of amide LA is the more important factor causing accumulation of bupivacaine than reduced protein binding capacity, particularly as protein levels tend to increase in response to surgery (Howard et al., 2012; see Table 27.9 for suggested maximum doses).

Case example: tonsillectomy pain

Adam, age 5, weight 20 kg has recurrent tonsillitis and is scheduled for adeno-tonsillectomy. The hospital he attends has an anaesthesia pre-assessment clinic, runs a programme of pre-admission visits to the hospital for children and their parents, and has an acute pain management service.

At *pre-assessment 2 weeks before surgery* Adam's health is found to be good except for mild asthma for which he takes salbutamol and beclomethasone by inhaler. The pre-assessment nurse asks if Adam has ever taken NSAIDs such as ibuprofen in the past, and his mother says that she has never given them to him because he has asthma. The nurse notes this, and mentions that it is sometimes OK to give NSAIDS to children with asthma. Adam's family are given a leaflet explaining the adeno-tonsillectomy surgery that includes discussion of postoperative pain and how it will be managed. As pain after tonsillectomy can persist for several days following discharge the need for analgesia at home, possibly for as long as 10 days, is noted. The leaflet includes a brief explanation of pain assessment procedures and an example of a self-report pain scale, using diagrams of faces.

One week prior to surgery Adam and his mother also attend the pre-admission visit where a further explanation of pain assessment takes place. A nurse instructs Adam in use of the faces pain self-report scale, and Adam's mother asks questions about what she will need to do for pain at home.

On the day of surgery the anaesthesiologist discusses the perioperative pain management plan with Adam and his mother during the pre-anaesthesia consultation. He explains that during the surgery the tonsillar fossa will be infiltrated with LA, which will be effective in the early postoperative period, but the effects will wear off after 1 or 2 h. Adam will also receive paracetamol (acetaminophen) and an opioid (fentanyl), during the surgery plus prophylactic medication for PONV. Analgesia will be given every few hours, and more will be available if needed.

Adam's mother is concerned about the potential use of NSAIDs, and the anaesthesiologist explains the risks and benefits of NSAIDS after tonsillectomy. Although risks are low, they decide not to use NSAIDs without further discussion. Adam wakes up in the post-anaesthesia care unit (PACU), feels disorientated, finds it difficult to swallow, and he is in pain. The PACU nurse administers IV morphine analgesia and Adam sleeps for a time, and then wakes up and is transferred to the ward area for the next few hours. After a while Adam's throat hurts a lot and it is difficult to swallow, and he indicates the penultimate face on the faces pain scale. He is given further paracetamol and some oral morphine, but also feels nauseous. As he continues to have pain, the nurse calls the anaesthesiologist who assesses Adam and discusses analgesic options with Adam's mother. The anaesthesiologist recommends giving a dose of ibuprofen (an NSAID) and Adam's mother agrees. About 45 min later, Adam seems much better and he is prescribed regular alternating doses of paracetamol and ibuprofen, and additional oral morphine if needed.

The next morning Adam is due to be discharged, but his mother is quite concerned about managing Adam's pain at home. A nurse explains that for 3 days she should continue to give regular medication (paracetamol and ibuprofen 'by the clock') unless any side effects occur, and thereafter to give analgesia at bedtime and according to pain assessments. Adam's mother is given written instructions and a telephone number to call if she needs further advice, and she is told that someone from the hospital will contact her the following day. After returning home Adam's mother speaks to a nurse as planned, she is asked about Adam's pain and is given advice, reassurance, and a reminder of who to contact if necessary. Adam recovers well and returns to school after a further week.

References

Akin, A., Ocalan, S., Esmaoglu, A., and Boyaci, A. 2010). The effects of caudal or intravenous clonidine on postoperative analgesia produced by caudal levobupivacaine in children. *Paediatr Anaesth*, 20, 350–355.

Allegaert, K., Palmer, G. M., and Anderson, B. J. (2011). The pharmacokinetics of intravenous paracetamol in neonates: size matters most. *Arch Dis Child*, 96, 575–580.

American Society of Anesthesiologists.(2012). Practice guidelines for acute pain management in the perioperative setting: an updated report by the American Society of Anesthesiologists Task Force on Acute Pain Management. *Anesthesiology*, 116, 248–273.

Anderson, B. and Palmer, G. (2006). Recent developments in the pharmacological management of pain in children. *Curr Opin Anaesthesiol*, 19, 285–292.

Anderson, B., Van Lingen, R., Hansen, T., Lin, Y., and Holford, N. (2002). Acetaminophen developmental pharmacokinetics in premature neonates and infants: a pooled population analysis. *Anesthesiology*, 96, 1336–1345.

Anghelescu, D. L., Burgoyne, L. L., Oakes, L. L., and Wallace, D. A. (2005). The safety of patient-controlled analgesia by proxy in pediatric oncology patients. *Anesth Analg*, 101, 1623–1627.

Berde, C. (1993). Toxicity of local anesthetics in infants and children. *J Pediatr*, 122, S14–20.

Bouwmeester, N. J., Anderson, B. J., Tibboel, D., and Holford, N. H. (2004). Developmental pharmacokinetics of morphine and its metabolites in neonates, infants and young children. *Br J Anaesth*, 92, 208–217.

Breau, L., Finley, G., McGrath, P., and Camfield, C. (2002). Validation of the Non-communicating Children's Pain Checklist-Postoperative Version. *Anesthesiology*, 96, 528–535.

Breau, L. M., and Burkitt, C. (2009). Assessing pain in children with intellectual disabilities. *Pain Res Manag*, 14, 116–120.

Broome, M. E., Richtsmeier, A., Maikler, V., and Alexander, M. (1996). Pediatric pain practices: A national survey of health professionals. *J Pain Symptom Manage*, 11, 312–320.

Buttner, W. and Fincke, W. (2000). Analysis of behavioural and physiological parameters for the assessment of postoperative analgesic demand in newborns, infants and young children. *Paediatr Anaesthe*, 10, 303–318.

Chambers, C., Reid, G., McGrath, P., and Finley, G. (1996). Development and preliminary validation of a postoperative pain measure for parents. *Pain*, 68, 307–313.

Dahmani, S., Michelet, D., Abback, P. S., Wood, C., Brasher, C., Nivoche, Y., *et al.* (2011). Ketamine for perioperative pain management in children: a meta-analysis of published studies. *Paediatr Anaesth*, 21, 636–652.

De Negri, P., Ivani, G., Visconti, C., De Vivo, P., and Lonnqvist, P. A. (2001). The dose-response relationship for clonidine added to a postoperative continuous epidural infusion of ropivacaine in children. *Anesth Analg*, 93, 71–76.

Disma, N., Frawley, G., Mameli, L., Pistorio, A., Alberighi, O. D., Montobbio, G., *et al.* (2011). Effect of epidural clonidine on minimum local anesthetic concentration (ED50) of levobupivacaine for caudal block in children. *Paediatr Anaesth*, 21, 128–135.

Ecoffey, C., Lacroix, F., Giaufre, E., Orliaguet, G., and Courreges, P. (2010). Epidemiology and morbidity of regional anesthesia in children: a follow-up one-year prospective survey of the French-Language Society of Paediatric Anaesthesiologists (ADARPEF). *Paediatr Anaesth*, 20, 1061–1069.

Elshammaa, N., Chidambaran, V., Housny, W., Thomas, J., Zhang, X., and Michael, R. (2011). Ketamine as an adjunct to fentanyl improves postoperative analgesia and hastens discharge in children following tonsillectomy—a prospective, double-blinded, randomized study. *Paediatr Anaesth*, 21, 1009–1014.

Engelman, E. and Marsala, C. (2012). Bayesian enhanced meta-analysis of post-operative analgesic efficacy of additives for caudal analgesia in children. *Acta Anaesthesiol Scand*, 56, 817–832.

Finley, G. A., Franck, L., Grunau, R., and Von Baeyer, C. L. (2005). *Why children's pain matters*, Seattle, WA: IASP.

Fitzgerald, M. and Walker, S. M. (2009). Infant pain management: a developmental neurobiological approach. *Nat Clin Pract Neurol*, 5, 35–50.

Franck, L. S., and Bruce, E. (2009). Putting pain assessment into practice: why is it so painful? *Pain Res Manag*, 14, 13–20.

Hicks, C., Von, B. C., Spafford, P., Van, K. I., and Goodenough, B. (2001). The Faces Pain Scale-Revised: toward a common metric in pediatric pain measurement. *Pain*, 93, 173–183.

Howard, R. (1997). Planning for pain relief. In S. Lindahl (ed.) *Clinical anaesthesiology: paediatric anaesthesia*, Vol. 10, pp. 65–676. London: Bailliere Tindall,

Howard, R. (2003). Current status of pain management in children. *JAMA*, 290, 2464–2469.

Howard, R., Carter, B., Curry, J., Jain, A., Liossi, C., Morton, N., *et al.* (2012). Good practice in postoperative and procedural pain management: guidelines from the Association of Paediatric Anaesthetists. *Paediatr Anaesth*, Suppl 1, 1–81.

Howard, R. F. (2010). Audits of postoperative analgesia: what have we learned and what should we do now? *Paediatr Anaesth*, 20, 117–118.

Howard, R. F., Lloyd-Thomas, A., Thomas, M., Williams, D. G., Saul, R., Bruce, E., *et al* (2010). Nurse-controlled analgesia (NCA) following major surgery in 10,000 patients in a children's hospital. *Paediatr Anaesth*, 20, 126–134.

Hunt, A., Goldman, A., Seers, K., Crichton, N., Mastroyannopoulou, K., Moffat, V., et al. (2004). Clinical validation of the paediatric pain profile. *Dev Med Child Neurol*, 46, 9–18.

Ivani, G. and Mossetti, V. (2010). Continuous central and perineural infusions for postoperative pain control in children. *Curr Opin Anaesthesiol*, 23, 637–642.

Karling, M., Renström, M., and Ljungman, G. (2002). Acute and postoperative pain in children: a Swedish nationwide survey. *Acta Paediatr*, 91, 660–666.

Karling, M., Stenlund, H., and Hagglof, B. (2007). Child behaviour after anaesthesia: associated risk factors. *Acta Paediatr*, 96, 740–747.

Kart, T., Christrup, L., and Rasmussen, M. (1997). Recommended use of morphine in neonates, infants and children based on a literature review: Part 2—clinical use. *Paediatr Anaesth*, 7, 93–101.

Kehlet, H. (1997). Multimodal approach to control postoperative pathophysiology and rehabilitation. *Br J Anaesth*, 78, 606–617.

Kehlet, H., Jensen, T., and Woolf, C. (2006). Persistent postsurgical pain: risk factors and prevention. *Lancet*, 367, 1618–1625.

Kelly, L. E., Rieder, M., Van Den Anker, J., Malkin, B., Ross, C., Neely, M. N., et al. (2012). More codeine fatalities after tonsillectomy in North American children. *Pediatrics*, 129(5), e1343–1347

Klamt, J. G., Garcia, L. V., Stocche, R. M., and Meinberg, A. C. (2003). Epidural infusion of clonidine or clonidine plus ropivacaine for postoperative analgesia in children undergoing major abdominal surgery. *J Clin Anesth*, 15, 510–514.

Kotiniemi, L., Ryhanen, P., and Moilanen, I. (1997a). Behavioural changes in children following day-case surgery: a 4-week follow-up of 551 children. *Anaesthesia*, 52, 970–976.

Kotiniemi, L., Ryhanen, P., Valanne, J., Jokela, R., Mustonen, A., and Poukkula, E. (1997b). Postoperative symptoms at home following day-case surgery in children: a multicentre survey of 551 children. *Anaesthesia*, 52, 963–969.

Llewellyn, N. and Moriarty, A. (2007). The national pediatric epidural audit. *Paediatr Anaesth*, 17, 520–533.

Lloyd-Thomas, A. and Howard, R. (1994). A pain service for children. *Paediatric Anaesthesia*, 4, 3–15.

Lynn, A., Nespeca, M., Bratton, S., and Shen, D. (2000). Intravenous morphine in postoperative infants: intermittent bolus dosing versus targeted continuous infusions. *Pain*, 88, 89–95.

Macintyre, P. E., Schug, S. A., Scott, D. A., Visser, E. J., and Walker, S. M. (2010). *APM:SE Working Group of the Australian and New Zealand College of Anaesthetists and Faculty of Pain Medicine. Acute pain management: scientific evidence* (3rd edn). Melbourne: ANZCA and FPM. Available at: <http://www.fpm.anzca.edu.au/resources/books-and-publications/publications-1/Acute%20Pain%20-%20final%20version.pdf>.

Macrae, W. A. (2008). Chronic post-surgical pain: 10 years on. *Br J Anaesth*, 101, 77–86.

Malviya, S., Voepel-Lewis, T., Burke, C., Merkel, S., and Tait, A. R. (2006). The revised FLACC observational pain tool: improved reliability and validity for pain assessment in children with cognitive impairment. *Paediatr Anaesth*, 16, 258–265.

Mathew, P. J., and Mathew, J. L. (2003). Assessment and management of pain in infants. *Postgrad Med J*, 79, 438–443.

Merkel, S. M. S., Voepel-Lewis, T., and Malviya, S. M. D. (2002). Pain Assessment in Infants and Young Children: The FLACC Scale: a behavioral tool to measure pain in young children. *AJN*, 102, 55–58.

Michelet, D., Andreu-Gallien, J., Bensalah, T., Hilly, J., Wood, C., Nivoche, Y., et al. (2012). A meta-analysis of the use of nonsteroidal antiinflammatory drugs for pediatric postoperative pain. *Anesth Analg*, 114, 393–406.

Morton, N. and Errera, A. (2010). APA national audit of pediatric opioid infusions. *Pediatr Anesth*, 20, 119–125.

Nelson, K. L., Yaster, M., Kost-Byerly, S., and Monitto, C. L. (2010). A national survey of American Pediatric Anesthesiologists: patient-controlled analgesia and other intravenous opioid therapies in pediatric acute pain management. *Anesth Analg*, 110, 754–760.

Peters, J., Schouw, R., Anand, K., Van Dijk, M., Duivenvoorden, H., and Tibboel, D. (2005). Does neonatal surgery lead to increased pain sensitivity in later childhood? *Pain*, 114, 444–454.

Power, N. M., Howard, R. F., Wade, A. M., and Franck, L. S. (2012). Pain and behaviour changes in children following surgery. *Arch Dis Child*, 97, 879–884.

Royal College of Nursing. (2009). *Clinical practice guidelines. The recognition and assessment of acute pain in children*. London: Royal College of Nursing. Available at: <www.rcn.org.uk/__data/assets/pdf_file/0004/269185/003542.pdf> (accessed 30 June 2012).

Rusy, L. M., Hainsworth, K. R., Nelson, T. J., Czarnecki, M. L., Tassone, J. C., Thometz, J. G., et al. (2010). Gabapentin use in pediatric spinal fusion patients: a randomized, double-blind, controlled trial. *Anesth Analg*, 110, 1393–1398.

Schmelzle-Lubiecki, B. M., Campbell, K. A., Howard, R. H., Franck, L., and Fitzgerald, M. (2007). Long-term consequences of early infant injury and trauma upon somatosensory processing. *Eur J Pain*, 11, 799–809.

Schnabel, A., Poepping, D. M., Kranke, P., Zahn, P. K., and Pogatzki-Zahn, E. M. (2011). Efficacy and adverse effects of ketamine as an additive for paediatric caudal anaesthesia: a quantitative systematic review of randomized controlled trials. *Br J Anaesth*, 107, 601–611.

Schnabel, A., Poepping, D. M., Pogatzki-Zahn, E. M., and Zahn, P. K. (2011). Efficacy and safety of clonidine as additive for caudal regional anesthesia: a quantitative systematic review of randomized controlled trials. *Paediatr Anaesth*, 21, 1219–1230.

Seth, N., Llewellyn, N., and Howard, R. (2000). Parental opinions regarding the route of administration of analgesic medication in children. *Paediatr Anaesth*, 10, 537–544.

Shapiro, B., Cohen, D., Covelman, K., Howe, C., and Scott, S. (1991). Experience of an interdisciplinary pediatric pain service. *Pediatrics*, 88, 1226–1232.

Stinson, J., Kavanagh, T., Yamada, J., Gill, N., and Stevens, B. (2006). Systematic review of the psychometric properties, interpretability and feasibility of self-report pain intensity measures for use in clinical trials in children and adolescents. *Pain*, 125, 143–157.

Stomberg, W. M., Lorentzen, P., Joelsson, H. K., Lindquist, H., and Halamje, H. (2003). Postoperative pain management on surgical wards-impact of database documentation of anesthesia organized services. *Pain Manage Nurs*, 4, 155–164.

Stratmann, G. (2011). Review article: neurotoxicity of anesthetic drugs in the developing brain. *Anesth Analg*, 113, 1170–1179.

Taylor, E. M., Boyer, K., and Campbell, F. A. (2008). Pain in hospitalized children: a prospective cross-sectional survey of pain prevalence, intensity, assessment and management in a Canadian pediatric teaching hospital. *Pain Res Manag*, 13, 25–32.

Tsui, B. C., and Suresh, S. (2010). Ultrasound imaging for regional anesthesia in infants, children, and adolescents: a review of current literature and its application in the practice of neuraxial blocks. *Anesthesiology*, 112, 719–728.

Turner, S. and Ford, V. (2004). Role of the selective cyclooxygenase 2 (COX-2) inhibitors in children. *Arch Dis Child Educ Pract Ed*, 89, ep46–ep49.

Van Dijk, M., De Boer, J. B., Koot, H. M., Duivenvoorden, H. J., Passchier, J., Bouwmeester, N., et al. (2001). The association between physiological and behavioral pain measures in 0-to 3-year-old infants after major surgery. *J Pain Symptom Manage*, 22, 600–609.

Van Dijk, M., Peters, J., Van Deventer, P., and Tibboel, D. (2005). The COMFORT Behavior Scale: a tool for assessing pain and sedation in infants. *Am J Nurs*, 105, 33–36.

Von Baeyer, C. and Spagrud, L. (2007). Systematic review of observational (behavioral) measures of pain for children and adolescents aged 3 to 18 years. *Pain*, 127, 140–150.

Von Baeyer, C. L. (2006). Children's self-report of pain intensity: scale selection, limitations and interpretation. *Pain Res Manage*, 11, 157–162.

Von Baeyer, C. L., Forsyth, S. J., Stanford, E. A., Watson, M., and Chambers, C. T. (2009a). Response biases in preschool children's ratings of pain in hypothetical situations. *Eur J Pain*, 13, 209–213.

Von Baeyer, C. L., Spagrud, L. J., McCormick, J. C., Choo, E., Neville, K., and Connelly, M. A. (2009b). Three new datasets supporting use of the Numerical Rating Scale (NRS-11) for children's self-reports of pain intensity. *Pain*, 143, 223–227.

Walker, S. and Howard, R. (2004). Neonatal pain. *Pain Reviews*, 9, 69–79.

Walker, S. M., Franck, L. S., Fitzgerald, M., Myles, J., Stocks, J., and Marlow, N. (2009). Long-term impact of neonatal intensive care and surgery on somatosensory perception in children born extremely preterm. *Pain*, 141, 79–87.

Walker, S. M., Westin, B. D., Deumens, R., Grafe, M., and Yaksh, T. L. (2010). Effects of intrathecal ketamine in the neonatal rat: evaluation of apoptosis and long-term functional outcome. *Anesthesiology*, 113, 147–159.

Walker, S. M., and Yaksh, T. L. (2012). Review article: neuraxial analgesia in neonates and infants: a review of clinical and preclinical strategies for the development of safety and efficacy data. *Anesth Analg*, 115, 638–662.

Walter-Nicolet, E., Annequin, D., Biran, V., Mitanchez, D., and Tourniaire, B. (2010). Pain management in newborns: from prevention to treatment. *Paediatr Drugs*, 12, 353–365.

Williams, D. G., Hatch, D. J., and Howard, R. F. (2001). Codeine phosphate in paediatric medicine. *Br J Anaesthes*, 86, 413–421.

Wolf, A. (1999). Tears at bedtime: a pitfall of extending paediatric day-case surgery without extending analgesia. *Br J Anaesth*, 82, 319–320.

Wong, D. and Baker, C. (1988). Pain in children: comparison of assessment scales. *Pediatr Nurs*, 14, 9–17.

CHAPTER 28

Pain in palliative care

Ross Drake and Renée McCulloch

Summary

Pain in palliative care for children is common and is often a result of different combinations of nociceptive (somatic and/or visceral) and neuropathic pain rather than being from a single aetiology. This pain is best addressed through a collaborative, interdisciplinary team employing a holistic approach to the child and their family. Medication, particularly opioids, has a central role in management but attempting to relieve pain without addressing the child's non-physical concerns is likely to lead to frustration. The expectation should be for exemplary control of pain bearing in mind some of the syndromes faced can be complex and may require quite sophisticated techniques to be managed appropriately including the use of surgical and anaesthetic procedures.

Introduction

Palliative care for children is the active total care of the child's body, mind, and spirit, and also involves giving support to the family. Health providers must evaluate and alleviate a child's physical, psychological, and social distress (World Health Organization (WHO), 1998) through the prevention and relief of suffering by early identification and impeccable assessment and treatment of pain (WHO, 1996).

Two aspects of this statement resonate loudly with health care professionals involved in palliative care: the reference to the multidimensional nature of assessment and management necessitating a collaborative, interdisciplinary team approach by paediatric trained professionals and the elevation of pain to a symptom requiring meticulous attention.

Pain is, arguably, the most feared symptom faced by children and their families during their palliative journey. Pain has a consistently high prevalence (Drake et al., 2003; Sirkia et al., 1998; Wolfe et al., 2000) but the ability to satisfactorily control pain can be quite variable (Sirkia et al., 1998; Wolfe et al., 2000) and changes over the final week of life (Drake et al., 2003).

A significant key to success involves effective communication just as much as choosing the right intervention. Open, honest discussion of assessment and treatment strategies provides the foundation of a trusting therapeutic relationship that, in turn, allows for dialogue about anxieties and misconceptions that can, if not addressed, hamper appropriate management.

Unfortunately, the evidence available to support therapeutic approaches to deal with children's pain during palliative care is sparse. This requires clinicians to use evidence from studies on acute pain in children and the literature of adult palliative care. This latter source demands cautious extrapolation to children, especially those with non-malignant conditions. Conditions experienced by children are quite different from adults as are the anatomy and physiology of the child and their cognitive responses to pain and pain therapies. However, even in the absence of evidence, safe and effective management can be achieved through a sensible, empirical approach centred on good observation and evaluation and an understanding of the disease process and therapeutics being used.

World Health Organization guidelines

The WHO has influenced the management of pain in children's palliative care through the publication in 1998 of a simple guideline outlining the rational stepwise approach to the management of cancer pain in children (WHO, 1998). The guidelines were effective in providing analgesia in this group (Zernikow et al., 2006). Clinically, their use was broadened to include children with non-malignant conditions although this expansion was never validated; an important factor as over half of children have a non-malignant condition (Drake et al., 2003; Feudtner et al., 2011).

In 2012 the WHO published a major review of the guidelines (WHO, 2012) with the new iteration based on the best available evidence and extended to cover persistent pain in children with medical illnesses. The analgesic ladder remains at the heart of the guidelines but the three-step ladder was reduced to two steps by removing the measure for mild to moderate pain. In effect, minor opioids are replaced with a low dose of a major opioid. The choice of analgesia is determined through 'impeccable assessment' and the point of entry established by the severity of pain.

The ladder is supported by three other 'rules' which remain unchanged to complete a logical framework for prescribing.

- By the clock—encourages the regular scheduling of analgesia to ensure a steady blood concentration and to reduce the peaks and troughs of intermittent dosing. This regular dosing should be supplemented with 'as needed' breakthrough doses for pain that may emerge.

- By the appropriate route—requires the least invasive route of administration to be used; the oral route is preferable in most circumstances.

- By the child—promotes individualized treatment according to the assessed need.

The reliance on opioids for pain management in palliative care is a distinguishing factor. However, there are occasions when children who could benefit from opioid therapy are, or their family are, unwilling to have the child take opioids. This is usually based on misconceptions about their use and the perception that opioids mark 'the beginning of the end'. These fears need to be explored and correct information provided. Unfortunately, reservations can be so powerful that a prescription for an alternative agent may be required even if it has, potentially, inferior efficacy. Simply, there is little point in prescribing the ideal drug if it is clear that the child and/or family will not comply with its administration. This makes the availability of effective alternatives (perceived to be safer) of real practical value.

Opioids are introduced once simple analgesia is no longer effective or if assessment indicates the child is having more than mild pain. The prescribing of opioids has been covered in depth by Strassels (Chapter 45, this volume), but in palliative care follows the 'by the clock' rule reaffirmed in the 2012 WHO guidelines with both continuous and 'as needed' or rescue analgesia being made available as highlighted in the following clinical case example.

Case example

A 10-year-old boy presents with relapsed, metastatic hepatoblastoma for which there are no further curative options. He has intermittent albeit frequent aching epigastric pain averaging 7/10 intensity. This equates to severe pain and an opioid in the form of oral morphine is commenced.

Initiation

An initial oral dose of 6 mg (0.2 mg/kg/dose) immediate-release morphine preparation is prescribed as a regular 4 h dose. An additional 6 mg rescue dose is advised to be taken as needed up to every hour (one-sixth of the total daily dose of 36 mg, i.e. 6 mg × 6 = 36 mg).

Titration

Day 1: the child requires 5 rescue doses (30 mg) in 24 h.

Day 2: the child requires 3 rescue doses (18 mg) in 24 h.

At the 48 h review he has averaged 4 rescue doses each day indicating the regular dose needs to be increased by 24 mg (i.e. 4 × 6 mg = 24 mg).

Regular dose: new total daily dose is 36 mg + 24 mg = 60 mg over 24 h or 10 mg every 4 h.

Breakthrough dose: remains one-sixth of total daily dose or 10 mg (60 mg ÷ 6) as needed up to every hour.

Day 3: the child requires 1 rescue dose (10mg) in 24 h.

Day 4: the child requires no rescue doses in 24 h.

At 48 h review the child has averaged less than 1 rescue dose each day indicating the regular dose does not need to be increased. The regular morphine dose can be converted to a long-acting preparation.

Regular dose: total daily dose is 60 mg or 30 mg twice daily of a slow-release morphine formulation.

Breakthrough dose: remains 10 mg of immediate-release morphine.

This example illustrates that the *titration* phase has ended and the *maintenance* phase begins. The maintenance phase starts when a reasonably stable dose of regular opioid has been reached and the total daily dose no longer needs adjustment. In reality this phase represents a period of slower titration where further increases may be required for disease-progression and, on occasion, opioid tolerance.

Continual assessment and review is required to ensure adequate analgesia is ongoing.

Challenging pain syndromes in palliative care

Episodic pain—breakthrough pain versus incident pain

Episodic pain in palliative care is usually seen in children with advanced cancer and equates to either 'breakthrough' or 'incident' pain. These are two distinct entities although the terms are often used, incorrectly, interchangeably.

Breakthrough pain has been defined as 'a transitory exacerbation of pain superimposed on a background of persistent usually well controlled pain' (Gomez-Batiste et al., 2002). The prevalence in children requiring palliative care is unknown although one study (Friedrichsdorf et al., 2006) indicated over 50% of children with cancer (n = 27) will experience one or more episodes. The solution is to adjust the dose of medication, usually an opioid, as described in the clinical case example. When the pain occurs at the end of a regular dose this is known as 'end-of-dose failure'. The remedy for this situation may simply be to increase the dose but failure (pain breakthrough) further away from the next dose may require shortening of the interval between doses. For example, consistent breakthrough pain at hour 9 of a 12 h sustained-release preparation may require 8-hourly dosing of the medication.

Incident pain refers to an intermittent or episodic, often severe, pain associated with specific events or activity such as weight bearing or coughing and escalation may be related to complications such as a pathological fracture. Management necessitates identifying, anticipating, and, if possible, avoiding the provoking factors. The requirement of any pharmacological intervention is for the medication to be immediately available, have a very rapid on- and off-set of action (Chu et al., 2008) and be highly potent. This can complicate management as analgesics are often too slow to be effective during the pain episode and cause toxicity as the agent becomes fully active when the pain naturally subsides.

The administration of parenteral short-acting opioids and nasal or buccal formulations come closest to the ideal. Interventional approaches should be contemplated especially when incident pain is unresponsive to medication. These range from simple measures such as a sling to immobilize the affected part to radiation therapy or chemotherapy to more sophisticated surgical or anaesthetic techniques.

Episodic pain—muscle spasm

Episodic pain may also reflect pain of a sporadic nature as seen with intestinal colic or muscle spasm. Muscle spasm is a potent source of significant discomfort for many children with severe neurological impairment, for example, cerebral palsy and neurodegenerative conditions, and often predates the involvement of palliative care. Management therefore requires collaboration and optimal use of non-pharmacological strategies and non-opioid medications before specific therapies needing specialist skill (i.e. surgical intervention, botulinum toxin, intrathecal drug delivery) are introduced.

Opioids should remain in consideration with anecdotal success reported by paediatric palliative care physicians in treating some children with opioids for severe chronic pain secondary to muscle spasm. A recent descriptive practice survey (Slater et al., 2010) appears to confirm the viability for using opioids in children with non-malignant conditions. However, regard must be given to the potential for children with non-malignant conditions to survive for many years and there should be regular review of the effectiveness of any opioid prescribed. Although anecdotal practice supports the use of opioid prescribing in children with non-malignant disorders, trial withdrawal of long-term opioids should be considered on a regular basis as the cause for the spasm may dissipate with time. Further information on the management of muscle spasm is available in Chapter 17 (Hickman et al., this volume).

Bone pain

Bone pain is typically a focal, deep-seated, and intense pain that a child may describe as 'boring' or 'like a drill'. The pain can start as intermittent but escalate to become constant and unremitting and may be complicated by spontaneous pain at rest and/or movement-related incident pain.

It appears to be a common symptom in children requiring palliative care and has been well documented in:

◆ Non-ambulatory children with chronic neurological conditions (Khoury and Szalay, 2007).

◆ Inherited metabolic disorders involving:

◆ primary defects of structural bone proteins—osteogenesis imperfect

◆ pathological involvement of bone from systemic disease—mucopolysaccharidosis (Rossi et al., 2011).

◆ Secondary distortion of the normal skeletal structures as an effect of systemic treatment, e.g. prolonged steroid use.

◆ Cancer-induced bone pain (CIBP) (Nathrath and Teichert von Lüttichau, 2009) from primary (Eyre et al., 2009), infiltrative bone marrow (Leeson et al., 1985), or metastatic disease or as a result of treatment (Sala and Barr, 2007).

Bone pain from chronic neurological conditions often results from low bone density for a variety of reasons and children are at an increased risk of non-traumatic fracture or fracture from minimal trauma when moved or handled (Henderson et al., 2004; Khoury and Szalay, 2007). The precise mechanism for CIBP continues to be debated with work implicating local inflammatory and neuropathic mechanisms as well as central mechanisms.

Management

The effective management of bone pain relies upon an individualized response tailored to the identified cause(s) and the child's clinical condition, life expectancy, and quality of life. As previously discussed, non-pharmacological methods and the WHO approach remain relevant.

Specific treatment involves using bisphosphonates while CIBP may require additional approaches.

Bisphosphonate therapy

There is extensive experience in bisphosphonate therapy in children with congenital and acquired forms of osteoporosis (Batch et al., 2003; Kotecha et al., 2010) with them appearing to be not only effective but safe, even with prolonged use (Bachrach et al., 2010; Henderson et al., 2002; Howe et al., 2010). In contrast use in adults has focused on treatment of painful metastatic malignant disease (Fulfaro et al., 1998) and malignant hypercalcaemia.

Bisphosphonates are analogues of inorganic pyrophosphate, a natural inhibitor for the formation of calcium phosphate crystals, and directly reduce bone resorption (Fleisch, 1998). This is achieved by

decreasing recruitment and function of osteoclasts and direct binding to hydroxyapatite crystals in bone, making it more resistant to resorption. They are available in intravenous and oral forms with second-generation aminobisphosponates like alendronate and pamidronate and third-generation agents such as ibandronate and zoledronic acid in regular use. Intravenous pamidronate has been the most frequently used agent, but intravenous clonidronate, ibandronate, alendronate, and zolendronate have all been shown to be as effective in cancer induced bone pain in adults and are often preferred as they are infused over a shorter time (15 min; Wardley et al., 2005).

Common side effects of bisphosphonate infusions include transient flu-like symptoms that occur 24 to 48 h after the first treatment but usually not in subsequent infusions and injection site reactions. The symptoms may be improved by prophylactic use of paracetamol or ibuprofen. Hypocalcaemia is an uncommon problem occurring within 72 h of infusion but this can be prevented by a daily intake of 1 to 1.5 g calcium. Renal toxicity is also a reported concern manifesting in patients with existing renal compromise.

Long-term adverse effects of osteonecrosis of the jaw (ONJ) and ocular inflammation have been reported. ONJ appears to be isolated to adults with cancer with recent studies (Baillargeon, 2011; Khan et al., 2008) concluding there was insufficient evidence to confirm a causal link between low-dose bisphosphonate use in the osteoporosis patient population and ONJ; the majority of children receive bisphosphonates for osteoporosis.

Other approaches for CIBP

Treatment of CIBP can require additional approaches such as radiotherapy to the painful site, procedures that immobilize bone particularly when associated with a fracture, and in some selected cases the use of radioisotopes and other minimally invasive techniques.

Radiotherapy

Radiotherapy plays an important role in the palliative treatment of bone metastases and remains the treatment of choice for localized disease (Falkmer et al., 2003; Hoegler, 1997; Steenland et al., 1999). This applies even to relatively radio-resistant tumours as a small reduction in the size of the lesion can have a significant modulating effect on pain. There are limited studies on the effectiveness of palliative radiotherapy in children but those that have been done are convincing (Caussa et al., 2011; Deutsch and Tersak, 2004; Gibbs et al., 2006).

The delivery of single fractions or short courses of radiotherapy are generally well tolerated by children. The acute toxicities are few and may include local erythema, pain, and itching at the site and the occurrence of nausea, vomiting, and tiredness. Revision of the child's opioid dose may be required as pain abates. Long-term toxicity is not a consideration given the child's prognosis.

Radiopharmaceuticals and interventional radioablative techniques

Radioactive bone-seeking agents are preferentially absorbed at areas of high bone turnover such as metastatic sites and are generally considered in the earlier stages of multisite disease, rather than being a last resort treatment. Several different radiopharmaceuticals are available with strontium-89 and samarium-153 approved and in common use. Evaluation in adult patients has indicated that radiopharmaceuticals are effective in reducing pain and analgesic requirements and improving quality of life. The onset of analgesia is within days to weeks and the duration of action varies according to the extent of metastatic bone disease. As such, it is not recommended in those with a life expectancy of less than approximately 4 weeks.

Different image-guided percutaneous techniques such as abla-tion, radiofrequency ionization, and cementoplasty can be used separately or in combination for palliation of symptoms in patients with primary or metastatic bone tumours. The therapeutic goal is managing pain through reduction in tumour volume, prevention and/or treatment of pathological fractures and decompression/debulking of bone tumours, specifically those protruding into the spinal canal. These treatments are gaining popularity in adult pal-liative medicine and several studies have shown success in lytic lesions refractory to conventional therapy (Belfiore et al., 2008; Thanos et al., 2008). Even newer treatment modalities such as mag-netic resonance-guided focused ultrasound (Liberman et al., 2009) have been reported to offer safe, non-invasive, and clinically effec-tive palliation of bone metastases.

Cancer pain

Cancer pain is detailed by Hickman et al. (Chapter 17, this vol-ume) and further discussion relates specifically to palliative care. Progressive cancer usually results in increasing illness burden and a myriad of complex and challenging symptoms with the evidence showing pain to be a distressing and prevalent symptom towards the end of life in children with this disease (Heath et al., 2010; Pritchard et al., 2008). In a recent study of 141 parents of children who died of cancer, more than 10% considered hastening their child's death; this was more likely if their child was in pain (Dussel et al., 2010). Anticipation and continuous planning of analgesic need is crucial to effective management particularly with the drive in many countries to provide as much care as possible outside of the hospital environment.

As disease progresses the goals of care alter to maximize qual-ity of life and minimize invasive treatments and procedures. Diagnoses regarding pain aetiology are based upon knowledge of disease pathology and clinical signs with minimal imaging and, fre-quently, the anticipation of pain or the assumption that pain must be present, particularly in the non-verbal child.

Not infrequently palliative chemotherapy may be offered in the hope of slowing disease progression and improving symptoms (Farah et al., 2011; Pui et al., 2011) but there is little solid evidence to show that it improves analgesia. There is clear data; however, that palliative radiotherapy with locally advanced disease can improve analgesic requirements, particularly when it is offered in combina-tion with other treatment modalities (Bhasker et al., 2008; Hechler et al., 2008).

Decision-making regarding palliative chemotherapy is complex. It is important to understand and acknowledge the multidimen-sional complexities surrounding these issues when considering additional treatments. One study has shown cancer-directed ther-apy at the time of death to be rated negatively by parents (Hechler et al., 2008). In contrast, a prospective study showed that parents strongly favoured aggressive treatment in the palliative phase com-pared with health professionals and ranked hope as a more impor-tant factor for making decisions about treatment (Tomlinson et al., 2011).

There is increasing experience with anaesthetic or neurosurgi-cal analgesic options, for example, epidural/intrathecal infusions or neurolytic blocks, when systemic analgesia has failed (Whyte and Lauder, 2012).

Epidural and peripheral nerve catheters can be used successfully despite typical contraindications (thrombocytopenia, fever, spinal

metastasis, vertebral fracture) and does not preclude patients from being cared for in their preferred setting (Anghelescu et al., 2010).

Polypharmacy and continual addition or increment of medica-tion, without consideration for withdrawal or efficacy of drugs, should be avoided. Of particular concern can be the phenomena of opioid-induced hypersensitivity (OIH). This may well go unrecog-nized and is significantly under reported in children in the litera-ture (Hallett and Chalkiadis, 2012; Heger et al., 1999).

OIH is most broadly defined as a state of nociceptive sensitization caused by exposure to opioids. The state is characterized by a para-doxical response whereby a person receiving opioids for the treatment of pain may become more sensitive to pain and is thought to be due to neuroplastic changes in the central and peripheral nervous system (Chu et al., 2008). It is important to note that OIH and analgesic tol-erance are two distinct pharmacological phenomena that can result in similar net effects on opioid requirements. However, increasing the dose of opioid in OIH will paradoxically aggravate the problem and worsen the patient's pain. Considerable diagnostic confidence is required to reduce the opioid consumption in a child with end-stage cancer. It is therefore recommended to rotate the opioid, potentially in combination with a N-methyl-D-aspartate (NMDA) receptor antagonist (Laulin et al., 2002; Mercadante and Arcuri, 2005; Sjøgren et al., 1994) and methadone has been reported to have efficacy in reducing high-dose OIH (Axelrod and Reville, 2007).

Cerebral irritation

Cerebral irritability is a term used to describe the clinical pres-entation of persistent, unremitting agitation and distress. In the paediatric palliative care setting it is most often associated with the non-verbal child with severe neurological impairment or the child with progressive, often neurodegenerative disorders such as adrenoleucodystrophy or AIDS encephalopathy and, occasionally, towards the end of life in children with malignancy. At the end of life most causes can be anticipated and planned for, such as hypoxia in respiratory failure or cerebral haemorrhage in bleeding disorders or brain tumours. Cerebral irritability may also be confused with an agitated delirium at the end of life although clinical management, at this stage, is very similar.

It is a commonly held belief that cerebral irritability in the neu-rologically impaired child, in the absence of new pathology, is due to an abnormal brain, and abnormal neurological processing (Klick and Hauer, 2010) and it can be difficult to know whether the child is experiencing pain. Morally and ethically, the assumption has to be that *pain is a feature of this condition* until proven otherwise.

Clinically, for most of these children behaviour deviates from their known non-distressed baseline and cerebral irritability can mimic previous pain behaviours for which a cause has been found (Breau et al., 2001; Stallard et al., 2002). Several papers have acknowledged that pain of unknown cause is often severe in chil-dren with impaired cognition (Breau et al., 2003; Hauer, 2010; Hauer et al., 2007).

The classical symptom in an infant or non-verbal child with severe neurological impairment is an unrelenting, high-pitched scream. However, a diverse range of pathologies can portray similar neurological pain-related behaviours (Figure 28.1) resulting in the child's distress. If symptoms present as an acute change in behav-iour, a full medical review may be required with appropriate inves-tigations to identify the aetiology and exclude a reversible cause. However, in the neurologically impaired child, the cause often

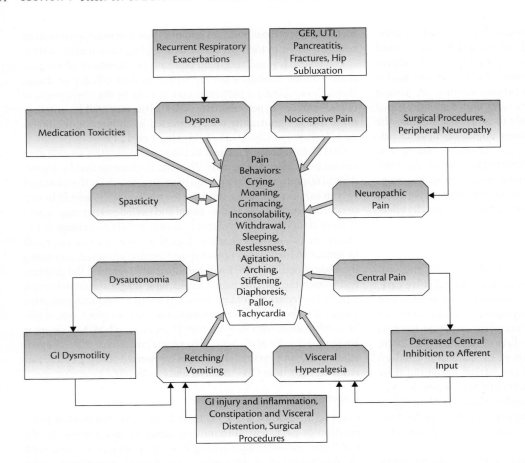

Figure 28.1 Potential sources of pain behaviour in children with severe neurological injury.
Reprinted from *Pediatric Palliative Care*, Volume 40, Issue 5, Jeffrey C. Klick and Julie Hauer, Current Problems in Pediatric and Adolescent Health Care, pp. 120–151, Copyright © 2010, with permission from Elsevier, http://www.sciencedirect.com/science/journal/15385442.

remains undefined and the behaviour frequently evolves with the condition and becomes a chronic pattern bringing about a significant burden for parents and carers with ensuing exhaustion and a sense of demoralization. Several hypotheses exist for this situation with two, central neuropathic pain and visceral hypersensitivity, well supported.

Central neuropathic pain

Central pain is a growing area of interest as improved understanding of pain pathways and processes makes it probable that it exists in infants and children with both non-malignant and malignant conditions.

Case example

A 13-year-old girl with early onset Huntingdon's chorea is persistently distressed whilst having her hair brushed or her head touched. Her parents are convinced that this response and her disordered sleeping are pain related. Examination, on multiple occasions, reveals a consistent behavioural distress to both brush and cold sensation testing over the scalp. Magnetic resonance imaging indicates bilateral lesions in the basal ganglia consistent with juvenile Huntingdon's chorea and a diagnosis of *central pain* is presumed. The girl was treated with and responded well to amitriptyline.

A recent definition suggests central neuropathic pain is 'pain arising as a direct consequence of a lesion or disease affecting the central somatosensory system' (Treede et al., 2008). It is triggered

by direct trauma or secondary damage by neurological disease or infection within the central nervous system (CNS) with disordered nociceptive processing at the molecular, cellular, and circuit level leading to system-wide changes in neuroexcitability that ultimately lead to central sensitization and an amplified pain experience (Hains and Vera-Portocarrero, 2011). Many metabolic, genetic, neurodegenerative, and neurological conditions in children could fulfil this definition by causing 'disease' or 'injury' of the CNS through diverse pathologies.

The concept of central pain was first introduced in 1891 (Edinger, 1891) and 15 years later, Dejerine and Roussy (1906) in their seminal paper 'Le Syndrome Thalamique', described a small case series of adult patients with a lesion in the thalamus and internal capsule causing 'severe, persistent, paroxysmal, often intolerable pain on the hemiplegic side not yielding to any analgesic treatment'. Central pain was hence termed 'thalamic pain' with the thalamus thought to play a key role, either as a generator of pain or by abnormal processing of ascending input (Craig et al., 1994; Wilkins and Brody, 1969). However, not all patients with a thalamic lesion suffered from pain and the spinothalamocortical pathway, important for temperature and pain sensibility, was also implicated (Boivie et al., 1989).

In adults the intensity of pain is reported to fluctuate and can be increased by internal or external stimuli such as stress or cold, and be alleviated by rest or distraction (Bowsher, 1996). Parallels can be found with infants and children with cerebral irritability as they have similar specific pain patterns, precipitating factors and they often respond well to sleep and sedation and, in some cases, distraction methods.

Strictly speaking, the newly proposed grading system to diagnose this condition requires a history suggestive of a relevant lesion, the presence of pain with a distinct sensory distribution in a corresponding body part, indication of negative or positive sensory signs within the area and confirmation of the lesion by a diagnostic test (Treede et al., 2008). Unfortunately, many children and infants with a possible diagnosis are not able to communicate making it very difficult to elicit sensory changes. However, if sensory disturbances like allodynia or dysaesthesia are consistently present then a strong indicator for central neuropathic pain is present.

The other challenge for paediatric clinicians caring for a non-verbal child with severe neurological impairment is that these children often have assorted types of pain. For instance, the complicated issue of whether spasticity is the primary cause of pain, or the result of pain from another source. Attention must be given to exploring and managing each pain type in a systematic way.

Visceral hypersensitivity

Visceral hypersensitivity or hyperalgesia is an altered response to visceral stimulation resulting in activation of pain sensation and has been regarded as a cause of functional gastrointestinal disease (Delgado-Aros and Camilleri, 2005). A recent review by Woolf reports that visceral pain hypersensitivity syndromes in the digestive system looks to have a component of central sensitization which is dynamically maintained by input from the gastrointestinal system (Woolf, 2011).

Gastrointestinal pain is commonly reported in children with severe cognitive impairment (Hauer, 2010; Hauer et al., 2007; Houlihan et al., 2004; Klick and Hauer, 2010) and chronic cerebral irritability in this group is often temporally related to gastrointestinal symptoms and signs including feed intolerance, flatus, retching, vomiting and pain. Development is thought to result from repeated painful gastrointestinal experiences in infancy; it is an outcome of sensitization not the underlying neurological injury. The consequence of these painful experiences is recruitment of previously silent nociceptors and sensitization of peripheral visceral afferent fibres causing pain (Hauer et al., 2007; Zangen et al., 2003). Such experiences might include a history of prolonged neonatal care, gastro-oesophageal reflux, constipation, gastrostomy feeding and fundoplication. Visceral pain has also been associated with motor abnormalities of the gut, exaggerated intraluminal pressures and pain sensation and an important factor in pain generation appears to be the presence of nociceptors in the gut wall that can be activated by a variety of modulators at lower, normally ineffective, intraluminal pressures (Buéno et al., 2000).

Management

Children with cerebral irritability present with their own individual narrative, symptoms, and signs. The most important step in the management is to obtain a detailed history and evaluation. In the case of chronic cerebral irritability, it may be necessary to request a symptom diary to establish temporal factors and understand the impact upon the child and family. This should be followed by the relevant investigations to exclude all other possible causes of pain and irritability. Treatment is then directed at the identified cause.

Pharmacological management directed at central neuropathic pain and visceral hypersensitivity has been poorly studied and, in adults, central neuropathic pain has been classically difficult to treat (Klit et al., 2009). Approaches with medication would usually involve a trial of adjuvant agents including tricyclic antidepressants, anticonvulsants, and NMDA receptor antagonists (Davis et al., 2009; Hauer et al., 2007; Zangen et al., 2003).

The paucity of paediatric data on this topic is striking considering the regular prescribing of anticonvulsants in paediatric practice. A single case report of a 3-month-old infant with neurological impairment and cerebral irritability detailed improvement in tone and disposition after the infant was treated with 5 mg/kg gabapentin at night following the failure of regular lorazepam and intermittent morphine to provide relief. Gabapentin was well tolerated and dose increases lead to further improvement (Behm and Kearns, 2001).

Opioids are not a first-line medication in this situation although they have been shown to improve pain in some central neuropathic pain conditions (Attal et al., 2010; Dworkin et al., 2007). They may be appropriate as a short-term control measure for acute neuropathic pain until other agents have been introduced and titrated to effect (Barrera-Chacon et al., 2011; O'Connor and Dworkin, 2009; Rowbotham et al., 2003). However, as the use of any analgesic medication for children with cerebral irritability may be necessary for a prolonged period of time the potential for long-term effects of using the medication must be given due consideration. In the case of a long-term opioid the development of tolerance or opioid-induced hyperalgesia is a concern. Despite these measures some children will have intractable symptoms and may require additional medications such as benzodiazepines, phenobarbitone, or agents such as levomepromazine and haloperidol.

Neural stimulation therapy including motor cortex stimulation (Fontaine et al., 2009), deep brain stimulation (Owen et al., 2006), and transcranial magnetic stimulation (Leung et al., 2009) have been reported to be successful in adults with treatment resistant central pain. There are no reports of any of these methods being used in children; however, the use of cortical brain stimulation is well established in children with refractory epilepsy and has a good therapeutic and safety profile.

Neuropathic pain

The cause of neuropathic pain is very dependent on the disease process and is often related to compression, direct invasion, or infection of the peripheral nerves or spinal cord and is detailed further in this volume by Walker (Chapter 21) and pharmacological treatment is described by Rastogi and Campbell (Chapter 48). In palliative care for children the mainstays of therapy involve the use of opioids and adjuvant analgesics. Although neuropathic pain is more likely than other types of pain to be partially or wholly opioid resistant (Collins et al., 1995), opioid responsiveness cannot be reliably predicted in individual patients solely on the basis of the type of pain (Cherny et al., 1994). Therefore, a trial of opioid therapy should not be withheld or limited solely on the basis of inferred pathophysiology.

Intractable pain

Palliative sedation in end of life care is an accepted but controversial means of providing relief from otherwise refractory and intolerable symptoms and distress (Chater et al., 1998; Manzini, 2011). The European Association for Palliative Care defines palliative sedation as the monitored use of medications intended to induce a state of decreased or absent awareness in order to relieve the burden of otherwise intractable suffering in an ethically acceptable manner (Cherny et al., 2009). The use of sedation in the setting of refractory pain assumes that all possible analgesic therapies have been employed and that there is no acceptable means of providing analgesia without compromising consciousness (Collins, 2010).

There is a considerable lack of information regarding palliative sedation in paediatrics; there are no international guidelines for children and little is known about the clinical effectiveness of sedation practice. A recent review of the paediatric literature offers some insight into practice by stating that sedation in children remains controversial and is influenced by educational, cultural, legal, moral, and health policy issues. Importantly, it highlighted that physical symptoms are described as an indication for practice but existential suffering must also be considered in the evaluation of refractoriness of symptoms (Kiman et al., 2011). Existential suffering of parents must also be acknowledged, as their distress behaviour may impact upon patient management and this was explored in the study by Dussell et al. (2010).

Reports of pain and suffering at the end of life are mainly described for children with end-stage cancer, but also recognized in HIV/AIDS (Bennett and Givens, 2011; Collins, 1995). Recent studies have shown that incidence may be higher than perhaps expected. A retrospective case series of children with end-stage cancer showed that 25 of 37 patients (68%) received 'palliative sedation' for unrelieved suffering, with pain being the most common symptom cited (Postovsky et al., 2007). Also, a survey (Pousset et al., 2011) of Belgian physicians signing death certificates of all children between the ages of 1 and 17 years found that continuous, deep, and persistent sedation was used in 21.8% of all deaths; 46.8% of all non-sudden deaths. Physicians had the explicit or concurrent intention of hastening death in one-quarter of cases. The incidence of continuous sedation in this study was higher than the 14.5% found in a comparable study of adults (Chambaere et al., 2010).

For the specific cohort who requires sedation for intractable pain, recommended therapeutic modalities include opioids, benzodiazepines, neuroleptic and anaesthetic agents such as propofol.

Conclusion

Managing pain is only one of the aspects of providing palliative care for children but in reality it is a core task as pain is one of the commonest symptoms experienced by dying children. It is encountered in every existential dimension and a child in severe pain cannot engage with carers in a way that allows meaningful exploration of wider fears or concerns. Even where the primary painful stimulus is physical, its perception and experience by a child will be dictated by the spiritual and psychosocial context in which it occurs. Good pain management therefore not only requires the use of appropriate analgesics but specific attention to psychosocial, cultural, spiritual, and other physical issues.

References

Anghelescu, D. L., Faughnan, L. G., Baker, J. N., Yang, J., and Kane, J. R. (2010). Use of epidural and peripheral nerve blocks at the end of life in children and young adults with cancer: the collaboration between a pain service and a palliative care service. *Paediatr Anaesth*, 20(12), 1070–1077.

Attal, N., Cruccu, G., Baron, R., Haanpää, M., Hansson, P., Jensen, T. S., *et al.* (2010). EFNS guidelines on the pharmacological treatment of neuropathic pain: 2010 revision. *Eur J Neurol*, 17(9), 1113–1123.

Axelrod, D. J., and Reville, B. (2007). Using methadone to treat opioid-induced hyperalgesia and refractory pain. *J Opioid Manage*, 3(2), 113–114.

Bachrach, S. J., Kecskemethy, H. H., Harcke, H. T., and Hossain, J. (2010). Decreased fracture incidence after 1 year of pamidronate treatment in children with spastic quadriplegic cerebral palsy. *Dev Med Child Neurol*, 52(9), 837–842.

Baillargeon, J. (2011). Osteonecrosis of the jaw in older osteoporosis patients treated with intravenous bisphosphonates. *Ann Pharmacother*, 45(10), 1199–1206.

Barrera-Chacon, J. M., Mendez-Suarez, J. L., Jáuregui-Abrisqueta, M. L., Palazon, R., Barbara-Bataller, E., and García-Obrero, I. (2011). Oxycodone improves pain control and quality of life in anticonvulsant-pretreated spinal cord-injured patients with neuropathic pain. *Spinal Cord*, 49(1), 36–42.

Batch, J. A., Couper, J. J., Rodda, C., Cowell, C. T., and Zachaarin, M. (2003). Use of bisphosphonate therapy for osteoporosis in children and adolescence. *J Paediatr Child Health*, 39, 88–92.

Behm, M. O., and Kearns, G. L. (2001). Treatment of pain with gabapentin in a neonate. *Pediatrics*, 108(2 II), 482–485.

Belfiore, G., Tedeschi, E., Ronza, F., Belfiore, M., Della Volpe, T., Zeppetella, G., *et al.* (2008). Radiofrequency ablation of bone metastases induces long-lasting palliation in patients with untreatable cancer. *Singapore Med J*, 49(7), 565–570.

Bennett, R. and Givens, D. (2011). Easing suffering for a child with intractable pain at the end of life. *J Pediatr Health Care*, 25(3), 180–185.

Bhasker, S., Bajpai, V., and Turaka, A. (2008). Palliative radiotherapy in paediatric malignancies. *Singapore Med J*, 49(12), 998–1001.

Boivie, J., Leijon, G., and Johansson, I. (1989). Central post-stroke pain. A study of the mechanisms through analyses of the sensory abnormalities. *Pain*, 37(2), 173–185.

Bowsher, D. (1996). Central pain: clinical and physiological characteristics. *J Neurol Neurosurg Psychiatry*, 61(1), 62–69.

Breau, L. M., Camfield, C., McGrath, P. J., Rosmus, C., and Finley, G. A. (2001). Measuring pain accurately in children with cognitive impairments: refinement of a caregiver scale. *J Pediatr*, 138(5), 721–727.

Breau, L. M., Camfield, C. S., McGrath, P. J., and Finley, G. A. (2003). The incidence of pain in children with severe cognitive impairments. *Arch Pediatr Adolesc Med*, 157(12), 1219–1226.

Buéno, L., Fioramonti, J., and Garcia-Villar, R. (2000). Pathobiology of visceral pain: molecular mechanisms and therapeutic implications. III Visceral afferent path-ways: a source of new therapeutic targets for abdominal pain. *Am J Physiol Gastrointest Liver Physiol*, 278(5), G670–676.

Caussa, L., Hijal, T., Michon, J., and Helfre, S. (2011). Role of palliative radiotherapy in the management of metastatic pediatric neuroblastoma: a retrospective single-institution study. *Int J Radiat Oncol*, 79(1), 214–219.

Chambaere, K., Bilsen, J., Cohen, J., Rietjens, J. A., Onwuteaka-Philipsen, B. D., Mortier, F., *et al.* (2010). Continuous deep sedation until death in Belgium: a nationwide survey. *Arch Intern Med*, 170(5), 490–493.

Chater, S., Viola, R., Paterson, J., and Jarvis, V. (1998). Sedation for intractable distress in the dying—a survey of experts. *Palliat Med*, 12(4), 255–269.

Cherny, N. I., Radbruch, L., Chasen, M., Coyle, N., Charles, D., Dean, M., *et al.* (2009). European Association for Palliative Care (EAPC) recommended framework for the use of sedation in palliative care. *Palliat Med*, 23(7), 581–593.

Cherny, N. I., Thaler, H. T., Friedlander-Klar, H., Lapin, J., Foley, K. M., Houde, R., *et al.* (1994). Opioid responsiveness of cancer pain syndromes caused by neuropathic or nociceptive mechanisms: a combined analysis of controlled, single-dose studies. *Neurology*, 44(5), 857–861.

Chu, L. F., Angst, M. S., and Clark, D. (2008). Opioid-induced hyperalgesia in humans: molecular mechanisms and clinical considerations. *Clin J Pain*, 24(6), 479–496.

Collins, J. J. (2005). Pain control options in palliative care: special considerations for children. *Am J Cancer*, 4(2), 77–85.

Collins, J. J. (2010). Symptom control in life-threatening illness in children. In G. Hanks, N. I. Cherny, N. A. Christakis, M. Fallon, S. Kaasa, and

R. K. Portenoy (eds) *Oxford textbook of palliative medicine*, pp. 1337–1347. Oxford: Oxford University Press.

Collins, J. J., Grier, H. E., Kinney, H.C., and Berde, C. B. (1995). Control of severe pain in children with terminal malignancy. *J Pediatr*, 126(4), 653–657.

Craig, A. D., Bushnell, M. C., Zhang, E. T., and Blomqvist, A. (1994). A thalamic nucleus specific for pain and temperature sensation. *Nature*, 372(6508), 770–773.

Davis, A. M., Bruce, A. S., Mangiaracina, C., Schulz, T., and Hyman, P. (2009). Moving from tube to oral feeding in medically fragile nonverbal toddlers. *J Pediatr Gastroenterol Nutr*, 49(2), 233–236.

Dejerine, J. R., and Roussy, G. (1906). Le syndrome thalamique. *Rev Neurol*, 12, 521–532.

Delgado-Aros, S. and Camilleri, M. (2005). Visceral hypersensitivity. *J Clin Gastroenterol*, 39(5 Suppl 3), S194–203.

Deutsch, M. and Tersak, J. (2004). Radiotherapy for symptomatic metastases to bone in children. *Am J Clin Oncol*, 27(2), 128–131.

Drake, R., Frost, J., and Collins, J. J. (2003). The symptoms of dying children. *J Pain Symptom Manage*, 26(1), 1–10.

Dussel, V., Joffe, S., Hilden, J. M., Watterson-Schaeffer, J., Weeks, J. C., and Wolfe, J. (2010). Considerations about hastening death among parents of children who die of cancer. *Arch Pediatr Adolesc Med*, 164(3), 231–237.

Dworkin, R. H., O'Connor, A. B., Backonja, M., Farrar, J. T., Finnerup, N. B., Jensen, T. S., et al. (2007). Pharmacologic management of neuropathic pain: evidence-based recommendations. *Pain*, 132(3), 237–251.

Edinger, L. (1891). Giebt es central antstehender schmerzen? *Dtsch Z Nervenheilk*, 1891, 1.

Eyre, R., Feltbower, R. G., Mubwandarikwa, E., Jenkinson, H., Parkes, S., Birch, J. M., et al. (2009). Incidence and survival of childhood bone cancer in northern England and the West Midlands, 1981–2002. *Br J Cancer*, 100(1), 188–193.

Falkmer, U., Jarhult, J., Wersall, P., and Cavallin-Stahl, E. (2003). A systematic overview of radiation therapy effects in skeletal metastases. *Acta Oncol*, 42(5–6), 620–633.

Farah, R. A., Nasser, S. C., Sabbagh, R. A., Dina, P. B., and Eid, T. A. (2011). Palliative tumor control by trabectedin in pediatric advanced sarcoma. *Curr Drug Ther*, 6(2), 97–99.

Feudtner, C., Kang, T. I., Hexem, K. R., Friedrichsdorf, S. J., Osenga, K., Siden, H., et al. (2011). Pediatric palliative care patients: a prospective multicenter cohort study. *Pediatrics*, 127(6), 1094–1101.

Fleisch, H. (1998). Bisphosphonates: mechanisms of action. *Endocr Rev*, 19(1), 80–100.

Fontaine, D., Hamani, C., and Lozano, A. (2009). Efficacy and safety of motor cortex stimulation for chronic neuropathic pain: critical review of the literature—Clinical article. *J Neurosurg*, 110(2), 251–256.

Friedrichsdorf, S. J., Finney, D., Bergin, M., Stevens, M., and Collins, J. J. (2006). Breakthrough pain in children with cancer. *J Pain Symptom Manage*, 34(2), 209–216.

Fulfaro, F., Casuccio, A., Ticozzi, C., and Ripamonti, C. (1998). The role of bisphosphonates in the treatment of painful metastatic bone disease: a review of phase III trials. *Pain*, 78(3), 157–169.

Gibbs, I. C., Tuamokumo, N., and Yock, T. I. (2006). Role of radiation therapy in pediatric cancer. *Hematol Oncol Clin N Am*, 20(2), 455–470.

Gomez-Batiste, X., Madrid, F., Moreno, F., Gracia, A., Trelis, J., Nabal, M., et al. (2002). Breakthrough cancer pain: prevalence and characteristics in patients in Catalonia, Spain. *J Pain Symptom Manage*, 24(1), 45–52.

Hains, B. and Vera-Portocarrero, L. P. (2011). *Animal models of central neuropathic pain*. New York: Springer.

Hallett, B. R., and Chalkiadis, G. A. (2012). Suspected opioid-induced hyperalgesia in an infant. *Br J Anaesth*, 108(1), 116–118.

Hauer, J. (2010). Identifying and managing sources of pain and distress in children with neurological impairment. *Pediatr Ann*, 39(4), 198–205.

Hauer, J. M., Wical, B. S., and Charnas, L. (2007). Gabapentin successfully manages chronic unexplained irritability in children with severe neurologic impairment. *Pediatrics*, 119(2), e519–522.

Heath, J. A., Clarke, N. E., Donath, S. M., McCarthy, M., Anderson, V. A., and Wolfe, J. (2010). Symptoms and suffering at the end of life in children with cancer: an Australian perspective. *Med J Aust*, 192(2), 71–75.

Hechler, T., Blankenburg, M., Friedrichsdorf, S. J., Garske, D., Hübner, B., Menke, A., et al. (2008). Parents' perspective on symptoms, quality of life, characteristics of death and end-of-life decisions for children dying from cancer. *Klinische Paediatrie*, 220(3), 166–174.

Heger, S., Maier, C., Otter, K., Helwig, U., and Suttorp, M. (1999). Morphine induced allodynia in a child with brain tumour. *Br Med J*, 319(7210), 627–628.

Henderson, R. C., Kairalla, J., Abbas, A., and Stevenson, R. D. (2004). Predicting low bone density in children and young adults with quadriplegic cerebral palsy. *Dev Med Child Neurol*, 46(6), 416–419.

Henderson, R. C., Lark, R. K., Kecskemethy, H. H., Miller, F., Harcke, H. T., and Bachrach, S. J. (2002). Bisphosphonates to treat osteopenia in children with quadriplegic cerebral palsy: a randomized, placebo-controlled clinical trial. *J Pediatr*, 141(5), 644–651.

Hoegler, D. (1997). Radiotherapy for palliation of symptoms in incurable cancer. *Curr Prob Cancer*, 21(3), 135–183.

Houlihan, C. M., O'Donnell, M. M., Conaway, M., and Stevenson, R. D. (2004). Bodily pain and health-related quality of life in children with cerebral palsy. *Dev Med Child Neurol*, 46(5), 305–310.

Howe, W., Davis, E., and Valentine, J. (2010). Pamidronate improves pain, wellbeing, fracture rate and bone density in 14 children and adolescents with chronic neurological conditions. *Dev Neurorehabil*, 13(1), 31–36.

Khan, A. A., Sandor, G. K.B, and Dore, E. (2008). Bisphosphonate associated osteonecrosis of the jaw. *J Rheumatol*, 36(3), 478–490.

Khoury, D. J., and Szalay, E. A. (2007). Bone mineral density correlation with fractures in nonambulatory pediatric patients. *J Pediatr Orthopaed*, 27(5), 562–566.

Kiman, R., Wuiloud, A. C., and Requena, M. L. (2011). End of life care sedation for children. *Current Opin Support Palliat Care*, 5(3), 285–290.

Klick, J. C., and Hauer, J. (2010). Pediatric palliative care. *Curr Prob Pediatr Adolescent Health Care*, 40(6), 120–151.

Klit, H., Finnerup, N. B., and Jensen, T. S. (2009). Central post-stroke pain: clinical characteristics, pathophysiology, and management. *Lancet Neurol*, 8(9), 857–868.

Kotecha, R. S., Powers, N., Lee, S. J., Murray, K. J., Carter, T., and Cole, C. (2010). Use of bisphosphonates for the treatment of osteonecrosis as a complication of therapy for childhood acute lymphoblastic leukaemia (ALL). *Pediatr Blood Cancer*, 54(7), 934–940.

Laulin, J. P., Maurette, P., Corcuff, J. B., Rivat C., Chauvin, M., and Simonnet, G. (2002). The role of ketamine in preventing fentanyl-induced hyperalgesia and subsequent acute morphine tolerance. *Anesth Analg*, 94(5), 1263–1269.

Leeson, M. C., Makley, J. T., and Carter, J. R. (1985). Metastatic skeletal disease in the pediatric population. *J Pediatr Orthop*, 5(3), 261–267.

Leung, A., Donohue, M., Xu, R., Lee, R., Lefaucheur, J. P., Khedr, E. M., et al. (2009). rTMS for suppressing neuropathic pain: a meta-analysis. *J Pain*, 10(12), 1205–1216.

Liberman, B., Gianfelice, D., Inbar, Y., Beck, A., Rabin, T., Shabshin, N., et al. (2009). Pain palliation in patients with bone metastases using MR-guided focused ultrasound surgery: a multicenter study. *Ann Surg Oncol*, 16(1), 140–146.

Manzini, J. L. (2011). Palliative sedation: ethical perspectives from Latin America in comparison with European recommendations. *Current Opin Support Palliat Care*, 5(3), 279–284.

Mercadante, S. and Arcuri, E. (2005). Hyperalgesia and opioid switching. *Am J Hospice Palliat Med*, 22(4), 291–294.

Nathrath, M. and Teichert von Lüttichau, I. (2009). Oncologic causes of bone pain. *Onkologische Ursachen von Knochenschmerzen*, 157(7), 655–660.

O'Connor, A. B., and Dworkin, R. H. (2009). Treatment of neuropathic pain: an overview of recent guidelines. *Am J Med*, 122(10 Suppl. 1), S22–32.

Owen, S. L.F, Green, A. L., Stein, J. F., and Aziz, T. Z. (2006). Deep brain stimulation for the alleviation of post-stroke neuropathic pain. *Pain*, 120(1–2), 202–206.

Postovsky, S., Moaed, B., Krivoy, E., Ofir, R., and Arush, M. W. B. (2007). Practice of palliative sedation in children with brain tumors and sarcomas at the end of life. *Pediatr Hematol Oncol*, 24(6), 409–415.

Pousset, G., Bilsen, J., Cohen, J., Mortier, F., and Deliens, L. (2011). Continuous deep sedation at the end of life of children in Flanders, Belgium. *J Pain Symptom Manage*, 41(2), 449–455.

Pritchard, M., Burghen, E., Srivastava, D. K., Okuma, J., Anderson, L., Powell, B., *et al.* (2008). Cancer-related symptoms most concerning to parents during the last week and last day of their child's life. *Pediatrics*, 121(5), e1301–1309.

Pui, C. H., Gajjar, A. J., Kane, J. R., Qaddoumi, I. A., and Pappo, A. S. (2011). Challenging issues in pediatric oncology. *Nature Rev Clin Oncol*, 8(9), 540–549.

Rossi, L., Zulian, F., Stirnemann, J., Billette de Villemur, T., and Belmatoug, N. (2011). Bone involvement as presenting sign of pediatric-onset Gaucher disease. *Joint Bone Spine*, 78(1), 70–74.

Rowbotham, M. C., Twilling, L., Davies, P. S., Reisner, L., Taylor, K., and Mohr, D. (2003). Oral opioid therapy for chronic peripheral and central neuropathic pain. *N Engl J Med*, 348(13), 1223–1232.

Sala, A. and Barr, R. D. (2007). Osteopenia and cancer in children and adolescents: the fragility of success. *Cancer*, 109(7), 1420–1431.

Sirkia, K., Hovi, L., Pouttu, J., and Saarinen-Pihkala, U. M. (1998). Pain medication during terminal care of children with cancer. *J Pain Symptom Manage*, 15, 220–226.

Sjøgren, P., Jensen, N. H., and Jensen, T. S. (1994). Disappearance of morphine-induced hyperalgesia after discontinuing or substituting morphine with other opioid agonists. *Pain*, 59(2), 313–316.

Slater, M. E., De Lima, J., Campbell, K., Lane, L., and Collins, J. (2010). Opioids for the management of severe chronic nonmalignant pain in children: a retrospective 1-year practice survey in a children's hospital. *Pain Med*, 11(2), 207–214.

Stallard, P., Williams, L., Velleman, R., Lenton, S., and McGrath, P. J. (2002). Brief report: behaviors identified by caregivers to detect pain in noncommunicating children. *J Pediatr Psychol*, 27(2), 209–214.

Steenland, E., Leer, J. W., van Houwelingen, H., Post, W. J., van den Hout, W. B., Kievit, J., *et al.* (1999). The effect of a single fraction compared to multiple fractions on painful bone metastases: a global analysis of the Dutch Bone Metastasis Study. *Radiother Oncol*, 52(2), 101–109.

Thanos, L., Mylona, S., Galani, P., Tzavoulis, D., Kalioras, V., Tanteles, S., *et al.* (2008). Radiofrequency ablation of osseous metastases for the palliation of pain. *Skeletal Radiol*, 37(3), 189–194.

Tomlinson, D., Bartels, U., Gammon, J., Hinds, P. S., Volpe, J., Bouffet, E., *et al.* (2011). Chemotherapy versus supportive care alone in pediatric palliative care for cancer: comparing the preferences of parents and health care professionals. *CMAJ*, 183(17), E1252–E1258.

Treede, R. D., Jensen, T. S., Campbell, J. N., Cruccu, G., Dostrovsky, J. O., Griffin, J. W., *et al.* (2008). Neuropathic pain: redefinition and a grading system for clinical and research purposes. *Neurology*, 70(18), 1630–1635.

Wardley, A., Davidson, N., Barrett-Lee, P., Hong, A., Mansi, J., Dodwell, D., *et al.* (2005). Zoledronic acid significantly improves pain scores and quality of life in breast cancer patients with bone metastases: a randomised, crossover study of community vs hospital bisphosphonate administration. *Br J Cancer*, 92(10), 1869–1876.

WHO. (1996). *Cancer pain relief with a guide to opioid availability* (2nd edn). Geneva: World Health Organization.

WHO. (1998). *Cancer pain relief and palliative care in children*. Geneva: World Health Organization.

WHO. (2012). *WHO guidelines on the pharmacological treatment of persisting pain in children with medical illnesses*. Geneva: World Health Organization.

Whyte, E. and Lauder, G. (2012). Intrathecal infusion of bupivacaine and clonidine provides effective analgesia in a terminally ill child. *Paediatr Anaesth*, 22(2), 173–175.

Wilkins, R. H., and Brody, I. A. (1969). The thalamic syndrome. *Arch Neurol*, 20(5), 559–562.

Wolfe, J., Grier, H. E., Klar, N., Levin, S. B., Ellenbogen, J. M., Salem-Schatz, S., *et al.* (2000). Symptoms and suffering at the end of life in children with cancer. *N Eng J Med*, 342(5), 326–333.

Woolf, C. J. (2011). Central sensitization: implications for the diagnosis and treatment of pain. *Pain*, 152(3 Suppl), S2–15.

Zangen, T., Ciarla, C., Zangen, S., Di Lorenzo, C., Flores, A. F., Cocjin, J., *et al.* (2003). Gastrointestinal motility and sensory abnormalities may contribute to food refusal in medically fragile toddlers. *J Pediatr Gastroenterol Nutr*, 37(3), 287–293.

Zernikow, B., Smale, H., Michel, E., Hasan, C., Jorch, N., and Andler, W. (2006). Paediatric cancer pain management using the WHO analgesic ladder: results of a prospective analysis from 2265 treatment days during a quality improvement study. *Eur J Pain*, 10(7), 587–595.

CHAPTER 29

Recurrent abdominal pain

Jennifer Verrill Schurman, Amanda
Drews Deacy, and Craig A. Friesen

Summary

Recurrent abdominal pain is a common complaint in children and adolescents; however, it has been historically understudied and not well understood. Recently, an improved diagnostic classification system has resulted in new research information being generated at an increasing rate. Although significant gaps in our knowledge remain, we are gradually coming to understand the complex aetiology of recurrent abdominal pain in children and are making strides in clinical treatment. However, specific clinical practice guidelines do not yet exist and evidence remains limited for most, if not all, of the common treatments employed. This chapter highlights current theory and evidence available to guide office-based assessment and intervention efforts, as well as promising directions for future research.

Introduction

Epidemiology

Recurrent abdominal pain has long been acknowledged to be one of the most common chronic pain entities in children. However, only recently has it been recognized as a global health problem. The prevalence has been estimated at 0.3% to 19% (median 8.4) in Western populations (Chitkara et al., 2005), with similar rates recently documented worldwide and including developing countries (Devanarayana et al., 2011; Zhou et al., 2011). Prevalence appears to peak in early school-age (4–6 years) and preadolescent children, with females somewhat overrepresented at older ages (Chitkara et al., 2005). Abdominal pain can persist for years with many children continuing to have problems with both abdominal pain and associated symptoms into adulthood (Gieteling et al., 2008).

History

In the late 1950s, Apley and Naish first described the entity which became known as recurrent abdominal pain of childhood or 'RAP' (Apley and Naish, 1958). RAP was described as three or more bouts of pain severe enough to affect activities that occurred over a period of at least 3 months. Less than 10% of the patients evaluated by Apley and Naish were determined to have an organic aetiology for their pain. Given the lack of diagnostics available during that time, it is likely that some children with organic disease were included under this heading. Even more important, children with a wide variety of clinical presentations and aetiologies were lumped under the single clinical 'diagnosis' of RAP. RAP was so inclusive as to be rendered useless to guide diagnosis or treatment. In recent years, there has been increasing effort to redefine RAP into more distinct groups to guide research and clinical decision-making. Continuing work began in 1990, the Rome II working group established discrete diagnostic criteria for several functional gastrointestinal disorders (FGIDs) in children (Rasquin-Weber et al., 1999). These were revised to the current Rome III diagnostic criteria in 2006 (Rasquin et al., 2006). As defined by the Rome criteria, the FGIDs are a set of diagnoses with specific symptom profiles in the absence of structural or biochemical abnormalities to explain the symptoms. FGIDs related to chronic or recurrent abdominal pain include irritable bowel syndrome (IBS), functional dyspepsia (FD), functional abdominal pain (FAP), and abdominal migraine (see Box 29.1 for symptom-based criteria). Both the American Academy of Pediatrics and the North American Society for Pediatric Gastroenterology, Hepatology, and Nutrition have supported this shift in diagnostic classification, calling for the term 'RAP' to be retired in 2005 (Di Lorenzo et al., 2005a). Although the Rome criteria have not been fully validated, there is evidence that the great majority of children who would have formerly been diagnosed with RAP meet criteria for at least one FGID, with IBS and FD being the two most common (Schurman et al., 2005; Walker et al., 2004). Although clinical experience would support the utility of Rome criteria, this utility has yet to be established in well-designed research studies. In addition, there is variability in how the Rome criteria are applied and the definition of 'organic disease' is not universal (Chogle et al., 2010). The diagnosis also can vary depending on who provides the history. For example, children and parents can vary greatly with regard to stool history (Schurman et al., 2005). While there is still work to be done to refine and validate the criteria, Rome III diagnoses represent the best available classification for children with recurrent abdominal pain and are the current basis for entry into most therapeutic trials.

Aetiology

FGIDs are probably best understood utilizing a biopsychosocial model which states that abdominal pain occurs as a result of varying contributions from, and interactions between, biological factors, psychological factors, and social factors. Each of these factors may initiate or contribute to the frequency, duration, or intensity of pain. Further, this model is dynamic; children are believed to achieve the same end result (i.e. abdominal pain) through different pathways.

Box 29.1 Rome III symptom criteria for functional gastrointestinal disorders related to abdominal pain in children

Functional dyspepsia

All of the following present at least once weekly for at least 2 months:

- Persistent or recurrent abdominal pain or discomfort centered in the upper abdomen.
- Pain not relieved by defecation or associated with a change in stool frequency or form.
- No evidence of an inflammatory, anatomic, metabolic, or neoplastic process to explain the symptoms.

Irritable bowel syndrome

All of the following present at least once weekly for at least 2 months:

- Abdominal discomfort or pain associated with two or more of the following:
  - improvement with defecation
  - onset associated with a change in stool frequency
  - onset associated with a change in stool form.
- No evidence of an inflammatory, anatomic, metabolic, or neoplastic process to explain the symptoms.

Functional abdominal pain

All of the following present at least once weekly for at least 2 months:

- Episodic or continuous abdominal pain.
- Does not meet criteria for another FGID.
- No evidence of an inflammatory, anatomic, metabolic, or neoplastic process to explain the symptoms.

Abdominal migraine

All of the following must have occurred at least twice in the preceding 12 months:

- Paroxysmal episodes of intense, acute periumbilical pain lasting at least 1 h.
- Intervening periods without pain lasting weeks to months.
- Pain which interferes with normal activities.
- Pain associated with at least two of the following:
  - anorexia
  - nausea
  - vomiting
  - headache
  - photophobia
  - pallor.
- No evidence of an inflammatory, anatomic, metabolic, or neoplastic process to explain the symptoms.

Reproduced with kind permission of the Rome Foundation, Copyright © Rome Foundation, Inc.

Biological factors

The biological factors most implicated in the generation of abdominal pain include motility disturbances, visceral hypersensitivity, and inflammation. A variety of motility disturbances have been well documented in adults with both IBS and FD. Although there are many fewer paediatric studies, the findings in children tend to parallel those in adults. IBS is associated with either rapid colonic transit typical of diarrhoea-predominant IBS (D-IBS) or delayed colonic transit typical of constipation-predominant IBS (C-IBS). However, transit is increased in only 48% of adults with D-IBS and decreased in only 20% of those with C-IBS (Camilleri and Di Lorenzo, 2012). FD has been associated with a wide array of electromechanical disturbances in adults including delayed gastric emptying, gastric electrical disturbances, impaired fundic accommodation (relaxation) with meals, and discoordinated gastroduodenal motility (Timmons et al., 2004). Delayed gastric emptying and gastric electrical disturbances have each been demonstrated in approximately 50% of children with FD (Friesen et al., 2006). Symptom severity also has been correlated with delayed emptying, gastric electrical abnormalities, impaired antral motility, and impaired accommodation in children with FD (Friesen et al., 2006; Devanarayana et al., 2008, 2012; Olafsdottir et al., 2000).

Visceral hypersensitivity is believed to be of central importance in the generation of pain in FGIDs in adults with similar, but somewhat conflicting, studies in children. In adults with IBS, increased rectal sensitivity to stretch has been reported in 21% to 95% of patients (Camilleri and Di Lorenzo, 2012). Rectal hypersensitivity has been demonstrated to have a sensitivity of 89% and a specificity of 83% in identifying children with IBS (Camilleri and Di Lorenzo, 2012). However, other studies have demonstrated much lower rates of hypersensitivity with no differences between paediatric patients with IBS and FAP. In adults with FD, visceral hypersensitivity to distension has been demonstrated in 34% to 65% of patients (Timmons et al., 2004). Hypersensitivity to acid has also been reported in adults with FD (Oshima et al., 2012). Water load volume, an indicator of visceral sensitivity, has been shown to differ between children with abdominal pain (including those specifically with FD) and controls (Anderson et al., 2008; Schurman et al., 2007).

The two main inflammatory cells which have been implicated in FGIDs are mast cells and eosinophils. In adults with IBS, mast cells are increased in the ileum and colon, are more likely to be in close proximity to nerves, and are more likely to be activated when near nerves; in addition, when near nerves, their density correlates with pain severity (Barbara et al., 2006; Park et al., 2003; Santos et al., 2005). Treatment with mast cell stabilizers has been shown to decrease the visceral hypersensitivity in IBS patients (Klooker et al., 2010). Mast cell density has been shown to be increased in the stomach of adults with FD and their activation is associated with visceral hypersensitivity (Hall et al., 2003; Hou et al., 2001). Duodenal eosinophils also have been highly implicated, with density significantly increased in adults with FD (Walker et al., 2011). Treatment directed at mucosal eosinophils has been shown to decrease pain in children with FD in association with duodenal eosinophilia (Friesen et al., 2004).

Stress response and biological factors

Stress in various forms predisposes adults to develop IBS and increases symptoms in children with FGIDs (Katiraei and Bultron, 2011; Walker et al., 2011). Anxiety and stress appear to interact with the gastrointestinal tract primarily through release of corticotrophin-releasing hormone (CRH) with secondary activation of mucosal mast cells. CRH mediates visceral sensitivity by activating mucosal mast cells with subsequent mediator sensitization of afferent sensory enteric nerves (Wood, 2004). An association has been reported between elevated rectal mast cells and anxiety in adults with IBS (Dunlop et al., 2002). Adults have demonstrated selective luminal release of tryptase and histamine from jejunal mast cells under cold stress; the magnitude of release was similar to that induced by allergen exposure in food allergic patients (Santos et al., 1998). The gastrointestinal response to stress can be mitigated by mast cell-stabilizing drugs (Moeser et al., 2007). An association between antral mast cell density and anxiety also has been demonstrated in children with FD (Schurman et al., 2010b).

Psychological factors

Children with FGIDs tend to have more concurrent symptoms of anxiety and depression than their peers (Di Lorenzo et al., 2005b). Further, early temperament markers of anxiety may predict a relative increased risk for the development of FGIDs in early school-age, while children with FGIDs appear to be at increased risk for anxiety and depression in the future (Di Lorenzo et al., 2005b; Ramchandani et al., 2006). While externalizing issues (e.g. aggression, conduct problems) may present in a subset of children with FGIDs, they are certainly far less common (Schurman et al., 2008). To date, however, there is no evidence that emotional or behavioural symptoms predict symptom severity, course, or response to treatment.

Social factors

While it is natural for parents to want to comfort their children when in pain, solicitous parenting behaviours have been found to predict prolonged illness, symptom reoccurrence, and increased disability in children with chronic medical conditions, including FGIDs (Brace et al., 2000; Walker and Zeman, 1992). Parental attention to the child's abdominal pain has been shown to increase verbal complaints in response to a water load task as compared to parental distraction; these behavioural changes were found despite children reporting similar levels of experienced pain across conditions (Walker et al., 2006). Parents of patients with FGIDs also tend to have more symptoms of anxiety and depression, as well as more physical complaints, leading to speculation that these parents may model more illness behaviour for their child, provide more attention to their child's physical symptoms, and/or bestow on the child a predisposition toward anxiety and/or gastrointestinal dysfunction (Ramchandani et al., 2006).

Other factors

While impractical to list all possible potential contributors to an individual child's abdominal pain experience, several additional areas merit specific mention. Sleep can play a major contributing role in the maintenance of chronic pain. Pain often results in increased stress and arousal that can interfere with the quality and quantity of a child's sleep, while decreased sleep quality and quantity have been found to predict increased pain the following day (Lewin and Dahl, 1999). Disrupted sleep has been found to result in increased emotional/behavioural problems that can, in turn, lower a child's pain tolerance, interfere with effective use of coping skills, and increase functional disability (Kundermann et al., 2004). Finally, adequate sleep appears to promote tissue healing, immune function, and the body's natural analgesic efforts, which can aid in both pain relief and recovery (Lewin and Dahl, 1999).

School can be very stressful for children with learning or social problems, particularly if these are not identified and treated effectively; escape from school may be very reinforcing for these children. One study found an inverse relationship between academic ability and number of visits to the school health office for physical complaints, including 'stomach ache,' such that regular education students with lower academic ability were 4.25 times more likely to visit the health office at school than students with high academic ability (Shannon et al., 2010). Similarly, in children with IBS, a stronger relationship between symptoms and disability has been documented for girls with lower perceived social competence and for boys with lower perceived athletic competence (Claar et al., 1999). More broadly, life event stress has been found to be higher in children with FGIDs, and the relationship between daily stressors and physical complaints is stronger, than in healthy control peers (Di Lorenzo et al., 2005b).

Even areas of difficulty that are clearly consequences of pain, arising secondary to pain onset, are important to consider in evaluation and treatment, as they may ultimately play a contributory role in pain maintenance and/or escalation. Functional disability is one such area. Children with frequent abdominal pain are at increased risk for social isolation and school absenteeism (Youssef et al., 2008). Children with FGIDs report quality of life lower than healthy peers and similar to that of children with inflammatory bowel disease (Youssef et al., 2006). However, recent research has highlighted the reciprocal nature of the relationship between pain and disability. While pain and disability are associated cross-sectionally, cutting back in normal daily activities on the current day appears to increase the subjective experience of pain and the likelihood of further activity cutbacks on the subsequent day (Schurman et al., 2011). Ultimately, over time, this may lead to an escalating cycle of pain and disability.

Implications for care

Evaluation

To date, no evidence-based guidelines exist for the evaluation of chronic abdominal pain, in general, or for any specific FGID related to pain in children. Currently, the presence of alarm signs and symptoms are accepted as indicators of potential organic disease and indications for further evaluations (Table 29.1). In the presence of alarm symptoms, blood tests, radiological evaluation, and endoscopy are reasonable evaluations and some recommendations are included in Table 29.1. In the absence of alarm symptoms, it is reasonable to make a diagnosis of a FGID without performing testing initially. In general, there is insufficient literature regarding the utility of any specific diagnostic tests in children with chronic abdominal pain including blood tests, ultrasound, or endoscopy (Di Lorenzo et al., 2005b). Despite the lack of studies, blood tests and endoscopy remain the most commonly performed 'standard' tests in the evaluation of dyspepsia in children in paediatric gastroenterologist practice (Schurman et al., 2010a). Ultimately, most children with chronic abdominal pain probably will not have an identified specific disease accounting for their symptoms. However, as discussed in the context of the biopsychosocial model, this does not mean that there are not biological contributors to the patient's pain. In fact, it is likely that there are biological contributors in the majority of cases and that, even in patients where symptoms are driven primarily by anxiety or stress (if we had a means to make

Table 29.1 Alarm signs and symptoms for chronic or recurrent abdominal pain with suggested initial workup

Signs/symptoms	Initial evaluation
1. Weight loss	CBC, albumin, ESR, CRP, and coeliac serology
2. Deceleration of linear growth	
3. Delayed puberty	
4. Significant vomiting	LFTs, amylase, lipase, UA, and abdominal ultrasound
5. RUQ pain/tenderness	
6. Haematemesis or haematochezia	CBC, ESR, CRP, coeliac serology, stool exam for pathogens, and endoscopy
7. RLQ pain/tenderness	
8. Chronic severe diarrhoea	
9. Perianal disease or oral lesions	
10. Systemic symptoms including unexplained fever, unexplained rash, or arthritis	
11. Family history of IBD or coeliac disease	
12. Dysphagia	Barium swallow and endoscopy

CBC = complete blood count; CRP = C-reactive protein; ESR = erythrocyte sedimentation rate; IBD= inflammatory bowel disease; LFT = liver function test; RLQ = right lower quadrant; RUQ = right upper quadrant; UA = urinalysis.

that determination), there is a biological pathway which translates the central stress response into gastrointestinal symptoms. It seems likely that, in the end, the value of testing will not be in making a diagnosis of an 'organic' disease but in identifying the biological factors (e.g. mucosal inflammation, dysmotility, and/or visceral hypersensitivity) contributing to the generation of symptoms and which might be amenable to specific treatments. This may account for recent findings that endoscopy results in a change in management in two-thirds of children with abdominal pain (Thakkar et al., 2011).

Identification of psychosocial factors that may be contributing to symptom generation, and that may be appropriate targets of treatment, also is pivotal as part of the initial clinical workup. To that end, brief self- and/or parent-report measures can be employed within a busy clinical setting to quickly screen for areas of concern and prioritize treatments as part of the initial clinical approach. Many validated questionnaires are available to assess issues common in children with FGIDs, such as psychological functioning, parent behaviour, sleep, and functional disability, among others (see supplementary material online for a list of questionnaires to consider by area). In addition, relevant information about school (e.g. attendance, perceived barriers, learning history) may be elicited quickly via a few targeted questions posed during the medical history.

Treatment

To date, no evidence-based guidelines exist for the treatment of chronic abdominal pain, in general, or for any specific FGID-related to pain in children. The current emphasis is on treating simultaneously as many of the identified biopsychosocial contributors as possible, with the belief that this provides the best opportunity to effectively break the pain cycle. In addition, the importance of early intervention cannot be overstated given the potential long-term consequences of functional disability on academic, social, and emotional development in children and adolescents. The following presents a stepped approach to care, beginning with what may be realistically accomplished within the primary care office setting, moving through referral for subspecialty collaboration, and ending with more intensive rehabilitation models for treatment.

Education and reassurance

Education is a vital foundational component of basic in-office care for children with FGIDs. Providing a clear explanation of FGIDs—including the reassuring messages that the child's pain is understood, that it is not dangerous, and that there is something that can be done about it—can be very helpful in decreasing anxiety and further healthcare seeking in both the parent and child (Di Lorenzo et al., 2005a). Further, clearly communicating the biopsychosocial nature of FGIDs helps provide a context for the multicomponent approach to treatment, thereby improving patient/family willingness to adhere to the recommended treatments and setting the stage for acceptance of later subspecialty referrals, if needed. In fact, there is some evidence that children whose parents accept a biopsychosocial conceptualization of abdominal pain and its treatment are more likely to experience symptom improvement (Scholl and Allen, 2007).

Medication

While education and reassurance are universal, medication management varies by specific FGID. However, evidence for most of the current medications in use has been obtained from studies in adults; only a small number of controlled studies in children currently exist.

In adults with IBS, tricyclic antidepressants (TCAs), selective serotonin reuptake inhibitors (SSRIs), and antispasmodics (including cimetropium/dicyclomine, peppermint oil, pinaverium, and trimebutine) targeting visceral hypersensitivity and/or dysmotility, but not bulking agents, are effective (Ford et al., 2009; Ruepert et al., 2011). There have been only two controlled paediatric trials assessing TCAs for FGIDs and no trials for SSRIs. Amitriptyline was ineffective in the larger trial which included FD, FAP, and IBS patients (Saps et al., 2009). In the other trial, which included only IBS patients, amitriptyline treatment was associated with decreased diarrhoea and pain (Bahar et al., 2008). Other than a single trial of peppermint oil, there are no controlled trials of antispasmodics in paediatric IBS (Kline et al., 2001). It appears that fibre has no significant effect on pain in children with IBS (Huertas-Ceballos et al., 2009). Antibiotics have been shown to be effective for non-constipated IBS in adults, but have not been evaluated in children (Basseri et al., 2011). Two controlled studies support the use of probiotics (*Lactobacillus rhamnosus* GG) in children with IBS (Francavilla et al., 2010; Gawrońska et al., 2007). Reasonable initial options based on the existing evidence would include daily low-dose TCAs (e.g. amitriptyline; 0.3 mg/kg given at bedtime) with antispasmodics (e.g. dicyclomine or peppermint oil) given on an as-needed basis, antibiotics directed at small bowel bacterial overgrowth (e.g. metronidazole or rifaximin), or probiotics for diarrhoea-predominant IBS and a laxative with an SSRI for constipation-predominant IBS.

Seventy-two per cent of paediatric gastroenterologists treat FD empirically (before endoscopy) with acid reduction therapy (Schurman et al., 2010a). H2 antagonists, proton pump inhibitors (PPIs), and prokinetics have been found to be superior to placebo in the treatment of FD in adults (Moayyedi et al., 2006). Only one small trial of acid suppression has been published in paediatric FD, in which famotidine was shown to be superior to placebo in global pain resolution (See et al., 2001). Prokinetics have not been evaluated for FD in children. Reasonable initial options based on the existing evidence would be an H2 antagonist or a PPI (especially if there are reflux symptoms) when pain is the predominant symptom or a prokinetic agent targeting dysmotility when pain is not the predominant symptom (e.g. more problems with nausea or bloating).

Outside of IBS and FD, there are two other controlled trials involving pain-associated FGIDs in children. Cyproheptadine was found to improve intensity and frequency of pain in children with FAP (Sadeghian et al., 2008). Pizotifen, which is not approved in the US, has been demonstrated to have efficacy in the treatment of abdominal migraine (Symon and Russell, 1995). Frequently prescribed medications for abdominal migraine include propranolol, cyproheptadine, and sumatriptan though these have not been evaluated in controlled trials in children.

Regardless of FGID, inflammation with eosinophils and/or mast cells represents a potential therapeutic target. Inflammation may be documented (e.g. duodenal eosinophils in FD) or suspected based on clinical profile (e.g. mast cells in an anxious D-IBS patient). Montelukast has been shown to be effective in children with FD in association with duodenal eosinophilia (Friesen et al., 2004). Other options targeting eosinophils and mast cells include combination of H1 and H2 antagonists (e.g. ranitidine and hydroxyzine) and oral cromolyn as a mast cell-stabilizing agent (Friesen et al., 2006; Stefanini et al., 1995).

Behavioural coaching

Parental education and skills training is a critical component of in-office care of chronic abdominal pain patients. Parents can be coached to maintain behavioural expectations for their child's participation in school and other activities (Scholl and Allen, 2007). Participating in normal daily activities, even when in pain, gives children a sense of control over the pain; as children feel more in control, anxiety (and the associated stress response) often will decrease. It is important to note that while some form of daily activity is critical to long-term health and recovery, overdoing it can complicate and prolong the symptom course. Emphasis should be placed on preventing further declines in functioning and on gradually and systematically increasing daily expectations from whatever point the child is currently. Parents should be taught to encourage and model good coping with pain symptoms (Scholl and Allen, 2007). Parents can gently remind and encourage children to use skills like deep breathing, distraction, relaxation, positive thinking, etc. during pain episodes, or before events that seem to trigger pain (e.g. eating, going to school, having a test). Parents can be encouraged to provide attention and praise (or other rewards) for children's demonstration of good coping and/or well behaviours (e.g. using relaxation, attending a portion of the school day), and to ignore and minimize attention paid to symptom complaints and non-verbal pain behaviours (Crushell et al., 2003). Related to this, providers can reassure parents that it is okay, and indeed preferable, not to regularly inquire about their child's pain. Pain is worse when children pay attention to it and better if they are distracted from it

(see supplementary material online for a handout covering a variety of behavioural coaching points).

School accommodation

Many children with chronic abdominal pain have school problems. They may miss school days (or even weeks) because of symptoms, doctors' visits, or hospitalizations. They also may get behind in daily school work, have a hard time paying attention in class, suffer social embarrassment related to frequent trips to the toilet, or feel overwhelmed by makeup work. Accommodations that can be helpful in terms of supporting patients' success at school and encouraging their regular attendance include: allowing easy access to the toilet, encouraging brief breaks for use of stress and pain management skills, allowing participation in clubs and sports while working on getting back to school, and carefully considering makeup work and the timeline for its completion. Helping families initiate a formal plan according to local regulations (e.g. Section 504 Plan in the US, Educational Statement in the UK) for a patient's health issues can be beneficial to formalize these accommodations and encourage consistent participation across all school staff. Additionally, when children have been out of school for a long period of time due to their abdominal pain and/or other physical symptoms, a gradual and structured return to the classroom may be an important part of the treatment plan. Approaching return to school in this fashion has the advantage of reducing patients' fear and avoidance, while reintegrating patients into age-appropriate academic/social activities and redirecting attention from symptoms toward functioning (Walker, 2004; Walker et al., 2009). Balancing demands with support is vitally important, as stress can increase pain and have an overall negative effect on the recovery process. Although variations on a graduated approach to school re-entry likely exist, the three key steps include: (1) choosing a block of time the patient is able to attend every day without increased symptoms, (2) the patient attending school for the agreed upon amount of time (no more, no less), regardless of pain, and (3) regularly evaluating the patient's progress to determine when and how much additional class time to add (see supplementary material online for a sample approach).

Collaboration with ancillary services

For a subset of children, in-office care will be insufficient to resolve the child's pain and/or disability. When this occurs, it may be helpful to refer the child for additional subspecialty treatment as part of the comprehensive treatment package. Maintenance of regular follow-up in the primary care office is vital, as is close collaboration with any subspecialty providers involved to ensure ongoing coordination of care and consistency of messages to the family. Some of these subspecialty services have an evidence base to support their use in children with FGIDs, while others are based on more theoretical or practical concerns.

The three ancillary services with the most, albeit still limited, empirical support are cognitive-behavioural therapy, hypnotherapy, and biofeedback-assisted relaxation training (BART; Brent et al., 2008). All three services, as applied to FGIDs, focus on changing thoughts and/or behaviours in the interest of alleviating physical symptoms. While these services also may help with subclinical anxiety, they primarily target pain management and behavioural activation; they are not geared to address major mental health disorders. When referring out for these services, it may be helpful to communicate expectations directly to the collaborating provider prior to, or at the onset, of care. Often, children with FGIDs do not have a diagnosable mental health disorder. As such, community providers without specific paediatric or health psychology training may not be certain of their role in the treatment plan and/or may not be experienced enough to know how to initiate treatment.

Certainly, when more substantial mental health issues are apparent, referral for individual therapy, psychiatry, and/or family therapy may be helpful. Even if these issues have arisen secondary to the onset of pain, mental health issues can be a significant source of emotional and social stress that may play a further contributory role in maintenance of pain and disability. Similarly, psychoeducational evaluation of learning issues may be helpful for a subset of children who have a history of academic performance concerns. More subtle learning issues may not be diagnosed until later in elementary school or beyond, as workload demands increase and exceed the individual's ability to compensate.

In some cases, in which children have been physically inactive for a prolonged period of time, or are resistant to increasing physical activity and engagement, a brief course of physical therapy may be beneficial to increase muscle tone, flexibility, and/or stamina. A home exercise plan based on the child's current level of physical conditioning and the desired activity goal (e.g. walking around the school building without difficulty, return to competitive sports) can be helpful in structuring the child's physical rehabilitation, as well as providing parents with tangible daily expectations that may be built into the behavioural contingency plan. Other alternative treatments, such as therapeutic massage and acupuncture, also may be beneficial in a subset of children with FGIDs to promote pain relief and recovery of function. Again, referral for many of these treatments will be based purely on practical concerns related to a given child, including the perceived acceptability of one treatment versus another, as the evidence base remains quite limited.

Intensive outpatient/inpatient rehabilitation

In the event that coordinated outpatient treatment as already described is not sufficient—that is, a child continues to experience significant pain symptoms and, more importantly, continues to suffer precipitous declines in his or her functioning—a higher level of treatment may be needed. Intensive day treatment or inpatient pain rehabilitation programmes may represent a useful model of care in these cases. Such programmes typically utilize all of the modalities previously described, albeit in a more structured, controlled environment to help patients and their parents to 'walk the walk' in real time and in the context of a supportive, therapeutic environment. The ultimate goal for these patients is to return to their homes, schools, and friends and transition back to their outpatient care team for monitoring and building upon gains made.

Unfortunately, only a few, uncontrolled studies have examined the effectiveness of such programmes. Results from three prospective studies of two different 3-week multidisciplinary inpatient programmes for paediatric chronic pain suggested improvements in pain intensity, pain-related disability, and school attendance, as well as in patients' emotional distress and pain-related coping (Eccleston et al., 2003; Hechler et al., 2009, 2010). A recent retrospective review of an inpatient paediatric pain treatment programme also documented improvements in school status, sleep, functional disability, physical mobility, and medication usage after a mean stay of 27 days (Maynard et al., 2010). While these results are encouraging and point to the possibility of inpatient treatment as a unique and effective treatment choice for children severely disabled by chronic pain, controlled treatment studies of intensive day treatment or inpatient pain rehabilitation remain sorely needed to justify the significant cost of these programmes.

Conclusion

With the current absence of specific clinical practice guidelines for assessment and treatment of paediatric recurrent abdominal pain, or FGIDs more specifically, the best available approach is one consistent with the widely accepted biopsychosocial model. Emphasis on early identification and treatment of all factors (i.e. biological, psychological, and social) that may be playing a contributory role in pain maintenance will provide the best opportunity for effective intervention and prevention of long-term issues. Additional research in this area—with particular emphasis on using current diagnostic classification systems to define samples, employing rigorous methodologies for execution of clinical trials, and attempting to identify the most powerful or necessary components of multicomponent treatment packages—will be necessary to improve the quality and consistency of care provided to this paediatric pain population.

Case example

Tyler, an 11-year-old boy, was evaluated for a 2-year history of daily abdominal pain, with associated complaints of nausea, bloating, and early satiety. His clinical history was positive for asthma, seasonal allergies, attention deficit hyperactivity disorder, and significant problems with sleep duration and quality. Tyler was being home-schooled and missed extracurricular/social activities several times per week due to pain. Past medical history included evaluation by a gastroenterologist and a naturopathic practitioner, with extensive laboratory testing plus upper and lower endoscopy. Review of Tyler's previous workup revealed normal lab findings, but increased duodenal eosinophil counts on endoscopic biopsies. He had been tried on multiple medications and followed a restricted diet without significant symptom relief.

Tyler's evaluation and initial treatment took place over a period of approximately 4 months. A few of the components considered pivotal in Tyler's treatment are highlighted here. Tyler was diagnosed with FD using the Rome III criteria. In addition to antihistamines and montelukast, he was prescribed oral cromolyn four times daily to address the identified inflammatory component of his abdominal pain. Tyler also was referred to a certified biofeedback practitioner near his home. He attended BART sessions three times per week initially and practised the skills several times per day at home. Tyler's family utilized a structured plan for graduated school re-entry, starting by attending one consistent class period daily and gradually adding time to his in-school schedule as stamina increased. During this process, Tyler also received instruction from a homebound teacher in the classes he was not yet attending. As specific classes were added to his in-school schedule, support for these classes was dropped from homebound and the amount of homebound instruction was reduced. Accommodations also were put in place that allowed Tyler to take breaks for BART practice and to use the toilet, as needed, during the school day.

Routine in-office follow-up continued on a regular basis to monitor progress, provide behavioural coaching, support continued engagement in treatment components, and modify the plan as needed. After 1 month of treatment, Tyler reported that BART was extremely helpful to him in terms of helping to manage his pain. After 4 months of treatment, Tyler reported having abdominal pain about once per week. His appetite, sleep, energy, and headaches also were improved. Within approximately 8 weeks of beginning graduated school re-entry, Tyler was attending school full time and participating in social activities with his peers.

It is important to convey the fact that Tyler's recovery was not perfectly linear, nor has it ended. Although not yet substantiated in the literature, clinical experience has suggested that eosinophilic inflammation within the gastrointestinal tract is especially sensitive to viral illnesses, seasonal allergies, and stress. Consistent with this, Tyler evidenced temporary symptom flares at predictable times during his treatment. While certainly disappointing for Tyler and his family, these setbacks provide important clues for preventing, or at least managing, flares when they occur. Proper hand washing to reduce transmission of viruses, aggressive treatment of seasonal allergies, and advance planning to reduce stress can be helpful in reducing the odds of a temporary increase in gastrointestinal inflammation and associated symptoms. Identifying and addressing potential triggers for future episodes can be an important part of long-term maintenance for an individual child.

References

Anderson, J. L., Acra, S., Bruehl, S., and Walker, L. S. (2008). Relation between clinical symptoms and experimental visceral hypersensitivity in pediatric patients with functional abdominal pain. *J Pediatr Gastroenterol Nutr*, 47, 309–315.

Apley, J. and Naish, N. (1958). Recurrent abdominal pain: a field survey of 1,000 school children. *Arch Dis Child*, 33, 165–170.

Bahar, R. J., Collins, B. S., Steinmetz, B., and Ament, M. E. (2008). Double-blind placebo-controlled trial of amitriptyline for the treatment of irritable bowel in adolescents. *J Pediatr*, 152, 685–689.

Barbara, G., Stanghellini, V., De Giorgio, R., and Corinaldesi, R. (2006). Functional gastrointestinal disorders and mast cells: implications for therapy. *Neurogastroenterol Motil*, 18, 6–17.

Basseri, R. J., Weitsman, S., Barlow, G. M., and Pimintel, M. (2011). Antibiotics for the treatment of irritable bowel syndrome. *J Gastroenterol Hepatol*, 7, 455–493.

Brace, M. J., Smith, M. S., McCauley, E., and Sherry, D. D. (2000). Family reinforcement of illness behavior: a comparison of adolescents with chronic fatigue syndrome, juvenile arthritis, and healthy controls. *J Dev Behav Pediatr*, 21, 332–339.

Brent, M., Lobato, D., and LeLeiko, N. (2008). Psychological treatmetns for pediatric functional gastrointestinal disorders. *J Pediatr Gastroneterol Nutr*, 48, 13–21.

Camilleri, M. and Di Lorenzo, C. (2012). The brain-gut axis: from basic understanding to treatment of irritable bowel syndrome and related disorders. *J Pediatr Gastroenterol Nutr*, 54(4), 446–453.

Chitkara, D. K., Rawt, D. J., and Talley, N. J. (2005). The epidemiology of childhood recurrent abdominal pain in Western countries: a systematic review. *Am J Gastroenterol*, 100, 1868–1875.

Chogle, A., Dhroove, G., Sztainberg, M., Di Lorenzo, C., and Saps, M. (2010). How reliable are the Rome III criteria for the assessment of functional gastrointestinal disorders in children? *Am J Gastroenterol*, 105, 2697–2701.

Claar, R. L., Walker, L. S., and Smith, C. A. (1999). Functional disability in adolescents and young adults with symptoms of irritable bowel syndrome: the role of academic, social, and athletic competence. *J Pediatr Psychol*, 24, 271–280.

Crushell, E., Rowland, M., Doherty, M., Gormally, S., Harty, S., and Bourke, B. E. (2003). Importance of parental conceptual model of illness in severe recurrent abdominal pain. *Pediatrics*, 1368–1372.

Devanarayana, N. M., De Silva, D. G. H., and De Silva, H. J. (2008). Gastric myoelectrical and motor abnormalities in children and adolescents with functional recurrent abdominal pain. *J Gastroenterol Hepatol*, 23, 1672–1677.

Devanarayana, N. M., Mettananda, S., Liyanarachchi, C., Nanayakkara, N., Perera, N., and Rajindrajith, S. (2011). Abdominal pain-predominant functional gastrointestinal diseases in children and adolescents: prevalence, symptomatology, and association with emotional stress. *J Pediatr Gastroenterol Nutr*, 53, 659–665.

Devanarayana, N. M., Rajindrajith, S., Rathnamalala, N., Samaraweera, S., and Benninga, M. A. (2012). Delayed gastric emptying rates and impaired antral motility in children fulfilling Rome III criteria for functional abdominal pain. *Neurogastroenterol Motil*, 24(5), 420–425.

Di Lorenzo, C., Colletti, R. B., Lehmann, H. P., Boyle, J. T., Gerson, W. T., Hyams, J. S., et al. (2005a). Chronic abdominal pain in children: a clinical report of the American Academy of Pediatrics and the North American Society for Pediatric Gastroenterology, Hepatology, and Nutrition. *J Pediatr Gastroenterol Nutr*, 40, 245–248.

Di Lorenzo, C., Colletti, R. B., Lehmann, H. P., Boyle, J. T., Gerson, W. T., Hyams, J. S., et al. (2005b). Chronic abdominal pain in children: a technical report of the American Academy of Pediatrics and the North American Society for Pediatric Gastroenterology, Hepatology, and Nutrition. *J Pediatr Gastroenterol Nutr*, 40, 249–261.

Dunlop, S. P., Jenkins, D., and Spiller, R. C. (2002). Elevated mast cells in rectal mucosa of IBS patients are associated with increased stress. *Neurogastroenterol Motil*, 14, 567–568.

Eccleston, C., Malleson, P., Clinch, J., Connell, H., and Sourbut, C. (2003). Chronic pain in adolescents: evaluation of a programme of interdisciplinary cognitive behaviour therapy. *Arch Dis Child*, 881–885.

Ford, A. C., Talley, N. J., Schoenfeld, P. S., Quigley, E. M., and Moayyedi, P. (2009). Efficacy of antidepressants and psychological therapies in irritable bowel syndrome: systematic review and meta-analysis. *Gut*, 58, 367–378.

Francavilla, R., Miniello, V., Magistà, A. M., De Canio, A., Bucci, N., Gagliardi, F., et al. (2010). A randomized controlled trial of Lactobacillus GG in children with functional abdominal pain. *Pediatrics*, 126, e1445–1452.

Friesen, C. A., Kearns, G. L., Andre, L., Neustrom, M., Roberts, C. C., and Abdel-Rahman, S. M. (2004). Clinical efficacy and pharmacokinetics of montelukast in dyspeptic children with duodenal eosinophilia. *J Pediatr Gastroenterol Nutr*, 38, 343–351.

Friesen, C. A., Lin, Z., Hyman, P., Andre, L., Welchert, E., Schurman, J. V., et al. (2006). Electrogastrography in pediatric functional dyspepsia: relationship to gastric emptying and symptom severity. *J Pediatr Gastroenterol Nutr*, 42, 265–269.

Friesen, C. A., Sandridge, L., Andre, L., Roberts, C. C., and Abdel-Rahman, S. M. (2006). Mucosal eosinophilia and response to H1/H2 antagonist and cromolyn therapy in pediatric dyspepsia. *Clinical Pediatrics*, 45, 143–147.

Gawrońska, A., Dziechciarz, P., Horvath, A., and Szajewska, H. (2007). A randomized double-blind placebo-controlled trial of Lactobacillus GG for abdominal pain disorders in children. *Aliment Pharmacol Ther*, 25, 177–184.

Gieteling, M. J., Bierma-Zeinstra, S. M., Passchier, J., and Berger, M. Y. (2008). Prognosis of chronic or recurrent abdominal pain in children. *J Pediatr Gastroenterol Nutr*, 47, 316–326.

Hall, W., Buckley, M., Crotty, P., and O'Morain, C. A. (2003). Gastric mucosal mast cells are increased in Helicobacter pylori-negative functional dyspepsia. *Clin Gastroenterol Hepatol*, 1, 363–369.

Hechler, T., Blankenburg, M., Dobe, M., Kosfelder, J., Hubner, B., and Zernikow, B. (2010). Effectiveness of a multimodal inpatient treatment for pediatric chronic pain: A comparison between children and adolescents. *Eur J Pain*, 97.e1–97.e9.

Hechler, T., Dobe, M., Kosfelder, J., Damschen, U., Hubner, B., Blankenburg, M., *et al.* (2009). Effectiveness of a 3-week multimodal inpatient pain treatment for adolescents suffering from chronic pain: Statistical and clinical significance. *Clin J Pain*, 156–166.

Hou, X.-H., Zhu, L.-R., Li, Q.-X., and Chen, J. D. (2001). Alterations in mast cells and 5-HT positive cells in gastric mucosa in functional dyspepsia patients with hypersensitivity. *Neurogastroenterol Motil*, 13, 398.

Huertas-Ceballos, A. A., Logan, S., Bennett, C., and Macarthur, C. (2009). Dietary interventions for recurrent abdominal pain (RAP) and irritable bowel syndrome (IBS) in childhood. *Cochrane Database Syst Rev*, 1, CD003019.

Katiraei, P., and Bultron, G. (2011). Need for a comprehensive medical approach to the neuro-immuno-gastroenterology of irritable bowel syndrome. *World J Gastroenterol*, 17, 2791–2800.

Kline, R. M., Kline, J. J., Di Palma, J., and Barbero, G. J. (2001). Enteric-coated, pH-dependent peppermint oil capsules for the treatment of irritable bowel syndrome in children. *J Pediatr*, 138, 125–128.

Klooker, T. K., Braak, B., Koopman, K. E., Welting, O., Wouters, M. M., van der Heide, S., *et al.* (2010). The mast cell stabilizer ketotifen decreases visceral hypersensitivity and improves intestinal symptoms in patients with irritable bowel syndrome. *Gut*, 59, 1213–1221.

Kundermann, B., Krieg, J.-C., Schrieber, W., and Lautenbacher, S. (2004). The effect of sleep deprivation on pain. *Pain Res Manag*, 9, 25–32.

Lewin, D. S., and Dahl, R. E. (1999). Importance of sleep in the management of pediatric pain. *J Dev Behav Pediatr*, 20, 244–252.

Maynard, C., Amari, A., Wiecorek, B., Christensen, J., and Slifer, K. (2010). Interdisciplinary behavioral rehabilitation of pediatric pain-associated disability: Retrospective review of an inpatient treatment protocol. *J Pediatr Psychol*, 128–137.

Moayyedi, P., Soo, S., Deeks, J., Delaney, B., Innes, M., and Forman, D. (2006). Pharmacological interventions for non-ulcer dyspepsia. *Cochrane Database Syst Rev*, 18, CD001960.

Moeser, A. J., Ryan, K. A., Nighot, P. K., and Blikslager, A. T. (2007). Gastrointestinal dysfunction induced by early weaning is attenuated by delayed weaning and mast cell blockade in pigs. *Am J Physiol—Gastrointest Liver Physiol*, 293, G413–G421.

Olafsdottir, E., Gilja, O. H., Aslaksen, A., Berstad, A., and Fluge, G. (2000). Impaired accommodation of the proximal stomach in children with recurrent abdominal pain. *J Pediatr Gastroenterol Nutr*, 30, 157–163.

Oshima, T., Okugawa, T., Tomita, T., Sakurai, J., Toyoshima, F., Watari, J., *et al.* (2012). Generation of dyspeptic symptoms by direct acid and water infusion into the stomachs of functional dyspepsia patients and healthy subjects. *Aliment Pharmacol Ther*, 35, 175–182.

Park, C. H., Joo, Y. E., Choi, S. K., Rew, J. S., Kim, S. J., and Lee, M. C. (2003). Activated mast cells infiltrate in close proximity to enteric nerves in diarrhea-predominant irritable bowel syndrome. *J Korean Med Sci*, 18, 204–210.

Ramchandani, P. G., Stein, A., Hotopf, M., and Wiles, N. J. (2006). Early parental and child predictors of recurrent abdominal pain at school age: results of a large populatino-based study. *J Am Acad Child Adolesc Psychiatry*, 45, 729–736.

Rasquin, A., Di Lorenzo, C. F., Guiralde, S., Hyams, J. S., Staiano, A., and Walker, L. S. (2006). Childhood functional gastrointestinal disorders: child/adolescent. *Gastroenterology*, 130, 1527–1537.

Rasquin-Weber, A., Hyman, P. E., Cucchiara, S., Fleisher, D. R., Hyams, J. S., Milla, P. J., *et al.* (1999). Childhood functional gastrointestinal disorders. *Gut*, 45 (Suppl II), II60–II68.

Ruepert, L., Quartero, A. O., de Wit, N. J., van der Heijden, G. J., Rubin, G., and Muris, J. W. (2011). Bulking agents, antispasmodics, and antidepressants for the treatment of irritable bowel syndrome. *Cochrane Database Syst Rev*, 8, CD003460.

Sadeghian, M., Farahmand, F., Fallahi, G. H., and Abbasi, A. (2008). Cyproheptadine for the treatment of functional abdominal pain in childhood: a double-blind randomized placebo-controlled trial. *Minerva Pediatr*, 60, 1367–1374.

Santos, J., Guilarte, M., Alonso, C., and Malagelada, J. R. (2005). Pathogenesis of irritable bowel syndrome: the mast cell connection. *Scand J Gastroenterol*, 40, 129–140.

Santos, J., Saperas, E., Nogueiras, C., Mourelle, M., Antolin, M., Cadahia, A., *et al.* (1998). Release of mast cell mediators into the jejunum by cold stress in humans. *Gastroenterology*, 114, 640–648.

Saps, M., Youssef, N., Miranda, A., Nurko, S., Hyman, P., Cocjin, J., *et al.* (2009). Multicenter, randomized, placebo-controlled trial of amitriptyline in children with functional gastrointestinal disorders. *Gastroenterology*, 137, 1261–1269.

Scholl, J., and Allen, P. (2007). A primary care approach to functional abdominal pain. *Pediatr Nurs*, 247–259.

Schurman, J. V., Connelly, M., Cushing, C. C., Wallace, D. P., and Drews, A. A. (2011, April). Multilevel modeling analysis of daily pain diary data: predictors of pain and functional impairment. Poster presented at the Society of Pediatric Psychology National Conference on Child Health Psychology. San Antonio, TX.

Schurman, J. V., Danda, C. E., Friesen, C. A., Hyman, P. E., Simon, S. D., and Cocjin, J. T. (2008). Variations in psychological profile among children with recurrent abdominal pain. *J Clin Psychol Med Sett*, 15, 241–251.

Schurman, J. V., Friesen, C. A., Andre, L., Welchert, E., Lavenbarg, T., Danda, C. E., *et al.* (2007). Diagnostic utility of the water load test in children with chronic abdominal pain. *J Pediatr Gastroenterol Nutr*, 44, 51–57.

Schurman, J. V., Friesen, C. A., Danda, C. E., Andre, L., Welchert, E., Lavenbarg, T., *et al.* (2005). Diagnosing functional abdominal pain with Rome II criteria: parent, child, and clinician agreement. *J Pediatr Gastroenterol Nutr*, 41, 291–295.

Schurman, J. V., Hunter, H. L., and Friesen, C. A. (2010a). Conceptualization and treatment of chronic abdominal pain in pediatric gastroenterology practice. *J Pediatr Gastroenterol Nutr*, 50, 32–37.

Schurman, J. V., Singh, M., Singh, V., Neilan, N., and Friesen, C. A. (2010b). Symptoms and subtypes in pediatric functional dyspepsia: relation to mucosal inflammation and psychological functioning. *J Pediatr Gastroenterol Nutr*, 51, 298–303.

See, M. C., Birnbaum, A. H., Schechter, C. B., Goldenberg, M. M., and Benkov, K. J. (2001). Double-blind, placebo-controlled trial of famotidine in children with abdominal pain and dyspepsia: global and quantitative assessment. *Digest Dis Sci*, 46, 985–992.

Shannon, R. A., Bergren, M. D., and Matthews, A. (2010). Frequent visitors: somatization in school-age children and implications for school nurses. *J School Nurs*, 26, 169–182.

Stefanini, G. F., Saggioro, A., Alvisi, V., Angelini, G., Capurso, L., di Lorenzo, G., *et al.* (1995). Oral cromolyn sodium in comparison to elimination diet in the irritable bowel syndrome, diarrheic type: multicenter study of 428 patients. *Scand J Gastroenterol*, 30, 535–541.

Symon, D. N., and Russell, G. (1995). Double-blind placebo-controlled trial of pizotifen syrup in the treatment of abdominal migraine. *Arch Dis Child*, 72, 48–50.

Thakkar, K., Dorsey, F., and Gilger, M. A. (2011). Impact of endoscopy on management of chronic abdominal pain in children. *Digest Dis Sci*, 56, 488–493.

Timmons, S., Liston, R., and Moriarty, K. J. (2004). Functional dyspepsia: motor abnormalities, sensory dysfunction, and therapeutic options. *Am J Gastroenterol*, 99, 739–749.

Walker, L. S. (2004). Helping the child with recurrent abdominal pain return to school. *Pediatr Ann*, 128–136.

Walker, L. S., and Zeman, J. L. (1992). Parental response to child illness behavior. *J Pediatr Psychol*, 17, 49–71.

Walker, L. S., Lipani, T. A., Greene, J. W., Caines, K., Stutts, J., Polk, D. B., *et al.* (2004). Recurrent abdominal pain: Symptom subtypes based on the Rome II criteria for pediatric functional gastrointestinal disorders. *J Pediatr Gastroenterol Nutr*, 38, 187–191.

Walker, L. S., Williams, S. E., Smith, C. A., Garber, J., Van Slyke, D. A., and Lipani, T. A. (2006). Parent attention versus distraction: impact on symptom complaints by children with and without chronic functional abdominal pain. *Pain*, 122, 43–52.

Walker, L., Beck, J., and Anderson, J. (2009). Functional abdominal pain and separation anxiety: Helping the child return to school. *Pediatr Ann*, 38, 267–271.

Walker, M. M., Warwick, A., Ung, C., and Talley, N. J. (2011). The role of eosinophils and mast cells in intestinal functional disease. *Curr Gastroenterol Rep*, 13, 323–330.

Wood, J. D. (2004). Enteric neuroimmunophysiology and pathophysiology. *Gastroenterology*, 127, 635–637.

Youssef, N. N., Atienza, K., Langseder, A. L., and Strauss, R. S. (2008). Chronic abdominal pain and depressive symptoms: analysis of the national longitudinal study of adolescent health. *Clin Gastroenterol Hepatol*, 6, 329–332.

Youssef, N. N., Murphy, T. G., Langseder, A. L., and Rosh, J. R. (2006). Quality of life for children with functional abdominal pain: a comparison study of patients' and parents perceptions. *Pediatrics*, 117, 54–59.

Zhou, H., Yao, M., Cheng, G., Chen, Y., and Li, D. (2011). Prevalence and associated factors of functional gastrointestinal disorders and bowel habits in Chinese adolescents; a school-based study. *J Pediatr Gastroneterol Nutr*, 53, 168–173.

CHAPTER 30

Chronic pelvic pain in children and adolescents

Susan L. Sager and Marc R. Laufer

Summary

Pain due to pelvic pathology in children and adolescents is often described as abdominal pain, and frequently coexists with gastrointestinal symptoms due to neuronal cross talk and viscero-viscero or viscero-somatic convergence of sensory afferents. Dysmenorrhea is highly prevalent among adolescents yet is underreported. Like many chronic conditions where repetitive noxious stimuli are present, dysmenorrhea can be associated with central sensitization of pain pathways and visceral hyperalgesia. In this chapter the components of a menstrual history, the importance of obtaining a menstrual history in adolescents with abdominopelvic pain, and the indications for referral to an adolescent gynaecologist are discussed. Endometriosis should be considered in the differential diagnosis of all females with chronic abdominopelvic pain of undetermined aetiology once the benchmark of thelarche has been met. Other overlooked causes of abdominopelvic pain include intercostal or subcostal neuralgias, nerve compression, and abdominal cutaneous nerve entrapment. A multidisciplinary approach to treatment of the patient with chronic abdominopelvic pain is discussed.

Introduction

Pelvic and abdominal pain is a common complaint in paediatric and adolescent primary care, and in some cases, persists into adulthood (Campo et al., 2001; Walker et al., 1995). Pelvic pain is a broad term that encompasses pain originating from viscera within the pelvic cavity, and from the myofascial and bony structures that comprise the pelvis. Pain due to pelvic pathology can be referred to other viscera, the back, abdominal wall, abdomen, hips, and upper thighs, reflecting a broad viscero-viscero and viscero-somatic distribution of the sensory and sympathetic afferent neurons of the lumbosacral plexus (Figure 30.1). For many young patients, the distinction between pelvic and abdominal pain is not well appreciated and descriptions of abdominopelvic pain can be highly variable. Accordingly, it is not uncommon for adolescents to describe pain due to pelvic pathology as 'stomach ache,' and also report symptoms of nausea, gastro-oesophageal reflux, constipation, and bloating in addition to abdominopelvic pain. Not surprisingly, many young adolescents with these non-specific symptoms are evaluated first by gastroenterologists and often have a diagnosis of irritable bowel

syndrome (IBS) or functional gastrointestinal disorder (FGID) prior to identifying other pelvic pathology.

Chronic pelvic pain is associated with changes in the neuronal processing of pain signals in the periphery, dorsal horn, and brain. Pain often persists long after the initiating pelvic inflammation or trauma is resolved. Patients referred for treatment of chronic pelvic pain may have histories that include visceral or musculoskeletal pathology but those initial inciting events have resolved or are being treated effectively by all measures. Further evaluations are often non-revealing of active pathology, and a functional disorder such as IBS becomes the referring diagnosis to the pain specialist. Central sensitization with development of visceral hyperalgesia can provide a framework for understanding why IBS is diagnosed so frequently in patients with pelvic pathology and why patients with pelvic pathology report gastrointestinal symptoms so frequently.

Causes of chronic pelvic pain

The differential diagnosis of abdominopelvic pain is extensive and includes orthopaedic, gastrointestinal, gynaecological, urological, traumatic, infectious, and neoplastic causes. A careful history will help direct the evaluation. Irritable bowel syndrome and stress are the most common diagnoses received by women with chronic pelvic pain, though many are diagnosed without any investigative tests (Zondervan et al., 2001). The most common causes of chronic pelvic pain in adolescent females are dysmenorrhea and constipation.

Dysmenorrhea

Dysmenorrhea is a syndrome characterized by recurrent, crampy, lower abdominal pain occurring during menses. Pain is often accompanied by nausea, vomiting, diarrhoea, headaches, and muscular cramps, and frequently co-occurs with other chronic pain conditions, including migraine, IBS, interstitial cystitis, fibromyalgia, and chronic fatigue syndrome (Alagiri et al., 1997). Dysmenorrhea affects up to 90% of post-menarchal adolescents, with 9% to 14% reporting pain as severe (Klein and Litt, 1981), and is the leading reason for missed school days and work in the adolescent population (Schroeder and Sanfilippo, 1999). Yet, underreporting of symptoms is common and many adolescents do not seek treatment for dysmenorrhea even when symptoms are severe and school days are missed (Klein and Litt, 1981). It is speculated

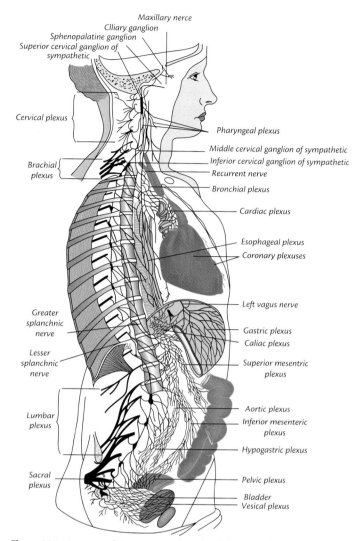

Figure 30.1 Anatomy of the nerve supply to the abdomen and pelvis. Reproduced from Henry Gray, *Anatomy of the Human Body*, 1918 edition, Copyright © 1918, with permission from Elsevier.

Central nervous system changes associated with dysmenorrhea lead to sensitization of other abdominopelvic viscera and somatic tissues, including bladder, intestine, abdominal wall, and back (Giamberardino et al., 1997). Animal studies have demonstrated that acute inflammation in one pelvic organ (uterus, colon or bladder) will induce inflammatory changes in either nearby or remote organs and affect the function of those organs (Berkley, 2005). This observation has been referred to as a 'cross-organ affect' and supports data from other studies demonstrating viscero-visceral convergence of sensory and sympathetic neurons in the spinal cord (Winnard et al., 2006).

Based on a history of pain with menses, the differential is limited. The majority of cases of dysmenorrhea in adolescents are primary, with normal ovulatory cycles and no associated pelvic pathology. Secondary dysmenorrhea refers to painful menstruation associated with pelvic abnormalities, which may be seen in about 10% of adolescents with dysmenorrhea. Referral to a gynaecologist is indicated for evaluation and treatment of severe dysmenorrhea and to rule out the possibility of an obstructive or partially obstructive anomaly such as a transverse vaginal septum, microperforate hymen, or obstructed hemivagina or hemiuterus. When a gynaecological exam is indicated, unlike in adults, the exam is often limited to a cotton swab inserted into the hymenal orifice to help determine if there is an anomaly of the vagina. If there is still concern a transabdominal ultrasound can be helpful.

Dysmenorrhea is typically initially treated with non-steroidal anti-inflammatory drugs (NSAIDs; Marjoribanks et al., 2010). If pain persists then hormonal therapy is used to lighten periods and decrease pain. This is achieved with either combination oestrogen/progestin hormonal pills or progestin-only therapy. Progestin-only therapy is typically utilized if there is a contraindication to the use of oestrogen such as in the case of migraine headaches with focal neurological symptoms or a history of a thrombophilia. If pain resolves with the use of NSAIDs and cyclic hormonal therapy then no further evaluation is usually needed. If pain persists on NSAIDs and hormonal therapy then laparoscopic evaluation is warranted to evaluate for the possibility of endometriosis as the underlying diagnosis. Approximately 70% of adolescents who have a persistence of pain on NSAIDs and 3 months of cyclic hormonal therapy who undergo a laparoscopy have endometriosis (Laufer et al., 1997).

Endometriosis

Endometriosis is a chronic inflammatory and painful condition defined as the presence of uterine glands and stroma outside the uterus. There is no clear understanding as to how endometriosis causes pain but proposed explanations include prostaglandin production, cytokine production, and adhesion formation. Endometriosis lesions can be found anywhere within the abdominal and pelvic cavity. Most lesions are seen on the ovaries, pelvic walls and cul-de-sac, but can also be found on bowel, bladder, ureters, liver, lung, and scar tissue. There are no laboratory tests or imaging studies diagnostic for endometriosis, and thus adolescent endometriosis is diagnosed by laparoscopic visualization.

In adult women, the most common cause of chronic pelvic pain is endometriosis (Fauconnier and Chapron, 2005), estimated to affect 4% to 17% of post-menarchal females (Ranney, 1980). Population studies of endometriosis in adolescents are likely to underestimate its prevalence due to underreporting of symptoms and failure to diagnose. In adolescents who seek treatment for unexplained

that many adolescents consider dysmenorrhea a variant of normal, which in part explains underreporting and why epidemiological data on treatment outcomes in young adolescents is lacking. In addition, many adolescents are hesitant to discuss gynaecological issues and have concerns that if they do verbalize their symptoms they may need a bimanual or speculum-assisted pelvic exam.

Dysmenorrhea is a cyclic pain, and recurrent nociceptive input from painful periods each month can lead to neuronal alterations at the level of the spinal cord and brain that persist throughout the menstrual cycle (Vincent et al., 2011). Studies in adults with dysmenorrhea have demonstrated central nervous system changes similar to those seen in other chronic pain conditions. Such changes include altered central processing of noxious stimuli (Vincent et al., 2011), metabolic and morphological changes in the brain as seen on imaging studies (Tu et al., 2009, 2010), alterations in hypothalamic–pituitary–adrenocortical axis function, and reduced quality of life (Vincent et al., 2011). Dysmenorrhea is therefore a cyclic pain that appears to develop features of a chronic neuropathic pain condition over time.

chronic pelvic pain, there is a 47% prevalence rate of endometriosis found at time of laparoscopy (Goldstein et al., 1979). Other studies have shown that 25% to 38% of adolescents with chronic pelvic pain who seek medical care and undergo laparoscopy have endometriosis (Kontoravdis et al., 1999; Vercellini et al., 1989). Empiric treatment with NSAIDs and oral contraceptives (for the treatment of dysmenorrhea as described earlier) can improve symptoms for many adolescents with chronic pelvic pain, but in cases where pain persists, greater than 70% of adolescents with chronic pelvic pain will be diagnosed with endometriosis (Laufer et al., 2003). In a more recent study, 97% of adolescents with persistence of pain on NSAIDs and combination hormonal therapy were found to have endometriosis on laparoscopic evaluation (Opoku-Anane and Laufer, 2012). The increase in prevalence from 70% to 97% may be due to the improvement of optics of laparoscopes with digital imaging.

Although commonly understood to be a disease of adult women, endometriosis can occur in adolescents and in pre-menarchal girls as early as 8 years of age (Marsh and Laufer, 2005). As endometriosis is an oestrogen-dependent disease, endometriosis should be considered in the differential diagnosis of all females with abdominal or pelvic pain once the benchmark of thelarche has been met (Economy and Laufer, 1999; Lubianca et al., 1998). More typically, women are diagnosed during their childbearing years when they seek medical treatment for infertility. However, data from the Endometriosis Association indicate that two-thirds of adult women with endometriosis reported onset of pelvic symptoms during adolescence, with 38% reporting symptom onset before age 15 years (Ballweg, 2004). On average there is a delay of 9 years from onset of symptoms to diagnosis of endometriosis, with longer delays (8–10 years) diagnosing adolescents compared to women in their 30s (<2 years; Ballweg, 2004, Hadfield et al., 1996). Adolescents under age 15 years with chronic pelvic pain saw an average of 4.2 doctors compared with women in their early 30s who saw an average of 2.6 doctors before diagnosis or referral (Ballweg, 2004).

Adolescent endometriosis can be a challenging diagnosis as signs and symptoms are often non-specific for gynaecological pathology and can differ from those reported by adults (Table 30.1). Adult women with endometriosis report gynaecological symptoms of abdominopelvic pain, severe dysmenorrhea, menorrhagia, irregular menses, subfertility or infertility, and acute adnexal pain due to

Table 30.1 Symptoms of adolescents with endometriosis

Presenting symptoms	Per cent
Acyclic and cyclic pain	62.5
Acyclic pain	28.1
Cyclic pain	9.4
Gastrointestinal pain	34.3
Urinary symptoms	12.5
Irregular menses	9.4
Vaginal discharge	6.3

Source: data from Laufer, M. et al., Prevalence of endometriosis in adolescent girls with chronic pelvic pain not responding to conventional therapy, *Journal of Pediatric and Adolescent Gynecology*, Volume 10, Issue 4, pp. 199–202, Copyright © 1997 North American Society for Pediatric and Adolescent Gynecology. Published by Elsevier Inc. All rights reserved.

ovarian cysts more frequently than controls without endometriosis (Ballard et al., 2008). Women experiencing these symptoms have a high risk of having endometriosis, especially if they experience more than one of these symptoms (Ballard et al., 2008). While adolescents may report similar symptoms as adults, 60% of adolescents with endometriosis report either abdominal or pelvic pain, and 90% report pain that occurs during menses (cyclic) as well as pain that is continuous throughout the menstrual cycle (acyclic) (Laufer et al., 1997).

Questioning adolescents about their menstrual history can identify markers associated with endometriosis (Chapron et al., 2011). A positive family history of endometriosis in a first-degree relative (odds ratio (OR) = 3.2; 95% confidence interval (CI): 1.2–8.8) school absenteeism during menstruation (OR = 1.7; 95% CI: 1–3), and use of oral contraceptive pills for treating severe primary dysmenorrhea in girls under18 years (OR = 4.2; 95% CI: 1.8–10.0) are predictive for endometriosis (Chapron et al., 2011).

Many women with endometriosis report a preponderance of gastrointestinal symptoms and have received a previous diagnosis of IBS or pelvic inflammatory disease (PID) which contributes to the delay in diagnosis of endometriosis in both adults and adolescents. In a consecutive series of 355 women undergoing laparoscopy for suspected endometriosis, 90% of the women with histologically confirmed endometriosis had gastrointestinal symptoms (bloating constipation, diarrhoea, nausea, vomiting). While bloating was the most frequent gastrointestinal symptom, reported by 83% of women, 71% also had other gastrointestinal symptoms (Maroun et al., 2009). Gastrointestinal symptoms are reported nearly as frequently as gynaecological symptoms in women with endometriosis (Maroun et al., 2009). Similarly, a national case–control survey from the UK concluded that 45% of women with endometriosis had a record of abdominal pain and only 15% had a record of pelvic pain (Ballard et al., 2008). Results from the same study also showed that women with endometriosis were 3.5 times more likely to have received a diagnosis of IBS and six times more likely to receive a diagnosis of PID than women without endometriosis (Seaman et al., 2008). There is no data specific for adolescents. The association between endometriosis and PID or IBS was less strong after the diagnosis of endometriosis was made, and these authors suggest some misdiagnosis among women with endometriosis, while posing the possibility of comorbidity between endometriosis and PID or IBS. Whether IBS coexists with endometriosis or is secondary to development of visceral hyperalgesia due to this chronic inflammatory disease is not known. Accordingly, endometriosis should be considered in the differential diagnosis of all females with abdominal or pelvic pain when a functional gastrointestinal disorder such as IBS is considered once the benchmark of thelarche has been met (Economy and Laufer, 1999).

Laparoscopic findings in adolescents also differ from adults, and a prior 'negative' laparoscopy should not rule out the possibility of endometriosis if a surgeon or gynaecologist unfamiliar with the appearance of adolescent endometriosis lesions performed the procedure. Under direct vision, endometriosis lesions in adolescents typically appear as red and clear lesions and the more classic black or brown lesions are more commonly seen in adult women (Laufer et al., 2003). The clear lesions can be difficult to visualize without the use of specialized surgical techniques. Endometriomas, a collection of endometriosis in the ovary, also commonly referred to as a 'chocolate cyst' are rarely seen in adolescents but have been reported (Wright and Laufer, 2010). A high index of suspicion and knowledge of the differences in presentation between adult women and adolescents is key to identifying and treating endometriosis. There is lack of long-term data on follow-up of endometriosis treatment. One long-term follow-up study shows that with early diagnosis and treatment, disease progression may be retarded (Doyle et al., 2009)

The pathogenesis of endometriosis remains unclear. Several theories have attempted to explain possible aetiologies, including developmental anomalies, retrograde menstruation, failure of endometrial cell apoptosis, immune and inflammatory disease, and genetics (Bulun, 2009). There is a 6.9% increased risk of endometriosis of first-degree relatives with endometriosis (Simpson et al., 1980). Other research suggests endometriosis, like migraine headache, is a neurovascular disease (Zhang et al., 2008), and indeed, compared to women without endometriosis, women with endometriosis have an increased density of sensory nerve fibres in the peritoneum and eutopic endometrium (Berkley et al., 2005; Tokushige et al., 2006).

Visceral hyperalgesia is a common finding in patients with endometriosis (Issa et al., 2012). The role of chronic inflammation in the development of visceral hyperalgesia and neuropathic pain was the subject of a recent review of endometriosis pain mechanisms (Evans et al., 2007). The authors identified research showing invasion of nociceptors into peritoneal endometriosis lesions and increased number of nerve terminals in endometriotic tissue, as well as activation of nociceptors by inflammatory mediators, sprouting of new nociceptors, and activation of silent nociceptors present in normal endometrium and peritoneum (Anaf et al., 2006; Berkley et al., 2005; Tokushige et al., 2006). The authors speculate that such nerve sprouting might be caused by increased levels of nerve growth factor (NGF), since expression of NGF in endometriotic tissue is reported to be higher than in eutopic endometrium (Anaf et al., 2006; Tokushige et al., 2006).

Increased signalling from visceral nociceptors to the spinal cord leads to sensitization of dorsal horn cells, convergence of visceral and somatic afferent pathways, and alterations in neural modulation of inhibitory and excitatory pain pathways throughout the central nervous system due to neuroplasticity (Bajaj et al., 2003; Berkley, 2005). Over time, pain spreads to other viscera (viscero-visceral hyperalgesia) and to the abdominal wall and back (viscera-somatic hyperalgesia) with somatic symptoms of cutaneous hypersensitivity to touch, i.e. allodynia (Giamberardino et al., 2010).

Currently there is no cure for endometriosis and treatment is aimed at controlling progression of disease and pain relief. Guidelines from the American College of Obstetricians and Gynecologists (ACOG) for management of adolescent endometriosis pain are extrapolated from the adult experience with endometriosis pain. Recommendations include surgical destruction and/or removal of visible lesions, hormonal suppression of ovulation and menstruation, and anti-inflammatory analgesics (ACOG, 2005). Surgical destruction of endometriosis and menstrual suppressive therapy can retard disease progression (Doyle et al., 2009). Yet, these interventions are variably effective and many adolescents continue to report pain despite anti-endometriosis therapy. Managing chronic pelvic pain due to endometriosis is a multidisciplinary endeavour and communication among clinicians across disciplines, including pain medicine, gynaecology, and psychology, is essential for good pain treatment outcomes.

Acute exacerbations in endometriosis pain may be surgical or non-surgical and an effort should be made to identify the cause of an acute increase in pain. Non-surgical causes of acute pain flares include a missed or delayed oral contraceptive pill, change in absorption of oral contraceptives due to medications, or change-over in hormonal therapy. Suspected ovarian torsion, tubal, or ovarian cysts, and adhesions require surgical evaluation. Close communication with the patient's gynaecologist is important to understanding the aetiology of episodic pain flares, and informs pain management.

Pelvic floor dysfunction

Pelvic floor dysfunction is being recognized more frequently as a cause of chronic pelvic pain in children and adolescents. In adults, pelvic floor dysfunction is associated increasing age and parity, and structural or mechanical changes in the pelvis (Baessler et al., 2004; Kepenekci et al., 2011; MacLellan et al., 2000). Injury to the sacrum, coccyx, pubis, and hip joints can be a cause of misalignment, tension, and inflammation of the attached ligaments, muscles, and nerves in the pelvis. Pain syndromes associated with pelvic floor dysfunction include interstitial cystitis/painful bladder syndrome (IC/PBS), chronic prostatitis/painful prostate syndrome (CP/PPS), vulvodynia, proctalgia fugax, coccyxdynia, piriformis syndrome, pudendal nerve entrapment, and others.

In children, pelvic floor tension myalgia is associated with voiding or elimination dysfunction, and spasm of the pelvic floor muscles. The typical presentation in children is night time awakening with severe lower abdominal or perineal pain. Urodynamic studies often identify high urethral pressures without structural obstruction of the outflow tract (Hoebeke et al., 2004). Conditions associated with pelvic floor dysfunction have been shown to respond well to biofeedback-assisted pelvic floor relaxation therapy (Li et al., 2006).

Chronic prostatitis/prostatic pain syndrome

In adolescent males, CP/PPS is defined by symptoms of voiding dysfunction (frequency, urgency, split stream and sense of residual urine) and pain (testicular, penile, scrotal, pelvic or rectal) as well as ejaculatory pain or discomfort. Males rarely exhibit these symptoms before puberty (Hoebeke et al., 2004; Tripp et al., 2009). However, in a study of North American adolescent males aged 16 to 19 years, the prevalence of CP was found to be 8.3%, comparable to adults (Tripp et al., 2009). Unlike adult CP, adolescents reported a preponderance of voiding symptoms, which led authors to conclude that CP in adolescents is most likely due to pelvic floor dysfunction (Li et al., 2006).

Interstitial cystitis/bladder pain syndrome

IC/BPS is a condition frequently occurring with endometriosis and IBS, and can be a related cause of chronic pelvic pain. Characteristic symptoms of IC include urinary frequency and urgency, usually with pelvic pain and nocturia, in the absence of bacterial infection or any other identifiable pathology. In adults, it is estimated that 85% of patients with chronic pelvic pain may have symptoms of IC (Parsons and Albo, 2002). The incidence of IC in children and adolescents is not known. In adults, IC is being identified more frequently with the use of the Interstitial Cystitis Symptom Index, a symptoms questionnaire (Clemons et al., 2002), and an intravesical potassium sensitivity test (PST; Chung et al., 2010). The PST is an office-based test useful for isolating the bladder as the source of pain and urgency symptoms. Potassium instilled into the bladder is a neuroirritant and causes an increase in pain symptoms. A positive PST suggests increased permeability of the bladder urothelium and lends support to the diagnosis of IC. Alternatively, instilling anaesthetic solution may also aid in the diagnosis of IC. The diagnosis is confirmed by cystoscopy. If IC is detected, then the patient can be treated for chronic pelvic pain of bladder origin. Urological therapy for IC has a high rate of success and often is best treated in a multidisciplinary setting.

Assessment

A careful history can help direct the workup and evaluation of patients with chronic pelvic pain. Quality and location of pain can help determine whether pain symptoms originate from viscera, are musculoskeletal, or from an entrapped nerve. Pain descriptors such as burning, aching, stabbing, spreading, or throbbing are common in patients with visceral hyperalgesia or neuralgia; inability to tolerate any tight fitting clothing and hypersensitivity of the abdominal wall or back to light touch or gentle pressure can indicate viscerosomatic convergence with referred pain to the abdomen or back. In addition to asking about location, onset, and frequency of pain symptoms, questioning for temporal association with injury or trauma such as an occult pelvic fracture, or suspected slipped capital femoral epiphysis, hip, or back injury can identify treatable orthopaedic conditions. Gastrointestinal and urinary symptoms often coexist with other pelvic pathology.

Obtaining a menstrual history and understanding norms for menstrual frequency, amount of bleeding, and severity of pain is important in order to determine whether further gynaecological investigation is needed when evaluating a patient referred for chronic abdominopelvic pain. For example, irregular periods are considered the norm for young teens because of anovulation; however, it is not well appreciated that during the early years after menarche, 90% of cycles will be within the range of 20 to 45 days even during the first gynaecological year (Popat et al., 2008). Cycles outside of the range of 20 to 45 days are statistically uncommon, even in young girls, and deserve evaluation for potential treatable causes.

A medication history may reveal that the patient is on an oral contraceptive pill. It is important to determine whether the pill was started for menstrual irregularities or pain, and note whether symptoms have improved since starting hormonal therapy. A family history of gynaecological disorders such as endometriosis, severe dysmenorrhea, or infertility can guide referral to an adolescent gynaecologist. A patient with a positive family history of endometriosis in a first-degree relative has a 6.9% increased risk of endometriosis in comparison with a 1% risk in controls (Simpson et al., 1980).

During the interview or exam, time should be set aside to speak confidentially with the patient about sexual activity, history of physical or sexual assault, and sexually transmitted infections as information on these sensitive subjects may be withheld in the presence of parents or guardians. In a systematic review of risk factors in women with and without chronic pelvic pain, Lathe et al identified a strong association between all types of chronic pelvic pain and pelvic pathology, history of childhood abuse, and psychological morbidity in adults (Latthe et al., 2006).

On physical exam, evaluation of the spine and pelvis looking for posture, gait, symmetry, range of motion, and tenderness to palpation may reveal biomechanical alterations. Leg-length discrepancy and pathology of the spine or hip can be referred to the groin and pelvis. A sensory exam of the back and abdomen to determine the presence of allodynia or hyperalgesia can provide evidence of central sensitization and neuropathic pain. Pain of visceral origin and associated viscero-somatic convergence may present as a non-dermatomal area of hyperalgesia or allodynia over the abdomen or back.

A dermatomal distribution of pain over the abdomen is suggestive of an intercostal or subcostal neuralgia, and may indicate pathology at any point along the nerve as it exits the spinal canal. Palpation of the area may reveal proximal and distal radiation along the course of the nerve, known as Valleix phenomenon. Neuroimaging of the spine is indicated if more proximal nerve involvement is suspected. Less commonly, tumour or herpes zoster is the cause.

Abdominal cutaneous nerve entrapment syndrome (ACNES) or an intercostal neuralgia can be overlooked causes of chronic abdominopelvic pain. The abdominal wall is innervated by the anterior rami of the lower six thoracic nerves (T7–T12) and the first lumbar nerve (L1–L2). Thoraco-abdominal nerves exit the spinal canal and terminate in posterior, lateral and anterior branches, providing sensory innervation to the abdominal wall and overlying skin. Similarly, L1 to L2 subcostal nerve involvement (ilioinguinal/iliohypogastric nerves) may present as vulvar or groin pain in girls or scrotal pain in boys. Terminal branches of these somatic nerves course through the lateral abdominal wall within a plane between the internal oblique and transversus abdominis muscles. The thoracic branches are anchored at various points through fibrous attachments within the wall which can tether or trap the nerve along its course as it passes to the superficial layers. The anterior cutaneous branch of an intercostal nerve is most vulnerable to entrapment because it makes a nearly 90-degree turn to enter a fibrous tunnel as it passes to the superficial tissues at the lateral border of the rectus abdominis muscle. A history of straining, coughing, or vomiting may be elicited as increased intra-abdominal pressure, intense muscle contraction, or blunt trauma to the abdominal wall can lead to nerve entrapment. Postoperatively, traction can be placed on the nerve by a scar.

On exam, one can look for a positive Carnett's sign. With the patient in the supine position, the examiner palpates along the lateral border of the rectus sheath and asks the patient to attempt a sit up. As the patient tenses the abdominal wall muscles, if entrapped, the anterior branch of the intercostal nerve becomes compressed between the examiner's finger and the taught abdominal muscles, resulting in worsening pain. If pain is from the viscera, tensing the muscles guards against more painful deeper palpation. Abdominal wall pain can be distinguished from visceral pain with a transversus abdominis plane (TAP) block, which numbs the abdominal wall. A rectus sheath block may relieve an abdominal cutaneous nerve entrapment; abdominal wall trigger points may have a similar presentation and can be identified with careful palpation.

General approach to treatment (Table 30.2)

When acute inflammatory pain is suspected, NSAIDs and opioid analgesics can provide good pain relief. It is known that non-steroidal anti-inflammatory analgesics are not as effective for treating neuropathic pain and visceral hyperalgesia (Cruccu et al., 2007;

Table 30.2 Approach to multidisciplinary treatment of pelvic pain in adolescents

Medications	NSAIDS
	Anticonvulsant
	Tricyclic antidepressants
	Tramadol/oxycodone
	Lidoderm patch
Nerve blocks	Trigger point injections
	Transversus abdominis plane (TAP)
	Pudendal nerve
	Ganglion impar
Physical therapy	Aquatherapy
	Pelvic floor retraining
	Core strengthening
	Endurance
	Flexibility
	TENS unit
Biobehavioural therapies	Cognitive behavioural therapy
	Biofeedback
	Guided imagery
	Treatment of depression and anxiety
	Assistance with school reentry
Complementary and alternative therapies	Acupuncture
	Acupressure
	Therapeutic massage

Dworkin et al., 2007). Development of central sensitization and chronic neuropathic pain may explain why pain continues despite treatment with standard anti-endometriosis therapies.

Neuropathic pain analgesics include tricyclic antidepressants and anticonvulsants. First-line agents most commonly used for treatment of neuropathic pain conditions include amitriptyline and gabapentin, typically chosen based on side effect profile as there is yet no data to support one class of drug over the other as far as pain relief efficacy. There is no data on the use of these drugs in patients with endometriosis.

Complicating the treatment of chronic pelvic pain is the observation that many adolescents with endometriosis and persistent pain have symptoms of anxiety and/or depression. Psychological support to develop pain coping strategies and to treat associated symptoms of depression or anxiety is part of a multidisciplinary approach to pain management. When medication is initiated, the selective serotonin re-uptake inhibitor class of antidepressants is frequently prescribed for depression and/or anxiety. When medication for anxiety or depression is a consideration, therapeutic dosing of amitriptyline as a neuropathic analgesic in the treatment of endometriosis pain can be limited due to concern for increased risk of serotonin syndrome. Additionally, many adolescents are concerned about weight gain, and have a history of IBS with constipation, both of which can be exacerbated by a tricyclic antidepressant and ultimately lead to medication non-compliance.

Patients benefit from physical therapy as part of a multidisciplinary approach to treatment of chronic pelvic pain. Prolonged periods of bed rest and compensatory postures can lead to myofascial pain and deconditioning, adding to the overall level of pain-related disability. When the patient has become homebound and no longer participates in athletic or after school activities the rationale for functional restoration is evident. Aquatherapy, gentle stretching, core and pelvic floor strengthening, and building endurance in a therapeutic setting can be the first steps toward re-engaging the patient in everyday activities.

Referred pain from the viscera, and viscero-somatic convergence of neural sensory pathways at the level of the spinal cord can result in allodynia and hyperalgesia of the abdominal wall. Transcutaneous electrical nerve stimulation (TENS) or topical application of a 5% lidocaine patch (Lidoderm®) can provide additional pain relief when the abdominal wall or back are tender. TENS involves stimulation of the skin using electrical currents at various pulse rates (frequencies) and intensities in order to provide pain relief. A conventional TENS emits pulses between 50 and 120 Hz at a low intensity producing a tapping or gentle buzzing sensation. It is speculated that TENS relieves pain by stimulating myelinated afferents, which in turn activate segmental inhibitory pathways, thereby altering the body's ability to receive or perceive pain signals. TENS units are the size of a small pager with attached electrodes that adhere to the skin at the site of pain. The units can be worn throughout the day, with the patient controlling the level of current for maximal comfort. Typically, physical therapists will trial a TENS unit over the abdomen and make recommendations for obtaining a unit for home use. The available data on high-frequency TENS suggest it is effective for the treatment of dysmenorrhea (Proctor et al., 2002; Walsh et al., 2009).

The use of acupuncture in managing painful periods is promising though data is limited. Findings should be interpreted with caution due to the small number of studies and study participants. No significant adverse effects were identified in this review (Smith et al., 2011).

When indicated, abdominal wall trigger point injections and TAP blocks can provide temporary pain relief, and help establish a diagnosis of abdominal wall neuralgia, a consideration when treating patients with abdominal incisions/scars, abdominal wall adhesions, or when nerve entrapment is suspected. Pain that is localized to the perineum may respond to a pudendal nerve or ganglion impar block.

Conclusions

Chronic pelvic pain is often described as abdominal pain in younger patients. Dysmenorrhea is more common in adolescents than adults and can be associated with changes in the central nervous system and other chronic pain conditions due to neuroplasticity. Central sensitization of visceral pain pathways can affect bowel and bladder function, and be associated with pelvic floor pain and dysfunction, which may be improved with physical therapy. In female adolescents with chronic abdominopelvic pain of undetermined aetiology, it is important to have a high index of suspicion for endometriosis, especially when a prior diagnosis of IBS is present. The diagnosis of endometriosis is commonly delayed until adulthood though symptoms start during adolescence. Adolescents with endometriosis can report either cyclic or acyclic pain and present with a preponderance of gastrointestinal symptoms. Obtaining a full menstrual history is an important aspect of the evaluation of female adolescents with chronic abdominopelvic pain.

Case example

A 14-year-old-female who has been to the emergency department (ED) many times over the past year for recurrent flare-ups of abdominal pain has received intravenous analgesia with ketorolac and morphine with transient relief. She has been thoroughly investigated for abdominal pain by multiple specialists from gastroenterology and general surgery over the preceding year. These investigations included computed tomography scans, abdominal and pelvic ultrasounds, HIDA (hepatobiliary iminodiacetic acid) scan and gall bladder emptying studies, and blood tests to rule out coeliac disease, infectious, and IBDs. Last year she underwent laparoscopic cholecystectomy for presumed gallbladder dysfunction, and at the same time had her appendix removed pre-emptively. The procedure was uneventful but she continued to report severe pain postoperatively. Repeated upper and lower endoscopies did not reveal abnormalities. She is being treated for IBS and gastro-oesophageal reflux disorder. At the time of her most recent ED visit, she presented with periumbilical and left lower quadrant pain which did not respond to repeated doses of intravenous morphine. The decision was made to admit the patient to the hospital for further evaluation of chronic abdominal pain and pain management.

Additional history revealed that her paediatrician has suggested she meet with a psychologist because of depressed mood and school avoidance. The patient started high school this year and has missed many days of school due to pain. She has stopped playing soccer and cheerleading due to pain, activities she previously enjoyed. She has withdrawn from peers and social activities. The patient spends most her time at home resting on the couch and worrying about undiagnosed serious illness. She feels that some healthcare providers no longer believe she has pain and view her as 'faking.' Sleep is difficult to initiate and non-restorative. She will probably have to repeat ninth grade due to absences.

The patient describes periumbilical and left lower quadrant pain that is present all the time to a variable degree. The pain symptoms developed gradually over the past 18 months. She cannot recall an inciting event or illness. The pain is described as a sharp, stabbing, and sometimes throbbing sensation that comes on randomly without obvious triggers. Any tight-fitting clothing over her abdomen worsens the pain. The pain is always present, but can range in intensity from 5 to 10/10 on a numerical rating scale. The pain is not related to food intake, bowel movements, or voiding, though sometimes these activities cause pain to increase. Pain is sometimes worse with menses but can occur any time of the month. She has occasional nausea but has not vomited. Bowel and bladder patterns have not changed. She has a history of constipation and is treated with Miralax®. She has an upcoming appointment with the Pain Treatment Clinic for evaluation of new low back pain.

Past medical history is significant for menarche at age 11 years. Menses are irregular and she takes an oral contraceptive pill. She is followed by GI for IBS, diagnosed at age 12 years with associated GERD which is treated with Prevacid® and constipation, treated with Miralax®. Previous surgeries include laparoscopic cholecystectomy and appendectomy. Family history reveals that her mother and aunts had difficulty conceiving.

On physical exam she is very anxious, lying on her right side, and crying. Vital signs: heart rate 93/min, regular; respiratory rate 15/min, crying; blood pressure 115/65; room air SpO_2 = 100%.

General physical and brief neurological examination revealed no abnormalities except for her abdominal examination: her abdomen was soft, non-distended, with decreased bowel sounds. Laparoscopic port sites located in the umbilicus, midline below the umbilicus, and left lower quadrant were well healed. The abdominal tenderness was diffuse, but greatest over the left lower quadrant and periumbilical area. Light touch or superficial palpation caused pain and she was unable to tolerate deep palpation. Carnett's test was negative. Abdominal examination otherwise was unremarkable.

Differential diagnosis:

- Visceral hyperalgesia due to central sensitization.
- Viscero-somatic convergence and referred pain from viscera.
- Abdominal cutaneous nerve entrapment (ACNE).
- Intercostal (T7–T12) or subcostal (L1) neuralgia.

Further history revealed that the patient had started taking oral contraceptives for irregular menses at the age of 13 years. She slept over a friend's house and forgot to take her pill the day before her pain developed. Her mother had a history of heavy and painful periods and both of her maternal aunts were diagnosed with endometriosis when they underwent laparoscopy as part of an infertility workup.

This patient was referred to an adolescent gynaecologist for evaluation. With her history of persistent abdominopelvic pain while on an oral contraceptive and positive family history of endometriosis, this patient has a high chance of being diagnosed with endometriosis.

At the time of laparoscopy she was found to have stage I endometriosis. The surgeon proceeded to cauterize visible lesions in the abdomen and pelvis. She was treated with a continuous oral contraceptive (without breaks or placebos for suppression of menses), and was started on gabapentin for treatment of the neuropathic component of her pain symptoms. Over the next 2 to 3 months, she had several episodes of painful spotting. Her pain symptoms flared and did not respond to NSAIDs. Her gynaecologist made some changes to her hormonal therapy to improve suppression of ovulation. She received a prescription for tramadol 25 to 50 mg every 8 h, with instructions to take no more than 3 to 5 days during the month.

Subsequently, with the combination of hormonal suppression, NSAIDs, gabapentin, and occasional tramadol, her pain symptoms subsided. She was able to return to school and began to work with a psychologist, and started taking an antidepressant for her mood symptoms. One month after her surgery, the patient was able to return to school for two classes a day, and within 2 weeks she was attending school full time, participating in gym class, and playing softball with her freshman team. She still has occasional severe cramping, but her pain is manageable on her current regimen and does not interfere with her desired activities.

References

Alagiri, M., Chottiner, S., Ratner, V., Slade, D., and Hanno, P. M. (1997). Interstitial cystitis: unexplained associations with other chronic disease and pain syndromes. *Urology*, 49, 52–57.

American College of Obstetricians and Gynecologists. (2005). ACOG Committee Opinion. Number 310, April 2005. Endometriosis in adolescents. *Obstet Gynecol*, 105, 921–927.

Anaf, V., Chapron, C., El Nakadi, I., De Moor, V., Simonart, T., and Noël, J. (2006). Pain, mast cells, and nerves in peritoneal, ovarian, and deep infiltrating endometriosis. *Fertil Steril*, 86, 1336–1343.

Baessler, K., Bircher, M. D., and Stanton, S. L. (2004). Pelvic floor dysfunction in women after pelvic trauma. *BJOG*, 111, 499–502.

Bajaj, P., Madsen, H., and Arendt-Nielsen, L. (2003). Endometriosis is associated with central sensitization: a psychophysical controlled study. *J Pain*, 4, 372–380.

Ballard, K. D., Seaman, H. E., De Vries, C. S., and Wright, J. T. (2008). Can symptomatology help in the diagnosis of endometriosis? Findings from a national case-control study—Part 1. *BJOG*, 115, 1382–1391.

Ballweg, M. L. (2004). Impact of endometriosis on women's health: comparative historical data show that the earlier the onset, the more severe the disease. *Best Pract Res Clin Obstet Gynaecol*, 18, 201–218.

Berkley, K. J. (2005). A life of pelvic pain. *Physiol Behav*, 86, 272–280.

Berkley, K. J., Rapkin, A. J., and Papka, R. E. (2005). The pains of endometriosis. *Science*, 308, 1587–1589.

Bulun, S. E. (2009). Endometriosis. *N Engl J Med*, 360, 268–279.

Campo, J. V., Di Lorenzo, C., Chiappetta, L., Bridge, J., Colborn, D. K., Gartner, J. C., *et al.* (2001). Adult outcomes of pediatric recurrent abdominal pain: do they just grow out of it? *Pediatrics*, 108, E1.

Chapron, C., Lafay-Pillet, M. C., Monceau, E., Borghese, B., Ngô, C., Souza, C., *et al.* (2011). Questioning patients about their adolescent history can identify markers associated with deep infiltrating endometriosis. *Fertil Steril*, 95, 877–881.

Chung, M. K., Butrick, C. W., and Chung, C. W. (2010). The overlap of interstitial cystitis/painful bladder syndrome and overactive bladder. *JSLS*, 14, 83–90.

Clemons, J. L., Arya, L. A., and Myers, D. L. (2002). Diagnosing interstitial cystitis in women with chronic pelvic pain. *Obstet Gynecol*, 100, 337–341.

Cruccu, G., Aziz, T. Z., Garcia-Larrea, L., Hansson, P., Jensen, T. S., Lefaucheur, J. P., *et al.* (2007). EFNS guidelines on neurostimulation therapy for neuropathic pain. *Eur J Neurol*, 14, 952–970.

Doyle, J. O., Missmer, S. A., and Laufer, M. R. (2009). The effect of combined surgical-medical intervention on the progression of endometriosis in an adolescent and young adult population. *J Pediatr Adolesc Gynecol*, 22, 257–263.

Dworkin, R. H., O'Connor, A. B., Backonja, M., Farrar, J. T., Finnerup, N. B., Jensen, T. S., *et al.* (2007). Pharmacologic management of neuropathic pain: evidence-based recommendations. *Pain*, 132, 237–251.

Economy, K. and Laufer, M. (1999). Pelvic pain. *Adolesc Med*, 10, 291–304.

Evans, S., Moalem-Taylor, G., and Tracey, D. J. (2007). Pain and endometriosis. *Pain*, 132 Suppl 1, S22–225.

Fauconnier, A. and Chapron, C. (2005). Endometriosis and pelvic pain: epidemiological evidence of the relationship and implications. *Hum Reprod Update*, 11, 595–606.

Giamberardino, M. A., Berkley, K. J., Iezzi, S., De Bigontina, P., and Vecchiet, L. (1997). Pain threshold variations in somatic wall tissues as a function of menstrual cycle, segmental site and tissue depth in non-dysmenorrheic women, dysmenorrheic women and men. *Pain*, 71, 187–197.

Giamberardino, M. A., Costantini, R., Affaitati, G., Fabrizio, A., Lapenna, D., Tafuri, E., *et al.* (2010). Viscero-visceral hyperalgesia: characterization in different clinical models. *Pain*, 151, 307–322.

Goldstein, D. P., Decholnoky, C., Leventhal, J. M., and Emans, S. J. (1979). New insights into the old problem of chronic pelvic pain. *J Pediatr Surg*, 14, 675–680.

Hadfield, R., Mardon, H., Barlow, D., and Kennedy, S. (1996). Delay in the diagnosis of endometriosis: a survey of women from the USA and the UK. *Hum Reprod*, 11, 878–880.

Hoebeke, P., Van Laecke, E., Renson, C., Raes, A., Dehoorne, J., Vermeiren, P., *et al.* (2004). Pelvic floor spasms in children: an unknown condition responding well to pelvic floor therapy. *Eur Urol*, 46, 651–654.

Issa, B., Onon, T. S., Agrawal, A., Shekhar, C., Morris, J., Hamdy, S., *et al.* (2012). Visceral hypersensitivity in endometriosis: a new target for treatment? *Gut*, 61, 367–372.

Kepenekci, I., Keskinkilic, B., Akinsu, F., Cakir, P., Elhan, A. H., Erkek, A. B., *et al.* (2011). Prevalence of pelvic floor disorders in the female population and the impact of age, mode of delivery, and parity. *Dis Colon Rectum*, 54, 85–94.

Klein, J. R., and Litt, I. F. (1981). Epidemiology of adolescent dysmenorrhea. *Pediatrics*, 68, 661–664.

Kontoravdis, A., Hassan, E., Hassiakos, D., Botsis, D., Kontoravdis, N., and Creatsas, G. (1999). Laparoscopic evaluation and management of chronic pelvic pain during adolescence. *Clin Exp Obstet Gynecol*, 26, 76–77.

Latthe, P., Mignini, L., Gray, R., Hills, R., and Khan, K. (2006). Factors predisposing women to chronic pelvic pain: systematic review. *Br Med J*, 332, 749–755.

Laufer, M., Goitein, L., Bush, M., Cramer, D., and Emans, S. (1997). Prevalence of endometriosis in adolescent girls with chronic pelvic pain not responding to conventional therapy. *J Pediatr Adolesc Gynecol*, 10, 199–202.

Laufer, M., Sanfilippo, J., and Rose, G. (2003). Adolescent endometriosis: diagnosis and treatment approaches. *J Pediatr Adolesc Gynecol*, 16, S3–11.

Li, Y., Qi, L., Wen, J. G., Zu, X. B., and Chen, Z. Y. (2006). Chronic prostatitis during puberty. *BJU Int*, 98, 818–821.

Lubianca, J. N., Gordon, C. M., and Laufer, M. R. (1998). 'Add-back' therapy for endometriosis in adolescents. *J Reprod Med*, 43, 164–172.

Maclellan, A. H., Taylor, A. W., Wilson, D. H., and Wilson, D. (2000). The prevalence of pelvic floor disorders and their relationship to gender, age, parity and mode of delivery. *BJOG*, 1460–1470.

Marjoribanks, J., Proctor, M., Farquhar, C., and Derks, R. S. (2010). Nonsteroidal anti-inflammatory drugs for dysmenorrhoea. *Cochrane Database Syst Rev*, 4, CD001751.

Maroun, P., Cooper, M. J., Reid, G. D., and Keirse, M. J. (2009). Relevance of gastrointestinal symptoms in endometriosis. *Aust N Z J Obstet Gynaecol*, 49, 411–414.

Marsh, E. E., and Laufer, M. R. (2005). Endometriosis in premenarcheal girls who do not have an associated obstructive anomaly. *Fertil Steril*, 83, 758–760.

Opoku-Anane, J. and Laufer, M. R. (2012). Prevalence of endometriosis in adolescent girls with chronic pelvic pain not responding to conventional therapy. *Have we underestimated? Presented at the North American Society of Pediatric and Adolescent Gynecology*, Miami, FL.

Parsons, C. L., and Albo, M. (2002). Intravesical potassium sensitivity in patients with prostatitis. *J Urol*, 168, 1054–1057.

Popat, V. B., Prodanov, T., Calis, K. A., and Nelson, L. M. (2008). The menstrual cycle: a biological marker of general health in adolescents. *Ann N Y Acad Sci*, 1135, 43–51.

Proctor, M. L., Smith, C. A., Farquhar, C. M., and Stones, R. W. (2002). Transcutaneous electrical nerve stimulation and acupuncture for primary dysmenorrhoea. *Cochrane Database Syst Rev*, 1, CD002123.

Ranney, B. (1980). Endometriosis: pathogenesis, symptoms, and findings. *Clin Obstet Gynecol*, 23, 865–874.

Schroeder, B., and Sanfilippo, J. S. (1999). Dysmenorrhea and pelvic pain in adolescents. *Pediatr Clin North America*, 46, 555–571.

Seaman, H. E., Ballard, K. D., Wright, J. T., and De Vries, C. S. (2008). Endometriosis and its coexistence with irritable bowel syndrome and pelvic inflammatory disease: findings from a national case-control study—Part 2. *BJOG*, 115, 1392–1396.

Simpson, J. L., Elias, S., Malinak, L. R., and Buttram, V. C. (1980). Heritable aspects of endometriosis. I. Genetic studies. *Am J Obstet Gynecol*, 137, 327–331.

Smith, C. A., Zhu, X., He, L., and Song, J. (2011). Acupuncture for primary dysmenorrhoea. *Cochrane Database Syst Rev*, 1, CD007854.

Tokushige, N., Markham, R., Russell, P., and Fraser, I. (2006). Nerve fibres in peritoneal endometriosis. *Hum Reprod*, 21, 3001–3007.

Tripp, D. A., Nickel, J. C., Ross, S., Mullins, C., and Stechyson, N. (2009). Prevalence, symptom impact and predictors of chronic prostatitis-like symptoms in Canadian males aged 16–19 years. *BJU Int*, 103, 1080–1084.

Tu, C. H., Niddam, D. M., Chao, H. T., Chen, L. F., Chen, Y. S., Wu, Y. T., *et al.* (2010). Brain morphological changes associated with cyclic menstrual pain. *Pain*, 150, 462–468.

Tu, C. H., Niddam, D. M., Chao, H. T., Liu, R. S., Hwang, R. J., Yeh, T. C., *et al.* (2009). Abnormal cerebral metabolism during menstrual pain in primary dysmenorrhea. *Neuroimage*, 47, 28–35.

Vercellini, P., Fedele, L., Arcaini, L., Bianchi, S., Rognoni, M. T., and Candiani, G. B. (1989). Laparoscopy in the diagnosis of chronic pelvic pain in adolescent women. *J Reprod Med*, 34, 827–830.

Vincent, K., Warnaby, C., Stagg, C. J., Moore, J., Kennedy, S., and Tracey, I. (2011). Dysmenorrhoea is associated with central changes in otherwise healthy women. *Pain*, 152, 1966–1975.

Walker, L. S., Garber, J., Vanslyke, D. A., and Greene, J. W. (1995). Long-term health outcomes in patients with recurrent abdominal-pain. *J Pediatr Psychol*, 20, 233–245.

Walsh, D. M., Howe, T. E., Johnson, M. I., and Sluka, K. A. (2009). Transcutaneous electrical nerve stimulation for acute pain. *Cochrane Database Syst Rev*, 2, CD006142.

Winnard, K. P., Dmitrieva, N., and Berkley, K. J. (2006). Cross-organ interactions between reproductive, gastrointestinal, and urinary tracts: modulation by estrous stage and involvement of the hypogastric nerve. *Am J Physiol Regul Integr Comp Physiol*, 291, R1592–1601.

Wright, K. N., and Laufer, M. R. (2010). Endometriomas in adolescents. *Fertil Steril*, 94, 1529.e7–9.

Zhang, G. H., Dmitrieva, N., Liu, Y., McGinty, K. A., and Berkley, K. J. (2008). Endometriosis as a neurovascular condition: estrous variations in innervation, vascularization, and growth factor content of ectopic endometrial cysts in the rat. *Am J Physiol Regul Integr Comp Physiol*, 294, R162–R171.

Zondervan, K. T., Yudkin, P. L., Vessey, M. P., Jenkinson, C. P., Dawes, M. G., Barlow, D. H., *et al.* (2001). Chronic pelvic pain in the community—symptoms, investigations, and diagnoses. *Am J Obstet Gynecol*, 184, 1149–1155.

CHAPTER 31

Headaches

Andrew D. Hershey

Introduction

A complaint of headache is one of the most common health complaints in children and adolescents with migraine representing one of the most common diseases of childhood. However, a complaint of headache is frequently ignored as a problem by patients, parents, teachers, and practitioners. Headaches are either due to an inciting event or illness (secondary headache) or can be a disease by itself (primary headache). Secondary headaches are due to an event or illness and can be recognized by their cause and effect association with this specific aetiology. Once the inciting event is treated or resolves, the headache should also resolve. When the headache persists, additional evaluation is needed. This cause and effect relationship can be confusing in patients with a primary headache. Oftentimes patients with primary headaches make an assumption that their headache is caused by other frequent problems in childhood including mild head injury, infections, and allergies. Furthermore, some of the secondary causes can exacerbate primary headaches in those patients prone to headaches. Lack of headache response to treatment of this presumed secondary cause, or recurrence of the headache without the associated secondary cause, is an indication that the incorrect secondary cause was identified, the incorrect treatment was chosen, or most likely that a primary headache was the actual aetiology.

Recurrent headaches, especially when episodic, are much more likely to represent primary headache disorders. Primary headaches are intrinsic to the nervous system and are the disease itself. Early recognition of the primary headaches in patients should result in improved response and outcome, minimizing the impact of the primary headaches and disability. Primary headaches can be grouped into migraine, tension-type headaches (TTHs), and trigeminal autonomic cephalalgia, and an additional grouping of rarer headaches without a secondary cause. The primary headache that has the greatest impact on a child's quality of life and disability is migraine and subsequently is the most frequent primary headache brought to the attention of parents, primary care providers, and school nurses (Figure 31.1).

Primary headaches

Migraine

Recurrent paediatric migraine has the most significant impact on a child's and parents' lives and consequentially will have the greatest potential improvement with optimal care. There remain many gaps in the recognition and management of migraine during childhood and often extrapolation from studies in adult headaches are incomplete or inaccurate when translated to children. Future studies should help to fill in the current gaps to further improve the lives of these children and their families.

Epidemiology

Bille reported the first extensive study of paediatric migraine's epidemiology in 1962 (Bille, 1962). This study used its own criteria for the definition of migraine in children that are no longer used. Even given that limitation, the study established the basis of paediatric migraine epidemiology recognizing that by age 15 nearly 75% of children will report having a significant headache with migraine in 3.9% of children age 7 to 15 years.

Epidemiology studies that have followed confirmed the high frequency of headaches in children and adolescents with migraines being the more disabling problem (reviewed by Winner and Hershey, 2007). The current standard for diagnosis used in scientific studies of headaches is the International Classification of Headache Disorders, second edition (ICHD-II; Headache Classification Subcommittee of the International Headache Society, 2004). These criteria have been widely utilized across a variety of countries with some degree of variation but consistently demonstrate the high prevalence of migraine during childhood.

Epidemiology studies have demonstrated a high frequency of self-reported headache with migraine occurring typically in one out of ten children. A study from Istanbul, Turkey found 46.2% of children age 5 to 13 years old (mean 8.2±2.4 years) reported a significant headache with 3.4% having migraine and an additional 8.7% having probable migraine (Isik et al., 2009). Another study from Turkey compared the prevalence of migraine and TTH using ICHD-II criteria and found migraine to be more common than TTH (21.3% versus 5.1%) with a further increase in the prevalence if the ICHD-II criteria of number of headaches and duration of the headaches were excluded (29.9% and 15.0%, respectively; Unalp et al., 2007). All headache types were found to be more common in females, with an increase in TTH in subjects with a temple location of their pain, having more than one sibling, and parent's education above high school. School absenteeism was higher in the migraine subjects.

Epidemiology studies of the transition from late adolescent to young adult years are rare. One relatively older study that focused on 15- to 19-year-olds found up to 28% of this age group had migraine with 19% having only migraine without aura and 9% having migraine with aura (Split and Neuman, 1999). There was an

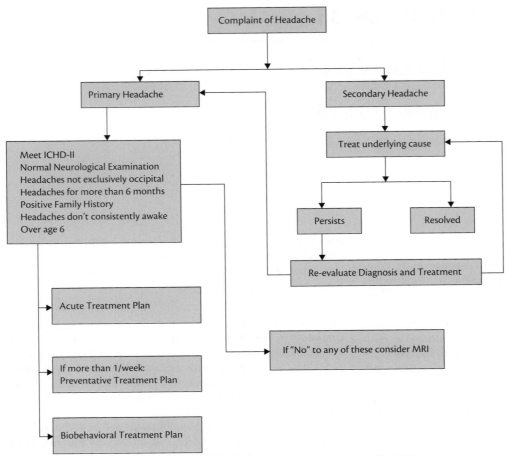

Figure 31.1 Schematic of diagnosis of evaluation of a child presenting with a complaint of headache.

increasing prevalence from age 15 to 19 with a female predominance for all ages. As this appears to be an area of growing prevalence, additional studies are needed to characterize these trends.

Pathophysiology

The pathophysiology of migraine in children and adolescents is likely the same as in adults, although the differences in headache characteristics in children need to be further investigated. The pathophysiology of migraine can be divided into the underlying biological risk factors for the expression of migraine and the specific biological processes that occur during the attack.

The predominant risk factor for the development of migraine is the inheritance of the genetic potential with the environmental influences contributing to the phenotypic expression of this genotype (Hershey, 2007; van de Ven et al., 2009; Wessman et al., 2007). Several models have demonstrated a genetic aetiology with shared environmental influence and the non-shared environmental influences. The best fitting model demonstrated a genetic influence of 60% to 70% with a non-shared environmental influence composing the remainder. This model suggests that migraine is a genetic disease, but with environmental factors significantly contributing to its expression.

The contribution of individual genes has begun to be identified. The identification of genes directly responsible for familial hemiplegic migraine—*CACNA1A* (Ophoff et al., 1996; Terwindt et al., 1998), *ATP1A2* (De Fusco et al., 2003; Vanmolkot et al., 2003),

and *SCN1A* (Dichgans et al., 2005), has provided insight into the importance of channels and astrocytes in migraine.

Several other biological process have been identified to be altered or associated with migraine in children and adults including immunological changes (Bockowski et al., 2009), increased levels of calcitonin gene-related peptide in migraine patients (Fan et al., 2009), decreased levels of coenzyme Q_{10} (Hershey et al., 2007), and hormonal changes (Crawford et al., 2009; Kroner-Herwig and Vath, 2009; Martin and Behbehani, 2006a, 2006b).

There also appears to be neurophysiological changes. In adult patients it has been found that interictally, patients with migraine have trigeminal sensitization as revealed by an altered blink reflex (De Marinis et al., 2003; Katsarava et al., 2002, 2003; Kaube et al., 2002), auditory response (Siniatchkin et al., 2003; W. Wang and Schoenen, 1998), and sensitization of the trigeminal vascular system (Burstein et al., 2005). In children, several studies have also identified similar neurophysiological and biological changes including alterations in the P100 visual response during visual-evoked potential testing (Unay et al., 2008), changes in the somatosensory-evoked potential with treatment of paediatric migraine (Vollono et al., 2010), habituation mismatch negativity and the P300 response (Valeriani et al., 2009), and impaired auditory response during an acute migraine using magnetic encephalography (Korostenskaja et al., 2011). In sum, these studies clearly demonstrate that during an acute migraine, there is brain dysfunction at the cellular and electrical level.

Cutaneous allodynia due to central sensitization has been studied as a clinical marker that reflects these neurophysiological changes in adults (Ashkenazi et al., 2007; Bigal et al., 2008; Burstein and Cutrer, 2000; Burstein et al., 2000; Jakubowski et al., 2005; Mathew et al., 2004). In subjects that have these symptoms during their migraine, there may be diminished response to treatment (Burstein and Jakubowski, 2004; Burstein et al., 2004; Jakubowski et al., 2005) and possible disease progression. In children this has only begun to be examined with limited findings (Eidlitz-Markus et al., 2007).

Diagnosis and evaluation

The International Headache Society has established diagnostic criteria for all headache subtypes including primary and secondary headaches—the ICHD-II (Headache Classification Subcommittee of the International Headache Society, 2004). These criteria have been widely used for both the clinical characterization of headaches and as a foundation for research in headaches. One of the keys to these criteria is the separation of those headaches thought to be intrinsic to the nervous system (primary headaches) and those headaches directly attributable to another cause (secondary headaches) with the first step in evaluation of recurrent headaches to eliminate the potential of a secondary headache. If a secondary aetiology is suspected, this should be initially evaluated and treated. If the suspected secondary aetiology is successfully treated, but the headache persists, diagnosis should be re-evaluated.

After the potential of secondary headache has been eliminated, a diagnosis of a primary headache can be made. The ICHD-II has three main categories of primary headaches and a fourth category for those rare headaches that are primary, but don't fall into one of these three main categories: migraine, TTHs, and trigeminal autonomic cephalalgias (including cluster headaches). In children, the most common types of primary headache are migraine and TTH.

Migraine can be subdivided into migraine without aura and migraine with aura, as well as additional migraine-related diagnoses including childhood periodic syndromes, retinal migraine, migraine complications, and probable migraine.

The ICHD-II criteria for migraine without aura and migraine with aura are undergoing revisions, but few changes are expected. For a migraine without aura the keys in the diagnosis include a recurrent headache disorder (at least five attacks) lasting 4 to 72 h, characterized by a focal, throbbing pain, that alters or worsens with activity and is of moderate to severe in intensity (two of four characteristics required) and associated with either nausea and/or vomiting or with photophobia and phonophobia (Headache Classification Subcommittee of the International Headache Society, 2004).

The ICHD-II addressed some of the unique issues related to childhood headaches resulting in an improvement in the specificity and sensitivity, although gaps do remain (Hershey et al., 2005; Lima et al., 2005; Rossi et al., 2008; Ruangsuwan and Sriudomkajorn, 2007): that childhood migraine tends to be of shorter duration (down to 1 h), that sleep should be included as part of the duration, that the location is more likely bilateral (typically frontal temporal), and that photophobia and phonophobia could be inferred by the parents and care providers based on the child's actions. The ICHD-II noted that if the location is exclusively occipital then additional workup is warranted.

Although the criteria do not completely recognize all children with migraine, these criteria should be used as a guideline for making the diagnosis. Use of standardized questionnaires with a semistructured interview can assist with assuring the completeness of this evaluation (Hershey et al., 1999). Such an approach has been shown to be very sensitive and specific in making the appropriate diagnosis of headache (Valentinis et al., 2009). This evaluation must incorporate the children's responses and not just be completed by the parents, as parents may be limited in their ability to characterize their children's headaches. In a study of 3461 parents and children (age 7 to 14 years), parents were accurate in reporting their child's headache frequency, but were less accurate recognizing other features associate with migraine (Kroner-Herwig et al., 2009).

Young children are also limited in their descriptive ability of their headaches and the use of children's drawings have been demonstrated to be both sensitive and specific in their diagnosis of paediatric headaches (Stafstrom et al., 2002, 2005; Wojaczynska-Stanek et al., 2008). In addition, very young children often will have additional variants of migraine such as the childhood periodic syndromes. The childhood periodic syndromes are thought to be precursors of migraine, are often first recognized as a child may not focus on the head pain, but rather on some of the abdominal symptoms (cyclic vomiting and abdominal migraine) or vertigo (benign paroxysmal vertigo of childhood). As the child ages they are better able to describe the head pain and the presence of migraine becomes more evident.

Evaluation guidelines have been developed by the collaboration of the American Academy of Neurology (AAN), Child Neurology Society, and the American Headache Society (Lewis et al., 2002). These guidelines reviewed the existing evidence for the evaluation of children with headaches and found that the neurological examination is the most critical test for identifying potential serious complications, while also confirming that the occipital location warranted further evaluation. When further evaluation is needed, a magnetic resonance imaging (MRI) study is the most sensitive test to identify structural abnormalities and should be the preferred neuroimaging test.

In addition to a complete history, general examination, and neurological examination, a comprehensive headache examination should also be performed (Linder, 2005). The comprehensive headache examination extends the neurological examination to examine for neck tenderness and stability, the stability of the temporomandibular joint, sinus and facial tenderness including peripheral nerve tenderness, and general cranial palpation. One useful test for sinus-related symptoms is Muller's sign in which the patient pressurizes their sinus and then coughs to create a brief vacuum, thus evaluating the openness of the sinuses. The applicability of this test at the bedside is very useful in dispelling any misperceptions of the headaches as sinus headaches.

As part of the history, the impact of the headache on a child's life needs to be assessed. The impact of a disease can be measured by its effect on the quality of life of the patients as well as the specific disability due to a disease. For paediatric migraine several instruments have begun to address these concerns. A review of the literature on the impact of paediatric migraine found 33 studies addressing this question and the tools used found that although the quality was inconsistent, the impact of migraine on a child's and family's lives was significant (Kernick and Campbell, 2009).

For quality of life one of the most widely administered tools for the assessment of the impact on paediatrics and adolescents' quality of life is the PedsQL 4.0 (Varni et al., 2001). This easily administered instrument address the quality of life in a disease-independent manner. The quality of life of children with headaches can be measured at a developmentally appropriate level and has an impact similar to other chronic disease (Powers et al., 2003, 2004). With treatment this impact improves, although there is preliminary evidence of a persistent impact even after successful treatment.

Disease-specific loss of function can be persistent in many chronic diseases. Headache and migraine is unique in its episodic nature and may therefore be more variable. For children and adolescents PedMIDAS has been developed (Hershey et al., 2001, 2004). This tool can be easily administered in clinical practice and used to assess the disability of an individual patient, the need for preventative medication, and the response to treatment.

The disability and impact of paediatric migraine in tertiary clinics is clear and it is becoming apparent that this also applies to paediatric and adolescent patients in the population. Assessing this can help guide the referral to specialty centres and measure the long-term outcome.

Comorbid conditions

The presence of additional diseases and conditions can complicate the diagnosis, management, and outcome of paediatric migraine. The common occurrence of secondary conditions that may directly contribute to headaches in children can confuse the underlying aetiology and delay the diagnosis of primary headaches while the impact of these comorbid conditions may also affect the underlying pathophysiological basis of children with migraine.

Several conditions have been demonstrated to have a comorbid relationship with migraine. These include asthma and allergic disorders (Gurkan et al., 2000; Ku et al., 2006), obesity (Hershey et al., 2009; Pinhas-Hamiel et al., 2008), epilepsy (Pellock, 2004; Piccinelli et al., 2006; Stevenson, 2006; Yamane et al., 2004), sleep disorders (Bruni et al., 1997; Gilman et al., Isik et al., 2007; 2007; Luc et al., 2006; Miller et al., 2003; Pakalnis et al., 2009), and psychological/emotional disorders (Kroner-Herwig et al., 2008; Pakalnis et al., 2007; Vannatta et al., 2008). The mechanism by which these comorbid conditions alter the expression of migraine and thus influence the underlying pathophysiology is largely unknown, but may be a consequence of the difficulty coping with multiple illnesses or may have a common pathway in brain pathology.

In adults one of the most frequently misdiagnosed headache is sinus headache (Cady and Schreiber, 2004; Schreiber et al., 2004). The presence of allergy and asthma symptoms in children may lead to the same confusion. In the screening of a large database of approximately 5000 children presenting to a tertiary headache centre, asthma was reported in 12.0% of these children. In contrast, using the same methodology to screen a tertiary asthma and allergy clinic, nearly 45.9% of these patients had recurrent headaches (Khurana Hershey et al., 2005). In comparing these two groups the patients referred primarily for a complaint of headache had the highest frequency and disability.

Head injury is another frequent event in children and adolescents. Many children can recall a significant or memorable head injury. When this occurs in a patient with a history of recurrent headache or migraine, it can often exacerbate the underlying primary headache disorder and complicate the evaluation and management and may affect the overall outcome.

With the increasing worldwide rate of obesity it has been noted that adults with migraine and obesity have a higher frequency and poorer response to treatment. This appears to also be present in adolescents.

In a multisite study of children with migraine it was found that children with a body mass index (BMI) percentile at the extremes (<5th percentile and >95th percentile) and children at risk of obesity (85th to 95th percentile) had a higher likelihood of increased frequency of headaches and disability. Intervention in the children that were obese or overweight through healthy weight control demonstrated a greater degree of improvement compared to children whose BMI remained high or increased (Hershey et al., 2009).

Sleep disturbances may increase the occurrence of migraine with sleep deprivation or altered sleep patterns triggering migraines. Furthermore, patients with migraine may also have comorbid sleep disorders. In a study of 1073 adolescents, the most frequent triggering factor for both migraine and non-migraine headaches was 'bad sleep' (Bruni et al., 2008). In a separate study, these sleep disturbances were identified as insufficient sleep (65.7%), daytime sleepiness (23.3%), difficulty falling asleep (40.6), and night waking (38%) (Gilman et al., 2007).

Psychological factors may play a complicated role in paediatric migraine that has been addressed in small studies that remain mixed in their findings (Powers et al., 2006). In a case–control designed study of 47 children (age 8–14 years), mothers perceived emotional and behavioural difficulties (Vannatta et al., 2008), while their classmates identified these same children with higher leadership and popularity (Vannattae al., 2008). The impact of psychological factors and school stressors have a significant impact on headaches with school phobia and anxiety exacerbating headache frequency (Fujita et al., 2009).

Headache may lead to suicidal ideation. A study of 3963 adolescents in Taiwan found that 8.5% had suicidal ideation, with an increased odds ratio of 2.9 for those adolescents with migraine and 4.6 in migraine with aura (S. J. Wang et al., 2009). This was impacted by both headache frequency and disability as measured by PedMIDAS.

Treatment

The treatment of paediatric migraine can be divided into pharmacological and biobehavioural medicine. Pharmacological treatments include both acute and preventative strategies to minimize the impact of the attacks, while biobehavioural treatment includes adherence strategies, coping skills, relaxation techniques, and healthy lifestyles. Goals of treatment should include rapid consistent treatment with a quick return to function (acute treatment), while also minimizing the frequency and impact of the migraine (preventative and biobehavioural treatment). These strategies often fail to be employed in general practice. In a study of 151 children age 10.4±3.2 years, only 30.2% were prescribed an appropriate dose of ibuprofen with only 26.5% instructed to treat the headache early (Cuvellier et al., 2007). In addition, lifestyle adjustments were recommended in less than 15% and only 8% were asked to keep a headache diary. Thus a critical component of paediatric headache management is education of the primary care providers as well as the patients and parents on the incorporation of all of these strategies.

Acute

The goal of acute treatment of paediatric migraine should be consistent response with minimal side effects and quick return to normal function. A detailed analysis and subsequent guidelines have been reported (Lewis et al., 2004). The effective acute medications fall into two broad groups—non-steroidal anti-inflammatory medications (NSAIDs) and triptans. The general principle is that NSAIDs (especially ibuprofen) are effective when used early in the attacks at an adequate dose (7.5–10.0 mg/kg/dose) and that triptans are effective when the NSAIDs are not completely effective, especially during the more severe attacks. Two triptans are currently approved by the US Food and Drug Administration (FDA) for children—almotriptan for ages 12 to 17 years and rizatriptan for ages 6 to 17 years.

One of the reasons for the limited number of positive studies and lack of wider US FDA approval of these medications is due to design of the studies that lead to a high placebo response rate ranging from 38% to 53% for pain relief and 17% to 26% for pain freedom at 2 h (Fernandes et al., 2008). When compared to adults, however, the overall response of the active medication in paediatric and adolescent studies was similar to the adult studies (Evers et al., 2009).

In a double-blind, placebo-controlled, three-way crossover study that included children down to age 6 (age 6–17 years old), rizatriptan was found to be consistently more effective than placebo at 2 h—74% for first treatment, 73% for second treatment versus 36% for placebo (Ahonen et al., 2006). This study used a 5 mg dose for children 20 to 39 kg and a 10 mg dose for those greater than 40 kg. Furthermore, rizatriptan was more effective at 1 h (50% and 55%) compared with placebo (29%).

Using a unique study design—a single-blind, 'placebo challenge,' randomized, double-blind, placebo-controlled, two-way, two-attack crossover, zolmitriptan nasal spray was studied in 248 adolescents (Lewis et al., 2007). Of the 171 patients that treated at least one attack, zolmitriptan nasal spray (5 mg) was found to be superior to placebo at 1 h with a 58.1% response for zolmitriptan compared to 43.3% for placebo. This study addressed many of the placebo response issue that had complicated previous studies, while also using a cross-over design.

A randomized, double-blind, placebo-controlled trial of almotriptan in with 866 adolescents (age 12–17 years) found a 2 h pain-relief rate that was significantly higher for all doses of almotriptan—6.25 mg (71.8%), 12.5 mg (72.9%), and 25 mg (66.7%) compared with placebo (55.3%) (Linder et al., 2008). Further analysis demonstrated superior sustained response with improvement in migraine-associated symptoms for almotriptan compared to placebo with the 12.5 mg dose associated with the most favourable response.

Ault studies have shown that combining NSAIDs with triptans is a highly effective way to improve the acute treatment of migraine (Brandes et al., 2007; Smith et al., 2005).

When acute treatment fails to relieve the headache, patients frequently visit the emergency department (Walker, 2008). A study of 432 children (2–18 years old, mean 8.9 years) visiting a paediatric emergency department found that headache was responsible for 0.8% of all the visits with respiratory disorders contributing 19.2% to the aetiology, migraines 18.5%, TTH 4.6%, post-traumatic headaches 5.5%, meningitis 4.1%, hydrocephalus 0.9%, and brain tumours 0.7% (Conicella et al., 2008). A study of 550 patients over a 12-month period, found headache to be responsible for 1.0% of the visits with primary headache representing 56.7% (9.6% migraine) and 42% as secondary headaches (Scagni and Pagliero, 2008). Viral illness contributed to 90.5% of the secondary headaches with a serious illness found in 4%. Only 40.5% of the patients received pharmacological treatment.

Treatment for children with headache in the emergency department, however, is often lacking. A Canadian study demonstrated that 44.2% received no treatment (23.3%), simple oral analgesics (with dopamine antagonist prescribed in 20.7%, opiates in 5.5%, ketorolac in 4.7%) and dihydroergotamine (DHE) in 1.0% (Richer et al., 2007). One of the most effective treatments for children in the emergency department is the combination of a dopamine antagonist (prochlorperazine) with ketorolac (Kabbouche and Linder, 2005; Kabbouche et al., 2001).

When these emergency department treatments are not successful, inpatient treatment may be necessary. In adults this has classically included the use of DHE and appears to be effective in children with 74.4% of the patients treated with DHE becoming headache free with a significant improvement in nearly all of the patients (Kabbouche et al., 2009). Nausea was the most common side effect, but otherwise the DHE was well tolerated.

Medication overuse is often a complicating factor in children with frequent headache but can be avoided with limitations in the number of times an acute medication is used. General guidelines are to limit the use of non-specific analgesics to less than two to three times per week, while limiting migraine specific agents to less than six times per month.

Preventative

When headaches are frequent (more than once a week) or disabling (PedMIDAS score above 30—Grade III or IV), preventative treatment should be considered. The goal of preventative treatment is to reduce the headache frequency (less than one to two per month) with decrease disability (PedMIDAS less than 10) for a sustained period of time (4 to 6 months). The presence of comorbid conditions may guide the treatment of choice. No medications are currently approved by the US FDA for the prevention of paediatric headaches and the AAN practice only identified flunarizine (not available in the US) as having sufficient evidence (Lewis et al., 2004).

Agents that have been used for paediatric migraine prevention include antidepressant medications, including amitriptyline (Hershey et al., 2000); antihypertensive medications, including propranolol (Forsythe et al., 1984; Ludvigsson, 1974; Olness et al., 1987); antihistamine/antiserotonergic medications, including cyproheptadine (Levinstein, 1991); and antiepileptic medications including valproic acid (Apostol et al., 2008, 2009a, 2009b; Serdaroglu et al., 2002) and topiramate (Lakshmi et al., 2007; Lewis et al., 2009; Winner et al., 2005).

Additionally, neutriceuticals may also be effective in treating paediatric headaches. Coenzyme Q_{10} appears to be deficient in a significant number of children and adolescents with frequent headaches (Hershey et al., 2007; Slater et al., 2011). Supplementation was noted to be associated with improvement in headache frequency in this open-labelled clinic observation study. Other agents that are also considered include butterbur—77% of children having a 50% or greater reduction in headache frequency in an open-label study (Pothmann and Danesch, 2005), riboflavin (Bruijn et al., 2010; O'Brien and Hershey, 2010), and magnesium (F. Wang et al., 2003).

Biobehavioural

Biobehavioural therapy, or the incorporation of adherence, education, lifestyle adjustment, and coping skills, is also essential to the management of paediatric migraine (Powers and Andrasik, 2005). Educating the patient and family on the proper use of their acute and preventative medication with a discussion about the importance of treatment and inclusion of the child in the decision-making process may greatly improve the adherence to the treatment approach. Adherence assessment has not yet been well studied in paediatric migraine, but is being recognized as an important component of the management of children with chronic or episodic disorders.

Incorporation of healthy lifestyle habits is also important to effective headache management. This includes adequate hydration with limited use of caffeine-containing beverages; a healthy, balanced diet while avoiding skipping meals; regular exercise; and sufficient sleep on a regular basis. As already discussed, sleep disturbances have begun to be studied as a significant contributor to paediatric migraine and treatment of the disturbances needs to be included in the treatment plan.

In order to attain this treatment several different approaches have recently been reported. Using telephone-assisted behavioural therapy, there was a trend to improvement in 34 adolescents after a 3- and 8-month period (Cottrell et al., 2007). Another study has begun to address the feasibility of using a CD-ROM to teach this behavioural therapy (Connelly et al., 2006).

Tension-type headaches

TTHS are generally thought of as mild recurrent headaches. Other names for this type of headache have included muscle contraction headache, idiopathic headache, and tension headache. They can be infrequent (less than one a month), frequent (more than once a month, but not more than half the month), and chronic (more than half the month). The headache severity is usually described as mild to moderate with the location being diffuse or in a band-like pattern and have a pressing pain quality. Similar to migraine, TTH is a primary headache disorder, and secondary aetiologies should be identified and the patient should have a normal neurological examination and comprehensive headache examination. As a primary headache, the most difficult component of making the diagnosis of TTH is separating it from migraine. This is largely due to the overlapping diagnostic characteristics, especially in severity (TTH as mild to moderate, migraine as moderate to severe) and associated symptoms (the allowance of nausea, photophobia, or phonophobia in TTH, but not vomiting).

The ICHD-II (Headache Classification Subcommittee of the International Headache Society, 2004) identifies four subtypes of TTH: ICHD 2.1 infrequent episodic tension-type headache, ICHD 2.2 frequent episodic tension-type headache, ICHD 2.3 chronic tension-type headache, and ICHD 2.4 probable tension-type headache. These are further subclassified according to the presence or absence of pericranial tenderness.

Diagnosis

Establishing a diagnosis of TTH in children is often difficult due to a lack of recognition of the headache characteristics, either due to a misunderstanding of the questions asked by the interviewer or separating the features from migraine. This may be heightened in TTH due to the lack of disease impact and disability, such that the patient and parent may not attend to these features as readily as they do for migraine.

As TTHs are often mild, the patient and parent may be vague in their descriptions with the parents unaware of the frequency of the headaches, especially if mild. Using standardized criteria such as the ICHD-II criteria, is useful in the diagnosis of paediatric

headaches and can serve to guide the interview process. Children's headache diagnosis is further complicated by the shorter duration of the headaches with spontaneous resolution, or response to rest, sleep, or behavioural therapies. Due to these issues, it may be necessary to observe the child over time and utilize diaries to identify the diagnostic characteristics.

The typical features that separate TTH from migraine are a lack of throbbing or pulsatile quality of the pain, a diffuse location, a mild severity, and lack of significant associated symptoms. Some researchers have argued that TTH and migraine are in a continuum (Cady et al., 2002), while others have argued that these are separate diseases with a broad spectrum of headaches represented by migraine (Lipton et al., 2000). Until biomarkers are available, this debate and the diagnosis of these two primary disorders will continue to have an overlapping difficulty.

Epidemiology

In adults, TTHs are thought to be the most common type of primary headache disorder, with a lifetime prevalence ranging from 30% to 78%. Yet TTHs remain the least well studied of the primary headache disorders. This is likely due to their low severity and lack of impact on a patient's quality of life and disability.

In children, all headache disorders have been less well studied and this is especially true for TTH (reviewed by Anttila, 2006). Epidemiology rates of TTH in children have been variable and have ranged from 0.9% (Abu-Arafeh and Russell, 1994) to 73% (Barea et al., 1996), with the most frequent range reported as 10% to 25% (Anttila, 2006). Using ICHD-I criteria, TTH are reported in 9.8% of 7- to 16-year-olds in Sweden (Laurell et al., 2004) and 12% of 12-year-olds in Finland (Anttila et al., 2002a). In the study from Finland, many of the children diagnosed with TTH had migrainous features with lack of muscle tenderness in children with TTH (Anttila et al., 2002). Both of these studies demonstrated an increasing frequency of TTH in girls over boys during adolescence. As this is also seen in migraine, there remains the possibility of an overlapping evolution of the diagnosis from migraine to TTH and vice versa.

The epidemiological identification of TTH, however, is hampered by the lack of attention paid to these headache disorders, especially when infrequent. Therefore, population-based epidemiology studies may underestimate the prevalence of TTH due to a recall bias, while the inaccuracies of the recall of individual features may overestimate the misclassified TTH that should actually be considered migraine. Regardless of these limitations, both migraine and TTH are common pain problems for both children and adults.

Treatment

Once it has been determined that a patient has TTH, a management plan needs to be developed. As is the case for most headache treatment studies in children, no large-scale treatment studies have been performed with a focus on TTH in children. For adults, several large studies that meet standard study guidelines have been performed (reviewed by Fumal and Schoenen, 2008) and the same basic principles of migraine management can be applied to TTH management—acute therapy, preventative therapy, and biobehavioural therapy with psychological intervention.

Acute

Episodic TTH may be self-limited and may be managed with simple analgesics such as acetaminophen and NSAIDs—ibuprofen or naproxen sodium. Both of these groups of medicines have been demonstrated to be effective in migraine in children and, by implication, may also be useful in TTH in children.

In addition, as TTH may be mild, but become frequent, the patient and family should be cautioned about the overuse of acute medication and subsequent medication overuse. This may be a major contributor to chronic daily headache. Since a mild TTH with no disability is often treated at home without or with limited medical professional intervention, this needs to be addressed at the initial use of acute medication.

When these simple analgesics are ineffective, the diagnosis should be re-evaluated and a consideration of migraine or other primary headache treatment initiated. This can include the triptans or indomethacin and may unmask an indomethacin responsive primary headache.

Preventative

When the TTH become frequent, preventative therapies may become necessary, especially if disability occurs. This is often the trigger for parents to seek medical attention for their child. For adults, amitriptyline has been demonstrated to be useful for prophylaxis of chronic TTH (Bedsten et al., 1996; Gobel et al., 1994). The preventative treatment of TTH in children is lacking and often gets overlapped with the treatment of chronic migraine or chronic daily headache. In adults with chronic TTH, the combination of amitriptyline and cognitive therapy may be even more effective than either one by itself.

Biobehavioural

Biobehavioural therapy includes adherence therapy, lifestyle adjustments, and specific psychological interventions including biofeedback-assisted relaxation therapy (BART) (Bussone et al., 1998) and cognitive-behavioural therapy. In a school-based study for the treatment of childhood headaches including TTH, adolescents responded well to relaxation therapies (Larsson et al., 2005). In children with TTH, biobehavioural therapy has been demonstrated to have prolonged effects over 3 years (Grazzi et al., 2001) and may be comparable to amitriptyline (Grazzi et al., 2004).

Overall, the treatment plan needs to incorporate all three components to be successful. With time, the TTH may also evolve into migraine or other primary headaches disorders and the treatment plan further adjusted (Kienbacher et al., 2006).

Secondary headaches

Secondary headaches are frequently diagnosed in children. Oftentimes this is a misdiagnosis of a primary headache, but needs to be ruled out and treated when suspected. A thorough review of secondary headaches can be found in *The Headaches* (3rd edition; Olesen et al., 2006) or *Wolff's Headaches and Other Head Pain* (8th edition; Silberstein et al., 2008). The remainder of this chapter will highlight a few secondary headaches that can be seen in children.

Medical-systemic causes of headache

Secondary headaches can occur as a symptom of other medical problems or to primary neurological disorders. This can include infections, metabolic disorders, renal problems, mitochondrial disorders, increased blood pressure, and haematological disorders. When a patient has a known medical condition either the condition itself or the treatment may induce headaches. It must be kept in mind that patients with known medical problems are not protected from primary headaches and if there is not a direct cause and effect and variation with treatment, a diagnosis and management of a primary headache disorder should be considered.

Vascular disorders

Vascular disorders can frequently have a headache as one of their symptoms (Roach and Riela, 1995). This can be attributed to ischaemia, haemorrhage, or diseases of the blood vessels including malformations, arteritis, injury to the vessels (i.e. dissection or surgical intervention), thrombosis, or genetic diseases of the blood vessels (i.e. CADASIL (cerebral autosomal dominant arteriopathy with subcortical infarcts and leucoencephalopathy), mitochondrial encephalomyopathy, lactic acidosis, and stroke-like episodes (MELAS)). These disorders for the most part are rare in children, but should be considered when other symptoms are present.

Cerebrovascular disease in children is rare occurring at a rate of 2.5/100 000. Symptoms of acute neurological changes occur at the same time of the headache. This needs to be considered on the first presentation of hemiplegic migraine, even in the setting of a family history.

Haemorrhage may be secondary to rupture of a vascular malformation or aneurysm or secondary to trauma. The presenting symptom is most often an acute severe headache ('worst headache of my life') associated with loss of consciousness, meningismus and local neurological symptoms. An underlying neurocutaneous disorder should be sought. If this diagnosis is suspected, imaging will usually show the haemorrhage. Angiography or venography may delineate the specific aetiology.

Vasculitis is being reported with increased frequency in children and adolescents but remains uncommon. Headaches occur in 40% to 70% of patients with primary central nervous system (CNS) vasculitis. It may occur in the setting of an autoimmune disorder such as systemic lupus erythematosus, polyarteritis, Wegener's granulomatosis, and Sjögren's syndrome. Although headaches may uncommonly be the initial symptom, other systemic symptoms have usually preceded the headache. The headaches may resemble either chronic TTH or migraine and usually exacerbate when the underlying autoimmune disorder worsens. Other neurological symptoms may include behavioural changes, cognitive dysfunction, seizures, and focal deficits. An MRI and magnetic resonance angiogram may show abnormalities. Cerebrospinal fluid (CSF) may be abnormal. Angiography may be required.

Emboli and thrombosis may be idiopathic or secondary trauma, coagulation disorders, autoimmune disorders, and congenital heart disease. Conditions such as moyamoya disease, fibromuscular dysplasia, arterial dissection, tumour, trauma, sickle cell anaemia, haemophilia, and dehydration may also cause secondary vascular disease.

Venous sinus thrombosis may occur in the presence of an underlying metabolic or systemic infection, a coagulation disorder, or patients who are dehydrated. The patients may present with headache, altered consciousness, lethargy, focal neurological symptoms and seizures. The neurological examination is usually abnormal and the MRI, as well as the magnetic resonance venogram, may show the thrombosed vessel and/or haemorrhage secondary to venous thrombosis. Consideration should be given to this diagnosis in the presence of a coagulopathy, systemic malignancy, and/or chemotherapy.

Neoplasms

Intracranial tumours are the second most common type of neo-plasm in children (Honig, 1982). In children younger than 15 years, the incidence is 2.4/100 000. Certain genetic syndromes such as neurofibromatosis, tuberous sclerosis, von Hippel–Lindau disease, and ataxia telangiectasis pose a greater risk for the development of neoplasms.

The fear of a brain tumour is one of the major concerns of parents bringing their children to the physician for evaluation of headache. However, the prevalence of primary headaches far outweighs the frequency of tumour-related headaches. There is a clear association between brain tumours and headaches with the majority of brain tumour having headache as one of the presenting manifestations.

The headache due to a brain tumour is the result of increased intracranial pressure due to the mass effect of the tumour or a block-age of cerebral spinal fluid drainage. In addition, the effects of the brain tumour on the surrounding tissue also induce changes in the neurological examination or neurological symptoms (Lewis et al., 2002). Other symptoms of brain tumour include seizures, ataxia, weakness, visual abnormalities, lethargy, and personality change in the majority of such patients—the course will be progressive. The neurological examination will be abnormal and the diagnosis can be confirmed by neuroimaging.

Due to the continued growth of the tumour, the headache pat-tern is usually chronic, progressive, with increases in frequency and severity over time. The rapidity of the growth of the tumour and the adaptability of the intracranial space to respond to this growth can modify the timing of the headache's presentation. It is frequently reported to occur in the morning due to a 'ball-valve' effect in which the CSF pressure builds in the recumbent position and is relieved by posture—the opposite of idiopathic intracranial hypertension.

Substance-induced headache

Prescribed medications, illicit drugs, dietary compounds, and tox-ins can cause headaches (Silberstein et al., 1998). These substances may initiate a headache, exacerbate a pre-existing headache, or cause headache on its withdrawal. A through history of exposure to medications and non-medications needs to be performed and removal or alteration of these substances, if possible, may be neces-sary before the headache responds. Stimulants used in the treat-ment of attention-deficit disorder may initiate headache, especially if they are restarted at maximum dosage after not having been taken for several days to weeks. One common stimulant used in children and adults is caffeine and caffeine addiction and its withdrawal can contribute to headache and exacerbate primary headaches.

Medication overuse headache (MOH) can occur with overuse of over-the-counter analgesic medication or prescription medica-tions. This has formerly been referred to as analgesic rebound head-ache. It is often associated with a gradual increase in frequency of medications that were successful or partially successful in headache treatment. These medications are typically taken at low doses or with repeated doses building to very frequent usage—up to daily. ICHD-II defines medication overuse as using prescription medica-tions more than ten times per month or over-the-counter analgesics more than 15 times per month, increasing the likelihood of MOH. Almost all medications used for the acute treatment of migraine can potentially cause MOH. If MOH is thought to be a contributor

to the development of frequent headaches, they should be limited for 4 to 6 weeks. At that point they can be re-introduced, but at a limited frequency.

Infectious disorders

Systemic infectious disorders or those localized to the CNS are com-monly associated with headache. The presence of an elevated tem-perature and tachycardia alone frequently give rise to a pounding headache which is often relieved when the temperature is lowered and the infection is treated. Among the common infections seen are sinusitis, otitis media, and pharyngitis. Among the infections affect-ing the CNS are meningitis, aseptic meningitis, and encephalitis (Bale, 1999). Brain abscess is uncommon. It occurs more commonly in children with cyanotic congenital heart disease, open head trauma, chronic ear infections, chronic pulmonary disease, post-neurosurgical procedures, and in the immunocompromised patient.

In any CNS infection, in addition to symptoms of increased intracranial pressure or progressive neurological disease, mening-ismus, rash, or elevated temperature may be present. Initial evalu-ation should include a brain imaging procedure to rule out a mass lesion. If at all possible, this should be performed prior to any lum-bar puncture.

Conclusion

The majority of recurrent headaches in children and adolescents are primary headaches. Secondary headaches, however, occur due to systemic or CNS disease. The history and physical examination should help identify whether a headache is primary or secondary with appropriate laboratory tests and neuroimaging confirming the suspicion. Ultimately, the diagnosis of the secondary headache will be the resolution of the headache once the secondary cause has been effectively treated, while persistence of recurrent headaches without the secondary cause helps confirm the diagnosis and man-agement of primary headaches.

References

Abu-Arafeh, I. and Russell, G. (1994). Prevalence of headache and migraine in schoolchildren. *Br Med J*, 309, 765–769.

Ahonen, K., Hamalainen, M. L., Eerola, M., and Hoppu, K. (2006). A randomized trial of rizatriptan in migraine attacks in children. *Neurology*, 67(7), 1135–1140.

Anttila, P. (2006). Tension-type headache in childhood and adolescence. *Lancet Neurol*, 5(3), 268–274.

Anttila, P., Metsahonkala, L., Aromaa, M., Sourander, A., Salminen, J., Helenius, H., *et al.* (2002a). Determinants of tension-type headache in children. *Cephalalgia*, 22(5), 401–408.

Anttila, P., Metsahonkala, L., Mikkelsson, M., Aromaa, M., Kautiainen, H., Salminen, J., *et al.* (2002b). Muscle tenderness in pericranial and neck-shoulder region in children with headache. A controlled study. *Cephalalgia*. 22(5), 340–344.

Apostol, G., Cady, R. K., Laforet, G. A., Robieson, W. Z., Olson, E., Abi-Saab, W. M., *et al.* (2008). Divalproex extended-release in adolescent migraine prophylaxis: results of a randomized, double-blind, placebo-controlled study. *Headache*, 48(7), 1012–1025.

Apostol, G., Lewis, D. W., Laforet, G. A., Robieson, W. Z., Fugate, J. M., Abi-Saab, W. M., *et al.* (2009a). Divalproex sodium extended-release for the prophylaxis of migraine headache in adolescents: results of a stand-alone, long-term open-label safety study. *Headache*, 49(1), 45–53.

Apostol, G., Pakalnis, A., Laforet, G. A., Robieson, W. Z., Olson, E., Abi-Saab, W. M., *et al.* (2009b). Safety and tolerability of divalproex sodium extended-release in the prophylaxis of migraine headaches: results of an open-label extension trial in adolescents. *Headache*, 49(1), 36–44.

Ashkenazi, A., Silberstein, S., Jakubowski, M., and Burstein, R. (2007). Improved identification of allodynic migraine patients using a questionnaire. *Cephalalgia*, 27(4), 325–329.

Bale, J. F. Jr. (1999). Human herpesviruses and neurological disorders of childhood. *Semin Pediatr Neurol*, 6(4), 278–287.

Barea, J. M., Tannhauser, M., and Rotta, N. T. (1996). An epidemiologic study of headache among children and adolescents of southern Brazil. *Cephalalgia*, 16, 545–549.

Bedsten, L., Jensen, R., and Olesen, J. (1996). A non-selective (amitriptyline), but not a selective (citalopram), serotonin reuptake inhibitor is effective in the prophylactic treatment of chronic tension-type headache. *J Neurol Neurosurg Psychiatry*, 61, 285–290.

Bigal, M. E., Ashina, S., Burstein, R., Reed, M. L., Buse, D., Serrano, D., et al. (2008). Prevalence and characteristics of allodynia in headache sufferers: a population study. *Neurology*, 70(17), 1525–1533.

Bille, B. (1962). Migraine in school children. *Acta Paediatr*, 51(suppl. 136), 16–151.

Bockowski, L., Sobaniec, W., and Zelazowska-Rutkowska, B. (2009). Proinflammatory plasma cytokines in children with migraine. *Pediatr Neurol*, 41(1), 17–21.

Brandes, J. L., Kudrow, D., Stark, S. R., O'Carroll, C. P., Adelman, J. U., O'Donnell, F. J., et al. (2007). Sumatriptan-naproxen for acute treatment of migraine: a randomized trial. *JAMA*, 297(13), 1443–1454.

Bruijn, J., Duivenvoorden, H., Passchier, J., Locher, H., Dijkstra, N., and Arts, W. F. (2010). Medium-dose riboflavin as a prophylactic agent in children with migraine: a preliminary placebo-controlled, randomised, double-blind, cross-over trial. *Cephalalgia*, 30(12), 1426–1434.

Bruni, O., Febrizi, P., Ottaviano, S., Cortesi, F., Giannotti, F., and Guidetti, V. (1997). Prevalence of sleep disorders in childhood and adolescence with headache: a case-control study. *Cephalalgia*, 1997, 17, 492–498.

Bruni, O., Russo, P. M., Ferri, R., Novelli, L., Galli, F., and Guidetti, V. (2008). Relationships between headache and sleep in a non-clinical population of children and adolescents. *Sleep Med*, 9(5), 542–548.

Burstein, R. and Cutrer, F. M. (2000). The development of cutaneous allodynia during a migraine attack: clinical evidence for the sequential recruitment of spinal and supraspinal nociceptive neurons in migraine. *Brain*, 123, 1703–1709.

Burstein, R. and Jakubowski, M. (2004). Analgesic triptan action in an animal model of intracranial pain: a race against the development of central sensitization. *Ann Neurol*, 55(1), 27–36.

Burstein, R., Collins, B., and Jakubowski, M. (2004). Defeating migraine pain with triptans: a race against the development of cutaneous allodynia. *Ann Neurol*, 55(1), 19–26.

Burstein, R., Levy, D., and Jakubowski, M. (2005). Effects of sensitization of trigeminovascular neurons to triptan therapy during migraine. *Rev Neurol (Paris)*, 161(6–7), 658–660.

Burstein, R., Yarnitsky, D., Goor-Aryeh, I., Ransil, B. J., and Bajwa, Z. H. (2000). An association between migraine and cutaneous allodynia. *Ann Neurol*, 47(5), 614–624.

Bussone, G., Grazzi, L., D'Amico, D., Leone, M., and Andrasik, F. (1998). Biofeedback-assisted relaxation training for young adolescents with tension-type headache: a controlled study. *Cephalalgia*, 18, 463–467.

Cady, R. K., and Schreiber, C. P. (2004). Sinus headache: a clinical conundrum. *Otolaryngol Clin North Am*, 37(2), 267–288.

Cady, R., Schreiber, C., Farmer, K., and Sheftell, F. (2002). Primary headaches: a convergence hypothesis. *Headache*, 42, 204–216.

Conicella, E., Raucci, U., Vanacore, N., Vigevano, F., Reale, A., Pirozzi, N., et al. (2008). The child with headache in a pediatric emergency department. *Headache*, 48(7), 1005–1011.

Connelly, M., Rapoff, M. A., Thompson, N., and Connelly, W. (2006). Headstrong: a pilot study of a CD-ROM intervention for recurrent pediatric headache. *J Pediatr Psychol*, 31(7), 737–747.

Cottrell, C., Drew, J., Gibson, J., Holroyd, K., and O'Donnell, F. (2007). Feasibility assessment of telephone-administered behavioral treatment for adolescent migraine. *Headache*, 47(9), 1293–1302.

Crawford, M. J., Lehman, L., Slater, S., Kabbouche, M. A., Lecates, S. L., Segers, A., et al. (2009). Menstrual migraine in adolescents. *Headache*, 49(3), 341–347.

Cuvellier, J. C., Fily, A., Joriot, S., Cuisset, J. M., and Vallee, L. (2007). French general practitioners' management of children's migraine headaches. *Headache*, 47(9), 1282–1292.

De Fusco, M., Marconi, R., Silvestri, L., Atorino, L., Rampoldi, L., Morgante, L., et al. (2003). Haploinsufficiency of ATP1A2 encoding the Na^+/K^+ pump alpha2 subunit associated with familial hemiplegic migraine type 2. *Nat Genet*, 33(2), 192–196.

De Marinis, M., Pujia, A., Natale, L., D'Arcangelo, E., and Accornero, N. (2003). Decreased habituation of the R2 component of the blink reflex in migraine patients. *Clin Neurophysiol*, 114(5), 889–893.

Dichgans, M., Freilinger, T., Eckstein, G., Babini, E., Lorenz-Depiereux, B., Biskup, S., et al. (2005). Mutation in the neuronal voltage-gated sodium channel SCN1A in familial hemiplegic migraine. *Lancet*, 366(9483), 371–377.

Eidlitz-Markus, T., Shuper, A., Gorali, O., and Zeharia, A. (2007). Migraine and cephalic cutaneous allodynia in pediatric patients. *Headache*, 47(8), 1219–1223.

Evers, S., Marziniak, M., Frese, A., and Gralow, I. (2009). Placebo efficacy in childhood and adolescence migraine: an analysis of double-blind and placebo-controlled studies. *Cephalalgia*, 29(4), 436–444.

Fan, P. C., Kuo, P. H., Chang, S. H., Lee, W. T., Wu, R. M., and Chiou, L. C. (2009). Plasma calcitonin gene-related peptide in diagnosing and predicting paediatric migraine. *Cephalalgia*, 29(8), 883–890.

Fernandes, R., Ferreira, J. J., and Sampaio, C. The placebo response in studies of acute migraine. *J Pediatr*, 152(4), 527–533, 33.e1.

Forsythe, W. I., Gillies, D., and Sills, M. A. (1984). Propanolol ('Inderal') in the treatment of childhood migraine, *Dev Med Child Neurol*. 26(6), 737–741.

Fujita, M., Fujiwara, J., Maki, T., Shibasaki, K., Shigeta, M., and Nii, J. (2009). Pediatric chronic daily headache associated with school phobia. *Pediatr Int*, 51(5), 621–625.

Fumal, A. and Schoenen, J. (2008). Tension-type headache: current research and clinical management. *Lancet Neurol*, 7(1), 70–83.

Gilman, D., Palermo, T. M., Kabbouche, M. A., Hershey, A. D., and Powers, S. W. (2007). Primary headache and sleep disturbances in adolescents. *Headache*, 47(8), 1189–1194.

Gobel, H., Hamouz, V., Hansen, C., Heininger, K., Hirsch, S., Lindner, V., et al. (1994). Chronic tension-type headache: amitriptyline reduces clinical headache-duration and experimental pain sensitivity but does not alter pericranial muscle activity readings. *Pain*, 59, 241–249.

Grazzi, L., Andrasik, F., D'Amico, D., Leone, M., Moschiano, F., and Bussone, G. (2001). Electromyographic biofeedback-assisted relaxation training in juvenile episodic tension-type headache: clinical outcome at three-year follow-up. *Cephalalgia*, 21(8), 798–803.

Grazzi, L., Andrasik, F., Usai, S., D'Amico, D., and Bussone, G. (2004). Pharmacological behavioural treatment for children and adolescents with tension-type headache: preliminary data. *Neurol Sci*, 25(Suppl 3), S270–271.

Gurkan, F., Ece, A., Haspolat, K., and Dikici, B. (2000). Parental history of migraine and bronchial asthma in children. *Allergol Immunopathol (Madr)*, 28(1), 15–17.

Headache Classification Subcommittee of the International Headache Society. (2004). The International Classification of Headache Disorders. *Cephalalgia*, 24(Supplement 1), 1–160.

Hershey, A. D. (2007). Genetics of migraine headache in children. *Curr Pain Headache Rep*, 11(5), 390–395.

Hershey, A. D., Powers, S. W., Bentti, A. L., and Degrauw, T. J. (2000). Effectiveness of amitriptyline in the prophylactic management of childhood headaches. *Headache*, 40(7), 539–549.

Hershey, A. D., Powers, S. W., Bentti, A.-L., and deGrauw, T. J. (1999). Standardized dosing of amitriptyline is highly effective in a pediatric headache center population. *Headache*, 39, 357–358.

Hershey, A. D., Powers, S. W., Nelson, T. D., Kabbouche, M. A., Winner, P., Yonker, M., *et al.* (2009). Obesity in the pediatric headache population: a multicenter study. *Headache*, 49(2), 170–177.

Hershey, A. D., Powers, S. W., Vockell, A. L., Lecates, S. L., Ellinor, P. L., Segers, A., *et al.* (2007). Coenzyme Q10 deficiency and response to supplementation in pediatric and adolescent migraine. *Headache*, 47(1), 73–80.

Hershey, A. D., Powers, S. W., Vockell, A. L., LeCates, S. L., Segers, A., and Kabbouche, M. A. (2004). Development of a patient-based grading scale for PedMIDAS. *Cephalalgia*, 24(10), 844–849.

Hershey, A. D., Powers, S. W., Vockell, A. L., LeCates, S., Kabbouche, M. A., and Maynard, M. K. (2001). PedMIDAS: development of a questionnaire to assess disability of migraines in children. *Neurology*, 57(11), 2034–2039.

Hershey, A. D., Winner, P., Kabbouche, M. A., Gladstein, J., Yonker, M., Lewis, D., *et al.* (2005). Use of the ICHD-II criteria in the diagnosis of pediatric migraine. *Headache*, 45(10), 1288–1297.

Honig, P. J., and Charney, E. B. (1982). Children with brain tumor headaches. Distinguishing features. *Am J Dis Child*, 136(2), 121–124.

Isik, U., Ersu, R. H., Ay, P., Save, D., Arman, A. R., Karakoc, F., *et al.* (2007). Prevalence of headache and its association with sleep disorders in children. *Pediatr Neurol*, 36(3), 146–151.

Isik, U., Topuzoglu, A., Ay, P., Ersu, R. H., Arman, A. R., Onsuz, M. F., *et al.* (2009). The prevalence of headache and its association with socioeconomic status among schoolchildren Instanbul, Turkey. *Headache*, 49(5), 697–703.

Jakubowski, M., Levy, D., Goor-Aryeh, I., Collins, B., Bajwa, Z., and Burstein, R. (2005). Terminating migraine with allodynia and ongoing central sensitization using parenteral administration of COX1/COX2 inhibitors. *Headache*, 45(7), 850–861.

Jakubowski, M., Silberstein, S., Ashkenazi, A., and Burstein, R. (2005). Can allodynic migraine patients be identified interictally using a questionnaire? *Neurology*, 65(9), 1419–1422.

Kabbouche, M. A., and Linder, S. L. (2005). Acute treatment of pediatric headache in the emergency department and inpatient settings. *Pediatr Ann*, 34(6), 466–471.

Kabbouche, M. A., Powers, S. W., Segers, A., LeCates, S., Manning, P., Biederman, S., *et al.* (2009). Inpatient treatment of status migraine with dihydroergotamine in children and adolescents. *Headache*, 49(1), 106–109.

Kabbouche, M. A., Vockell, A. L., LeCates, S. L., Powers, S. W., and Hershey, A. D. (2001). Tolerability and effectiveness of prochlorperazine for intractable migraine in children. *Pediatrics*, 107(4), E62.

Katsarava, Z., Giffin, N., Diener, H. C., and Kaube, H. (2003). Abnormal habituation of 'nociceptive' blink reflex in migraine—evidence for increased excitability of trigeminal nociception. *Cephalalgia*, 23(8), 814–819.

Katsarava, Z., Lehnerdt, G., Duda, B., Ellrich, J., Diener, H. C., and Kaube, H. (2002). Sensitization of trigeminal nociception specific for migraine but not pain of sinusitis. *Neurology*, 59(9), 1450–1453.

Kaube, H., Katsarava, Z., Przywara, S., Drepper, J., Ellrich, J., and Diener, H. C. (2002). Acute migraine headache: possible sensitization of neurons in the spinal trigeminal nucleus? *Neurology*, 58(8), 1234–1248.

Kernick, D., and Campbell, J. (2009). Measuring the impact of headache in children: a critical review of the literature. *Cephalalgia*, 29(1), 3–16.

Khurana Hershey, G., Stevenson, M., Grube, E., and Hershey, A. (2005). Characterization of headache presenting to a tertiary allergy clinic. *Cephalalgia*, 25(10), 1004.

Kienbacher, C., Wober, C., Zesch, H. E., Hafferl-Gattermayer, A., Posch, M., Karwautz, A., *et al.* (2006). Clinical features, classification and prognosis of migraine and tension-type headache in children and adolescents: a long-term follow-up study. *Cephalalgia*, 26(7), 820–830.

Korostenskaja, M., Pardos, M., Kujala, T., Rose, D. F., Brown, D., Horn, P., *et al.* (2011). Impaired auditory information processing during acute migraine: a magnetoencephalography study. *Int J Neurosci*, 121(7), 355–365.

Kroner-Herwig, B. and Vath, N. (2009). Menarche in girls and headache—a longitudinal analysis. *Headache*, 49(6), 860–867.

Kroner-Herwig, B., Morris, L., and Heinrich, M. (2008). Biopsychosocial correlates of headache: what predicts pediatric headache occurrence? *Headache*, 48(4), 529–544.

Kroner-Herwig, B., Morris, L., Heinrich, M., Gassmann, J., and Vath, N. (2009). Agreement of parents and children on characteristics of pediatric headache, other pains, somatic symptoms, and depressive symptoms in an epidemiologic study. *Clin J Pain*, 25(1), 58–64.

Ku, M., Silverman, B., Prifti, N., Ying, W., Persaud, Y., and Schneider, A. (2006). Prevalence of migraine headaches in patients with allergic rhinitis. *Ann Allergy Asthma Immunol*, 97(2), 226–230.

Lakshmi, C. V., Singhi, P., Malhi, P., and Ray, M. (2007). Topiramate in the prophylaxis of pediatric migraine: a double-blind placebo-controlled trial. *J Child Neurol*, 22(7), 829–835.

Larsson, B., Carlsson, J., Fichtel, A., and Melin, L. (2005). Relaxation treatment of adolescent headache sufferers: results from a school-based replication series. *Headache*, 45(6), 692–704.

Laurell, K., Larsson, B., and Eeg-Olofsson, O. (2004). Prevalence of headache in Swedish schoolchildren, with a focus on tension-type headache. *Cephalalgia*, 24(5), 380–388.

Levinstein, B. (1991). A comparative study of cyproheptadine, amitriptyline, and propranolol in the treatment of adolescent migraine. *Cephalalgia*, 11, 122–123.

Lewis, D. W., Ashwal, S., Dahl, G., Dorbad, D., Hirtz, D., Prensky, A., *et al.* (2002). Practice parameter: evaluation of children and adolescents with recurrent headaches: report of the Quality Standards Subcommittee of the American Academy of Neurology and the Practice Committee of the Child Neurology Society. *Neurology*, 59(4), 490–498.

Lewis, D. W., Winner. P., Hershey, A. D., and Wasiewski, W. W. (2007). Efficacy of zolmitriptan nasal spray in adolescent migraine. *Pediatrics*, 120(2), 390–396.

Lewis, D., Ashwal, S., Hershey, A., Hirtz, D., Yonker, M., and Silberstein, S. (2004). Practice Parameter: pharmacological treatment of migraine headache in children and adolescents: Report of the American Academy of Neurology Quality Standards Subcommittee and the Practice Committee of the Child Neurology Society. *Neurology*, 63(12), 2215–2224.

Lewis, D., Winner, P., Saper, J., Ness, S., Polverejan, E., Wang, S., *et al.* (2009). Randomized, double-blind, placebo-controlled study to evaluate the efficacy and safety of topiramate for migraine prevention in pediatric subjects 12 to 17 years of age. *Pediatrics*, 123(3), 924–934.

Lima, M. M., Padula, N. A., Santos, L. C., Oliveira, L. D., Agapejev, S., Padovani, C. (2005). Critical analysis of the international classification of headache disorders diagnostic criteria (ICHD I-1988) and (ICHD II-2004), for migraine in children and adolescents. *Cephalalgia*, 25(11), 1042–1047.

Linder, S. L. (2005). Understanding the comprehensive pediatric headache examination. *Pediatr Ann*, 34(6), 442–446.

Linder, S. L., Mathew, N. T., Cady, R. K., Finlayson, G., Ishkanian, G., and Lewis, D. W. (2008). Efficacy and tolerability of almotriptan in adolescents: a randomized, double-blind, placebo-controlled trial. *Headache*, 48(9), 1326–1336.

Lipton, R. B., Stewart, W. F., Cady, R., Hall, C., O'Quinn, S., Kuhn, T., *et al.* (2000). Sumatriptan for the range of headaches in migraine sufferers: results of the Spectrum Study. *Headache*, 40, 783–791.

Luc, M. E., Gupta, A., Birnberg, J. M., Reddick, D., and Kohrman, M. H. (2006). Characterization of symptoms of sleep disorders in children with headache. *Pediatr Neurol*, 34(1), 7–12.

Ludvigsson, J. (1974). Propranolol used in prophylaxis of migraine in children. *Acta Neurol Scand*, 50, 109–115.

Martin, V. T., and Behbehani, M. (2006a). Ovarian hormones and migraine headache: understanding mechanisms and pathogenesis—part 2. *Headache*, 46(3), 365–386.

Martin, V. T., and Behbehani, M. (2006b). Ovarian hormones and migraine headache: understanding mechanisms and pathogenesis—part I. *Headache*, 46(1), 3–23.

Mathew, N. T., Kailasam, J., and Seifert, T. (2004). Clinical recognition of allodynia in migraine. *Neurology*, 63(5), 848–852.

Miller, V. A., Palermo, T. M., Powers, S. W., Scher, M. S., and Hershey, A. D. (2003). Migraine headaches and sleep disturbances in children. *Headache*, 43(4), 362–368.

O'Brien, H. L., and Hershey, A. D. (2010). Vitamins and paediatric migraine: riboflavin as a preventative medication. *Cephalalgia*, 30(12), 1417–1418.

Olesen, J., Goadsby, P., Ramadan, N., Tfelt-Hansen, P., and Welch, K. (2006). *The headaches* (3rd edn). Philadelphia, PA: Lippincott, Williams & Wilkins.

Olness, K., MacDonald, J. T., and Uden, D. L. (1987). Comparison of self-hypnosis and propranolol in the treatment of juvenile classic migraine. *Pediatrics*, 79(4), 593–597.

Ophoff, R. A., Terwindt, G. M., Vergouwe, M. N., van Eijk, R., Oefner, P. H., Hoffman, M. G., et al. (1996). Familial hemiplegic migraine and episodic ataxia type-2 are caused by mutations in the Ca^{2+} channel gene CACNL1A4. *Cell*, 87, 544–552.

Pakalnis, A., Butz, C., Splaingard, D., Kring, D., and Fong, J. (2007). Emotional problems and prevalence of medication overuse in pediatric chronic daily headache. *J Child Neurol*, 22(12), 1356–1359.

Pakalnis, A., Splaingard, M., Splaingard, D., Kring, D., and Colvin, A. (2009). Serotonin effects on sleep and emotional disorders in adolescent migraine. *Headache*, 49(10), 1486–1492.

Pellock, J. M. (2004). Understanding co-morbidities affecting children with epilepsy. *Neurology*, 62(5 Suppl 2), S17–23.

Piccinelli, P., Borgatti, R., Nicoli, F., Calcagno, P., Bassi, M. T., Quadrelli, M., et al. (2006). Relationship between migraine and epilepsy in pediatric age. *Headache*, 46(3), 413–421.

Pinhas-Hamiel, O., Frumin, K., Gabis, L., Mazor-Aronovich, K., Modan-Moses, D., Reichman, B., et al. (2008). Headaches in overweight children and adolescents referred to a tertiary-care center in Israel. *Obesity*, 16(3), 659–663.

Pothmann, R., and Danesch, U. (2005). Migraine prevention in children and adolescents: results of an open study with a special butterbur root extract. *Headache*, 45(3), 196–203.

Powers, S. W., and Andrasik, F. (2005). Biobehavioral treatment, disability, and psychological effects of pediatric headache. *Pediatr Ann*, 34(6), 461–465.

Powers, S. W., Gilman, D. K., and Hershey, A. D. (2006). Headache and psychological functioning in children and adolescents. *Headache*, 46(9), 1404–1415.

Powers, S. W., Patton, S. R., Hommel, K. A., and Hershey, A. D. (2003). Quality of life in childhood migraines: clinical impact and comparison to other chronic illnesses. *Pediatrics*, 112(1 Pt 1), e1–5.

Powers, S. W., Patton, S. R., Hommel, K. A., and Hershey, A. D. (2004). Quality of life in paediatric migraine: characterization of age-related effects using PedsQL 4.0. *Cephalalgia*, 24(2), 120–127.

Richer, L., Graham, L., Klassen, T., and Rowe, B. (2007). Emergency department management of acute migraine in children in Canada: a practice variation study. *Headache*, 47(5), 703–710.

Roach, E. and Riela, A. (1995). *Pediatric cerebrovascular disorders* (2nd edn). New York: Futura.

Rossi, L. N., Vajani, S., Cortinovis, I., Spreafico, F., and Menegazzo, L. (2008). Analysis of the International Classification of Headache Disorders for diagnosis of migraine and tension-type headache in children. *Dev Med Child Neurol*, 50(4), 305–310.

Ruangsuwan, S., and Sriudomkajorn, S. (2007). 375 childhood primary headache: clinical features, the agreement between clinical diagnosis and diagnoses using the international classification of headache disorders in Thai children. *J Med Assoc Thai*, 90(7), 1309–1316.

Scagni, P. and Pagliero, R. (2008). Headache in an Italian pediatric emergency department. *J Headache Pain*, 9(2), 83–87.

Schreiber, C. P., Hutchinson, S., Webster, C. J., Ames, M., Richardson, M. S., and Powers, C. (2004). Prevalence of migraine in patients with a history of self-reported or physician-diagnosed 'sinus' headache. *Arch Intern Med*, 164(16), 1769–1772.

Serdaroglu, G., Erhan, E., Tekgul, H., Oksel, F., Erermis, S., Uyar, M., et al. (2002). Sodium valproate prophylaxis in childhood migraine. *Headache*, 42(8), 819–822.

Silberstein, S., Lipton, R., and Dodick, D. (2008). *Wolff's headaches and other head pain* (8th edn). New York: Oxford University Press.

Silberstein, S. D., Lipton, R. B., and Goadsby, P. J. (1998). *Headache in clinical practice*. Oxford: Isis Medical Media, Ltd.

Siniatchkin, M., Kropp, P., and Gerber, W. D. (2003). What kind of habituation is impaired in migraine patients? *Cephalalgia*, 23(7), 511–518.

Slater, S. K., Nelson, T. D., Kabbouche, M. A., Lecates, S. L., Horn, P., Segers, A., et al. (2011). A randomized, double-blinded, placebo-controlled, crossover, add-on study of CoEnzyme Q10 in the prevention of pediatric and adolescent migraine. *Cephalalgia*, 31(8), 897–905.

Smith, T. R., Sunshine, A., Stark, S. R., Littlefield, D. E., Spruill, S. E., and Alexander, W. J. (2005). Sumatriptan and naproxen sodium for the acute treatment of migraine. *Headache*, 45(8), 983–991.

Split, W. and Neuman, W. (1999). Epidemiology of migraine among students from randomly selected secondary schools in Lodz. *Headache*, 39, 494–501.

Stafstrom, C. E., Goldenholz, S. R., and Dulli, D. A. (2005). Serial headache drawings by children with migraine: correlation with clinical headache status. *J Child Neurol*, 20(10), 809–813.

Stafstrom, C. E., Rostasy, K., and Minster, A. (2002). The usefulness of children's drawings in the diagnosis of headache. *Pediatrics*, 109(3), 460–472.

Stevenson, S. B. (2006). Epilepsy and migraine headache: is there a connection? *J Pediatr Health Care*, 20(3), 167–171.

Terwindt, G. M., Ophoff, R. A., Haan, J., Vergouwe, M. N., van Eijk, R., Frants, R. R., et al. (1998). Variable clinical expression of mutations in the P/Q-type calcium channel gene in familial hemiplegic migraine. *Neurology*, 50, 1105–1110.

Unalp, A., Dirik, E., and Kurul, S. (2007). Prevalence and clinical findings of migraine and tension-type headache in adolescents. *Pediatr Int*, 49(6), 943–949.

Unay, B., Ulas, U. H., Karaoglu, B., Eroglu, E., Akin, R., and Gokcay, E. (2008). Visual and brainstem auditory evoked potentials in children with headache. *Pediatr Int*, 50(5), 620–623.

Valentinis, L., Valent, F., Mucchiut, M., Barbone, F., Bergonzi, P., and Zanchin, G. (2009). Migraine in adolescents: validation of a screening questionnaire. *Headache*, 49(2), 202–211.

Valeriani, M., Galli, F., Tarantino, S., Graceffa, D., Pignata, E., Miliucci, R., et al. (2009). Correlation between abnormal brain excitability and emotional symptomatology in paediatric migraine. *Cephalalgia*, 29(2), 204–213.

Van de Ven, R. C., Kaja, S., Plomp, J. J., Frants, R. R., van den Maagdenberg, A. M., and Ferrari, M. D. (2007). Genetic models of migraine. *Arch Neurol*, 64(5), 643–646.

Vanmolkot, K. R., Kors, E. E., Hottenga, J. J., Terwindt, G. M., Haan, J., Hoefnagels, W. A., et al. (2003). Novel mutations in the Na^+, K^+-ATPase pump gene ATP1A2 associated with familial hemiplegic migraine and benign familial infantile convulsions. *Ann Neurol*, 54(3), 360–366.

Vannatta, K., Getzoff, E. A., Gilman, D. K., Noll, R. B., Gerhardt, C. A., Powers, S.W., et al. (2008). Friendships and social interactions of school-aged children with migraine. *Cephalalgia*, 28(7), 734–743.

Vannatta, K., Getzoff, E. A., Powers, S. W., Noll, R. B., Gerhardt, C. A., and Hershey, A. D. (2008). Multiple perspectives on the psychological functioning of children with and without migraine. *Headache*, 48(7), 994–1004.

Varni, J. W., Seid, M., and Kurtin, P. S. (2001). PedsQL 4.0: reliability and validity of the Pediatric Quality of Life Inventory version 4.0 generic core scales in healthy and patient populations. *Med Care*, 39(8), 800–812.

Vollono, C., Ferraro, D., Miliucci, R., Vigevano, F., and Valeriani, M. (2010). The abnormal recovery cycle of somatosensory evoked potential components in children with migraine can be reversed by topiramate. *Cephalalgia*, 30(1), 17–26.

Walker, D. M., and Teach, S. J. (2008). Emergency department treatment of primary headaches in children and adolescents. *Curr Opin Pediatr*, 20(3), 248–254.

Wang, F., Van Den Eeden, S. K., Ackerson, L. M., Salk, S. E., Reince, R. H., and Elin, R. J. (2003). Oral magnesium oxide prophylaxis of frequent migrainous headache in children: a randomized, double-blind, placebo-controlled trial. *Headache*, 43(6), 601–610.

Wang, S. J., Fuh, J. L., Juang, K. D., and Lu, S. R. (2009). Migraine and suicidal ideation in adolescents aged 13 to 15 years. *Neurology*, 72(13), 1146–1152.

Wang, W., and Schoenen, J. (1998). Interictal potentiation of passive 'oddball' auditory event-related potentials in migraine. *Cephalalgia*, 18(5), 261–265.

Wessman, M., Terwindt, G. M., Kaunisto, M. A., Palotie, A., and Ophoff, R. A. (2007). Migraine: a complex genetic disorder. *Lancet Neurol*, 6(6), 521–532.

Winner, P. and Hershey, A. D. (2007). Epidemiology and diagnosis of migraine in children. *Curr Pain Headache Rep*, 11(5), 375–382.

Winner, P., Pearlman, E. M., Linder, S. L., Jordan, D. M., Fisher, A. C., and Hulihan, J. (2005). Topiramate for migraine prevention in children: a randomized, double-blind, placebo-controlled trial. *Headache*, 45(10), 1304–1312.

Wojaczynska-Stanek, K., Koprowski, R., Wrobel, Z., and Gola, M. (2008). Headache in children's drawings. *J Child Neurol*, 23(2), 184–191.

Yamane, L. E., Montenegro, M. A., and Guerreiro, M. M. (2004). Comorbidity headache and epilepsy in childhood. *Neuropediatrics*, 35(2), 99–102.

CHAPTER 32

Persisting pain in childhood medical illness

Martha Mherekumombe and John J. Collins

Summary

Persisting pain in the context of medical illness has been recognized recently as a global problem by the World Health Organization (WHO, 2012). Whilst the epidemiology of medical illness varies throughout the world, the general principles of pain management are applicable to most medical illnesses in children and are effective. Successful pain management for most children is contingent on the availability of the WHO model list of essential medicines for children (WHO, 2011), although regrettably not all medicines are available in every country in the world.

Introduction

Pain is commonly experienced by children in the context of medical illness. This may be due to acute or short-lived pain related to procedures for diagnostic, treatment, or surgical interventions. Persisting pain refers to any long-term pain and medical illnesses refers to specific situations of ongoing tissue damage where there is a clear role for pharmacological treatment. Persisting pain in childhood illness implies the duration of pain is lasting beyond what would be expected from an acute injury. This latter is currently the subject of a WHO initiative to improve management of persisting pain in children due to medical illness (WHO, 2012). This chapter discusses persisting pain in the context of non-malignant disease (HIV/AIDS, cystic fibrosis, neurofibromatosis, neuromuscular disease, cerebral palsy) and confines itself to a discussion of pharmacological management. The reader is referred to other sections of this book for the issues and management of persisting pain due to other conditions and for non-pharmacological strategies for pain management.

The pharmacological management of persisting pain in children with non-malignant illnesses

The principles of pain management in the context of paediatric medical illness are broadly applicable to most disease processes. The correct use of analgesic medicines will relieve pain in most children with persisting pain due to medical illness and relies on the following key concepts (Box 32.1):

- The availability of medicines on the WHO model list of essential medicines for children (WHO, 2011b).

- Using a two-step strategy for analgesic prescription: simple analgesics for mild pain (step 1), opioids for moderate to severe pain (step 2).

- Dosing of analgesics at regular intervals when pain is constant ('by the clock'). It is also recommended that children with persisting pain have medicines available for breakthrough pain. As there is insufficient evidence to recommend a particular opioid or route of administration for breakthrough pain in children, there is a need to make an appropriate choice of treatment modality based on clinical judgement, medicine availability, pharmacological considerations, and patient related factors.

- Using the simplest route of administration and avoiding the intramuscular route ('by the mouth'). The choice of alternative routes of administration when the oral route is not possible should be based on clinical judgement, availability, feasibility, and patient preference.

- Tailoring treatment to the individual child ('by the individual').

Among other WHO recommendations, paracetamol and ibuprofen are the medicines of choice in the first step (mild pain) and morphine is recommended as the first-line strong opioid for the treatment of persisting moderate to severe pain in children with medical illnesses. The selection of alternative opioid analgesics to morphine should be guided by considerations of safety, availability, cost, and suitability, including patient-related factors. Switching opioids and/or route of administration in children is recommended in the presence of inadequate analgesic effect with intolerable side effects. Routine rotation of opioids is not recommended (WHO, 2012).

Opioids for the management of non-malignant pain in childhood

Data on the management of severe pain using opioids in children with non-malignant disease is limited. One retrospective review studied opioid prescription for chronic severe non-malignant pain in a multidisciplinary paediatric pain clinic. During a 12-month period, 104 patients were seen in the clinic, of which 49 received an opioid as part of their pain management; 11 received an opioid for more than 3 months, and five of these were still receiving an opioid at the end of the study period. Overall, there appeared to be better

Box 32.1 WHO key concepts: the pain management of persisting pain in children with medical illness

1. Using a two-step strategy for analgesic prescription, simple analgesics for mild pain (step 1), opioids for moderate to severe pain (step 2).

2. Dosing at regular intervals when pain is constant ('by the clock'). It is also recommended that children with persisting pain have medicines available for breakthrough pain.

3. Using the simplest route of administration ('by the mouth') and avoiding the intramuscular route. The choice of alternative routes of administration when the oral route is not possible should be based on clinical judgement, availability, feasibility, and patient preference.

4. Tailoring treatment to the individual child ('by the individual').

pain control and improved function in these patients while receiving opioid therapy in the context of prescription in a multidisciplinary pain clinic with a multisystem approach to pain management. More data are needed to know if such therapy is safe and beneficial on a longer-term basis (Slater et al., 2010).

Adjuvant analgesics for management of persisting pain in children with medical illness

An adjuvant analgesic is a medicine that has a primary indication other than pain, but is analgesic in some painful conditions. This excludes medicines administered primarily to manage adverse effects associated with analgesics, such as laxatives and antiemetics. The WHO recently reviewed the evidence for the use of adjuvant analgesic medicines in pain management for children (WHO, 2012). The use of corticosteroids as adjuvant medicines is not recommended for the treatment of persisting pain in children with medical illnesses, nor is the use of bisphosphonates for the treatment of bone pain in children due to the low quality of evidence. Although frequently used for the management of neuropathic pain in children, it was not possible to make evidence-based recommendations for or against the use of tricyclic antidepressants (TCAs), selective serotonin reuptake inhibitors (SSRIs), or anticonvulsants as adjuvant medicines. In addition, recommendations regarding the risks or benefits of ketamine or systemic local anaesthetics as adjuvants to opioids for the treatment of neuropathic pain in children, or for the use of benzodiazepines and/or baclofen as adjuvants in the management of pain associated with muscle spasm and spasticity, could not be made based on the current literature. The quality of current evidence, and risks and benefits of different treatments are summarized in the WHO document, and the need for further analgesic research in children with persistent pain and medical illness to establish the role of these medicines in paediatric pain treatment is emphasized (WHO, 2012).

WHO health system recommendations for a global strategy to improve pain management in children

In an effort to ensure the universal application of the general principles and clinical recommendations, the WHO also makes health system recommendations acknowledging that lack of access to the correct treatment for persisting pain is often related to issues in the

health system (WHO, 2012). It recommends the education of health professionals in the standardized management of persisting pain in children with medical illnesses and in the handling of the necessary medicines, including opioid analgesics. Further, health professionals should be allowed to handle opioids within their scope of practice or professional role based on their general professional licence without any additional licensing requirements. Individual countries may consider, subject to their situation, allowing other professions to diagnose, prescribe, administer, and/or dispense opioids for reasons of flexibility, efficiency, increased coverage of services, and/or improved quality of care. The conditions under which such permission is granted would be based on the demonstration of competence, sufficient training, and personal accountability for professional performance (WHO, 2012).

Human immunodeficiency virus and acquired immunodeficiency syndrome

Human immunodeficiency virus (HIV) causes immunosuppression by infecting the immune system, in particular CD4 (cluster of differentiation 4, a glycoprotein expressed on the surface of T helper cells, monocytes, macrophages, and dendritic cells) lymphocytes. Immunosuppression from the viraemia results in variable disease manifestations and disease progression (Luzuriaga and Sullivan, 1998).

A growing number of children and young adults in the world are infected with HIV, with the majority of these in developing countries. Approximately 3.4 million children under the age of 15 are living with HIV worldwide, and there were an estimated 390 000 newly infected children in 2010 (UNAIDS, 2011). The majority of these children live in sub-Saharan Africa where skilled clinicians, medications, and technology limit the provision of optimal care (De Baets et al., 2007). In 2010 the estimated number of children with acquired immunodeficiency disease (AIDS) who died in Sub-Saharan Africa was 230 000, 14 000 in South and South East Asia compared to less than 100 in North America, and Western and Central Europe (UNAIDS, 2011). The introduction of antiretroviral medication has dramatically changed the course of HIV and children are surviving longer. In the absence of antiretroviral therapy (ART), HIV disease in children is more aggressive, with a significant proportion of children presenting with severe disease. The rate of ART use in children under 15 years in developing countries as estimated by WHO in 2010 was 23%, with between 3% to 29% in Africa (WHO, 2011a). Without ART paediatric HIV is usually more aggressive and most of the children die before the age of 5 years (WHO, 2011a).

Effective pain management is also hindered by limited availability of opioids in developing countries. One study conducted in Africa showed approximately half of the children dying of AIDS received no analgesia (De Baets et al., 2007). It has been hypothesized that pain may be a unique manifestation of HIV and report of pain has been associated with a higher mortality (Gaughan et al., 2002). Effective pain management could also be hindered by potential drug interactions, and difficulties in differentiating ongoing disease and treatment side effects (Strafford et al., 1991).

Prevalence of pain in children with HIV/AIDS

Pain in children with HIV is highly prevalent (Gray et al., 2010) but is commonly unrecognized, inadequately treated, and not prioritized (Norval et al., 2006). Earlier in the course of HIV, pain can be transient in nature (Oleske, 2007), but as HIV progresses and the CD4 cell count decreases, pain can be severe (AIDSinfo, 2008). With the fall in the CD4 cell count, children with progressive disease have more pain, which can become chronic and severe (De Baets et al., 2007; Gaughan et al., 2002; Lolekha et al., 2004).

The prevalence of pain in children with HIV and AIDS is uncertain due to limited literature reports and few studies specifically related to in HIV-related paediatric pain. Reported prevalence of pain in children ranges from 20% (Gaughan et al., 2002) to 60% (Hirschfeld et al., 1996). Lolekha's cross-sectional study of a paediatric outpatient population found 44% of children with HIV complained of pain and 6.6% of these children had pain lasting more than 3 months and occurring twice or more per week (Lolekha et al., 2004). A higher incidence of pain (67%) with associated sleep disturbance has been reported in younger children (67%) (Hirschfeld et al., 1996). Serchuck et al also reported a higher incidence of pain in young children, and in girls (Serchuck et al., 2010). Gender differences are thought to be influenced by communication skills and cultural bias (Gaughan et al., 2002). Overall, the prevalence of pain in children with HIV/AIDS is comparable to that of paediatric cancer pain (between 37% to 78%; Hirschfeld et al., 1996).

Although pain is a frequent symptom, it unfortunately often continues to be poorly treated (Yaster and Schechter, 1996). Some of the reasons include: lack of confidence among health care professionals in assessing and managing pain in children and misconceptions surrounding opioid use in children (AIDSinfo, 2008). Persisting pain can be also associated with increased mortality, a decreased quality of life (AIDSinfo, 2008), and increase in hospital admissions (Josephs et al., 2010).

Causes of pain in HIV/AIDS

HIV/AIDS pain is multifactorial and can arise from: complications of the disease (e.g. infections, inflammation, neoplasms), adverse drug reactions, and compromised immune status. Pain may be exacerbated by: psychological factors such as stress, clinical depression, anxiety, and fear; greater socioeconomic stresses (Serchuck et al., 2010); and also by poor nutritional status (AIDSinfo, 2008; Berg et al., 2009; De Baets et al., 2007; Gaughan et al., 2002; Hirschfeld et al., 1996; Serchuck et al., 2010).

Disease-related pain can affect many organs, predominately the gastrointestinal, neurological, pulmonary, and dermatological systems (AIDSinfo, 2008; Strafford et al., 1991). The most frequent cause of pain in children with HIV was gastrointestinal or limb pain (Hirschfeld et al., 1996). Other causes of somatic pain include painful disorders of the skin, connective tissue, muscle, bone, and visceral pain. Somatic pain tends to be well localized, sharp, and acute whilst visceral pain is less localized and is often described as deep, dull, aching, gnawing or spasmodic pain (Amery et al., 2009). More generalized bodily pain, headache, chest or neuropathic pain can also occur. A survey of ambulatory adult patients with HIV in the US reported somatic pain in 45% of cases, visceral pain in 15%, neuropathic pain in 19%, and in 4% of cases the causes of pain were unknown (Hewitt et al., 1997).

Gastrointestinal pain in children with HIV/AIDS

Immunosuppression causing infection and consequent pain can manifest in any part of the gastrointestinal system. Pain can result from oropharyngeal candidiasis, dental caries, gingivitis, aphthous ulcers, herpetic stomatitis and oesophagitis from candida, cytomegalovirus (CMV), herpes simplex virus (HSV), or mycobacterium (New York State Department of Health AIDS Institute, 2001; Wilcox,

2010; Yaster and Schechter, 1996; Yogev, 2011). Candida oesophagitis is a common problem and risk factors for developing it include prior oral candidiasis, a low CD4 count, and antibiotic use. Pain can manifest as odynophagia (painful swallowing) or retrosternal pain.

Infectious gastroenteritis from bacteria, parasites, viruses, or fungal agents can cause small and large bowel enteritis and severe abdominal pain (Wilcox, 2010). Atypical infections such as *Mycobacterium avium-intracellulare* (MAI) can cause abdominal pain, usually related to the accompanying lymphadenopathy (Wilcox, 2010). Patients with a CD4 count less than 100/microlitre are more susceptible to CMV, fungi, *Mycobacterium avium* complex (MAC), and unusual protozoa infections. CMV infection can cause pain through gastritis, a focal ulcer, gastric outlet obstruction, or gastric mass. It can also cause enteritis, small and large bowel perforation, colitis, appendicitis, hepatitis, cholecystitis, cholangitis, and pancreatitis. *Cryptosporidium* causes gastritis, gastric outlet obstruction, small bowel enteritis, appendicitis, cholecystitis and hepatitis. Conversely, patients with a CD4 count greater than 400/microlitre are more likely to have common bacterial infections or neoplasia (Wilcox, 2010).

Another rare cause of abdominal pain is gastrointestinal lymphoma (Yaster and Schechter, 1996) which may present as a mass causing obstruction, hepatic, splenic, or mesenteric infiltration (New York State Department of Health AIDS Institute, 2001; Wilcox 2010; Yogev, 2011).

Nucleoside reverse transcriptase inhibitors (NRTIs) used in therapy can cause mitochondrial toxicity, hepatic steatosis, and abdominal pain, and there are limited reported cases in children (McComsey and Leonard, 2004). Complications from ART (didanosine, or lamivudine) include pancreatitis with or without abdominal pain and hepatitis.

Neuropathic pain in children with HIV/AIDS

The nervous system is major target for HIV infection, which can affect both the central and the peripheral nervous systems. The nervous system can be affected in multiple ways: as a direct consequence of opportunistic infections or malignancies occurring because of immunosuppression, from treatment-related neurotoxic effects, or systemic complications of HIV on brain function (Dobalian et al., 2004). Possible HIV-related immunological mechanisms include antigen–antibody immune complex deposition in blood vessels, causing a vasculitis in small, medium, and large vessels. Evidence supporting this includes the demonstration of HIV p24 antigen in endoneurial blood vessels, HIV replication in nerve biopsies, and the presence of HIV in cultures of nerve tissue (Brinley et al., 2001; Epstein et al., 1986).

Peripheral neuropathy

Peripheral neuropathy is reported to occur in about 13% to 34% of children with HIV/AIDS (AIDSinfo, 2011; Araujo et al., 2000). Approximately 34% of children in early or later stages of HIV report symptoms and signs of peripheral neuropathy in the absence of potential neurotoxic ARV drugs (Serchuck et al., 2010; Van Dyke et al., 2008). However, there is a higher prevalence of peripheral neuropathy in children with encephalopathy and symptomatic AIDS. Peripheral neuropathy in children is often not as severe, frequent, or debilitating as that which occurs in adults (Araujo et al., 2000; Floeter et al., 1997). It is unclear whether the peripheral nervous system of children is more resilient to neuropathic insults associated with HIV infection or whether few reports reflects an under diagnosis of peripheral neuropathy in this patient group (Floeter et al., 1997).

The incidence of ART-associated neuropathy is 0.1% with use of stavudine, lamivudine, and nevirapine (AIDSinfo, 2011). The toxicity of non-reverse transcriptase inhibitor (NRTI) therapy is thought to result from mitochondrial toxicity resulting in peripheral neuropathy, myopathy, lactic acidosis, hepatitis, hepatitis steatosis, cardiomyopathy and lipoatrophy/lipodystrophy. Not all children on combination ART, which includes an NRTI, develop peripheral neuropathy (Araujo et al., 2000; Floeter et al., 1997). HIV-positive adult Caucasian patients who have the mitochondrial haplo-group T have an increased risk of peripheral neuropathy (Hulgan et al., 2005; Van Dyke et al., 2008). Van Dyke and colleagues postulated that the mitochondrial DNA polymorphism that predisposes to NRTI-induced mitochondrial toxicity is uncommon in children from an African American or Hispanic background (Van Dyke et al., 2008). Modest rates of toxicity have also been observed in younger children although not fully defined in paediatrics.

Neuropathic pain predominately occurs in the distal lower limbs, particularly in the feet (Araujo et al., 2000; Floeter et al., 1997). The pain is usually described as aching, burning, or painful numbness (AIDSinfo, 2011). Some experience hyperalgesia and allodynia. Paradoxical hyperalgesia in association with escalating drug requirements has been reported in children undergoing prolonged intensive and invasive care (AIDSinfo, 2011; Gray et al., 2010). However, neuropathic pain can be fluctuating in nature and may not interfere with daily activities. Chronic sensory symptoms predominate, with bilateral and distal pain and paraesthesia, similar to reports in adults (Araujo et al., 2000).

Headache in children with HIV/AIDS

Headache in HIV/AIDS can result from meningitis or meningoencephalitis opportunistic infections. Bacterial meningitis commonly presents with headache (Gumbo et al., 2002). Other causes of headache include sinusitis, central nervous system (CNS) lymphoma, viral encephalopathy, and rarely toxoplasmosis, and *Cryptococcus neoformans*. Opportunistic infections from toxoplasmosis, and CMV are uncommon in children, as infection is usually from reactivation of a previously acquired infection.

Although meningoencephalitis from *Cryptococcus neoformans* is rare in children living with AIDS compared to adult patients, there may be an increasing number of African children affected (Gumbo et al., 2002). The other causes of headache include complications of ART such as zidovudine, causing an adverse reaction. Tension headaches and migraine are reported in adults but the frequency in children is unknown. Dihydroergotamine or ergotamine should not be co-administered with protease inhibitors as this may cause ergot toxicity resulting in nausea, vomiting, and sustained vasoconstriction with local tissue hypoxia and ischemic injury. Children with HIV/AIDS can develop spasticity and rigidity due to CNS complications of infection causing considerable pain and immobility. Management of this pain involves a multidisciplinary approach help improve comfort and mobility of these patients (AIDSinfo, 2011).

Musculoskeletal pain in children with HIV/AIDS

Bone pain in children with HIV/AIDS can be due to multiple causes that include: osteopenia as a result of bone loss and altered bone metabolism, cancer, and infections such as osteomyelitis or septic arthritis. Decreased bone mineral density is seen in children with HIV/AIDS (Fortuny et al., 2008), the pathogenesis of which is likely to be multifactorial including mineral and vitamin deficiency.

Bisphosphonates have been used to treat this type of pain and should be considered despite limited use in ARV treated HIV-infected children. Another bone problem seen in children is avascular necrosis or osteonecrosis presenting as hip pain (McComsey and Leonard, 2004). When bone pain occurs, the recommended first-line therapy is generally a non-steroidal anti-inflammatory (NSAID) provided there are no contraindications to its use.

Idiopathic polymyositis, myositis secondary to zidovudine (AZT) toxicity, and infectious pyomyositis can cause muscular pain in HIV-infected children (Lane, 1998). Muscular pain from AZT may occur as a result of an idiosyncratic reaction causing muscle weakness and elevation of muscle enzymes and can occur at all CD4 levels. Discontinuing or reducing AZT dose may reduce pain severity.

Procedural pain and its impact in children with HIV/AIDS

Children with HIV/AIDS may experience many painful procedures such as venepuncture, bone marrow aspirate, lumbar puncture, or nasogastric tube insertion. An early report documented a total of 193 painful procedures in 22 children with AIDS (Strafford et al., 1991). The heightened pain experience from repeated painful procedures may contribute to a higher pain report in younger children (Serchuck et al., 2010). Procedural pain management is essential to minimize the experience of pain. Comprehensive guidelines are available which outline pharmacological and non-pharmacological approaches to common procedures, including preprocedure preparation (Amery et al., 2009; Schiff et al., 2001). (Additional information related to procedural pain management is included in Chapter 18 (Palmer and Babl), Chapter 19 (Taddio), and Chapter 47 (Zempsky) in this volume.)

Special considerations for pain management in children with HIV/AIDS

Management of HIV/AIDS-related pain may be complex. It is important to recognize pain, assess its severity, and develop treatment goals for managing pain in the context to the HIV symptomatology (New York State Department of Health AIDS Institute, 2001). The availability of medications also has an impact on pain management. Poorly controlled HIV-related pain can affect a child's quality of life, interfering with activity and sleep (AIDSinfo, 2008).

Treating pain in HIV/AIDS requires a multimodal approach. Diagnosing and treating the cause of pain is vital, particularly as lowering the viral load could contribute to an improved response to analgesics (AIDSinfo, 2008). The goals of treatment should also be focused on reducing the incidence and severity of treatment-related pain. Age-appropriate pain severity measurement scales should be used and implementation of the principles of pain management as recently outlined by the WHO (WHO, 2012).

Generally, mild pain is treated with simple analgesia such as paracetamol and NSAIDs. However, NSAIDs should be used with caution as they may exacerbate bone marrow suppression and worsen gastrointestinal symptoms in patients with HIV and have potential drug–drug interactions with ARV (Gray et al., 2010).

Protease inhibitors (PIs), NNRTI or NRTIs can have significant drug interactions with analgesics, including buprenorphine, codeine, dextropropoxyphene, diamorphine, fentanyl, mefenamic acid, pethidine, tramadol, and ketamine. The simultaneous use of these medications may result in increased plasma drug concentrations, toxicity, or relative overdose of the pain medications. These interactions can be managed by altering the drug dosage or timing of administration as well as therapeutic drug monitoring (TDM). For example, cautious use of methadone is employed in patients on PIs and NNRTIs as these drugs can induce the metabolism of methadone and lead to withdrawal symptoms. Dosing of methadone therefore need to be increased whilst on these ARV. Conversely, methadone toxicity has been reported with the discontinuation of PIs or NNRTIs (AIDSinfo, 2008).

In addition to this, the hepatic isoenzyme changes induced by these pain medications can alter PI or NNRTI pharmacokinetics (AIDSinfo, 2008). Conservative dosing is therefore recommended, with titration against individual response. Dosing guidelines exist for adults for antiretroviral drug interactions (Ammann, 2009) and interactions can be managed by altering the drug dosage or timing of administration as well as TDM. However, there is no universal rule for ARV dose calculation in children that can be considered accurate under all circumstances. Body weight is the most accessible and widely used metric, but is also the mostly likely to result in inaccurate dosing. Body surface area (BSA) is recommended as it more closely meets the efficacy and safety requirements for infants and children (Norval et al., 2006). However, as BSA does not take height into account, dosing based on the BSA should be used with caution in children with malnutrition. Careful monitoring of organ function through appropriate laboratory diagnostic tests, a patient's clinical status, weight gain, increased growth and development, decreased opportunistic infections, increased CD4 counts, and decreased viral loads can be used to confirm efficacy of the ART (Norval et al., 2006).

Special considerations for pharmacotherapy in HIV/AIDS

Excessive activation of the N-methyl-D-aspartate (NMDA) receptor occurs in the presence of gp120, a protein found on the outer envelope of HIV (AIDSinfo, 2008). It is thought that this may contribute to increased pain severity potentially requiring escalating opioid and sedative requirements. Both dextromethorphan and ketamine block the NMDA receptor, but their use can be limited by an unfavourable side effect profile. Ketamine has anecdotally been associated with severe cardiac rhythm disturbance, electrolyte abnormalities, and even cardiac arrest in children with advanced HIV and AIDS (AIDSinfo, 2008). Adult literature suggests that methadone administration may be associated with lower CD4 cell count and CD4/CD8 cell ratios and in vitro studies also suggest an increase in HIV replication in human blood monocyte-derived macrophages exposed to methadone (AIDSinfo, 2008).

Myopathic pain is managed by firstly addressing the underlying cause, decreasing inflammation, and maximizing ART. Neuropathic pain and peripheral neuropathy due to medication is managed by stopping medications that produce neuropathy, and using analgesics as per the WHO recommendations (WHO, 2012). Neuropathic pain may also be managed with γ-aminobutyric acid agonists (GABA) such as baclofen, ART, NMDA receptor blockade, and anticonvulsants (AIDSinfo, 2008). Abdominal pain from inflammatory processes such as pancreatitis, infection, gall bladder and biliary tract disease, malabsorption syndromes, tumours, and medication side effects can all cause persisting pain in children with HIV/AIDS. Mouth pain from aphthous ulcers and dysphagia are managed by using mouth washes, a soft brush, having soft food, and appropriate analgesia. Candidiasis should be treated with antifungals such as miconazole, fluconazole, and topical anaesthetics for local pain relief. Aphthous ulcers have also been managed with prednisolone and dexamethasone mouth washes.

Case example: human immunodeficiency virus and acquired immunodeficiency syndrome

Moses is a 4-year-old with AIDS whose parents had recently died from the same diagnosis. He was admitted to hospital in Africa with vomiting, diarrhoea, and pain. He was noted to have mouth ulcers, severe oral thrush, a cough, and noted to be underweight with signs of malnutrition, and clinically dehydrated. He was distressed and in severe pain, but unable to localize the pain. His initial management included oral morphine (which he vomited), intravenous fluids, antibiotics, and topical oral antifungals. His pain worsened and his hospital had access to an intravenous morphine preparation, as recommended by the WHO model list of essential medicines for children (WHO, 2011b). A regular schedule of subcutaneous morphine was started for the management of constant severe pain. His pain severity decreased and eventually his pain was well managed with a regular schedule of oral morphine once his vomiting stopped. Further investigations showed he also had tuberculosis (TB) and anti-TB therapy was commenced.

Cystic fibrosis

Cystic fibrosis (CF) is an inherited multisystem disorder, and the primary defect relates to dysfunction of the cystic fibrosis transmembrane conductance regulator protein (CFTR). CF is characterized by obstruction and infection of airways and by maldigestion and its consequences. As a result, CF is the major cause of severe chronic lung disease in children, and of most cases of exocrine pancreatic insufficiency in early life (Egan, 2011). Due to the wide array of presenting symptoms and complications, CF enters the differential diagnosis of many paediatric conditions (Egan, 2011). CF is the most common life-limiting recessive genetic trait among white people, with a prevalence of approximately 1/3500 live births in northern Europe, North America, and Australia and New Zealand. The prognosis for children living with CF has improved dramatically over the last few decades. This is due to several factors including improved nutrition and improved treatment of respiratory infections. Notwithstanding this improvement in prognosis, this illness is still associated with significant morbidity, but there has been little evaluation of the extent and impact of pain on children with CF.

Pain in cystic fibrosis

Recognition that pain is a common symptom in children with CF was first established in the 1990s. A retrospective chart review at a tertiary care hospital was conducted summarizing the end-of-life care of US patients more than 5 years of age and dying from CF (Robinson et al., 1997). Twenty-five per cent of these patients had been receiving opioids for the treatment of chronic headache and/or chest pain for more than their last 3 months of life. When opioids were used for the treatment of breathlessness and/or chest pain, the proportion increased to 86%. When pain was present, it was described as 'serious' pain with chest, head, extremity, abdomen, and back being the more common locations.

The incidence of chronic pain in children with CF increases sharply in the last 6 months of life (Ravilly et al., 1996). Headaches (55% of patients) and chest pain (65%) were frequently reported, although back pain (19%), abdominal pain (19%), and limb pain

(16%) were also common. In patients with headache, the main aetiologies were hypercarbia or hypoxia, migraine, and sinusitis. The majority of chest pain was musculoskeletal, with pleuritis, pneumothorax, and rib fracture also reported.

A recent comparative study of children and adults with CF examined the prevalence of pain in CF and the consequences to activities of daily living (Sermet-Gaudelus et al., 2009). The study included 73 children (1–18 years) and 110 adults (18–52 years); 59% of the children and 89% of the adults reported at least one episode of pain during the previous month. Pain was significantly more intense and lasted significantly longer among adults, but incidence did not differ significantly between the two populations, and was not related to the severity of CF. In this study the most prevalent locations were the abdomen for children, and the back, head, and chest for adults. Although pain significantly limited physical activity, only 15% of patients reported that it caused absenteeism, and 27% reported that it negatively affected their family life. The mean intensity of greatest pain during the past month, rated on a 0 to 10 visual analogue scale was 4.9 (2) (mean [standard deviation]) for children and 6 (2) for adults. Only 40% and 50%, respectively, of those with pain reported the use of analgesic treatment, mainly paracetamol. At least one episode of procedural pain during the previous month was reported by 85% of children and 78% of adults. This study demonstrates the high incidence of undertreated pain in CF patients throughout their lives and indicates the need for a thorough assessment of pain in children with CF.

Reported interventions for pain in CF have included a variety of non-pharmacological and pharmacological therapies (Ravilly et al., 1996). Forty-one patients (53%) had pain severe enough to require opioid treatment, and ten patients (13%) received opioids for more than 3 months. In eight patients with more severe pain, regional analgesia was found to be particularly effective (Ravilly et al., 1996).

Case example: cystic fibrosis

A 14-year-old adolescent with CF was admitted to hospital with severe left-sided chest pain exacerbated by deep inspiration. A chest X-ray revealed a fracture of the right anterior seventh rib and associated osteopenia. The patient was admitted to hospital for analgesia and chest physiotherapy. Analgesia consisted of intravenous opioid analgesia self-administered via a patient-controlled analgesia (PCA) pump through a central venous access device. The young patient was encouraged to administer the opioid prior to chest physiotherapy and instructed to support his chest wall when coughing. A TENS unit was used and gave improved analgesia. Osteoclast inhibitor therapy was commenced, following endocrinology review, to correct the osteopenia and reduce the chance of spontaneous fracture in the future. This patient was discharged home 2 weeks later with a regular schedule of oral analgesia for management of his persisting pain.

Neurofibromatoses

Nerofibromatoses are autosomal dominant disorders that that cause tumours to grow on nerves and are associated with other abnormalities such as skin changes and bone deformities. There are specific diagnostic criteria for neurofibromatosis type 1 (NF1) and neurofibromatosis 2 (NF2; Sahin, 2011). NF1 is more common and has a better prognosis with a lower incidence of CNS tumours than NF2, but may still be associated with significant morbidity.

Pain in neurofibromatosis

Neurofibromas typically involve the skin, but may also be situated along peripheral nerves and blood vessels or within viscera, and can produce pain in children (Sahin, 2011). The lesions characteristically appear during adolescence as small rubbery lesions with a slight discolouration of the overlying skin. Neurofibromas may be associated with swelling and local pain ('pins and needles' or 'shooting' pain) and dysaesthesia in the nerve distribution. Plexiform neurofibromas are often present at birth and frequently located in the orbital or temporal region of the face, result from diffuse thickening of nerve trunks (Sahin, 2011). Plexiform neurofibromas may produce overgrowth of an extremity and the deformity of the corresponding bone may cause pain.

A neurofibroma occasionally differentiates into a malignant nerve cell tumour and the incidence of phaeochromocytoma, rhabdomyosarcoma, leukaemia, and Wilms' tumour is higher than the general population (Sahin, 2011). The possibility of a malignant change in a neurofibroma should be considered in the patient with pain which is persisting despite analgesic treatment.

Scoliosis is a common complication found in 10% of patients with neurofibromatosis (Sahin, 2011), and this skeletal abnormality may also be a source of pain. In addition, pathological fracture is occasionally associated with pseudoarthrosis, and should be considered in this setting if pain is of sudden onset, severe, and persisting.

Case example: neurofibromatosis

A 16-year-old boy presented to the paediatric pain clinic with neurofibromatosis which was diagnosed at the age of 10 years. He presented with intermittent 'sharp, shooting' pain in his arm and this followed a C5, C6 nerve distribution. His imaging studies demonstrated multiple neurofibromas along C5 and C6 nerves, but none suggestive of malignant change. Initially well controlled on a combination of simple analgesics and gabapentin as a treatment for neuropathic pain, his pain escalated over several months to become severe, constant, and precluded sleep. This change necessitated an increase in his analgesia to include an opioid given on a regular basis and the continuation of the gabapentin. A nerve biopsy was performed which diagnosed a peripheral nerve sheath tumour. Despite treatment with chemotherapy, the tumour progressed in size and caused further pain necessitating the parenteral administration of an opioid and referral for palliative care.

Neuromuscular diseases

Neuromuscular diseases are disorders of the motor unit, which consists of the motor neuron, its axon, the neuromuscular junction, and the muscle fibres innervated by the motor neuron. Paediatric neuromuscular conditions that may be associated with pain include: developmental disorders of muscle (e.g. nemaline and central core disease), muscular dystrophies (e.g. Duchenne's), spinal muscular atrophies, and Guillain–Barré syndrome (GBS).

Pain in neuromuscular disorders

Although the neuromuscular diseases of childhood are a heterogeneous group of conditions, there is often a similarity in the causation of pain. Muscle weakness is common and sometimes associated with cramps, which can be distressing and for which simple remedies, such as massage, seem to be the most effective. Most persisting pain in neuromuscular disease is a consequence of the orthopaedic complications of muscle weakness. In particular, pain associated with hip dislocation and progressive scoliosis. Pain can initially be mild in these orthopaedic conditions and simple analgesics sufficient for treatment. With progression, surgical options are often considered and may be more effective for pain relief in the longer term. Occasionally, a few young patients with neuromuscular conditions may require surgery to correct scoliosis or hip dislocation causing severe pain. If surgical options are precluded due to anaesthetic risk, long-term opioid therapy for the management of severe pain may be warranted.

Case example: neuromuscular diseases

A 16-year-old boy with Duchenne's muscular dystrophy and severe persisting back pain due to severe scoliosis was reviewed in a pain clinic for children. Corrective surgery was scheduled; however, severe and persisting pain necessitated the administration of a regular schedule of opioid medication. Prior to starting the opioid he was reviewed by his respiratory team as he was being treated with nocturnal non-invasive ventilation for the treatment of hypercapnia. The respiratory team repeated a sleep study which demonstrated the effectiveness of his non-invasive ventilation. The opioid therapy was effective and was commenced under close supervision in hospital. His surgery was completed a few days later and initially he was closely monitored in the paediatric intensive care unit. His postoperative analgesia accounted for the fact that he was needing opioid prior to surgery. His course was uneventful and at the time of discharge simple analgesics were only required for adequate pain control.

Guillain–Barré syndrome

GBS is an acute immune-mediated polyradiculoneuropathy comprising a broad spectrum of clinical variants (Ruts et al., 2010). It often occurs following a non-specific viral infection and usually results in an ascending paralysis. In developed countries it is the most common cause of flaccid paralysis in children (47%), followed by transverse myelitis (19%), and then a variety of causes, including encephalomyelitis, tick-bite paralysis, and infantile botulism (Morris et al., 2003).

Pain in Guillain–Barré syndrome

Data from a prospective study in adult patients with GBS indicated one-third had pain in the 2 weeks prior to the onset of weakness, two-thirds had pain in the acute phase, and 38% overall had persisting pain at 12 months' follow-up (Ruts et al., 2010). Low back and proximal muscle pain, radicular limb pain, peripheral dysaesthesiae, and arthralgias are common in adults; and multiple pain patterns may coexist and overlap, which complicates clinical assessment (Gorson, 2010). Whilst paraesthesiae are commonly

described in children with GBS (Morris et al., 2003), the epidemiology of pain experienced by children with GBS is less well described and the literature is confined to the occasional case report (Pier et al., 2010).

The pathophysiology of pain in GBS is poorly understood. Putative mechanisms include irritation of the nervi nervorum innervating nerve trunks and the dorsal rami, demyelinating of large sensory nerve fibres causing pain dysaesthesiae, and dysfunction of small nerve fibres. Animal studies have suggested a role for T-cell-mediated inflammation and the release of pro-inflammatory cytokines producing thermal hyperalgesia and allodynia (Gorson, 2010). Musculoskeletal pain related to prolonged immobility may also be a contributing factor (Gorson, 2010).

Case example: Guillain–Barré

A 10-year-old boy was transferred from a regional hospital to a tertiary children's hospital with a history of weakness in his hands and feet and a complaint of an uncomfortable 'burning' sensation in his hands and feet. The weakness progressed in his limbs proximally and a diagnosis of GBS was made. Concern about progressive respiratory muscle weakness necessitated admission to the paediatric intensive care unit for close monitoring of his respiratory status, but invasive ventilation was avoided and he was discharged from intensive care within 7 days. In the ward he complained of increasing pain related to the dysaesthesiae in his limbs, which was not responsive to simple analgesics. Given the neuropathic quality of his pain he was administered gabapentin. Within 1 week of starting this medication his pain decreased and this greatly facilitated his rehabilitation programme.

Cerebral palsy

Cerebral palsy (CP) is a diagnostic term to describe a group of permanent, but non-progressive, disorders of movement and posture causing activity limitation. CP may be attributed to a range of disturbances in the developing fetal or infant brain, for example, genetic, metabolic, ischaemic, and infectious causes (Johnston, 2011). The motor disorders are often accompanied by disturbances of communication, sensation, perception, cognition, and behaviour, in addition to epilepsy and secondary musculoskeletal problems (Johnston, 2011).

Pain in cerebral palsy

Pain in children with CP is common (Engel et al., 2005) and is associated with a lower quality of life and self-perception (Russo et al., 2008). Therefore, clinicians should enquire about pain in every child with CP and consider appropriate pain management (Riquelme et al., 2011). A recent cross-sectional multicentre European study determined the prevalence and associations of self-reported and parent-reported pain in children with CP of all severities (Parkinson et al., 2010). Children aged 8 to 12 years were randomly selected from population-based registers of children with CP in eight European regions and a further region recruited 75 children from multiple sources. Data on pain in the weeks prior to the survey were available from 490 children who gave self-report and parents of 806 children (who could not self-report) gave their perception of their child's pain. The estimated population prevalence of self-reported pain in the previous week was 60% (95% confidence interval (CI): 54–65%) and that of parent-reported pain in the previous 4 weeks was 73% (95% CI: 69–76%). Older children reported more pain, but pain was not significantly associated with severity of impairment. In parental reports, severity of child impairment, seizures, and parental unemployment were associated with more frequent and severe pain.

There are many causes of pain in children with cerebral palsy, which can be categorized as:

* Gastrointestinal (e.g. dysphagia, gastro-oesophageal reflux, constipation).

* Orthopaedic (e.g. hip subluxation and dislocation, equinus valgus deformities of knee and ankle, scoliosis, kyphosis, contractures).

* Neuromuscular (e.g. pain related to spasticity, nerve entrapments).

* Rehabilitative (e.g. pain related to the physical therapy activities of stretching and bracing).

Pain treatment strategies should be directed at the specific causes listed and if analgesic agents are needed, the general principles outlined at the beginning of this chapter are applicable. The diagnostic process may be difficult, and a case has been made to obtain a whole-body technetium bone scan in children with CP for whom there is no obvious case, as occasionally occult fractures may be identified (Bajelidze et al., 2008). Novel treatments for pain related to spasticity include botulinum toxin type A injections (Lundy et al., 2009) and intrathecal baclofen (Hoving et al., 2009a, 2009b).

Case example: cerebral palsy

A 12-year-old girl with severe CP presented to the ED with behaviours indicating to her care-givers that she had severe pain. Normally a happy child she had a 48 h history of inconsolable crying and grimacing facial expressions. Previously diagnosed comorbidity included gastro-oesophageal reflux which was being treated with a proton pump inhibitor and subluxed hips for which surgery was not intended in the near future. Apart from demonstrating signs consistent with severe CP her clinical examination revealed severe hip adductor muscle spasm. The centrally acting muscle relaxant baclofen was administered regularly and her pain behaviours improved dramatically.

References

AIDSinfo. (2008). *Managing complications of HIV infection in HIV infected children on antiretroviral therapy. Guidelines for the use of antiretroviral agents in pediatric HIV infection* [Online]. Available at: <http//www.aidsinfo.nih.gov>.

AIDSinfo. (2011). *Panel on antiretroviral therapy and medical management of HIV-infected children. Guidelines for the use of antiretroviral agents in pediatric HIV infection* [Online]. Available at: <http://aidsinfo.nih.gov/ContentFiles/PediatricGuidelines.pdf>.

Amery, J., Meiring, M., Albertyn, R., and Jassal, S. (2009). Pain. In J. Amery, (ed.) *Children's palliative care in Africa*, pp. 97–124. Oxford: Oxford University Press.

Ammann, A. (2009). *Antiretroviral drug dosing for infants and children: calculation by weight or body surface area, global strategies for HIV prevention.* [Online]. <http://www.womenchildrenhiv.org/wchiv?page=wx-resource&root=typ&cat=05%subcat=prrv&rid=21039> (accessed 21 January 2009).

Araujo, A. P., Nascimento, O. J., and Garcia, O. S. (2000). Distal sensory polyneuropathy in a cohort of HIV-infected children over five years of age. *Pediatrics*, 106, E35.

Bajelidze, G., Belthur, M. V., Littleton, A. G., Dabney, K. W., and Miller, F. (2008). Diagnostic evaluation using whole-body technetium bone scan in children with cerebral palsy and pain. *J Pediatr Orthop*, 28, 112–117.

Berg, K. M., Cooperman, N. A., Newville, H., and Arnsten, J. H. (2009). Self-efficacy and depression as mediators of the relationship between pain and antiretroviral adherence. *AIDS Care*, 21, 244–248.

Brinley, F. J.Jr., Pardo, C. A., and Verma, A. (2001). Human immunodeficiency virus and the peripheral nervous system workshop. *Arch Neurol*, 58, 1561–1566.

De Baets, A. J., Bulterys, M., Abrams, E. J., Kankassa, C., and Pazvakavambwa, I. E. (2007). Care and treatment of HIV-infected children in Africa: issues and challenges at the district hospital level. *Pediatr Infect Dis J*, 26, 163–173.

Dobalian, A., Tsao, J. C., and Duncan, R. P. (2004). Pain and the use of outpatient services among persons with HIV: results from a nationally representative survey. *Med Care*, 42, 129–138.

Egan, M. (2011). Cystic fibrosis. In R. M. Kleigman, B. F. Stanton, N. F. Schor, J. W. St. Geme, and R. E. Behrman (eds) *Nelson textbook of pediatrics*, pp. 1481–1496. Philadelphia, PA: Saunders.

Engel, J. M., Petrina, T. J., Dudgeon, B. J., and McKearnan, K. A. (2005). Cerebral palsy and chronic pain: a descriptive study of children and adolescents. *Phys Occup Ther Pediatr*, 25, 73–84.

Epstein, L. G., Sharer, L. R., Oleske, J. M., Connor, E. M., Goudsmit, J., Bagdon, L., *et al.* (1986). Neurologic manifestations of human immunodeficiency virus infection in children. *Pediatrics*, 78, 678–687.

Floeter, M. K., Civitello, L. A., Everett, C. R., Dambrosia, J., and Luciano, C. A. (1997). Peripheral neuropathy in children with HIV infection. *Neurology*, 49, 207–212.

Fortuny, C., Noguera, A., Alsina, L., Villaronga, M., Vidal-Sicart, S., and Sanchez, E. (2008). Long-term use of bisphosphonates in the treatment of HIV-related bone pain in perinatally infected pediatric patients. *AIDS*, 22, 1888–1890.

Gaughan, D. M., Hughes, M. D., Seage, G. R.3rd, Selwyn, P. A., Carey, V. J., Gortmaker, S. L., *et al.* (2002). The prevalence of pain in pediatric human immunodeficiency virus/acquired immunodeficiency syndrome as reported by participants in the Pediatric Late Outcomes Study (PACTG 219). *Pediatrics*, 109, 1144–1152.

Gorson, K. C. (2010). This disorder has some nerve: chronic pain in Guillain-Barre syndrome. *Neurology*, 75, 1406–1407.

Gray, G. E., Laher, F., and Lazarus, E. (2010). The management of pain in adults and children living with HIV/AIDS. In A. Kopf and N. B. Patel (eds) *Guide to pain management in low-resource settings*. IASP. [Online]. Available at: <http://www.iasp-pain.org/AM/Template.cfm?Section=Home&SECTION=Home, Home, Home, Home&CONTENTID=11669&TEMPLATE=/CM/HTMLDisplay.cfm> (accessed 12 January 2012).

Gumbo, T., Kadzirange, G., Mielke, J., Gangaidzo, I. T., and Hakim, J. G. (2002). Cryptococcus neoformans meningoencephalitis in African children with acquired immunodeficiency syndrome. *Pediatr Infect Dis J*, 21, 54–56.

Hewitt, D. J., McDonald, M., Portenoy, R. K., Rosenfeld, B., Passik, S., and Breitbart, W. (1997). Pain syndromes and etiologies in ambulatory AIDS patients. *Pain*, 70, 117–123.

Hirschfeld, S., Moss, H., Dragisic, K., Smith, W., and Pizzo, P. A. (1996). Pain in pediatric human immunodeficiency virus infection: incidence and characteristics in a single-institution pilot study. *Pediatrics*, 98, 449–452.

Hoving, M. A., Van Raak, E. P., Spincemaille, G. H., Palmans, L. J., Becher, J. G., and Vles, J. S. (2009a). Efficacy of intrathecal baclofen therapy in children with intractable spastic cerebral palsy: a randomised controlled trial. *Eur J Paediatr Neurol*, 13, 240–246.

Hoving, M. A., Van Raak, E. P., Spincemaille, G. H., Van Kranen-Mastenbroek, V. H., Van Kleef, M., Gorter, J. W., et al. (2009b). Safety and one-year efficacy of intrathecal baclofen therapy in children with intractable spastic cerebral palsy. *Eur J Paediatr Neurol*, 13, 247–256.

Hulgan, T., Haas, D. W., Haines, J. L., Ritchie, M. D., Robbins, G. K., Shafer, R. W., et al. (2005). Mitochondrial haplogroups and peripheral neuropathy during antiretroviral therapy: an adult AIDS clinical trials group study. *AIDS*, 19, 1341–1349.

Johnston, M. V. (2011). Encephalopathies. In R. M. Kleigman, B. F. Stanton, N. F. Schor, J. W. St. Geme, and R. E. Behrman (eds) *Nelson textbook of pediatrics*, pp. 2061–2068. Philadelphia, PA: Saunders.

Josephs, J. S., Fleishman, J. A., Korthuis, P. T., Moore, R. D., and Gebo, K. A. (2010). Emergency department utilization among HIV-infected patients in a multisite multistate study. *HIV Med*, 11, 74–84.

Lane, N. (1998). *Rheumatologic and musculoskeletal manifestations of HIV* [Online]. Available at: <http://hivinsite.ucsf.edu/InSite?page=kb-04-01-15> (accessed 21 January 2012).

Lolekha, R., Chanthavanich, P., Limkittikul, K., Luangxay, K., Chotpitayasunodh, T., and Newman, C. J. 2004. Pain: a common symptom in human immunodeficiency virus-infected Thai children. *Acta Paediatr*, 93, 891–898.

Lundy, C. T., Doherty, G. M., and Fairhurst, C. B. (2009). Botulinum toxin type A injections can be an effective treatment for pain in children with hip spasms and cerebral palsy. *Dev Med Child Neurol*, 51, 705–710.

Luzuriaga, K. and Sullivan, K. L. (1998). Viral and immunopathogenesis of vertical HIV-1 infection. In P. A. Pizzo, and C. M. Wilfert (eds) *Pediatric AIDS*, pp. 89–104. Baltimore, MD: Williams and Wilkins.

McComsey, G. A., and Leonard, E. (2004). Metabolic complications of HIV therapy in children. *AIDS*, 18, 1753–1768.

Morris, A. M., Elliott, E. J., D'Souza, R. M., Antony, J., Kennett, M., and Longbottom, H. (2003). Acute flaccid paralysis in Australian children. *J Paediatr Child Health*, 39, 22–26.

Norval, D., O' Hare, B., and Matusa, R. (2006). HIV/AIDS. In A. Goldman, R. Hain, and S. Liben, (eds) *Oxford textbook of palliative care for children*, pp. 467–480. Oxford: Oxford University Press.

Oleske, J. (2007). *Pain relief for children with HIV/AIDS: a global imperative*. [Online]. <http://www.whocancerpain.wisc.edu> (accessed 28 November 2011).

Parkinson, K. N., Gibson, L., Dickinson, H. O., and Colver, A. F. (2010). Pain in children with cerebral palsy: a cross-sectional multicentre European study. *Acta Paediatr*, 99, 446–451.

Pier, D. B., Hallbergson, A., and Peters, J. M. (2010). Guillain-Barre syndrome in a child with pain: lessons learned from a late diagnosis. *Acta Paediatr*, 99, 1589–1591.

Ravilly, S., Robinson, W., Suresh, S., Wohl, M. E., and Berde, C. B. (1996). Chronic pain in cystic fibrosis. *Pediatrics*, 98, 741–747.

Riquelme, I., Cifre, I., and Montoya, P. (2011). Age-related changes of pain experience in cerebral palsy and healthy individuals. *Pain Med*, 12, 535–545.

Robinson, W. M., Ravilly, S., Berde, C. B., and Wohl, M. E. (1997). End-of-life care in cystic fibrosis. *Pediatrics*, 100, 205–209.

Russo, R. N., Miller, M. D., Haan, E., Cameron, I. D., and Crotty, M. (2008). Pain characteristics and their association with quality of life and self-concept in children with hemiplegic cerebral palsy identified from a population register. *Clin J Pain*, 24, 335–342.

Ruts, L., Drenthen, J., Jongen, J. L., Hop, W. C., Visser, G. H., Jacobs, B. C., et al. (2010). Pain in Guillain–Barre syndrome: a long-term follow-up study. *Neurology*, 75, 1439–1447.

Sahin, M. (2011). Neurofibromatosis. In R. M. Kleigman, B. F. Stanton, N. F. Schor, J. W. St. Geme, and R. E. Behrman (eds) *Nelson textbook of pediatrics*, pp. 2046–2048. Philadelphia, PA: Saunders.

Schiff, W. B., Holtz, K. D., Peterson, N., and Rakusan, T. (2001). Effect of an intervention to reduce procedural pain and distress for children with HIV infection. *J Pediatr Psychol*, 26, 417–427.

Serchuck, L. K., Williams, P. L., Nachman, S., Gadow, K. D., Chernoff, M., and Schwartz, L. (2010). Prevalence of pain and association with psychiatric symptom severity in perinatally HIV-infected children as compared to controls living in HIV-affected households. *AIDS Care*, 22, 640–648.

Sermet-Gaudelus, I., De Villartay, P., De Dreuzy, P., Clairicia, M., Vrielynck, S., Canoui, P., et al. (2009). Pain in children and adults with cystic fibrosis: a comparative study. *J Pain Symptom Manage*, 38, 281–290.

Slater, M. E., De Lima, J., Campbell, K., Lane, L., and Collins, J. (2010). Opioids for the management of severe chronic nonmalignant pain in children: a retrospective 1-year practice survey in a children's hospital. *Pain Med*, 11, 207–214.

Strafford, M., Cahill, C., Schwartz, T., Yee, J., Sethna, N., and Berde, C. (1991). Recogition and treatment of pain in pediatric patients with AIDS. *J Pain Symptom Manage*, 6, 146.

UNAIDS. (2011). *World AIDS day report*. Geneva: UNAIDS.

Van Dyke, R. B., Wang, L., and Williams, P. L. (2008). Toxicities associated with dual nucleoside reverse-transcriptase inhibitor regimens in HIV-infected children. *J Infect Dis*, 198, 1599–1608.

World Health Organization. (2011a). *Global HIV/AIDS response: epidemic update and health sector towards universal access, progress report 2011* [Online]. Available at: <www.who.int/hiv/pub/progress_report2011/en/index.html>.

World Health Organization. (2011b). *WHO model list of essential medicines for children* [Online]. Available at: <http://whqlibdoc.who.int/hq/2011/a95054_eng.pdf>.

World Health Organization. (2012). *WHO guidelines on the pharmacological treatment of persisting pain in children with medical illnesses*. [Online]. Available at: <http://whqlibdoc.who.int/publications/2012/9789241548120_Guidelines.pdf>

Wilcox, C. (2010). Gastrointestinal consequences of infection with human immunodeficiency virus. In M. Feldman, L. S. Friedman, and L. J. Brandt, (eds) *Sleisenger and Fordtran's gastrointestinal and liver disease*, pp. 523–536. Philadelphia, PA: Saunders.

Yaster, M. and Schechter, N. (1996). Pain and human immunodeficiency virus infection in children. *Pediatrics*, 98, 455–456.

Yogev, R. C., and Chadwick, E. G. (2011). Acquired immunodeficiency syndrome. In R. M. Kleigman, B. F. Stanton, N. F. Schor, J. W. St. Geme, and R. E. Behrman (eds) *Nelson textbook of pediatrics*, 1157–1176. Philadelphia, PA: Saunders.

CHAPTER 33

Common pain problems in the outpatient setting

F. Ralph Berberich and Neil L. Schechter

Summary

This chapter will review key concepts pertaining to paediatric pain relief in office settings. Included are general principles important to achieve pain reduction, pain attributed to normative developmental processes such as teething, colic, and 'growing pains', pain from infections such as otitis media and pharyngitis, and pain from minor procedures.

Introduction

Unfortunately, many advances in paediatric pain management have not been applied to the paediatric office (Berberich and Schechter, 2012). For example, despite their exponential increase in number, immunizations are often still administered in a manner similar to the way they were 40 years ago, continuing to contribute to a rate of needle phobia of 10% or more. Furthermore, little research has been done on relieving the pain of otitis or pharyngitis, common problems which are a significant source of discomfort. The reasons for this are manifold but certainly due at least in part to the less dramatic and often ephemeral nature of pain in the office. There exists additional concern that systematically addressing these issues might reduce office productivity and efficiency. Despite these barriers, addressing pain may prevent some of its short- and long-term consequences. Additionally, attention to pain is likely to enhance the relationship between the physician and the child and his or her family (Schechter et al., 2007).

General principles

The office based clinician, who typically has a long-term relationship with the child and family, and is well versed in child development, is in position to incorporate the principles of pain reduction into the practice setting. By doing so, he or she can lower the cumulative impact and memory of repeated 'minor' painful insults (Von Baeyer et al., 2004). He or she can perhaps prevent the development of needle phobia, teach parents to provide comfort for their children, and reduce the anticipatory fear and anxiety that often surrounds visits to a health care professional (Schechter et al., 2010). Development of a paediatric office that routinely employs the following principles will improve the quality of life not only for the child and his or her family but also for the paediatric office staff (Schechter et al., 2010).

There is enormous individual variability in response to a painful stimulus

Pain is a complex multifactorial phenomenon with enormous variation from person to person. There is no predictable level of pain response for a given nociceptive stimulus. The pain experience for any child is a composite of various factors including temperament, age, previous experience, parental response, social modelling, genetic predispositions, and psychological state (Blount et al., 2008; McMurtry et al., 2010; Schechter et al., 2007, 2010). A clinician who knows the child and family well can anticipate how the child might respond based on unique attributes of the child and his or her previous response to painful procedures. Clinicians also can benefit from the parent's in-depth knowledge of the child. Awareness of prior reactions, temperamental characteristics, and family dynamics may suggest non-pharmacological strategies and stave off more aggressive interventions.

Explanation and guidance regarding pain may help reduce it

Anticipatory guidance has become a cornerstone of paediatric practice. Although children display significant individual differences, they develop, in general, predictable sequences that allow us to anticipate what their challenges will be. Routinely incorporating information about pain into well child visits may allow children and families to prepare for, and appropriately cope with, the painful experiences that arise during childhood. This includes identifying helpful individualized strategies as well as recognizing when analgesics may be of value, and how best to use them. Two of the constructs are discussed in the following two sections.

Anticipate and/or prevent pain whenever possible

The importance of anticipating pain and the prompt use of pain reduction strategies should be emphasized at the outset of the physician–patient relationship. Pain may be more easily controlled if it can be prevented or addressed early on. Clinicians should give information about medication dosing and safe intervals between doses. Parents should understand that pain medication can be given proactively in anticipation of pain after injury or during illness or before procedures such as venepuncture. When a medication is appropriate for either pain or fever, parents should be instructed not to omit that medication 'because there is no fever'.

Promote self-mastery in the child

Teaching children techniques that can allow them to control their pain decreases the helplessness that they may feel when confronted with a painful situation. The clinician periodically can support and reinforce the importance of participatory distraction and encourage parents to identify the most appropriate and effective coping measures for their child. They best know their child's temperament, and the strategies that have been effective previously. Measures such as singing a song together, reading a story, watching a video, are ways to reduce the 'bother' and trauma of a painful or frightening event. These techniques, as well as others incorporated into an immunization sequence, can diminish the pain response and its associated anxiety (Berberich and Landman, 2009). Many of these techniques could be practised at home to enhance their mastery. As the child grows, the clinician can remind parents to bring along stuffed animals, books, or smartphones and to help engage in self-calming non-procedural talk and activities. Parents should learn that it helps to look forward to something pleasurable, i.e. 'When we've finished here, then we can . . .'

Attention to the language and demeanour of the clinician and the parent is critical

Language and demeanour have a critical role in shaping the child's experience of, and response to, painful situations. Children readily read verbal and non-verbal signals, such as facial expressions, tone, pitch of voice, whether a sentence rises or falls, and the degree of confidence and security displayed by a parent (Blount et al., 2008). If the content of what is said is at odds with the non-verbal message, the child may be confused and suffer uncertainty and paradoxical anxiety. Parental demeanour projecting excessive worry and a sense of catastrophe often will cause exaggerated responses in children (Vervoort et al., 2011a, 2011b). Parental modelling can contribute to the development of fear and enduring phobias (de Roznay et al., 2006). Therefore, parents should be advised to be cognizant of their own attitudes towards pain and how any negative prejudice or anxiety might be transmitted to their child.

Words uttered in the doctor's office have greater than expected impact (Berberich, 2007). Parents and clinicians should be aware that children might take to heart what may seem like relatively 'innocent' analogies such as 'like a bee sting' (Berberich and Schechter, 2011) or statements that conflict with what the child is thinking, such as 'It's OK' or 'Don't worry'. It is far better to instruct parents, pointing out the nuances of language as well as the possible contradiction between intent and effect when speaking to children. In particular, a frightened child may hear as a threat what is actually intended only as a light-hearted parental tease, so the clinician should respond appropriately to comments of this kind. Curiously, there is evidence indicating that excessive reassurance is not always reassuring and over-empathizing may actually increase anxiety and discomfort rather than diminishing them (Schechter et al., 2010).

Parents have a critical role to play in pain reduction

Parents should be encouraged to be active, supporting participants in every medical encounter and be informed how they can be most helpful. We have learned that parents, when properly informed and respected, can play an essential role in the reduction of the pain problems. Parents can help us identify the type and timing of preparation that seems most effective. They can practise now-familiar distraction techniques at home and use these to coach the child through painful procedures in the office. When medically safe, upright comfort positioning, often on a parent's lap, is the best choice for the examination or any procedure that could be seen as invasive (Lacey et al., 2008; Schechter et al., 2007; Sparks et al., 2007). If restraint on an exam table is required, positioning a parent near the child's head and seeking cooperative possibilities reduces anxiety.

Analgesics in the outpatient setting

The judicious use of pharmacological agents remains a mainstay of successful pain treatment. Acetaminophen (paracetamol, APAP) and non-steroidal anti-inflammatory drugs (NSAIDs), typically ibuprofen, constitute the primary first line agents. They are considered to be equally safe although ibuprofen may be a bit more effective (Pierce and Voss, 2010). Until there is sufficient evidence to support one agent over another, a step wise approach, similar to the World Health Organization pain ladder, seems reasonable when pain persists despite a properly administered single agent. This entails adding one agent to the other at safe dose intervals (Wright and Liebelt, 2007). While there seems to be no antipyretic advantage to an 'alternating' 3 h acetaminophen/ibuprofen schedule other than its perceived simplicity (Wright and Liebelt, 2007), analgesia may be enhanced by utilizing both in combination (Ong et al., 2010). To avoid confusion, written administration plans are advisable (Wright and Liebelt, 2007). Physicians need to prepare parents so that they completely understand how to use these medications and neither overdose nor underdose. Handouts or office web sites for parents are often helpful.

The clinician may face situations in which pain is not treated adequately with acetaminophen or NSAIDs. Oxycodone and hydrocodone deliver predictable and potent levels of analgesia and are available in liquid preparations. Despite the lack of clinical trials and potential concerns about opioid abuse, fear of untoward outcomes, and lack of published guidelines, paediatricians and family physicians should be prepared to consider these opioids when faced with moderate to severe pain. Tramadol (Ultram™) is an atypical opioid that has been used safely and effectively in children at an oral dose of 1 to 2 mg/kg every 6 h. Those who treat children should not prescribe codeine-containing medications because of its ineffectiveness in many children and toxicity in some. Inert codeine is metabolized to its active metabolite, morphine at a 10:1 ratio in 'normal' metabolizers. However, there are clinically significant, even fairly large, numbers in whom the CYP2D6 enzyme responsible for that metabolism is genetically altered. In many individuals, up to 30% of the general population, this enzyme variant of CYP2D6 results in poor metabolism, which translates to ineffectiveness. In others, especially those of North African descent, ultrarapid conversion to morphine may result in toxic levels and a risk of mortality (Kelly et al., 2012). All opioids tend to produce constipation and this side effect is best anticipated with consideration of stool softening and laxative agents. Pruritis, hallucinations and dreams, and somnolence should be encountered relatively less frequently in outpatients receiving appropriate doses and short courses.

Table 33.1 lists step-up groupings of common pain medications applicable to the paediatric office setting. These will have a variety of trade names and formulations. Opioids are regulated in most countries and may require special prescription forms. One must be especially cautious when prescribing combination opioid medications that may include other analgesics, decongestants, or

Table 33.1 Paediatric oral pain medications (formulations may vary)

Drug	Dose (mg/kg)	Interval (h)	Suspensions (mg/ml)	Tabs (mg)
APAP	15	4–6	160/1 160/5	160, 325, 500
Ibuprofen	10	6–8	100/5	200, 400 600
Tramadol	1–2	4–6	N/A (US)	50, 100–300
Hydrocodone	0.1–0.2	4–6	2.5/5	2.5, 5, 10
Hydromorphone	0.05	4–6	5/5	5
Oxycodone	0.1	4–6	1/1	5

antitussives. For example, Lortab® elixir contains hydrocodone 2.5 mg per 5ml, but also has APAP 167 mg, requiring dose adjustment of any concurrent APAP for pain or fever. It also contains 7% alcohol. In addition, any condition that affects drug metabolism or concurrent medication such as diphenhydramine, atropine, or some psychotropic drugs may compound or mask common side effects such as somnolence, nausea, and pruritis.

It is important to alert families to formulation variance, idiosyncratic dropper markings, expiration dates, the importance of closing childproof containers, and proper disposal of unused opioid medication. Parents should be encouraged to consider pain apart from its cause and an independent symptom that calls for independent attention. It is still the case that parents sometimes withhold pain medication for fear that important symptoms may be masked and the validity of the physical examination compromised (Bromberg and Goldman, 2007). It may be appropriate to introduce general guidelines for analgesic medications early, perhaps coinciding with immunizations at 2 months of age. Periodic reinforcement can be provided at intervals during well child visits.

Pain associated with specific conditions

In the following section, specific pain problems will be reviewed. These include pain arising from the evaluation and treatment of specific disease states, pain that stems from normative processes, and pain from commonly performed procedures. Needle procedures are discussed elsewhere in this text (Taddio, Chapter 19).

Pain stemming from specific disease processes

Otitis and otalgia

Acute otitis media (AOM) is the most common cause of childhood physician visits in the US, generating 16 million outpatient encounters and 13 to 15 million prescriptions per year, as well as significant financial costs (Woodwell and Cherry, 2004). Additionally, about 2.4 million US healthcare visits occur for the treatment of acute otitis externa (AOE) (Centers for Disease Control and Prevention (CDC) 2011a).

Common to both entities is otalgia, which is often quite intense (Narcy et al., 2006). The structures of the external canal, middle ear, and tympanic membrane contain a wealth of nociceptive innervation responsive to inflammation and pus under pressure (Zempsky and Schechter, 2000). Antibiotics do not have a rapid or profound effect on the resolution of pain (Spiro et al., 2008). While controversy continues to surround recommendations for the institution and choice of antibiotics, the treatment of otalgia remains a pressing concern, especially for parents confronted with crying children and sleepless nights.

Systemic oral analgesics are recommended first. Most commonly, these are acetaminophen, ibuprofen, or combinations of both, as previously described. It may take up to an hour for acetaminophen and ibuprofen to become noticeably effective. In the case of AOM without perforation, local analgesic therapy may bridge this gap and allow for rapid comfort. In the US, Auralgan® (antipyrine, benzocaine, and glycerine) is popular for this purpose, although definitive benefit remains to be established. A double blind, randomized, placebo-controlled paediatric study using topical aqueous 2% lignocaine showed a 50% reduction in pain scores from baseline at 10 and 30 min (Bolt et al., 2008) but the validity of the study has been challenged (Bharti and Bharti, 2008). In a non-controlled multicentre observational study of a little over 400 children, most of whom had AOM, another comparable analgesic, procaine with phenazone yielded physician rated efficacy of 'good' or 'very good' in more than 95% (Adam et al., 2009). However, an earlier Cochrane review found insufficient evidence to support the effectiveness of either topical analgesia or naturopathic herbal eardrops (Foxlee et al., 2006). Clinicians confronted with intractable otalgia should be prepared to utilize opioids, as they are likely to be effective.

In AOE, it seems clear that antibiotic ear drops with or without hydrocortisone plus suspension of water exposure leads to the most rapid resolution of pain as well as the infection (Roland et al., 2008). A variety of warm oils and hot compress applications may provide transient symptomatic relief, but have not been tested rigorously.

Otalgia is a common occurrence and parents should be educated about pain treatment in advance of the first ear infection. In a report describing an education program at the 15-month well-child examination, to which was added a proactive prescription for antipyrine-benzocaine otic drops (Auralgan®), the study group experienced reductions of 80% emergency room, 40% urgent care, and 28% primary care visits for otalgia (McWilliams et al., 2008).

Acute pharyngitis

In a sample of 160 families that included approximately 240 children, 41% experienced at least one episode of acute sore throat in a 16-month prospective study period (Danchin et al., 2007). Bacterial infection, notably by group A *Streptococcus* accounts for roughly 20% to 35% of pharyngeal infections (Shaikh, et al., 2010). While the literature is replete with articles about group A streptococcal disease, evidence-based pain management protocols are lacking. This persists despite the observation that antibiotics do little to ablate pharyngeal pain.

Pain control here as with many other conditions begins with the administration of oral analgesics, specifically acetaminophen and ibuprofen. Medication may be harder to give because of pain and dysphagia, or from illness-associated vomiting. When either is prominent, rectal acetaminophen may be the better choice. Although most pharyngeal pain resolves by 48 h, prescribing around-the-clock analgesic increases that resolution from 55% to more than 70% (Bertin et al., 1991). Tramadol or opioid-ibuprofen/acetaminophen combinations may be indicated to relieve refractory pain and maintain hydration.

The treatment of mononucleosis-associated exudative tonsillitis may require maximum analgesia efforts. Once a presumptive diagnosis is established, a short course of steroids may provide relatively rapid relief. Steroids have been found effective for other forms of severe pharyngitis as well (Korb et al., 2010). In two randomized clinical trials in which paediatric patients received dexamethasone, 0.3 mg/kg to 15 mg maximum (Roy et al., 2004), or 0.6 mg/kg single dose to 10 mg maximum (Olympia et al., 2005), versus placebo, sore throat resolved earlier and faster, whether or not patients tested positive for group A *Streptococcus* or mononucleosis.

Lozenges and cough drops designed to soothe throats are not advised for children under the age of 4 years or for others in whom there is an aspiration risk. A transient benefit for older children may be presumed to represent benign intervention, but no studies actually exist to demonstrate pain relief or significant soothing. A randomized clinical trial in adults undertaken in the UK showed about 2 h relief from amylmetacresol/2,4 dichlorobenzoyl alcohol lozenges (McNally et al., 2010.) Some practitioners or parents may favour herbal preparations or a variety of home remedies, but their safety and efficacy likewise still need to be tested.

Gingivostomatitis

In children, stomatitis, faucal ulcers and gum swelling, are commonly associated with primary herpes simplex or herpangina due to Coxsackie infections. A majority of children will have had primary herpes simplex or another form of viral pharyngitis by age 5 years. Pain and reluctance to eat and drink are the primary symptoms of concern, as the illnesses themselves typically run a benign course.

Analgesic medications, acetaminophen and ibuprofen, may be prescribed around the clock and timed to reach peak effect at mealtimes. If dehydration or inadequate oral intake result, opioid combinations or intravenous rehydration may be necessary. Acidic foods such as citrus or vinegar may cause pain. Milk-based shakes or their equivalent may be preferred to solid food. Depending on the location of lesions, drinking through a large straw may be accepted.

Acyclovir may shorten the duration and thus indirectly affect pain (Faden, 2006). A number of topical medications can be prescribed, most of them derived from experience with chemotherapy and radiation-induced stomatitis. The rationale behind these agents is to coat exposed ulcers. Thus either diphenhydramine-bismuth subsalicylate (Kaopectate®), or diphenhydramine-aluminium/magnesium hydroxide is often used on an anecdotal basis. There are no published prospective trials comparing the treatment options.

Viscous xylocaine 2% is attractive for its numbing properties but carries a theoretical risk for aspiration and the possibility of a child biting his own buccal mucosa. There have been documented toxicities, some fatal, due to overdose or swallowing rather than 'swish and spit' (Curtis et al., 2009). Application of the lidocaine directly to the lesions may be safer, but saliva is likely to carry at least some throughout the oropharynx and therefore entail the same risks.

Pain associated with normal growth and development

Certain events are so often encountered during the course of normal growth and development that it is hard to consider them abnormal. However frequency does not dismiss the significance and validity of the pain experienced. Few interventions have been identified as efficacious for these problems and reassuring parents of their benign nature and supporting them through them these episodes is perhaps the most valuable contribution that the clinician can make.

Colic

Colic was defined almost half a century ago by the rule of 3s, coined by Wessel as excessive crying and fussing for more than 3 h per day, more than 3 days a week, for more than 3 weeks' duration. Colic is one of childhood's most disconcerting, yet physiologically benign, conditions, occurring in up to 20% of infants (Shergill-Bonner, 2010). There are those who maintain that colic is not painful, but rather a state of pain-unrelated excessive crying without identified cause (Lucassen and Assenfelft, 2001). Despite its unknown aetiology, there seems to be agreement that abdominal distress is associated with amplifying aerophagia and distension. No medication resolves colic and there also is no other proven standard therapy (Hall et al., 2011). Herb teas and similar preparations such as fennel-containing gripe water are often suggested, but none have been studied systematically. Other approaches such as formula alterations, probiotics, acupuncture, chiropractic manipulations, and massage have been advocated by some (Arikan et al., 2008), but remain unsupported by evidence.

Measures undertaken by clinicians currently seek to minimize parental distress, maintain bonding, and offer reassurance as to the absence of long-term consequences (Keefe et al., 2006). Dietary alterations only help if there is an identified intolerance. (Shergill-Bonner, 2010). Interruption of breastfeeding or multiple formula changes may be undesirable consequences of well-intentioned interventions. Given the frustration of parents, a variety of unproven interventions such as gentle rocking while pacing, long rides in the car, swaddling and 'shushing' (Karp, 2007), competing noise such as that generated by a vacuum cleaner, and parental ear plugs, all continue to be suggested.

Teething

A variety of behaviours, such as irritability, intermittent crying, and increased chewing may indicate teething during the first 6 months of life (Feldens et al., 2010), although the caveat is that these may also be part of normal development. Much is falsely blamed on tooth eruption, especially by parents surrounded by teething lore (Owais et al., 2010). Prospective cohort studies have revealed only weak association with previously reported symptoms, and no association with severe illness (Ramos-Jorge et al., 2011). Local pain and low-grade fever may be attributed to teething legitimately only by a process of elimination.

Oral ibuprofen and acetaminophen have long been used to treat teething pain, especially when it interferes with sleep. Opioids are not recommended because there is no evidence for efficacy in the setting of a relatively mild, yet protracted condition. Parents may be cautioned that a baby who immediately soothes when picked up may not be suffering from teething pain. There is no evidence that topical and homeopathic preparations, ice pack massages, or frozen foods applied locally provide effective relief. However, frozen solid, non-phthalate containing teething rings, hard apples, frozen bagels, are popular. Agents containing lidocaine, benzocaine or comparable anaesthetics can be toxic, rarely associated with methaemoglobinaemia, even occasionally lethal (Curtis et al., 2009). Some teething gels have been associated with salicylate toxicity (Williams et al., 2011). Although widely available, there is no evidence to support herbal and other over-the-counter teething remedies.

Growing pains

The term describes a poorly understood syndrome of recurring bilateral lower limb discomfort, typically occurring at night in active children during the pre-pubertal growth years. The incidence is estimated at 10% to 20% between the ages of 3 to 12 years, with a peak occurrence between ages 4 to 8 years (Goodyear-Smith and Arroll, 2006). The pain may be sufficient to awaken the child. Characteristically, there are no physical findings and no other limbs or muscle groups are involved. Children are asymptomatic during the day. The diagnosis is made by exclusion; yet the recurring nature of symptoms without anatomic explanation may arouse anxiety on the part of parents and this in turn my intensify symptom reports. A recent literature search disclosed the absence of evidence to endorse any particular form of therapy (Evans, 2008). Systemic oral analgesics such as ibuprofen or acetaminophen may be administered in conjunction with local measures such as massage, stretching, and warmth. The latter may be accomplished with heavy-duty cotton, wool, or polyester socks that extend over the calf. To enhance warmth, these can be preheated in the dryer. Microwaved heat packs may be useful, but need to be assessed for hot spots before being applied.

Pain associated with common procedures

Circumcision

Surgical removal of the penile foreskin is probably the most common, and controversial perinatal procedure in paediatrics. In the US, roughly half or 1.2 million male newborns are circumcised each year. For about one-fifth of the world's population, circumcision is a religious expectation. There is recent data suggesting circumcision may contribute to a reduction in the incidence of HIV/sexually transmitted infections (Bailey et al., 2007) and this may in turn signal an increase in its acceptance (CDC, 2011b). Medical, ethical, and legal pros and cons aside, the issue of pain management persists, whether circumcision is carried out in the office, hospital, or elsewhere.

Recently, the American Academy of Pediatrics issued a policy statement, which reaffirms the appropriateness and specifics of proper analgesia (American Academy of Pediatrics, 2012). The American Academy of Family Physicians (AAFP), American College of Obstetricians and Gynecologists, Canadian Pediatric Society, British Medical Association, and the British Association of Paediatric Urologists have issued comparably supportive policy statements. Without analgesia, circumcision causes physiological signs of marked distress, such as elevated heart rate, blood pressure, and plasma cortisol, increased crying, and augmented reactions to painful stimuli in infancy (Taddio et al., 1997).

Taddio summarized the influence of circumcision technique and topical and local anaesthetics on the attenuation of this distress. Circumcisions were performed with one of three clamps, the Gomco, Plastibell, or Mogen. Local anaesthesia infiltration consisted of dorsal penile nerve block (DPNB), ring block, or topical anaesthesia. DPNB is carried out in a fairly standardized manner with 1% lidocaine without adrenaline 0.2 to 0.5 ml delivered at the 10:00 and 02:00 position subcutaneously at the base of the penis penetrating Buck's fascia (Kirya and Werthman, 1978). A circumferential ring block is performed with the same lidocaine injected mid-shaft or behind the corona.

Choice of clamp may reflect operator training, degree of comfort, or perceived risk of performing the procedure as much as evidence-based data. In combination with DPNB, the Mogen clamp entails less pain and a shorter procedure time than the Gomco clamp (Kurtis et al., 1999).

Taddio has summarized the substantial data confirming the effectiveness and safety of DPNB (Taddio, 2001) versus placebo or no treatment. A 1997 randomized clinical trial compared pain using a ring block, DPNB, and topical lidocaine-prilocaine cream. The study showed an advantage for ring block in that it alone was effective for the foreskin separation and incision phases of circumcision (Lander et al., 1997).

What topical analgesia gains by being simple to use, effective, and portable, it loses as it provides relatively poor analgesia during the brief probe lysis of glans adhesions. The duration of the pre-procedure application of topical anaesthetics influences the clinical outcome. Taddio has cited a range of 45 to 90 min as well as a dosage range of 0.5 to 5 g (Taddio, 2001). However, the depth of anaesthetic effect relates to the duration of application and is greater with longer wait times of up to 120 min in at least one adult study (Wahlgren and Quiding, 2000). There does exist the theoretical potential for methaemoglobinaemia related to prilocaine, however the clinically significant risk has been estimated to be 0% (Taddio, 2001). Liposomal lidocaine cream (LMX-4) also has been shown to be safe and effective, comparable to lidocaine-prilocaine cream in a randomized trial (Lehr et al., 2005).

A Cochrane Review evaluated 35 trials involving 1997 newborn males to generate best evidence conclusions regarding efficacy of pain interventions (Brady-Fryer et al., 2004). The meta-analysis indicated that DPNB and lidocaine-prilocaine cream both reduce circumcision pain when compared to placebo and that DPNB is relatively more effective than lidocaine-prilocaine cream applied for 60 to 90 min. However, strict comparability of studies was rare as the choice of clamp utilized and length of wait time varied.

Additional measures to lessen discomfort include non-nutritive sucking, sucrose, and having the baby securely and properly held by a person as opposed to a plastic moulded restraint (Stang et al., 1997; Taddio, 2001). Acetaminophen may be effective postoperatively, but has little effect before the procedure (Taddio, 2001).

Cerumen impaction

Excessive earwax may impede the accurate diagnosis of middle ear disease. Its mechanical removal can cause pain, trauma, and bleeding. A 2004 literature review and meta-analysis of adult and paediatric studies showed a 40% clearance rate when water or oil-based otic cerumenolytic agents were instilled for several days. A 2009 Cochrane review indicated that while otic wax removal drops were more effective than water, none stood out as being superior to any other (Burton and Doree, 2009). In order to avoid being confronted with an acute need to remove cerumen, a clinician can begin dealing with it whenever it is noted. Instilling over-the-counter cerumenolytics several times a week during sleep may prove useful, as long as there is no otorrhoea. Faced with blocked ear canals in the office, irrigation with saline, plain water or a 50:50 hydrogen peroxide/water mixture has been found to be effective; however, electric irrigators produce noise that may frighten some children and the sensation of water flooding the external canal may prove unpleasant for others. Preceding irrigation with a 10 min instillation of liquid ducosate sodium (Colace®) may aid cerumenolysis, but this method has not been studied systematically. Published guidelines do not indicate a preference or endorse one removal method over another (Hand and Harvey, 2004; Roland et al., 2008). There is no demonstrable efficacy to support a variety of folk remedies such as the instillation of oils and garlic. Others, such as candling are ineffective and can cause injury (Zackaria and Aymat, 2009).

Urinary catheterization

Despite its imperfections sterile catheterization remains the gold standard to diagnose urinary tract infection (UTI; Wingerter and Bachur, 2011). Suprapubic aspiration is associated with pain and a tendency towards more procedure failures than urinary catheterization (El-Naggar et al., 2010). In a randomized controlled trial, the administration of oral sucrose reduced pain scores and showed a relatively more rapid return to baseline in infants less than 30 days of age (Rogers et al., 2006). However, this beneficial effect was not apparent beyond the first month of life.

In addition to catheterization for UTI diagnosis, this procedure is an integral part of the voiding cystourethrogram (VCUG). New guidelines could reduce the necessity for VCUGs (Schroeder et al., 2011), but not entirely eliminate them. Topical 2% lidocaine gel instillation may reduce catheterization pain (Vaughan et al., 2005), although the evidence is mixed in clinical trials. Even though VCUGs are not conducted in the paediatric office, the clinician may become involved by preferentially referring patients to institutions that attend to the associated discomfort. A 2005 randomized study reported effectiveness of hypnotic relaxation in children who had a prior VCUG and were more than 4 years of age (Butler et al, 2005). Successful sedation with 70% nitrous oxide (Zier et al., 2007), intranasal fentanyl (Chung et al., 2010), and midazolam (Herd, 2008) has been reported, although others question whether it is beneficial for the properly prepared child (Sandy et al, 2011). The decision might best be individualized by the physician who actually knows the patient. For some, offering preparation, procedural narration and distraction (Salmon et al., 2006), often the province of child life specialists, may be an appropriate stand alone or supplemental choice.

Cauterization and foreign body removal

Intranasal silver nitrate cauterization for epistaxis can cause discomfort. This and nasal swabbing are both swift, but the stinging and sneezing can be quite unpleasant. Clinicians often are faced with having to retrieve a pea or bead from a nostril. Similarly, obtaining a nasopharyngeal sample by means of a swab may be considered invasive. Where indicated in a fearful child, topical 4% lidocaine delivered by means of a reusable bottle metered dose atomizer with a disposable applicator (MADomizer™) may be acceptable prior to instrumentation. Alternatively, anaesthetic solutions can be compounded 50:50 with a nasal decongestant containing oxymetazoline.

Tick removal

Some children may be disturbed by the sensation of skin tenting during removal by traction. Others may seek rapid removal knowing an insect has attached and burrowed into their skin. A 4 to 10 sec spray of vapocoolant (PainEase®) may relieve pain and provide kinaesthetic distraction as well.

Ocular foreign body and corneal abrasion

Proxymetacaine anaesthetic drops can facilitate examination and provide a more accurate diagnosis of foreign body (Sklar et al., 1989). A temporary burning sensation may still be experienced. Anaesthetic drops are instilled only for diagnosis, and not for treatment, because of toxicity and sensitization risks. Patching the eye often stops the pain.

Subungual hematoma

Subungual hematomas cause pain secondary to pressure, which can be relieved by creating a hole in the affected nail. This may provoke anxiety, but should not be painful when accomplished by means of a hand-held single-use cautery (Bovie®). The cautery tip is gently applied to the nail over the hematoma in short bursts, following the manufacturer's safety directions, until sufficient penetration allows the underlying blood to extrude. A trephining drill or rotating needle can accomplish drainage as well, but some pressure is required and this itself causes pain and potential anxiety, while other associations such as drill with needle may arouse fear or panic. Children should be told in advance and shown that the nail feels no pain.

The 'pain-sensitive' office

By systematically incorporating the previously described principles and strategies into practice, the burden of pain in the paediatric office can be reduced significantly. Additionally, attention to the office environment, physician and staff participation and a general declared emphasis on pain reduction can make a difference.

Office environment

It is stands to reason that the best paediatric office milieu is one that is cheerful and non-threatening, or better yet, calming, both in its physical surroundings and in the demeanour of its personnel. Most practitioners assume that age appropriate toys, books, and media that utilize innate curiosity can do much to put children at ease. Given the relationship between anxiety and pain perception, environmental props and office flow policies that generate a mood of calm could be expected to have an impact on that anxiety, for better or for worse. Yet there is no data establishing precise formulas for how those are to be constituted.

As most children often wait in examination rooms after leaving the waiting area, the same kind of props should be available in that location. There is no direct evidence favouring one colour scheme or set of books and magazines over another, and this would be hard to come by as cultural, age, and individual preferences all vary widely, and gender also influences choices. It nevertheless remains a worthy goal to seek the means to divert the child's attention from preoccupation with the pending examination, immunizations, and other disquieting procedures or treatment (Berberich and Landman 2009; Du et al., 2008; Schechter et al., 2007).

An environment rich in distracting materials may be helpful in shifting focus, especially as it allows, even encourages, parents to engage in non-procedural talk (Schechter et al., 2007). Although supporting data are lacking, the choice of wall colour, posters and images likely can do much to support a sense of comfort and familiarity and engage the child. When choosing the elements that will characterize the office and examination rooms, the suggestibility of children should be kept in mind although the evidence for positive effect is mixed (Berberich and Landman, 2009; Kohen and Olness, 2011). By posting photographs of patients and families, children can recognize themselves, perhaps their friends, and be given an anxiety-tempering message of normalcy and familiarity. Similarly, posters of animals or amusing cartoons provide suggestions of levity and arouse interest.

Children's affinity for animals, how they uniquely relate to them, and their assignment of animals to characters and 'personality' traits are themselves subjects of study (Melson, 2005). Some may be associated with bravery (lions, tigers), others with nurturing (birds in a nest, mother bears and cubs), and yet others with coziness (puppies, kittens). Children readily absorb the messages that such stories and images provide. Further, they may use associations and implications to change behaviours (Wansink et al., 2012). Since so many children gravitate towards inanimate representations of animals to provide emotional support and security (Triebenbacher, 1998), having a stuffed, easy-to-wipe-down, office 'mascot' to cuddle may provide yet another useful prop.

Office Pain 'Champion'

Even if an office has committed itself to being 'pain sensitive', it is helpful to identify a pain champion who can recruit the ongoing participation of colleagues and staff, remain current by reviewing paediatric pain literature, and set the tone for staff commitment to foster comfort (Kuttner, 2010; Schechter, 2008). That dedicated clinician can generate appropriate literature for parents and educate the office staff in order to maintain a pain minimizing focus. For patients with chronic pain conditions, pertinent books and web site links can be made available. In complex situations, the office pain champion can become an in office consultant and guide appropriate referral to a paediatric pain specialist (Berberich and Schechter, 2012).

Proactive pain management

Because of the negative conditioning effect of pain, and simply because it causes distress, its infliction should be avoided wherever possible, especially in very young children (Schechter, 2008; Zempsky and Schechter, 2003). A proactive approach might be termed anticipatory anticipation! A prime example would be to prescribe 2.5% lidocaine-prilocaine cream or 4% Lidocaine (LMX-4®) cream together with instructions for a 90–120 min covered application before elective blood draws such as lead level determinations. Parents can apply these agents at home, eliminating the need for office application and the wait time, and thus reducing barriers to their use. Similarly, parents of infants can be reminded before the 2-, 4-, and 6-month visits about acetaminophen or ibuprofen administration after immunizations, as well as how to apply local measures such as cool compresses. At the 12-month visit, when toddlers begin to walk and stumble and injure themselves, the clinician can remind parents to use local measures and medicate early for 'minor' pain. Because the crying associated with pain is so unnerving, repetition serves to embed the parents' responses in a way that these become more automatic and prompt. Teaching appropriate consolation could shorten the distress associated with injections, inducing more rapid resolution of pain and possibly

affecting the degree of negative conditioning that result from it (Harrington et al., 2012). The development and dissemination of evidence-based, online, video, and written material instructing parents how to approach medical office visits and uncomfortable procedures would be most welcome.

Attention to comfort

In the pain-sensitive office, comfort measures such as nursing, non-nutritive sucking, and sucrose administration are supported (Pillai Riddell, et al., 2011). Easy access to oral 24% sucrose (Sweetease™) or topical anaesthetics will promote their use. Respect for a child's autonomy tempers fear as does parental proximity. Until it becomes a yes or no option for a curious child, the examination table is best avoided unless absolutely necessary. Being supine with a physician hovering over you can be intimidating. The timesaving importance of allowing children to adopt positions of security has been identified in the context of IV placement (Sparks et al., 2007). Most paediatricians become quite adept at demonstrating instruments and creating games as part of the physical examination. They will already have learned to save the most invasive parts of the exam for last. The active participation of the child is one of the best routes to cooperation. Areas of pain are best approached gradually and with careful attention to facial expression and body language. Posting signs and web site information indicating that the office is committed to addressing pain emphasizes commitment.

Communication about pain

There is no uniform agreement as to what constitutes authenticity and honesty when kids ask about procedures that may cause discomfort. Deceit and trickery permanently destroy trust. Yet 'informing' can be phrased as a negative or positive suggestion, even taking into account the unpredictable individuality of each child. Therapeutic language is that which is crafted to elicit positive coping responses. That skill is taught, among others, by experts in the field of paediatric hypnosis, which, together with biofeedback, can be useful for procedures (Butler et al., 2005) and for acute and chronic pain (Kohen and Olness, 2011). In the United States, the National Pediatric Hypnosis Institute and the American Society for Clinical Hypnosis currently provide training workshops. The Milton Erickson Society of Germany is also active in promoting paediatric hypnosis instruction.

Conclusion

In this chapter, we have sought to coalesce some of the limited available information on pain treatment in paediatric outpatient facilities. While recognizing the need for additional research, uniform application of what we already know will go a long way toward reducing the burden of outpatient pain. Despite perceived obstacles and past patterns of indifference, pain in paediatric offices can and should receive the attention it deserves. What is required is a long view, one that acknowledges the significance of the 'little' insults that can be avoided with a bit of effort and the expenditure of a small amount of time. Attention to pain can improve the doctor/patient/family relationship by rendering a child more cooperative and less frightened. That leads to an adult who feels more comfortable within the medical system rather than fearful and avoiding of it. Every clinic setting deserves a pain 'champion' to prod all those delivering the health care at that facility to be mindful of, and proactive in, dealing with pain.

Case examples, with and without a pain-sensitive approach

A 2-year-old girl presents crying with an earache and a temperature of 39°C having slept poorly and received a single dose of acetaminophen during the previous night. The doctor examines the patient and finds the ear canal occluded by cerumen. He takes a plastic curette and places it in the external canal to remove earwax. The child jerks her head and cries out in pain. The child appears upset and her mother asks, 'Did that hurt her?'. He tries again and notices that there is some bleeding in the external canal. Still unable to see, he orders an ear wash. The child cries throughout. When the doctor returns, he is still unable to visualize the tympanic membrane, and the child writhes and cries loudly each time he approaches to insert the otoscope. He prescribes a course of amoxicillin, telling the parent that the child likely has an ear infection.

A 2-year-old girl presents crying with an earache, having slept poorly and received a single dose of acetaminophen during the previous night. While waiting for the doctor, she is given a dose of acetaminophen at the paediatrician's request. The tympanic membrane cannot be visualized due to impacted cerumen. The paediatrician instils 'magic' docusate drops and places a cotton wick 'furry ball' in the external canal. As his patient lies in her mother's lap, she reads some stories and plays a smartphone game with her daughter while he attends to another patient. After 10 min, the medical assistant comes in, explains to the child that her ear is going to have a little bath so the doctor can see better and she gently irrigates the ear. The doctor returns, thanks the child for helping him by being brave and wicks the canal dry revealing an inflamed and retracted, but non-bulging tympanic membrane. He chooses to treat with analgesics alone, explaining around the clock administration of ibuprofen to the parent and presenting her with a written step-up plan based on the addition of acetaminophen. He also prescribes Auralgan® drops in the event pain returns before the next dose of analgesia is due. The parent is given a dose sheet upon which the per-weight ibuprofen and acetaminophen doses appropriate for the child are indicated and circled. A follow-up parental phone report is arranged.

References

Adam, D., Federspil P., Lukes, M., and Petrowicz, O. (2009). Therapeutic properties and tolerance of procaine and phenazone containing eardrops in infants and very young children. *Arzneimittelforschung*, 59, 504–512.

American Academy of Pediatrics. (2012). Circumcision policy statement. *Pediatrics*, 130(3), 585–586.

Arikan, D., Alp, H., Goezuem, S., Orbak, Z., and Cifci, E. K. (2008). Effectiveness of massage, sucrose solution, herbal tea, or hydrolyzed formula in the treatment of infantile coli. *J Clin Nurs*, 17(13), 1754–1761.

Bailey, R. C., Moses, S., Parker, C. B., Agot, K., MacLean, I., Krieger, J. N., et al. (2007). Male circumcision for HIV prevention in young men in Kisumu, Kenya: a randomized controlled trial. *Lancet* 369, 657–666.

Berberich, F. R. (2007). Pediatric suggestions: using hypnosis in the routine examination of children. *Am J Clin Hypn*, 50(2), 121–129.

Berberich, F. R., and Landman, Z. (2009). Reducing immunization discomfort in 4- to 6-year-old children: a randomized clinical trial. *Pediatrics*, 124(2), e203–209.

Berberich, F. R., and Schechter, N. L. (2012). Pediatric office pain: crying for attention. *Pediatrics*, 129(4), e1057–1059.

Bertin, L., Pons, G., d'Athis, P., Lasfargues, G., Maudelonde, C., Duhamel, J. F., et al. (1991). Randomized, double-blind, multicenter, controlled trial of ibuprofen versus acetaminophen (paracetamol) and placebo for treatment of symptoms of tonsillitis and pharyngitis in children. *J Pediatr*, 119(5), 811–814.

Bharti, B. and Bharti, S. (2008). Is topical lignocaine for pain relief in acute otitis media really effective? *Arch Dis Child*, 93(8), 714.

Bolt, P., Barnett, P., Babl F. E., and Sharwood L. N. (2008). Topical lignocaine for pain relief in acute otitis media: results of a double-blind placebo-controlled randomised trial. *Arch Dis Child*, 93, 40–44.

Blount, R. L., Devine, K. A., Cheng, P. S., Simons, L. E., and Hayutin, L. (2008). The impact of adult behaviors on infant distress during immunizations. *J Pediatr Psychol*, 33(10), 1163–1174

Brady-Fryer, B., Wiebe, N., and Lander, J. A. (2004). Pain relief for neonatal circumcision. *Cochrane Database Syst Rev*, 4, CD004217.

Bromberg, R. and Goldman, R. D. (2007). Does analgesia mask diagnosis of appendicitis among children? *Can Fam Physician*, 53, 39–41.

Burton, M. J., and Doree, C. (2009). Ear drops for the removal of ear wax. *Cochrane Database Syst Rev*, 1, CD004326.

Butler, L. D., Symons B. K., Henderson, S. L., Shortliffe, L. D., and Spiegel, D. (2005). Hypnosis reduces distress and duration of an invasive medical procedure for children. *Pediatrics*, 115(1), e77–85.

Centers for Disease Control and Prevention (CDC). (2011a). Estimated burden of acute otitis externa—United States, 2003–2007. *MMWR Morb Mortal Wkly Rep*, 60(19), 605–609.

Centers for Disease Control and Prevention (CDC). (2011b). Trends in in-hospital newborn male circumcision--United States, 1999–2010. *MMWR Morb Mortal Wkkly Rep*, 60(34), 1167–1168.

Chung, S., Lim, R., and Goldman, R. D. (2010). Intranasal fentanyl versus placebo for pain in children during catheterization for voiding cystourethrography. *Pediatr Radiol*, 40(7), 1236–1240.

Curtis, L. A., Dolan, T. S., and Seibert, H. E. (2009). Are one or two dangerous? Lidocaine and topical anesthetic exposures in children. *J Emerg Med*, 37(1), 32–39.

Danchin, M. H., Rogers, S., Kelpie, L., Selvaraj, G., Curtis, N., Carlin, J. B., et al. (2007). Burden of acute sore throat and group A streptococcal pharyngitis in school-aged children and their families in Australia. *Pediatrics*, 120(5), 950–995.

De Roznay, M., Cooper, P. J., Tsigaras, N., and Murray, L. (2006). Transmission of social anxiety from mother to infant: an experimental study using a social referencing paradigm. *Behav Res Ther*, 44(8), 1165–1175.

Du, S., Jaaniste, T. G., Champion, G., and Yap, C. S. L. (2008). Theories of fear acquisition: the development of needle phobia in children. *Pediatr Pain Lett*, 10 (2).

El-Naggar, W., Yiu, A., Mohamed, A., Shah, V., Manley, J., McNamara, P., et al. (2010). Comparison of pain during two methods of urine collection in preterm infants. *Pediatrics*, 125(6), 1224–1229.

Evans, A. M. (2008). Growing pains: contemporary knowledge and recommended practice. *J Foot Ankle Res*, 1(1), 4.

Faden, H. (2006). Management of primary herpetic gingivostomatitis in young children. *Pediatr Emerg Care*, 22(4), 268–269.

Feldens, C. A., Faraco, I. M., Ottoni, A. B., Feldens, E. G., and Vítolo, M. R. (2010). Teething symptoms in the first year of life and associated factors: a cohort study. *J Clin Pediatr Dent*, 34(3), 201–6.

Foxlee, R., Johansson, A., Wejfalk, J., Dawkins, J., Dooley, L., and Del Mar, C. (2006). Topical analgesia for acute otitis media. *Cochrane Database Syst Rev*, 3, CD005657.

Goodyear-Smith, F. and Arroll, B. (2006). Growing pains. *Br Med J*, 333 (7566), 456–457.

Hand, C. and Harvey, I. (2004). The effectiveness of topical preparations for the treatment of earwax: a systematic review. *Br J Gen Pract*, 54(508), 862–867.

Hall, B., Chesters, J., and Robinson, A. (2011). Infantile colic: a systematic review of medical and conventional therapies. *J Paediatr Child Health*, 48(2), 128–137

Harrington, J. W., Logan, S., Harwell, C., Gardner, J., Swingle, J., McGuire, E., et al. (2012). Effective analgesia using physical interventions for infant immunizations. *Pediatrics*, 129(5), 815–822.

Herd, D. W. (2008). Anxiety in children undergoing VCUG: sedation or no sedation? *Adv Urol*, 2008, 498614.

Karp, H. (2007). Swaddling and excessive crying. *J Pediat*, 151(1), e2–3; author reply e3.

Kelly, L. E., Rieder, M., van den Anker, J., Malkin, B., Ross, C., Neely, M. N., *et al.* (2012). More codeine fatalities after tonsillectomy in North American children. *Pediatrics*, 129(5), 1343–1347.

Kirya, C. and Werthmann, M. W. Jr. (1978). Neonatal circumcision and penile dorsal nerve block—a painless procedure. *J Pediatr*, 92, 998–1000.

Keefe, M. R, Kajrlsen, K. A., Lobo M. L., Kotzer, A. M., and Dudley, W. N. (2006). Reducing parenting stress in families with irritable infants. *Nurs Res*, 55(3), 198–205.

Kohen, D. P., and Olness, K. (2011). *Hypnosis and hypnotherapy with children* (4th edn). New York: Routledge; Taylor & Francis Group.

Korb, K., Scherer, M., and Chenot, J. F., (2010). Steroids as adjuvant therapy for acute pharyngitis in ambulatory patients: a systematic review *Ann Fam Med*, 8(1), 58–63.

Kurtis, P. S., DeSilva, H. N., Bernstein, B. A. Malakh, L., and Schechter, N. L (1999). A comparison of the Mogen and Gomco clamps in combination with dorsal penile nerve block in minimizing the pain of neonatal circumcision. *Pediatrics*, 103(2), e23.

Kuttner, L. (2010). *A child in pain*. Bethel, CT: Crown House.

Lacey, C. M., Finkelstein, M., and Thygeson, M. V. (2008). The impact of positioning on fear during immunizations: supine versus sitting up. *J Pediatr Nurs*, 23(3), 195–200.

Lander J., Brady-Fryer B., Metcalfe, J. B., Nazarali, S., and Muttitt, S. (1997). Comparison of ring block, dorsal penile nerve block, and topical anesthesia for neonatal circumcision: a randomized controlled trail. *JAMA*, 278(24), 2157–2162.

Lucassen, P. L., and Assendelft, W. J. (2001). Systematic review of treatments for infant colic. *Pediatrics*, 108(4), 1047–1048.

Lehr, V. T., Cepeda, E., Fratterelli, D. A., Thomas, R., LaMothe, J., and Aranda, J. V. (2005). Lidocaine 4% cream compared with lidocaine 2.5% and prilocaine 2.5% or dorsal penile nerve block for circumcision. *Am J Perinatol*, 22(5), 231–237.

McNally, D., Simpson, M., Morris, C., Shephard, A., and Goulder, M. (2010). Rapid relief of acute sore throat with AMC/DCBA throat lozenges: randomised controlled trial. *Int J Clin Pract*, 64(2), 194–207.

McWilliams, D. B., Jacobson, R. M., Van Houten, H. K., Naessens, J. M., and Ytterberg, K. L. (2008). A program of anticipatory guidance for the prevention of emergency department visits for ear pain. *Pediatr Adolesc Med*, 162, 151–156.

Melson, G. F. (2005). *Why the wild things are. Animals in the lives of children.* Cambridge. MA: Harvard University Press.

Narcy, P., Reinert, R., and Olive, G. (2006). Therapeutic management and objective evaluation of pain in children consulting for acute otitis media (abstract). 7th International Symposium on Pediatric Pain, Vancouver, Canada.

Ong, C. K., Seymour, R. A., Lirk, P., and Merry, A. F. (2010). Combining paracetamol (acetaminophen) with non-steroidal anti-inflammatory drugs: a qualitative systemic review of analgesic efficacy for acute postoperative pain. *Anesth Analg*, 110, 1170–1179.

Olympia, R. P, Khine, H., and Avner, J. R. (2005). Effectiveness of oral dexamethasone in the treatment of moderate to severe pharyngitis in children. *Arch Pediatr Adolesc Med*, 159 (3), 278–282.

Owais, A. I., Zawaideh, F., and Bataineh, O. (2010). Challenging parents' myths regarding their children's teething. *Int J Dent Hyg*, 8(1), 28–34. Erratum in: *Int J Dent Hyg*, 8(4), 324.

Pierce, C. A., and Voss, B. (2010). Efficacy and safety of ibuprofen and acetaminophen in children and adults: a meta-analysis and qualitative review. *Ann Pharmacother*, 44(3), 489–506.

Pillai Riddell, R. R., Racine, N. M., Turcotte, K., Uman, L.S., Horton, R. E., Din Osmun, L., *et al.* (2011). Non-pharmacological management of infant and young child procedural pain. *Cochrane Database Syst Rev*, 5, CD006275.

Ramos-Jorge, J., Pordeus, I. A., Ramos-Jorge, M. L., and Paiva, S. M. (2011). Prospective longitudinal study of signs and symptoms associated with primary tooth eruption. *Pediatrics*, 128(3), 471–476.

Rogers, A. J., Greenwald, M. H., Deguzman, M. A., Kelley, M. E., and Simon, H. K. (2006). A randomized controlled trial of sucrose analgesia in infants younger than 90 days of age who require bladder catheterization in the emergency department. *Acad Emerg Med*, 13(6), 617–622.

Roland, P. S., Smith, T. L., Schwartz, S. R., Rosenfeld, R. M., Ballachanda, B., Earll, J. M., *et al.* (2008). Clinical practice guideline: cerumen impaction. *Otolaryngol Head Neck Surg*, 139(3 Suppl 2), S1–S21.

Roy, M., Bailey, B., Amre, D. K., Girodias, J. B., Bussières, J. F., and Gaudreault, P. (2004). Dexamethasone for the treatment of sore throat in children with suspected infectious mononucleosis: a randomized, double-blind, placebo-controlled, clinical trial. *Arch Pediatr Adolesc Med*, 158(3), 250–254.

Salmon, K., McGuigan, F., and Pereiera, J. K. (2006). Brief report: optimizing children's memory and management of an invasive procedure: the influence of procedural narration and distraction. *J Pediatr Psychol*, 31(5), 522–527.

Schechter, N. L. (2008). From the ouchless place to comfort central: the evolution of a concept. *Pediatrics*, 122(Suppl 3), S154–160.

Schechter, N. L., Bernstein, B. A., and Beck, A. (1991). Individual differences in children's response to pain: the role of temperament and parental characteristics. *Pediatrics*, 87, 171–177.

Schechter, N. L., Bernstein, B. A., Zempsky, W. T., Bright, N. S., and Willard, A. K. (2010). Educational outreach to reduce immunization pain in office settings. *Pediatrics*, 126(6), e1514–1521.

Schechter, N. L., Zempsky, W. T., Cohen, L. L., McGrath, P. J., McMurtry, C. M., and Bright, N. S. (2007). Pain reduction during pediatric immunizations: evidence-based review and recommendations. *Pediatrics*, 119(5), e1184–e1198.

Schroeder, A. R., Abidari, J. M., Kirpekar, R., Hamilton, J. R., Kang, Y. S., Tran, V., *et al.* (2011). Impact of a more restrictive approach to urinary tract imaging after febrile urinary tract infection. *Arch Pediatr Adolesc Med*, 165(11), 1027–1032.

Shaikh, N., Leonard, E., and Martin, J. M. (2010). Prevalence of streptococcal pharyngitis and streptococcal carriage in children: a meta-analysis. *Pediatrics*, 126(3), e557–564.

Shergill-Bonner, R. (2010). Infantile colic: practicalities of management, including dietary aspects. *J Fam Health Care*, 20(6), 206–209.

Sklar, D. P., Lauth, J. E., and Johnson, D. R. (1989). Topical anesthesia of the eye as a diagnostic test. *Ann Emerg Med*, 18(11), 1209–1211.

Sparks, L. A., Setlik, J., and Luhman, J. (2007). Parental holding and positioning to decrease IV distress in young children: a randomized clinical trial. *J Pediatr Nurs*, 22(6), 440–447.

Spiro, D. M., Arnold, D. H., and Meckler, G. D. (2008). The concept and practice of a wait-and-see approach to acute otitis media. *Curr Opin Pediatr*, 20(1), 72–78.

Stang, H. J., Snellman, L. W., Condon, L. M., Conroy, M. M., Loiebo, R., Brodersen, L., *et al.* (1997). Beyond dorsal penile nerve block: a more humane circumcision. *Pediatrics*, 100(2), e3.

Taddio, A. (2001). Pain management for neonatal circumcision. *Paediatr Drugs*, 3(2), 101–111.

Taddio, A., Stevens, B., Craig, K., Rastogi, P., Ben-David, S., Shennan, A., *et al.* (1997). Efficacy and safety of lidocaine-prilocaine cream for pain during circumcision. *N Engl J Med*, 336, 1197–1201

Triebenbacher, S. L. (1998). Pets as transitional objects: their role in children's emotional development. *Psychol Rep*, 82(1), 191–200.

Vaughan, M., Paton, E.A., Bush, A., and Pershad, J. (2005). Does lidocaine gel alleviate the pain of bladder catheterization in young children? A randomized, controlled trial. *Pediatrics*, 116(4), 917–920.

Vervoor, T., Caes, L., Trost, Z., Sullivan. M., Vangronsveld, K., and Goubert, L. (2011a). Social modulation of facial pain display in high-catastrophizing children: an observational study in schoolchildren and their parents. *Pain*, 152(7), 1591–1599.

Vervoort, T., Huguet, A., Verhoeven, K., and Goubert, L. (2011b). Mothers' and fathers' responses to their child's pain moderate the relationship between the child's pain catastrophizing and disability. *Pain*, 152(4), 786–793.

Von Baeyer, C. L., Marche, T. A., Rocha, E. M., and Salmon, K. (2004). Children's memory for pain: overview and implications for practice. *J Pain*, 5(5), 241–249.

Wahlgren, C. F., and Quiding, H. (2000). Depth of cutaneous analgesia after application of a eutectic mixture of the local anesthetics lidocaine and prilocaine (EMLA cream). *J Am Acad Dermatol*, 42(4), 584–588.

Wansink, B., Shimizu, M., and Camps, G. (2012). What would batman eat?: priming children to make healthier fast food choices. *Pediatr Obes*, 7(2), 121–123.

Williams, G. D., Kirk, E. P., Wilson, C. J., Meadows, C. A., and Chan, B. S. (2011). Salicylate intoxication from teething gel in infancy. *Med J Aust*, 194(3), 146–148.

Wingerter, S. and Bachur, R. (2011). Risk factors for contamination of catheterized urine specimens in febrile children. *Pediatr Emerg Care*, 27(1), 1–4.

Woodwell, D. A., and Cherry, D. K. (2004). National ambulatory medical care survey: 2002 summary. *Adv Data*, 26(346), 1–44.

Wright, A. D., and Liebelt, E. L. (2007). Alternating antipyretics for fever reduction in children: an unfounded practice passed down to parents from pediatricians. *Clin Pediatr*, 46(2), 146–150.

Zackaria, M., and Aymat, A. (2009). Ear candling: a case report. *Eur J Gen Pract*, 15(3), 168–169.

Zier, J. L., Kvam, K. A., Kurachek, S. C., and Finkelstein, M. (2007). Sedation with nitrous oxide compared with no sedation during catheterization for urologic imaging in children. *Pediatr Radiol*, 37(7), 679–684.

Zempsky, W. T., and Schechter, N. L. (2000). Office-based pain management. *Pediatr Clin North Am*, 47(3), 601–615.

Zempsky, W. T., and Schechetr, N. L. (2003). What's new in the management of pain in children. *Pediatr Rev*, 24(10), 337–348

Supplementary online materials

Figure 33.1 Office poster.

CHAPTER 34

Effective management of children's pain and anxiety in the emergency department

Robert M. (Bo) Kennedy

Summary

Effective management of children's pain and anxiety during emergency department (ED) visits facilitates medically necessary care and procedures and increases patient, family, and health care provider satisfaction. This chapter will review evidence-based techniques for achieving this goal. A significant focus is upon non-pharmacological strategies to relieve children's anxiety because high levels of anxiety exacerbate sensitivity to pain and disrupt coping mechanisms of the child and parent. In addition, advances in techniques for pain relief for specific procedures will be detailed. Aspects of procedural sedation and analgesia that are especially pertinent to the ED will also be reviewed along with two recommended regimens for moderate and deep sedation.

Introduction

Pain due to injury or illness and fear of painful medical procedures are common experiences for most children seeking care in the ED (Drendel et al., 2006; Zempsky et al., 2004a). Although the truly 'Ouchless ED' (Kennedy and Luhmann, 1999) is more a philosophical concept than a concrete goal, there are many strategies to reduce pain and distress in this setting. Poorly managed pain is distressful for children, their parents, and health care providers and may produce physiological and psychological reactions that have acute and long-term consequences in children of all ages (Pate, 1996; Taddio et al., 1997; von Baeyer et al., 2004; Weisman et al., 1998). Inadequate pain control is also a significant cause of dissatisfaction with emergency care (R. W. Smith et al., 2007). Finally, effective management of children's pain and anxiety facilitates accurate physical exam assessments, performance of necessary medical procedures, and compliance with recommendations.

A child's perception of pain is significantly affected by his emotional state, temperament, prior painful experiences, and coping skills, as well as by parent and health care provider interactions (Khan and Weisman, 2007). Anxiety, exacerbated by the unknown and frightening ED environment, often interferes with a child's and his parent's coping mechanisms. Approaching the child with a calm, playful style can significantly reduce both the child's and parent's apprehension. Redirecting the child's attention away from his pain and impending medical care can significantly reduce distress. Family members can aid in these distraction strategies but may need specific guidance (Bauchner et al., 1994; see Cohen et al., Chapter 53, this volume)

Most children desire to have their parent present during medical care, even when they know their parent cannot reduce their pain (Ross and Ross, 1984). In addition, most parents wish to be with their child in these situations because they believe they can help reduce their child's distress and be helpful to the health care providers (Bauchner et al., 1989). Allowing young children to assume 'positions of comfort' when feasible, e.g. suggesting the child lay in his parent's lap during suturing or sitting chest-to-chest with the parent giving a gentle but controlling hug during a venous catheter insertion reduces distress in young children and their parents, when local anaesthesia is also used (Sparks et al., 2007).

Analgesics in the ED

Painful conditions are usually identified when the child is initially triaged upon presentation to the ED. Interventions can be initiated at this time for many patients, including for anticipated painful medical interventions. Placement of topical local anaesthetics which require 30 to 60 min absorption time to be effective also can improve efficiency of care. Examples include instillation of lidocaine-epinephrine (adrenaline)-tetracaine (LET) gel into lacerations (Priestley et al., 2003) or application of anaesthetic skin creams on a child who is likely to require venous cannulation. When a fracture is suspected, splinting the injury and administering oral oxycodone at triage prior to sending the child for radiographs safely reduces the child's pain, including during manipulation of the injured extremity for the radiographs (Charney et al., 2008). Rapid initiation of pain relief for other painful conditions such as burns or sickle-cell vaso-occlusive episodes can also be achieved with administration of oxycodone at triage. Standing orders for nurse initiation of these strategies greatly facilitates this practice.

Acetaminophen (paracetamol) and ibuprofen are frequently used oral analgesic medications for mild to moderate pain, whereas ketorolac and opioids are commonly administered intravenously (IV) for more severe pain. Because some people poorly metabolize codeine to its active form and others experience increased adverse effects from relatively small doses when they ultra-rapidly metabolize the drug, codeine is considered an unreliable analgesic agent (Gasche et al., 2004; Williams et al., 2002). Oxycodone is an effective and safe oral analgesic for significant pain (Charney et al., 2008).

Acetaminophen (paracetamol) is administered at 10 to 15 mg/kg/dose orally every 4 to 6 h, not to exceed five doses in 24 h; maximum daily dose: 4000 mg/day.

Ibuprofen is administered orally 75 mg/kg/day not to exceed 3750 mg/day. Administration with food or milk decreases gastrointestinal upset. Ibuprofen 10 mg/kg provided similar reduction in fracture-related pain as oxycodone 0.1 mg/kg (Koller et al., 2007) or acetaminophen with codeine (Friday et al., 2009) and better than acetaminophen or codeine alone (Clark et al., 2007).

Ketorolac is usually administered IV for moderate to severely painful conditions such as migraine headache (Brousseau et al., 2004). For children aged 2 to 16 years and those older than 16 years who weigh less than 50 kg, the recommended dose is 0.5 mg/kg as a single dose; maximum dose: 15 mg. For children older than 16 years and greater than 50 kg, the recommended dose is 30 mg.

Morphine (0.05–0.1 mg/kg IV) is the mainstay for potent analgesia in the paediatric ED. It reliably provides sustained relief for most painful conditions. However, other medications may have advantages in specific conditions.

Fentanyl (1–2 mcg/kg IV), unlike morphine, does not cause clinically significant histamine release and thus is preferred in patients who have increased potential for hypotension, e.g. trauma or sepsis. Its rapid onset facilitates titration to effective analgesia. Intranasal (IN) administration of fentanyl (1.5–2 mcg/kg) has been shown to provide similar analgesia as intravenously administered morphine for fracture-related pain (Borland et al., 2007). It can also be used to augment sedation for painful procedures, e.g. with nitrous oxide (N_2O) for abscess incision and drainage or fracture reduction (Seith et al., 2012). IN administration is facilitated by devices that create a fine mist to increase broad distribution of the drug onto nasal mucosa (Wolfe, 2007).

Oxycodone is an opioid analgesic medication that is readily absorbed by the oral route and is often administered for painful conditions when no IV access is established, e.g. at triage for possible fractures or burns (Charney et al., 2008). It can also be used to augment sedation for painful procedures without vascular access, e.g. with N_2O. For out-of-hospital analgesia 0.05–0.15 mg/kg is recommended. For ED analgesia, 0.2 mg/kg administered at triage to children with painful injuries caused tiredness but not sedation or clinically apparent changes in ventilation or oxygenation (Charney et al., 2008). For procedural analgesia, 0.2 mg/kg may be administered along with N_2O for minor fracture reduction, burn debridement, or abscess drainage.

Local anaesthesia

Effective local anaesthesia greatly reduces anxiety and the need for procedural sedation, particularly when topical and nearly painless placement of anaesthetics can be achieved (Pierluishi and Terndrup,

1989) and behavioural interventions are used (see also Zempsky, Chapter 47, this volume).

Gels containing 4% lidocaine, 0.1% epinephrine (adrenaline), and 0.5% tetracaine (LET), when instilled for at least 30 min into an open wound, are sufficiently absorbed to provide local anaesthesia (Eidelman et al., 2011; G. A. Smith et al., 1997). These gels provide complete anaesthesia for 70% to 90% of facial and scalp lacerations and about half of extremity lacerations (Singer and Stark, 2001; G. A. Smith et al., 1997). Thus, supplemental injected anaesthetic is often necessary. Application of gel formulations directly into the wound is more effective than placement of gauze soaked with anaesthetic solution atop, perhaps due to improved contact of the anaesthetics with the wound (Resch et al., 1998). Because topical anaesthetics can cause toxicity due to rapid absorption when applied on mucosal membranes and large abrasions, only small amounts should be applied on these wounds, e.g. use a cotton swab to apply a drop of LET into a lip laceration (Bonadio, 1996). Application of LET to fingers for 45 min is effective and safe (White et al., 2004).

Numerous studies confirm local anaesthetics significantly reduce the pain of needle puncture during IV catheter insertion, blood sampling, and intramuscular vaccine injections (Schechter et al., 2007; Zempsky, 2008). Topical anaesthetic creams containing lidocaine-prilocaine (EMLA®), tetracaine (amethocaine; Ametop®), or liposomized lidocaine (L.M.X.$_4$®) reduce venepuncture pain but require 30 to 90 min for penetration (Eidelman et al., 2005). A topical patch uses warming to hasten onset of topical anaesthesia (Synera®; Sethna et al., 2005). These anaesthetics may be applied in triage when it is clear the child will need venepuncture or IV insertion.

Buffering lidocaine, lidocaine with adrenaline, or bupivacaine to a neutral pH significantly reduces the pain of infiltration without impacting effectiveness (Christoph et al., 1988; McKay et al., 1987). Adding 1 ml of sodium bicarbonate (8.4%) per 10 ml of anaesthetic brings the pH of the solution to 7.2 to 7.4. Because buffered lidocaine begins to degrade after 2 to 4 weeks, it must be mixed locally or purchased from specialty pharmaceutical companies. To assure effective local anaesthesia in lacerations, consider injecting buffered lidocaine through the wound after 30 to 45 min of application of LET (see Box 34.1). Buffered lidocaine can be injected through a 30-gauge needle with minimal pain and achieves immediate deep local anaesthesia for IV catheter insertion (Klein et al., 1995; Luhmann et al., 2004; McNaughton et al., 2009). Because of the rapid onset and effectiveness of anaesthesia, lack of need for special equipment and low cost, this technique is used for more than 85% of IV insertions in children in the author's ED (unpublished data). Of note, use of local anaesthetics has been found by some to improve success rate on the first attempt (74% with 4% lidocaine cream versus 55% for placebo; Taddio et al., 2005) and 84% with EMLA versus 65% with nothing (Baxter et al., 2005). The J-tip® device can be used to drive lidocaine through intact skin without use of a needle (Jimenez et al., 2006).

Pain management for ED procedures

Procedures commonly performed in the ED that are considered intensely painful by paediatric ED health care providers, with most painful first, are suprapubic aspiration, intramuscular injection, lumbar puncture, IV catheter insertion, urethral catheterization,

Box 34.1 Methods to minimize pain of local anaesthesia (LA) injection

1. Distract patient.
2. Use topical anaesthetic gel prior to infiltration of additional LA.
3. Warm LA to body temperature.
4. Buffer LA to neutral pH (add 1 ml of 8.4% sodium bicarbonate to 9 ml of anaesthetic).
5. Use fine needle (27–30 gauge).
6. Inject slowly.
7. Use smallest effective volume.
8. Infiltrate through wound, not skin.
9. Inject 'looser', deeper subdermal layer before 'tighter' dermal tissues.
10. Block individual nerves when possible.

Adapted by permission from BMJ Publishing Group Limited. *Emergency Medicine Journal*, O. Quaba et al., A users guide for reducing the pain of local anaesthetic administration, Volume 22, Issue 3, pp. 188–189, Copyright © 2005, http://emj.bmj.com/.

and nasogastric (NG) tube insertion (Babl et al., 2008a). Effective pain management or alternative procedures can be achieved for most of these procedures. Ceftriaxone can be reconstituted with buffered lidocaine to reduce injection pain when that antibiotic is administered by the intramuscular route (Hayward et al., 1996). Strategies for the remaining procedures are addressed in the following sections.

Venous access

Venepuncture to obtain blood samples for medical tests or to insert indwelling catheters is the most common painful procedure performed in the ED (see also Taddio, Chapter 19; Zempsky, Chapter 47, this volume). Needle-sticks cause significant pain, distress, and negative memories for children of all ages (Humphrey et al., 1992). Among medical procedures during hospital encounters, needle-sticks are a separate, critical, and distressful event for most children (Fradet et al., 1990). Despite guidelines and increasing evidence highlighting the importance of pain associated with venous access procedures, management of this pain is often inadequate (Bhargava and Young, 2007; MacLean et al., 2007; Zempsky et al., 2004a).

Increasing evidence suggests infants experience needle-stick pain more intensely than older children (Anand and Scalzo, 2000; Kennedy et al., 2008). Furthermore, increased distress during needle-sticks, including in newborns and older infants (Peters et al., 2003; Taddio et al., 2002), has been associated with negative memory and greater distress during future procedures and avoidance of future medical care (Davey, 1989; Pate, 1996; von Baeyer et al., 2004).

Poorly managed venous access pain also impacts the child's family members. Increases in heart rate, blood pressure, and anxiety have been measured in parents who observed their child receiving a venepuncture in the ED (R. W. Smith et al., 2007). In a prospective ED survey of parents of children younger than 8 years of age, 65% were willing to stay an extra hour, 77% were willing to spend an extra $15, and 37% were willing to pay an extra $100 to ensure that the procedure was painless (Walsh and Bartfield, 2006).

Health care providers find performing venous access procedures in fearful and anxious children to be stressful. The morale of nurses has been negatively impacted by perceptions that they cause significant procedural pain (Nagy, 1998). Nurses in our paediatric ED reported a significant reduction in their distress associated with IV insertion after they began using comfort techniques and a protocol that empowered them to initiate use of local anaesthesia (Luhmann et al., 1999).

Even with complete anaesthesia (see 'Local anaesthetics'), anxiety related to needle use causes distress in many kids, thus local anaesthetic techniques are considerably augmented by concurrent use of non-pharmacological techniques to reduce anxiety. In addition to distraction simply allowing young children to sit upright on their parent's lap during IV insertion, instead of being held supine on a stretcher, can significantly lower distress, increase parent satisfaction, and does not alter the number of IV attempts needed (Sparks et al., 2007).

Lacerations

Children presenting to the ED for care of lacerations are typically frightened and anxious. These moderately painful injuries cause concern in the patients and their parents about additional pain during repair as well as cosmetic and functional outcomes. As previously discussed application of topical anaesthetic gels and use oxycodone at the time of triage immediately begins to address the child's pain and can improve efficiency of care (Charney et al., 2008; Priestley et al., 2003). Use of injected anaesthetics is discussed in the 'Analgesics in the ED' section.

Many small lacerations may not need to be closed. In an intriguing study, patients (primarily adults) with uncomplicated lacerations of the hand that would normally be sutured (full thickness, <2 cm, without tendon, joint, fracture, or nerve complications), were randomized to either being sutured or conservative treatment (tap water irrigation, antibiotic ointment, and gauze dressing for 1–2 days; Quinn et al., 2002). Both groups had similar time to resumption of normal activities and cosmetic appearance with the conservative treatment faster and less painful. In the author's ED most parents quickly accept the advantages of this 'common-sense' approach for minor hand/finger and foot/toe lacerations when reminded of how they likely treated their own similar minor injuries. Although initially worrisome in appearance, tongue lacerations very rarely need closure, including gaping lacerations extending to the tongue's edge (Patel, 2008).

Surface skin adhesives (octyl- or butyl-cyanoacrylates) and adhesive-strips have been used for many years to close clean minor wounds in areas where there is little tension or motion (Farion et al., 2003; Zempsky et al., 2004b). Cosmetic outcomes have been similar to closures with sutures and with reduced procedure pain and time. Careful approximation of irregular wound edges during gluing can be challenging in restless children, but a newly evaluated adhesive mesh used for initial approximation may make this easier and a stronger closure (Singer et al., 2011). Staples, while enabling rapid closure of wounds, require special tools and a return visit to health care for removal, making this a less desirable technique than absorbable sutures, glue, or adhesive strips.

Use of absorbable sutures obviates the need for a second distressful health care visit for suture removal. Suture materials that degrade significantly by 3 to 10 days, e.g. 6–0 fast-absorbing or plain gut or irradiated 5–0 polyglactin 910 (Vicryl Rapide™), are used for facial laceration closure with similar cosmetic outcomes to closure with nylon (Al-Abdullah et al., 2007; Karounis et al., 2004; Luck et al., 2008). Slightly longer lasting materials, e.g. 4–0 chromic gut or Vicryl Rapide™ are used for closure of trunk or extremity lacerations. As an adjunct, the tissue adhesives may be used to cover, protect and reinforce fragile rapidly absorbed gut sutures, thus allowing children to shower.

Lumbar puncture

Lumbar puncture (LP) is commonly performed in infants and toddlers without local anaesthesia or other pain management, despite this being the standard in older children and adults. A 2004 survey found two-thirds of academic paediatric emergency physicians do not routinely use local anaesthesia for neonatal LPs (Baxter et al., 2004). In a 2007 survey of paediatric and emergency medicine residents across Canada, paediatric residents reported performing LPs with no local anaesthetic much more frequently than their emergency medicine counterparts (Breakey et al., 2007). Slightly more encouraging, a 2011 prospective study found that local anaesthetics were administered in 54% of infants less than 12 months of age and in 99% of toddlers 12 to 24 months of age undergoing LP for suspected meningitis in the ED or paediatric units at a university hospital (Gorchynski and McLaughlin, 2011). Emergency physicians exclusively used injected 1% lidocaine while paediatric physicians preferred a topical anaesthetic. However, a 2011 survey of ED faculty and paediatric emergency medicine fellows at five Midwestern US hospitals, with approximately half of respondents trained in general emergency medicine, found that although 78% of the physicians believed pain intervention is worthwhile for infant LPs, less than one-third regularly use pharmacological interventions to reduce LP pain in this age group (Hoyle et al., 2011).

There is a surprising lack of literature on the effectiveness of local anaesthesia in reducing the pain of LP in neonates (Madsen, 2009). In a randomized double-blind comparison of the topical anaesthetic cream EMLA® to placebo cream in newborns undergoing LP, all the newborns had evidence of pain (Pinheiro et al., 1993). However, compared with placebo, EMLA® significantly attenuated the pain response as shown by lower heart rates and behavioural scores. This and other studies demonstrate that infants typically cry and struggle when simply positioned for a LP, whether or not topical or injected local anaesthesia is used, and that reduction in distress associated with use of a local anaesthetic may be difficult to discern clinically (Porter et al., 1991). Administration of oral sucrose and use of non-nutritive sucking, in addition to local anaesthetic, provides additional reduction of distress.

Common rationales for not using injected lidocaine in infants include that its use makes the infant suffer 'two sticks instead of one' and that the injected lidocaine makes the LP more difficult by obscuring landmarks. However, a 1993 study of neonates undergoing LP found that while the infants struggled when infiltrated with lidocaine, those who received lidocaine struggled significantly less during the spinal needle insertion (Pinheiro et al., 1993). Consistent with these findings, a 2006 prospective observational study of infants in a university ED found LPs performed with local anaesthetic were twice as likely to be successful and atraumatic (Baxter et al., 2006). Finally, a 2007 prospective evaluation of 1459 children, median age of 3 months, who were undergoing LPs in a single ED, found that not using a local anaesthetic was a significant independent predictor of traumatic or unsuccessful LP on the first attempt (35%; Nigrovic et al., 2007). These studies suggest use of local anaesthetics in infants reduces distress and struggling and increases the likelihood of a successful atraumatic LP.

What is the most effective local anaesthetic technique in older children also remains an open question. No clinical trials of local anaesthesia were found in non-infant children undergoing LP in the ED. Reduction of pain with EMLA® prior to lumbar puncture has been found in children with cancer when the LP was successful on first but not subsequent attempts (Holdsworth et al., 1997). Double-blinded randomized trials in older children undergoing LP in the ED are needed to evaluate the effectiveness of newer options such as buffered lidocaine, injection with 30-gauge needles, and liposomal lidocaine cream.

Many children benefit from sedation during elective LP but children undergoing LP in the ED are often ill and may have compromised cardiopulmonary function, worsened by being held in a maximally flexed position for the procedure, thus increasing the risk of adverse events associated with procedural sedation. For these patients, administration of an anxiolytic dose of midazolam or 50% N_2O may improve patient tolerance of the procedure with minimal sedation and lessen the likelihood of respiratory depression. This strategy may also make children more amenable to distraction. Effective local anaesthesia is crucial to this strategy.

Recommendations for ED patients undergoing LP are as follows:

Infants: anaesthetic cream (e.g. EMLA®, LMX®, Ametop®) followed by slow injection of buffered lidocaine via 30-gauge needle, along with nutritive suckling (pacifier, with sucrose for <6 weeks of age).

Toddlers and older children: anxiolysis with midazolam (IV, PO, IN) along with topical anaesthetic cream (e.g. EMLA®, LMX®, Ametop®), distraction by Child Life Specialist or instructed family member or ED staff, slow injection of buffered lidocaine via 30-gauge needle. If N_2O is available, may substitute or combine with midazolam, monitoring oxygenation with pulse oximetry. If child is very distressed and has good cardiopulmonary function, may consider moderate or deep sedation.

Urethral catheterization

Urethral catheterization (UC) is considered by children and adults to be one of the most painful and distressing common procedures performed in the ED, with males reporting more pain than females (Babl et al., 2008a; Kozer et al., 2006; Singer et al., 1998). Lubricating anaesthetic gel is widely recommended in adults to reduce the pain caused by the friction and pressure from the catheter's passage through the urethra into the bladder, but this adjunct is rarely used in paediatric ED patients, perhaps due to time constraints and because of only moderate reduction of distress (MacLean et al., 2007; Vaughan et al., 2005).

UC has been found in infants to cause less pain and be more likely successful in obtaining urine for analysis and culture, compared to suprapubic aspiration, without increased adverse events (Pollack et al., 1994; Tobiansky and Evans, 1998). In a study of febrile full-term infants, less than 2 months of age, suprapubic aspiration through skin anaesthetized by EMLA® was also found to be more painful than UC using a 5-French feeding tube lubricated with sterile 2% lidocaine gel (Kozer et al., 2006).

In older infants and toddlers, behavioural pain scores were high and did not differ during UC in children less than 2 years of age when 1 to 2 ml of either non-anaesthetic or 2% lidocaine gel was applied topically to the genital mucosa for 2 to 3 min before catheterization and the remainder of the gel used as lubricant on the catheter (Vaughan et al., 2005). However, others found reduced distress when 2% lidocaine gel was applied topically for 2 min then instilled into the urethra for 2 more minutes when compared to non-anaesthetic gel in febrile 2- to 24-month-old ED patients (Mularoni et al., 2009).

In children between 4 and 11 years of age, use of 2% lidocaine gel was associated with significantly less pain and distress during UC for cystograms compared to non-anaesthetic gel when the lidocaine gel was applied with sufficient time to provide anaesthesia (Gerard et al., 2003). A cotton ball soaked with either lidocaine or placebo lubricant was placed on the urethral meatus and held in place for 1 to 2 min. Then, dependent upon the size of the child, 0.5 to 2.0 ml lubricant or lidocaine gel was instilled into the urethra. The instillation was repeated twice more, with 2 min intervals between each instillation. A child life specialist provided distraction and support during the procedure and rated the child's distress. The group receiving 2% lidocaine gel had significantly lower self-report pain and observed distress.

Because significant pain and distress occurs with UC despite use of anaesthetic gel, alternative adjuncts have been investigated. Oral *sucrose* solution (24%) administered 2 min prior to UC reduced pain scores and crying in infants less than but not older than 30 days of age (Rogers et al., 2006). Midazolam 0.6 mg/kg orally induced complete amnesia for UC in 60% and partial amnesia in 31% of very anxious children (mean age 4.4 years; Elder and Longenecker, 1995) and intranasal midazolam 0.2 mg/kg significantly reduced distress in children median age 2 to 3 years (Stokland, 2003). Intranasal fentanyl, 2 mcg/kg, of note, did not reduce UC pain in children 4 to 8 years of age (Chung et al., 2010). Most successfully, N_2O 50% to 70% has been found to reduce distress behaviour and need for restraint in children during UC compared to non-sedated controls or to those receiving oral midazolam (Keidan et al., 2005; Zier, 2007).

Nasogastric intubation

Although emergency physicians and nurses acknowledge the marked discomfort, NG tube insertion is typically performed without any form of pain relief other than a lubricant in children (Juhl et al., 2005; Stock et al., 2008). Studies in adults designed to find an effective local anaesthetic technique for NG tube insertion have primarily focused upon use of 2% to 10% lidocaine as a gel, nasal spray, or nebulized mist (Gallagher, 2004; Kuo et al., 2010). Cetacaine and cocaine have also been investigated but are not recommended due to associated toxicities (US Food and Drug Administration, 2011). A systematic review of five randomized controlled trials in adults concluded that administration of nebulized or atomized lidocaine before NG tube insertion can decrease pain by 60% (Kuo et al., 2010). Two more recent randomized controlled trials in adults likewise found benefit from lidocaine spray (Chan and Lau, 2010) and gel (Uri et al., 2011).

In contrast to the studies in adults, Babl and colleagues, in a well-designed comparison of nebulized 2% lidocaine at 4 mg/kg to saline placebo in children between 1 to 5 years of age in the ED, found distress scores were very high in both groups during NG tube insertion and terminated the study early (Babl et al., 2009). No child demonstrated any evidence of lidocaine toxicity but, of note, the trachea was inadvertently intubated in one child in each group, emphasizing the need for confirmation of gastric placement by pH, radiograph, or other means (Kuo et al., 2010). Further investigations in children are needed to determine how best to reduce the pain of NG tube insertion. Perhaps as important, clinicians may reconsider whether NG tube insertion can be avoided (Witting, 2007).

When considering the available evidence, it is recommended clinicians administer intranasal 2% lidocaine at 4 mg/kg (0.2 ml/kg of 2%) as a gel or atomized spray to children at least 5 min prior to NG tube insertion. Oxymetazoline or phenylephrine nasal sprays may be co-administered to shrink the nasal mucosa and reduce epistaxis. Most children will show signs of distress during the administration of the lidocaine and NG tube insertion but it is likely a significant portion of the pain of the procedure will have been abated. Blunting of protective airway reflexes may occur with these techniques.

Abdominal pain

Abdominal pain is a common nonspecific complaint in children seeking medical evaluation in the ED (Reynolds and Jaffe, 1992; Scholer et al., 1996). Acute cramping abdominal pain from self-limited minor illnesses such as gastroenteritis or viral infections is not effectively reduced by analgesic medications and may be prolonged by opioids that exacerbate intestinal ileus. Many systemic illnesses may cause abdominal pain, including diabetic ketoacidosis, haemolytic uremic syndrome, Henoch–Schönlein purpura, hepatitis, and myocarditis, the diagnosis of which are usually made with a careful history and physical exam, and, occasionally, specific ancillary tests. Some causes of abdominal pain may require antibiotic treatment including lower lobe pneumonias, urinary tract infections, streptococcal pharyngitis, and pelvic inflammatory disease. It is also important to evaluate for conditions that may require urgent surgical intervention such as trauma, volvulus, intussusception, ovarian torsion, incarcerated hernia, or appendicitis. For many of these conditions, administration of an analgesic medication after a diagnosis or further evaluation or therapeutic intervention is begun will provide some patient relief without obscuring the diagnosis or increasing management errors (Ranji et al., 2006). The best studied example is when the diagnosis of appendicitis is being considered, administration of morphine or buccal oxycodone has been found not to interfere with clinical diagnosis while reducing pain preoperatively and facilitates diagnostic techniques such as abdominal ultrasound (Sharwood and Babl, 2009). However, this practice is frequently underutilized (Goldman et al., 2006; Kim et al., 2003).

Headache

Headache is a common chief complaint in children presenting to the ED (Burton et al., 1997; Kan et al., 2000; Lewis and Qureshi, 2000). The majority of these children are diagnosed with viral illnesses or migraine headaches. After viral infections, rebound headaches from chronic daily use of ibuprofen or acetaminophen (Vasconcellos et al., 1998), and rare but life-threatening causes of headache, including meningitis, encephalitis, intracranial abscess or haemorrhage, hydrocephalus, hypertension, or brain tumour are excluded by a careful history, neurological exam, and, if necessary, intracranial imaging (Kan et al., 2000; King, 2012), the diagnosis of migraine headache should be considered (Lewis, 2009). Migraine headaches in children are defined as recurrent headaches with pain-free intervals and at least three of the following six symptoms: (1) an aura; (2) unilateral location; (3) throbbing or pulsatile pain; (4) nausea, vomiting, or abdominal pain; (5) relief after sleep; and (6) a family history of migraines (Lewis, 2009; Prensky and Sommer, 1979).

Pharmacological treatment of migraine headaches in children in the emergency setting is primarily based upon trials in adults due to few paediatric studies (Lewis et al., 2004). As with other painful conditions, the therapeutic goal is reduction in pain, nausea, and other symptoms to a level which the patient can tolerate; complete abolition of symptoms is uncommon. If the patient has not already taken an effective dose prior to ED presentation, an oral dose of ibuprofen, 10 to 15 mg/kg, or acetaminophen 15 mg/kg may provide relief (Damen et al., 2005; Lewis et al., 2004). Triptans, although not formally approved for use in children, have been shown to reduce migraine-related pain in this age group with benefit best demonstrated in use of nasal sumatriptan 10 to 20 mg (Damen et al., 2005; Eiland, 2010; Lewis et al., 2004). Because triptans induce vasoconstriction, their use with basilar artery and hemiplegic migraine may worsen symptoms.

The combination of intravenous hydration, ketorolac, and prochlorperazine may be an effective treatment for paediatric migraine headaches (Damen et al., 2005; Lewis et al., 2004). A randomized double-blind trial in 62 children aged 5 to 18 years presenting to the ED with a migraine headache compared IV ketorolac (0.5 mg/kg; maximum 30 mg) to prochlorperazine (0.15 mg/kg; maximum 10 mg), after normal saline 10 ml/kg infused over 30 min (Brousseau et al., 2004). By 60 min, 55% of those who received ketorolac and 85% of those who received prochlorperazine had a 50% or greater reduction in pain scores; neither group experienced significant adverse effects. Unfortunately, IV preparations of prochlorperazine are in short-supply or unavailable in the US. Alternative antiemetics that may be effective but little studied include promethazine, chlorpromazine, metoclopramide, and ondansetron.

Paediatric procedural sedation and analgesia (PSA) in the ED

When effective local anaesthesia is not possible for intensely painful ED procedures or when distress-related behaviours will interfere with accomplishment of the procedure, sedation may be necessary. Many advances in PSA for non-elective procedures in non-fasted children in the ED have been developed (Kennedy, 2011). This section will review aspects especially pertinent to paediatric PSA in the ED (see also Cravero, Chapter 20, this volume).

PSA in children receiving emergency care has greater inherent risks than elective sedation. Patients frequently have not fasted and thus may have 'full stomachs' (Agrawal et al., 2003; Babl et al., 2005; Roback et al., 2004). More importantly, gastric emptying unpredictably may slow or stop due to ileus caused by painful injury or serious illness and is delayed further by opioids administered for pain management. Thus, brief postponement of sedation may have little impact. Compounding this issue, children undergoing painful or anxiety provoking procedures typically require deeper levels of sedation than adults or teenagers to control their behaviour.

Furthermore, unanticipated arrival or deterioration of other critical ED patients may demand sedating team members' immediate attention. These possibilities impact ED PSA choices.

Goals of ED PSA are the same as for elective PSA, with the foremost being assurance of the patient's safety and welfare during sedation and recovery. Aspects with particular pertinence to ED PSA include:

(1) Most children undergoing ED PSA are ASA Physical Status Class I and II and at low risk for serious adverse events when closely monitored and simple rescue interventions quickly applied (Green et al., 200; Peña and Krauss, 1999). However, children with acute illnesses may have less cardiopulmonary reserve and more likely to have adverse responses to sedative and analgesic medications, but perhaps less so when ketamine is used (Green et al., 2009). A focused physical exam immediately prior to sedation should be repeated to detect any changes in the child's physiological status such as acute onset of wheezing or fever which may increase risk for adverse events.

(2) Fasting is a well-established consensus-based practice to reduce aspiration risk during elective general anaesthesia. However, little clinical data has been published to help determine risk of adverse events when children undergoing ED PSA have not fasted or whether postponing PSA for a short period reduces risk (Green et al., 2007; Mace et al., 2008). Protective airway reflexes are generally preserved during moderate sedation (American Society of Anesthesiologists Task Force on Sedation and Analgesia by Non-Anesthesiologists, 2002) and relatively intact during deep sedation or even light general anaesthesia with ketamine, the most commonly used drug for ED PSA in children (Green et al., 2011). However, these reflexes are likely blunted during deep sedation with opioids, benzodiazepines, barbiturates, and propofol, especially during periods of apnoea (American Society of Anesthesiologists Task Force on Sedation and Analgesia by Non-Anesthesiologists, 2002; Oberer et al., 2005). Intubation of the trachea, rarely performed for ED PSA, likely increases the risk of pulmonary aspiration due to pharmacological abolition of protective reflexes to facilitate intubation and mechanical interference with glottis closure during passage of the endotracheal tube; thus elective intubation for ED PSA may increase risk of aspiration. Routine administration of antacids or pharmacological agents to increase gastric motility prior to general anaesthesia is not beneficial (American Society of Anesthesiologist Task Force on Preoperative Fasting, 1999); this likely holds true for ED PSA.

The incidence of pulmonary aspiration during ED PSA is not well established but appears to be very low. Pooling of the available data in the literature suggests the incidence of clinically apparent pulmonary aspiration during ED PSA is no more frequent than 1:2000 paediatric patient encounters (Mace et al., 2008).

Vomiting, usually during recovery, is a common adverse event during ED PSA in children, occurring in as much as 25% of patients when opioids are co-administered prior to sedation (Luhmann et al., 2006; Wathen et al., 2000). No correlation was found between the length of preprocedural fasting and vomiting in children receiving ketamine or N_2O (Agrawal et al., 2003; Babl et al., 2005; Roback et al., 2004). Coadministration of ondansetron reduced vomiting associated with ketamine ED PSA from 12.6% to 4.7% with 13 patients needing to be treated to prevent one episode of vomiting

(Langston et al., 2008). Fortunately, protective airway reflexes are likely present during active vomiting. Passive regurgitation of gastric contents due to relaxed gastro-oesophageal sphincter tone, e.g. during apnoea, however, may be associated with pulmonary aspiration.

When local anaesthesia or effective analgesia can be achieved, safety may be enhanced and some children may prefer lighter levels of sedation without loss of awareness, e.g. N_2O with a fracture haematoma block.

In many smaller EDs, the only physician present must be responsible for performing both the sedation and the procedure. In these situations, there must be a second staff member at the bedside who has been trained in sedation and resuscitation techniques. This second person is responsible for monitoring the patient's cardiopulmonary status and the need for interventions to manage adverse events. This individual may, for moderate sedation, assist with minor, interruptible tasks once the patient's level of sedation and cardiopulmonary functions have stabilized, provided adequate monitoring of the patient is maintained (American Academy of Pediatrics Committee on Drugs, 1992; American Society of Anesthesiologists Task Force on Sedation and Analgesia by Non-Anesthesiologists, 2002; Godwin et al., 2005). *For deep sedation*, this second staff member should have no other responsibilities than monitoring the patient and recording. This usually means a third provider is needed if assistance in performing the procedure is expected. The responsible physician must be able to easily interrupt performance of the procedure to assist with or assume management of adverse events.

ED PSA technique recommendations for children

Many PSA techniques for ED paediatric procedures have been reported (Kennedy, 2011). It is recommended that the provider become knowledgeable and experienced with a limited number when initially gaining experience with paediatric ED PSA. Use of N_2O or ketamine enables safe and effective ED PSA in children for most ED procedures. Techniques that have greater frequency of adverse cardiopulmonary effects, e.g. fentanyl + propofol or midazolam, should be used only by experienced sedation providers.

N2O 50% to 70% induces mild to moderate sedation with anxiolysis, moderate analgesia, and partial amnesia. Its advantages include no need for venous access, rapid onset and offset (within 2–5 min), and few adverse effects other than vomiting or occasional dysphoria. Delivery of the gas via full face mask rather than a dental-style nasal hood is more effective for ED PSA. Deeper sedation can be achieved by co-administration of opioids with N_2O but the risk of adverse effects, especially vomiting, is increased (Luhmann et al., 2006; Seith et al., 2012).

At a specific concentration of N_2O, depth of sedation can vary considerably. Babl found 90% of children receiving 50% to 70% N_2O were mildly sedated, whereas moderate or deep sedation occurred in 3% receiving 70% N_2O and in none receiving 50% (Babl et al., 2008b). When administered along with IN fentanyl or oral oxycodone, 50% N_2O induced deep sedation in 15% to 20% (Luhmann et al., 2006; Seith et al., 2012). As much as 10% of children may be poorly sedated during ED PSA with N_2O (Babl 2008b, 2008c; Luhmann et al., 2001). Augmentation of N_2O analgesic effects by concurrent use of local anaesthesia and/or systemic analgesia for painful procedures is also crucial (Babl et al., 2008c). Since children are partially aware during N_2O sedation, strategies to enhance the gas's anxiolytic, dissociative, and euphoric effects are vital to

successful use. Guided imagery significantly augments N_2O's efficacy and helps allay anxiety. Children naïve to intoxication are frequently frightened by the floating or tingling sensations caused by the gas, but they usually accept these effects when incorporated into non-frightening story-telling (Clark and Brunick, 2007b; Clark et al., 2006). N_2O can safely be administered by specially trained nurses to healthy children for ED PSA (Frampton et al., 2003).

N_2O is effective for brief painful ED procedures, especially when local anaesthesia is used—examples include lacerations, lumbar puncture, IV placement, urethral catheterization, and abscess incision and drainage (Babl et al., 2008b; Keidan et al., 2003; Luhmann et al., 2001). Oxycodone 0.2 mg/kg PO (or fentanyl IN 2 mcg/kg) provides additional analgesia in young children with injuries that are difficult to fully locally anaesthetize and may result in deep sedation (Seith et al., 2012).

For displaced mid to distal forearm fractures, a combination of N_2O + oxycodone or intranasal fentanyl + lidocaine haematoma block reduces patient distress as effectively as ketamine, avoids need for venous access, and results in rapid recovery (Luhmann et al., 2006). An effective haematoma block (2.5 mg/kg, maximum 100 mg buffered 1% lidocaine) is critical for this technique. For simple greenstick fractures, the haematoma block is less reliable but significant analgesia is provided and residual pain during reduction is often ameliorated by partial amnesia (Hennrikus et al., 1995).

Ketamine induces dissociative deep sedation or light general anaesthesia within 60 sec of IV administration with little significant respiratory depression or blunting of protective airway reflexes and causes a mild increase in heart rate and blood pressure (Green et al., 2011). It more effectively reduces pain and distress and causes less adverse cardiopulmonary effects than regimens using fentanyl with midazolam or propofol (Godambe et al., 2003; Kennedy et al., 1998). Because of these attributes, ketamine is the most widely used technique for ED PSA in children. Nonetheless, respiratory depression or apnoea, usually brief, may rarely occur (Green et al., 2009). Complete lack of responsiveness to painful stimuli is unnecessary with ketamine as it is also a potent amnestic agent (Kennedy et al., 1998).

Laryngospasm has been reported to occur in as many as 0.3% of children undergoing ketamine PSA, often during recovery (Green et al., 2009). Providers must be prepared to manage laryngospasm by initiating continuous positive airway pressure along with jaw thrust-head tilt to open the airway. These interventions likely will be sufficient, but if obstruction persists, succinylcholine (0.1–1 mg/kg IV) may be required to break the laryngospasm (Hampson-Evans et al., 2008). Most laryngospasm will be brief but relapses have been reported (Cohen and Krauss, 2006). Febrile upper respiratory infections may increase risk for laryngospasm (Olsson and Hallen, 1984).

Conclusion

Pain assessment and management in the ED is a vital component of care. Sometimes that involves systemic analgesia, sometimes local anaesthesia, sometimes distraction, sometimes sedation, but often, all of these. Effective management of pain and distress improves patient outcomes by protecting the children psychologically and physiologically, and by enabling us to perform more accurate examinations and necessary painful therapeutic and diagnostic procedures. Furthermore, it improves health care provider credibility, parental satisfaction, and compliance with recommendations. In this evidence-based review, proven techniques to achieve these goals have been highlighted and areas where further research is needed to develop improved safe and effective methods have been identified.

Case example

A 3-year-old boy sustained a gaping 3 cm laceration to his forehead when he fell on the playground. Topical anaesthetic LET gel has been applied during triage. He is fearful and resists your exam. His mother thinks he will not be still during suturing. You consider sedation with ketamine but wonder whether there are alternatives that will require less time and fewer ED resources. The following strategies are suggested.

This child has been frightened by his injury and is worried that the treating ED staff, strangers to him, will cause additional pain during repair. Several techniques may help him feel less threatened by refocusing his attention away from his injury. First, chat in a relaxed manner with his parent. One then might play a brief game with younger patients, e.g. offering a palm-up 'give me five' hand-slap greeting but quickly move the hand when the child tries to give the slap, causing him to miss. Surprised by a doctor playing a familiar game, many children break into a smile, as do their parents. Alternatively, initially asking the child about her shoes, toy, or some object other than their injury, helps many relax by transferring their attention to something familiar and non-frightening. Likewise, when preparing to suture, one may ask the young child to tell about his last birthday party, colour a picture, recite the 'ABCs' or sing a favourite bedtime lullaby. Playing an interactive game on a computer tablet can be an extremely effective distraction. Family members can aid in these distraction strategies but may benefit from specific guidance. Suturing as the young child sits in his parent's lap can be very reassuring. With school-aged or teenage children, a simple joke, e.g. 'So, your sister/brother/girlfriend, etc, had nothing to do with this (injury), right?!' may help them relax. Getting the child and parent to laugh usually eases their tension.

In addition, effective painless local anaesthesia is critical. Instil LET gel directly into the wound and cover for at least 30 min. Application of LET at the time of triage provides time for absorption and immediately addresses the child's pain. If time permits, returning several times to the child's treatment room to re-apply the LET without causing pain helps desensitize the anxious child to one's presence and to manipulation of his wound. Because complete anaesthesia may not be achieved with LET, especially in non-facial lacerations, augment the local anaesthesia by injecting buffered lidocaine using a short very fine needle, e.g. ½ inch 30 gauge. Show the child the syringe without the needle, tell him you will put some medicine into his 'owie' (the wound), that 'it might feel really cold' and ask him to let you know if you are 'pushing too hard' as you apply the medicine. This helps the child interpret the sensation in a non-frightening manner. Avoid alarming language such as, 'a little stick', 'burning', or 'hurt'. Obscure the syringe and needle by keeping it close to the child's face making it difficult for the child to see the needle. Inject slowly through the wound. Finally, consider administering oral oxycodone, 0.2 mg/kg, to reduce the tenderness of the bruise surrounding the injury; this often also causes children to feel tired and more relaxed. Using these techniques, the need to sedate children for laceration repair can be significantly reduced.

References

Agrawal, D., Manzi, S. F., Gupta, R., and Krauss, B. (2003). Preprocedural fasting state and adverse events in children undergoing procedural sedation and analgesia in a pediatric emergency department. *Ann Emerg Med*, 42(5), 636–646.

Al-Abdullah, T., Plint A. C., and Fergusson, D. (2007). Absorbable versus nonabsorbable sutures in the management of traumatic lacerations and surgical wounds: a meta-analysis. *Pediatr Emerg Care*, 23(5), 339–344.

American Academy of Pediatrics Committee on Drugs. (1992). Guidelines for monitoring and management of pediatric patients during and after sedation for diagnostic and therapeutic procedures. *Pediatrics*, 89(6 Part 1), 1110–1115.

American Society of Anesthesiologists Task Force on Sedation and Analgesia by Non-Anesthesiologists. (2002). Practice guidelines for sedation and analgesia by non-anesthesiologists. *Anesthesiology*, 96(4), 1004–1017.

American Society of Anesthesiologist Task Force on Preoperative Fasting. (1999). Practice guidelines for preoperative fasting and the use of pharmacologic agents to reduce the risk of pulmonary aspiration: application to healthy patients undergoing elective procedures. *Anesthesiology*, 90(3), 896–905.

Anand, K. J., and Scalzo, F. M. (2000). Can adverse neonatal experiences alter brain development and subsequent behavior? *Biol Neonate*, 77(2), 69–82.

Babl, F. E., Goldfinch, C., Mandrawa, C., Crellin, D., O'Sullivan, R., and Donath, S. (2009). Does nebulized lidocaine reduce the pain and distress of nasogastric tube insertion in young children? A randomized, double-blind, placebo-controlled trial. *Pediatrics*, 123, 1548–1555.

Babl, F. E., Mandrawa, C., O'Sullivan, R., and Crellin, D. (2008a). Procedural pain and distress in young children as perceived by medical and nursing staff. *Pediatr Anesth*, 18(5), 412–419.

Babl, F. E., Puspitadewi, A., Barnett, P., Oakley, E., and Spicer, M. (2005). Preprocedural fasting state and adverse events in children receiving nitrous oxide for procedural sedation and analgesia. *Pediatr Emerg Care*, 21(11), 736–743.

Babl, F. E., Oakley, E., Puspitadewi, A., and Sharwood, L. N. (2008c). Limited analgesic efficacy of nitrous oxide for painful procedures in children. *Emerg Med J*, 25, 11, 717–721.

Babl, F. E., Oakley, E., Seaman, C., Barnett, P., and Sharwood, L. N. (2008b). High-concentration nitrous oxide for procedural sedation in children: adverse events and depth of sedation. *Pediatrics*, 121(3), e528–532.

Bauchner, H., Vinci, R., and Waring, C. (1989). Pediatric procedures: do parents want to watch? *Pediatrics*, 84, 907–909.

Bauchner, H., Vinci, R., and May, A. (1994). Teaching parents how to comfort their children during common medical procedures. *Arch Dis Child*, 70, 548–550.

Baxter, A. L., Welch, J. C., Burke, B. L., and Isaacman, D. J. (2004). Pain, position, and stylet styles infant lumbar puncture practices of pediatric emergency attending physicians. *Pediatr Emerg Care*, 20(12), 816–820.

Baxter, A. L., Ewing, P., Evans, N., Manworren, R., Ware, A., and Mix, A. (2005). EMLA application in ED triage increases venipuncture success. Pediatric Academic Societies, 2902. Available at: <http://www.abstracts2view.com/pasall>.

Baxter, A. L., Fisher, R., Burke, B. L., Goldblatt, S., Isaacman, D. J., and Lawson, M. (2006). Local anesthetic and stylet styles: factors associated with resident lumbar puncture success. *Pediatrics*, 117, 876–881.

Bhargava, R. and Young, K. D. (2007). Procedural pain management patterns in academic pediatric emergency departments. *Acad Emerg Med*, 14(5), 479–482.

Bonadio, W. (1996). Safe and effective method for application of tetracaine, adrenaline, and cocaine to oral lacerations. *Ann Emerg Med*, 28, 396–398.

Borland, M., Jacobs, I., King, B., and O'Brien, D. (2007). A randomized controlled trial comparing intranasal fentanyl to intravenous morphine for managing acute pain in children in the emergency department. *Ann Emerg Med*, 49, 335–340.

Breakey, V. R., Pirie, J., and Goldman, R. D. (2007). Pediatric and emergency medicine residents' attitudes and practices for analgesia and sedation during lumbar puncture in pediatric patients. *Pediatrics*, 119, e631–636.

Brousseau, D. C., Duffy, S. J., Anderson, A. C., and Linakis, J. G. (2004). Treatment of pediatric migraine headaches: a randomized, double-blind trial of prochlorperazine versus ketorolac. *Ann Emerg Med*, 43, 256–262.

Burton, L. J., Quinn, B., Pratt-Cheney, J. L., and Pourani, M. (1997). Headche etiology in a pediatric emergency department. *Pediatr Emerg Care*, 13, 1–4.

Chan, C. P., and Lau, F. L. (2010). Should lidocaine spray be used to ease nasogastric tube insertion? A double-blind, randomised controlled trial. *Hong Kong Med J*, 16, 282–286.

Charney, R. L., Yan, Y., Schootman, M., Kennedy, R. M., and Luhmann, J. D. (2008). Oxycodone versus codeine for triage pain in children with suspected forearm fracture: a randomized controlled trial. *Pediatr Emerg Care*, 24(9), 595–600.

Christoph, R. A., Buchanan, L., Begalia, K., and Schwartz, S. (1988). Pain reduction in local anesthetic administration through pH buffering. *Ann Emerg Med*, 17, 117–120.

Chung, S., Lim, R., and Goldman, R. (2010). Intranasal fentanyl versus placebo for pain in children during catheterization for voiding cystourethrography. *Pediatr Radiol*, 40, 1236–1240.

Clark, M. S., Campbell, S. A., and Clark, A. M. (2006). Technique for the administration of nitrous oxide/oxygen sedation to ensure psychotropic analgesic nitrous oxide (PAN) effects. *Int J Neurosci*, 116(7), 871–877.

Clark, E., Plint, A. C., Correll, R., Gaboury, I., and Passi, B. (2007). A randomized, controlled trial of acetaminophen, ibuprofen, and codeine for acute pain relief in children with musculoskeletal trauma. *Pediatrics*, 119, 460–467.

Clark, M. and Brunick, A. (2007). *Handbook of nitrous oxide and oxygen sedation* (3rd edn). St Louis, MO: Elsevier Health Sciences.

Cohen, V. G., and Krauss, B. (2006). Recurrent episodes of intractable laryngospasm during dissociative sedation with intramuscular ketamine. *Pediatr Emerg Care*, 22(4), 247–9.

Damen, L., Bruijn, J. K. J., Verhagen, A. P., Berger, M. Y., Passchier, J., and Koes, B. W. (2005). Symptomatic treatment of migraine in children: a systematic review of medication trials. *Pediatrics*, 116, e295–302.

Davey, G. C. (1989). Dental phobias and anxieties: evidence for conditioning processes in the acquisition and modulation of a learned fear. *Behav Res Ther*, 27, 51–58.

Drendel, A. M., Brousseau, D. C., and Gorelick, M. H. (2006). Pain assessment for pediatric patients in the emergency department. *Pediatrics*, 117, 1511–1518.

Eidelman, A., Weiss, J. M., Lau, J., and Carr, D. B. (2005). Topical anesthetics for dermal instrumentation: a systematic review of randomized, controlled trials. *Ann Emerg Med*, 46(4), 343–351.

Eidelman, A., Weiss, J. M., Baldwin, C. L., Enu, I. K., McNicol, E. D., and Carr, D. B. (2011). Topical anaesthetics for repair of dermal laceration. *Cochrane Database Syst Rev*, 6, CD005364.

Eiland, L. S., and Hunt, M. O. (2010). The use of triptans for pediatric migraines. *Paediatric Drugs*, 12(6), 379–89.

Elder, J. S., and Longenecker, R. (1995). Premedication with oral midazolam for voiding cystourethrography in children: safety and efficacy. *Am J Roentgenol*, 164, 1229–1232.

Farion, K. J., Osmond, M. H., Hartling, L., Russell, K. F., Klassen, T. P., Crumley, E., et al. (2003). Tissue adhesives for traumatic lacerations: a systematic review of randomized controlled trials. *Acad Emerg Med*, 10, 110–118.

Fradet, C., McGrath, P. J., Kayd, J., Adams, J., and Lukec, B. (1990). A prospective survey of reactions to blood tests by children and adolescents. *Pain*, 40, 53–60.

Frampton, A., Browne, G. J., Lam, L. T., Cooper, M. G., and Lane, L. G. (2003). Nurse administered relative analgesia using high concentration nitrous oxide to facilitate minor procedures in children in an emergency department. *Emerg Med J*, 20(5), 410–413.

Friday, J. H., Kanegaye, J. T., McCaslin. I., Zheng, A., and Harley, J. R. (2009). Ibuprofen provides analgesia equivalent to acetaminophen–codeine in the treatment of acute pain in children with extremity injuries: a randomized clinical trial. *Acad Emerg Med*, 16, 711–716.

Gallagher, E. J. (2004). Nasogastric tubes: hard to swallow. *Ann Emerg Med*, 44(2), 138–141.

Gasche, Y., Daali, Y., Fathi, M., Chiappe, A., Cottini, S., Dayer, P., et al. (2004). Codeine intoxication associated with ultrarapid CYP2D6 metabolism. *N Engl J Med*, 351(27), 2827–2831.

Gerard, L., Cooper, C., Duethman, K., Gordley, B., and Kleiber, C. (2003). Effectiveness of lidocaine lubricant for discomfort during pediatric urethral catheterization. *J Urol*, 170, 564–567.

Godambe, S. A., Elliot, V., Matheny, D., and Pershad, J. (2003). Comparison of propofol/fentanyl versus ketamine/midazolam for brief orthopedic procedural sedation in a pediatric emergency department. *Pediatrics*, 112, 116–123.

Godwin, S. A., Caro, D. A., Wolf, S. J., Jagoda A. S., Charles, R., Marett, B. E., et al. (2005). Clinical policy: procedural sedation and analgesia in the emergency department. *Ann Emerg Med*, 45(2), 177–196.

Goldman, R. D., Crum, D., Bromberg, R., Rogovik, A., and Langer, J. C. (2006). Analgesia administration for acute abdominal pain in the pediatric emergency department. *Pediatr Emerg Care*, 22, 18–21.

Gorchynski, J. and McLaughlin, T. (2011). The routine utilization of procedural pain management for pediatric lumbar punctures: are we there yet? *J Clin Med Res*, 3(4), 164–167.

Green, S. M., Roback, M. G., Miner, J. R., Burton, J. H., and Krauss, B. (2007). Fasting and emergency department procedural sedation and analgesia: a consensus-based clinical practice advisory. *Ann Emerg Med*, 49(4), 454–461.

Green, S. M., Roback, M. G., Krauss, B. Brown, L., McGlone, R. G., Agrawal, D., et al. (2009). Predictors of airway and respiratory adverse events with ketamine sedation in the emergency department: an individual-patient data meta-analysis of 8,282 children. *Ann Emerg Med*, 54, 158–168.

Green, S. M., Roback, M. G., Kennedy, R. M., and Krauss, B. (2011). Clinical practice guideline for emergency department ketamine dissociative sedation: 2011 update. *Ann Emerg Med*, 57, 449–461.

Hampson-Evans, D., Morgan, P., and Farrar, M. (2008). Pediatric laryngospasm. *Paediatr Anaesth*, 18(4), 303–307.

Harrison, D., Bueno, M., Yamada, J., Adams-Webber, T., and Stevens, B. (2010). Analgesic effects of sweet-tasting solutions for infants: current state of equipoise. *Pediatrics*, 126, 894–902.

Hayward, C., Nafziger, A., Kohlhepp, S., and Bertino, J. (1996). Investigation of bioequivalence and tolerability of intramuscular ceftriaxone injections by using 1% lidocaine, buffered lidocaine, and sterile water diluents. *Antimicrob Agents Chemother*, 40(2), 485–487.

Hennrikus, W. L., Shin, A. Y., and Klingelberger, C. E. (1995). Self-administered nitrous oxide and a hematoma block for analgesia in the outpatient reduction of fractures in children. *J Bone Joint Surg* A-77(3), 335–339.

Holdsworth, M. T., Raisch, D. W., Winter, S. S., Chavez, C. M., Leasure, M. M., and Duncan, M. H. (1997). Differences among raters evaluating the success of EMLA cream in alleviating procedure-related pain in children with cancer. *Pharmacotherapy*, 17(5), 1017–1022.

Hoyle, J. D., Rogers, A. J., Reischman, D. E., Powell, E. C., Borgialli, D. A., Mahajan, P. V., et al. (2011). Pain intervention for infant lumbar puncture in the emergency department: physician practice and beliefs. *Acad Emerg Med*, 18, 140–144.

Humphrey, G. B., Boon, C. M., van Linden van den Heuvell, G. F., and van de Wiel, H. B. (1992). The occurrence of high levels of acute behavioral distress in children and adolescents undergoing routine venipunctures. *Pediatrics*, 90, 87–91.

Jimenez, N., Bradford, H., Seidel, K. D., Sousa, M., and Lynn, A. M. (2006). A comparison of a needle-free injection system for local anesthesia versus EMLA for intravenous catheter insertion in the pediatric patient. *Anesth Analg*, 102(2), 411–414.

Juhl, G. A., and Conners, G. P. (2005). Emergency physicians' practices and attitudes regarding procedural anaesthesia for nasogastric tube insertion. *Emerg Med J*, 22, 243–245.

Kan, L., Nagelberg, J., and Maytal, J. (2000). Headaches in a pediatric emergency department: etiology, imaging, and treatment. *Headache*, 40(1), 25–29.

Karounis, H., Gouin, S., Eisman, H., Chalut, D., Pelletier, H., and Williams, B. (2004). Randomized, controlled trial comparing long-term cosmetic outcomes of traumatic pediatric lacerations repaired with absorbable plain gut versus nonabsorbable nylon sutures. *Acad Emerg Med*, 11, 730–735.

Keidan, I., Zaslansky, R., Yusim, Y., Ben-Ackon, M., Rubinstien, M., Perel, A., *et al.* (2003). Continuous flow 50:50 nitrous oxide:oxygen is effective for relief of procedural pain in the pediatric emergency department. *Acute Pain*, 5, 25–30.

Keidan, I., Zaslansky, R., Weinberg, M., Ben-Shlush, A., Jacobson, J. M., Augarten, A. *et al.* (2005). Sedation during voiding cystourethrography: comparison of the efficacy and safety of using oral midazolam and continuous flow nitrous oxide. *J Urology*, 174, 1598–1601.

Kennedy, R. M. (2011). Sedation in the emergency department: a complex and multifactorial challenge. In K. Mason, (ed.) *Pediatric sedation outside of the operating room: a multispecialty international collaboration*, pp. 263–331. New York: Springer.

Kennedy, R. M., and Luhmann, J. D. (1999). The 'ouchless emergency department' getting closer: advances in decreasing distress during painful procedures in the emergency department. *Pediatr Clin North Am*, 46(6), 1215–1247.

Kennedy, R. M., Luhmann, J., and Zempsky, W. T. (2008). Clinical implications of unmanaged needle-insertion pain and distress in children. *Pediatrics*, 122, S130–133.

Kennedy, R. M., Porter, F. L., Miller, J. P., and Jaffe, D. M. (1998). Comparison of fentanyl/midazolam with ketamine/midazolam for pediatric orthopedic emergencies. *Pediatrics*, 102(4), 956–963.

Khan, K. A., and Weisman, S. (2007). Nonpharmacologic pain management strategies in the pediatric department. *Clin Pediatr Emerg Med*, 8, 240–247.

Kim, M. K., Galustyan, S., Sato, T. T., Bergholte, J., and Hennes, H. M. (2003). Analgesia for children with acute abdominal pain: a survey of pediatric emergency physicians and pediatric surgeons. *Pediatrics*, 112, 1122–116.

King, C. (2012). Emergent evaluation of headache in children. Available at: <http://www.uptodate.com/contents/emergent-evaluation-of-headache-in-children> (accessed 28 October 2012).

Klein, E. J., Shugerman, R. P., Leigh-Taylor, K., Schneider, C., Portscheller, D., and Koepsell, T. (1995). Buffered lidocaine: analgesia for intravenous line placement in children. *Pediatrics*, 95, 709–712.

Koller, D. M., Myers, A. B., Lorenz, D., and Godambe, S. A. (2007). Effectiveness of oxycodone, ibuprofen, or the combination in the initial management of orthopedic injury-related pain in children. *Pediatr Emerg Care*, 23(9), 627–33.

Kozer, E., Rosenbloom, E., Goldman, D., Lavy, G., Rosenfeld, N., and Goldman, M. (2006). Pain in infants who are younger than 2 months during suprapubic aspiration and transurethral bladder catheterization: a randomized, controlled study. *Pediatrics*, 118, e51–56.

Kuo, Y., Yen, M., Fetzer, S., and Lee, J. (2010). Reducing the pain of nasogastric tube intubation with nebulized and atomized lidocaine: a systematic review and meta-analysis. *J Pain Symptom Manage*, 40, e613–620.

Langston, W. T., Wathen, J. E., Roback, M. G., and Bajaj, L. (2008). Effect of ondansetron on the incidence of vomiting associated with ketamine sedation in children: a double-blind, randomized, placebo-controlled trial. *Ann Emerg Med*, 52(1), 30–34.

Lewis, D., Ashwal, S., Hershey, A., Hirtz, D., Yonker, M., and Silberstein, S. (2004). Practice Parameter: Pharmacological treatment of migraine headache in children and adolescents: Report of the American Academy of Neurology Quality Standards Subcommittee and the Practice Committee of the Child Neurology Society. *Neurology*, 63, 2215–2224.

Lewis, D. W. (2009). Pediatric migraine. *Neurol Clin*, 27, 481–501.

Lewis, D. W., and Qureshi, F. (2000). Acute headache in children and adolescents presenting to the emergency department. *Headache*, 40, 200–203.

Luck, R. P., Flood, R., Eyal, D., Saludades, J., Hayes, C., and Gaughan, J. (2008). Cosmetic outcomes of absorbable versus nonabsorbable sutures in pediatric facial lacerations. *Pediatr Emerg Care*, 24(3), 137–142.

Luhmann, J. D., Hurt, S., Shootman, M., and Kennedy, R. M. (2004). A comparison of buffered lidocaine versus Ela-Max® before peripheral intravenous catheter insertions in children. *Pediatrics*, 113(3), e217–220.

Luhmann, J. D., Kennedy, A. H., and Kennedy, R. M. (1999). Reducing distress associated with pediatric IV insertion. *Pediatrics*, 103S, 240.

Luhmann, J. D., Kennedy, R. M., Porter, F. L., Miller, J. P., and Jaffe, D. M. (2001). A randomized clinical trial of continuous- flow nitrous oxide and midazolam for sedation of young children during laceration repair. *Ann Emerg Med*, 37(1), 20–27.

Luhmann, J. D., Shootman, M., Luhmann, S. J., and Kennedy, R. M. (2006). A randomized comparison of nitrous oxide plus hematoma block versus ketamine plus midazolam for emergency department forearm fracture reduction in children. *Pediatrics*, 118(4), e1078–1086.

Mace, S. E., Brown, L. A., Francis, L., Godwin, S. A., Hahn, S. A., Howard, P. K., *et al.* (2008). Clinical policy: critical issues in the sedation of pediatric patients in the emergency department. *Ann Emerg Med*, 51(4), 378–399.

MacLean, S., Obispo, J., and Young, K. (2007). The gap between pediatric emergency department procedural pain management treatments available and actual practice. *Pediatr Emerg Care*, 23, 2.

Madsen, S. (2009). Towards evidence based emergency: best BETs from the Manchester Royal Infirmary medicine: topical anaesthetic and pain associated with lumbar puncture in neonates. *Emerg Med J*, 26, 57.

McKay, W., Morris, R., and Mushlin, P. (1987). Sodium bicarbonate attenuates pain on skin infiltration with lidocaine, with or without epinephrine. *Anesth Analg*, 66, 572–574.

McNaughton, C., Zhou, C., Robert, L., Storrow, A., and Kennedy, R.M. (2009). A randomized, crossover comparison of injected buffered lidocaine, lidocaine cream, and no analgesia for peripheral intravenous cannula insertion. *Ann Emerg Med*, 54, 214–220.

Mularoni, P., Cohen, L., DeGuzman, M., Mennuti-Washburn, J., Greenwald, M., and Simon, H. (2009). A randomized clinical trial of lidocaine gel for reducing infant distress during urethral catheterization. *Pediatr Emerg Care*, 25, 439–443.

Nagy, S. (1998). A comparison of the effects of patients' pain on nurses working in burns and neonatal intensive care units. *J Adv Nurs*, 27(2), 335–340.

Nigrovic, L. E., Kuppermann, N., and Neuman, N. (2007). Risk factors for traumatic or unsuccessful lumbar punctures in children. *Ann Emerg Med*, 49, 762–771.

Oberer, C., von Ungern-Sternberg, B. S., Frei, F. J., and Erb, T. O. (2005). Respiratory reflex responses of the larynx differ between sevoflurane and propofol in pediatric patients. *Anesthesiology*, 103, 1142–1148.

Olsson, G. L., and Hallen, B. (1984). Laryngospasm during anaesthesia—a computer-aided incidence study in 136,929 patients. *Acta Anaesthesiol Scand*, 28, 567–575.

Pate, J. T., Blount, R. L., Cohen, L. L., and Smith, A. J. (1996). Childhood medical experience and termperament as predictors of adult functioning in medical situations. *Child Healthcare*, 25(4), 281–298.

Patel, A. (2008). Tongue lacerations. *Br Dent J*, 204(7), 355.

Peña, B. M. G., and Krauss, B. (1999). Adverse events of procedural sedation and analgesia in a pediatric emergency department. *Ann Emerg Med*, 34, 483–491.

Peters, J. W., Koot, H. M., de Boer, J. B., Passchier, J., Bueno-de-Mesquita, J. M., de Jong, F. H., *et al.* (2003). Major surgery within the first 3 months of life and subsequent biobehavioral pain responses to immunization at later age: a case comparison study. *Pediatrics*, 111(1), 129–135.

Pierluishi, G. J., and Terndrup, T. E. (1989). Influence of topical anesthesia on the sedation of pediatric emergency department patients with lacerations. *Pediatr Emerg Care*, 5, 211–215.

Pinheiro, J., Furdon, S., and Ochoa, L. (1993). Role of local anesthesia during lumbar puncture in neonates. *Pediatrics*, 91(2), 379–382.

Pollack, C. V., Pollack, E. S., and Andrew, M. E. (1994). Suprapubic bladder aspiration versus urethral catheterization in ill infants: success, efficiency and complication rates. *Ann Emerg Med*, 23, 225–230.

Porter, F. L., Miller, J. P., Cole, F. S., and Marshall, R. E. (1991). A controlled clinical trial of local anesthesia for lumbar punctures in newborns. *Pediatrics*, 88, 663–669.

Prensky, A. L., and Sommer, D. (1979). Diagnosis and treatment of migraine in children. *Neurology*, 29, 506–510.

Priestley, S., Kelly, A. M., Chow, L., Powell, C., and Williams, A. (2003). Application of topical local anesthetic at triage reduces treatment time for children with lacerations: a randomized controlled trial. *Ann Emerg Med*, 42, 34–40.

Quaba, O., Huntley, J. S., Bahia, H., and McKeown, D. W. (2005). A users guide for reducing the pain of local anaesthetic administration. *Emerg Med J*, 22, 188–189.

Quinn, J., Cummings, S., Callaham, M., and Sellers, K. (2002). Suturing versus conservative management of lacerations of the hand: randomised controlled trial. *Br Med J*, 325(7359), 299–300.

Ranji, S. R., Goldman, L. E., Simel, D. L., and Shojania, K. G. (2006). Do opiates affect the clinical evaluation of patients with acute abdominal pain? *JAMA*, 296, 1764–1774.

Resch, K., Schilling, C., Borchert, B. D., Klatzko, M., and Uden, D. (1998). Topical anesthesia for pediatric lacerations: a randomized trial of lidocaine-epinephrine-tetracaine solution versus gel. *Ann Emerg Med*, 32, 693–697.

Reynolds, S. L., and Jaffe, D. M. (1992). Diagnosing abdominal pain in a pediatric emergency department. *Pediatr Emerg Care*, 8, 126–128.

Roback, M. G., Bajaj, L., Wathen, J. E., and Bothner, J. (2004). Preprocedural fasting and adverse events in procedural sedation and analgesia in a pediatric emergency department: are they related? *Ann Emerg Med*, 44(5), 454–459.

Rogers, A. J., Greenwald, M., DeGuzman, A. M., Kelley, M., and Simon, H. (2006). A randomized, controlled trial of sucrose analgesia in infants younger than 90 days of age who require bladder catheterization in the pediatric emergency department. *Acad Emerg Med*, 13, 617–622.

Ross, D. M., and Ross, S. A. (1984). Childhood pain: the school-aged child's viewpoint. *Pain*, 20(2), 179–191.

Schechter, N. L., Zempsky, W. T., Cohen, L. L., McGrath, P. J., McMurtry, C. M., and Bright, N. S. (2007). Pain reduction during pediatric immunizations: evidence-based review and recommendations. *Pediatrics*, 119(5), e1184–1198.

Scholer, S. J., Pituch, K., Orr, D. P., and Dittus, R. S. (1996). Clinical outcomes of children with acute abdominal pain. *Pediatrics*, 98, 680–685.

Seith, R. W., Theophilos, T., and Babl, F. E. (2012). Intranasal fentanyl and high-concentration inhaled nitrous oxide for procedural sedation: a prospective observational pilot study of adverse events and depth of sedation. *Acad Emerg Med*, 19, 31–36.

Sethna, N. F., Verghese, S. T., Hannallah, R. S., Solodiuk, J. C., Zurakowski, D., and Berde, C. B. (2005). A randomized controlled trial to evaluate S-Caine Patch™ for reducing pain associated with vascular access in children. *Anesthesiology*, 102, 403–408.

Sharwood, L. N., and Babl, F. E. (2009). The efficacy and effect of opioid analgesia in undifferentiated abdominal pain in children: a review of four studies. *Pediatr Anesth*, 19, 445–451.

Singer, A. J., Chale, S., Giardano, P., Hocker, M., Cairns, C., Hamilton, R., et al. (2011). Evaluation of a novel wound closure device: a multicenter randomized controlled trial. *Acad Emerg Med*, 18, 1060–1064.

Singer, A. J., Kowalska, A., Richman, P. B., Hollander, J. E., Nashed, A. H., McCuskey, C., et al. (1998). Gender differences in pain associated with urethral catheterization [abstract]. *Acad Emerg Med*, 5, 535.

Singer, A. J., and Stark, M. J. (2001). LET versus EMLA for pretreating lacerations: a randomized trial. *Acad Emerg Med*, 8, 223–230.

Smith, G. A., Strausbaugh, S. D., Harbeck-Wegger, C., Cohen, D. M., Shields, B. J., and Powers, J. D. (1997). New non-cocaine-containing topical anesthetics compared with tetracaine-adrenaline-cocaine during repair of lacerations. *Pediatrics*, 100, 825–830.

Smith, R. W., Shah, V., Goldman, R. D., and Taddio, A. (2007). Caregivers' responses to pain in their children in the emergency department. *Arch Pediatr Adolesc Med*, 161, 578–582.

Sparks, L. A., Setlik, J., and Luhman, J. (2007). Parental holding and positioning to decrease iv distress in young children: a randomized controlled trial. *J Pediatr Nurs*, 22(6), 440–447.

Stock, A., Gilbertson, H., and Babl, F. (2008). Confirming nasogastric tube position in the emergency department: pH testing is reliable. *Pediatr Emerg Care*, 24(12), 805–809.

Stokland, E., Andréasson, S., Jacobsson, B., Jodal, U., and Ljung, B. (2003). Sedation with midazolam for voiding cystourethrography in children: a randomized double-blind study. *Pediatr Radiol*, 33, 247–249.

Taddio, A., Katz, J., Ilersich, A. L., and Koren, G. (1997). Effect of neonatal circumcision on pain response during subsequent routine vaccination. *Lancet*, 349, 599–603.

Taddio, A., Shah, V., Gilbert-MacLeod, C., and Katz, J. (2002). Conditioning and hyperalgesia in newborns exposed to repeated heel lances. *JAMA*, 288(7), 857–861.

Taddio, A., Soin, H. K., Schuh, S., Koren, G., and Scolnik, D. (2005). Liposomal lidocaine to improve procedural success rates and reduce procedural pain among children: a randomized controlled trial. *Can Med Assoc J*, 172(13), 1691–1695.

Tobiansky, R. and Evans, N. (1998). A randomized controlled trial of two methods for collection of sterile urine in neonates. *J Paediatr Child Health*, 34, 460–462.

US Food and Drug Administration. (2011). *FDA safety alert: benzocaine topical products: sprays, gels and liquids—risk of methemoglobinemia*. Available at: <http://www.fda.gov/Safety/MedWatch/SafetyInformation/SafetyAlertsforHumanMedicalProducts/ucm250264.htm>.

Uri, O., Yosefov, L., Haim, A., Behrbalk, E., and Halpern P. (2011). Lidocaine gel as an anesthetic protocol for nasogastric tube insertion in the ED. *Am J Emerg Med*, 29, 386–390.

Vasconcellos, E., Piña-Garza, J. E., Millan, E. J., and Warner, J. S. (1998). Analgesic rebound headache in children and adolescents. *J Child Neurol*, 13, 443–447.

Vaughan, M., Paton, E., Bush, A., and Pershad, J. (2005). Does lidocaine gel alleviate the pain of bladder catheterization in young children? A randomized, controlled trial. *Pediatrics*, 116, 917–920.

Von Baeyer, C. L., Marche, T. A., Rocha, E. M., and Salmon, K. (2004). Children's memory for pain: overview and implications for practice. *J Pain*, 5(5), 241–249.

Walsh, B.M. and Bartfield, J.M. (2006). Survey of parental willingness to pay and willingness to stay for 'painless' intravenous catheter placement. *Pediatr Emerg Care*, 22(11), 699–703.

Wathen, J. E., Roback, M. G., Mackenzie, T., and Bothner, J. P. (2000). Does midazolam alter the clinical effects of intravenous ketamine sedation in children? A double-blind, randomized, controlled, emergency department trial. *Ann Emerg Med*, 36(6), 579–588.

Weisman, S. J., Bernstein, B., and Schechter, N. L. (1998). Consequences of inadequate analgesia during painful procedures in children. *Arch Pediatr Adolesc Med*, 152, 147–149.

White, N. J., Kim, M. K., Brousseau, D. C., Bergholte, J., and Hennes, H. (2004). The anesthetic effectiveness of lidocaine-adrenaline-tetracaine gel on finger lacerations. *Pediatr Emerg Care*, 20(12), 812–815.

Williams, D. G., Patel, A., and Howard, R. F. (2002). Pharmacogenetics of codeine metabolism in an urban population of children and its implications for analgesic reliability. *Br J Anaesth*, 89(6), 839–845.

Witting, M. D. (2007). 'You wanna do what?!' Modern indications for nasogastric intubation. *J Emerg Med*, 33(1), 61–64.

Wolfe, T. (2007). Intranasal fentanyl for acute pain: techniques to enhance efficacy. *Ann Emerg Med*, 49(5), 721–722.

Zempsky, W. T. (2008). Pharmacologic approaches for reducing venous access pain in children. *Pediatrics*, 122, S140–153.

Zempsky, W. T., Cravero, J. P., American Academy of Pediatrics Committee on Pediatric Emergency Medicine, and Section on Anesthesiology and Pain Medicine. (2004a). Relief of pain and anxiety in pediatric patients in emergency medical systems. *Pediatrics*, 114, 1348–1356.

Zempsky, W. T., Parrotti, D., Grem, C., and Nichols, J. (2004b). Randomized controlled comparison of cosmetic outcomes of simple facial lacerations closed with Steri Strip* skin closures or Dermabond* Tissue Adhesive. *Pediatr Emerg Care*, 20(8), 519–524.

Zier, J. L., Kvam, K. A., Kurachek, S. C., and Finkelstein, M. (2007). Sedation with nitrous oxide compared with no sedation during catheterization for urologic imaging in children. *Pediatr Radiol*, 37, 678–684.

SECTION 5

Measurement of pain

CHAPTER 35

Neonatal and infant pain assessment

Grace Y. Lee and Bonnie J. Stevens

Introduction

Pain assessment in neonates and infants is challenging. Although clinicians and scientists have benefited from impressive increases in research on developmental neurobiology, behaviour, and physiology of infant pain capabilities and responses, there is no 'gold standard' infant pain indicator, measure, or approach. Therefore, pain is inferred from the observed responses. These responses are not easily interpretable as they are: (1) modified by contextual factors (e.g. previous experience with pain) and individual infant characteristics (e.g. gestational age (GA), postnatal age (PNA), gender, health status); (2) dependent on the attitudes, beliefs, knowledge, and observational skills of care providers; and (3) reliant on the availability of psychometrically sound assessment measures. Inferring pain is not unique to infants; in adults, for example, self-report is not a direct unbiased measure of this subjective phenomenon—rather it is influenced by a multiplicity of factors and is thus, an indirect measure. In fact, some would suggest that no direct measure of pain has been validated to date.

Pain assessment is an essential foundation for instituting pain relieving interventions to mitigate pain and its consequences in the developing child. Effective pain management is frequently considered an indicator of quality health care practice (Sidani, 2003). Therefore, accurate, timely and feasible pain assessment needs to be featured in policies, guidelines, and procedures at the institutional and policy implementation levels. However, the measurement of pain in neonates and infants may be imprecise and inadequate. This dilemma begs the question as to whether it is possible to develop the perfect measure for this population. In the meantime, we advocate using the best measures available while addressing the existing measurement issues.

This chapter encompasses: (1) the conceptualization of infant pain within a particular biopsychosocial and developmental context; (2) a comprehensive evaluation of existing neonatal/infant pain assessment measures and indicators (e.g. biomarkers and cortical indicators); (3) integration of recommendations on pain assessment measures and practices within clinical practice guidelines, policies, and procedures; and (4) challenges associated with neonatal and infant pain assessment in terms of research, clinical and knowledge translation (KT) issues.

Conceptualization of pain in neonates and infants

Pain and nociception

Pain is an elusive phenomenon that poses unique measurement challenges. For adults, pain measurement usually encompasses the verbal response of the individual experiencing it. However, the inability to communicate verbally does not preclude the individual from pain or negate their need for pain-relieving treatment; thus, behavioural and physiological indicators are commonly used as proxies in assessing pain in infants. However, due to the infant's developmental stage and associated vulnerability, they are completely dependent on their caregivers to observe and interpret these indicators. Their expression of pain and experience are intrinsically intertwined with the caregiver and the sociocultural context in which pain is experienced.

Pain is often conceptualized within the biomedical model of care where the focus is on the sensory processes of nociception and the transmission of signals originating from peripheral nociceptors to receptors in the brain. This model is limited in understanding pain in infants and is an incomplete representation of pain in humans (Sullivan, 2008). Given the importance attributed to the psychosocial context and the processes of development and interaction with the infant's environment, theories such as the systems-based synactive theory of development (Als, 1982) and the social communication model (SCM) of infant pain (Craig, 2009) are extremely relevant.

The synactive theory of development

The synactive theory of development (Als, 1982) focuses on the evolving, continuous, and dynamic relationship between key subsystems within the developing infant organizational structure (e.g. autonomic, motor, state organizational, attentional-interactive, and self-regulatory) and salient aspects of the environment. Als asserts that the infant alternates between stabilizing (e.g. smooth well-regulated functioning) and integrating responses to facilitate functional competence. The caregiver's role is to protect the infant (especially preterm newborns) against external sources of stress and mitigating its effects. The Neonatal Individualized Developmental

Care and Assessment (NIDCAP) programme with a central focus on the social processes involved in protecting and maintaining the stability of the infant within a particular external environment has evolved from this theory. The Assessment of Preterm Infants' Behaviour (APIB) instrument (Als et al., 1982) provides a systematic profile for assessing the individual infant's behavioural cues as a measure of their system capacity and regulatory abilities. Preventing and/or minimizing stressful procedures, assisting the infant to maintain and regulate organized behavioural state and instituting developmentally specific strategies to mitigate the effects of stressful events are hallmark interventions. These physical (e.g. positioning, bundling), tactile (e.g. kangaroo care, non-nutritive sucking), and behavioural (e.g. distraction) strategies are also used as pain-relieving interventions.

The social communication model of pain

The SCM (Craig, 2009) promotes understanding of the complex interactions between biological, psychological, and social features of pain. Craig asserts that pain is a sequence of complex interdependent stages, characterized by feedback loops among sequential stages. Assessing infant pain is construed as a dynamic, interactive process between child and caregiver (e.g. health professional, family or others) who are uniquely influenced by family, community, and culture. Infants almost invariably react to acute tissue stress and damage in a manner that distinguishes 'pain' from 'non-pain' states. These reactions provide a means for caregivers to decode the pain expression and infer the infant's subjective state from biological and behavioural correlates.

This model is unique in its focus on interaction with the caregiver encompassing their cognitive and affective capabilities that support complex social interactions and processes. Once pain is expressed by the infant, caregivers interpret that the infant is in pain. This attribution of pain is influenced by the caregiver's (1) sensitivities, (2) knowledge level (e.g. of the specific child or alternatives to distress), (3) attitudes and beliefs, and (4) prior relationship to the child. The stage is then set for implementing and evaluating pain-relieving interventions.

While the SCM of infant pain addresses the broader context of pain, our current knowledge is primarily centred on acute tissue-damaging or nociceptive pain, with little clarity on the infant's experience and expression of more prolonged acute (e.g. postoperative), persistent (e.g. recurrent), or chronic pain. This understanding is important as the basis for the development and validation of pain assessment indicators and measures in these domains. A more detailed exploration of the SCM is provided by Pillai Riddell et al. (Chapter 9, this volume).

Pain assessment measures and indicators

Acute versus chronic

Neonatal and infant pain assessment measures have been developed for both acute and chronic pain. *Acute pain* signals a specific nociceptive event, injury, or illness, is usually of sudden onset, and is limited to a short period of time. Acute pain typically subsides with effective management after the painful event (e.g. heel lance) or when the illness or injury resolves; it can be persistent and re-occur in multiple episodes over time. Most research on infant pain assessment has used tissue damaging stimuli as the paradigm for

determining behavioural and physiological responses; multidimensional and composite measures are almost exclusively comprised of indicators from acute pain studies. A typical behavioural response depicting the behavioural facial action acute pain response in infants is shown in Figure 35.1.

Chronic pain is frequently defined as pain that has persisted beyond the normal tissue healing time. However, the temporal delineation of 'healing time' is debated as somewhere between 3 and 6 months. The temporal delineation presents additional dilemmas when considering prolonged pain in infants. In addition to the issue of total life span, which may be less than 3 or 6 months, infants have limited time comprehension abilities and cannot fully appreciate past, present, and future or process information in a moment by moment fashion. Researchers have largely ignored chronic pain assessment and its complexities in infants focusing almost exclusively on acute pain, with only a few measures addressing this more prolonged phenomenon (see Table 35.1).

Unidimensional versus multidimensional

Infant pain measures can also be classified as either *unidimensional* (one global item or a multiple items within a single domain) or *multidimensional* (multiple items with multiple domains/composite measures) where *dimension* refers to an aspect of a phenomenon and *domain* is the set of possible dimensions within the phenomenon. Applying these definitions to pain, unidimensional single item measures capture one dimension of the experience (e.g. visual analogue scale capturing pain intensity) whereas unidimensional single domain measures include: (1) multiple items (e.g. brow bulge, eye squeeze) from a single domain (e.g. facial expression) within a single dimension (e.g. behavioural), for example, the Neonatal Facial Coding System (Grunau and Craig 1987); or (2) multiple items (e.g. brow bulge, hand movement, high pitch cry) from multiple domains (e.g. facial expression, movement, cry) within a single dimension (e.g. behavioural), for example, Douleur Aigue du Nouveau-ne (Carbajal et al., 1997).

Multidimensional (composite) measures include multiple items (e.g. brow bulge, heart rate, gestational age) from multiple domains (e.g. facial expression, biomarker,) within multiple dimensions (e.g. behavioural, physiological,), such as the Premature Infant Pain Profile (Stevens et al., 1996). The issue of combining dimensions in multidimensional measures is frequently raised by measurement critics, who suggest mixing poorly correlated dimensions in total scores is unjustified and may lead to ineffective or incomplete management. Conversely, proponents suggest dissociation between indicators is common in a complex entity and therefore taking all dimensions into account is necessary to capture the full scope of the phenomenon for well-informed decision-making (McDowell, 2006).

Existing neonatal and infant pain measures

Approximately four dozen measures have been developed to assess pain in neonates and infants over the past three decades. Several have been extensively validated, although their feasibility and clinical utility are infrequently addressed. The most well-validated measures are multidimensional behavioural indicators or composite measures. Only a few measures incorporate individual infant characteristics or contextual factors. Furthermore, the current body of neonatal pain measures is comprised of a narrow and finite cadre of behavioural and physiological items. Recommendations to expand this repertoire and to explore potential new indicators

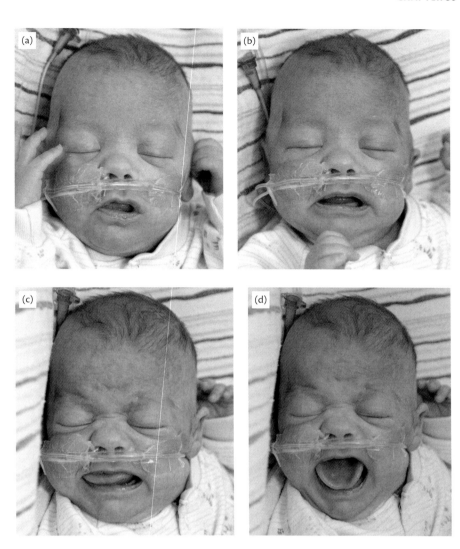

Figure 35.1 Example of a typical behavioural response depicting the behavioural facial action acute pain response in infants.

(e.g. cortical indices) or biomarkers (e.g. cortisol) and their relationship to observed behavioural indicators have only recently been considered. A critical appraisal of unidimensional and multidimensional neonatal and infant pain measures with demonstrated reliability and validity is summarized in Table 35.1.

Individual pain indicators

Given the issues associated with observation of behavioural and physiological pain indicators in neonates and infants, researchers have begun to investigate potential biomarkers and neurocognitive/physiological indicators.

Biomarkers

Several researchers have conducted studies examining the use of cortisol as a biomarker of stress as a pain indicator during/after an invasive procedure. While some reported an increases of cortisol (Franck et al., 2011; Grunau et al., 2010), others found no differences (Cignacco et al., 2009; Gibbins et al., 2008a). These conflicting results may be associated with the heterogeneity of study designs, sample size, intensity of the painful procedure, severity of illness, and method of cortisol collection.

Heart rate variability (HRV) is another biomarker that has been substantially studied, especially in the extremely low birth weight infant population. For example, Grunau and colleagues (2001) demonstrated a heightened cardiac sympathetic activity during heel lance where the most significant factors associated with altered behavioural and autonomic pain reactivity at 32 weeks PCA (greater number of previous invasive procedures since birth and GA at birth) were related to a dampened response. After controlling for these variables, exogenous steroid exposure independently contributed to the behavioural and autonomic pain scores, also dampening the response. A summary of recent studies on biomarkers in infant pain is included in Table 35.2.

Cortical indicators

There is growing interest on the role of the brain in pain mechanism and transmission of noxious stimuli from the periphery to the central nervous system. The majority of research has been conducted with animals. However, newer non-invasive neuroimaging techniques including electrophysical methods (electroencephalogram—EEG), radiological methods (positron emission tomography—PET), magnetic resonance techniques (magnetic resonance

Table 35.1 Unidimensional and multidimensional composite measures for acute pain and persistent/ prolonged/ chronic pain

Pain scale	Dimension/ domain	Type of pain	Age level	Indicators	Psychometric properties
Unidimensional single-domain measures					
ABC Scale (Bellieni et al., 2005, 2007)	Behavioural	Acute (procedural)	Preterm/full-term infants	Cry: (a) Pitch of first cry (b) Rhythmicity of bout of crying (c) Cry constancy	*Term infants:* Interrater reliability: (Cohen's K = 0.83) Intrarater reliability: (Cohen's K = 0.85) Specificity: analgesic/non-analgesic (P <0.0001); pain/ sham (P <0.0001) Sensitivity: high correlation between ABC and DAN Concurrent validity: (Spearman r = 0.91) Internal consistency: (Cronbach's alpha = 0.76) Practicality: nurses scored as 'good' *Preterm infants:* Interrater reliability (K = 0.70) Concurrent validity: (r = 0.68; r2 = 0.45; p <0.0001) between ABC and PIPP
Neonatal Facial Coding System (NFCS) (Grunau and Craig, 1987)	Behavioural	Acute (procedural and postoperative)	> 25 weeks GA—term infants	Facial actions Brow bulge Eye squeeze Naslabial furrow Open lips Horizontal mouth Vertical mouth Lips pursed Taut tongue Chin quiver Tongue protrusion	*Acute pain:* Interrater reliability: (r = 0.60–1.00) Intrarater reliability: (r = 0.88) Content and face validity Construct validity: (r = 0.79, P <0.001; Lilley et al., 1997) *Postoperative pain:* Interrater reliability: (r = 0.84–1.0) Concurrent validity with VAS and COMFORT-B scale: (with VAS (P <0.001) and COMFORT-B (P <0.001). With HR mean (P <0.001), BP mean (P <0.001), HRV (P <0.001), and BPV (P= 0.007) (Peters et al., 2003)
Unidimensional multiple-domains measures					
Behavioral Indicators of Infant Pain (BIIP) Scale (Holsti and Grunau, 2007a)	Behavioural	Acute (procedural)	23–32 weeks GA	State Facial actions Hand actions	Internal consistency: (r = 0.82) Interrater reliability: (r = 0.80–0.92) Construct validity: (F[1, 86] = 85.9, p <0.0001) Concurrent validity with NIPS: (earlier born <29 weeks (EB) r = 0.64, p < 0.0001; later born 29–32 weeks (LB) r = 0.60, p <0001). Correlations between the BIIP and mean heart rate (EB r = 0.33, p <0.05; LB r = 0.50, p <0.001)
Bernese Pain Scale for Neonates (BPSN) (Cignacco et al., 2004)	Behavioural	Acute (procedural)	27–41 weeks GA with/ without ventilation	Alertness Duration of crying Time to calm Skin colour, Eyebrow bulge with eye squeeze, Posture Breathing pattern Interrater reliability: (r = 0.86–0.97)	Intrarater reliability: (r = 0.98–0.99) Construct validity: (P <0.0001) Concurrent and convergent validity: BPSN compared to VAS and PIPP (r = 0.86, and r = 0.91, P <0.0001, respectively)
Children's and Infants' Postoperative Pain Scale (CHIPPS) (Büttner and Finke, 2000)	Behavioural	Prolonged (postoperative)	Birth–4 years	Crying Facial expression Posture of trunk and legs Motor restlessness	Internal consistency: (>1 year) (Cronbach's alpha = 0.96) Interrater reliability: (>3 years) (r = 0.64–0.77) Content validity Construct and concurrent validity in older subsample (P <0.001)

(Continued)

Table 35.1 (*Continued*)

Pain scale	Dimension/domain	Type of pain	Age level	Indicators	Psychometric properties
Douleur Aigue du Nouveau-ne (DAN) (Carbajal et al., 1997, 2005)	Behavioural	Acute (procedural)	24–41 weeks GA	Facial expression Limb movement Vocalizations/attempt at vocalizations	Internal consistency: (Cronbach's alpha = 0.88) Interrater reliability: (r = 0.91) Content validity
Face, Legs, Activity, Cry, Consolability (FLACC) scale (Manworren and Hynan, 2003; Merkel et al., 1997)	Behavioural	Acute (procedural)	Birth to adolescents (also for children with disabilities)	Face Legs Activity Cry Consolability	Interrater reliability (K = 0.61) Content validity Concurrent validity (P <0.001)
Modified Behavioural Pian Scale (MBPS) (Taddio et al., 1995)	Behavioural	Acute (procedural)	2–6 months	Facial expression Cry Body movement	Interrater reliability: (ICC = 0.95) Internal consistency: (r = 0.55–0.66) Test-rest reliability: (r = 0.95) Content validity Construct validity: (P <0.01) Concurrent validity: (r = 0.68–0.74)

Multidimensional composite measures

Pain scale	Dimension/domain	Type of pain	Age level	Indicators	Psychometric properties
Cardiac Analgesic Assessment Scale (CAAS) (Suominen et al., 2004)	Behavioural, Physiological	Prolonged (postoperative)	Birth–mean age = 2.5 years	Papillary size Heart rate Blood pressure Respiratory and motor response	Interrater reliability: (r = 0.86–1.0) Content validity Convergent validity: (K = 0.33; P <0.05 pre-post bolus)
Crying Requires oxygen Increased vital signs Expression Sleep (CRIES) Scale (Krechel and Bildner, 1995)	Behavioural, physiological	Prolonged (postoperative)	28 weeks GA–6 years	Crying Requires O$_2$	Convergent validity (with PIPP and VAS) Concurrent validity: with NIPS and CHIPPS (range r = 0.30–0.38)
Increased vital signs Expression Sleep (CRIES) Scale (Krechel and Bildner, 1995)				Increased vital signs Expression Sleepless	Construct validity and predictive validity: (sensitivity and specificity >90%) Interrater reliability: (r = 0.98) Feasibility: global rating for routine use was low (20%) Rated as moderately feasible for clinical practice
COMFORT scale (Ambuel et al., 1992)	Behavioural, physiological	Acute, acute (prolonged), chronic and level of sedation	0–17 years	Alertness, calmness respiratory response Crying Physical movement Muscle tone Facial tension Blood pressure (MAP) baseline Heart rate baseline VAS	Interrater reliability: (Kappa = 0.54- 0.93) Internal consistency: (Cronbach's α= 0.92, ICC = 0.82–0.85, r = 0.90–0.92) Concurrent validity (r = 0.75, P <0.01) Content validity Convergent validity: with clinician judgement (r = 0.89–0.96) Concurrent validity: with VAS (r = 0.44–0.96)
Echelle Douleur Inconfort Nouveau-né (EDIN) (Debillon et al., 2001)	Behavioural, physiological	Prolonged (postoperative)	26–36 weeks GA	Facial expression Movement Sleep Consoliability	Interrater reliability: (k = 0.69, r = 0.59–0.74) Internal consistency: (Cronbach's α= 0.92) Content validity Construct validity: (P <0.000)

(Continued)

Table 35.1 (*Continued*)

Pain scale	Dimension/ domain	Type of pain	Age level	Indicators	Psychometric properties
EVENDOL (Moreaux, 2010)	Behavioural, physiological	Acute (pain in emergency)	1 month– 6 years	Complaint Grimace Movements Postures Interaction with surroundings	Interrater reliability: (r >0.9, weighted kappa 0.7 to 0.9) Construct validity: before /after nalbuphine (p < 0.0001), at mobilization (p = 0.0011) Concurrent validity: between VAS and EVENDOL >0.8 (p <0.0001); between EVENDOL and other scales (EDIN, CHEOPS, FLACC, TPPPS): 0.5 to 0.93 Content validity: (Cronbach coefficient = 0.83 to 0.92).
Faceless acute neonatal pain scale (FANS) (Milesi et al., 2010)	Behavioural, physiological	Acute (procedural)	Preterm infants	Heart rate variation Acute discomfort Limb movements Vocal expressions	Inter-rater agreement: (r = 0.92) Internal consistency: (Cronbach's α = 0.72) Concurrent validity: FANS and DAN (ICC = 0.88)
Hartwig Score (Hünseler et al., 1991)	Behavioural, physiological	Acute	Infants	Motor response Grimacing Eyes Respiration Aspiration	Interrater reliability: (ICC = 0.934) Internal consistency: all items (Cronbach's alpha = 0.867) Concurrent validity: between Hartwig Score and VAS: mean of the differences of 0.77 (0.77); 95% CI of 0.508–1.03 (0.411; 1.129) and levels of agreement from −1.76 to 3.23 (−1.74 to 3.0); between Hartwig Score and Comfort scale: mean differences of 0.15 (0.34); 95% CI of 0.013–0.287 (0.104; 0.576) and levels of agreement from −1.49 to 1.77 (−1.13 to 1.82) (Hünseler et al., 2011)
Liverpool Infant Distress Scale (LIDS) (Horgan and Choonara, 1996; Horgan et al., 2002)	Behavioural, physiological	Prolonged (postoperative)	Neonates	Facial expression Sleep pattern Cry quantity and quality, Spontaneous movement and excitability Flexion of fingers, toes, Tone	Internal consistency: (r = 0.84–0.94) Interrater reliability: (r = 0.74–0.88) Intrarater reliability: (r = 0.1 = 0.96) Content validity Discriminant validty: (P = 0.004–0.0000)
Multidimensional Assessment of Pain Scale (MAPS) (Ramelet et al., 2007a, 2007b)	Behavioural, physiological	Prolonged (postoperative)	0–31 months	Vital signs Breathing pattern Facial expressions Body movement State of arousal	Internal consistency: (Cronbach's alpha = 0.62 at baseline, 0.80 at 15 min, 0.37 at 30 min, 0.26 at 60 min. When 'vital signs' was deleted, internal consistency at baseline, 15, 30, and 60 min improved r = 0.64, 0.79, 0.67, and 0.71) Concurrent validity: between MAPS and FLACC: mean of differences 0.44 (CI: 0.18–0.71); limits of agreement = −1.22 to 2.09; between MAPS and VAS: mean of differences 0.25 (CI of 0.02–0.49); limits of agreement −1.24 to 1.74 Clinical utility: reported as useful in preverbal children (median 2, IQR1) and moderately simple (median 2, IQR 0). Median observation time was 2 min (IQR 4) and mean assessment time was 35.3 (±26) sec
Modified Infant Pain Scale (MIPS) (Buchholz et al., 1998)	Behavioural, physiological	Prolonged (postoperative)	4–30 weeks PNA	Sleep Facial expression Quality of cry Spontaneous motor activity, Excitability/ responsiveness to stimulation, Flexion fingers/toes,	Interrater reliability: (r = 0.85) Content validity Convergent validity: in dichotomous rating (P <0.0001)

(Continued)

Table 35.1 (*Continued*)

Pain scale	Dimension/domain	Type of pain	Age level	Indicators	Psychometric properties
				Sucking Overall tone, Consolability, Sociability, Change in HR, BP Fall in O_2 saturation	
Modified Postoperative Comfort Score (Guinsburg et al., 1998)	Behavioural, physiological	Prolonged (mechanical ventilation)	< 32 weeks GA	Sleep Facial expression Sucking Hyper-reactivity Agitation Hypertonicity Toes/fingers flexion Consolability	Convergent validity: in bedside (P <0.00001) and laboratory video coding (P = 0.02) Content validity Divergent validity: placebo and analgesic samples (P <0.05)
Modified Postoperative Comfort Score (Guinsburg et al., 1998)	Behavioural, physiological	Prolonged (postoperative)	Preterm infants	Sleep Facial expression Activity Tone Consolibility Cry Sociability	Content validity Discriminant validity: (P <0.0001)
Napean Neonatal Intensive Care Unit Pain Assessment Tool (NNICUPAT) (Marceau, 2003)	Behavioural, physiological, and contextual	Acute (procedural)	Ventilated infants 25–36 weeks GA	Facial expression Body movement Colour Saturation Respiration Heart rate Nurse perception of pain	Content validity Interrater reliability: before and during procedure (r = 0.88) Interrater reliability: after procedure (r = 0.48) Concurrent validity: during procedure (0.01)
Neonatal Infant Pain Scale (NIPS) (Lawrence et al., 1993)	Behavioural, physiological	Acute (procedural)	Preterm and full-term	Facial expression Cry Breathing patterns Arm movement Leg movement State of arousal	Interrater reliability: (r = 0.92–0.97) Internal consistency: (0.87–0.95) Content validity Concurrent validity: (r = 0.53–0.83)
Neonatal Pain, Agitation and Sedation Scale (N-PASS) (Hummel et al., 2003, 2008, 2010)	Behavioural, physiological	Acute (procedural) and prolonged (mechanical ventilation)	23–40 weeks GA	Crying/irritability Behavioural state Facial expression Extremities/tone Vital signs (HR, RR, BP, O_2 saturation)	Interrater reliability: (r = 0.85–0.95) Intrarater reliability: (Spearman's rho r = 0.874, P <0.0001). Construct (discriminate) validity: (Z=-6.429, P <0.0001) Internal consistency: (Cronbach's alpha = 0.84–0.89) Convergent validity: with PIPP (r = 0.83 with high pain scores, r = 0.61 with low pain scores)
Riley Infant Pain Scale (RIPS) (Schade et al., 1996)	Behavioural, physiological	Prolonged (postoperative)	<3 years or children unable to verbalize pain	Facial expression Body movement Sleep Verbal/vocal Consolability Response to movement/touch	Interrater reliability: (ICC = 0.53–0.83; lower <1 month age group) Internal consistency: (r = 0.73–0.88) Content validity Discriminant validity: (P<0.001)

(Continued)

Table 35.1 (*Continued*)

Pain scale	Dimension/domain	Type of pain	Age level	Indicators	Psychometric properties
Pain Assessment in Neonates Scale (PAIN) (Hudson-Barr et al., 2002)	Behavioural, physiological	Acute (procedural)	26–47 weeks GA	Facial expression Cry Breathing patterns Extremity movement State arousal O_2 saturation Increased heart rate	Content validity Concurrent validity: (r = 0.93)
Pain Assessment Tool (PAT) (Hodgkinson et al., 1994)	Behavioural, physiological and contextual	Prolonged (postoperative)	27 weeks to full-term	Posture/tone Sleep pattern Expression Colour Cry Respirations Heart rate O_2 saturations Blood pressure Nurse perception	Interrater reliability: (r = 0.85) Content validity Convergent validity: (r = 0.38) Concurrent validity: (r = 0.76) (Spence et al., 2005)
Postoperative Pain Score (POPS) for Infants (Barrier et al., 1989)	Behavioural, physiological	Prolonged (postoperative)	1–7 months	Infant sleep during the preceding hour Facial expression Cry Motor activity Excitability Flexion Sucking Tone Consolability	Interrater reliability: (r = 0.79–0.88) Content validity Discriminant validity: (P < 0.0001)
Premature Infant Pain Profile (PIPP) (Stevens et al., 1996)	Behavioural, physiological, and contextual	Acute (procedural)	Term and preterm neonates	GA Behavioural state Heart rate O_2 saturation Brow bulge Eye squeeze Nasolabial furrow	Interrater reliability: (r >0.89 for total score) Intrarater reliability scores: (r = 0.95) Internal consistency: (alpha = 0.59–0.76) Construct validity: (P <0.05) Convergent validity: between PIPP and CRIES: (r=0.447; P <0.001; r = 0.292 to 0.472; P <0.005, respectively; ICC=0.6139; 95% CI: 0.4–0.76); between PIPP and FLACC: (r=0.462 to 0.521; P <0.01); between PIPP and N-PASS: (r = 0.81 to 0.83) during severe pain and (r=0.61) for minimal-to-moderate pain. Feasibility: staff nurses able to use after a brief explanation and practice session. (Jonsdottir and Kristjansdottir, 2005). Clinical utility: Schiller (1999) examined the PIPP and the CRIES. Both measures were rated as clinically useful: PIPP rated higher on acceptability and the CRIES rated higher on completion time and cost.
Premature Infant Pain Profile–Revised (PIPP–R) (Gibbins, 2008b; Stevens et al., 2012)	Behavioural, physiological, and contextual	Acute (procedural)	Term and preterm neonates	Same as PIPP but GA and behavioural state scored only when subtotal score of behavioural and physiological indicators > 0	Convergent validity: between PIPP and PIPP–R: (R^2 = 0.93, p <0.0001) for ELBW infants during diaper change (R^2 = 0.91, p <0.0001) and heel lance (R^2 = 0.98, p <0.0001) conditions. PIPP and PIPP-R scores were highly correlated (R^2 = 0.98, p <0.001) for infants 25–41 weeks GA

Table 35.1 (*Continued*)

Pain scale	Dimension/ domain	Type of pain	Age level	Indicators	Psychometric properties
					Construct validity: PIPP–R scores were significantly lower during diaper change [mean 8.3(SD = 2.9)] compared to heel lance [mean 9.9 (SD= 3.1); (t (95) = 4.51, p = 0.036)]. Feasibility: Mean scores on each feasibility scale (median of 4/of 5).
Scale for Use in Newborns (SUN) (Blauer and Gerstmann, 1998)	Behavioural, physiological (movement, facial expression biomarkers, biomarkers)	Prolonged (excluded postoperative)	24–40 weeks GA	Central nervous system state Breathing Movement Tone, face Heart rate Mean blood pressure	Content validity Discriminant validity: (p < 0.05–0.01)

Table 35.2 Biomarker indicators of neonatal/ infant pain

Indicator(s)	Reference	Study design/methods	Main results
Cortisol			
Behavioural Biochemical	Cignacco et al., 2009	Single group, exploratory repeated measures design exploring the variability in pain response in preterm infants who received sucrose during routine heel stick (n = 9)	72–94% within-subject variability No significant differences in cortisol before and after the heel sticks (p = 0.55). A general gradual decrease of cortisol levels across time
Behavioural Physiological Biochemical	Franck et al., 2011	Prospective observational study comparing indices of pain in critically ill full-term neonates following cardiac surgery (n = 81)	A 27% difference in COMFORT scores between tissue damaging and non-tissue damaging procedures (P <0.001). COMFORT score and the high-frequency HRV showed inverse correlations with opioid dose and plasma levels over the first 48 h postoperatively; after accounting for clinical variables, only COMFORT score remained significant (P <0.001). Both behavioural and physiological variables accounted for 45% and 15% respectively of the variance in COMFORT scores (P <0.001). Plasma cortisol increased postoperatively but no change in urinary cortisol
Physiological Behavioural Biochemical	Gibbins et al., 2008a	Prospective crossover design comparing physiological, behavioural and biochemical responses to painful and non-painful procedures in ELGA infants (n = 50)	Facial actions—brow bulge (t = −4.6, p <0.001), eye squeeze (t = −3.5, p <0.002), nasolabial furrow (t = −3.3, p <0.002) and vertical mouth stretch (t = −2.6, P <0.01), increased post heel lance. No changes in physiology, body movement, or cortisol following the heel lance
Behavioural Physiological Biochemical	Grunau et al., 2010	Prospective cohort study examining cortisol reactivity during immunization in preterm (n = 99) and full-term (n = 39) infants at corrected age 4 months	Cortisol (P = 0.011), facial activity (P <0.0001), and HR increased (P <0.0001) during immunizations. Cortisol was lower in preterm ELGA and VLGA boys, compared with full-term boys (P = 0.006)
Behavioural Biochemical	Holsti et al., 2007b	Randomized cross-over design examining facial responses, adrenocorticotropic hormone (ACTH) and cortisol levels in preterm infants during routine nursing procedures (n = 90 preterm infants: extremely low gestational age (ELGA: 28 weeks); very low gestational age (VLGA: 29–31 weeks))	Facial actions increased significantly from baseline during clustered care (p = 0.001), and continued during the recovery phase. The correlation between ACTH and cortisol differed significantly between the two GA groups. During clustered care, ELGA infants showed no relationship between ACTH and cortisol, whereas VLGA infants showed a significant correlation (r = 0.62, p = 0.0001)
Biochemical	Schaffer et al., 2009	Prospective cohort study comparing salivary cortisol and cortisone levels during rest and a pain-induced stress event in small for gestational age (SGA) and appropriate for gestational age (AGA) neonates 34 weeks of gestation (n = 58)	In AGA neonates, salivary cortisol and cortisone levels significantly increased after the stress event (P <0.05) while SGA infants exhibited a blunted response

(Continued)

Table 35.2 *(Continued)*

Indicator(s)	Reference	Study design/methods	Main results
Biochemical	Yamada et al., 2007	Prospective cohort study to determine differences between (a) hair cortisol levels in term and preterm infants exposed to stress in the NICU and (b) hair cortisol levels and severity of illness (n = 60 infants >25 weeks GA)	No significant differences between the hair cortisol levels in hospitalized term and preterm infants. Hospitalized infants had significantly higher hair cortisol levels than healthy term infants (t (76) = 2.755, p = 0.004) Term NICU infants showed a statistically significant association between total number of ventilator days and hair cortisol levels: for every extra day on the ventilator, hair cortisol levels increased on average by 0.2 mol/g (p = 0.03)
Heart rate variability (HRV)			
Behavioural Physiological	Faye et al., 2010	Prospective cohort study exploring HRV to pain in the full-term newborn (n = 28). Postoperative pain assessed using EDIN scale at the end of the 2 h recording period	Mean EDIN scores were 21 and 72 in respectively the groups 'Low EDIN' and 'High EDIN'. HFVI was significantly lower in the 'High EDIN' group than in the 'Low EDIN' (0.70.2 vs. 1.20.3, respectively; P <0.01). An HFVI <0.9 predicted an EDIN score 5, with a sensitivity of 90%, and a specificity of 75%
Physiological	Padhye et al., 2009	Prospective repeated measures cohort study to characterize the HRV response of high-risk very low birth weight infants (<1500 g) from 23–38 weeks GA (n = 38 infants) to heel lance procedure and venepuncture	HRV in both bands decreased during pain (P<0.001), followed by a recovery to near-baseline levels (P = 0.166). Venepuncture and mechanical ventilation attenuated the HRV response to pain (P= 0.024 and P=0.001 respectively). HRV at the baseline increased with GA but the growth rate of high-frequency power was reduced in mechanically ventilated infants
Physiological Behavioural	Stevens et al., 2007	Prospective observational cohort study comparing pain responses to heel lance from infants at high (Cohort A, n = 54), moderate (Cohort B, n = 45) and low (Cohort C, n = 50) risk for NI (n = 149)	A significant cohort by phase interaction for total facial action (F(6, 409) = 3.50, p = 0.0022) and 4 individual facial actions existed; with Cohort C demonstrating the most facial action. A significant Phase effect existed for increased maximum HR (F(3, 431) = 58.1, p = 0.001), minimum HR (F(3, 431) = 78.7, p = 0.001), maximum O_2 saturation (F(3, 425) = 47.6, p = 0.001), and minimum O_2 saturation (F(3, 425) = 12.2, p = 0.001) with no cohort differences Cohort B had significantly higher minimum (F(2, 79) = 3.71, p = 0.029), and mean (F(2, 79) = 4.04, p = 0.021) fundamental cry frequencies A significant phase effect for low/high-frequency HRV ratio (F(2, 216) = 4.97, p = 0.008) was found with the greatest decrease in Cohort A. Significant cohort by phase interactions existed for low- and high-frequency HRV

imaging—MRI), and near-infrared spectroscopy (NIRS), have been explored to try and better understand structural, biochemical, or functional neuronal activity in the brain's response to noxious stimulation. A summary of the most recent studies are included in Table 35.3.

Recently, Brummelte et al. (2012), using MRI, three-dimensional magnetic resonance spectroscopic imaging, and diffusion tensor imaging demonstrated that greater numbers of skin-breaking procedural pain indicators may contribute to impaired brain development in preterm infants. Fabrizi and colleagues (2011) systematically mapped the maturation of tactile and nociceptive activity in the developing human brain using EEG signals. Specific neural circuits for discrimination between touch and nociception emerged from 35 to 37 weeks GA in the human brain.

Although, biomarkers, cortical indicators and cognitive mapping provide novel and objective means to exploring the infant's response to pain, decoding their complex and variable patterns and comparing them to behavioural pain indicators and composite measures has not been sufficiently explored. Carefully designed measurement studies comparing cognitive indicators with established

measures in appropriate designs are needed. For example, for randomized controlled trials, a measure of methodological quality such as the CONsolidated Standards of Reporting Trials (CONSORT, 2010) statement that includes whether a validated measure, appropriate randomization, and follow-up of outcomes are used should be incorporated as a guideline for reporting the methodological quality of published studies and responsible external generalization of the results.

Current clinical practice guidelines, policies, and procedures

An important aspect of improving clinical outcomes is to ensure that the most recent evidence is effectively translated into clinical practice. This translation needs to be supported by inclusion of recommendations for pain assessment within wider pain management guidelines. To date, several published guidelines from professional organizations have included recommendations on pain assessment and management (see Table 35.4). The majority do not focus on children, although there are a few that are specific to children

Table 35.3 Cognitive indicators of neonatal/infant pain

Indicator	Reference	Study design/methods	Main results
Magnetic resonance imaging (MRI)	Brummelte et al., 2012	Prospective cohort study (n = 86 preterm infants 24–32 weeks GA) to examine relationship between procedural pain and early brain development	Greater numbers of painful procedures were associated with reduced white matter (p = 0.028) and reduced subcortical grey matter (p = 0.004) after adjusting for multiple clinical factors
Electro-encephalography (EEG)	Fabrizi et al., 2011	Prospective cohort study (N = 18 infants 37–45 weeks GA; and N = 41 infants 28–45 weeks GA (born at 24–41 weeks GA)) comparing touch or heel lance	Occurrence in the preterm infants was significantly less than in the full-term infants (p = 0.01tactile potential; p = 0.01 nociceptive-specific potential). Latencies of tactile and nociceptive-specific potentials were shorter in full-term infants than in premature infants. Neuronal bursts were significantly greater in preterm infants than term infants whether evoked by touch (p = 0.048) or noxious lance (p <0.001) Neural circuits for discrimination between touch and nociception emerge from 35–37 weeks GA in the human brain
	Slater et al., 2010	Pilot prospective cohort study to determine whether cortical neurons are specifically activated by noxious stimuli in newborns (N = 10 infants 35–39 weeks PMA) using EEG recording following a routine heel lance	The potential was observed in the central electrodes and characterized by a positivity that occurs at approximately 560 msec post-stimulus The magnitude of the nociceptive-specific potential was not dependent on sleep state, whereas an earlier potential, which was sleep-state dependent, was evoked by both noxious and non-noxious stimulation Researchers report that results provide the first direct evidence of specific noxious-evoked neural activity in the infant brain
Electro-myography (EMG)	Schasfoort et al., 2008	Prospective cohort study to determine the feasibility of long-term, objective, and continuous measurement of peripheral motor parameters to discriminate between pain and no pain in hospitalized pre-verbal infants during (a) acute painful procedure: n = 9 (5–175 days of age): and (b) postoperative pain: n = 14 infants (age range 45–400 days for age) measured for prolonged periods (mean 7 h) using acceleration sensors on one arm and both legs, and two muscle activity parameters derived from EMG sensors	*Acute painful procedure:* the accelerometry-based parameters legs activity and overall extremity activity (i.e. mean of arm and legs) was significantly higher during heel lance than before or after lance (p ≤0.001) *Post-operative pain:* relationships existed between accelerometry-based overall extremity activity and COMFORT scale (r = 0.76, p <0.001), and between EMG-based wrist flexor activity and COMFORT (r = 0.55, p <0.001, for a subgroup of 7 infants) Researchers conclude that long-term, objective, and continuous measurement of peripheral motor parameters is feasible, has high potential, and is promising to assess pain in preverbal hospitalized infants
Near-infrared spectroscopy (NIRS)	Bartocci et al., 2006	Prospective cohort study to study patterns of supraspinal pain processing in neonates (N = 40 preterm neonates at 28–36 weeks GA) and at 25–42 h following standardized tactile (skin disinfection) and painful (venepuncture) stimuli. Changes were monitored by NIRS over both somatosensory cortices in 29 newborns, and over the contralateral somatosensory and occipital areas in 11 newborns. HR and peripheral O$_2$ saturation (SaO$_2$) were recorded simultaneously with NIRS parameters: oxygenated (HbO$_2$), deoxygenated, and total haemoglobin were also measured	Tactile stimulation produced no changes in HR or SaO$_2$ HR increased in the first 20 sec (p < 0.001), while SaO$_2$ decreased during the 40 sec after venepuncture (p <0.0001). Following tactile or painful stimulation, [HbO$_2$] increased bilaterally (p <0.0001) Pain-induced [HbO$_2$] increases in the contralateral somatosensory cortex (p <0.05) were not mirrored in the occipital cortex (p >0.1) Pain-related [HbO$_2$] increases were significantly more pronounced in male neonates, inversely correlated with GA and directly correlated with PNA. Researchers concluded that painful and tactile stimuli elicit specific haemodynamic responses in the somatosensory cortex, implying conscious sensory perception in preterm neonates
	Slater et al., 2006	Prospective cohort study to determine whether premature infants process pain at a cortical level (N = 18 infants 25 and 45 weeks PMA) assessed by changes in cerebral oxygenation over the somatosensory cortex in response to noxious stimulation using real-time NIRS	Noxious stimulation produced a clear cortical response, measured as an increase in total haemoglobin concentration [HbT] in the contralateral somatosensory cortex, from 25 weeks. Cortical responses were significantly greater in awake versus sleeping infants. In awake infants, the response in the contralateral somatosensory cortex increased with age while latency decreased with age. Researchers concluded that noxious information is transmitted to the preterm infant cortex from 25 weeks, highlighting the potential for both higher-level pain processing and pain-induced plasticity in the human brain

(Continued)

Table 35.4 Pain assessment guidelines and recommendations for neonates and infants

Guideline source/association	Content	Pain assessment measures recommended	Feasibility/clinical utility
Assessment and management of acute pain in the newborn—Web continuing education resource (Association of Women's Health, Obstetric and Neonatal Nurses (AWHONN), Canada, 2002)	Acute pain and consequences Validity and reliability of pain assessment measures Selection of newborn pain assessment tools Practice exercises	PIPP CRIES NIPS FLACC CDSVN RIPS POPS BPS EDIN NFCS PAIN	27 pages No specific recommendations for timing or documentation of pain assessment
Assessment of acute pain in children: development of evidence-based guidelines United Kingdom (Stapelkamp et al., 2011)	Appraisal of tools for (a) children with or without cognitive impairment and (b) neonates, infants and verbal children, and non-verbal children with cognitive impairment Practice recommendations Practice points	NFCS NNICUPAT NIPS OPS PAT PIPP	12 pages Recommendation of timing and documentation: (a) assess, record and re-evaluate pain at regular intervals; (b) frequency of assessment determined according to the individual needs of the child and setting; (c) language, ethnicity and cultural factors may influence expression and assessment of pain Clear tables outlining recommendations. Effective use of symbols to illustrate features of pain assessment measures
Best Practice Clinical Guideline Assessment and Management of Neonatal Pain (Australian and New Zealand Neonatal Network, 2007)	Key recommendations listed Audit tool Algorithms for procedural pain and pain assessment	No specific pain measures recommended.	14 pages Overall strategies for timing and frequency of assessment: (a) at beginning of the shift, (b) prior to/end of a painful procedure, (c) at least once/shift (every 4–6 h) and when analgesia is being used, and (d) during weaning and 48 h following weaning Specific actions based on assessment score
Consensus Statement for the Prevention and Management of Pain in the Newborn (Anand and the International Evidence-Based Group for Neonatal Pain, 2001)	General principles for the prevention and management of pain in newborns Painful procedures in the NICU Methods for pain assessment pain in newborns Recommended analgesic doses for neonates, adverse effects	PIPP NFCS NIPS CRIES	8 pages Recommended timing: concomitantly with the vital signs, undertaken and documented every 4–6 h or as indicated by the pain scores or clinical condition of the neonate Other recommendations: (a) pain assessment instruments should be sensitive and specific for infants of different GA and/or pain types; (b) Pain assessment should be comprehensive and multidimensional, including contextual, behavioural, and physiological indicators
Evidenced-based clinical practice guideline for management of newborn pain Australia (Spence et al., 2010)	Key recommendations Audit tool Algorithms for procedural pain and pain assessment	General recommendation for using validated measures but no specific measures recommended.	Recommended timing: (a) baseline pain assessment on admission and with a substantial change in health status; (b) during routine care, at least once per shift or when infant seems uncomfortable Table with guide for use of an assessment tool
Guideline statement: management of procedure-related pain in neonates Australia (Paediatrics & Child Health Division, The Royal Australasian College of Physicians, 2006)	Pain and its consequences, responses of infants to pain, general principles for the prevention and management of pain in neonates Summary of current evidence in prevention and management of pain with specific procedures (e.g. venepuncture, ROP exam)	PIPP NFCS NIPS CRIES	9 pages No specific recommendations for timing or documentation of pain assessment More emphasis with management of pain

(Continued)

Table 35.4 (*Continued*)

Guideline source/association	Content	Pain assessment measures recommended	Feasibility/clinical utility
Nursing Best Practice Guideline—Assessment & Management of Pain Canada (Registered Nurses Association of Ontario 2002; revised 2007)	Guideline development Process and responsibilities Interpretation of evidence Definition of terms Practice, education, organization and policy Recommendations Evaluation and monitoring	PIPP NIPS	174 pages Guideline for all populations across the lifespan Recommended timing: (a) at least once a day, (b) on a regular basis according to the type and intensity of pain and the treatment plan. Recommended documentation: (a) on a standardized form specific to the population and setting; (b) include initial, comprehensive and re-assessment; (c) document regularly and routinely on forms that are accessible to all clinicians; (d) teach individuals and families (as proxy recorders) to document pain assessment on the appropriate tools
Pain Assessment in the Nonverbal Patient: Position Statement with Clinical Practice Recommendations United States (American Society for Pain Management Nursing, 2006)	Discusses pain assessment in all non-verbal patients Background information on pain assessment in neonates	CHEOPS CHIPPS COMFORT CRIES DSVNI PIPP RIPS UWCH	9 pages Recommended timing and documentation; (a) Pain should be routinely monitored, assessed, reassessed, and documented clearly to facilitate treatment and communication; (b) after intervention and regularly over time, and (c) documented in a readily visible and consistent manner that is accessible to all health care providers
Prevention and Management of Pain in the Neonate: An Update (American Academy of Pediatrics, Committee on Fetus and Newborn and Section on Surgery, Section on Anesthesiology and Pain Medicine, Canadian Paediatric Society and Fetus and Newborn Committee, 2006)	Pain and stress in the neonate Pain assessment Recommendations	CRIES COMFORT PIPP NIPS N-PASS NFCS PAT SUN EDIN BPSN	Specific to neonates Focused and easy to read Age appropriateness of measures indicated Recommended timing: neonates should be assessed for pain routinely and before and after procedures No specific recommendations for documentation of pain assessment

and even fewer for neonates and infants. The major content areas covered in these guidelines include background material on pain and its consequences, summaries of current evidence in prevention and management of pain with specific procedures (e.g. heel lance) and recommendations for implementation. From a systematic review of pain assessment guidelines using Medical Subject Headings (MeSH) terms *Pain Measurement*, *Pain Management*, exp *Pain/cl, di [Classification, Diagnosis]*, *Guideline or practice guideline*, *Intensive Care Units*, *Neonatal* and limited to newborn, English language from 1946 to present, only seven guidelines included specific recommendations of neonatal or infant pain assessment measures; the PIPP and NFCS were most commonly recommended. Six guidelines recommended specified timing and frequency of pain assessment. The recommendations were generally consistent across timing of assessments and documentation every 4 to 6 h or as indicated by the pain scores or clinical condition of the neonate. Overall, although great efforts have been made by researchers to consolidate evidence into practice guidelines, several gaps remain. Also, although some guidelines are clear with user-friendly tables and flow diagrams, many require more concrete recommendations.

For example, more specific directives (e.g. care paths or care plans) that include clear, succinct statements on pain assessment with visual decision-making aids and specific recommendation for timing, documentation of assessment measures utilized and scores, and action plans to follow with assessment results targeted specifically for the neonatal and infant populations are needed.

Challenges and controversies associated with neonatal and infant pain assessment

There has been a long history of neglect of pain during infancy. Although many improvements have been achieved in the wake of ever-increasing knowledge expansion in the past few decades, future advancement will depend on adequately addressing and resolving current theoretical, clinical, research, and KT challenges and controversies.

Theoretical challenges and controversies

Science, as a social institution, has not stimulated adequate support for a comprehensive understanding of the interpersonal and social aspects of pain within the infant. The current focus has been more on the biology of pain with diminished importance placed on the psychological aspects (Craig, 2009). Clearly defining pain in infants in accurate terms that are broadly applicable to the neonatal and infant population is essential. Without this definition, terms such as nociception, pain, stress, distress, as well as analgesia, calming, and comfort are often used interchangeably or incorrectly and may result in inadequate measurement and erroneous conclusions regarding pain management.

The *absence of a behavioural pain response* to stimulation which would normally be painful (e.g. heel lance) is particularly in need of exploration in relation to pain in infants. Absence of pain response as measured by behavioural or a composite of behavioural and physiological indicators, has been reported to occur in approximately 20% of infants (Johnston et al 1999). This may be because: (1) the response is so weak that it escapes observer detection, (2) the infant may be incapable of mounting any response due to extenuating circumstances (e.g. severity of illness, extreme prematurity), or (3) the infant does not perceive the stimulus as painful. Regardless of the reason, this is a serious situation because pain behaviour in response to tissue damage is such a universal response in other populations and makes evolutional sense. It is also difficult to dispute the importance of behavioural indicators in particular given their consistency across populations, situations, and contexts. Furthermore, it places infants in a vulnerable situation where they are completely dependent on the judgement of caregivers to make accurate conclusions surrounding their care and pain management.

Similarly, *absence of a physiological (e.g. heart rate (HR)) or cortical response (e.g. EEG)* to nociceptive stimulation also does not necessarily indicate absence of pain (or analgesia, if an intervention is being evaluated). It may indicate that an inappropriate response was measured or that the sensitivity of the measure or the analyses was questionable. These issues illustrate the need for sensitive and valid indicators of pain and clarity surrounding the terms 'pain', 'nociception', and 'analgesia' in infants amongst clinicians and researchers in relation to pain assessment. Future investigation needs to focus on whether a relationship exists between behavioural observational indicators of pain (e.g. facial action) and biomarkers or cortical indicators associated with noxious stimulation, and under what conditions.

Progress has been primarily made in the conceptualization and assessment of acute pain in neonates and infants. Further consideration of unique developmental and communication processes requires further attention. Key unanswered questions relate to (1) how repeated pain at certain stages of the infant's development influences pain expression and (2) what are the crucial elements from the infant's interaction with the environment and caregivers that influence pain expression and assessment by caregivers?

Progress towards the optimal management of pain during infancy also demands an exploration of pain beyond the acute-procedural (e.g. immunization pain), acute-repetitive (e.g. multiple heel lances), or acute-prolonged (e.g. postoperative pain) domains. Examination of the existence of a pathological pain state, whereby pain continues beyond expectation or persists for a significant portion of the infant's existence is crucial. Knowing that the human nervous system is extremely malleable in response to noxious environmental influences during infancy suggests that steps taken to manage pain need to be varied and tailored to the individual infant's needs.

Clinical challenges and controversies

Clinical challenges in pain assessment relate to the integration of knowledge into practice or KT. From the measurement perspective, difficulty in identifying a criterion ('gold standard') for determining the validity of the phenomenon, lacking the subjective, unique and private nature of the symptom is paramount (Sidani, 2003). Behavioural and physiological variables often correlate inconsistently and poorly with each other and with other indicators (e.g. correlation is often around 0.3). This incongruence and the lack of the patient's self-report, often brings into question the validity of the measure or indicator, creates controversies on the benefits and disadvantages of unidimensional verses multidimensional measurement approaches, and may affect judgement about pain intensity and decision-making about the effectiveness of interventions. The multidimensionality of the pain phenomenon in measurement is often vigorously debated; whereas some lobby for the simplicity of a single indicator of pain, many feel a multidimensional approach is essential for a comprehensive understanding of the experience that informs individualized and effective interventions. Supporters of a more unidimensional approach, fail to articulate how scores on individual indicators or groups of indicators can be viewed to comprehensively provide accurate information to the clinician making decisions at the bedside. Pain intensity is most often the only dimension reported, when occurrence, frequency, duration, impact, meaning, and response are other important information required.

With the development of a broad array of measures for assessing acute pain, selection of the 'best' pain measure becomes a challenge. Developing clearly articulated selection criteria for choosing a measure for clinical and/or research purposes is essential. These criteria could include: (1) validity (measuring accurately the phenomenon of interest; being responsive to changes in the phenomenon), (2) reliability (measuring with the least amount of measurement error so that the score is reliable and reproducible across raters and time), (3) feasibility (ease of scoring, time, cost, clarity of instructions), and (4) clinical utility (ability to use pain scores for a particular infant, in a particular setting, in a meaningful way to make decisions on future pain management strategies).

Despite the plethora of existing pain measures, there is still a paucity of validated measures for the most vulnerable groups of infants who are most critically ill, paralysed, and preterm, at the end of life or with severe neurological impairments. For example, few measures have been validated with the most preterm or extremely low gestational age (ELGA) infants. Because of their immature pain processing, stress-response systems, and development, these infants' responses may be different or at least more subtle and difficult to detect than those of more mature neonates. In addition, non-painful touch and pain responses are often similar. This phenomenon is thought to be due to the wide receptive fields that do not allow for differentiation between these two types of stimuli, thus making it difficult for the care provider to discern whether the infant is experiencing pain or not or whether a targeted intervention is effective. Yet these infants have large numbers of painful events for diagnosis and treatment. Thus, there is an urgent need to develop new measures or validate existing measures for this population.

Routine pain assessment using validated measures is generally purported to be the basis of timely and effective pain management and quality care. These pain practices represent a key component in pain guidelines, policies, and professional standards; yet, pain assessment in infants is not universal or even well integrated into clinical care. Franck and Bruce (2009) suggest that there is insufficient evidence to evaluate the effectiveness of standardized pain assessment in terms of process or clinical outcomes. More research on the efficacy, effectiveness, and cost benefit of standardized pain assessment in relation to clinical and process outcomes needs to be considered as existing research on the use of standardized pain assessment tools has limited evidence for improved process or patient outcomes. Furthermore, a misalignment may exist between the necessity of engaging care providers in accurate assessment of pain in the non-verbal individual and their ability and motivation to do so: 'Poor compliance with pain assessment guidelines may not simply be an issue of the "research-to-practice gap", but it may indicate unspoken resistance to use of methods that are overly simplistic, burdensome to patients, often inaccurate and perhaps even disrespectful of clinical expertise and experience' (Franck and Bruce, 2009, p. 19).

Research and KT challenges and controversies

Several areas for future research have been indicated to improve and expand pain assessment in neonates and infants. Unanswered questions continue to be posed on the most optimal measurement approach as well as the feasibility and clinical utility of existing measures and indicators. Without seeing clinical benefit of pain assessment for the infants, there is little hope for engaging clinicians in this most important aspect of quality patient care. There is clear debate on the value and limitations of unidimensional and multidimensional approaches to measurement and potential ways to resolve these issues. Pain is well entrenched within the biomedical model of providing health care and future research needs to explore the influence of the context of pain assessment in relation to individual (e.g. their capacity and sensitivity to detect pain in others) and system (e.g. culture of unit, priority of pain management, leadership, timeliness, busyness, expectations) factors that may influence assessing and management of pain. Strategies to facilitate the translation of what we 'know' into what we 'do' for infants and their families in relation to assessment and management of pain is also lacking. KT strategies that include reminders, education and educational outreach, and audit and feedback need to be better incorporated into changing behaviours or health care professionals to enable pain practice changes and ultimately clinical outcomes.

Summary

Pain assessment in neonates and infants is complex and challenging. Although a broad variety of pain measures have been developed and validated, many fall short of meeting the needs of this population; especially those who are most vulnerable, preterm, ill, or cognitively or developmentally challenged. Lack of a gold standard continues to plague pain assessment in infants; yet clinically there is a need to use the best measures available to attempt optimal pain management. Biomarkers and cortical indicators are currently being investigated to expand our understanding of pain and its effects in infants. The need to move beyond acute procedural pain and concentrate on accurately assessing pain that is prolonged, persistent, or palliative is crucial. Integrating the science of measurement with clinical excellence remains a challenge for clinicians and researchers alike.

Case example

Baby C was born at 27 weeks, is now 15 days old and presented with necrotizing enterocolitis (NEC) and bowel perforation. Her condition is unstable with poor perfusion. She is intubated, ventilated, and is being stabilized for the operation room (OR). A peripheral arterial line insertion was attempted but unsuccessful. She is lethargic with minimal spontaneous movement. The vital signs are: heart rate (HR) 179, respiratory rate (RR) 60, blood pressure (BP) 50/32 (25), oxygen saturation 92, ventilation rate 40/min, pressures 18/7 O_2 55%O_2. The nurse suspects the baby is in pain, because when she checks the abdominal girth she notices that the baby is wincing. She does not have time to complete a formal assessment using a validated pain measure.

The surgery was completed. Upon return from the OR, the baby was not reversed from anaesthetic and displayed minimal movement. The vital signs were HR 180, BP 56/26 (30), O_2 sat 95 in 70% O_2. The baby's colour is pale. The PIPP score is 9. A morphine infusion of 10 mcg/kg/min is started. The vital signs 1 h later are: HR 165, BP 60/32 (40), O_2 sat 92 in 40% O_2.

During rounds the next day, pain assessment of the baby was reviewed with the following discussion:

1. A pain assessment score should be completed on admission as per hospital pain guidelines. Clinicians need to think about pain as the fifth vital sign. Although the nurse was extremely busy, it was important to complete a pain score and inform the doctor that she suspected the baby was in pain with a validated pain score.

2. A morphine infusion could have been started prior to the OR to reduce the baby's pain.

3. Postoperative guidelines were reviewed and a plan for frequent monitoring of pain was posted at the bedside as per the guidelines.

References

Als, H. (1982). Towards a synactive theory of development: promise for the assessment and support of infant individuality. *Infant Ment Health J*, 3, 229–243.

Als, H., Lester, B. M., Tronick, E. C., and Brazelton, T. B. (1982). Manual for the assessment of preterm infants' behavior (APIB). Appendix to Als, H., Lester, B. M., Tronick, E. C., and Brazelton, T. B. Towards a research instrument for the assessment of preterm infants' behavior. In H. E. Fitzgerald, B. M. Lester, and M. W. Yogman (eds) *Theory and research in behavioral pediatrics, Vol 1*, pp. 65–132. New York: Plenum Publishers.

Ambuel, B., Hamlett, K. W., Marx, C. M., and Blumer, J. L. (1992). Assessing distress in pediatric intensive care environments: the COMFORT scale. *J Pediatr Psychol*, 17(1), 95–109.

American Academy of Pediatrics Committee on Fetus and Newborn, American Academy of Pediatrics Section on Surgery, Canadian Paediatric Society Fetus and Newborn Committee, Batton, D. G., Barrington, K. J., and Wallman, C. (2006). Prevention and management of pain in the neonate: an update. [Erratum appears in *Pediatrics*, 2007; 119(2), 425]. *Pediatrics*, 118(5), 2231–2241.

American Academy of Pediatrics. Committee on Psychosocial Aspects of Child and Family Health. Task Force on Pain in Infants, Children and Adolescents. (2001). The assessment and management of acute pain in infants, children, and adolescents. *Pediatrics*, 108(3), 793–797.

Anand, K. J. and International Evidence-Based Group for Neonatal Pain. (2001). Consensus statement for the prevention and management of pain in the newborn. *Arch Pediatr Adolesc Med*, 155(2), 173–180.

Association of Women's Health, Obstetric and Neonatal Nurses (AWHONN). (2002). Assessment and management of acute pain in the newborn— Web continuing education resource. Available at: <http://motherbaby. weebly.com/uploads/4/9/7/6/4976511/neonatal_pain.pdf>.

Australian and New Zealand Neonatal Network (ANZNN). (2007). *Best practice clinical guideline assessment and management of neonatal pain.* Sydney: ANZNN.

Barrier, G., Attia, J., Mayer, M. N., Amiel-Tison, C., and Shnider, S. M. (1989). Measurement of post-operative pain and narcotic administration in infants using a new clinical scoring system. *Intens Care Med*, 15(Suppl 1), S37–39.

Bartocci, M., Bergqvist, L. L., Lagercrantz, H., and Anand, K. J. (2006). Pain activates cortical areas in the preterm newborn brain. *Pain*, 122(1–2), 109–117.

Bellieni, C., Maffei, M., Ancora, G., Cordelli, D., Mastrocola, M., Faldella, G., et al. (2007). Is the ABC pain scale reliable for premature babies? *Acta Paediatr*, 96(7), 1008–1010.

Bellieni, C. V., Bagnoli, F., Sisto, R., Neri, L., Cordelli, D., and Buonocore, G. (2005). Development and validation of the ABC pain scale for healthy full-term babies. *Acta Paediatr*, 94(10), 1432–1436.

Blauer, T. and Gerstmann, D. (1998). A simultaneous comparison of three neonatal pain scales during common NICU procedures. *Clin J Pain*, 14(1), 39–47.

Brummelte, S., Grunau, R. E., Chau, V., Poskitt, K. J., Brant, R., Vinall, J., et al. (2012). Procedural pain and brain development in premature newborns. *Ann Neurol*, 71, 385–396.

Buchholz, M., Karl, H. W., Pomietto, M., and Lynn, A. (1998). Pain scores in infants: a modified infant pain scale versus visual analogue. *J Pain Symptom Manage*, 15(2), 117–124.

Buttner, W. and Finke, W. (2000). Analysis of behavioural and physiological parameters for the assessment of postoperative analgesic demand in newborns, infants and young children: a comprehensive report on seven consecutive studies. *Paediatr Anaesth*, 10(3), 303–318.

Carbajal, R., Lenclen, R., Jugie, M., Paupe, A., Barton, B. A., and Anand, K. J. S. (2005). Morphine does not provide adequate analgesia for acute procedural pain among preterm neonates. *Pediatrics*, 115(6), 1494–1500.

Carbajal, R., Paupe, A., Hoenn, E., Lenclen, R., and Olivier-Martin, M. (1997). [APN: evaluation behavioral scale of acute pain in newborn infants]. *Arch Pediatrie*, 4(7), 623–628.

Cignacco, E., Denhaerynck, K., Nelle, M., Buhrer, C., and Engberg, S. (2009). Variability in pain response to a non-pharmacological intervention across repeated routine pain exposure in preterm infants: a feasibility study. *Acta Paediatr*, 98(5), 842–846.

Cignacco, E., Mueller, R., Hamers, J. P., and Gessler, P. (2004). Pain assessment in the neonate using the Bernese Pain Scale for Neonates. *Early Hum Dev*, 78(2), 125–131.

CONSORT. (2012, 31 January). *Transparent reporting of trials* [Online]. Available at: <http://www.consort-statement.org/consort-statement/overview0/>.

Craig, K. D. (2009). The social communication model of pain. *Can Psychol*, 50(1), 22–32.

Debillon, T., Zupan, V., Ravault, N., Magny, J. F., and Dehan, M. (2001). Development and initial validation of the EDIN scale, a new tool for assessing prolonged pain in preterm infants. *Arch Dis Child Fetal Neonatal Ed*, 85(1), F36–41.

Fabrizi, L., Slater, R., Worley, A., Meek, J., Boyd, S., Olhede, S., et al. (2011). A shift in sensory processing that enables the developing human brain to discriminate touch from pain. *Curr Biol*, 21(18), 1552–1558.

Faye, P. M., De Jonckheere, J., Logier, R., Kuissi, E., Jeanne, M., Rakza, T., et al. (2010). Newborn infant pain assessment using heart rate variability analysis. *Clin J Pain*, 26(9), 777–782.

Franck, L. S., and Bruce, E. (2009). Putting pain assessment into practice: why is it so painful? *Pain Res Manag*, 14(1), 13–20.

Franck, L. S., Ridout, D., Howard, R., Peters, J., and Honour, J. W. (2011). A comparison of pain measures in newborn infants after cardiac surgery. *Pain*, 152(8), 1758–1765.

Gibbins, S., Stevens, B., Beyene, J., Chan, P. C., Bagg, M., and Asztalos, E. (2008a). Pain behaviours in extremely low gestational age infants. *Early Hum Dev*, 84(7), 451–458.

Gibbins, S., Stevens, B., McGrath, P., Dupuis, A., Yamada, J., Beyene, J., et al. (2008b). Changes in physiological and behavioural pain indicators over time in preterm and term infants at risk for neurologic impairment. *Early Hum Dev*, 84(11), 731–738.

Grunau, R. E., and Craig, K. D. (1987). Pain expression in neonates: facial action and cry. *Pain*, 28(3), 395–410.

Grunau, R. E., Tu, M. T., Whitfield, M. F., Oberlander, T. F., Weinberg, J., Yu, W., et al. (2010). Cortisol, behavior, and heart rate reactivity to immunization pain at 4 months corrected age in infants born very preterm. *Clin J Pain*, 26(8), 698–704.

Guinsburg, R., Kopelman, B.I., Anand, K.J., De Almeida, M.F., Peres Cde, A. and Miyoshi, M.H. (1998). Physiological, hormonal, and behavioral responses to a single fentanyl dose in intubated and ventilated preterm neonates. *J Pediatr*, 132(6), 954–959.

Hartwig, S., Roth, B., and Theisohn, M. (1991). Clinical experience with continuous intravenous sedation using midazolam and fentanyl in the pediatric intensive care unit. *Eur J Pediatr*, 150, 784–788.

Herr, K., Coyne, P. J., Key, T., Manworren, R., McCaffery, M., Merkel, S., et al. (2006). Pain assessment in the nonverbal patient: position statement with clinical practice recommendations. *Pain Manage Nurs*, 7(2), 44–52.

Hodgkinson, K., Bear, M., Thorn, J., and Van Blaricum, S. (1994). Measuring pain in neonates: evaluating an instrument and developing a common language. *Aust J Adv Nurs*, 12(1), 17–22.

Holsti, L. and Grunau, R. E. (2010). Considerations for using sucrose to reduce procedural pain in preterm infants. *Pediatrics*, 125(5), 1042–1047.

Holsti, L. and Grunau, R. E. (2007a). Initial validation of the Behavioral Indicators of Infant Pain (BIIP). *Pain*, 132(3), 264–272.

Holsti, L., Weinberg, J., Whitfield, M. F., and Grunau, R. E. (2007b). Relationships between adrenocorticotropic hormone and cortisol are altered during clustered nursing care in preterm infants born at extremely low gestational age. *Early Hum Dev*, 83(5), 341–348.

Horgan, M. and Choonara, I. (1996). Measuring pain in neonates: an objective score. *Paediatr Nurs*, 8(10), 24–27.

Horgan, M. F., Glenn, S., and Choonara, I. (2002). Further development of the Liverpool Infant Distress Scale. *J Child Health Care*, 6(2), 96–106.

Hudson-Barr, D., Capper-Michel, B., Lambert, S., Palermo, T. M., Morbeto, K., and Lombardo, S. (2002). Validation of the Pain Assessment in Neonates (PAIN) scale with the Neonatal Infant Pain Scale (NIPS). *Neonatal Netw*, 21(6), 15–21.

Hummel, P., Lawlor-Klean, P., and Weiss, M. G. (2010). Validity and reliability of the N-PASS assessment tool with acute pain. *J Perinatol*, 30(7), 474–478.

Hummel, P., Puchalski, M., Creech, S. D., and Weiss, M. G. (2003). N-PASS: neonatal pain agitation and sedation scale: reliability and validity. Poster presented at the Pediatric Academic Societies 2003 Annual Meeting, 6 May 2003, Seattle, WA.

Hummel, P., Puchalski, M., Creech, S. D., and Weiss, M. G. (2008). Clinical reliability and validity of the N-PASS: neonatal pain, agitation and sedation scale with prolonged pain. *J Perinatol*, 28(1), 55–60.

Hunseler, C., Merkt, V., Gerloff, M., Eifinger, F., Kribs, A., and Roth, B. (2011). Assessing pain in ventilated newborns and infants: Validation of the Hartwig score. *Eur J Pediatri*, 170(7), 837–843.

International Association for the Study of Pain. (2003). *IASP Task Force on Taxonomy: ASP pain terminology*. Available at: <http://www.iasp-pain.org/terms-p.html>.

Johnston, C. C., Stevens, B. J., Franck, L. S., Jack, A., Stremler, R., and Platt, R. (1999). Factors explaining lack of response to heel stick in preterm newborns. *J Obstet Gynecol Neonatal Nurs*, 28(6), 587–594.

Jonsdottir, R. B., and Kristjansdottir, G. (2005). The sensitivity of the premature infant pain profile-PIPP to measure pain in hospitalized neonates. *J Eval Clin Pract*, 11, 598–605.

Krechel, S. W., and Bildner, J. (1995). CRIES: a new neonatal postoperative pain measurement score. Initial testing of validity and reliability. *Paediatr Anaesth*, 5(1), 53–61.

Lawrence, J., Alcock, D., McGrath, P., Kay, J., MacMurray, S.B., and Dulberg, C. (1993). The development of a tool to assess neonatal pain. *Neonatal Netw*, 12(6), 59–66.

Lilley, C. M., Craig, K. D., and Grunau, R. E. (1997). The expression of pain in infants and toddlers: developmental changes in facial action. *Pain*, 72, 161–170.

Manworren, R. C., and Hynan, L. S. (2003). Clinical validation of FLACC: preverbal patient pain scale. *Pediatric Nurs*, 29(2), 140–146.

Marceau, J. (2003). Pilot study of a pain assessment tool in the Neonatal Intensive Care Unit. *J Paediatr Child Health*, 39(8), 598–601.

McDowell, I. (2006). *Measuring health: a guide to rating scales and questionnaires* (3rd edn). New York: Oxford University Press.

Merkel, S. I., Voepel-Lewis, T., Shayevitz, J. R., and Malviya, S. (1997). The FLACC: a behavioral scale for scoring postoperative pain in young children. *Pediatr Nurs*, 23(3), 293–297.

Milesi, C., Cambonie, G., Jacquot, A., Barbotte, E., Mesnage, R., Masson, F., *et al.* (2010). Validation of a neonatal pain scale adapted to the new practices in caring for preterm newborns. *Arch Dis Child Fetal Neonatal Ed*, 95(4), F263–6.

Moreaux, T. (2010). [Evendol, a pain assessment scale for pediatric emergency departments]. *Soins Pediatrie, Puericulture, Puericulture* (256), 32–34.

Padhye, N. S., Williams, A. L., Khattak, A. Z., and Lasky, R. E. (2009). Heart rate variability in response to pain stimulus in VLBW infants followed longitudinally during NICU stay. *Dev Psychobiol*, 51(8), 638–649.

Paediatrics & Child Health Division, The Royal Australasian College of Physicians. (2006). Guideline statement: management of procedure-related pain in neonates. *J Paediatr Child Health*, 42(Suppl 1), S31–39.

Peters, J. W., Koot, H. M., Grunau, R. E., De Boer, J., Van Druenen, M. J., Tibboel, D., *et al.* (2003). Neonatal Facial Coding System for assessing postoperative pain in infants: item reduction is valid and feasible. *Clin J Pain*, 19(6), 353–363.

Registered Nurses Association of Ontario (RNAO). (2007). Assessment and management of pain: supplement. Available at: <http://www.rnao.org/Storage/29/2351_BPG_Pain_and_Supp.pdf>.

Ramelet, A., Rees, N., McDonald, S., Bulsara, M., and Abu-Saad, H. H. (2007a). Development and preliminary psychometric testing of the Multidimensional Assessment of Pain Scale: MAPS. *Paediatr Anaesth*, 17(4), 333–340.

Ramelet, A. S., Rees, N. W., McDonald, S., Bulsara, M. K., and Huijer Abu-Saad, H. (2007b). Clinical validation of the Multidimensional Assessment of Pain Scale. *Paediatr Anaesth*, 17(12), 1156–1165.

Schade, J. G., Joyce, B. A., Gerkensmeyer, J., and Keck, J. F. (1996). Comparison of three preverbal scales for postoperative pain assessment in a diverse pediatric sample. *J Pain Symptom Manage*, 12(6), 348–359.

Schaffer, L., Muller-Vizentini, D., Burkhardt, T., Rauh, M., Ehlert, U., and Beinder, E. (2009). Blunted stress response in small for gestational age neonates. *Pediatr Res*, 65(2), 231–235.

Schasfoort, F. C., Formanoy, M. A., Bussmann, J. B., Peters, J. W., Tibboel, D., and Stam, H. J. (2008). Objective and continuous measurement of peripheral motor indicators of pain in hospitalized infants: a feasibility study. *Pain*, 137(2), 323–331.

Schiller, C.-J. (1999). Clinical utility of two neonatal pain assessment measures. (Unpublished Master of Science thesis). University of Toronto Graduate Department of Nursing Science, ON.

Sidani, S. (2003). Symptom management. In D. Doran, (ed.) *Nursing-sensitive outcomes state of the science*, pp. 115–177. Sudbury, MA: Jones and Bartlett Publishers.

Slater, R., Cantarella, A., Gallella, S., Worley, A., Boyd, S., Meek, J., *et al.* (2006). Cortical pain responses in human infants. *J Neurosci*, 26(14), 3662–3666.

Slater, R., Worley, A., Fabrizi, L., Roberts, S., Meek, J., Boyd, S., *et al.* (2010). Evoked potentials generated by noxious stimulation in the human infant brain. *Eur J Pain*, 14(3), 321–326.

Spence, K., Gillies, D., Harrison, D., Johnston, L., and Nagy, S. (2005). A reliable pain assessment tool for clinical assessment in the neonatal intensive care unit. *J Obstet Gynecol Neonatal Nurs*, 34(1), 80–86.

Spence, K., Henderson-Smart, D., New, K., Evans, C., Whitelaw, J., Woolnough, R., *et al.* (2010). Evidenced-based clinical practice guideline for management of newborn pain. *J Paediatr Child Health*, 46(4), 184–192.

Stapelkamp, C., Carter, B., Gordon, J., and Watts, C. (2011). Assessment of acute pain in children: development of evidence-based guidelines. *Int J Evid Based Healthcare*, 9(1), 39–50.

Stevens, B., Franck, L., Gibbins, S., McGrath, P. J., Dupuis, A., Yamada, J., *et al.* (2007). Determining the structure of acute pain responses in vulnerable neonates. *Can J Nurs Res*, 39(2), 32–47.

Stevens, B., Johnston, C., Petryshen, P., and Taddio, A. (1996). Premature Infant Pain Profile: development and initial validation. *Clin J Pain*, 12(1), 13–22.

Sullivan, M. J. L. (2008. Toward a biopsychomotor conceptualization of pain: implications for research and intervention. *Clin J Pain*, 24, 281–290.

Suominen, P., Caffin, C., Linton, S., McKinley, D., Ragg, P., Davie, G., and Eyres, R. (2004). The cardiac analgesic assessment scale (CAAS): a pain assessment tool for intubated and ventilated children after cardiac surgery. *Paediatr Anaesth*, 14(4), 336–343.

Taddio, A., Goldbach, M., Ipp, M., Stevens, B., and Koren, G. (1995). Effect of neonatal circumcision on pain response during vaccination in boys. *Lancet*, 345, 291–2.

Yamada, J., Stevens, B., De Silva, N., Gibbins, S., Beyene, J., Taddio, A., *et al.* (2007). Hair cortisol as a potential biologic marker of chronic stress in hospitalized neonates. *Neonatology*, 92(1), 42–49.

Supplementary online materials

Figure 35.2 Neonatal Facial Coding System.
Reproduced from Grunau, R and Craig, K, Pain expression in neonates: facial action and cry, *PAIN*®, Volume 28, pp. 395–410, Copyright © 1987. This figure has been reproduced with permission of the International Association for the Study of Pain® (IASP). The figure may NOT be reproduced for any other purpose without permission.

Figure 35.3 Behavioural Indicators of Infant Pain (BIIP): preterm and full term.
Reproduced from Holsti, L. and Grunau, R.E, Initial validation of the Behavioral Indicators of Infant Pain (BIIP), *PAIN*®, Volume 132, pp. 264–272, Copyright © 2007.

This figure has been reproduced with permission of the International Association for the Study of Pain® (IASP). The figure may not be reproduced for any other purpose without permission.

Figure 35.4 PIPP-R: the Premature Infant Pain Profile-Revised (PIPP-R).
Reproduced from Bonnie Stevens, Sharyn Gibbins, Janet Yamada, et al, The Premature Infant Pain Profile-Revised (PIPP-R): Initial Validation and Feasibility, *The Clinical Journal of Pain*, Published Ahead-of-Print, Copyright © 2013, with permission from Lippincott Williams & Wilkins, Inc. DOI: 10.1097/AJP.0b013e3182906aed.

CHAPTER 36

Self-report: the primary source in assessment after infancy

Carl L. von Baeyer

Summary

Self-report is the primary source of information for assessment of pain and measurement of its intensity in children age 3 years and older. This chapter provides an overview of the variables addressed in assessment, specific tools used to obtain self-reports, and interpretation of pain scores. Challenges include establishing whether children are able to understand and use self-report scales and interpreting self-reported pain scores when they conflict with clinicians' observation. New developments in self-report assessment are introduced, such as new support for the use of numerical rating scales and development of computer and smartphone self-report tools. Recommendations are provided supporting integration of self-report of pain in pain management.

Statement of aims

Using information in this chapter, clinicians will be able to choose, administer, understand, and interpret appropriate self-report tools to assess and measure pain in children 3 years of age and older.

Introduction

The nature of self-report

A self-report is an oral, written, or non-verbal account or portrayal of a person's own thoughts, feelings, or actions. Self-report is the principal means by which one can learn about someone else's experience. Because pain is primarily an internal experience (Merskey and Bogduk, 1994), self-report, when available, is widely considered to be the primary source for assessment and measurement of pain, taking priority over observation, reports by proxies such as family members, physiological data, and knowledge of the clinical context (Pasero and McCaffery, 2011). However, describing self-report as 'the gold standard' is misleading (Craig, 2009; Craig and Badali, 2004). A gold standard score is a score which, in the presence of conflicting data, must be regarded as the correct one. But there are many circumstances under which self-reports of pain may be distorted or misunderstood, as detailed later in this chapter.

In young children such as normally developing 2-year-olds, self-report may be limited to vocalization and pointing to indicate the presence of pain in parts of their body. Starting around age 3 years, children can learn to quantify the intensity of their pain (small, medium, big) and to describe its location and its temporal and sensory qualities. By early adolescence, the ability to use self-report measures is similar to that of adults.

Complementing this chapter, several other detailed discussions of assessment of paediatric pain by self-report are available (Champion et al., 1998; Cohen et al., 2008; Huguet et al., 2010; Ruskin et al., 2011; Stinson et al., 2006; von Baeyer, 2006, 2009a).

Background

Assessment versus measurement

Measurement is assigning a number to a quantity and is most often done for pain intensity, although other aspects of pain such as its unpleasantness and its temporal features can also be quantified. Assessment is a broader enterprise: collecting and appraising qualitative as well as quantitative information, often from multiple sources, and taking the context into account. Measurement is often part of assessment. Assessment includes appraisal of the developmental, psychosocial, and medical factors that trigger, exacerbate, and relieve the pain.

The purposes of *assessment* include diagnosis of the cause of the pain, selection and evaluation of treatments, goal setting, and allocation of resources such as laboratory investigations. The purposes of *measurement* of pain intensity include quantifying pain before analgesic treatment and evaluating the effects of that treatment, both for individuals and in clinical trials.

Domains of assessment

Describing pain only in terms of its intensity is like describing music only in terms of its loudness: it is a gross oversimplification of the complexity of pain experience (von Baeyer, 2006). That oversimplification is needed to make decisions about pain management and to evaluate their outcome. However, numerous other aspects of pain can be assessed by self-report, as reviewed and systematized by the Initiative on Methods, Measurement and Pain Assessment in Clinical Trials (IMMPACT, <http://www.immpact.org>). This is a multidisciplinary project to improve clinical trials of treatments for pain based on expert consensus and commissioned reviews of literature. The paediatric IMMPACT project (McGrath et al., 2008) identifies domains that would be important to assess not only in clinical trials but in many clinical situations. (The word 'domain' is used here in the sense used in the adult and paediatric IMMPACT reports, that is, meaning the different aspects or dimensions of pain, including intensity, location, sensory qualities, etc. The word is used with a different sense by Lee and Stevens (Chapter 35, this volume).) Self-report is an important source of information on each one. The domains include, among others, those listed in Table 36.1. The functional measures include measurement of interference caused by pain with physical, cognitive, emotional and social functioning (e.g. school participation and performance), as well as coping.

As shown in Table 36.1, a mnemonic for domains of assessment that is widely accepted and used among emergency and other nurses is PQRST. The mnemonic is represented in many slightly differing forms on the Web, adapted here.

Table 36.1 Domains of assessment of pain[a]

Ped-IMMPACT	PQRST mnemonic
♦ Pain intensity	♦ P = Provocation and Palliation. What started the pain? What makes it worse? What makes it better?
♦ Symptoms and adverse events	
♦ Physical functioning	♦ Q = Quality. What are the sensory qualities of the pain (aching, stabbing, pricking, burning, etc.)?
♦ Emotional functioning	
♦ Role functioning	♦ R = Region and Radiation. Where is the pain located? Does it spread?
♦ Sleep	♦ S = Severity. Score the pain intensity using a self-report or observational scale.
	♦ T = Timing and Type of onset. When did it begin? How often does it occur? Is it sudden or gradual? How long does it last?

Other

♦ Past pain experiences: surgery, accident, illness
♦ Family members' pain histories and pain behaviour
♦ Other pains in addition to the presenting problem
♦ For each type of pharmacological, physical, and psychological treatment used in the past: effectiveness, adherence, and adverse effects

[a]Ped-IMMPACT refers to the paediatric project of the Initiative on Methods, Measurement and Pain Assessment in Clinical Trials, <http://www.immpact.org>. Categories listed under 'Other' are particularly relevant to recurrent and chronic pain.

Data on these domains should be recorded in patient charts and flow sheets. A frequent concern, however, is that most flow sheets and electronic medical records allow for only a single number for a pain intensity score (parallel to the boxes for vital signs such as temperature). Thus the domains of assessment might be covered on admission, for example, in an Initial Pain Assessment Tool (<http://www.partnersagainstpain.com/printouts/A7012AF4.pdf>), but might not be followed up systematically in subsequent assessments, although information can be placed in narrative notes.

Age-appropriate measurement of pain intensity

The ability to self-report internal states normally develops starting around age 3 years, with particularly rapid increases in the preschool years (Besenski et al., 2007; Spagrud et al., 2003). This developmental change is illustrated in Figure 36.1, which is based on the assumptions that an age-appropriate self-report tool is used and that children are trained in use of the tool when not in acute distress. The developmental course in this ability is parallel with advances in other language and cognitive skills, and is influenced by experience with pain (von Baeyer et al., 2011).

Age 8 years and older: visual analogue scale; numerical rating scale

The most commonly administered scale, the numerical rating scale (NRS; <http://www.usask.ca/childpain/NRS>), is well supported by recent studies for use in children 8 years and older (Bailey et al., 2010; Miró et al., 2009; von Baeyer et al., 2009). An alternate name for the NRS, when it is administered entirely verbally, is verbal numeric scale (VNS): this name has the advantage of distinguishing the tool from scales administered on paper or electronically. There are no established or validated verbal descriptors for the maximal pain on the NRS or VNS (e.g. most hurt, worst pain, worst possible pain, most pain you could imagine), but these anchor phrases have a marked influence on pain intensity scores (von Baeyer, 2009b). Moreover, intermediate numbers have no fixed meaning across individuals: a 6 out of 10 might mean moderate pain for some people and severe for others. Difficulties often encountered with the VNS include using numbers above the top of the scale and reporting fractional numbers. Reduction of these difficulties has been achieved for adults by showing the patient a visual aid, that is, a printed page showing the numbers from 0 through 10 with verbal anchors at each end (Pasero and McCaffery, 2011) while requesting a verbal response.

The visual analogue scale (VAS) is a well-established tool for obtaining self-report of pain intensity in normally developing children 8 years and older (Stinson et al., 2006), with some studies suggesting that it can be used for younger children in the 5 to 7-year age range. Variants of the VAS have been explored, notably the coloured analogue scale (McGrath et al., 1996) which has been extensively validated and used in research.

Figure 36.1 Faces Pain Scale—Revised (FPS-R). Instructions in about 40 languages are available at <http://www.iasp-pain.org/FPSR>. Reproduced from Hicks et al., The Faces Pain Scale—Revised: toward a common metric in pediatric pain measurement, *PAIN*®, Volume 93, Issue 2, pp. 173–83, Copyright © 2001. This figure has been reproduced with permission of the International Association for the Study of Pain® (IASP). The figure may NOT be reproduced for any other purpose without permission.

For quick use, or for individuals who have difficulty with these scales, simple word descriptors of intensity sometimes suffice: for example, 'a little bit' of hurt, 'medium', 'a lot', 'a real lot' for young children, or 'slight', 'mild', 'moderate', 'strong', and 'intense' for older children (Ruskin et al., 2011, p. 231). No standardized sets of these words have been evaluated and they cannot be recorded on the popular 0 to 10 common metric for pain intensity scales. Similarly, for informal use, the rapid and simple finger span scale is available: pain intensity is indicated by the distance between the tip of the thumb and the tip of the index finger (Merkel 2002) with more space signifying more pain. The finger span scale has the advantages of requiring no equipment, nor speech by the child, though the scale may be psychometrically inferior to faces and visual analogue scales (Goodenough et al., 2005).

As represented in Figure 36.1, some normally-developing individuals over the age of 12, including perhaps 8% to 10% of adults, find that pain intensity scales such as NRS and VAS do not make sense to them, and thus cannot make use of these tools, reflecting the complex and idiosyncratic nature of pain scales (Williams et al., 2000).

Age 3 years and older: faces scales, Pieces of Hurt

The VAS and the NRS are presumed to require the child to have some competence in seriation (putting things in order) and magnitude estimation, as well as counting in the case of the NRS. These skills are not well developed in most children before age 6 or 7. By contrast, faces scales, in principle, require only matching one's own state of distress to one of the pictures, without necessarily having to estimate quantities along a numerical or spatial dimension (Champion et al., 1998). These limited cognitive demands make faces scales more suitable for children of preschool age than the VAS and NRS.

Dozens of faces scales have been created; of these, three have emerged as the predominant and best validated choices (Tomlinson et al., 2010): the Faces Pain Scale–Revised (FPS-R; Figure 36.2; <http://www.iasp-pain.org/FPSR>) (Hicks et al., 2001); the OUCHER (Beyer et al., 1992; <http://www.oucher.org>); and the Wong-Baker FACES Pain Rating Scale (Whaley and Wong 1991; <http://www.wongbakerfaces.org>). Each of these was developed

independently starting in the 1980s. Each has six faces and is scored 0–2–4–6–8–10, using the widely accepted 0 to 10 common metric (von Baeyer and Hicks, 2000). The scales are otherwise quite different from each other. There has been debate over the psychometric properties, utility, and preference among these three faces scales (e.g. Chambers and Craig, 1998). The FPS-R has most often been recommended as the scale to use in research due to its explicit interval scale properties, its neutral rather than smiling lower anchor, its lack of tears at the upper anchor, its validation in several countries, and the availability of instructions in many languages (Tomlinson et al., 2010).

The Pieces of Hurt tool comprises four poker chips, checkers, or similar game pieces (Hester 1979). Children are asked to indicate how many 'pieces of hurt' they have, from 0 to 4 years. Various sets of instructions have been published. The tool was originally referred to as the Poker Chip Tool but this has elicited some resistance from parents who do not want their child exposed to gambling, so the more acceptable phrase 'Pieces of Hurt' is commonly used. Although the research on this tool has been done primarily with 5- and 6-year-olds, it has been recommended for use with children as young as 3 years (Stinson et al., 2006).

Other simplifications of pain intensity scales adapted for preschool-aged children have been proposed but not yet adequately studied. For example, one could ask whether the child has any hurt (using a word the child knows). If the answer is no, the score is 0. If yes, then a modified faces scale comprising three faces—small, medium, and large pain intensity—is administered (von Baeyer et al., 2011, 2013). The faces would be redrawn to suit the preference and comprehension of young children.

Interpretation of self-reported pain intensity scores

In general, comparisons of pain intensity scores across time within an individual are more valid than comparisons of such scores across different children. In other words, the score 8/10 might mean something quite different to one child than to another. However, within individuals, an increase or decrease over time can be interpreted as an index of the efficacy of pain management efforts.

Despite these limitations in interpretation of self-report scores, there have been efforts to create and validate algorithms governing analgesic administration by pain scores, whereby drugs and dosages are selected following rules based on the intensity and duration of pain (e.g. Falanga et al., 2006). Data on effects of such algorithms are mixed.

Children's pain intensity scores do not always make sense to adults. Children sometimes assign high scores to their pain intensity when they are assumed to be in no or little pain (e.g. before a needle or operation); at other times they assign low scores when they are believed to be in severe pain. Caregivers might not understand the numerous possible reasons for these discrepancies.

♦ Young children might not understand the scale, so they often use a variety of irrelevant strategies to answer the caregiver's question (von Baeyer et al., 2009). For example, up to one-third of children aged 3 and 4 use only the bottom and top of pain scales, treating them as dichotomous (pain or no pain) rather than graded scales.

♦ A variety of cognitive skills are required for accurate use of self-report scales, as catalogued by Besenski et al. (2007). These skills

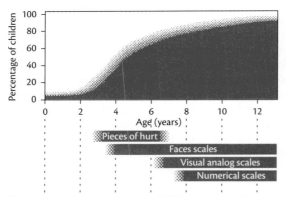

Figure 36.2 Estimated percentage of children who are able to provide valid self-report of pain intensity as a function of age.
Adapted from Lara Spagrud et al., Children's Self-Report of Pain Intensity: The Faces Pain Scale–Revised, *American Journal of Nursing*, Volume 103, Issue 12, pp. 62–64, Copyright © 2003 C. L. von Baeyer, with permission of the author. This figure has been reproduced with permission of the International Association for the Study of Pain® (IASP). The figure may not be reproduced for any other purpose without permission.

develop gradually, with a majority of children but not all acquiring the necessary skills by age 7 or 8.

♦ Children sometimes locate their pain within a body part, not in themselves, thus in a sense separating themselves from the pain and producing lower than expected pain ratings (Wennstrom and Bergh, 2008).

♦ Adults have experience with a variety of mental models (Halford, 1993) for rating quantities. They have encountered volume controls to adjust loudness; thermometers, weight scales, and rulers; and star systems for rating quality of hotels or movies. Young children have far less experience with such mental models, though they have encountered staircases (low to high steps), toys that can be placed in order from small to large, and pictures of small and larger numbers of objects. Such analogies can be useful in measurement of pain intensity, as for example in the Pieces of Hurt tool.

♦ Children probably have a very different understanding of the top scale anchor (a hypothetical maximal level of pain) than adults, as children have less direct and vicarious experience of severe pain. Moreover, young children might not be able simultaneously to think of their own pain and a hypothetical maximal pain for comparison of the two, a characteristic termed 'centration' in Piaget's accounts of cognitive development (Gelman and Baillargeon, 2003).

♦ Children might be inclined to deny or minimize their pain because they believe, accurately or not, that something bad will happen as a result of giving a high score, e.g. having to undergo further unpleasant diagnostic procedures, or disappointing their family, or not being allowed to do a desired activity.

♦ Children might be motivated to provide high pain intensity scores because they anticipate some benefit, e.g. being allowed to stay home from school, or avoiding chores, or eliciting increased parental care and concern, or obtaining desired medications.

When a child's self-report pain scores do not seem to make sense to the caregiver, additional efforts to resolve discrepancies are needed, as discussed in the following sections.

The place of self-report in a hierarchy of pain assessment techniques

Pasero and McCaffery (2011, p. 123) present a five-step strategy for assessment that starts with (1) eliciting self-report if possible. If the patient is unable to give a self-report, then the following steps are followed in order. (2) Identify pathological conditions and events or procedures that might cause pain. (3) Observe for behaviours expressing pain, possibly using an observational tool. (4) Solicit information from caregivers and family members. (5) Attempt a trial of physical, psychological, and/or pharmacological means of pain relief, to see if the observed behaviours reflect reduced pain.

Interpreting self-report scores when they conflict with observation and context

A child might give a low self-report pain score when the context and the child's behaviour suggest that pain intensity is high, or the converse (see case example). The correlation between self-report and observational scales of pain intensity in children is usually statistically significant but modest. For example, in a study

of postoperative pain in children aged 3 to 7 years (Beyer et al., 1990), the median correlation between concurrent scores on an observational measure, the Children's Hospital of Eastern Ontario Pain Scale (CHEOPS), and the Oucher was $r = 0.41$, and between the CHEOPS and a mechanical VAS it was $r = 0.35$. Similarly, in a study of 5-year-olds undergoing immunization injections (Cassidy et al., 2001), Spearman correlations between a faces pain score and the CHEOPS during and after the needle were $r_s = 0.47$ and $r_s = 0.33$. In other words, in many cases the self-report scores were at variance with observers' scores on a well-established behavioural measure.

The modest observer–child concordance, and the lack of a gold standard measure of pain intensity, lead to a dilemma for clinicians. There is no validated way to combine and balance estimates of pain intensity from different sources, nor to adjust self-report scores to bring them into line with observation and knowledge of the clinical context. Yet several studies have shown that nurses often do so: they alter patients' self-reported pain scores when recording them in medical charts (Pasero and McCaffery, 2011, p. 18), or fail to ask for self-report and substitute their own informal rating. Pasero and McCaffery suggest that when patients' self-report scores are not accepted and acted upon, 'chaos quickly ensues' (p. 21) because each clinician has different impressions, standards, and biases in judging patients' pain. On the other hand, sometimes self-reports conflict with other sources of information (see case example). In this case example, much additional information is required beyond the simple pain intensity score.

One source of the difficulty is the campaign to treat pain scores, particularly self-report pain scores, as the 'fifth vital sign.' In practical terms, that means recording a single pain intensity score similar to a temperature, blood pressure, or heart rate score. Unlike the true vital signs, such pain scores represent a massive oversimplification. To make valid decisions about pain management requires a variety of additional information. Berde and McGrath (2009) stated that 'it remains a clinical art to combine patients' reports, behavioral observation, and physiologic measurement with the history, physical exam, laboratory information, and overall clinical context in guiding clinical judgments and therapeutic interventions' (p. 474). An example of a situation evoking the need for skill in this 'clinical art' is outlined in the case example.

Case example: an implausible self-report pain score

Clinical question: a 6-year-old male patient has emerged from anaesthesia following hernia repair and is being prepared for transfer to the paediatric ward. The intraoperative anaesthetic is presumed to be past its half-life at this time. The patient's body is rigid in an antalgic position (legs drawn up), he is whimpering, and he has a high heart rate. His facial expression appears to express strong pain. He is shown a faces scale to obtain his self-reported pain intensity. He points to the no-pain (0/10) face. Should this be accepted as indicating that he has no pain, leading to a decision to defer or minimize analgesic treatment?

Interpretation: the self-report score of 0/10 in this instance cannot be regarded as 'the gold standard,' that is, a score which, in the presence of contradictory information, must be taken as correct. The self-report conflicts with (1) knowledge of the clinical context, namely, the fact that the child has had an operation which in most individuals produces pain, and the fact that the intraoperative analgesic is likely to be wearing off; and with (2) observation of his behaviour, including his facial expression, vocalization, and physical rigidity. Alternate explanations for the 0/10 score include the following: the child (1) did not understand or fully attend to the faces scale, or (2) did not want to upset his parent by reporting pain, or (3) was afraid of having to stay in hospital longer, or of having something painful done such as an injection if he admitted to pain on the faces scale.

Good clinical practice would be to continue the assessment process as follows. (1) Ask the parents to assist with assessment based on pain behaviours they have noted in their child in the past. (2) Note the child's response to his parents' efforts to distract or comfort him. (3) Administer intravenous analgesia and note the response after an appropriate interval (analgesic trial). (4) Make notes in the medical record of this information, not only a pain score but also the narrative of additional information, for transfer with the patient to the ward. (5) Recommend that a ward nurse or parents discuss the pain scale with the child later on when he is in less distress, so that he can use the scale in subsequent pain management.

Temporal characteristics of pain

It is common to ask for ratings of pain 'right now' or at the time of a painful procedure, in addition to ratings of pain intensity 'at its worst' and 'at its least' over a specified time period. Particularly with recurrent and chronic pain, questions are needed to assess the frequency and duration of pain episodes: 'How often did you have this kind of pain in the last week/month?'; 'How long did this pain usually last each time you had it?'. More reliable answers to these questions can be obtained via self-report pain diaries, discussed later in this chapter.

Pain interference

Measures of pain interference assess the extent to which pain impairs child and family quality of life, attendance and performance at school, leisure and social functioning, maintenance of positive mood and mental attention or concentration, and other variables reflecting general functioning. These are relevant both to acute pain (e.g. interference with postoperative ambulation) and chronic pain. An example of such a measure is the brief eight-item PROMIS Pediatric Pain Interference Scale (Varni et al., 2010), which contains items such as 'I had trouble moving around when I had pain' and 'it was hard for me to pay attention when I had pain'. (For further information see Tham et al., Chapter 41, this volume.)

Comfort-function goal: setting a target level of pain

With children older than about 8 to 10 years, it may be helpful in making decisions on analgesic administration to inquire about the highest severity of pain that would still allow the patient to carry out valued activities (e.g. socializing, exercising, or attending school). The question itself communicates that pain relief might not be complete, and that the patient has a role in balancing the desired effects of medications with their side effects. For example, a child might have severe current pain of 8/10, requiring intervention, but might feel able to go to school when a target pain severity

of 3/10 can be achieved. However, there appears to be no research with children and adolescents on their understanding and utilization of comfort-function goals.

Location of pain

Patients, including children, often fail to report parts of the body that hurt besides the primary presenting problem or the operative site, so specific inquiry is recommended. For example, children in the postoperative period are sometimes more bothered by an intravenous catheter than by pain at the site of the operation. Self-report of the location of pain can be elicited by verbal questioning, or by asking the child to point to the affected parts, or by providing a checklist of body parts, or by utilizing a body diagram (also referred to as a pain chart, manikin, or pain drawing). The latter methods are reviewed by von Baeyer et al. (2011). Research presently available supports the ability of most children age 8 years and over to complete a pain chart unassisted, while younger children may be able to do so with adult support. Also promising for locating pain symptoms in younger children are picture boards as used in assistive and augmentative communication with children with handicaps; these require only pointing to one among an array of pictures (Mesko et al., 2011).

Pain qualities

Sensory characteristics of pain, such as burning, aching, or pricking, may be of diagnostic importance, particularly in differentiating neuropathic from nociceptive sources of pain. The Adolescent Pediatric Pain Tool (Savedra et al., 1993) includes a list of adjective descriptors for this purpose, adapted from the McGill Pain Questionnaire. The list includes words such as: annoying, bad, horrible (among affective descriptors); crushing, itching, burning (among sensory descriptors); comes and goes, constant (among temporal descriptors). Patients are asked to circle the words that apply to their pain. It is designed for children age 8 and over.

Desirable features of self-report measures of pain

Tools for collection of self-report should have as many as possible of the features listed in Box 36.1 (Hester et al., 1998; Pasero and McCaffery 2011; von Baeyer 2006). The self-report scales recommended in this chapter have most or all of these characteristics.

How are self-report measures validated?

Validation of self-report measures is inherently problematic because self-report reflects internal experience that is not accessible by other means. Articles about pain assessment often describe a scale simply as 'reliable and valid'. This reflects a misunderstanding of the nature of validation, which is not a one-time occurrence but a gradual process of accruing and weighing evidence for the ability of the scale to make accurate predictions or discriminations in a variety of clinical contexts and with different clinical populations. In systematic reviews, a scale is generally considered adequately validated for research and clinical use in a particular context if multiple studies of good methodological quality from different research groups have demonstrated one or more types of validity for that context.

Several lines of evidence are commonly used to establish that a pain scale is reliable and valid for a particular clinical application

---

Box 36.1 Desirable features of self-report measures of pain

+ Evidence for validity and reliability in the current clinical context.

+ Developmentally and culturally appropriate, that is, within the child's cognitive, language, and social skills.

+ Easily and quickly understood, and well accepted by patients and clinicians.

+ Easily used with the patient to set pain management or functional goals (e.g. use the scale to indicate a target pain intensity as a guide for pain management or for planning physical exercise).

+ Places low burden on clinician to administer, score, and record.

+ Free or inexpensive and easy to obtain, reproduce, and distribute (e.g. on the Internet).

+ Where physical materials are needed, these should be easily disinfected or disposable.

+ Available in multiple languages.

Source: data from Pasero and McCaffery, *Pain assessment and pharmacologic management*, Elsevier Mosby, St Louis, Missouri, USA, Copyright © 2011, and Hester et al, Putting pain measurement into clinical practice, in *Measurement of pain in infants and children* (ed.) Finley and McGrath, International Association for the Study of Pain Press, Seattle, USA, pp. 179–198, Copyright © 1998.

Box 36.2 Lines of evidence for validity of pain scales. Examples of studies employing each line of evidence to support self-report measures of pain intensity are cited by von Baeyer (2006)

+ Correlations (or similar measures of association) of self-report ratings with other validated self-report scales administered at the same time. Such validity correlations are typically high, and it is good practice to set an a priori minimum such as $r \geq 0.7$ in validating a new scale. (Simply indicating statistical significance is not adequate, because in large samples very small associations are statistically significant but are not meaningful indications of validity.)

+ Correlations (or similar measures of association) of self-report ratings with validated observational pain scales administered at the same time. These correlations are typically moderate, and it is good practice to set an a priori minimum such as $r \geq 0.4$ in validating a new scale.

+ Accurate ranking of hypothetical no pain, moderate-pain, and high-pain events depicted in pictures or stories.

+ Increased pain ratings in response to painful clinical or experimental procedures.

+ Decreased pain ratings in response to analgesic interventions or less painful ways of performing a procedure.

+ Decreased pain ratings over successive minutes, hours, or days of postprocedure, postoperative, or postinjury recovery.

Source: data from von Baeyer, C. L, Children's self-reports of pain intensity: Scale selection, limitations and interpretation, *Pain Research and Management*, Volume 11, Issue 3, pp. 157–62, Copyright © 2006, Pulsus Group Inc.

(Box 36.2). Validity of assessment tools is best demonstrated by multiple lines of evidence from multiple research groups in multiple and diverse clinical samples, as compiled in systematic reviews (e.g. Cohen et al., 2008).

Children with mild developmental delay or communication impairment

Estimation of pain intensity in children with moderate to severe neurological impairment relies primarily on observational measures (see Belew et al., Chapter 16; MacLaren Chorney and McMurtry, Chapter 37, this volume). Few studies have examined self-report measurement in this population (Benini et al., 2004). Children with mild impairment, or a mental age above 4 years, can sometimes use self-report measures designed for young children (Fanurik et al., 1998). However, nurses often overestimate the ability of cognitively-impaired children to use self-report scales (Fanurik et al., 1998). Children with mild cognitive impairment should, in general, be given a chance to use self-report scales suitable for their mental age, and the resulting scores can be supplemented or supported by observational measures.

Measurement in chronic versus acute pain

Self-report assumes special importance in chronic and recurrent pain, because the overt behavioural expressions of pain attenuate over time without necessarily being associated with decreases in the internal experience of pain. In other words, patients with chronic pain commonly report high levels of pain without showing overt expressions of pain, unless the latter are triggered by social or physical cues. Assessment of chronic pain includes an emphasis on its consequences, including physical, emotional, and social functioning, thus requiring multidimensional pain questionnaires and interview protocols.

Multidimensional pain scales, that is, scales that measure different dimensions, domains, or aspects of pain at the same time, are used mostly with recurrent and chronic pain conditions. Such scales are available in both self-report and parent-report forms, including the Varni/Thompson Pediatric Pain Questionnaire (Varni et al., 1987) and the Bath Adolescent Pain Questionnaire (Eccleston et al., 2005). The Adolescent Pediatric Pain Tool (Savedra et al., 1993) similarly provides a body outline, a rating scale for pain intensity, and a checklist of descriptive words. Self-report measures of pain have also been published for some specific recurrent and chronic disorders such as abdominal pain (Malaty et al., 2005) and headache (Budd et al., 1994).

Tools to elicit self-reports of pain intensity are generally similar for acute and chronic pain. Pain diaries are used to track fluctuations in pain intensity, interference and coping over time (Palermo, 2009; Stinson, 2009).

Gender and cultural issues

While sex differences are widely reported in the prevalence and intensity of pain, no studies to date suggest that pain must be assessed using different methods in boys versus girls. The most salient sex difference in the pain assessment process reported to date may be the ability of girls to discriminate between pain intensity and pain unpleasantness at a somewhat younger age (around 8 years) than boys (around 10 years) (Goodenough et al., 1999).

By contrast, much research has focused on adaptation of self-report tools to different cultural, ethnic, or racial groups. Commentary on pain assessment in sub-Saharan Africa is provided by Walters (2009). One of the best-known faces scales, the OUCHER, is published in separate versions displaying Caucasian, African American, Hispanic, Asian, and First Nations (North American Aboriginal) children. The Faces Pain Scale–Revised and the Wong-Baker FACES Pain Rating Scale have both been used around the world; psychometric studies on the FPS-R have been carried out in Australia, Brazil, Canada, Spain, Thailand, and USA. Inuit children and adolescents in the Canadian Arctic prefer the standard Wong-Baker FACES Pain Rating Scale to a version with pictures adapted for the Inuit culture, although older adults prefer the latter (Ellis et al., 2011). The three most-researched faces scales appear to have acceptable utility in many cultures and countries.

Self-report using new technologies

Rapid development is occurring in the use of smart phones, computers, and web-based applications to elicit, record, and analyse self-reports of pain (Stinson, 2009; Stinson et al., 2008). Documented advantages of such technologies include the following.

- In numerous studies, adolescents and children as young as 4 years prefer computer over paper-and-pencil measures. For example, in a study of hospitalized children, 87% of those who expressed a preference preferred a handheld computer over paper for administration of the Faces Pain Scale–Revised (Wood et al., 2011).

- These technologies reduce the burden on caregivers in administration and scoring of measures.

- They reduce or eliminate backfilling, that is, the common tendency for people to skip diary entries and then fill them in later.

- They lend themselves to integration in electronic medical records (EMR) and automated databases: scores can be uploaded automatically using Web or cell phone communication. A caveat in this context is that EMR systems often provide only a single data field for a pain score at a particular time point in time, making it difficult to deal with (a) discrepant estimates from different sources (self-report, parent observation, staff observation, clinical context), and (b) multiple ratings over time that come from a pain diary.

Future research on self-report

It is generally assumed that assessing pain using pain scales improves pain management outcomes, but evidence supporting this assumption is scant (Franck and Bruce 2009). Further research is needed on this topic, as discussed by Lee and Stevens (Chapter 35, this volume).

While the NRS is now well established for children 8 years of age and older, the validity and reliability of this tool in the hands of younger children who can count, at least by age 6 and 7, require further investigation (Castarlenas et al., 2013).

Preschool-aged children, 3 to 5 years of age, are often not asked for self-reports because their responses, even on simple pain intensity scales, are frequently eccentric and hard to understand (Champion et al., 1998; von Baeyer 2006). Moreover, asking questions is thought to be a poor way to get information from young children, especially for strangers (Wilkinson 2003). Instead, it takes extra time and special skill to interact with young children in order

Box 36.3 Recommendations for clinical practice, education, and research

- Use self-report measures as the *primary source* in a hierarchy of pain assessment methods (Pasero and McCaffery, 2011) (followed by consideration of probable sources of pain, observation of behaviour, obtaining parents' report of pain behaviours, and conducting a trial of pain-relieving treatment.).

- To the extent that the clinical situation requires and permits, obtain self-report on all of the relevant domains of assessment (see Table 36.1).

- Obtain and record the child's self-report of pain intensity, location, and temporal and sensory features on initial assessment and at intervals following treatment.

- For measurement of pain intensity, use a validated scale, e.g. the NRS from age 8 up, one of three faces scales from age 4 up, or the Pieces of Hurt for age 3 to 6.

- Use consistent verbal anchor phrases for maximal pain, such as 'most pain' or 'worst pain you could have,' without embellishment or variation between patients.

- For children with mild developmental delay, use self-report measures suitable for their mental age.

- Compare pain intensity scores across time within individuals, not across children, because the scores have different meanings for different people.

- Institutions should select a small set of scales for regular use by staff that covers the range of ages and clinical conditions typically encountered. Such a set might include NRS for older children, a faces scale for younger children, and one or two appropriate observational scales. For chronic pain, one or two multidimensional questionnaires or interviews should be selected.

- Remember that pain assessment is more than measurement of intensity: location, temporal, sensory and emotional features, and functional consequences of pain also require assessment.

- Take self-reports of pain into account when planning pain treatment and evaluating its effects.

to develop an 'ideal discourse' in which the children's thoughts can be expressed without fear of giving a 'wrong answer' or being judged or criticized. The social and cognitive barriers to effective communication with preschool-aged children about pain, and targets for research on these issues, are discussed by Champion et al. (1998).

Key recommendations

Recommendations for clinical practice, education, and research on self-report assessment of pain in children are offered in Box 36.3.

Conclusion

Self-report is the primary source of information for assessment and measurement of pain, to be obtained whenever possible. But getting valid self-reports from children presents special challenges, particularly those younger than 6 to 8 years.

This chapter has emphasized interpretation of the meaning of self-report scores in the context of many biological, social, cognitive, and developmental influences. Tools suited for different ages are cited. An agenda for future research is suggested.

Self-reports of pain can be compared within individuals across time, but not between individuals. Their meaning is often idiosyncratic and may not agree with estimates of pain intensity based on other sources, that is, observation of behaviour and knowledge of the clinical context. This chapter concludes with a structured process to follow when self-reports of pain or the absence of pain are not supported by information from other sources.

Acknowledgements

The author thanks the following for their suggestions regarding an earlier version of this chapter: C. T. Chambers, D. Lake, L. Oakes, and C. Pasero.

References

Bailey, B., Daoust, R., Doyon-Trottier, E., Dauphin-Pierre, S., and Gravel, J. (2010). Validation and properties of the verbal numeric scale in children with acute pain. *Pain*, 149, 216–221.

Benini, F., Trapanotto, M., Gobber, D., Agosto, C., Carli, G., Drigo, P., et al. (2004). Evaluating pain induced by venipuncture in pediatric patients with developmental delay. *Clin J Pain*, 20, 156–163.

Berde, C. and McGrath, P. (2009). Pain measurement and Beecher's challenge: 50 years later. *Anesthesiology*, 111, 473–444.

Besenski, L. J., Forsyth, S. J., and von Baeyer, C. L. (2007). Screening young children for their ability to use self-report pain scales. *Pediatr Pain Lett*, 9, 1–7. Available at: <http://childpain.org/ppl>.

Beyer, J. E., Denyes, M. J., and Villarruel, A. M. (1992). The creation, validation, and continuing development of the Oucher: a measure of pain intensity in children. *J Pediatr Nurs*, 7, 335–346.

Beyer, J. E., McGrath, P. J., and Berde, C. B. (1990). Discordance between self-report and behavioral pain measures in children aged 3–7 years after surgery. *J Pain Symptom Manage*, 5, 350–356.

Budd, K. S., Workman, D. E., Lemsky, C. M., and Quick, D. M. (1994). The Children's Headache Assessment Scale (CHAS): factor structure and psychometric properties. *J Behav Med*, 17, 159–179.

Cassidy, K. L., Reid, G. J., McGrath, P. J., Finley, G. A., Smith, D. J., Morley, C., et al. (2001). Watch needle, watch TV: audiovisual distraction in preschool immunization. *Pain Med*, 3, 108–118.

Castarlenas, E., Miró, J., and Sánchez-Rodríguez, E. (2013). Is the verbal numerical rating scale a valid tool for assessing pain intensity in children below 8 years of age? *J Pain*, 14, 297–304.

Chambers, C. T., and Craig, K. D. (1998). An intrusive impact of anchors in children's faces pain scales. *Pain*, 78, 27–37.

Champion, G. D., Goodenough, B., von Baeyer, C. L. and Thomas, W. (1998). Measurement of pain by self-report. In G. A. Finley, and P. J. McGrath (eds) *Measurement of pain in infants and children progress in pain research and management, Vol 10*, pp. 123–160. Seattle, WA: IASP Press.

Cohen, L. L., Lemanek, K., Blount, R. L., Dahlquist, L. M., Lim, C. S., Palermo, T. M., et al. (2008). Evidence-based assessment of pediatric pain. *J Pediatr Psychol*, 33, 939–955.

Craig, K. D. (2009). The social communication model of pain. *Can Psychol*, 50, 22–32.

Craig, K. D., and Badali, M. A. (2004). Introduction to the special series on pain deception and malingering. *Clin J Pain*, 20, 377–382.

Eccleston, C., Jordan, A., McCracken, L. M., Sleed, M., Connell, H., and Clinch, J. (2005). The Bath Adolescent Pain Questionnaire (BAPQ): development and preliminary psychometric evaluation of an instrument to assess the impact of chronic pain on adolescents. *Pain*, 118, 263–270.

Ellis, J. A., Ootoova, A., Blouin, R., Rowley, B., Taylor, M., Decourtney, C., et al. (2011). Establishing the psychometric properties and preferences for the Northern Pain Scale. *Int J Circumpolar Health*, 229, 274–285.

Falanga, I. J., Lafrenaye, S., Mayer, S. K., and Tétrault, J. (2006). Management of acute pain in children: Safety and efficacy of a nurse-controlled algorithm for pain relief. *Acute Pain*, 8, 45–54.

Fanurik, D., Koh, J. L., Harrison, R. D., Conrad, T. M., and Tomerlin, C. (1998). Pain assessment in children with cognitive impairment: an exploration of self-report skills. *Clin Nurs Res*, 7, 103–124.

Franck, L. S., and Bruce, E. (2009). Putting pain assessment into practice: why is it so painful? *Pain Res Manag*, 14, 13–20.

Gelman, R. and Baillargeon, R. (2003). A review of some Piagetian concepts. In J. H. Flavell, and E. M. Markman (eds) *Handbook of child psychology*, pp. 167–230. New York: Wiley.

Goodenough, B., Piira, T., von Baeyer, C., Chua, K., Wu, E., Trieu, J. D. H., et al. (2005). Comparing six self-report measures of pain intensity in children. *Suffering Child*, 1–25. Available at: <http://www.usask.ca/childpain/research/6scales/6scales.pdf>.

Goodenough, B., Thomas, W., Champion, G. D., Perrott, D., Taplin, J. E., von Baeyer, C. L., et al. (1999). Unravelling age effects and sex differences in needle pain: ratings of sensory intensity and unpleasantness of venipuncture pain by children and their parents. *Pain*, 80, 179–190.

Halford, G. S. (1993). *Children's understanding: the development of mental models*. Hillsdale, NJ: Erlbaum Associates.

Hester, N. K. (1979). The preoperational child's reaction to immunization. *Nurs Res*, 28, 250–255.

Hester, N. O., Foster, R. L., Jordan-Marsh, M., Ely, E., Vojir, C. P., and Miller, K. L. (1998). Putting pain measurement into clinical practice. In G. A. Finley, and P. J. McGrath (eds) *Measurement of pain in infants and children*, pp. 179–198. Seattle, WA: IASP Press (as in Champion et al., 1998).

Hicks, C. L., von Baeyer, C. L., Spafford, P. A., van Korlaar, I., and Goodenough, B. (2001). The Faces Pain Scale–Revised: toward a common metric in pediatric pain measurement. *Pain*, 93, 173–183.

Huguet, A., Stinson, J. N., and McGrath, P. J. (2010). Measurement of self-reported pain intensity in children and adolescents. *J Psychosom Res*, 68, 329–336.

Malaty, H. M., Abudayyeh, S., O'Malley, K. J., Wilsey, M. J., Fraley, K., Gilger, M. A., et al. (2005). Development of a multidimensional measure for recurrent abdominal pain in children: population-based studies in three settings. *Pediatrics*, 115, e210–215.

McGrath, P. A., Seifert, C. E., Speechley, K. N., Booth, J. C., Stitt, L., et al. (1996). A new analogue scale for assessing children's pain: an initial validation study. *Pain*, 64, 435–443.

McGrath, P. J., Walco, G. A., Turk, D. C., Dworkin, R. H., Brown, M. T., Davidson, K., et al. (2008). Core outcome domains and measures for pediatric acute and chronic/recurrent pain clinical trials: PedIMMPACT recommendations. *J Pain*, 9, 771–783.

Merkel, S. (2002). Pain assessment in infants and young children: the finger span scale: the finger span scale provides an estimate of pain intensity in young children. *Am J Nurs*, 102, 55–56.

Merskey, H. and Bogduk, N. (1994). *Classification of chronic pain: descriptions of chronic pain syndromes and definitions of pain terms*. Seattle, WA: IASP Press.

Mesko, P. J., Eliades, A. B., Christ-Libertin, C., and Shelestak, D. (2011). Use of picture communication aids to assess pain location in pediatric postoperative patients. *J Perianesth Nurs*, 26, 395–404.

Miró, J., Castarlenas, E., and Huguet, A. (2009). Evidence for the use of a numerical rating scale to assess the intensity of pediatric pain. *Eur J Pain*, 13, 1089–1095.

Palermo, T. M. (2009). Assessment of chronic pain in children: current status and emerging topics. *Pain Res Manag*, 14, 21–26.

Pasero, C. and McCaffery, M. (2011). *Pain assessment and pharmacologic management*. St Louis, MO: Elsevier Mosby.

Ruskin, D., Amaria, K., Warnock, F., and McGrath, P. (2011). Assessment of pain in infants, children and adolescents. In D. C. Turk, and R. Melzack (eds) *Handbook of pain assessment* (3rd edn), pp. 213–241. New York: Guilford.

Savedra, M. C., Holzemer, W. L., Tesler, M. D., and Wilkie, D. J. (1993). Assessment of postoperative pain in chidren and adolescents using the Adolescent Pediatric Pain Tool. *Nurs Res*, 42, 5–9.

Spagrud, L. J., Piira, T., and von Baeyer, C. L. (2003). Children's self-report of pain intensity. *Am J Nurs*, 103, 62–64.

Stinson, J. N. (2009). Improving the assessment of pediatric chronic pain: harnessing the potential of electronic diaries. *Pain Res Manag*, 14, 59–64.

Stinson, J. N., Kavanagh, T., Yamada, J., Gill, N., and Stevens, B. (2006). Systematic review of the psychometric properties, interpretability and feasibility of self-report pain intensity measures for use in clinical trials in children and adolescents. *Pain*, 125, 143–157.

Stinson, J. N., Stevens, B. J., Feldman, B. M., Streiner, D., McGrath, P. J., Dupuis, A., *et al.* (2008). Construct validity of a multidimensional electronic pain diary for adolescents with arthritis. *Pain*, 136, 281–292.

Tomlinson, D., von Baeyer, C. L., Stinson, J. N., and Sung, L. (2010). A systematic review of faces scales for the self-report of pain intensity in children. *Pediatrics*, 126, e1168–1198.

Varni, J. W., Stucky, B. D., Thissen, D., Dewitt, E. M., Irwin, D. E., Lai, J. S., *et al.* (2010). PROMIS Pediatric Pain Interference Scale: an item response theory analysis of the pediatric pain item bank. *J Pain*, 11, 1109–1119.

Varni, J. W., Thompson, K. L., and Hanson, V. (1987). The Varni/Thompson Pediatric Pain Questionnaire. I. Chronic musculoskeletal pain in juvenile rheumatoid arthritis. *Pain*, 28, 27–38.

von Baeyer, C. L. (2006). Children's self-reports of pain intensity: scale selection, limitations and interpretation. *Pain Res Manage*, 11, 157–162.

von Baeyer, C. L. (2009a). Children's self-report of pain intensity: what we know, where we are headed. *Pain Res Manag*, 14, 39–45.

von Baeyer, C. L. (2009b). Numerical rating scale for self-report of pain intensity in children and adolescents: Recent progress and further questions. *Eur J Pain*, 13, 1005–1007.

von Baeyer, C. L., Chambers, C. T., Forsyth, S. J., Eisen, S., and Parker, J. A. (2013). Developmental data supporting simplification of self-report measures of pain for preschool-age children. *J Pain*, in press.

von Baeyer, C. L., Forsyth, S. J., Stanford, E. A., Watson, M., and Chambers, C. T. (2009). Response biases in preschool children's ratings of pain in hypothetical situations. *Eur J Pain*, 13, 1005–1007.

von Baeyer, C. L., and Hicks, C. L. (2000). Support for a common metric for pediatric pain intensity scales. *Pain Res Manage*, 5, 157–160.

von Baeyer, C. L., Lin, V., Seidman, L. C., Tsao, J. C. I., and Zeltzer, L. K. (2011). Pain charts (body maps or manikins) in assessment of the location of pediatric pain. *Pain Manage*, 1, 61–68.

von Baeyer, C. L., Spagrud, L. J., McCormick, J. C., Choo, E., Neville, K., and Connelly, M. A. (2009). Three new datasets supporting use of the Numerical Rating Scale (NRS-11) for children's self-reports of pain intensity. *Pain*, 143, 223–227.

von Baeyer, C. L., Uman, L. S., Chambers, C. T., and Gouthro, A. (2011). Can we screen young children for their ability to provide accurate self-reports of pain? *Pain*, 152, 1327–1333.

Walters, M. A. (2009). Pain assessment in sub-Saharan Africa. *Pediatr Pain Lett*, 13, 22–26. Available at: <http://www.childpain.org/ppl>.

Wennstrom, B. and Bergh, I. (2008). Bodily and verbal expressions of postoperative symptoms in 3- to 6-year-old boys. *J Pediatr Nurs*, 23, 65–76.

Whaley, L. F., and Wong, D. L. (1991). *Nursing care of infants and children*. St Louis, MO: Mosby-Year Book.

Wilkinson, S. R. (2003). *The child's world of illness: the development of health and illness behaviour*. New York: Cambridge University Press.

Williams, A. C., Davies, H. T. O., and Chadury, Y. (2000). Simple pain rating scales hide complex idiosyncratic meanings. *Pain*, 85, 457–463.

Wood, C., von Baeyer, C. L., Falinower, S., Moyse, D., Annequin, D., and Legout, V. (2011). Electronic and paper versions of a faces pain intensity scale: concordance and preference in hospitalized children. *BMC Pediatr*, 11, 87.

CHAPTER 37

Behavioural measures of pain

Jill MacLaren Chorney and
C. Meghan McMurtry

Introduction

Measurement is the process of assigning numbers to things (Bakeman and Gottman, 1986) and can be as familiar as using a ruler to measure length and a scale to measure weight. We also use measurement to characterize internal states and experiences. In the context of pain, we can use numerical or facial expression scales to translate one's own or another's experience into a given value. Using behavioural tools, we seek to measure, or assign numbers to, observable behaviours. Behaviours that are measured may be motoric (body movements), vocal (sounds), or verbal (words) and observed behaviours can be further characterized (e.g. tone of voice, intensity of movement).

This chapter will review the current state of evidence on behavioural measures of pain in children and adolescents including a brief discussion of future directions. To demonstrate the utility of behavioural scales, we also include a clinical case example at the end of this chapter. A few limits of coverage should be noted. First, although some of the measures included in this chapter may have been used for infants, we will not review measures that are only validated for infants as these measures are covered by Lee and Stevens (Chapter 35, this volume)). Second, given that there are no well-established behavioural measures of chronic pain, this chapter will focus on measures that are relevant to acute and procedural pain and will also not cover other pain-related outcome measures (e.g. functional disability, quality of life). Finally, multidimensional composite scales containing behavioural and physiological items will not be reviewed (e.g. COMFORT; Ambuel et al., 1992). There are recent, good quality reviews published in the area of behavioural measures of pain (Cohen et al., 2008; von Baeyer and Spagrud, 2007). As with any assessment tool, the psychometrics of behavioural measures are critical; thus, tools deemed well established or approaching well established in these reviews will be included. Coverage of tools that are not well established can be found in the relevant reviews (Cohen et al., 2008; von Baeyer and Spagrud, 2007). We make one notable exception: the existing reviews did not specifically identify measures that are relevant to children with developmental delays or cognitive impairments. We see measures for this population as particularly important and therefore include a brief review here.

Background

Why use behaviour as a measure of pain?

Given the subjective and personal nature of pain, self-report has generally been considered to be the gold standard of measurement. Despite the recognition of its importance, in some cases self-report may not be feasible, possible, or the best choice for measuring pain (Schiavenato and Craig, 2010). For example, children who do not communicate verbally or who have cognitive impairments may have difficulty providing self-report. Children who are sedated or in severe distress may also have difficulty providing self-report and behavioural observation is less intrusive. Even in situations in which self-report is possible, other forms of measurement may be beneficial. For example, in some cases children may be motivated to under-report their pain to appear brave or to avoid receiving needles. In these cases, observing behaviour as a measurement of pain may be helpful in determining whether the child is in need of further assessment or treatment. In fact, a child's behaviour may be the first signal to a caregiver that the child is in pain (McGrath, 1998). Observation of behaviour is also particularly useful when the goal is to examine interactions between individuals and understand the bidirectional relationships between the social context and experience of pain (Schiavenato and Craig, 2010).

Characteristics of behavioural measures

Behavioural measures may vary on several dimensions, including the level of granularity with which they capture observations. At one end are global measures of pain such as numerical rating scales or visual analogue scales. These scales are clinically-feasible, but individual behaviours determining the score may not be well understood and children demonstrating very different behaviours may be given the same rating (von Baeyer and Spagrud, 2007). In contrast to global measures are those that characterize behaviours at a very precise level such as the Child–Adult Medical Procedure Interaction Scale (Blount et al., 1989). These systems are useful, but are time consuming to administer and generally require high-quality video recordings of behaviours.

Behavioural measures also vary based on whether they characterize the intensity and/or frequency of behaviours. Measures can be categorized as dichotomous (present/absent), ordinal (more, less), and interval (frequency over time). Although easiest to collect, dichotomous checklists are limited in the extent to which they capture gradations of behaviour and infer intensity from number of behaviours endorsed in a given time period. Rating scales are more specific with scores usually considered on Likert-type scales (e.g. none/absent, a little, frequently). Interval scales generally capture data over time and can vary in their level of specificity.

Time sampling may also vary. Some measures are designed to record behaviours at one point in time, but in this way capture only a snapshot of a child's behaviour. Other measures define an observation interval that may be based on time (e.g. 15 sec, 24 h) or event (e.g. phase of procedure). This method captures a longer sample of children's behaviour but risks distortion. For example, in a 24 h observation interval, a child who cries for only 30 min receives the same score as a child who cries for the entire period. Continuous recording is also sometimes used. In this method of recording, observers note any instance when a behaviour occurs; this coding allows various metrics including proportions of behaviours (e.g. target behaviour/total behaviours), proportions of time (e.g. behaviours/time interval), or rates (e.g. behaviours/minute) of behaviours. Continuous recording can also be used to report information on timing of when behaviours occurred (time-sequential) or simply the order of behaviours (event-sequential). Continuous recording provides the most representative data, but is time intensive to collect, although this has been made easier with recent advances in computer recording.

An understanding of differences between behavioural measures is critical and the previous list of characteristics (e.g. granularity, time sampling) is intended to be illustrative rather than exhaustive. There is no measure that is perfect for all situations; each type of measure has its own strengths and weaknesses and these are important to acknowledge and understand when choosing a scale to use and interpreting resulting data.

Behavioural measures of pain in children

Measures reviewed are organized based on the context in which they have been typically used (e.g. procedures, postoperative). Consideration is given to the time and equipment requirements for each of these measures. For example, several of the measures require video recording, training, and detailed coding and, although they offer important information for research, they may not be practical in clinical settings due to high burden. Alternatively, some measures can be administered in the moment while behaviour is occurring and therefore are more feasible in clinical settings. Further discussion is also provided regarding the type of rater who administers these scales. Tables 37.1 and 37.2 provide an overview of reviewed measures including original reference and context.

Procedural or brief pain episodes

Children's Hospital of Eastern Ontario Pain Scale (CHEOPS)
The CHEOPS (McGrath et al., 1985), originally developed to measure postoperative pain, has been used in a variety of painful contexts and is now considered a well-established measure of brief pain episodes (Cohen et al., 2008; von Baeyer and Spagrud, 2007). The CHEOPS is administered using a time-sampling procedure with a

5 sec observation period and a 25 sec recording period (McGrath et al., 1985). In some protocols, this sampling procedure has been repeated four times over a 2 min period and an average of scores has been used (Beyer et al., 1990). The CHEOPS consists of six items each rated on a three-point scale (e.g. cry ranges from 1 = no cry to 3 = scream), with total scores ranging from 4 to 13 points for each period. Although the initial validation of the scale did not provide descriptors for ranges of scores, subsequent researchers have done so. For example, Disma and colleagues (2009) described scores between 4 and 6 as minimal pain, 7 to 9 as mild pain, and 10 to 13 as severe pain. The CHEOPS was designed to be clinically feasible and can be completed relatively quickly.

The CHEOPS was developed using nurses' reports of common behaviours exhibited by post-surgical children (McGrath et al., 1985). After piloting and refinement, the scale showed excellent initial interrater reliability (average per cent agreement ranged from 90% to 99.5%) and good internal consistency (inter-correlations among items ranged from 0.35 to 0.81). Convergent validity was demonstrated with moderate to high correlations with nurse and researcher-completed (unblinded) visual analogue scale ratings (total score correlations of 0.81 and 0.86 respectively) (McGrath et al., 1985). CHEOPS scores were also responsive to analgesic intervention (although ratings were unblinded). Subsequently, comparison of the CHEOPS with two self-report measures of pain demonstrated that scores on the CHEOPS tend to underestimate pain over time after surgery (Beyer et al., 1990). To date, the CHEOPS has been used extensively in a variety of painful contexts (e.g. surgery, immunizations, venepunctures, fracture reduction) and countries.

Face, Legs, Activity, Cry, and Consolability scale (FLACC)
The FLACC (Merkel et al., 1997), originally developed for postoperative pain, has been classified as a well-established measure for both postoperative and brief pain episodes (von Baeyer and Spagrud, 2007). Although based in part on behaviours contained in the CHEOPS, each of the five behaviours on this scale is scored on a consistent 0 to 2 metric, yielding a total score between 0 and 10 with higher scores indicating greater pain. The FLACC is used as a point assessment, although the observation period has not been specified. It was designed to be clinically-feasible with low burden. Despite the 0 to 10 metric, it should be noted that, as the interval properties of the tool have not been firmly established, the score cannot be considered equivalent to a 0 to 10 self-report scale (von Baeyer and Spagrud, 2007).

The original study of the FLACC (Merkel et al., 1997) showed adequate interrater reliability (average $r = 0.94$ for 30 children at three separate time periods; kappa values for each FLACC category were acceptable and ranged from 0.52 to 0.82). Supporting convergent validity, a moderate correlation ($r = 0.41$) was found between the FLACC scores and a global nurse rating of pain and a strong positive correlation ($r = 0.80$) was found with another measure of pain (Objective Pain Scale). The FLACC also demonstrated responsiveness to analgesic intervention (albeit with unblinded raters) (Merkel et al., 1997). Subsequent research has continued to support the interrater reliability, construct validity, internal consistency, specificity and sensitivity of the FLACC (Voepel-Lewis et al., 2010). Since its development, the FLACC has been used in a variety of different acute pain contexts (Bable et al., 2009) and age ranges (Marmo and Fowler, 2010). Several language translations

Table 37.1 Review of behavioural measures of pain

Measure	Rater	Number and format of items	Behaviours included	Scoring method	Scoring details
CHEOPS	◆ Health care professional ◆ Researcher	6 items with various rating scales (e.g. 0 to 2, 1 to 3, 1 to 2)	One scale (Cry, Facial, Child verbal, Torso, Touch, Legs)	◆ Interval scoring ◆ 5-sec interval (one time)	Range: 4–13
FLACC	◆ Health care professional ◆ Researcher	Five items all rated 0 to 2	One scale (Face, Legs, Activity, Cry, Consolability)	◆ Point scoring ◆ Interval time not defined	Range: 0–10
CFCS	Researcher	13 items: 10 ratings and 3 dichotomously scored	Three subscales: ◆ Eyes (e.g. brow furrow) ◆ Nose (e.g. nasiolabial furrow) ◆ Mouth (e.g. mouth stretch)	◆ Interval scoring ◆ 1- to 2-sec interval (repeated)	Scoring methods has varied. Often mean intensity, mean frequency, or total intensity
PPPM	Parent	15 items all dichotomously scored	One scale (e.g. Cry more easily than usual, Refuse to eat, Eat less than usual, Groan or moan more than usual)	◆ Interval scoring ◆ Interval based on daytime events (breakfast to lunch, lunch to supper, supper to bed time)	Range: 0–15
PBRS	◆ Health care professional ◆ Researcher	13 items (later revised to 11) all dichotomously scored	One scale (e.g. Cry, Cling, Fear verbal, Pain verbal, Flail, Muscular rigidity)	◆ Interval scoring ◆ Intervals based on procedural events (e.g. preprocedure, procedure, recovery)	Range: 0–13 (or 0–11 for revised) for each procedural phase. Add to derive total score
PBCL	◆ Health care professional ◆ Researcher	Eight items all rated 1 to 5	One scale (e.g. Muscle tension, Screaming, Crying, Restraint used, Pain verbalized)	◆ Interval scoring ◆ Intervals based on procedural events (e.g. pre-procedure, procedure, recovery)	Range: 8–40 for each procedural phase. Add to derive total score.
OSBD	◆ Health care professional ◆ Researcher	11 items (later revised to 8 items) all dichotomously scored	One scale (e.g. Information seeking, Cry, Scream, Verbal pain, Flail)	◆ Interval scoring ◆ 15-sec interval (repeated over 4 procedural phases)	◆ Each item is assigned a weight between 1 and 4 (e.g. Scream weighted as 4.0, Cry weighted as 1.5) ◆ Range 0–28 for 11 item version
CAMPIS	Researcher	35 items all dichotomously scored	Four subscales: ◆ Adult to adult (e.g. procedural talk, humour) ◆ Adult to child (e.g. reassuring comment to child; non-procedural talk) ◆ Child distress (e.g. crying) ◆ Child coping (e.g. humour)	Continuous event scoring	Rates (behaviour/minute) or proportions (behaviour/total behaviours)
CAMPIS-R	Researcher	Six items (item represents category of behaviour) all dichotomously scored	Six items/subscales: ◆ Adult neutral, Adult coping-promoting, Adult distress-promoting, Child distress, Child coping, Child neutral	◆ Continuous or interval scoring ◆ Intervals based on procedural events	Rates (behaviour/minute) or proportions (behaviour/total behaviours) interval
CAMPIS-SF	Researcher	Four items (item represents category of behaviour) all rated 1 to 5	Four items/subscales ◆ Adult coping promoting ◆ Adult distress promoting ◆ Child coping ◆ Child distress	◆ Interval scoring ◆ Intervals based on procedural events (e.g. preprocedure, procedure, recovery)	Range 1–5 for each item/subscale for each interval

(Continued)

Table 37.1 (*Continued*)

Measure	Rater	Number and format of items	Behaviours included	Scoring method	Scoring details
NCCPC	◆ Primary caregiver	◆ 30 items all dichotomously scored	Seven subscales: ◆ Vocal Behaviour (e.g. whining) ◆ Social (e.g. withdrawn) ◆ Facial Expression (e.g. grimacing) ◆ Activity (e.g. less active) ◆ Body and Limbs (e.g. stiff, spastic) ◆ Physical signs (e.g. change in colour) ◆ Eating/Sleeping (e.g. increase in sleep)	◆ Interval scoring ◆ Interval time not defined	Range: 0–30
NCCPC-Revised	Primary caregiver	30 items all rated 0 to 3	Same as original NCCPC	◆ Interval scoring ◆ Interval time not defined	Range 0–90
NCCPC-Postoperative	Primary caregiver or researcher	6 subscales with items rated 0–3 each	Same as original NCCPC with Eating/Sleeping scale removed	◆ Interval scoring ◆ 10-min interval	Range 0–60

Table 37.2 Review of original references for behavioural measures of pain

Measure	Primary reference	Population	Context
CHEOPS	McGrath et al. (1985)	*Original:* 1–7-year-old Canadian children	*Original:* post-surgical (variety of surgeries)
		Subsequent: Age range has included 4 months–18 years	*Subsequent contexts have included:* perioperative (anaesthesia induction, post-surgical); various medical procedures (acupuncture, venepuncture, intramuscular injections, immunizations, fracture reductions, dental, bone marrow aspirations, laceration repair); severe pain from fractures or sickle cell disease
		Samples have included: American, Canadian, Chinese, Czech, Dutch, French, Indian, Iranian, Italian, Korean, Scottish, Singaporean, Spanish, Swedish, Turkish, Thai, and Trinidadian children and adolescents	
FLACC	Merkel et al. (1997)	*Original:* 2-month–7-year-old American children	*Original:* post-surgical in the PACU
		Subsequent: Age range has included 15 days to adults over 80 years	*Subsequent contexts have included:* perioperative (including post-dental surgery); critically ill, ventilated and minimally conscious individuals; various medical procedures (e.g. immunizations, urethral catheterization, temperature assessment, nasogastric tube insertion, venepunctures or subcutaneous venous port access, laceration repair, chest drain removal, fracture reduction)
		Samples have included: American, Austrian, Australian, Belgian, Brazilian, British, Canadian, Egyptian, Finnish, French, Indian, Iranian, Israeli, Italian, Korean, Swedish, Taiwanese, Thai, and Turkish children and adults	
		Has been modified for children with cognitive impairment	
CFCS	Chambers et al. (1996a)	*Original:* 13–74-month old Canadian infants and children	*Original:* post-surgical (variety of surgeries)
	Gilbert et al. (1999)		
		Subsequent: Age range has included: 4–14 years	*Subsequent contexts have included:* immunizations; stretching exercises; experimental pain
		Has been used in children with cerebral palsy and significant neurological impairment	
PPPM	Chambers et al. (1996b)	*Original:* 7–12-year-old Canadian children	*Original:* post-surgical (variety of surgeries)
		Subsequent: Age range has included 6 months–18 years	*Subsequent contexts have included:* everyday pains; post fracture reductions; chronic pain; burn injuries

Table 37.2 *(Continued)*

Measure	Primary reference	Population	Context
		Samples have included: American, British, Dutch, Finnish, German, Indian, and Korean children and adolescents	
PBRS	Katz et al. (1980)	*Original:* 8 month–17-year-old American children and adolescents	*Original:* bone marrow aspirations
	Revised: Katz et al. (1987)		
		Subsequent: Age range has included 8 months–18 years	*Subsequent contexts have included:* perioperative; various medical procedures (lumbar punctures, immunizations, venepunctures, burn injury treatment, chemotherapy, and others)
		Samples have included: American, Canadian, and Dutch children and adolescents	
PBCL	LeBaron and Zeltzer (1984)	*Original:* 6–17-year-old American children and adolescents	*Original:* bone marrow aspirations
		Subsequent: Age range has included 0.1–19 years	*Subsequent:* various medical procedures (intravenous port access, lumbar punctures, bone marrow aspirations, nasendoscopy, venepuncture, fracture reductions, laceration repairs, VCUG, paediatric assessments)
		Samples have included American, Australian, Canadian, French, Greek, Italian, New Zealander, and Swedish children and adolescents	
OSBD	Original: Jay et al. (1983)	*Original:* 2–20-year-old American children and adolescents	*Original:* bone marrow aspirations
	Revised: Elliott et al. (1987)		
		Subsequent: Age range has included 1–18 years	*Subsequent:* perioperative; medical examinations and other examinations/procedures (bone marrow aspirations, lumbar punctures, immunizations, venepunctures, venous cannulations, dressing changes, exercise and play for children with burn injuries, fracture reduction, laceration repair)
		Samples have included American, Australian, British, Italian, and New Zealander children	
CAMPIS	Blount et al. (1989)	*Original:* 5–13-year-old American children	*Original:* bone marrow aspirations and lumbar punctures
CAMPIS-R	Blount et al. (1990)		
CAMPIS-SF	Blount et al. (2001)	*Subsequent: Age range has included* 2–18 years	*Subsequent:* various medical procedures (immunizations, bone marrow aspirations, lumbar punctures, venepunctures, intramuscular injections, venous cannulations, stretching during physiotherapy, voiding cystourethrograms); cold pressor task.
		Samples have included American, Australian, Canadian, British, and Portuguese children and adolescents. Modified versions have been used with Australian and Austrian samples	
			Revised versions have also been used in other laboratory analogues of child pain and/or discomfort
NCCPC	McGrath et al. (2008)	*Original NCCPC:* 3–44-year-old Canadian individuals with severe to profound cognitive impairments	*Original NCCPC:* Mixed pain episodes (every day or procedural pain)
NCCPC-Revised	Breau et al. (2002)		*Original NCCPC-PV:* postsurgical
NCCPC-Post-operative	Breau et al. (2002)	*Original NCPCC-PO:* 3–19-year-old Canadian children and adolescents with cognitive impairments	*Subsequent:* postsurgical (NCCPC); every day pains; acute pain in hospital
		Subsequent: Age range has included: 40 months to adult	
		Samples have included French, Swiss-German, and Swedish infants, children, and adults.	

are available (Voepel-Lewis et al., 2010) and the scale has been used in many countries around the world.

Child Facial Coding System (CFCS)

The CFCS (Chambers et al., 1996a) is a measure of children's facial movements and was categorized as an approaching well-established measure by Cohen et al. (2008). The CFCS assigns ratings to ten facial muscle movements and dichotomous scoring to three others. All 13 movements are grouped into three categories (eyes, nose, mouth). A 1 or 2 sec interval coding system is used and each facial action is coded within each interval (Gilbert et al., 1999). Scoring metrics of mean intensity and frequency (Breau et al., 2001) and total intensity (Gilbert et al., 1999) have been used. The CFCS is a high-burden measure and thus is not feasible for clinical use.

The CFCS is a modification of the well-established Facial Action Coding System (Ekman et al., 2002) and Neonatal Facial Action Coding System (Grunau and Craig, 1987). The first validation study of the CFCS examined pain in the recovery room following surgery in preschool children (Gilbert et al., 1999). Results showed good concurrent validity; CFCS scores significantly correlated with global observer visual analogue ratings of pain over various 2 min time blocks (r ranged from 0.33 to 0.73). There was also a significant negative correlation between CFCS score and time in the recovery room ($r = -0.46$). Two other studies examined responsivity of the CFCS to pain. Breau et al. (2001) found a change in facial action following an immunization. Cassidy et al. (2002) found no difference in CFCS scores between distraction and standard care for children undergoing immunizations. It is unclear whether this intervention was not successful or whether the CFCS was not sensitive to this difference.

Postoperative pain

Parents' Postoperative Pain Measure (PPPM)

The PPPM (Chambers et al., 1996b) was developed to be completed by parents for their children at home following surgery and has been recommended for this use (von Baeyer and Spagrud, 2007). The PPPM is a 15-item dichotomous checklist designed to be easy to complete with minimal training. The majority of items ask parents to compare current to typical behaviour of the child. Example items include: whine or complain more than usual, play less than usual, hold sore part of body, and want to be close to parent more than usual. A cut-off score of 6 out of 15 has been shown to have excellent sensitivity and specificity (>80% each for day 1 and day 2 in Chambers et al., 1996b). The checklist uses an observation interval tied to daytime routines (i.e. between breakfast and lunch, lunch and supper, or supper and bedtime).

The PPPM was designed from the results of Reid et al. (1995) who asked parents for the cues they used to assess children's postoperative pain following surgery. In the original validation study (Chambers et al., 1996b) a 29-item version was reduced to 15 items using item correlations and factor analysis. Good construct validity was demonstrated through relatively high correlations with child self-report of pain ($r = 0.61$ day 1 and 2), moderate correlations with child self-report of emotional distress ($r = 0.39$ and 0.27 day 1 and 2), and decreases in scores from postoperative day 1 one to day 2. Internal consistency was also very good (Cronbach's alpha coefficients for day 1: 0.88 and day 2: 0.87) (Chambers et al., 1996b). Additional validation of the measure by Finley et al. (2003) further supported the tool's construct validity. The PPPM has also been successfully modified for everyday pains (Francke et al., 2010) and burn injuries (Patterson et al., 2002). Ten translated versions are reportedly available (von Baeyer et al., 2011). Recently, a short-form version of the scale using the common 0 to 10 metric of pain intensity was developed by von Baeyer and colleagues (PPPM-SF; von Baeyer et al., 2011). The PPPM-SF is made up of two factors (functional interference, pain behaviours) and shows strong consistency with the original scale ($r = 0.98$), high internal consistency (Cronbach's alpha = 0.85), and scores were unrelated to child sex or age. Promising construct validity of the total score was demonstrated through significantly lower scores on the second postoperative day compared to the first as well as moderate correlations with child self-report of pain intensity on both postoperative days ($r = 0.54$ on day 1 and $r = 0.53$ on day 2).

The FLACC (described earlier) has been identified as a well-established measure of in-hospital postoperative pain (von Baeyer and Spagrud, 2007).

Measures of procedural distress and interactions

Procedure Behavioral Rating Scale (also referred to as the Procedural Behavior Rating Scale; PBRS)

One of the first observational measures of child distress during painful medical procedures was the PBRS (Katz et al., 1980). The PBRS has been described as a promising assessment of distress and pain-related fear by von Baeyer and Spagrud (2007) and an approaching well-established assessment of pain and behavioural distress by Cohen et al. (2008). The PBRS originally included 13 operationally defined behaviours and was later revised to include 11 items (the two items removed were reportedly more indicative of anxiety) (Katz et al., 1987). Observers indicate the presence (or absence) of each of the behaviours for phases of the procedure (pre-procedure, procedure, recovery); scores are the sum of behaviours displayed in each phase and across all phases. The PBRS (original or revised) is relatively fast to score, but the score does not capture frequency data beyond the gross level for each phase.

The first study with the PBRS included children with cancer undergoing bone marrow aspirations (Katz et al., 1980). Interrater reliability was high across procedural phases (95% agreement; correlations ranged from $r = 0.88$ to 0.91 with a grand total score correlation of $r = 0.94$) and scores revealed a pattern consistent with mounting pre-procedural anxiety that peaked during the procedure and reduced somewhat during recovery. Nurses' ratings of child anxiety showed moderate to strong positive correlations with PBRS phase and total scores (ranging from $r = 0.36$ to 0.69; Katz et al., 1982). Younger children received higher scores than older children. Subsequent research has used the original and modified versions of the PBRS to capture child distress during a variety of painful procedures including lumbar punctures (Katz et al., 1982), burn treatments (Tarnowski et al., 1987), venepunctures and immunizations (Schechter et al., 1991).

Procedure Behavior Checklist (PBCL)

The PBCL (LeBaron and Zeltzer, 1984) was designed for use with children and adolescents undergoing bone marrow aspirations. The PBCL has been categorized as an approaching well-established assessment measure for distress and pain-related fear (von Baeyer and Spagrud, 2007), a well-established observational measure of pain and behavioural distress (Cohen et al., 2008), and has been recommended as an outcome measure of procedural distress in paediatric pain clinical trials (McGrath et al., 2008). The PBCL includes eight operationally defined behaviours which parallel the items on the PBRS (Katz et al., 1980). Each behaviour is rated from 1 (very mild) to 5 (extremely intense) during each of three procedural phases (preprocedure, procedure, recovery) (LeBaron et al., 1984). In general, there are two forms of the scale used most commonly: the original eight-item scale (Heden et al., 2011) and a modified version including ten items (addition of groaning and flinching) (Liossi et al., 2007). The two additional behaviours were captured and reported by LeBaron and Zeltzer (1984) in their original paper but not formally as part of the PBCL.

In the original study, interrater reliability was adequate to good (ranged from $r = 0.64$ to 0.86 across the three time periods, with percent agreement ranging from 72% to 94% and overall agreement of 84%; LeBaron and Zeltzer, 1984). No sex differences emerged but younger children were more likely to score higher on the PBCL during the procedure due to an increase in demonstrative distress behaviours compared to older children. The pattern of relationships between ratings on the PBCL with observer and self-report ratings of pain indicated that the PBCL related more strongly to anxiety (versus pain) and to observer (versus self-report) ratings. For example, the relationships between the PBCL and child self-report of pain were: pre-procedure $r = 0.26$, procedure $r = 0.44$, and postprocedure $r = -0.09$. The parallel correlations between the PBCL and child self-reported anxiety were: pre-procedure $r = 0.49$, procedure $r = 0.53$, and post-procedure $r = 0.21$. Observer ratings of child anxiety were moderately to highly correlated with PBCL scores across time points (r ranged from 0.59 to 0.74). Observer ratings of child pain were moderately related to PBCL scores across time points (r ranged from 0.42 to 0.65) (LeBaron and Zeltzer 1984). Use of the PBCL to assess pain and distress behaviours has continued in a broad age range of children (Freyer et al., 1997), in a number of different medical contexts, and by researchers in a variety of countries.

Observation Scale of Behavioral Distress (OSBD)

According to Jay et al. (1983), the OSBD is a revised version of the PBRS (Katz et al., 1980). Deemed a well-established measure by Cohen et al. (2008), the original version of OSBD contained 11 behaviours consistent with distress (pain and anxiety). A later revision of the measure eliminated three items that were infrequent or negatively related to total distress scores, leaving an eight-item scale (Elliott et al., 1987). Each behaviour is operationally-defined and the medical procedure is divided into four phases. In contrast to the PBRS procedural phases, behaviours are recorded on the OSBD as present or absent in 15 sec intervals. Each category of behaviour is also assigned an intensity weighting (e.g. screaming is weighted 4.0 whereas nervous behaviour is weighted 1.0). These intensity weightings were derived based on the average ratings provided by three health care professionals familiar with the procedure on which the measure was validated (bone marrow aspirations).

In the original study of the OSBD, interrater reliability was generally high (r ranged 0.72 to 0.99 over the phases, with the total $r = 0.99$; percent agreements similarly ranged from 80% to 91% with a total agreement of 84%; Jay et al., 1983). Construct validity was supported through a variety of significant positive correlations with related constructs including children's trait anxiety ($r = 0.63$), children's anticipated and experienced levels of procedural pain ($r = 0.76$ and 0.62, respectively), as well as parental ratings of child

anxiety during the clinic visit and anxiety symptoms in the preceding 24 h (both at $r = 0.38$) (Jay et al., 1983). However, child state anxiety was not significantly related to OSBD scores (Jay et al., 1983). There were no reliable overall sex differences; however, similar to research with the PBRS, overall scores of the OSBD decreased with age ($r = -0.76$). The OSBD and revised versions have shown sensitivity to both pharmacological and non-pharmacological pain interventions (Dahlquist et al., 1985; Jay et al., 1987). Versions of the OSBD have been used in a wide range of medical contexts including venepunctures (Dahlquist et al., 1985), dressing changes (Kanagasundaram et al., 2001), and fracture reduction (Kennedy et al., 1998).

The major limitation with the OSBD and its versions, as with several other scales of a similar nature, is the length of time required for training and coding. In addition, many studies using the OSBD have differed in their definitions and timing of phases. Some authors have pointed out that the length of phase may have little to do with child behaviour but may change the overall score of the measure (Tucker et al., 2001).

Child Adult Medical Procedure Interaction Scale (CAMPIS)

Partially based on the OSBD (Jay et al., 1983), the CAMPIS (Blount et al., 1989) was designed to capture adult behaviour and the full spectrum of child behaviour including coping. Cohen and colleagues (2008) categorized the CAMPIS and its revisions as well established in measuring pain and behavioural distress. The original version of the CAMPIS has 35 operationally-defined verbalizations by children (16 codes) and adults (19 codes), and is administered using a continuous recording strategy. (Additional information including manuals can be accessed at: <http://psychology.uga.edu/people/bios/faculty/BlountDoc/Blount-CAMPIS%20&%20CAMPIS-R%20no%20affect.pdf>.) Although the CAMPIS manual includes a Likert-type scale of vocal affect coding, this has not typically been used in published studies. Overall interrater reliabilities were excellent for child and adult behaviours (kappas of 0.92 and 0.80 respectively; Blount et al., 1989).

The CAMPIS was later revised to group adult and child behaviours on empirical and conceptual bases (Blount et al., 1990). Note, however, that validation of this revision was on the same sample as the original tool (Blount et al., 1989). In the CAMPIS-R, the original 35 codes are collapsed into six categories: child distress, child coping, child neutral, adult distress promoting, adult coping promoting, and adult neutral. Continuous or interval coding can be used. In a paper exploring the validity of the CAMPIS-R, interrater reliability was good to excellent for each of the behaviour categories (e.g. child coping; kappas ranged from 0.65 to 0.92; Blount et al., 1992). Supporting construct validity, the code groupings showed most of the expected relationships with observational, self-report, and adult report measures of child fear and pain (Blount et al., 1997). For example, child coping was positively related to staff ratings of child cooperation ($r = 0.37$) and inversely related to child distress on the OSBD ($r = -0.49$) and child self-report of pain ($r = -0.22$). Similarly, child distress behaviour was positively related to OSBD distress scores ($r = 0.57$), child self-report of pain ($r = 0.34$), and parent ratings of child pain ($r = 0.25$). Adult behaviour categories showed most of the expected relationships. Parent distress promoting behaviour was related to increased child self-report of pain ($r = 0.21$), OSBD distress ($r = 0.64$), and inversely to staff ratings of child cooperation ($r = -0.43$). Parent coping promoting behaviours were only weakly related to staff ratings of child cooperation ($r = 0.22$) and were not significantly related to child self-report of pain, fear, or OSBD distress (Blount et al., 1997). Of note, adult 'neutral' behaviours were weakly related to some outcomes. For example, parent neutral behaviours were inversely related to OSBD distress ($r = -0.37$; Blount et al., 1997).

The CAMPIS-R has demonstrated sensitivity to changes in parent and/or child behaviour following intervention (Blount et al., 1992). Use of the CAMPIS and its revised version can provide exceptionally rich interactional data and description for research; these data are achieved through extensive effort however, including recording the interactions, followed by detailed post hoc transcription and coding, making the burden likely too high for clinical use.

The CAMPIS-short form (CAMPIS-SF; Blount et al., 2001) was designed to be an alternative to the CAMPIS-R that can be administered in real-time. The CAMPIS-SF removes the neutral codes and retains the child and adult distress (promoting) and coping (promoting) groups. For each phase of the procedure, behaviour groups are scored on a five-point Likert scale (e.g. 1 = none/one, 5 = maximum or nearly continuous). Initial training takes approximately 1.5 to 2 days, following which videos can be coded in real time. In the initial study, good to excellent interrater reliability was achieved (kappas ranged from 0.74 to 1.0) (Blount et al., 2001). Correlations between CAMPIS-SF child behaviours and other measures of child distress were in the expected directions (e.g. CAMPIS-SF child distress was positively correlated with OSBD distress, $r = 0.84$, child coping was negatively correlated with OSBD distress, $r = -0.40$).

In addition to its development for lumbar punctures and bone marrow aspirations (Blount et al., 1989), the CAMPIS has been used in various forms in many procedural settings including immunizations (Blount et al., 1992; Cohen et al., 1999), venepunctures (McMurtry et al., 2010), and voiding cystourethrograms (Salmon and Pereira, 2002). The CAMPIS has also been translated into Portuguese (Pedro et al., 2010).

Behavioural measures of pain in children with intellectual disabilities

Children with intellectual disabilities are a population for whom behavioural measurement may be particularly beneficial. Although children in this group who are higher functioning may be able to provide some degree of self-report, observation is often relied upon as a standard of measurement. A full systematic review and synthesis is beyond the scope of this chapter, but we review two scales that have been the most consistently used and demonstrate good psychometric properties with this population.

Non-communicating Children's Pain Checklist (NCCPC)

The most widely validated behavioural tool for assessing pain in children with intellectual disabilities is the NCCPC. The original checklist included 30 dichotomous items grouped into seven subscales and was completed by primary caregivers (McGrath, 2008). The checklist showed good internal consistency, test–retest reliability, and convergent and divergent validity (Breau et al., 2000). A revised version was published and, although the measure continues to be called a checklist, the use of ordinal ratings (zero to three) results in this new measure now being better described as a rating scale (Breau et al., 2002). The new scale (range of 0–90), still completed by primary caregivers, continued to be internally consistent (Chronbach's alpha = 0.93) and showed good concurrent validity with parent-rated numerical rating scales ($r = 0.46$) (Breau et al., 2002). A cut-off of 7 was found to have the best balance of sensitivity (84%) and specificity (68%). The observation time for administering the NCCPC-R is somewhat unclear. In the validation studies, caregivers reported on painful events that lasted from 1 min to 24 h and presumably provided ratings on the basis of the entire event.

A postoperative version of the NCCPC (NCCPC-Post operative; NCCPC-PO) retains the ordinal ratings of the NCCPC-R, but removes the eating/sleeping subscale (Breau et al., 2002). In an attempt to examine whether individuals other than primary caregivers could provide valid ratings using this scale, the measure was administered by both primary caregivers and research assistants. This scale further improved on the NCCPC-R by specifying an observation interval of 10 min. Similar to the NCCPC-R, the postoperative version showed good internal consistency and convergent validity (Breau et al., 2002). Excellent interrater reliability was found between caregivers and research assistants (ICC = 0.82 pre-surgery and 0.79 post-surgery), and research assistant NCCPC scores showed good convergent validity with visual analogue scale (VAS) ratings of pain ($r = 0.72$ between NCCPC and caregiver VAS). A cut-off of 11 was deemed to be the best balance of sensitivity (88%) and specificity (81%) on the NCCPC-PO. Since its original publication, the NCCPC has been translated and validated in several other languages including French (Zabalia et al., 2011) and Swedish (Johansson et al., 2010). Further discussion of pain assessment and management in children with disabilities can be found in Chapter 16 (Belew et al., this volume).

Face, Legs, Activity, Cry, Consolability scale–Revised (FLACC–R)

The FLACC scale has been used in its original form and has also been revised to measure pain behaviour in children with cognitive impairment. In the first study using the FLACC with this population (Voepel-Lewis et al., 2002), nurses administered the FLACC postoperatively using an observation interval of 2 to 3 min before and after analgesic administration. FLACC scores were significantly correlated with parent global ratings of children's pain ($r = 0.65$) and the FLACC was responsive to analgesic administration (5.3 ± 2.8 before analgesic, 2.0 ± 1.4 after analgesic). Intraclass correlations between independent raters were significant (range 0.51–0.78), but more stringent interrater reliability analyses (exact agreement, kappa) showed some evidence of lower reliability, especially in the Legs and Activity categories (range 0.27–0.50). In a follow-up study, Malviya et al. (2006) revised the FLACC scale by adding additional behavioural descriptors within each category. Similar to the original scale, FLACC–R scores were significantly correlated with parent global ratings of children's pain ($r = 0.74$). An improvement on inter-rater reliability was evident with the revised scale; intraclass correlations (range 0.75–0.90) and kappa values (0.44–0.57) were higher than those reported with the original tool.

In addition to the two scales described here, a number of other tools have been proposed to assess pain in children with cognitive impairment including the recently published Individualized Numerical Rating Scale (Solodiuk et al., 2010). Facial expression has also been suggested to evaluate pain in specific populations (e.g. children with autism; Messmer et al., 2008).

Areas of special consideration

Cross cultural considerations

Several of the scales reviewed have been used by researchers around the world (e.g. FLACC, CHEOPS). However, the vast majority of behavioural measures of pain have been developed and validated in English speaking populations within largely Western cultures. Although some may argue that pain behaviours should be universal, the utility of behavioural measures has recently been questioned in groups that speak languages other than English or have different cultural backgrounds (Finley et al., 2009). This argument is supported by a small body of research examining some differences in pain behaviour across infants from different cultural groups (Lewis et al., 1993; Rosmus et al., 2000). Literature on cultural considerations in behavioural measurement of pain in older children is limited. One study used the CAMPIS-R (Blount et al., 1990) to study behavioural interactions in 3- to 6-year-old Portuguese children receiving immunizations (Pedro et al., 2010). This study found that new adult behaviours were important to add in this population (e.g. intimidation, reward promise, rationalization). Literature on cultural differences in children's pain behaviour is limited, but suggests that caution be used in applying currently available measures outside of the population in which they were developed. Sweeping conclusions on the impact of culture on these measures will likely not be useful; instead, it will be important to consider individual differences in socialization and history of pain in order to best interpret pain behaviour. A detailed discussion of culture, communication and pain can be found in Chapter 11 (Clemente, this volume).

Pain versus distress

It is important to note that not all of the behaviours included in the scales previously discussed are necessarily specific to pain. In fact, there have been questions about the utility of differentiating pain from other negative emotions especially around acute procedures (Blount and Loiselle, 2009). For example, cry is a common behaviour included on many pain measures, but this same behaviour can be indicative of a range of emotions including fear, anxiety, sadness, or anger. This is particularly evident in studies of invasive procedures in which the same scale is used to measure anticipatory distress/fear/anxiety and procedural pain. There is an implied assumption that behaviours displayed before the procedure are indicative of distress and those displayed during and after the procedure are indicative of pain, but there are clear similarities in behaviours across all phases. However, distinguishing between pain and other negative emotions such as fear may be important for appropriate intervention; the ability of children, caregivers, and researchers to accurately tease apart these constructs has implications for our understanding of the pain context, accurate measurement, and targeted intervention and should be explored in future research (Bird and McMurtry, 2012).

Modification of scales

It is clear that many scales that were developed and validated in one context have subsequently been used in other contexts. For example, the CHEOPS was originally developed for postoperative pain but has since been used in other painful procedures. In some cases, use of a measure in another context requires modification of the scale. This is particularly evident in studies using the CAMPIS where investigators have added or removed behaviours from the measure (Caldwell-Andrews et al., 2005; Chorney et al., 2012). Although this process is not necessarily problematic, it is important that modifications are well described and further psychometric testing is completed.

Conclusion

Although self-report is often considered the gold standard of pain measurement, authors have recently pointed out the limitations of this approach (Schiavenato and Craig, 2010). Young children and those with significant cognitive impairments may not be able to provide self-report and even in older children, self-report may not always be reliable. Contextual factors can influence children's reports of pain and may result in children over or underreporting their experience. Measures to quantify overt behaviour are an important addition to a thorough pain assessment. Several well-validated measures are available for acute pain including procedural and postoperative contexts. One measure is available for parents as raters, but the majority of measures are designed to be administered by healthcare professionals or researchers. Some measures can be administered at the bedside, whereas others need to be administered using video recordings. There are currently two well-validated behavioural measures of pain in children with developmental delays, one of which can be administered by parents.

Although data on behavioural pain measurement are strong, a few limitations should be noted. First, most of the studies have been completed in English-speaking populations from Western cultures and the applicability of these scales outside the population in which they were originally validated is questionable. Second, although all of these scales include behaviours that have been identified by consensus and validation to be related to painful stimuli, it is important to note that none of these behaviours are specific to pain. Children may cry, grimace, or show physical tension with a range of other negative emotions.

Despite these limitations, behavioural measurement of pain is an integral part of thorough pain assessment and, in some cases, may be the most valid measure available. The availability of measures of pain behaviour and accompanying adult behaviour opens new doors to examine contextual influences on children's pain and distress. Future work in this area needs to continue to consider clinical utility and develop decision metrics around the use of these scales, particularly around decisions to treat. It is also important to acknowledge individual differences and contextual influences on pain expression and consider these in treatment decisions. Finally, given the relatively high prevalence and burden of recurrent/chronic pain in children and adolescents (King et al., 2011) further development of the understanding of the role of behavioural measurement in this area is critical.

Case example

Molly is a 7-year-old girl who is on the medical surgical ward of a tertiary care children's hospital following an emergency appendectomy. Molly had surgery yesterday and today her nurse, Tim, has noticed that she seems to be quiet and tearful.

Molly has around the clock dosing of analgesics, but Tim suspects that she might still be having pain. Tim is aware that children in this age range can usually provide self-report of their pain, and uses a validated tool (the Faces Pain Scale–Revised) to ask Molly to rate her pain. Molly does not talk or make eye contact with Tim when he is explaining the scale and reaches for her mother. Her mother encourages Molly to use the scale and Molly quickly points to the first face (indicating no pain). Tim and Molly's mother explain the scale again and remind Molly to point to the face that matches how she feels. Molly again points to the first face on the scale.

Outside the room, Molly's mother tells Tim that she believes Molly is having pain. She says that Molly doesn't like to take medicine and she wonders if Molly is rating her pain as very low to avoid taking medication. Tim agrees that this is possible and suggests that they use some additional ways of assessing Molly's pain. Tim knows that he will be in Molly's room for a short period of time, so wants a scale that he can administer based on a short observation. He chooses the FLACC because this scale has been validated for children in Molly's age range and in postoperative pain. Using this scale, Tim observes that Molly's face is grimaced and her jaw is clenched, her legs are tensed and restless and she is squirming in her bed, she is whimpering, but is consoled by her mother sitting in her bed with her. Using FLACC scoring, Molly scores a six out of ten. Tim takes this as additional evidence that Molly is experiencing pain. He pages the physician on call who recommends titrating Molly's medication on the basis of Tim's information. Tim discusses this plan with Molly and her mother and addresses Molly's potential concerns about taking more medication (she was worried that she would need to get another needle). He also offers to get a movie for Molly so she can be distracted. About a half hour later, Tim again assesses Molly's pain using the FLACC. Her score has decreased to one out of ten. Molly appears generally relaxed, but shifts in her bed once while Tim is observing. Tim discusses this score with Molly and her mother and Tim again asks Molly to rate her pain using the FPS–R. Molly chooses the first face of the FPS–R and Molly's mother reports that she feels Molly's pain is now well managed. Tim remind Molly and her mother to call if they feel Molly's pain is increasing again and notes that he will be back to check on them in a few hours.

References

Ambuel, B., Hamlett, K. W., Marx, C. M., and Blumer, J. L. (1992). Assessing distress in pediatric intensive care environments: The COMFORT scale. *J Pediatr Psychol*, 17, 95–109.

Bable, F. E., Goldfinch, C., Mandrawa, C., Crellin, D., O'Sullivan, R., and Doanth, S. (2009). Does nebulized lidocaine reduce the pain and distress of nasogastric tube insertion in young children? A randomized, double-blind, placebo-controlled trial. *Pediatrics*, 123, 1548–1555.

Bakeman, R. and Gottman, J. M. (1986). *Observing interaction: an introduction to sequential analysis*. Cambridge University Press: Cambridge.

Beyer, J. E., McGrath, P. J., and Berde, C. B. (1990). Discordance between self-report and behavioral pain measures in children aged 3–7 years after surgery. *J Pain Symptom Manage*, 5, 350–356.

Bird, L. and McMurtry, C. M. (2012). Fear in pediatric acute pain: role and measurement. *Pain Manage*, 2, 527–529.

Blount, R. L., Bachanas, P. J., Powers, S. W., Cotter, M. C., Franklin, A., Chaplin, W., *et al*. (1992). Training children to cope and parents to coach them during routine immunizations: Effects on child, parent, and staff behaviors. *Behav Ther*, 23, 689–705.

Blount, R. L., Bunke, V., Cohen, L. L., and Forbes, C. J. (2001). The Child-Adult Medical Procedure Interaction Scale-Short Form (CAMPIS-SF):

validation of a rating scale for children's and adults' behaviors during painful medical procedures. *J Pain Symptom Manage*, 22, 591–599.

Blount, R. L., Cohen, L. L., Frank, N. C., Bachanas, P. J., Smith, A. J., Manimala, M. R., *et al*. (1997). The Child-Adult Medical Procedure Interaction Scale—Revised: an assessment of validity. *J Pediatr Psychol*. 22, 77–88.

Blount, R. L., Corbin, S. M., Sturges, J. W., Wolfe, V. V., Prater, J. M., and James, L. D. (1989). The relationship between adults' behavior and child coping and distress during BMA/LP procedures: a sequential analysis. *Behav Ther*, 20, 585–601.

Blount, R. L., and Loiselle, K. A. (2009). Behavioural assessment of pediatric pain. *Pain Res Manag*, 14, 47–52.

Blount, R. L., Sturges, J. W., and Powers, S. W. (1990). Analysis of child and adult behavioral variations by phase of medical procedure. *Behav Ther*, 21, 33–48.

Breau, L. M., McGrath, P. J., Camfield, C., Rosmus, C., and Finley, G. A. (2000). Preliminary validation of an observational pain checklist for persons with cognitive impairments and inability to communicate verbally. *Dev Med Child Neurol*, 42, 609–616.

Breau, L. M., McGrath, P. J., Camfield, C. S., and Finley, G. A. (2002) Psychometric properties of the non-communicating children's pain checklist-revised. *Pain*, 99, 349–357.

Breau, L. M., McGrath, P. J., Craig, K. D., Santor, D., Cassidy, K., and Reid, G. J. (2001). Facial expression of children receiving immunizations: a principal components Analysis of the Child Facial Coding System. *Clin J Pain*, 17, 178–186.

Caldwell-Andrews, A. A., Blount, R. L., Mayes, L. C., and Kain, Z. N. (2005). Behavioral interactions in the perioperative environment: a new conceptual framework and the development of the perioperative child-adult medical procedure interaction scale. *Anesthesiology*, 103, 1130–1135.

Cassidy, K., Reid, G. J., McGrath, P. J., Finley, G. A., Smith, D. J., Morley, C., *et al*. (2002). Watch needle, watch TV: audiovisual distraction in preschool immunization. *Pain Med*, 3, 108–118.

Chambers, C. T., Cassidy, K. L., McGrath, P. J., Gilbert, C. A., and Craig, K. D. (1996a). Child Facial Coding System manual. Halifax, Nova Scotia: Dalhousie University and University of British Columbia. Unpublished manuscript.

Chambers, C. T., Reid, G. J., McGrath, P. J., and Finley, G. A. (1996b). Development and preliminary validation of a postoperative pain measure for parents. *Pain*, 68, 397–413.

Chorney, J. M., Tan, E. T., Martin, S. R., Fortier, M. A., and Kain, Z. N. (2012). Children's behavior in the postanesthesia care unit: the development of the Child Behavior Coding System-PACU (CBCS-P). *J Pediatr Psychol*, 37(3), 338–347.

Cohen, L. L., Blount, R. L., Cohen, R. J., Schaen, E. R., and Zaff, J. F. (1999) Comparative study of distraction versus topical anesthesia for pediatric pain managment during immunizations. *Health Psychol*, 18, 591–598.

Cohen, L. L., Lemanek, K., Blount, R. L., Dahlquist, L. M., Lim, C. S., Palermo Tonya, M., *et al*. (2008). Evidence-based assessment of pediatric pain. *J Pediatr Psychol*, 33, 939–955.

Dahlquist, L. M., Gil, K. M., Armstrong, F. D., Ginsberg, A., and Jones, B. (1985). Behavioral management of children's distress during chemotherapy. *J Behav Ther Exp Psychiatry*, 16, 325–329.

Disma, N., Tuo, P., Pellegrino, S., and Astuto, M. (2009). Three concentrations of levobupivacaine for ilioinguinal/iliohypogastric nerve block in ambulatory pediatric surgery. *J Clin Anesthes*, 21, 389–393.

Ekman, P., Friesen, W. V., and Hager, J. C. (2002). *The Facial Action Coding System* (2nd edn). London: Weidenfeld & Nicolson.

Elliott, C. H., Jay, S. M., and Woody, P. (1987). An observation scale for measuring children's distress during medical procedure. *J Pediatr Psychol*, 12, 543–551.

Finley, G. A., Chambers, C. T., McGrath, P. J., and Walsh, T. M. (2003). Construct validity of the parents' postoperative pain measure. *Clin J Pain*, 19, 329–334.

Finley, G. A., Kristjansdottir, O., and Forgeron, P. A. (2009). Cultural influences on the assessment of children's pain. *Pain Res. Manage*, 14, 33–37.

Francke, E. I., Demetropoulos, C. K., Agabegi, S. S., Truumees, E., and Herkowitz, H. N. (2010). Distractive force relative to initial graft compression in an in vivo anterior cervical discectomy and fusion model. *Spine*, 35, 526–530.

Freyer, D. R., Schwanda, A. E., Sanfilippo, D. J., Hackbarth, R. M., Hassan, N. E., Kopec, J. S., an *et al.* (1997). Intravenous methohexital for brief sedation of pediatric oncology outpatients: physiologic and behavioral responses. *Pediatrics*, 99, 1–7.

Gilbert, C. A., Lilley, C. M., Craig, K. D., McGrath, P. J., Court, C. A., Bennett, S. M., *et al.* (1999). Postoperative pain expression in preschool children: validation of the child facial coding system. *Clin J Pain*, 15, 192–200.

Grunau, R. and Craig, K. D. (1987). Pain expression in neonates: facial action and cry. *Pain*, 28, 395–410.

Heden, L. E., von Essen, L., and Ljungman, G. (2011). Effect of morphine in needle procedures in children with cancer. *Eur J Pain*, 15, 1056–1060.

Jay, S. M., Elliott, C. H., Katz, E., and Siegel, S. E. (1987). Cognitive–behavioral and pharmacologic interventions for children's distress during painful medical procedures. *J Consult Clin Psychol*, 55, 860–865.

Jay, S. M., Ozolins, M., Elliott, C. H., and Caldwell, S. (1983). Assessment of children's distress during painful medical procedures. *Health Psychol*, 2, 133–147.

Johansson, M., Carlberg, E. B., and Jylli, L. (2010). Validity and reliability of a Swedish version of the Non-Communicating Children's Pain Checklist—Postoperative Version. *Acta Paediatrica*, 99, 929–933.

Kanagasundaram, S. A., Lane, L. J., Cavalletto, B. P., Keneally, J. P., and Cooper, M. G. (2001). Efficacy and safety of nitrous oxide in alleviating pain and anxiety during painful procedures. *Arch Dis Child*, 84, 492–495.

Katz, E. G. Kellerman, J., and Ellenberg, L. (1987). Hypnosis in the reduction of acute pain and distress in children with cancer. *J Pediatr Psychol*, 12, 379–394.

Katz, E. R., Kellerman, J., and Siegel, S. E. (1980). Behavioral distress in children with cancer undergoing medical procedures: developmental considerations. *J Consult Clin Psychol*, 48, 356–365.

Katz, E. R., Sharp, B., Kellerman, J., Marston, A. R., Hershman, J. M., and Siegel, S. E. (1982). Beta-endorphin immunoreactivity and acute behavioral distress in children with leukemia. *J Nervous Mental Dis*, 170, 72–77.

Kennedy, R. M., Porter, F. L., Miller, P., and Jaffe, D. M. (1998). Comparison of fentanyl/midazolam with ketamine/midazolam for pediatric orthopedic emergencies. *Pediatrics*, 102, 956–963.

King, S., Chambers, C. T., Huguet, A., MacNevin, R. C., McGrath, P. J., Parker, L., *et al.* (2011). The epidemiology of chronic pain in children and adolescents revisited: a systematic review. *Pain*, 152, 2729–2738.

LeBaron, S. and Zeltzer, L. (1984). Assessment of acute pain and anxiety in children and adolescents by self-reports, observer reports, and a behaviour checklist. *J Consult Clin Psychol*, 52, 729–738.

Lewis, M., Ramsay, D. S., and Kawakami, K. (1993). Differences between Japanese infants and Caucasian American infants in behavioral and cortisol response to inoculation. *Child Dev*, 64, 1722–1731.

Liossi, C., White, P., Franck, L., and Hatira, P. (2007). Parental pain expectancy as a mediator between child expected and experienced procedure-related pain intensity during painful medical procedures. *Clin J Pain*, 23, 392–399.

Malviya, S., Voepel-Lewis, T., Burke, C., Merkel, S., and Tait, A. R. (2006). The revised FLACC observational pain tool: improved reliability and validity for pain assessment in children with cognitive impairment. *Ped Anesthesia*, 16, 258–265.

Marmo, L. and Fowler, S. (2010). Pain assessment tool in the critically ill post-open heart surgery patient population. *Pain Manage Nurs*, 11, 134–140.

McGrath, P. J. (1998). Behavioral measures of pain. In G. A. Finley, and P. J. McGrath (eds) *Measurement of pain in infants and children*, pp. 83–102. Seattle: IASP Press.

McGrath, P. J., Johnston, G., Goodman, J. T., Dunn, J., and Chapman, J. (1985). CHEOPS: a behavioral scale for rating postoperative pain in children. In

H. L. Fields, R. Dubner, and F. Cervero (eds) *Advances in pain research and therapy*, Vol. 9, pp. 395–402. New York: Raven,

McGrath, P. J., Walco, G. A., Turk, D. C., Dworkin, R. H., Brown, M. T., Davidson, K., *et al.* (2008). Core outcome domains and measures for pediatric acute and chronic/recurrent pain clinical trials: PedIMMPACT recommendations. *J Pain*, 9, 771–783.

McMurtry, C. M., Chambers, C. T., McGrath, P. J., and Asp, E. (2010). When 'don't worry' communicates fear: children's perceptions of parental reassurance and distraction during a painful medical procedure. *Pain*, 150, 52–58.

Merkel, S. I., Voepel-Lewis, T., Shayevitz, J. R., and Malviya, S. (1997). The FLACC: A behavioral scale for scoring postoperative pain in young children. *Pediatr Nurs*, 23, 293–297.

Messmer, R. L., Nader, R., and Craig, K. D. (2008). Brief report: judging pain intensity in children with autism undergoing venepuncture: the influence of facial activity. *J Autism Dev Disord*, 38, 1391–1394.

Patterson, D., Ptacek, J., Carrougher, G., Heimbach, D., Sharar, S., and Honari, S. (2002). PRN vs regularly scheduled opioid analgesics in pediatric burn patients. *J Burn Care Rehabil*, 23, 424–430.

Pedro, H., Barros, L., and Moleiro, C. (2010). Brief report: parents and nurses' behaviors associated with child distress during routine immunization in a Portuguese population. *J Pediatr Psychol*, 35, 602–610.

Reid, G. J., Hebb, J., McGrath, P. J., Finley, G. A., and Forward, S. P. (1995). Cues parents use to assess postoperative pain in their children. *Clin J Pain*, 11, 229–235.

Rosmus, C., Johnston, C. C., Chan-Yip, A., and Yang, F. (2000). Pain response in Chinese and non-Chinese Canadian infants: is there a difference? *Soc Sci Med*, 51, 175–184.

Salmon, K. and Pereira, J. K. (2002). Predicting children's response to an invasive medical investigation: the influence of effortful control and parent behavior. *J Pediatr Psychol*, 27, 227–233.

Schechter, N. L., Bernstein, B. A., Beck, A., Hart, L., and Scherzer, L. (1991). Individual differences in children's response to pain—role of temperament and parental characteristics. *Pediatrics*, 87, 171–177.

Schiavenato, M. and Craig, K. D. (2010). Pain assessment as a social transaction beyond the gold standard. *Clin J Pain*, 26, 667–676.

Solodiuk, J. C., Scott-Sutherland, J., Meyers, M., Myette, B., Shusterman, C., Karian, V. E., *et al.* (2010). Validation of the Individualized Numeric Rating Scale (INRS): a pain assessment tool for nonverbal children with intellectual disability. *Pain*, 150, 231–236.

Tarnowski, K. J., McGrath, M. L., Calhoun, M. B., and Drabman, R. S. (1987). Pediatric burn injury—self mediated versus therapist mediated debridement. *J Pediatr Psychol*, 12, 567–579.

Tucker, C. L., Slifer, K. J., and Dahlquist, L. M. (2001). Reliability and validity of the Brief Behavioral Distress Scale: a measure of children's distress during invasive medical procedures. *J Pediatr Psychol*, 26, 513–523.

Voepel-Lewis, T., Zanotti, J., Dammeyer, J. A., and Merkel, S. (2010). Reliability and validity of the face, legs, activity, cry, consolability behavioural tool in assessing acute pain in critically ill patients. *Am J Crit Care*, 19, 55–61.

Voepel-Lewis, T., Merkel, S., Tait, A. R., Trzcinka, A., and Malviya, S. (2002). The reliability and validity of the face, legs, activity, cry, consolability observational tool as a measure of pain in children with cognitive impairment. *Anesth Analg*, 95, 1224–1229.

von Baeyer, C. L., Chambers, C. T., and Eakins, D. M. (2011). Development of a 10-item short form of the Parents' Postoperative Pain Measure: the PPPM-SF. *J Pain*, 12, 401–406.

von Baeyer, C. L., and Spagrud, L. J. (2007). Systematic review of observational (behavioral) measures of pain for children and adolescents aged 3 to 18 years. *Pain*, 127, 140–150.

Zabalia, M., Breau, L. M., Wood, C., Leveque, C., Hennequin, M., Villeneuve, E., *et al.* (2011). Validation of the French version of the non-communicating children's pain checklist-postoperative version. *Can J Anaesth*, 58, 1016–1023.

Supplementary online materials

Figure 37.1 Parents' postoperative pain measure (PPPM).
Reproduced with permission from Chambers, C. T., Reid, G. J., McGrath, P. J., and Finley, G. A., Development and preliminary validation of a postoperative pain measure for parents, *PAIN*®, Volume 68, pp. 307–313, Copyright © 1996. This figure has been reproduced, with permission of the International Association for the Study of Pain® (IASP). The figure may NOT be reproduced for any other purpose without permission.

Figure 37.2 Parents' postoperative pain measure short form (PPPM-SF).
Reprinted from *The Journal of Pain*, Volume 12, Issue 3, Carl L. von Baeyer, Christine T. Chambers, and Darby M. Eakins, Development of a 10-Item Short Form of the Parents' Postoperative Pain Measure: The PPPM-SF, pp. 401–406, Copyright © 2011 American Pain Society, published by Elsevier Inc. All rights reserved, http://www.sciencedirect.com/science/journal/15265900.

Figure 37.3 Children's Hospital of Eastern Ontario Pain Scale (CHEOPS).
Reproduced from McGrath P, Johnson G, Goodman J, Schillinger J, Dunn J, Chapman J, CHEOPS: A behavioral scale for rating postoperative pain in children, in H. Fields, R. Dubner, F. Cervero (eds) *Advances in Pain Research and Therapy*, Volume 9, pp. 395–402, Copyright © 1985, with permission of the author.

Figure 37.4 NCCPCR (Non Communicating Children's Pain Scale).
Reproduced from Breau, L. M., McGrath, P. J., Camfield. C. S., and Finley, G.A. Psychometric properties of the non-communicating children's pain checklist-revised, *PAIN*®, Volume 99, Issue 1–2, pp. 349–357, Copyright © 2002. This table/questionnaire has been reproduced with permission of the International Association for the Study of Pain® (IASP). The table may NOT be reproduced for any other purpose without permission..

CHAPTER 38

Biomarkers of pain: physiological indices of pain reactivity in infants and children

Susanne Brummelte, Tim F. Oberlander, and Kenneth D. Craig

Summary

Biomarkers are common in all areas of clinical work, health research, and are critical indicators of diseases and physiological states. Preferably, a biomarker should be non-invasively accessible, low in cost, highly specific, sensitive, and easy to interpret. Due to the complexity of the pain system, no unidimensional reliable biomarker for pain has been identified to date. Developmental changes and delayed maturation of the involved physiological systems add another layer of complexity to the use of biomarkers in the paediatric population. Nevertheless, readily available and reliable biomarkers of pain would greatly enhance timely and appropriate treatment of pain, especially in infants and verbally or cognitively challenged children. This chapter examines currently available markers, their use, and limitations.

Introduction

Biomarkers of health or stress reactivity are widely used in all areas of pain medicine, typically adding meaning to self-report and non-verbal measures. They are of critical importance when access to pain experience is difficult, such as in preverbal infants and in children with developmental disabilities with limited communication and social expression. The neural substrate and related endocrine, immune, and genetic components of the pain system offer a wide variety of potential biomarkers (Goldman and Koren, 2002; Oberlander and Saul, 2002). However, physiological, contextual, and developmental factors, as well as methodological factors related to the acquisition and analysis of physiological signals or biomarkers, add challenges to the use of these biological responses in infants and children. Importantly, changes in biomarker levels must be considered in the context of an infant or child's neurobiological development and environmental contexts, such as preterm birth, neonatal intensive care unit (NICU) care, pharmacological and non-pharmacological interventions, and health and disease status (e.g. neurological injury).

No single validated unidimensional physiological marker has emerged that satisfactorily reflects painful events in children. While the expectation that a sensitive and specific marker will be discovered drives research in this field, research integrating the biological with the social-emotional nature of pain may ultimately become the most successful approach to understanding this universal but highly subjective human experience.

Defining biomarkers and pain reactivity

Biomarkers have been defined as 'a characteristic that is objectively measured and evaluated as an indicator of normal biologic processes, pathogenic processes or pharmacological responses to a therapeutic intervention' (Biomarkers Definitions Working Group, 2001, p. 91). Biomarkers typically can be found in everyday clinical management of health and disease; however, as the pain experience is such a subjective, multidimensional phenomenon, identification of biomarkers in this setting has been challenging (Marchi et al., 2009). To date, the focus has been on complex neurobiological system indicators that might provide reliable links between biology and pain-related experience and behaviour, such as variations in cardiac autonomic variability, immune function, brain blood flow, neuroimaging, and neuroendocrine stress hormone responses. Here, we focus on markers of particular promise, including those that have been studied sufficiently in a paediatric population. Mainly, these are measures of autonomic nervous system (ANS) function, reflected in measures of heart rate (HR) or heart rate variability (HRV), activity in the hypothalamic–pituitary–adrenal (HPA) axis (cortisol), the endogenous opioid system, in particular beta endorphin, and genetic, inflammatory, and neuroimaging substrates with potential as biomarkers.

These physiological measures are recognized here as indices of homeostatic changes that follow a painful event. The measures seek to be specific to the nociceptive system, but invariably engage all physiological systems reactive to pain and stress, thereby typically not serving as exclusive indicators of painful responses. Access to sensitive markers of pain is of great value to clinicians, even though specificity remains an elusive objective. The properties and caveats of biomarkers need to be considered before examining in detail the multiple potential pain system markers. This perspective is offered to encourage avoidance of thinking about these indices as 'measures of pain'.

Setting the scene

In the first instance, having readily available and reliable non-invasive biomarkers would greatly facilitate timely recognition of pain in infants and children. While the sensitivity and specificity of a response may be questioned, physiological responses may be considered evidence of pain reactivity and should not be discounted as a 'surrogate measure' of pain in infants, regardless of the physiological repertoire available (Anand and Craig, 1996). The question of whether the response is specific to pain often requires clarification, with context (e.g. injury or invasive procedure) typically providing the necessary confirmation. The reactions also are important because they verify the individual's *capacity* to mount and regulate a response in the face of a painful stimulus. 'Pain biomarkers' should be regarded as an index of a physiological process of 'reactivity' that reflects how one or more systems 'behave' or respond to a painful event and a capacity for recovery and not a direct measure of pain per se. These markers directly reflect features of systems that respond to stressors, and increases or decreases in the magnitude or rates of change indicate disease processes.

Secondly, biomarkers are used as *outcome measures* to quantify the effect of pharmacological or psychological interventions. HR, stress hormones, or catecholamine responses may be blunted by interventions, such as the use of analgesics (Anand and Hickey, 1992) or local anaesthetics (Lindh et al., 2000). Diminished reactivity presumably reflects less biological distress, thereby suggesting treatment effectiveness. However, an analgesia-induced decrease in a biomarker does not by itself indicate that pain is reduced and this needs to be verified through an association with reduced subjective distress.

Thirdly, biomarker responses are used as predictors of health and developmental outcome. For instance, higher baseline vagal or parasympathetic modulation in full-term infants predicts greater cortisol response to a heel stick at 6 months of age (Gunnar et al., 1995) and in former low birth weight infants, low biobehavioural pain reactivity at 32 weeks predicts poorer motor function at 8 months (Grunau et al., 2006). Further, more neonatal procedural pain in preterm infants in the NICU is associated with reduced white and subcortical grey matter maturation (Brummelte et al., 2012b). In this sense, features of pain exposure itself provide biomarkers that predict later development. In line with this, it is important to note that repeated exposure to painful procedures may also influence the response of a biomarker as children may transform to the repeated or continuous exposure with altered pain sensitivity (see Grunau, Chapter 4, this volume).

Biomarker characteristics

Ideally, physiological markers would provide a meaningful biological signal with high sensitivity and specificity (Figure 38.1), such as low haemoglobin as an index of anaemia. From this perspective, a perfect biomarker for pain would be reactive to the experience and able to distinguish pain from non-noxious stressful or non-stressful events. Other desirable characteristics include availability in a fast, easy, non-invasive, and inexpensive manner and empiric validity. While HR or cortisol changes can be easily and inexpensively obtained, they are non-specific indices. Neuroimaging or genetic analysis typically are not available or even feasible and pose problems for interpretability.

The pain system is multifaceted and typically engages a broad range of complex and interrelated biological activities that are not easily quantified. The complexity of pain experience is also reflected in self-report (Melzack, 1975) and non-verbal expression (Craig et al., 2010) measurements. The highly diverse physiological systems subserving pain include central and peripheral neural components, genes, inflammatory and endocrine markers, all of which have been studied as indices of pain reactivity (Anand and Hickey, 1987; Borsook et al., 2011a; Goldman and Koren, 2002; Peterson and Servinsky, 2007). Biomarkers reflect different levels/stages of the pain perception pathway (Figure 38.2) and it is important to understand what the index indicates for the pain experience of an individual. It may indicate features of afferent nociceptive input, but fail to account for affective and cognitive features of pain experience. Further, biomarkers considered to be related to a painful condition, may not necessarily indicate the presence of pain. For example, cystatin C can be elevated during labour pain (Mannes et al., 2003), but also during pain-controlled Caesarean sections (Eisenach et al., 2004), suggesting that this marker may disclose tissue damage rather than pain per se. Importantly, non-noxious processes such as general arousal, stress or tissue damage may all contribute to changes in potential biomarkers. In addition, markers may differ for different sources of pain, as preclinical studies suggest that inflammatory and neuropathic pain, for instance, have distinct markers (for review, see Marchi et al., 2009). Thus, pain biomarkers can be characterized as cellular, molecular, and physiological indices of processes involved in pain and pain-related generalized stress responses, but while pain is invariably stressful, not all stress is painful.

Conceptual Model of a Pain Biomarker

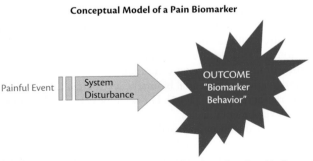

Figure 38.1 Ideal concept of a biomarker. Physiological markers ideally provide a meaningful biological signal with high sensitivity and specificity. Image courtesy of Tim Oberlander.

Biomarker response patterns

Decoding complex and variable patterns of potential biomarker activity into measurable and identifiable components is frequently challenging. The response patterns reflect processes which maintain the function of homeostatic physiological systems within a relatively narrow range. Deconstructing the complexity is typically

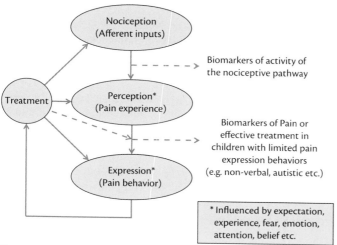

Figure 38.2 Biomarkers along the pain pathway. Pathway from pain perception to pain expression in humans and potential for biomarkers of pain at each level. Adapted from Eija Kalso, Biomarkers for pain, *PAIN*°, Volume 107, Issue 3, pp. 199–201, Copyright © 2004. This figure has been reproduced with permission of the International Association for the Study of Pain® (IASP). The figure may not be reproduced for any other purpose without permission.

accomplished as follows. First, key features are identified that reflect both the amount of change from baseline, or reactivity (*intensity*), and return to baseline, the regulation phase (*recovery*) (Figure 38.3). Quantification is typically represented by a mean of multiple measures of *change scores* (simple time 1 minus time 2), along with the standard deviation. The capacity to upregulate or downregulate the response can be represented by the *slope* of the change from baseline to maximal stress or stress to recovery (Linden et al., 1997), calculated using regression coefficients. An area under the curve (AUC) measure has gained attention as a meaningful cumulative measure of reactivity and recovery, as, for instance, for the cortisol awakening response (Pruessner et al., 2003). More organized patterns of rhythmic physiological signals, such as HR, signal a greater capacity to respond to environmental demands. Rather than signalling pain, measures of changes in autonomic and central nervous system activity may reflect the neural capacity to mount a pain response and an appropriate physiological reaction to a painful stimulus.

Comparisons of responses between two or more groups require consideration of baseline levels. The Law of Initial Values asserts that the size of a psychophysiological response is dependent on the initial baseline level of the measure (Berntson et al., 1994; Wilder, 1962). Differences between groups in responses to painful events may reflect differing baselines rather than a variable impact of the noxious event itself. For example, ceiling effects have been observed; infants already in an aroused state at the onset of a noxious event may demonstrate a smaller increase in sympathetic arousal and a smaller decrease in parasympathetic withdrawal (Grunau et al., 2001).

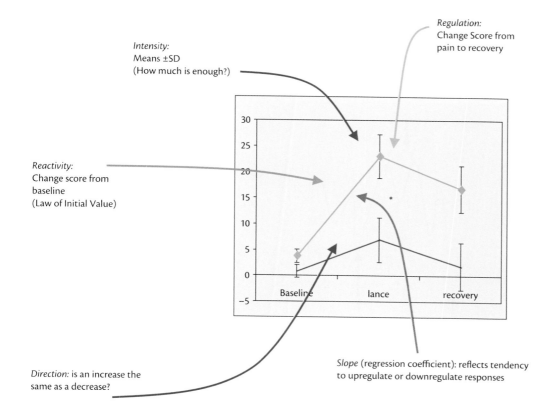

Figure 38.3 Quantifying components of the patterns of response to a painful event. Hypothetical reactivity patterns comparing responses in Group A vs. Group B. Patterns include measures of: *Intensity (magnitude), Reactivity, Regulation, Direction,* and *Slope.* Image courtesy of Tim Oberlander.

Other limits on biomarkers have been reported. A static or slow responding system or one that has a limited range of responses is less likely to provide satisfactory biomarkers than a dynamic one. Systems with inherent rhythms, such as the HPA diurnal pattern, may bias against observing an acute response to a painful event if one samples during a morning cortisol peak period. A predictable response pattern is easier to observe when the signal returns to a baseline compared with a response pattern that remains elevated (continuous response) or has an unpredictable or paroxysmal pattern following a stressful event (see Figure 38.4). Thus, consideration must be given to a biomarker's typical response pattern and contextual influences to appreciate its behaviour in a painful context.

Heart rate and heart rate variability

The ANS plays a key part in the homeostatic response to internal demands and external challenges (stress). Thus, measures of ANS function such as HR or HRV are well suited as biomarkers as these are biological signals that reflect components of the stress and/or pain response systems. HRV reflects variation in the time between heart beats and is a natural occurring physiological phenomenon. ANS function can be easily studied via non-invasive methods and displays a fast (within seconds) response and recovery pattern that can be quantified to yield measures of magnitude, variability, and direction of the signal (see Figures 38.3 and 38.4). Effects are mediated via two branches, parasympathetic and sympathetic, and responses can be quantified to yield discrete continuous and bi-directional indexes of relationships between both branches (Berntson et al., 1997; Grossman, 1992).

HR, particularly variations linked to respiratory patterns (vagal tone), provides commonly used autonomic biomarkers (Porges, 1992). Systems that control autonomic aspects of cardiovascular function are closely linked to systems that modulate pain reactivity (Randich and Maixner, 1984) and activation of vagal afferents can both facilitate and inhibit nociception (Lovick, 1993).

Developmental maturation of the ANS has to be taken into account when investigating HR and HRV. Typically, mean basilar HR among term-born infants increases to a maximum in the first 2 months of life and then decreases through infancy (Doussard-Roosevelt et al., 1997). In contrast, HRV undergoes opposite changes, and after the first 2 months of life is generally positively correlated with age (Finley and Nugent, 1995; Massin and von Bernuth, 1997). HR typically shows an immediate increase following the noxious event (Craig et al., 1993; Oberlander and Saul, 2002) and a decline during recovery. However, in infants a short decrease in HR has been described 3 to 5 sec after a vaccine, followed by the characteristic increase (Johnston and Strada, 1986).

Further, critical measurement and contextual caveats need to be considered in using HRV measures. HRV varies with the length of the HR epoch assessed and proximity to the noxious event. HRV increases as the length of the record increases (McIntosh et al., 1993; Oberlander et al., 2000; Saul et al., 1988). See Voss et al. (2009) for a review of methodological considerations in the use of HRV.

Cortisol measures

Cortisol is the predominant glucocorticoid in humans and it regulates homeostatic stress responses by mobilizing energy to meet the body's needs, such as elevating blood glucose levels. In response to a stressor, the HPA axis releases cortisol from the adrenal cortex, thus offering a key stress biomarker reflecting both central and peripheral reactivity.

Salivary cortisol can be non-invasively obtained and has been more widely studied as a biomarker of affective and behavioural responses to stress than pain per se (for review, see Dickerson

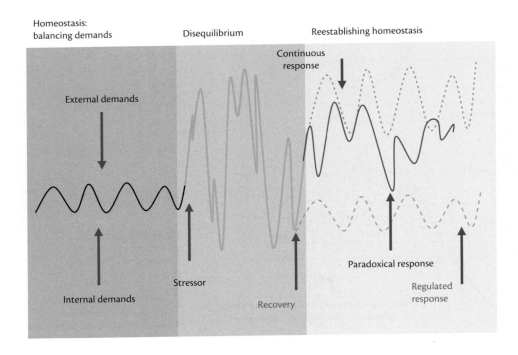

Figure 38.4 Phases and patterns of biomarker reactivity. Hypothetical characteristic behaviours of a stress/pain biomarkers extending from an undisturbed baseline condition to acute response phase (reactivity) to recovery (regulation of response) period. Image courtesy of Tim Oberlander.

and Kemeny, 2004; Hellhammer et al., 2009). Importantly, cortisol increases take minutes before they can be observed in saliva or blood, thus cortisol is a rather slow or 'long-acting' component of stress reactivity.

The cortisol awakening response has been associated with experimental pain ratings in adults (e.g. Goodin et al., 2012). Pain or stressful events reliably elicit a cortisol increase in men and women aged 18 or older; however, in children or adolescents, stressful situations or painful experiences such as inoculations or blood draws do not always lead to significant increases in cortisol levels (for review, see Gunnar et al., 2009). It has been suggested that pain- or stress-induced HPA axis activation in children may vary with the social environment, such as comforting or distracting parental behaviour (McCarthy et al., 2011), demonstrating central regulation of the HPA axis and thus explaining diminished or absent increases in cortisol in certain situations (Gunnar et al., 2009). Thus, cortisol may not be a reliable diagnostic marker for pain experience in a paediatric population.

However, cortisol patterns associated with pain exposure early in life may serve as a biomarker for predicting subsequent HPA axis stress function. Greater cumulative neonatal pain exposure in preterm infants was associated with higher basal cortisol levels during a visual novelty task at 8 months of age (Grunau et al., 2004) and early pain exposure, even when controlling for morphine exposure, predicts cortisol levels up to school age in children born preterm (Brummelte et al., 2012a). These studies suggest that exposure to multiple painful events during the preterm period may contribute to 'resetting' subsequent basal arousal systems, which may regulate the HPA axis system. There is increasing recognition that early experience at critical time periods, perhaps manifesting itself through epigenetic effects and brain neuroplasticity, can change neurocognitive development (Meaney, 2010; Neville and Bavelier, 2002).

Endogenous opioids as markers of pain

Endogenous opioids are an important component of the anti-nociceptive system (Millan, 2002). Plasma beta endorphin (BE) levels are easy to obtain and are often examined as they relate to acute and chronic pain outcomes (Bruehl et al., 2012). It has been suggested that elevated resting plasma BE levels may be a potential biomarker for reduced endogenous opioid analgesic capacity (Bruehl et al., 2012). BE produces analgesia by binding to opioid receptors (particularly of the mu subtype) at both pre- and postsynaptic nerve terminals in the peripheral nervous system. Through a cascade of interactions, binding of BE results in inhibition of the release of tachykinins, particularly substance P, a key protein involved in the transmission of pain (Stein, 1995). In adults, it has been shown that the degree of pain experienced by a surgical patient during and after a procedure correlates with plasma BE levels (Sprouse-Blum et al., 2010). Further, both pre- and postoperative plasma BE levels correlate positively with postoperative pain severity for various major surgeries (Matejec et al., 2003). Thus, BE levels can be elevated in response to increased pain, probably as a result of increased endogenous analgesia, but increases have also been found in response to exogenous analgesia (El-Sheikh and Boswell, 2004), which makes the interpretation of this signal challenging.

In neonates, infants and children, BE levels did not increase significantly after (pain-controlled) surgery (Mirilas et al., 2010),

although levels were greater preoperatively compared to non-surgical patients in neonates and school-age children. This lack of increase has been interpreted as a protection from surgical stress and postoperative pain by fentanyl/propofol anaesthesia (Mirilas et al., 2010). Further, one study found significantly lower BE levels in juvenile patients suffering from migraines or headaches compared to healthy controls (Battistella et al., 1996), while another study found significantly increased levels in a group of children suffering from a painful atopic dermatitis (pruritus) compared to controls or children with healed (non-painful) dermatitis (Georgala et al., 1994). Similarly, positive and negative associations between pain ratings and BE concentrations in children undergoing painful procedures have been reported (Bachiocco et al., 1995; Katz et al., 1982). More studies are needed to better understand the BE response to acute and chronic pain in children.

Other biomarkers: skin conductance

In response to pain, as well as other sources of stress, skin sympathetic nerves release acetylcholine, which acts on muscarine receptors leading to increases in skin conductance. Changes in skin conductance react immediately and are described as continuous, objective, and more sensitive and specific than other currently available biomarkers for assessing pain (Storm, 2008). They have been reported to have a high sensitivity to pain (about 90%) and moderately high specificity (about 60%) in both children and adults (Hullett et al., 2009; Ledowski et al., 2007), at least for moderate to severe pain (Breimhorst et al., 2011; Loggia et al., 2011b; Munsters et al., 2012; Pereira-da-Silva et al., 2012). Studies have demonstrated associations between self-reported pain and skin conductance fluctuations in postoperative paediatric patients aged 1 to 16 years (Hullett et al., 2009), as well as poor correlation of skin conductance with self-reported pain scores (Choo et al., 2010).

Recent studies have raised concern about the reliability (Breimhorst et al., 2011) and specificity of electrodermal activity. For instance, central sympathetic inhibitory drugs and sympathetic nerve activation like nausea, vomiting, and anxiety may influence the skin conductance index (Storm, 2008). Importantly, abundant tactile stimulation and high-sound levels in the neonatal units yield stress responses similar to heel stick when monitored using plasma catecholamine and skin conductance (Bremner and Fitzgerald, 2008; Hellerud and Storm, 2002; Lagercrantz et al., 1986), questioning its specificity. In addition, a recent study by Valkenburg et al. (2012) demonstrated that skin conductance peaks could result from changes in vital parameters such as skin temperature and may thus be unrelated to pain. Skin conductance may provide an additional easy to use and non-invasive tool, but more research is needed to confirm its specificity and to determine the clinical applicability of the method.

Inflammatory and genetic markers

Inflammatory markers have been associated with pain. However, most of these cytokines are not specific to pain, but are released in response to inflammation or tissue damage. Nevertheless, altered cytokine levels have been associated with chronic pain. For instance, Slade et al. (2011) identified monocyte chemoattractant peptide (MCP)-1, interleukin (IL)-1ra, IL-8, and transforming growth factor (TGF)β1 as potential diagnostic markers and therapeutic targets for pain in patients with temporomandibular disorder. Animal models suggest that alterations in specific cytokine levels and their receptors contribute to the development and maintenance of chronic pain (e.g. Abbadie et al., 2009). Therefore, these markers may represent novel targets for therapeutic intervention. More research is needed to confirm this association and its specificity for pain, especially in children.

Recent research on genetic variability and the association of certain genotypes with altered drug metabolism underlines the importance of taking genetic variants into account when analysing or interpreting biomarkers. Evidence is evolving demonstrating the increased risk of certain genotypes for developing chronic pain. For instance, Diatchenko and colleagues (2005) demonstrated that variants of the gene encoding catecholamine-O-methyltransferase (COMT), an enzyme that controls levels of adrenaline and other chemicals and is released in response to stress, influenced both human pain perception and sensitivity and the risk for developing a chronic pain condition. Intriguingly, the COMT genotype was a stronger predictor of overall pain severity than burn size, burn depth, or time from admission to pain interview assessment in individuals hospitalized after thermal burn injury (Orrey et al., 2012). A case–control study of children suffering from chronic tension-type headache (CTTH) investigating the Val158Met polymorphism of the COMT gene found that children expressing the Met/Met genotype showed a longer headache history and lower pressure pain thresholds compared with those with Met/Val or Val/Val genotype, but no increased predisposition to suffer from CTTH in children (Fernandez-de-las-Penas et al., 2011). Studies have demonstrated altered ANS activity (e.g. heart rate changes) and cortisol levels in children in response to stressors depending on the COMT or serotonin transporter genotype (Armbruster et al., 2011; Mueller et al., 2011). Gene–environment interactions have been investigated (e.g. Mueller et al., 2011), with recent studies in adults suggesting that the Val158Met polymorphism contributes to interindividual differences in neural pain-processing by affecting cognitive aspects of pain processing (Loggia et al., 2011a; Schmahl et al., 2012). However, further research with children is needed on this topic. More genetic variants have been identified in recent years (e.g. in the gene encoding the P2X7 receptor; Sorge et al., 2012) or the endothelin-receptor A (EDNRA; Kleiber et al., 2007), but their potential as markers of pain and as novel targets for therapeutics, particularly in the paediatric population, remains unknown. These studies broaden our understanding of individual differences in pain sensitivities and may help to identify children at risk for developing chronic pain.

Neuroimaging as a biomarker

Neuroimaging applications allow the study of human brain function *in vivo*. Techniques have been developed which offer different temporal, spatial, or spectral resolutions. These methods have identified which brain areas are activated during a painful procedure in the adult human brain and indicate that touch and pain display uniquely different evoked potentials (Apkarian et al., 2011). The major challenge for using neuroimaging as a marker of pain or pain intensity is that most of the available techniques, such as electroencephalography (EEG), advanced magnetic imaging, or magnetoencephalography (MEG), require complex instrumentation that is very costly and not easily accessible for everyday

clinical procedures. These methods have been valuable however in understanding long-term changes and neural plasticity in response to acute and chronic pain in the developing brain. As functional imaging offers a non-invasive 'window' into the developing brain, these applications provide promising tools to assess the nature of the pain experience in infants and in children with chronic pain and to provide insights into potential treatments for pain (Borsook et al., 2011b; Holsti et al., 2011; Ranger et al., 2011; Sava et al., 2009). However, not unlike the concern with other biomarkers of pain, the specificity of the marker, i.e. the specificity of the cognitive activation map in response to pain is still an issue, as there is again overlap with other physiological systems such as arousal or stress.

Biomarkers in special populations

Premature care and early infancy

Contextual variables inherent to the painful event have important implications for selection and use of biomarkers (Sellam et al., 2011). In a NICU setting, greater exposure to painful procedures, sex, and ventilation have been associated with physiological response to heel sticks (Sellam et al., 2013). Health status of the infant demonstrably alters the 'performance' of biomarkers (Goldstein et al., 1998). Similarly, mechanical ventilation, reduced lung compliance, neurological compromise from birth asphyxia, intraventricular haemorrhage, or periventricular leucomalacia have all been associated with altered HRV and parasympathetic function (Hanna et al., 2000; Prietsch et al., 1994; van Ravenswaaij-Arts et al., 1995).

Not surprisingly, opioid analgesia may influence a biomarker's response to a painful stimulus. In preterm and term infants, opioids reduce HR responses to noxious events. In neonates, opioids decrease cardiovascular responses to surgical stress (Anand and Hickey, 1992). However, response to opioid analgesics varies with the basal state of the infant. When not in pain, opioids produce tachycardia and increased ventricular contractility by way of reflex sympathetic activation. These adverse side effects can be prevented by beta-adrenergic blockade (Franz et al., 1982; Vatner et al., 1975). In contrast, under conditions of high initial sympathetic activity such as pain or stress, opioids decrease blood pressure by a centrally mediated sympatholysis (Lowenstein et al., 1969). These differing, contrary and context-based opioid-mediated effects make it essential to account for these factors when interpreting an infant's clinical pain response. Interestingly, even simple procedures such as routine tactile nursing procedures can modulate HR and behavioural reactivity to pain in very preterm infants if they are preformed shortly before a painful procedure, suggesting that a heightened state of arousal affected modulation of HR in response to pain (Holsti et al., 2006). Further, a recent study by Slater et al. (2012) showed that preterm infants undergoing a tissue-damaging procedure had higher concentrations of uric acid and malondialdehyde in plasma compared to infants not experiencing any tissue damage, indicating elevated oxidative stress. Malondialdehyde levels were also significantly correlated with pain scores measured with the Premature Infant Pain Profile, suggesting a relationship between procedural pain and oxidative stress in preterm infants. Such an association may prove helpful to determine preterm infants' pain levels in the future, but more research is needed on this topic.

Among preterm infants, sympathetic control appears to dominate, while parasympathetic influences become predominant near term and beyond. Thus, in preterm infants, HRV increases with age but remains lower at term compared with term-born infants, suggesting continued maturational delay (Porges, 1992). Importantly, small for gestational age infants may have a higher HR and lower HRV when compared with appropriate for gestational age term-born infants (Spassov et al., 1994), suggesting that trends in maturation of cardiac autonomic control may be related to both gestational age and level of neurological maturity. Similarly, the HPA axis is still immature in preterm infants and cortisol levels are often inappropriately low in infants in the NICU (Fernandez et al., 2008; Hanna et al., 1993; Kari et al., 1996). Further, it is challenging to obtain blood or sufficient saliva from these infants to measure cortisol in a timely pattern.

Conceptual age and early pain experience are also important modifiers. Preterm infants (<28 weeks) have been shown to be more responsive to procedures as they progress towards term (i.e. their HR responses become increasingly more vigorous) (Porter et al., 1999). Maximum HR response to a heel lance in infants born at 28 weeks, but studied at 4 weeks of extrauterine life, was higher when compared with infants born at 32 weeks' gestational age (Johnston et al., 1996). Differences in HR, HRV, and cortisol at various ages may be due to the early adverse experiences such as repeated pain exposure (Grunau et al., 2005) and may reflect a permanent reprogramming of the ANS or HPA axis, which needs to be taken into consideration when trying to interpret a biomarker's level or response.

Pain biomarkers in the context of developmental disabilities

Children with profound intellectual or developmental disabilities are often non-verbal or otherwise communicatively impaired which makes it difficult to reliably assess pain status through conventional means (i.e. self-report). In these cases, facial action coding has been used to successfully identify painful experiences during invasive procedures (Grunau et al., 1990; LaChapelle et al., 1999; Nader et al., 2004; Oberlander et al., 1999). Some studies indicate that prior reports of reduced pain sensitivity in these populations arose from failure to use appropriate assessment procedures rather than insensitivity in these populations (Tordjman et al., 2009). For instance, it was believed that sensory processing is reduced and pain is absent or blunted among individuals with intellectual and related neurodevelopmental disorders (IDDs) and chronic self-injurious behaviour (SIB), but new data suggests higher (not lower) levels of reactivity to an array of calibrated sensory stimuli for individuals with chronic SIB (Symons, 2011). Similarly, Tordjam et al. (2009) reported greater heart rate response to venepuncture and the elevated plasma beta-endorphin levels in individuals with autism, which reflects enhanced physiological and biological stress responses. This is consistent with the findings of Nader et al. (2004) demonstrating more vigorous facial displays during venepuncture in children with autism. These results indicate that children with autism are sensitive to pain, despite prior reports of reduced pain sensitivity (Tordjman et al., 2009). These studies underline the need for reliable physiological biomarkers of pain, which can be used in addition to conventional measures and behavioural observations. Children with cognitive or emotional impairments may have different modes of expressing their pain, and having physiological indices of nociception or pain perception available would be a tremendous asset to help reduce the suffering of these patients.

Conclusion

While multiple biomarkers are readily available for use in studies of pain reactivity, no single biomarker characterizes all aspects of paediatric pain. Pain system function early in life has complex interrelationships with other developmentally sensitive stress reactivity systems and drawing a single conclusion about 'pain biomarker responses' based on the observation of function of one system is questionable. Typical childhood contexts vary and influence a marker to 'behave' differently under different contextual and illness conditions.

From an evolutionary point of view, behavioural responses such as facial expression and crying are still the best indicators of pain, as mothers did not, and still do not, carry around heart rate monitors or EEG equipment. Modern techniques help us to better understand pain perception and consequences of chronic pain in a population-based model, but are often not reliable in predicting individual responses or outcomes. In contrast, genetic variations such as the COMT or hepatic metabolic factors may prove to be valuable predictors of pain sensitivity in adults and hold future promise for individualized anaesthesia models and pain treatments.

It is important to recognize that while pain may be a universal human experience it is by nature a complex and variable phenomenon (Melzack, 1975), both within individuals, over time, and across populations. Understanding the pain of another person requires considerable careful judgement, including the need to integrate various sources of information, such as self-report, non-verbal expression and evidence of injury or disease. While all experience has biological substrates, the challenge of identifying and measuring biomarkers for such a diverse experience as pain is significant, as many factors, such as the cost, non-invasive accessibility, dependence on environmental factors, the specificity, sensitivity, and speed of the response pattern, as well as developmental changes and/or delayed maturation of the involved physiological systems need to be considered.

Taken together, we are in urgent need of 'better' physiological biomarkers of pain to reliable assess pain in non-verbal or otherwise challenged children that would work towards identifying the best multidimensional approach to understand and effectively treat pain in the paediatric patients.

Case example: irritability of unknown origin—making sense of biomarker pain signals?

George is a 12-year-old with multiple developmental disabilities associated with a significant neurological impairment of an unknown genetic-metabolic disorder. He has multiple cognitive, language, and motor impairments, is fed via a gastrostomy tube, has infrequent seizures, and has been treated for gastro-oesophageal reflux. He has a ventriculoperitoneal shunt for hydrocephalus and is thought to have recurrent headaches—there is a family history of migraines.

George's medications include valproic acid, ranitidine, and lactulose, with glycerine suppositories, phosphate enemas, acetaminophen, and lorazepam, as needed. His parents and caregivers rely on a variety of non-specific verbal and hand and head movements to understand his communication of pleasure or discomfort. Increasingly, he engages in SIB. His symptoms have increased in frequency, duration, and intensity and particularly troubling are his continuous facial grimacing. In the rare moments when he is not crying his parents report that he becomes irritable and typical sensory experiences that had been pleasant were now ineffective or even aversive. One night, George awoke crying with increased vigour. Finding that he had no fever, but his HR was 150/min at rest and he was breathing rapidly (>40/min), his father stopped an overnight feed. Because of increased generalized arousal and irritability, which his mother thinks reflects a severe painful condition, he was brought to his local emergency department.

On examination he was agitated and engaged in SIB (hitting his left ear) coupled with a grimace. He was afebrile but responsive to touch and his heart rate was 80/min and regular, and respiratory rate was 15/min. Laboratory investigations revealed a white blood count of 18 000, with a left shift and erythrocyte sedimentation rate of 45. Chest X-ray was typical and consistent with previous images. The residents who examined him were puzzled—he appeared to all as if he might be in pain, but his cardiorespiratory status was telling a different story—where were the 'pain signals', they asked?

References

Abbadie, C., Bhangoo, S., De Koninck, Y., Malcangio, M., Melik-Parsadaniantz, S., and White, F. A. (2009). Chemokines and pain mechanisms. *Brain Res Rev*, 60, 125–134.

Anand, K. J., and Craig, K. D. (1996). New perspectives on the definition of pain. *Pain*, 67, 3–6.

Anand, K. J., and Hickey, P. R. (1987). Pain and its effects in the human neonate and fetus. *N Engl J Med*, 317, 1321–1329.

Anand, K. J., and Hickey, P. R. (1992). Halothane-morphine compared with high-dose sufentanil for anesthesia and postoperative analgesia in neonatal cardiac surgery. *N Engl J Med*, 326, 1–9.

Apkarian, A. V., Hashmi, J. A., and Baliki, M. N. (2011). Pain and the brain: specificity and plasticity of the brain in clinical chronic pain. *Pain*, 152, S49–64.

Armbruster, D., Mueller, A., Strobel, A., Lesch, K. P., Brocke, B., Kirschbaum, C., et al. (2011). Children under stress—COMT genotype and stressful life events predict cortisol increase in an acute social stress paradigm. *Int J Neuropsychopharmacol*, 1–11.

Bachiocco, V., Gentili, A., and Bortoluzzi, L. (1995). Beta-endorphin and 'overt' pain measures in children. *J Pain Symptom Manage*, 10, 1–3.

Battistella, P. A., Bordin, A., Cernetti, R., Broetto, S., Corra, S., Piva, E., et al. (1996). Beta-endorphin in plasma and monocytes in juvenile headache. *Headache*, 36, 91–94.

Berntson, G. G., Bigger, J. T. Jr, Eckberg, D. L., Grossman, P., Kaufmann, P. G., Malik, M., et al. (1997). Heart rate variability: origins, methods, and interpretive caveats. *Psychophysiology*, 34, 623–648.

Berntson, G. G., Uchino, B. N., and Cacioppo, J. T. (1994). Origins of baseline variance and the Law of Initial Values. *Psychophysiology*, 31, 204–210.

Biomarkers Definitions Working Group. (2001). Biomarkers and surrogate endpoints: preferred definitions and conceptual framework. *Clin Pharmacol Ther*, 69, 89–95.

Borsook, D., Becerra, L., and Hargreaves, R. (2011a). Biomarkers for chronic pain and analgesia. Part 1: the need, reality, challenges, and solutions. *Discov Med*, 11, 197–207.

Borsook, D., Becerra, L., and Hargreaves, R. (2011b). Biomarkers for chronic pain and analgesia. Part 2: how, where, and what to look for using functional imaging. *Discov Med*, 11, 209–219.

Breimhorst, M., Sandrock, S., Fechir, M., Hausenblas, N., Geber, C., and Birklein, F. (2011). Do intensity ratings and skin conductance responses reliably discriminate between different stimulus intensities in experimentally induced pain? *J Pain*, 12, 61–70.

Bremner, L. R., and Fitzgerald, M. (2008). Postnatal tuning of cutaneous inhibitory receptive fields in the rat. *J Physiol*, 586, 1529–1537.

Bruehl, S., Burns, J. W., Chung, O. Y., and Chont, M. (2012). What do plasma beta-endorphin levels reveal about endogenous opioid analgesic function? *Eur J Pain*, 16, 370–380.

Brummelte, S., Chau, C. M., Synnes, A., Cepeda, I. L., Weinberg, J., and Grunau, R. E. (2012a). Neonatal pain predicts cortisol levels at age 7 years in children born preterm. Pediatric Academic Societies Meeting, Boston, MA, Abstract 3640.2.

Brummelte, S., Grunau, R. E., Chau, V., Poskitt, K. J., Brant, R., Vinall, J., et al. (2012b). Procedural pain and brain development in premature newborns. *Ann Neurol*, 71, 385–396.

Choo, E. K., Magruder, W., Montgomery, C. J., Lim, J., Brant, R., and Ansermino, J. M. (2010). Skin conductance fluctuations correlate poorly with postoperative self-report pain measures in school-aged children. *Anesthesiology*, 113, 175–182.

Craig, K. D., Versloot, J., Goubert, L., Vervoort, T., and Crombez, G. (2010). Perceiving pain in others: automatic and controlled mechanisms. *J Pain*, 11, 101–108.

Craig, K. D., Whitfield, M. F., Grunau, R. V., Linton, J., and Hadjistavropoulos, H. D. (1993). Pain in the preterm neonate: behavioural and physiological indices. *Pain*, 52, 287–299.

Diatchenko, L., Slade, G. D., Nackley, A. G., Bhalang, K., Sigurdsson, A., Belfer, I., et al. (2005). Genetic basis for individual variations in pain perception and the development of a chronic pain condition. *Hum Mol Genet*, 14, 135–143.

Dickerson, S. S., and Kemeny, M. E. (2004). Acute stressors and cortisol responses: a theoretical integration and synthesis of laboratory research. *Psychol Bull*, 130, 355–391.

Doussard-Roosevelt, J. A., Porges, S. W., Scanlon, J. W., Alemi, B., and Scanlon, K. B. (1997). Vagal regulation of heart rate in the prediction of developmental outcome for very low birth weight preterm infants. *Child Dev*, 68, 173–186.

Eisenach, J. C., Thomas, J. A., Rauck, R. L., Curry, R., and Li, X. (2004). Cystatin C in cerebrospinal fluid is not a diagnostic test for pain in humans. *Pain*, 107, 207–212.

El-Sheikh, N. and Boswell, M. V. (2004). Plasma beta-endorphin levels before and after relief of cancer pain. *Pain Physician*, 7, 67–70.

Fernandez, E. F., Montman, R., and Watterberg, K. L. (2008). ACTH and cortisol response to critical illness in term and late preterm newborns. *J Perinatol*, 28, 797–802.

Fernandez-de-las-Penas, C., Ambite-Quesada, S., Rivas-Martinez, I., Ortega-Santiago R, de-la-Llave-Rincón, A. I., Fernández-Mayoralas, D. M., et al. (2011). Genetic contribution of catechol-O-methyltransferase polymorphism (Val158Met) in children with chronic tension-type headache. *Pediatr Res*, 70, 395–399.

Finley, J. P., and Nugent, S. T. (1995). Heart rate variability in infants, children and young adults. *J Auton Nerv Syst*, 51, 103–108.

Franz, D. N., Hare, D. B., and McCloskey, K. L. (1982). Spinal sympathetic neurons: possible sites of opiate-withdrawal suppression by clonidine. *Science*, 215, 1643–1645.

Georgala, S., Schulpis, K. H., Papaconstantinou, E. D., and Stratigos, J. (1994). Raised beta-endorphin serum levels in children with atopic dermatitis and pruritus. *J Dermatol Sci*, 8, 125–128.

Goldman, R. D., and Koren, G. (2002). Biologic markers of pain in the vulnerable infant. *Clin Perinatol*, 29, 415–425.

Goldstein, B., Fiser, D. H., Kelly, M. M., Mickelsen, D., Ruttimann, U., and Pollack, M. M. (1998). Decomplexification in critical illness and injury: relationship between heart rate variability, severity of illness, and outcome. *Crit Care Med*, 26, 352–357.

Goodin, B. R., Quinn, N. B., King, C. D., Page, G. G., Haythornthwaite, J. A., Edwards, R. R., et al. (2012). Enhanced cortisol increase upon awakening is associated with greater pain ratings but not salivary cortisol or soluble tumor necrosis factor-alpha receptor II responses to acute pain. *Clin J Pain*, 28, 291–299.

Grossman, P. (1992). Respiratory and cardiac rhythms as windows to central and autonomic biobehavioral regulation: selection of window frames, keeping the panes clean and viewing the neural topography. *Biol Psychol*, 34, 131–161.

Grunau, R. E., Holsti, L., Haley, D. W., Oberlander, T., Weinberg, J., Solimano, A., *et al.* (2005). Neonatal procedural pain exposure predicts lower cortisol and behavioral reactivity in preterm infants in the NICU. *Pain*, 113, 293–300.

Grunau, R. E., Oberlander, T. F., Whitfield, M. F., Fitzgerald, C., and Lee, S. K. (2001). Demographic and therapeutic determinants of pain reactivity in very low birth weight neonates at 32 weeks' postconceptional age. *Pediatrics*, 107, 105–112.

Grunau, R. E., Weinberg, J., and Whitfield, M. F. (2004). Neonatal procedural pain and preterm infant cortisol response to novelty at 8 months. *Pediatrics*, 114, e77–84.

Grunau, R. E., Whitfield, M. F., Fay, T., Holsti, L., Oberlander, T., and Rogers, M. L. (2006). Biobehavioural reactivity to pain in preterm infants: a marker of neuromotor development. *Dev Med Child Neurol*, 48, 471–476.

Grunau, R. V., Johnston, C. C., and Craig, K. D. (1990). Neonatal facial and cry responses to invasive and non-invasive procedures. *Pain*, 42, 295–305.

Gunnar, M. R., Porter, F. L., Wolf, C. M., Rigatuso, J., and Larson, M. C. (1995). Neonatal stress reactivity: predictions to later emotional temperament. *Child Dev*, 66, 1–13.

Gunnar, M. R., Talge, N. M., and Herrera, A. (2009). Stressor paradigms in developmental studies: what does and does not work to produce mean increases in salivary cortisol. *Psychoneuroendocrinology*, 34, 953–967.

Hanna, B. D., Nelson, M. N., White-Traut, R. C., Silvestri, J. M., Vasan, U., Rey, P. M., *et al.* (2000). Heart rate variability in preterm brain-injured and very-low-birth-weight infants. *Biol Neonate*, 77, 147–155.

Hanna, C. E., Keith, L. D., Colasurdo, M. A., Buffkin, D. C., Laird, M. R., Mandel, S. H., *et al.* (1993). Hypothalamic pituitary adrenal function in the extremely low birth weight infant. *J Clin Endocrinol Metab*, 76, 384–387.

Hellerud, B. C., and Storm, H. (2002). Skin conductance and behaviour during sensory stimulation of preterm and term infants. *Early Hum Dev*, 70, 35–46.

Hellhammer, D. H., Wust, S., and Kudielka, B. M. (2009). Salivary cortisol as a biomarker in stress research. *Psychoneuroendocrinology*, 34, 163–171.

Holsti, L., Grunau, R. E., and Shany, E. (2011). Assessing pain in preterm infants in the neonatal intensive care unit: moving to a 'brain-oriented' approach. *Pain Manag*, 1, 171–179.

Holsti, L., Grunau, R. E., Whifield, M. F., Oberlander, T. F., and Lindh, V. (2006). Behavioral responses to pain are heightened after clustered care in preterm infants born between 30 and 32 weeks gestational age. *Clin J Pain*, 22, 757–764.

Hullett, B., Chambers, N., Preuss, J., Zamudio, I., Lange, J., Pascoe, E., *et al.* (2009). Monitoring electrical skin conductance: a tool for the assessment of postoperative pain in children? *Anesthesiology*, 111, 513–517.

Johnston, C. C., Stevens, B., Yang, F., and Horton, L. (1996). Developmental changes in response to heelstick in preterm infants: a prospective cohort study. *Dev Med Child Neurol*, 38, 438–445.

Johnston, C. C., and Strada, M. E. (1986). Acute pain response in infants: a multidimensional description. *Pain*, 24, 373–382.

Kalso, E. (2004). Biomarkers for pain. *Pain*, 107, 199–201.

Kari, M. A., Raivio, K. O., Stenman, U. H., and Voutilainen, R. (1996). Serum cortisol, dehydroepiandrosterone sulfate, and steroid-binding globulins in preterm neonates: effect of gestational age and dexamethasone therapy. *Pediatr Res*, 40, 319–324.

Katz, E. R., Sharp, B., Kellerman, J., Marston, A. R., Hershman, J. M., Siegel, S. E. (1982). Beta-endorphin immunoreactivity and acute behavioral distress in children with leukemia. *J Nerv Ment Dis*, 170, 72–77.

Kleiber, C., Schutte, D. L., McCarthy, A. M., Floria-Santos, M., Murray, J. C., and Hanrahan, K. (2007). Predictors of topical anesthetic effectiveness in children. *J Pain*, 8, 168–174.

LaChapelle, D. L., Hadjistavropoulos, T., and Craig, K. D. (1999). Pain measurement in persons with intellectual disabilities. *Clin J Pain*, 15, 13–23.

Lagercrantz, H., Nilsson, E., Redham, I., and Hjemdahl, P. (1986). Plasma catecholamines following nursing procedures in a neonatal ward. *Early Hum Dev*, 14, 61–65.

Ledowski, T., Bromilow, J., Wu, J., Paech, M. J., Storm, H., and Schug, S. A. (2007). The assessment of postoperative pain by monitoring skin conductance: results of a prospective study. *Anaesthesia*, 62, 989–993.

Linden, W., Earle, T. L., Gerin, W., and Christenfeld, N. (1997). Physiological stress reactivity and recovery: conceptual siblings separated at birth? *J Psychosom Res*, 42, 117–135.

Lindh, V., Wiklund, U., and Hakansson, S. (2000). Assessment of the effect of EMLA during venipuncture in the newborn by analysis of heart rate variability. *Pain*, 86, 247–254.

Loggia, M. L., Jensen, K., Gollub, R. L., Wasan, A. D., Edwards, R. R., and Kong, J. (2011a). The catechol-O-methyltransferase (COMT) val158met polymorphism affects brain responses to repeated painful stimuli. *PLoS One*, 6, e27764.

Loggia, M. L., Juneau, M., and Bushnell, M. C. (2011b). Autonomic responses to heat pain: Heart rate, skin conductance, and their relation to verbal ratings and stimulus intensity. *Pain*, 152, 592–598.

Lovick, T. A. (1993). Integrated activity of cardiovascular and pain regulatory systems: role in adaptive behavioural responses. *Prog Neurobiol*, 40, 631–644.

Lowenstein, E., Hallowell, P., Levine, F. H., Daggett, W. M., Austen, W. G., Laver, M. B. (1969). Cardiovascular response to large doses of intravenous morphine in man. *N Engl J Med*, 281, 1389–1393.

Mannes, A. J., Martin, B. M., Yang, H. Y., Keller, J. M., Lewin, S., Gaiser, R. R., *et al.* (2003). Cystatin C as a cerebrospinal fluid biomarker for pain in humans. *Pain*, 102, 251–256.

Marchi, A., Vellucci, R., Mameli, S., Rita Piredda, A., and Finco, G. (2009). Pain biomarkers. *Clin Drug Investig*, 29(Suppl 1), 41–46.

Massin, M. and von Bernuth, G. (1997). Normal ranges of heart rate variability during infancy and childhood. *Pediatr Cardiol*, 18, 297–302.

Matejec, R., Ruwoldt, R., Bodeker, R. H., Hempelmann, G., and Teschemacher, H. (2003). Release of beta-endorphin immunoreactive material under perioperative conditions into blood or cerebrospinal fluid: significance for postoperative pain? *Anesth Analg*, 96, 481–486.

McCarthy, A. M., Hanrahan, K., Scott, L. M., Zembldge, N., Kleiber, C., and Zimmerman, M. B. (2011). Salivary cortisol responsivity to an intravenous catheter insertion in children with attention-deficit/hyperactivity disorder. *J Pediatr Psychol*, 36, 902–910.

McIntosh, N., Van Veen, L., and Brameyer, H. (1993). The pain of heel prick and its measurement in preterm infants. *Pain*, 52, 71–74.

Meaney, M. J. (2010). Epigenetics and the biological definition of gene x environment interactions. *Child Dev*, 81, 41–79.

Melzack, R. (1975). The McGill Pain Questionnaire: major properties and scoring methods. *Pain* 1, 277–299.

Millan, M. J. (2002). Descending control of pain. *Prog Neurobiol*, 66, 355–474.

Mirilas, P., Mentessidou, A., Kontis, E., Antypa, E., Makedou, A., and Petropoulos, A. S. (2010). Serum beta-endorphin response to stress before and after operation under fentanyl anesthesia in neonates, infants and preschool children. *Eur J Pediatr Surg*, 20, 106–110.

Mueller, A., Armbruster, D., Moser, D. A., Canli, T., Lesch, K. P., Brocke, B., *et al.* (2011). Interaction of serotonin transporter gene-linked polymorphic region and stressful life events predicts cortisol stress response. *Neuropsychopharmacology*, 36, 1332–1339.

Munsters, J., Wallstrom, L., Agren, J., Norsted, T., and Sindelar, R. (2012). Skin conductance measurements as pain assessment in newborn infants born at 22–27 weeks gestational age at different postnatal age. *Early Hum Dev*, 88, 21–26.

Nader, R., Oberlander, T. F., Chambers, C. T., and Craig, A. D. (2004). Expression of pain in children with autism. *Clin J Pain*, 20, 88–97.

Neville, H. and Bavelier, D. (2002). Human brain plasticity: evidence from sensory deprivation and altered language experience. *Prog Brain Res*, 138, 177–188.

Oberlander, T. and Saul, J. P. (2002). Methodological considerations for the use of heart rate variability as a measure of pain reactivity in vulnerable infants. *Clin Perinatol*, 29, 427–443.

Oberlander, T. F., Gilbert, C. A., Chambers, C. T., O'Donnell, M. E., and Craig, K. D. (1999). Biobehavioral responses to acute pain in adolescents with a significant neurologic impairment. *Clin J Pain*, 15, 201–209.

Oberlander, T. F., Grunau, R. E., Whitfield, M. F., Fitzgerald, C., Pitfield, S., and Saul, J. P. (2000). Biobehavioral pain responses in former extremely low birth weight infants at four months' corrected age. *Pediatrics*, 105, e6.

Orrey, D. C., Bortsov, A. V., Hoskins, J. M., Shupp, J. W., Jones, S. W., Cicuto, B. J., *et al.* (2012). Catechol-O-methyltransferase genotype predicts pain severity in hospitalized burn patients. *J Burn Care Res*, 33(4), 518–523.

Pereira-da-Silva, L., Virella, D., Monteiro, I., Gomes, S., Rodrigues, P., Serelha, M., *et al.* (2012). Skin conductance indices discriminate nociceptive responses to acute stimuli from different heel prick procedures in infants. *J Matern Fetal Neonatal Med*, 25, 796–801.

Peterson, N. C., and Servinsky, M. D. (2007). Development of molecular and cellular biomarkers of pain. *Comp Med*, 57, 554–562.

Porges, S. W. (1992). Vagal tone: a physiologic marker of stress vulnerability. *Pediatrics*, 90, 498–504.

Porter, F. L., Wolf, C. M., and Miller, J. P. (1999). Procedural pain in newborn infants: the influence of intensity and development. *Pediatrics*, 104, e13.

Prietsch, V., Knoepke, U., and Obladen, M. (1994). Continuous monitoring of heart rate variability in preterm infants. *Early Hum Dev*, 37, 117–131.

Pruessner, J. C., Kirschbaum, C., Meinlschmid, G., and Hellhammer, D. H. (2003). Two formulas for computation of the area under the curve represent measures of total hormone concentration versus time-dependent change. *Psychoneuroendocrinology*, 28, 916–931.

Randich, A. and Maixner, W. (1984). Interactions between cardiovascular and pain regulatory systems. *Neurosci Biobehav Rev*, 8, 343–367.

Ranger, M., Johnston, C. C., Limperopoulos, C., Rennick, J. E., and du Plessis, A. J. (2011). Cerebral near-infrared spectroscopy as a measure of nociceptive evoked activity in critically ill infants. *Pain Res Manag*, 16, 331–336.

Saul, J. P., Albrecht, P., Berger, R. D., and Cohen, R. J. (1988). Analysis of long term heart rate variability: methods, 1/f scaling and implications. *Comput Cardiol*, 14, 419–422.

Sava, S., Lebel, A. A., Leslie, D. S., Drosos, A., Berde, C., Becerra, L., *et al.* (2009). Challenges of functional imaging research of pain in children. *Mol Pain*, 5, 30.

Schmahl, C., Ludascher, P., Greffrath, W., Kraus, A., Valerius, G., Schulze, T. G., *et al.* (2012). COMT val158met polymorphism and neural pain processing. *PLoS One*, 7, e23658.

Sellam, G., Engberg, S., Denhaerynck, K., Craig, K. D., and Cignacco, E. L. (2013). Contextual factors associated with pain response of preterm infants to heel-stick procedures. *Eur J Pain*, 17(2), 255–263.

Sellam, G., Cignacco, E. L., Craig, K. D., and Engberg, S. (2011). Contextual factors influencing pain response to heelstick procedures in preterm infants: what do we know? A systematic review. *Eur J Pain*, 15, 661.e1–661.15.

Slade, G. D., Conrad, M. S., Diatchenko, L., Rashid, N. U., Zhong, S., Smith, S., *et al.* (2011). Cytokine biomarkers and chronic pain: association of genes, transcription, and circulating proteins with temporomandibular disorders and widespread palpation tenderness. *Pain*, 152, 2802–2812.

Slater, L., Asmerom, Y., Boskovic, D. S., Bahjri, K., Plank, M. S., Angeles, K. R., *et al.* (2012). Procedural pain and oxidative stress in premature neonates. *J Pain*, 13, 590–597.

Sorge, R. E., Trang, T., Dorfman, R., Smith, S. B., Beggs, S., Ritchie, J., *et al.* (2012). Genetically determined P2X7 receptor pore formation regulates variability in chronic pain sensitivity. *Nat Med*, 18, 595–599.

Spassov, L., Curzi-Dascalova, L., Clairambault, J., Kauffmann, F., Eiselt, M., Médigue, C., *et al.* (1994). Heart rate and heart rate variability during sleep in small-for-gestational age newborns. *Pediatr Res*, 35, 500–505.

Sprouse-Blum, A. S., Smith, G., Sugai, D., and Parsa, F. D. (2010). Understanding endorphins and their importance in pain management. *Hawaii Med J*, 69, 70–71.

Stein, C. (1995). The control of pain in peripheral tissue by opioids. *N Engl J Med*, 332, 1685–1690.

Storm, H. (2008). Changes in skin conductance as a tool to monitor nociceptive stimulation and pain. *Curr Opin Anaesthesiol*, 21, 796–804.

Symons, F. J. (2011). Self-injurious behavior in neurodevelopmental disorders: relevance of nociceptive and immune mechanisms. *Neurosci Biobehav Rev*, 35, 1266–1274.

Tordjman, S., Anderson, G. M., Botbol, M., Brailly-Tabard, S., Perez-Diaz, F., Graignic, R., *et al.* (2009). Pain reactivity and plasma beta-endorphin in children and adolescents with autistic disorder. *PLoS One*, 4, e5289.

Valkenburg, A. J., Niehof, S. P., van Dijk, M., Verhaar, E. J., and Tibboel, D. (2012). Skin conductance peaks could result from changes in vital parameters unrelated to pain. *Pediatr Res*, 71, 375–379.

van Ravenswaaij-Arts, C. M., Hopman, J. C., Kollee, L. A., Stoelinga, G. B., and van Geijn, H. P. (1995). The influence of artificial ventilation on heart rate variability in very preterm infants. *Pediatr Res*, 37, 124–130.

Vatner, S. F., Marsh, J. D., and Swain, J. A. (1975). Effects of morphine on coronary and left ventricular dynamics in conscious dogs. *J Clin Invest*, 55, 207–217.

Voss, A., Schulz, S., Schroeder, R., Baumert, M., and Caminal, P. (2009). Methods derived from nonlinear dynamics for analysing heart rate variability. *Philos Transact A Math Phys Eng Sci*, 367, 277–296.

Wilder, J. (1962). Basimetric approach (law of initial value) to biological rhythms. *Ann N Y Acad Sci*, 98, 1211–1220.

CHAPTER 39

The neurophysiological evaluation of nociceptive responses in neonates

Ravi Poorun and Rebeccah Slater

Summary

Human pain and suffering is most often communicated by language. The ability to communicate verbally puts adults and older children at a distinct advantage over our young counterparts. Infants and newborns cannot talk—which makes the reliable subjective measurement of pain difficult in this population. In neonates, we have traditionally relied on objective measurements of physiological and behavioural responses to noxious stimulation (Stevens et al., 2007), and research continues to search for the best measures of pain in neonates (Stevens and Franck, 2001; see also Lee and Stevens, Chapter 35, this volume).

In this chapter we review the use of quantitative neurophysiological techniques to evaluate nociceptive responses in the central nervous system of the neonate. We will discuss how:

+ electromyography (EMG) can be used to measure flexion reflex withdrawal.

+ near-infrared spectroscopy (NIRS) and electroencephalography (EEG) can be used to measure brain activity evoked by noxious stimulation.

+ magnetic resonance imaging (MRI) may be exploited to investigate the development of nociceptive processing in the neonatal and infant brain.

The appropriate use of these techniques may help us understand how the functional development of the human brain enables processing of nociceptive stimuli.

Introduction

It was once a long-held belief that due to the immaturity of the peripheral and central nervous systems, neonates did not feel pain. Coupled with limited data regarding the safety and efficacy of analgesia in neonates, minimal analgesia was often administered for procedures that would most certainly be painful in adults (Anand et al., 1987). Over the past 30 years, the study of childhood and infant pain has evolved to become a subject of active research (McGrath and Unruh, 2002). It is now accepted that human infants process noxious stimuli, and that this information is transmitted to the brain. However, while the use of neurophysiological and neuroimaging techniques has been extensively used in the study of adult pain, these techniques have had relatively limited use in evaluating the response to nociceptive stimuli in neonates and infants. Neurophysiological measures in older children are discussed by Hermann (Chapter 40, this volume).

Key stages of anatomical development have been identified in the human infant brain, such as:

+ The growth of thalamocortical axons into the cortical plate from 26 gestational weeks (Kostovic and Judas, 2002).

+ The elaboration of terminals and onset of cortical differentiation from 31 weeks.

+ The formation of callosal and association pathways from 34 weeks (Kostovic and Judas, 2010).

However, almost nothing is known about the functional correlates of these events. Through investigation of the developing human nervous system we can try to ask 'What is the pattern of brain activity that underpins the human experience of pain?'. In the adult brain, numerous structures are involved in the experience of pain, including the brainstem, thalamus, and a rich variety of cortical areas, which includes the somatosensory cortex, cingulate cortex, insula, and amygdale (Tracey and Mantyh, 2007). However, the extent to which these structures are involved in infant pain is unknown. Direct measurement of brain activity, using a variety of techniques, will further our understanding of how noxious events are processed by the infant nervous system. In this chapter we will highlight some of the important advances that have been made using neurophysiological measures to study responses to noxious and non-noxious stimuli in early life.

Electromyography

Electromyography (EMG) records the electrical activity produced by skeletal muscle. In neonates, surface EMG is preferred over the more-invasive intramuscular EMG techniques, and is most often used to monitor the flexion reflex withdrawal activity of the underlying biceps femoris in the posterior thigh, or tibialis anterior in the anterolateral lower leg. The flexion withdrawal reflex (Sherrington, 1910) has been used in adult subjects to study the spinal processing of nociceptive stimuli (Willer, 1977) and analgesic sensitivity (Willer, 1985). In both preterm and term neonates, the flexion reflex can be evoked by mechanical or electrical stimulation (Andrews and Fitzgerald, 1994, 1997, 1999; Fitzgerald et al., 1989). However, the stimulus intensity or threshold or for eliciting reflex activity is lower than in adults (Hugon, 1973), and reflexes can be elicited by non-painful stimuli. Increasing age sees a gradual reorganization and decrease in spinal cord excitability (Jennings and Fitzgerald, 1996, 1998; see also Walker and Baccei, Chapter 6, this volume), which is accompanied by a rise in threshold of the neonatal withdrawal reflex (Andrews and Fitzgerald, 1994; Fitzgerald et al., 1988). Below 35 weeks postconceptual age, preterm infants display sensitization to innocuous stimuli and a reduction in threshold (Andrews and Fitzgerald, 1994) whilst older infants display habituation to the same non-noxious stimuli. Habituation is characterized by a reduction in the number of observed reflex withdrawal responses but with no alteration in withdrawal threshold following repeated stimulation (Andrews and Fitzgerald, 1994; Fitzgerald et al., 1988). Similarly, habituation of reflex responses can be seen in adults with intact or divided spinal cords (Dimitrijević and Nathan, 1970; Dimitrijević et al., 1972).

Over the postnatal period, somatosensory and motor pathways in the central nervous system (CNS) are continually maturing (Fitzgerald, 2005). While EMG techniques cannot tell us anything about the subjective experience or perception of pain, they are extremely useful in understanding the development of spinal nociceptive processing.

Near-infrared spectroscopy

Near-infrared spectroscopy (NIRS) can be used to measure blood and tissue oxygenation. The method is based on spectroscopic measurements of oxygenated and deoxygenated haemoglobin concentration and depends on the transparency of biological tissue to near-infrared light. It uses the optical property that the absorption of near-infrared light is dependent on the amount of oxygenated and deoxygenated haemoglobin present in the tissue (Owen-Reece et al., 1999). Source and detector pairs can be placed on the surface of the skull and local changes in the intensity of the emitted and absorbed light can quantify changes in tissue oxygenation. In addition, absolute parameters such as blood flow and cerebral blood volume can be calculated. The measurement of changes in haemodynamic activity—as a proxy measure of functional brain activity—is based on the assumption that increased tissue oxygenation represents an increase in regional cerebral blood flow, associated with an increase in underlying neural activity (Logothetis et al., 2001).

NIRS is widely used in neonatal research to measure functional activation of the cortex (Kusaka et al., 2004). Recently, this technique has been used in neonatal studies investigating cerebral responses following noxious stimulation. Cortical haemodynamic activity has been recorded in infants in response to noxious events, including heel lance, venepuncture, and endotracheal tube suctioning and repositioning (Bartocci et al., 2006; Limperopoulos et al., 2008; Slater et al., 2006, 2008). These studies suggest that an increase in haemoglobin concentration can be observed in the somatosensory cortex in preterm neonates from approximately 25 weeks of gestation. The magnitude of this activity is dependent on the infant's age, but is also influenced by other clinical features, such as the sleep state of the infants. Similar changes in haemoglobin concentration in the somatosensory cortex were not found when non-skin-breaking tactile stimuli were applied to the surface of the skin, even though reflex withdrawal responses were observed, suggesting the observed changes in brain activity were related to the noxious input.

Using NIRS for clinical bedside pain assessment remains challenging because movement artefacts can interfere with the quality of the recorded signal and there is an extremely high attrition rate for recording of high-quality data. However, with secure optode placement, movement artefacts can be minimized, and careful control of the infants' environment can improve the quality and accuracy of the recordings. Further NIRS studies have demonstrated that following noxious stimuli there is a good correlation between the magnitude of the haemodynamic changes recorded in the contralateral somatosensory cortex and the more classically recorded change in neonatal facial expression (Slater et al., 2009). Other experimental and clinical conditions have also been shown to alter the size of the haemodynamic response, such as the location of the stimulus and the number of prior painful procedures (Ozawa et al., 2010, 2011; Slater et al., 2006). Importantly, all these studies lead to the conclusion that infants who are exposed to noxious stimuli during this immature developmental period, process this information at the level of the cortex, even though some infants do not manifest an observable behavioural response (Slater et al., 2008).

These studies provide some evidence that preterm and newborn infant responses to noxious stimulation are not purely reflexive, but the information is transmitted to the infant cortex. While this does not provide evidence of the perception of pain and cannot tell us what an infant feels, it is likely that activity in higher-level cortical regions of the brain is necessary, though maybe not sufficient, for the perception of pain.

Electroencephalography and evoked potentials

Electroencephalography (EEG) has been extensively used to investigate neurological function in neonates and infants. The technique provides an opportunity to record the electrical activity generated by large populations of cerebral neurons. An EEG represents fluctuating electrical field potentials as a function of time, and the deflections represent changes in voltage and polarity. By recording from multiple electrode sites, it is possible to obtain a representation of the spatial distribution of the electric field recorded over the scalp. EEG is often characterized by the frequency and amplitude of the recorded activity and during the early neonatal period the characteristic patterns of EEG activity change rapidly with gestational age (André et al., 2010). For example, throughout early developmental there is a reduction in the discontinuity observed in the EEG recordings. In addition, an increase in characterized rhythmical patterns of activity, such as delta brushes and temporal sawtooth waveforms, is observed, followed by their subsequent disappearance (Dreyfus-Brisac and Monod, 1972). The identification of these characteristic patterns of EEG activity during this developmental period is often used in the clinical assessment of neonatal cerebral function.

EEG can be used to measure specific patterns of brain activity recorded in response to known stimuli. These evoked patterns of activity are referred to as evoked or event-related potentials. In neonatal pain research, specific changes in EEG activity have been recorded in response to acute noxious stimulation, such as a clinically essential heel lance (Slater et al., 2010a, 2010b). By considering the features of the evoked activity, such as the polarity, timing, and topography, inference can be made about the how the brain processes noxious sensory information.

An event-locking technique has been developed to enable the evoked neuronal activity following a single clinical noxious event to be recorded (Fabrizi et al., 2011; Worley et al., 2012). Use of this technique has provided electrophysiological evidence that the immature infant brain can discriminate between acute noxious and non-noxious stimulation from 35 gestational weeks (Slater et al., 2010a). These electrophysiological measures of nociceptive-specific brain activity are useful for understanding how the developing human brain responds to nociceptive stimuli, and may potentially be useful to test the ability of analgesic treatments in neonates to suppress these increases in brain activity. Nevertheless, these experimental studies are challenging and require specialist data acquisition and analysis skills (Fabrizi et al., 2011; Vanhatalo et al., 2009; Worley et al., 2012).

Investigation of the maturation of EEG responses to peripheral stimuli in infants from 28 weeks of gestation has shown that these evoked patterns of activity only become dominant after approximately 35 weeks of gestation (Fabrizi et al., 2011). There appears to be a gradual shift with advancing maturity, from non-specific bursts of neuronal activity to modality-specific activity that is discriminative between noxious and non-noxious events. A further study that has investigated clinical factors that modulate this activity demonstrates that infants born preterm (24–32 weeks of gestation) who have reached their due date have a larger evoked response following noxious stimulation than normal term-born infants (Slater et al., 2010b). In contrast, there is no difference in the magnitude of the evoked response following non-noxious simulation. Although it cannot be concluded that prior pain experience specifically alters the subsequent processing of nociceptive information, it is clear that some aspect of being born preterm differentially alters the cerebral response to nociceptive stimuli compared with non-noxious tactile stimuli. Recent magnetic resonance imaging (MRI) data supports this observation and suggests that early procedural pain in very preterm infants contributes to impaired brain development (Brummelte et al., 2012; see also Grunau, Chapter 4, this volume). It is possible that the anatomical alterations observed in infants exposed to excessive nociceptive inputs may underpin some of the functional differences in subsequent nociceptive processing.

Magnetic resonance imaging

MRI has revolutionized the way we approach pain research. Being non-invasive and non-ionizing, MRI is the ideal technique to investigate the anatomical (e.g. structure and maturation) and functional (e.g. activity and connectivity) networks of the brain involved in the CNS processing of sensory stimulation during early human development.

The transient subplate zone (Kostovic and Molliver, 1974) is one of the main signs of cortical immaturity (Kostovic and Vasung, 2009) and is significant for the normal development of the human telencephalon, which subsequently develops into the cerebral cortex and basal ganglia (Kostovic and Rakic, 1990; see also Fitzgerald, Chapter 8, this volume). From the subplate grows the thalamo-cortical and cortico-cortical connections (Kostovic and Rakic, 1990), with its neurons contributing to the first evoked potentials from 24 weeks of gestation (Hrbek et al., 1973). Standard MRI techniques allow for the assessment of brain development in infants. Highly sensitive assessment of grey and white matter and the differentiation of myelination in white matter can be visualized. *In vivo*, the transient subplate zone can be seen as an area of hypointensity on magnetic resonance images (Prayer et al., 2006), but after 32 weeks of gestation, the transient subplate zone becomes less visible (Kostovic and Vasung, 2009).

Functional MRI (fMRI) is a non-invasive technique that assesses cortical activation. The most commonly used contrast method is blood oxygen level-dependent (BOLD) imaging. BOLD measures the magnetic change in haemoglobin between the oxygenated and deoxygenated states that accompany neuronal activity (Logothetis and Pfeuffer, 2004; Ogawa et al., 1998), but it is important to be aware that BOLD measures dynamic changes in blood flow and is not directly linked to neural activity. In newborns, most fMRI studies have focused on the visual system, and have demonstrated that visual activation can be obtained in sedated infants (Souweidane et al., 1999). The ability to view abnormal decreases in visual activity (Panigrahy and Bluml, 2007), asymmetric, or absent activations (Bernal and Altman, 2004) makes fMRI a feasible tool to view the visual cortex in disease (Seghier and Hüppi, 2010). This could be extrapolated to other neonatal conditions, possibly including the assessment of pain. The non-invasive nature of fMRI allows for repeated scanning in children and longitudinal studies investigating the development of neural networks can be achieved.

In the MRI scanner, neonates and infants are asleep, either naturally or with sedation, and this is one of the major limitations of fMRI—due to the lack of cooperation, tasks involving active participation cannot be performed (Souweidane et al., 1999). However, even asleep, infants show distinct brain activations to cognitive (Redcay et al., 2008) and sensory (Seghier et al., 2006) passive tasks. A more recent discovery is the fluctuation in BOLD fMRI response to intrinsic neuronal activity (Fox and Raichle, 2007). Collecting fMRI data during periods of quiet rest (i.e. without any task) have revealed strong anatomical and functional connections forming a resting-state network (RSN) in the absence of external stimuli (Raichle and Snyder, 2007). Resting-states in infants born preterm or at term have found five consistent RSN cortical 'hubs': the primary visual cortex; bilateral sensorimotor areas; bilateral auditory cortex; a network including the precuneus area, lateral parietal cortex, and the cerebellum; as well as an anterior network that incorporated the medial and dorsolateral prefrontal cortex (Fransson et al., 2007). With resting-state networks being identified in healthy infants there is a growing interest in evaluating network alterations in infants with brain injury (Seghier and Hüppi, 2010).

In neonates, there is great potential for the various MRI techniques to elucidate the higher CNS processing of noxious stimuli. RSNs in healthy neonates do not entirely correspond to those commonly found in adults (Fransson et al., 2011). Assuming that the cortical hubs denote areas involved in tasks requiring high information processing (Sporns et al., 2007) some reorganization of RSNs must occur between birth and adulthood. It is proposed that cortical hubs in infants may be dominated by processes involving reflexive behaviour, and those in adults centred toward complex, adaptive behaviour (Fransson et al., 2011).

While MRI has been extensively used in adult pain studies, and specific network disruptions have been described in several adult pathologies including chronic back pain (Baliki et al., 2008), its application in children has only recently begun and to date has not been used to advance our understanding of infant pain. In adults, pain studies utilizing fMRI have involved healthy volunteers or patients. Despite the variability in individual experience, a central 'pain matrix' has been described with some areas of the brain showing consistent patterns of activation following noxious stimulation (Seifert and Maihofner, 2009). These brain areas include, but are not limited to, the thalamus, primary somatosensory cortex (S1), secondary somatosensory cortex (S2), insula, forebrain, and anterior cingulate cortex (ACC) (Tracey and Mantyh, 2007) and involves areas traditionally involved in modulating the cognitive (Apkarian et al., 2004) and emotional (Becerra et al., 2001) aspects of pain perception.

To date, there is only one MRI study investigating the processing of noxious stimuli in children (Hohmeister et al., 2010). Cerebral pain response in children and adolescents aged 11 to16 years were compared in children with experience of a neonatal intensive care unit (NICU) born preterm or at term, and term born children without NICU experience. Preterm but not term NICU children displayed an exaggerated noxious-specific response compared with controls when stimulated with moderately painful heat stimuli. Brain regions, which classically form part of the adult pain matrix, were activated during noxious stimulation but were not observed during non-painful warmth stimulation. Further, ex-preterm children displayed an increased sensitization to painful stimuli without habituation. This would suggest that in the long term, previous experience of NICU might cause neurodevelopmental changes and cause an alteration in some aspects of nociceptive processing (see also Hermann, Chapter 40, this volume).

A recent imaging development may begin to disclose the reorganization of cortical hubs. Diffusion tensor imaging (DTI) makes it possible to visualize the connections between different brain regions by measuring changes in the diffusion of water in white matter tracts (Alexander et al., 2007). DTI can identify differences between normal and abnormal tracts, and when combined with fMRI studies can help understand the structural connectivity between different brain regions (Hüppi and Dubois, 2006). With resting-state functional connectivity being based, but not exclusively, on direct anatomical connections (Damoiseaux and Greicius, 2009), the assessment of the functional and structural relationships in the infant brain may begin to be investigated.

Conclusion

The measurement of evoked brain activity in response to nociceptive stimuli in preterm and term born infants may help validate existing behavioural, somatic motor, and autonomic measures of nociception. In addition, these techniques may help in the development of more robust clinical tools for measuring infant pain. This brain-oriented approach to understanding nociception must be considered alongside the existing body of literature that characterizes the clearly observable neonatal behavioural and physiological responses to noxious stimulation. It would be ideal to develop a specific neural biomarker that is a direct correlate of pain experience, however, in the absence of language this is out of our grasp.

Any measure of activity in the CNS following a noxious input in non-verbal patients, be it behavioural, autonomical, or neurophysiological is ultimately a surrogate measure of the experience and cannot tell us what an infant feels. Nevertheless, direct measurement of brain activity may further our understanding of how noxious events are processed by the infant nervous system.

References

Alexander, A. L., Lee, J. E., Lazar, M., and Field, A. S. (2007). Diffusion tensor imaging of the brain. *Neurotherapeutics*, 4, 316–329.

André, M., Lamblin, M. D., d'Allest, A. M., Curzi-Dascalova, L., Moussalli-Salefranque, F., Nguyen The Tich, S., *et al.* (2010). Electroencephalography in premature and full-term infants. Developmental features and glossary. *Neurophysiol Clin*, 40(2), 59–124.

Anand, K. J., Sippell, W. G., and Aynsley-Green, A. (1987). Randomised trial of fentanyl anaesthesia in preterm babies undergoing surgery: effects on the stress response. *Lancet*, 1(8527), 243–248.

Andrews, K. A., and Fitzgerald, M. (1994). The cutaneous withdrawal reflex in human neonates: sensitization, receptive fields, and the effects of contralateral stimulation. *Pain*, 56, 95–101.

Andrews, K. A., and Fitzgerald, M. (1997). A comparison of the mechanically and electrically evoked flexion reflex as a quantifiable measure of responses to innocuous and noxious skin stimulation in human neonates. *J Physiology*, 501.P, 98P.

Andrews, K. A., and Fitzgerald, M. (1999). The cutaneous flexion reflex in human neonates: a quantitative study of threshold and stimulus/response characteristics, following single and repeated stimuli. *Dev Med Child Neurol*, 41, 696–703.

Apkarian, A. V., Sosa, Y., Krauss, B. R., Thomas, P. S., Fredrickson, B. E., Levy, R. E., *et al.* (2004). Chronic pain patients are impaired on an emotional decision-making task. *Pain*, 108, 129–136.

Baliki, M. N., Geha, P. Y., Apkarian, A. V., and Chialvo, D. R. (2008). Beyond feeling: chronic pain hurts the brain, disrupting the default-mode network dynamics. *J Neurosci*, 28, 1398–1403.

Bartocci, M., Bergqvist, L. L., Lagercrantz, H., and Anand, K. J. (2006). Pain activates cortical areas in the preterm newborn brain. *Pain*, 122(1–2), 109–117.

Becerra, L., Breiter, H. C., Wise, R., Gonzalez, R. G., and Borsook, D. (2001). Reward circuitry activation by noxious thermal stimuli. *Neuron*, 32, 927–946.

Bernal, B. and Altman, N. (2004). Visual functional magnetic resonance imaging in patients with Sturge-Weber syndrome. *Pediatr Neurol*, 31, 9–15.

Brummelte, S., Grunau, R. E., Chau, V., Poskitt, K. J., Brant, R., Vinall, J., *et al.* (2012). Procedural pain and brain development in premature newborns. *Ann Neurol*, 71(3), 385–396

Damoiseaux, J. S., and Greicius, M. D. (2009). Greater than the sum of the parts: a review of studies combining structural and resting-state functional connectivity. *Brain Struct Funct*, 213, 525–533.

Dimitrijević, M. R., Faganel, J., Gregoric, M., Nathan, P. W., and Trontelj, J. K. (1972). Habituation: effects of regular and stochastic stimulation. *J Neurol Neurosurg Psychiatry*, 35, 234–242.

Dimitrijević, M. R., and Nathan, P. W. (1970). Studies of spasticity in man. IV: changes in flexion reflex with repetitive cutaneous stimulation in spinal man. *Brain*, 93, 743–768.

Dreyfus-Brisac, C. and Monod, N. (1972). The electroencephalogram of fulterm newborns and premature infants. In A. Remond, and G. C. Lairy (eds) *Handbook of electroencephalography and clinical neurophysiology*, pp. 6–23. Amsterdam: Elsevier.

Fabrizi, L., Slater, R., Worley, A., Meek, J., Boyd, S., Olhede, S., *et al.* (2011). A shift in sensory processing that enables the developing human brain to discriminate touch from pain. *Curr Biology*, 21(18), 1552–1558.

Fabrizi, L., Worley, A., Patten, D., Holdridge, S., Cornelissen, L., Meek, J., *et al.* (2011). Electrophysiological measurements and analysis of nociception in human infants. *J Vis Exp*, 58, 3118.

Fitzgerald, M. (2005). The development of nociceptive circuits. *Nature Rev Neurosci*, 6, 507–520.

Fitzgerald, M., Millard, C., and MacIntosh, N. (1989). Cutaneous hypersensitivity following peripheral tissue damage in newborn infants and its reversal with topical anaesthesia. *Pain*, 39, 31–36.

Fitzgerald, M., Shaw, A., and Macintosh, N. (1988). The postnatal development of the cutaneous flexor reflex: comparative study of preterm infants and newborn rat pups. *Dev Med Child Neurol*, 30, 520–526.

Fox, M. D., and Raichle, M. E. (2007). Spontaneous fluctuations in brain activity observed with functional magnetic resonance imaging. *Nature Rev Neurosci*, 8, 700–711.

Fransson, P., Aden, U., Blennow, M., and Lagercrantz, H. (2011). The functional architecture of the infant brain as revealed by resting-state fMRI. *CerebCortex*, 21(1), 145–154.

Fransson, P., Skiöld, B., Horsch, S., Nordell, A., Blennow, M., Lagercrantz, H., *et al.* (2007). Resting-state networks in the infant brain. *Proc Natl Acad Sci U S A*, 104, 15531–15536.

Hohmeister, J., Kroll, A., Wollgarten-Hadamek, I., Zohsel, K., Demirakça, S., Flor, H., *et al.* (2010). Cerebral processing of pain in school-aged children with neonatal nociceptive input: an exploratory fMRI study. *Pain*, 150(2), 257–267.

Hrbek, A., Karlberg, P., and Olsson, T. (1973). Development of visual and somatosensory evoked responses in pre-term newborn infants. *Electroencephalogr Clin Neurophysiol*, 34, 225–232.

Hugon, M. (1973). Exteroceptive reflexes to stimulation of the sural nerve in normal man. In J. E. Desmedt, (ed.) *New developments in electromyography and clinical neurophysiology. Vol. 3*, pp. 713–729. Basel: Karger.

Hüppi, P. S., and Dubois, J. (2006). Diffusion tensor imaging of brain development. *Semin Fetal Neonat Med*, 11, 489–497.

Jennings, E. and Fitzgerald, M. (1996). C-Fos can be induced in the neonatal rat spinal cord by both noxious and innocuous peripheral stimulation. *Pain*, 68, 301–306.

Jennings, E. and Fitzgerald, M. (1998). Postnatal changes in responses of rat dorsal horn cells to afferent stimulation: a fibre induced sensitisation. *J Physiol*, 509, 859–867.

Kostovic, I. and Judas, M. (2002). Correlation between the sequential ingrowth of afferents and transient patterns of cortical lamination in preterm infants. *Anat Rec*, 267(1), 1–6.

Kostovic, I. and Judas, M. (2010). The development of the subplate and thalamocortical connections in the human foetal brain. *Acta Paediatr*, 99, 1119–1127.

Kostovic, I. and Molliver, M. E. (1974). A new interpretation of the laminar development of the cerebral cortex: synaptogenesis in different layers of neopallium in the human fetus. American Association of Anatomists. Eighty seventh annual session. *Anat Rec*, 178, 395.

Kostovic, I. and Rakic, P. (1990). Developmental history of the transient subplate zone in the visual and somatosensory cortex of the macaque monkey and human brain. *J Comp Neurol*, 297, 441–470.

Kostovic, I. and Vasung, L. (2009). Insights from in vitro fetal magnetic resonance imaging of cerebral development. *Semin Perinatol*, 33, 220–233.

Kusaka, T., Kawada, K., Okubo, K., Nagano, K., Namba, M., Okada, H., *et al.* (2004). Noninvasive optical imaging in the visual cortex in young infants. *Hum Brain Mapp*, 22(2), 122–132.

Limperopoulos, C., Gauvreau, K. K., O'Leary, H., Moore, M., Bassan, H., Eichenwald, E. C., *et al.* (2008). Cerebral hemodynamic changes during intensive care of preterm infants. *Pediatrics*, 122(5), e1006–1013.

Logothetis, N. K., Pauls, J., Augath, M., Trinath, T., and Oeltermann, A. (2001). Neurophysiological investigation of the basis of the fMRI signal. *Nature*, 412(6843), 150–157.

Logothetis, N. K., and Pfeuffer, J (2004). On the nature of the BOLD fMRI contrast mechanism. *Magn Res Imaging*, 22, 1517–1531.

McGrath, P. J., and Unruh, A. M. (2002). The social context of neonatal pain. *Clin Perinatol*, 29(3), 555–572.

Ogawa, S., Menon, R. S., Kim, S. G., and Ugurbil, K. (1998). On the characteristics of functional magnetic resonance imaging of the brain. *Annu Rev Biophys Biomol Struct*, 27, 447–474.

Owen-Reece, H., Smith, M., Elwell, C. E., and Goldstone, J. C. (1999). Near infrared spectroscopy. *Br J Anaesth*, 82(3), 418–426.

Ozawa, M., Kanda, K., Hirata, M., Kusakawa, I., and Suzuki, C. (2010). Effect of gender and hand laterality on pain processing in human neonates. *Early Hum Dev*, 87(1), 45–48.

Ozawa, M., Kanda, K., Hirata, M., Kusakawa, I., and Suzuki, C. (2011). Influence of repeated painful procedures on prefrontal cortical pain responses in newborns. *Acta Paediatr*, 100(2), 198–203.

Panigrahy, A. and Bluml, S. (2007). Advances in magnetic resonance neuroimaging techniques in the evaluation of neonatal encephalopathy. *Top Magn Res Imaging*, 18, 3–29.

Prayer, D., Kasprian, G., Krampl, E., Ulm, B., Witzani, L., Prayer, L., *et al.* (2006). MRI of normal fetal brain development. *Eur J Radiol*, 57, 199–216.

Raichle, M. E., and Snyder, A. Z. (2007). A default mode of brain function: a brief history of an evolving idea. *Neuroimage*, 37, 1083–1090.

Redcay, E., Haist, F., and Courchesne, F. (2008). Functional neuroimaging of speech perception during a pivotal period in language acquisition. *Dev Sci*, 1, 237–252.

Seghier, M. L., and Hüppi, P. S. (2010). The role of functional magnetic resonance imaging in the study of brain development, injury, and recovery in the newborn. *Semin Perinatol*, 34(1), 79–86.

Seghier, M. L., Lazeyras, F., and Hüppi, P. S. (2006). Functional MRI of the newborn. *Semin Fetal Neonat Med*, 11, 479–488.

Seifert, F. and Maihofner, C. (2009). Central mechanisms of experimental and chronic neuropathic pain: findings from functional imaging studies. *Cell Mol Life Sci*, 66(3), 375–390.

Sherrington, C. S. (1910). Flexion reflex of the limb, crossed extension reflex, and reflex stepping and standing. *J Physiol*, 40, 28–121.

Slater, R., Cantarella, A., Franck, L., Meek, J., and Fitzgerald, M. (2008). How well do clinical pain assessment tools reflect pain in infants? *PLoS Med*, 5(6), e129.

Slater, R., Cantarella, A., Gallella, S., Worley, A., Boyd, S., Meek, J., *et al.* (2006). Cortical pain responses in human infants. *J Neurosci*, 26(14), 3662–3666.

Slater, R., Cantarella, A., Yoxen, J., Patten, D., Potts, H., Meek, J., *et al.* (2009). Latency to facial expression change following noxious stimulation in infants is dependent on postmenstrual age. *Pain*, 146(1–2), 177–182.

Slater, R., Fabrizi, L., Worley, A., Meek, J., Boyd, S., and Fitzgerald, M. (2010a). Premature infants display increased noxious-evoked neuronal activity in the brain compared to healthy age-matched term-born infants. *Neuroimage*, 52(2), 583–589.

Slater, R., Worley, A., Fabrizi, L., Roberts, S., Meek, J., Boyd, S., *et al.* (2010b). Evoked potentials generated by noxious stimulation in the human infant brain. *Eur J Pain*, 14(3), 321–326.

Souweidane, M. M., Kim, K. H., McDowall, R., Ruge, M. I., Lis, E., Krol, G., *et al.* (1999). Brain mapping in sedated infants and young children with passive-functional magnetic resonance imaging. *Pediatr Neurosurg*, 30, 86–89.

Sporns, O., Honey, C. J., and Kötter, R. (2007). Identification and classification of hubs in brain networks. *PLoS One*, 2(10), e1049.

Stevens, B. J., and Franck, L. S. (2001). Assessment and management of pain in neonates. *Paediatr Drugs*, 3, 539–558.

Stevens, B. J., Pillai Riddell, R. R., Oberlander, T. E., and Gibbins, S. (2007). Assessment of pain in neonates and infants. In K. J. Anand, B. J. Stevens, and P. J. McGrath, (eds) *Pain in neonates and infants* (3rd edn), pp. 67–90. Edinburgh: Elsevier.

Tracey, I. and Mantyh, P. W. (2007). The cerebral signature for pain perception and its modulation. *Neuron*, 55(3), 377391.

Vanhatalo, S., Jousmäki, V., Andersson, S., and Metsäranta, M. (2009). An easy and practical method for routine, bedside testing of somatosensory systems in extremely low birth weight infants. *Pediatr Res*, 66(6), 710–713.

Willer, J. C. (1977). Comparative study of perceived pain and nociceptive flexion reflex in man. *Pain*, 3, 69–80.

Willer, J. C. (1985). Studies on pain: the effects of morphine on a spinal nociceptive flexion reflex and related pain sensation in man. *Brain Res*, 331, 105–114.

Worley, A., Fabrizi, L., Boyd, S., and Slater, R. (2012). Multi-modal pain measurements in infants. *J Neurosci Methods*, 205, 252–257.

CHAPTER 40

Sensory processing and neurophysiological evaluation in children

Christiane Hermann

Summary

Traditionally, pain in children is assessed by behavioural observation and by self-report with a focus on perceived pain intensity. In this chapter, more recently developed standardized psychophysical procedures to assess abnormalities in sensory and pain processing and non-invasive neurophysiological methods to unravel the neuronal mechanisms underlying the experience of pain are described and how they have been used for investigating paediatric pain. For both sensory and neurophysiological assessment methods, the underlying assumptions and theoretical underpinnings are outlined. Following a brief overview of commonly used measures and methods, methodological issues are addressed that need to be considered when planning to use such methods and when interpreting the obtained findings. Finally, empirical examples are reviewed that highlight the use of these techniques for addressing major research questions such as the development of pain processing and changes in sensory and pain processing associated with chronic paediatric pain.

Introduction

The International Association for the Study of Pain (IASP) defines pain 'as an unpleasant sensory and emotional experience associated with actual or potential tissue damage, or described in terms of such damage' (Merskey and Bogduk, 1994, p. 210). Accordingly, sensory processing represents a core component of the pain experience. Pain needs to be distinguished from nociception. Nociception entails all physiological processes involved in the transduction of nociceptive (i.e. noxious or potentially tissue-damaging) input by receptors, and the peripheral and central neuronal activity involved in the subsequent processing of nociceptive input. By contrast, pain is a complex subjective experience that is correlated with nociceptive activity, but is not fully accounted for by it. Dating back to the nineteenth century, psychophysics has evolved as the scientific study of the relationship between physical stimuli (e.g. visual, auditory) and the subjective perception they induce. For the sensory evaluation in pain states, a variety of psychophysical methods, often referred to as quantitative sensory testing, have been developed that allow quantification of an individual's subjective response to painful and non-painful stimuli. Although abnormal psychophysical findings have been related to specific neuronal mechanisms, such interpretations remain putative as the neuronal substrate is not directly assessed.

For investigating neuronal mechanisms of pain, many neurophysiological methods ranging from single-cell or nerve fibre recordings to neuroimaging are available. Here, the focus lies on non-invasive neuroimaging methods such as near-infrared spectroscopy (NIRS), electroencephalography (EEG), and functional magnetic resonance imaging (fMRI) which have been used for studying paediatric pain. Neurophysiological methods for the diagnosis of disease-related pathology will not be addressed.

Quantitative sensory testing

Over the past 25 years, quantitative sensory testing (QST) has been developed as a method to systematically assess the functioning of sensory and pain pathways. Interest in QST originally grew from efforts for a better diagnosis and mechanism-based understanding of neuropathic pain. Neuropathic pain is of neurogenic origin and arises as a direct consequence of lesions or diseases of the somatosensory system (Treede et al., 2008; see Walker Chapter 21, this volume). It is characterized by various symptoms and signs such as sensory loss, paraesthesias, spontaneous onging or paroxysmal pain, and stimulus-evoked pain presumably resulting from pathophysiological somatosensory functioning. The traditional clinical exam of these symptoms has limitations as it is mostly qualitative in nature and lacks standardization of stimulation and measurement (Hansson et al., 2007).

QST has been derived from experimental psychophysical methods. Traditionally, psychophysical procedures can be divided into two broad classes depending on whether it is the stimulus or the response that is the primary dependent variable (Gracely, 2006). Response-dependent methods assess individuals' variable responses to a predefined set of stimuli. Examples are almost all methods used for measuring suprathreshold pain such as rating scales. Stimulus-dependent psychophysical methods entail the administration of varying stimuli with a fixed response and it is stimulus intensity that is measured. Typically, such stimulus-dependent methods are used for determining thresholds. Yet, they also allow suprathreshold pain assessment such as pain tolerance. For determining thresholds, three classical psychophysical procedures are established.

Method of limits (MLI): this method entails the administration of stimuli of varying intensity until the subject notes a certain sensation and indicates this verbally or behaviourally. Usually, stimuli are delivered in ascending series, the subject's response stops further increase in intensity. Sensory detection and pain thresholds are defined as the stimulus intensity required to evoke a given sensation (e.g. touch, warmth) or pain, respectively. Whereas sensory detection thresholds rely on discriminating the presence versus absence of a specific sensation, pain thresholds are not only influenced by perceptual sensitivity, but also by the given verbal label and the subject's pain labelling behaviour and the ensuing response bias (Gracely, 2006). In order to reduce expectancy or habituation effects, it is often recommended to use both ascending and descending series. MLI is reaction-time dependent (Yarnitsky and Ochoa, 1990). Most likely, this accounts for thermal thresholds being about 1.5°C higher when determined by MLI as compared to reaction-time independent methods (e.g. Defrin et al., 2006; children: Meier et al., 2001). Despite this limitation, MLI is frequently used because instructions are simple and it is less time-consuming than other procedures. There are reaction time-independent MLI variants. The method of levels entails the administration of stimuli with pre-defined intensity and the subject's response is recorded. Depending on the subject's positive or negative response, stimulus intensity is systematically either decreased (following a positive response) or increased (following a negative response) until it converges onto the threshold (Meier et al., 2001; Yarnitsky et al., 1990). Stimulus intensity can either be changed in absolute steps or in steps of modality-specific, just noticeable, differences (Yarnitsky, 1997). Reaction-time independent measures are more reliable than reaction-time dependent measures, but require more trials (Yarnitsky, 1997).

Method of constant stimuli: similar to MLI, the subject is exposed to a set of stimuli with predefined intensity above and below the threshold of interest. However, these stimuli are presented randomly and the subject is asked to indicate whether or not the stimulus evoked a certain sensation. The threshold is defined as the intensity that the subject reports as the sensation of interest in 50% of the trials.

Method of adjustment: unlike MLI, this method requires the subject to directly adjust stimulus intensity until a certain sensation occurs. This procedure has to be repeated many times. Aside from the long duration, it is disadvantageous in that some of the stimulation devices for certain pain modalities do not allow the subject to control stimulus intensity.

In most cases, QST protocols exclusively rely on MLI for determining sensory detection and pain thresholds; mostly for practical reasons, such as keeping the duration of the testing within reasonable limits. Length of testing is an issue because the subject should be alert and awake and motivated to cooperate with the experimenter.

QST measures

Sensory modalities

Quantitative sensory testing does not refer to defined set of measures. QST measures can broadly be categorized as static or dynamic (Arendt-Nielsen and Yarnitsky, 2009). Threshold measures (e.g. detection, pain) and pain magnitude ratings for a given stimulus are typically considered as 'static' and are used for assessing the basal state of the somatosensory system. Threshold determination

is helpful for detecting sensory losses and gains such as altered pain sensitivity (hyperalgesia, allodynia, hyperpathia). Including suprathreshold stimuli is important because hypersensitivity can be observed if thresholds are reduced, elevated, or unchanged. 'Dynamic' measures require activation of the pain system such that possible changes in specific mechanisms of pain processing become evident. For example, sensitization to nociceptive input is a key factor in the development of chronic pain. Such sensitization occurs in the peripheral and the central nervous system (Woolf, 2011). In humans, temporal summation (i.e. the increase in perceived pain intensity upon prolonged or repetitive painful stimulation), is considered to represent a perceptual correlate primarily of central sensitization (e.g. Granot et al., 2006). Accordingly, some QST protocols include measures of temporal summation. The testing of descending pain inhibitory mechanisms using procedures of painful counter-irritation is another example of a dynamic QST measure.

Comprehensive QST protocols usually include the testing of different sensory modalities such as thermal, touch, pressure, and vibratory stimuli. For obvious reasons of impracticability and problems of standardization, chemical stimulation is not included. Testing different sensory modalities allows the assessment of the integrity of different types of receptors, peripheral nerve fibres and information integration within the central nervous system. Mechanical stimuli such as light touch, pressure, or punctate stimuli activate Aß, Aδ, and C fibres (see Table 40.1; Walk et al., 2009). The processing of warm and heat stimuli is dependent on C-fibre activation, cold sensations and noxious cold involve Aδ-fibre and C-fibre activity, respectively. The processing of painful stimuli is mediated both by modality-specific and convergent pathways (Craig, 2003). Hence, pain sensation is the result of central integration of sensory non-nociceptive information and nociceptor input (Defrin et al., 2002). Accordingly, correlations between (supra-)threshold measures across modalities are typically low (e.g. Bhalang et al., 2005). Indeed, factor analyses of different pain modality measures (e.g. heat, ischaemic, pressure, electrical) revealed separate factors each representing a sensory modality (Hastie et al., 2005; Neziri et al., 2011a). In addition, measures of temporal summation loaded on a separate factor, supporting the distinction between static and dynamic measures (Hastie et al., 2005).

Sensory testing site

When performing QST, the choice of testing sites is important. The obtained values vary considerably between different body regions (e.g. Defrin et al., 2006; children: Hogeweg et al., 1996; Meier et al., 2001; Meh and Denislic, 1994). In one of the most comprehensive studies in healthy adults, QST was performed bilaterally on the face, and at the hand and foot (Rolke et al., 2006b). Similarly, in children, while no left–right differences were observed, sensitivity was highest in the face and lowest in the foot and, with intermediate values in the hand (Blankenburg et al., 2010). Presumably, this region-specific sensitivity is accounted for by differences in innervation and/or thickness of the epidermis. However, these differences, at least for thresholds obtained by MLI, may also be a result of reaction-time-dependent threshold determination. If the method of levels rather than MLI was used, differences in sensitivity between body regions such as foot versus upper body were no longer observed, at least for thermal stimuli (Defrin et al., 2006). Although, in healthy subjects, thermal pain sensitivity does not

Table 40.1 Overview of the QST measures included in the German Research Network on Neuropathic Pain (DFNS) QST protocol (Rolke et al., 2006) as used in a large sample of healthy children and adolescents for determining normative reference values (Blankenburg et al., 2010)

Static measures	QST parameter	Peripheral nerve fibre	Testing procedure	Testing device
Thermal				
Cold	Detection threshold (CDT)	Aδ	MLI (descending)	Computer-controlled contact heat probe (e.g. TSA II, MEDOC, Israel, or MSA, SOMEDIC, Sweden)
	Pain threshold (CPT)	C, Aδ	MLI (descending)	
Warm/heat	Detection threshold (WDT)	C	MLI (ascending)	
	Pain threshold (HPT)	C, Aδ	MLI (ascending)	
Cold/warm	Thermal sensory limen (TSL)	C, Aδ	Alternating warm/cold stimuli	
	Paradoxical heat sensations (during TSL)		Verbal report	
Mechanical				
Cutaneous punctate				
blunt	Detection threshold (MDT)	Aß	MLI (ascending + descending)	von Frey filaments
sharp	Pain threshold (MPT)	Aδ, C	MLI (ascending + descending)	Calibrated pinpricks (N=7; 8–512 mN)
Deep pressure	Pain threshold (PPT)	Aδ, C	MLI (ascending)	Pressure algometer
Vibration	Detection threshold (VDT)	Aß	MLI (descending)	Tuning fork
Dynamic and other measures				
Mechanical				
Sharp	Pain sensitivity	Aδ, C	Numerical pain intensity ratings for all 7 pinpricks (5 repetitions each in pseudo-randomized order)	Calibrated pinpricks (N = 7 with intensities 8–512 mN)
	Wind-up ratio (temporal summation)	Aδ, C	Mean pain rating of 5 series of repetitive stimuli relative to mean pain rating of 5 single stimuli	
Dynamic light touch	Dynamic mechanical allodynia	Aß	Mean numerical pain rating for the 3 touch intensities	3 levels of force: cotton wisp, cotton wool tip, brush

MLI = method of limits.

seem to vary between different parts of the hand (i.e. dorsum, finger, thenar eminence), its interindividual variability is lowest at the thenar eminence, thus facilitating use of this site for normative reference data (Hagander et al., 2000).

Comprehensive standardized QST protocol example

QST in research and in clinical practice requires standardized procedures that promise sufficient reliability, allow comparisons across studies, and reference to norms (e.g. Walk et al., 2009). Most recently, the German Research Network on Neuropathic Pain (DFNS) compiled a battery of tests for sensory loss (small and large fibres) and sensory gain (hyperalgesia, allodynia, hyperpathia) (Rolke et al., 2006b). In two sensory modalities (mechanical, thermal), and bilaterally at three measurement sites (face, hand, foot), both static (detection and pain thresholds) and dynamic (e.g. temporal summation) QST parameters are assessed in a fixed order within one session with detection thresholds determined prior to pain thresholds and suprathreshold measures. Table 40.1 gives a more detailed overview of the obtained QST parameters. The DFNS QST battery is unique as it is the only QST battery for which data in healthy adults, different pain populations and children (Blankenburg et al., 2010, 2011) have been obtained.

Psychometric considerations: normative QST data

The clinical usefulness of QST depends on relating individual QST findings to reference data. For the DFNS QST battery, normative data are available for both healthy adults (Rolke et al., 2006b; for a similar protocol see Neziri et al., 2011b) and children (Blankenburg et al., 2010). These data for children compare fairly well with previous reports for selected measures in healthy children using similar instructions and devices (e.g. Hilz et al., 1996, 1998a, 1998b; Meier et al., 2001). However, values can differ when compared to studies using at least slightly different procedures and smaller samples with a greater age range (e.g. Thibault et al., 1994; Walker et al., 2009). By comparing the patient's profile of sensory losses and gains to such normative data, absolute references can be made (Magerl et al., 2010). Alternatively, relative references are possible. Neuropathic pain often affects only one side of the body. In light of the lack of left–right differences in healthy individuals, the unaffected side can then be used as a within-subject (relative) reference and allows characterization of the pattern of disturbed sensory functioning on the affected side (e.g. Kemler et al., 2000).

Psychometric considerations: reliability of QST

Aside from the availability of normative data, adequate reliability is another prerequisite for validity and clinical usefulness of QST. In their review of the literature, Siao and Cros (2003) concluded that reproducibility of QST findings varied greatly across studies depending on study methodology, sample size, type of study sample, number of examiners, and retest interval. More recently, in healthy adults and patients, retest reliability both for comprehensive QST batteries or thermal measures was reported as good, at least for retest intervals ranging between 1 to 2 days and up to 3 weeks (e.g. Agostinho et al., 2009; Geber et al., 2011; Heldestad et al., 2010; Moloney et al., 2011; Wylde et al., 2011). In children, retest reliability has not been systematically investigated in sufficiently large healthy and patient samples. Determination of pressure pain thresholds has excellent retest reliability in children with orthopaedic disorders, at least when measured on the same day (Nikolajsen et al., 2011). Similarly, retest reliability for sensory detection thresholds is good (Hilz et al., 1996; Thibault et al., 1994).

In most studies, retest reliability has been determined by computing correlations, the coefficient of variation, or by comparing the means for test–retest measurements. However, these statistical procedures only determine the strength of association, but not agreement (Bland and Altman, 1986). In addition, these tests are based on groups and cannot be applied when deciding on the clinical significance of findings. Derived from the Bland–Altmann graphical procedure for determining agreement between measurement methods, the coefficient of repeatability is a measure of normal day-to-day variability, thus providing limits of normal variation (Bland et al., 1986). For example, in a study in healthy adults, normal limits for heat pain threshold (thenar) ranged between 39.5°C and 51.9°C and the coefficient of repeatability was 5.6 °C, i.e. a difference between heat pain thresholds measured on different occasions in the same subject must exceed this magnitude in order to be considered a true difference (Sand et al., 2010).

Since QST is performed by an examiner, interrater reliability is also important. In adults, for the DFNS QST battery, good interrater reliability has been demonstrated both for computer-assisted (thermal) and manually obtained (mechanical) QST parameters (Geber et al., 2011). Notably, the experimenters had undergone extensive training at one centre. In other studies, interrater reliability was substantially lower (e.g. Peters et al., 2003). Similarly, in healthy children, interrater reliability for pressure pain is satisfactory, but lower than retest reliability (Nikolajsen et al., 2011).

Overall, both retest and interrater reliability of QST in children and adolescents requires systematic empirical evaluation. In order to maximize reliability, examiners should follow a highly standardized measurement protocol and be sufficiently trained.

Modulating influences on QST measurement outcomes

Being a psychophysical procedure, QST relies on the subject's perception and response behaviour. Hence, procedural, contextual and interindividual factors may influence the outcome of QST and further underline the necessity for standardization.

Procedural and methodological influences

QST parameters are typically determined by calculating the mean of several (N = 3–7) trials in order to yield more reliable estimates. In one of the few studies testing this assumption, cold, but not warm detection and cold pain thresholds significantly decreased from the first to the second trial with no further change across six additional trials (Agostinho et al., 2009). Heat pain threshold strongly increased from the first to the sixth trial; such habituation to painful heat is mediated by peripheral and central processes (Greffrath et al., 2007). The order of the tests may also be relevant. For example, mechanical pain sensitivity was higher and mechanical pain threshold lower when thermal testing preceded mechanical testing as opposed to when mechanical testing was

performed first (Grone et al., 2012). For the thermal modality, no order effects were observed. Initial assessment of pain threshold may also exert a confounding influence on the determination of detection thresholds, at least for thermal stimuli (Heldestad et al., 2010). Especially for thermal testing using contact heat, starting temperature (e.g. Hilz et al., 1995), rate of the temperature increase (e.g. Yarnitsky et al., 1990) and size of skin area (e.g. Khalili et al., 2001) influence the obtained values due to spatial and temporal summation (cf. Jorum and Arendt-Nielsen, 2003). Furthermore, room and skin temperature can have an effect (Hilz et al., 1995; Strigo et al., 2000).

Contextual influences

While it is well established that pain responses are modulated by the psychosocial context in which they occur, surprisingly little is known about how these factors impact on QST findings. We observed that mothers' presence during QST testing decreased children's pain sensitivity although mothers only observed the testing from a distance and did not interact with their children (Hohmeister et al., 2009; Zohsel et al., 2006). This modulating influence could be accounted for by perceived social support and/or by distraction. Situationally induced anxiety may also exert a modulating influence. For example, in children undergoing thermal, pressure, and cold pain tasks anticipatory anxiety accounted for about 30% of variance in pain report across tasks (Tsao et al., 2004). By contrast, pain-related coping including catastrophizing does not affect QST results in children (Blankenburg et al., 2011). Biological variables such as circadian rhythms may also modulate QST findings. Very few systematic studies exist, but did not confirm robust circadian patterns of heat pain thresholds (e.g. Bachmann et al., 2011).

Interindividual age-related differences

In adults, age and gender influence QST results (e.g. Neziri et al., 2011b). Healthy participants older than 40 years of age as compared to younger participants had significantly higher detection and pain thresholds except for mechanical pain sensitivity measures (Rolke et al., 2006a; see also Hilz et al., 1998a; Meh et al., 1994). Whether sensory and pain sensitivity undergoes a developmental change during childhood and adolescence is less clear. In a first study using the DFNS QST battery, young children (6–8 years) had higher thermal and detection thresholds and lower heat, pressure and mechanical pain thresholds when compared to older children (9–12 years) and adolescents (13–16 years) with the latter two groups not differing significantly (Blankenburg et al., 2010). Yet, in a follow-up study comparing exclusively 7- and 14-year-olds (Blankenburg et al., 2011), the age effect for warmth and mechanical detection thresholds was not confirmed, an age-related increase in pain thresholds was again observed and is consistent with previous reports (e.g. Haslam, 1969; Hogeweg et al., 1996). Earlier studies also found detection thresholds to be age-insensitive; however, most of these studies focused on only one sensory modality, and were limited in sample size and age range (e.g. Hilz et al., 1996; Meh et al., 1994; Thibault et al., 1994). Undoubtedly, somatosensory and pain processing undergoes functional maturation, especially during the first year of life (Fitzgerald, 2005). Whether such developmental changes in somatosensory functioning and pain processing continue during childhood and adolescence, is less clear. Importantly, it cannot fully be ruled out that QST in young children may also be less reliable due to the reaction-time dependence of many QST measures, and due to the fact that QST parameters do not only reflect sensory sensitivity, but also entail a response bias component (Gracely, 2006). Possibly, this response bias, rather than the actual sensitivity, may change throughout childhood and adolescence.

Interindividual sex-related differences

In healthy adults undergoing QST, females have significantly lower pain thresholds than men, whereas no effect of sex on detection thresholds was observed (Rolke et al., 2006a). This sex-related difference in pain sensitivity is consistent with conclusions of an earlier meta-analysis on sex-related differences in pain sensitivity (Riley et al., 1998). In youth, few studies have systematically addressed this issue. In a large cohort of about 175 healthy children and adolescents between 6 and 16 years old, girls had significantly lower detection for thermal, pressure, and vibratory stimuli and lower thermal and pressure pain thresholds, whereas no sex-related differences with regard to mechanical stimuli was observed (Blankenburg et al., 2010). By contrast, in a follow-up study of 7- and 14-year olds, no sex differences in pain sensitivity emerged, girls had only lower warmth detection thresholds (Blankenburg et al., 2011). Similarly, no sex differences with regard to pressure pain thresholds were observed in children with orthopaedic disorders (Nikolajsen et al., 2011). Blankenburg et al. speculated that puberty and the concomitant hormonal changes presumably account for the emerging sex differences in pain sensitivity in adulthood. However, a recent meta-analysis of the experimental literature concluded that even in healthy adults, there is no clear and consistent pattern of sex differences in pain sensitivity (Racine et al., 2012a). One explanation may be that rather than biological sex differences, it is psychosocial factors that determine whether or not sex differences are observed (Racine et al., 2012b). Specifically, gender role stereotypes may be particularly important in determining one's response to painful stimulation (Alabas et al., 2012). This could at least partially explain why sex differences in pain sensitivity are not consistently found both in adults and in youth.

Related to the issue of possible sex difference, it has been suggested that subjects' responses especially to painful stimuli may depend on the sex of the experimenter. While such an influence of experimenter sex has been documented in some studies, Racine et al. (2012b) concluded that the available empirical literature in adults does not support a clear and consistent pattern of influence. In children and adolescents, the issue of experimenter sex influencing QST measurements has not been systematically addressed.

Use of QST in children and adolescents

QST is feasible in children as young as 6 years of age (Blankenburg et al., 2010; Hogeweg et al., 1996). Thermal detection thresholds have even been measured in preschool children at the age of 4 years (Hilz et al., 1996). In children, QST studies have focused on three research questions. Specifically, altered sensory and pain processing has been studied in the context of:

♦ Chronic pain problems with or without putative sensory abnormalities.

♦ Diseases with an increased risk for neuropathic pain.

♦ Delineating the impact of neonatal pain.

Chronic paediatric pain is associated with enhanced pain sensitivity as indicated by lowered pain thresholds and augmented temporal summation which, however, does not necessarily affect all sensory modalities (e.g. Walco et al., 1990; Zohsel et al., 2006).

Moreover, QST can be helpful to determine how generalized such altered pain responding is. For example, children with recurrent abdominal pain did not show altered threshold or sensitization in response to somatic pain stimuli as opposed to previously demonstrated visceral pain hypersensitivity (Zohsel et al., 2008b). QST has been performed in children suffering from growing pains. Sensory thresholds for innocuous brush, cold, vibration and deep pressure stimuli were normal, thus there was no evidence for dysfunctional peripheral nerves (Pathirana et al., 2011). Interestingly, children with growing pains perceived these non-painful stimuli as more intense, and had lowered pressure pain thresholds which may reflect disturbed somatosensory processing (Hashkes et al., 2004). Thus far, neuropathic pain in children has not been systematically evaluated using QST. QST can be useful for early detection of peripheral neuropathy in children with diabetes even in the absence of clinical symptoms (Blankenburg et al, 2012; Heimans et al., 1987).

QST measurements have rather consistently revealed that repeated pain experiences during the neonatal period result in long-term altered functioning of the somatosensory and pain systems (e.g. Hermann et al., 2006; Schmelzle-Lubiecki et al., 2007; Walker et al., 2009). QST may also be useful for detecting hypo- or hypersensitivity to normal sensory stimulation which presumably underlies sensory modulation disorder (Bar-Shalita et al., 2009).

Neurophysiological evaluation

Neurophysiological methods and especially neuroimaging have played a pivotal role in unravelling the neural substrates of pain. Due to the complex nature of pain, it is not surprising that activation of a large distributed functional network of brain regions, often referred to as the 'pain matrix' underlies the experience of pain. According to a meta-analysis of neuroimaging data, experimental pain is most commonly associated with activations in the primary and secondary somatosensory cortex, thalamus, insula, anterior cingulate and prefrontal region (Apkarian et al., 2005). Depending on type of stimulation, task, and other contextual and individual factors, regions such as amygdala, hippocampus, parietal and temporal areas, the cerebellum, and brainstem areas can also be activated. The neural representation of chronic pain differs from that of experimental pain, and chronic pain modulates brain responses to acute pain (e.g. Baliki et al., 2010). For example, the neuronal signature of chronic pain includes brain areas such as the medial prefrontal cortex which is involved in the processing of self-relevant information (for a review, see Apkarian et al., 2009). Neurophysiological methods have helped to identify the neuronal mechanisms of pain modulation by cognitive processes such as attention or pain-related expectations and by emotions (e.g. Tracey and Mantyh, 2007; Wiech and Tracey, 2009; Wiech et al., 2008). Moreover, these methods have been crucial for confirming neuronal plasticity, i.e. changes in the functioning and/or structure of the nervous system, as a core mechanism in chronic pain (Tracey and Bushnell, 2009; Woolf, 2011).

Most recently, in various chronic pain conditions, structural changes such as decreased grey matter density have been observed which, aside from syndrome-specific alterations, seem to commonly affect brain regions such as cingulate cortex, orbitofrontal cortex, insula, and dorsal pons which are involved in sensory-emotional-motivational integration processes and pain regulation (Apkarian et al., 2009; May, 2008). These structural changes are likely to be consequence of repeated pain and can be reversed by successful treatment (Rodriguez-Raecke et al., 2009; Seminowicz et al., 2011). While there is a wealth of data in adults, relatively few studies have used these methods to study pain processing during childhood. To some extent, this may be explained by not all neurophysiological techniques being easy to use in children.

Neurophysiological methods used for the study of paediatric pain

In the past two decades, an unprecedented progress in the development of neuroimaging techniques occurred. A thorough review of these techniques is beyond the scope of this chapter. Here, the focus is on methods that have been used for studying paediatric pain.

Neuroimaging

Generally, neuroimaging methods can be subdivided into those assessing structural, and those assessing functional, changes in the brain. Structural changes (e.g. grey matter density) or changes in structural connectivity between brain regions are measured by voxel-based morphometry and diffusion tensor imaging, respectively (Sava et al., 2009). Functional imaging techniques differ with regard to the parameter that is measured as a proxy of neural activity.

Electrophysiological techniques

Techniques such as EEG or magnetoencephalography directly measure electrical activity of neuronal assemblies with high temporal resolution (Pizzagalli, 2007). EEG activity recorded on the scalp is presumably generated by excitatory and inhibitory postsynaptic potentials in cortical neurons, hence EEG is not well suited for measuring subcortical activity, and does not yield whole-brain imaging data. Spatial information about the source of the electrical activity has to be inferred by computational models. Due to the high temporal resolution, it is possible to separate event-related, i.e. time-locked brain activity from background EEG oscillation. These event-related potentials (ERPs) are characterized by distinct components, i.e. negative and positive peaks in the EEG waveform, which reflect different aspects of stimulus processing. For example, in response to painful stimulation, somatosensory ERPs typically show an initial negative peak at about 150 ms post-stimulus followed by a positive peak at about 260 ms (N150–P260). The absolute value of this negative-positive vertex response correlates positively with subjective pain intensity (Garcia-Larrea et al., 1997). Later ERP components (e.g. P300) reflect cognitive processes such as attention and memory (Fabiani et al., 2007). Typically, ERPs are derived based on averaging many trials such that time-locked EEG changes can be discriminated from random variations of EEG activity. However, statistical methods (e.g. principal component analysis) can be applied for single trial analysis such as the cortical response to a heel lance (Slater et al., 2010c).

Indirect measures of neural activity: metabolism, oxygen consumption, and blood flow

Another approach is to record changes in metabolism, oxygen consumption, and blood flow based on the assumption that these are closely related to neural activity. FMRI is based on measuring changes in the ratio of oxygenated to deoxygenated haemoglobin in the blood and, therefore, is referred to as a blood oxygen level-dependent (BOLD) imaging technique. Oxygen consumption due to increased neuronal activity is followed by an increase in blood flow and blood volume that leads to reduced concentration of deoxygenated haemoglobin and a concomitant increase in the BOLD signal (e.g. Wager et al., 2007). Major advantages of fMRI are the relatively high spatial resolution for localizing changes in cortical, subcortical, brainstem, and even spinal activity, and non-invasiveness that permits its use in children. Nonetheless, fMRI studies in children are challenging because the scanner environment is likely to be experienced as mildly anxiety-provoking, at least initially. Moreover, fMRI recordings are highly subject to movement artefacts and, therefore, require the subject to lie still during the scanning. This can be a difficult task, especially for younger children. The processing of fMRI data requires that individual data are related to a standard template of common spatial coordinates in order to anatomically localize brain activations. The human brain not only grows in size, but also undergoes structural changes from infancy through childhood until adulthood (e.g. Johnson, 2001). Only recently, MRI atlas templates for different age groups have become available that are based on MRI recordings in larger and more representative samples of children and adolescents (Fonov et al., 2011).

Similar to fMRI, near-infrared spectroscopy (NIRS) is a non-invasive imaging technique based on measuring shifts in (de-)oxygenated haemoglobin. Whereas fMRI uses the different paramagnetic properties as recording signal, NIRS relies on the different optical properties in the visible and near-infrared light range (Bunce et al., 2006). Light administered to the scalp is absorbed by tissue and scattered back to the surface. Oxygenated and deoxygenated haemoglobin differ in their absorption sensitivity depending on the wavelength of the light. By using wavelengths maximizing the absorption by (de)oxygenated haemoglobin, measuring the light scattered back to the surface can be used to infer brain activity. NIRS is an especially promising technique for use in children and even infants because it is safe, non-invasive, and can even be performed as part of a clinical exam (Ranger et al., 2011).

Understanding paediatric pain—evidence from neurophysiological studies

Evaluation in early life

Neurophysiological methods have fundamentally contributed to unravelling the development of pain processing, especially during early infancy (e.g. Fabrizi et al., 2011; see also Chapter 40 40 Poorun and Slater, Chapter 39, this volume). In 2006, using NIRS, two studies were the first to demonstrate that, as early as 25 weeks postmenstrual age, an invasive painful medical procedure (e.g. heel lance, venepuncture) as compared to non-painful touch elicits a distinct haemodynamic response in the contralateral somatosensory cortex, hence at this developmental stage thalamocortical pathways are sufficiently mature for cortical processing of nociceptive input (Bartocci et al., 2006; Slater et al., 2006). Also, different intensive care procedures are accompanied by significant cerebral haemodynamic changes (Limperopoulos et al., 2008). Extending these findings, time-locked EEG recordings in infants undergoing heel lance revealed a distinct component consisting of a negative and positive deflection at about 500 ms (N420–P560) at electrode sites above the somatosensory cortex that is specific for nociceptive input and is larger in preterm compared to full-term-born infants (Slater et al., 2010b, 2010c). Such direct measuring of cortical activity is especially promising for evaluating the efficacy of (non-)pharmacological treatments for infants given that, at this age, pain measurement usually relies exclusively on behavioural observations and physiological parameters (e.g. heart rate, oxygen saturation). For example, in infants, oral sucrose as compared to water did not reduce the cortical response to a painful heel stick despite resulting in an attenuated behavioural pain response (Slater et al., 2010a). Using fMRI, we studied the long-term impact of neonatal pain experiences on brain activation in response to heat pain in school-aged preterm and full-term-born children having undergone treatment in a neonatal intensive care unit (NICU) and control children (Hohmeister et al., 2010). In all three groups, tonic heat pain led to significant activations of brain regions typically involved in pain processing (see Figure 40.1). The preterm, but not the full-term NICU children exhibited significant activations in a number of brain regions (thalamus, anterior cingulate cortex, cerebellum, basal ganglia, and periaqueductal grey) that were not significantly activated in controls. Moreover, the preterms showed significantly higher activations than controls in primary somatosensory cortex, anterior cingulate cortex, and insula. Hence, exposure to pain at a vulnerable stage of the developing pain circuitry, may affect both sensory and affective processing of pain later in life.

Chronic pain

In chronic paediatric pain, EEG has been used to study cognitive aspects of pain processing and specific pathophysiological mechanisms. In children with migraine and children with recurrent abdominal pain, we recorded somatosensory-evoked potentials in response to painful and non-painful mechanical stimuli which had to be ignored while performing a primary task (Hermann et al., 2008; Zohsel et al., 2008a). Painful stimuli elicited a significantly larger vertex potential (N150–P260) compared to non-painful stimuli. In both pain groups, the P300 in response to both painful and non-painful stimuli was significantly greater than in the controls (see Figure 40.2). This suggests that chronic pain in children is associated with automatic attention to painful and potentially painful stimuli. In migraine, heightened cortical excitability and altered cortical sensory processing have been proposed as pathogenetic mechanisms. Consistent with such concepts, in children with migraine, both cross-sectional and longitudinal studies entailing the measurement of ERPs to sensory stimuli (e.g. visual) and slow cortical potentials suggest altered maturation of cortical information processing (Oelkers-Ax et al., 2008; Siniatchkin et al., 2010). Thus far, only one study has used fRMI in chronic paediatric pain. Children with complex regional pain syndrome (CRPS) were exposed to non-noxious thermal and mechanical stimulation during the acute pain phase and after recovery (Lebel et al., 2008; see also Clinch, Chapter 24, this volume). In the acute pain phase, patients experienced allodynia in the affected extremity and, consistently,

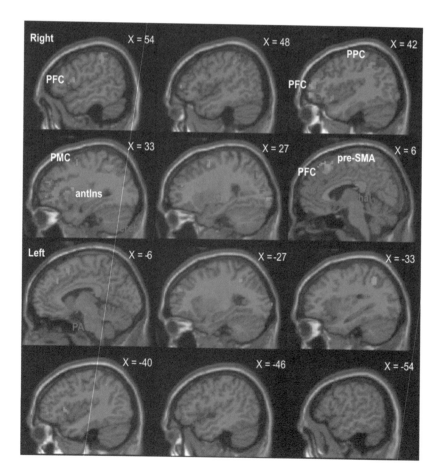

Figure 40.1 Significant brain activations ($p < 0.001$, $k \geq 10$) during painful tonic heat stimulation in NICU-preterms (red), NICU-full-terms (blue), and the controls (green), superimposed on a normalized $T1$-weighted brain. X-coordinates of brain slices (in mm) refer to the Montreal Neurological Institute standard brain. PFC = prefrontal cortex; PPC = posterior parietal cortex; PMC = premotor cortex; antIns = anterior insula; Cereb = cerebellum; BG = basal ganglia; pre-SMA = pre-supplementary motor area; ACC = anterior cingulate cortex; Thal = thalamus; PAG = periaqueductal grey.

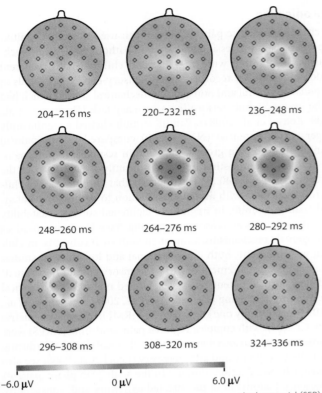

204–216 ms   220–232 ms   236–248 ms

248–260 ms   264–276 ms   280–292 ms

296–308 ms   308–320 ms   324–336 ms

−6.0 μV   0 μV   6.0 μV

Figure 40.2 Between-group difference somatosensory evoked potential (SEP) maps for painful stimuli within the P3 latency window (200–340 msec) comparing children with RAP and healthy controls. The children underwent an oddball paradigm with auditory stimuli as rare targets and painful mechanical stimuli administered to the index finger of the non-dominant hand. The grey shades indicates the difference in magnitude of SEP amplitude between the two groups. Reproduced from Hermann, C. et al., Cortical correlates of an attentional bias to painful and innocuous somatic stimuli in children with recurrent abdominal pain, PAIN®, Volume 136, Issue 3, pp. 397–406, Copyright © 2008. This figure has been reproduced with permission of the International Association for the Study of PAIN® (IASP). The figure may NOT be reproduced for any other purpose without permission.

non-noxious stimuli induced activation of brain regions involved in sensory and cognitive-emotional pain processing. Intriguingly, even after symptomatic recovery, brain activations in response to stimulation of the affected versus the unaffected extremity differed suggesting long-term alterations in the functioning of sensory and pain pathways.

Conclusion

Psychophysical methods such as QST allow reliable and valid assessment of sensory and pain processing in children and are suitable for bedside examination. Psychophysical measures are useful for characterizing altered sensory and pain processing in chronic pain states and following exposure to painful events. Due to its cognitive demands, psychophysical testing requires children to be at least 6 years of age; hence investigating early development of pain processing is precluded. Here, neurophysiological techniques have substantially advanced our understanding as they allow measurement of neuronal activity without requiring a behavioural response from the child. Nonetheless, neurophysiological studies are still scarce, especially those aiming at unravelling the neuronal mechanisms of chronic paediatric pain. Aside from methodological issues,

this is most likely accounted for by ethical considerations given the relatively high demand on children's compliance with instructions and measurement requirements.

References

Agostinho, C. M. S., Scherens, A., Richter, H., Schaub, C., Rolke, R., Treede, R. D., *et al.* (2009). Habituation and short-term repeatability of thermal testing in healthy human subjects and patients with chronic non-neuropathic pain. *Eur J Pain*, 13, 779–785.

Alabas, O. A., Tashani, O. A., Tabasam, G., and Johnson, M. I. (2012). Gender role affects experimental pain responses: a systematic review with meta-analysis. *Eur J Pain*, 16(9), 1211–1223.

Apkarian, A. V., Bushnell, M. C., Treede, R.-D., and Zubieta, J.-K. (2005). Human brain mechanisms of pain perception and regulation in health and disease. *Eur J Pain*, 9, 463–484.

Apkarian, A. V., Baliki, M. N., and Geha, P. Y. (2009). Towards a theory of chronic pain. *Prog Neurobiol*, 87, 81–97.

Arendt-Nielsen, L. and Yarnitsky, D. (2009). Experimental and clinical applications of quantitative sensory testing applied to skin, muscles and viscera. *J Pain*, 10, 556–572.

Bachmann, C. G., Nitsche, M. A., Pfingsten, M., Gersdorff, N., Harder, C., Baier, P. C., *et al.* (2011). Diurnal time course of heat pain perception in healthy humans. *Neurosci Lett*, 489, 122–125.

Baliki, M. N., Geha, P. Y., Fields, H. L., and Apkarian, A. V. (2010). Predicting value of pain and analgesia: nucleus accumbens response to noxious stimuli changes in the presence of chronic pain. *Neuron*, 66, 149–160.

Bar-Shalita, T., Vatine, J. J., Seltzer, Z., and Parush, S. (2009). Psychophysical correlates in children with sensory modulation disorder (SMD). *Physiol Behav*, 98, 631–639.

Bartocci, M., Bergqvist, L. L., Lagercrantz, H., and Anand, K. J. (2006). Pain activates cortical areas in the preterm newborn brain. *Pain*, 122, 109–117.

Bhalang, K., Sigurdsson, A., Slade, G. D., and Maixner, W. (2005). Associations among four modalities of experimental pain in women. *J Pain*, 6, 604–611.

Bland, J. M., and Altman, D. G. (1986). Statistical methods for assessing agreement between two methods of clinical measurement. *Lancet*, 1, 307–310.

Blankenburg, M., Boekens, H., Hechler, T., Maier, C., Krumova, E., Scherens, A., *et al.* (2010). Reference values for quantitative sensory testing in children and adolescents: developmental and gender differences of somatosensory perception. *Pain*, 149, 76–88.

Blankenburg, M., Kraemer, N., Hirschfeld, G., Krumova, E. K., Maier, C., Hechler, T., *et al.* (2012). Childhood diabetic neuropathy: functional impairment and non-invasive screening assessment. *Diabet Med*, 29, 1425–1432

Blankenburg, M., Meyer, D., Hirschfeld, G., Kraemer, N., Hechler, T., Aksu, F., *et al.* (2011). Developmental and sex differences in somatosensory perception—a systematic comparison of 7- versus 14-year-olds using quantitative sensory testing. *Pain*, 152, 2625–2631.

Bunce, S. C., Izzetoglu, M., Izzetoglu, K., Onaral, B., and Pourrezaei, K. (2006). Functional near-infrared spectroscopy. *IEEE Eng Med Biol Mag*, 25, 54–62.

Craig, A. D. (2003). Pain mechanisms: labeled lines versus convergence in central processing. *Annu Rev Neurosci*, 26, 1–30.

Defrin, R., Ohry, A., Blumen, N., and Urca, G. (2002). Sensory determinants of thermal pain. *Brain*, 125, 501–510.

Defrin, R., Shachal-Shiffer, M., Hadgadg, M., and Peretz, C. (2006). Quantitative somatosensory testing of warm and heat-pain thresholds: the effect of body region and testing method. *Clin J Pain*, 22, 130–136.

Fabiani, M., Gratton, G., and Federmeier, K. D. (2007). Event-related brain potentials: methods, theory, and applications. In J. T. Caccioppo, L. G. Tassinary, and G. G. Berntson, *Handbook of psychophysiology*, pp. 85–120. New York: Cambridge University Press.

Fabrizi, L., Slater, R., Worley, A., Meek, J., Boyd, S., Olhede, S., *et al*. (2011). A shift in sensory processing that enables the developing human brain to discriminate touch from pain. *Curr Biol*, 21, 1552–1558.

Fitzgerald, M. (2005). The development of nociceptive circuits. *Nat Rev Neurosci*, 6, 507–520.

Fonov, V., Evans, A. C., Botteron, K., Almli, C. R., McKinstry, R. C., and Collins, D. L. (2011). Unbiased average age-appropriate atlases for pediatric studies. *Neuroimage*, 54, 313–327.

Garcia-Larrea, L., Peyron, R., Laurent, B., and Mauguiere, F. (1997). Association and dissociation between laser-evoked potentials and pain perception. *NeuroReport*, 8, 3785–3789.

Geber, C., Klein, T., Azad, S., Birklein, F., Gierthmuhlen, J., Huge, V., *et al*. (2011). Test-retest and interobserver reliability of quantitative sensory testing according to the protocol of the German Research Network on Neuropathic Pain (DFNS): a multi-centre study. *Pain*, 152, 548–556.

Gracely, R. H. (2006). Studies of pain in human subjects. In S. B. McMahon, and M. Koltzenburg (eds) *Textbook of pain* (5th edn), pp. 267–291. Philadelphia, PA: Elsevier Churchill Livingstone.

Granot, M., Granovsky, Y., Sprecher, E., Nir, R. R., and Yarnitsky, D. (2006). Contact heat-evoked temporal summation: tonic versus repetitive-phasic stimulation. *Pain*, 122, 295–305.

Greffrath, W., Baumgartner, U., and Treede, R. D. (2007). Peripheral and central components of habituation of heat pain perception and evoked potentials in humans. *Pain*, 132, 301–311.

Grone, E., Crispin, A., Fleckenstein, J., Irnich, D., Treede, R. D., and Lang, P. M. (2012). Test order of quantitative sensory testing facilitates mechanical hyperalgesia in healthy volunteers. *J Pain*, 13, 73–80.

Hagander, L. G., Midani, H. A., Kuskowski, M. A., and Parry, G. J. (2000). Quantitative sensory testing: effect of site and skin temperature on thermal thresholds. *Clin Neurophysiol*, 111, 17–22.

Hansson, P., Backonja, M., and Bouhassira, D. (2007). Usefulness and limitations of quantitative sensory testing: clinical and research application in neuropathic pain states. *Pain*, 129, 256–259.

Hashkes, P. J., Friedland, O., Jaber, L., Cohen, H. A., Wolach, B., and Uziel, Y. (2004). Decreased pain threshold in children with growing pains. *J Rheumatol*, 31, 610–613.

Haslam, D. R. (1969). Age and the perception of pain. *Psychonomic Sci*, 15, 86–87.

Hastie, B. A., Riley, J. L. III, Robinson, M. E., Glover, T., Campbell, C. M., Staud, R., *et al*. (2005). Cluster analysis of multiple experimental pain modalities. *Pain*, 116, 227–237.

Heimans, J. J., Bertelsmann, F. W., de Beaufort, C. E., de Beaufort, A. J., Faber, Y. A., and Bruining, G. J. (1987). Quantitative sensory examination in diabetic children: assessment of thermal discrimination. *Diabet Med*, 4, 251–253.

Heldestad, V., Linder, J., Sellersjo, L., and Nordh, E. (2010). Reproducibility and influence of test modality order on thermal perception and thermal pain thresholds in quantitative sensory testing. *Clin Neurophysiol*, 121, 1878–1885.

Hermann, C., Hohmeister, J., Demirakca, S., Zohsel, K., and Flor, H. (2006). Long-term alteration of pain sensitivity in school-aged children with early pain experiences. *Pain*, 125, 278–285.

Hermann, C., Zohsel, K., Hohmeister, J., and Flor, H. (2008). Cortical correlates of an attentional bias to painful and innocuous somatic stimuli in children with recurrent abdominal pain. *Pain*, 136, 397–406.

Hilz, M. J., Axelrod, F. B., Hermann, K., Haertl, U., Duetsch, M., and Neundorfer, B. (1998a). Normative values of vibratory perception in 530 children, juveniles and adults aged 3–79 years. *J Neurol Sci*, 159, 219–225.

Hilz, M. J., Glorius, S., and Beric, A. (1995). Thermal perception thresholds: influence of determination paradigm and reference temperature. *J Neurol Sci*, 129, 135–140.

Hilz, M. J., Glorius, S. E., Schweibold, G., Neuner, I., Stemper, B., and Axelrod, F. B. (1996). Quantitative thermal perception testing in preschool children. *Muscle Nerve*, 19, 381–383.

Hilz, M. J., Stemper, B., Schweibold, G., Neuner, I., Grahmann, F., and Kolodny, E. H. (1998b). Quantitative thermal perception testing in 225 children and juveniles. *J Clin Neurophysiol*, 15, 529–534.

Hogeweg, J. A., Kuis, W., Oostendorp, R. A., and Helders, P. J. (1996). The influence of site of stimulation, age, and gender on pain threshold in healthy children. *Phys Ther*, 76, 1331–1339.

Hohmeister, J., Demirakca, S., Zohsel, K., Flor, H., and Hermann, C. (2009). Responses to pain in school-aged children with experience in a neonatal intensive care unit: cognitive aspects and maternal influences. *Eur J Pain*, 13, 94–101.

Hohmeister, J., Kroll, A., Wollgarten-Hadamek, I., Zohsel, K., Demirakca, S., Flor, H., *et al*. (2010). Cerebral processing of pain in school-aged children with neonatal nociceptive input: an exploratory fMRI study. *Pain*, 150, 257–267.

Johnson, M. H. (2001). Functional brain development in humans. *Nat Rev Neurosci*, 2, 475–483.

Jorum, E. and Arendt-Nielsen, L. (2003). Sensory testing and clinical neurophysiology. In H. Breivik, W. Campbell, C. Eccleston (eds) *Clinical pain management: practical applications and procedures*, pp. 27–38. London: Arnold Publishers.

Kemler, M. A., Schouten, H. J., and Gracely, R. H. (2000). Diagnosing sensory abnormalities with either normal values or values from contralateral skin: comparison of two approaches in complex regional pain syndrome I. *Anesthesiology*, 93, 718–727.

Khalili, N., Wendelschafer-Crabb, G., Kennedy, W. R., and Simone, D. A. (2001). Influence of thermode size for detecting heat pain dysfunction in a capsaicin model of epidermal nerve fiber loss. *Pain*, 91, 241–250.

Lebel, A., Becerra, L., Wallin, D., Moulton, E. A., Morris, S., Pendse, G., *et al*. (2008). FMRI reveals distinct CNS processing during symptomatic and recovered complex regional pain syndrome in children. *Brain*, 131, 1854–1879.

Limperopoulos, C., Gauvreau, K. K., O'Leary, H., Moore, M., Bassan, H., Eichenwald, E. C., *et al*. (2008). Cerebral hemodynamic changes during intensive care of preterm infants. *Pediatrics*, 122, e1006–e1013.

Magerl, W., Krumova, E. K., Baron, R., Tolle, T., Treede, R. D., and Maier, C. (2010). Reference data for quantitative sensory testing (QST): refined stratification for age and a novel method for statistical comparison of group data. *Pain*, 151, 598–605.

May, A. (2008). Chronic pain may change the structure of the brain. *Pain*, 137, 7–15.

Meh, D. and Denislic, M. (1994). Quantitative assessment of thermal and pain sensitivity. *J Neurol Sci*, 127, 164–169.

Meier, P. M., Berde, C. B., DiCanzio, J., Zurakowski, D., and Sethna, N. F. (2001). Quantitative assessment of cutaneous thermal and vibration sensation and thermal pain detection thresholds in healthy children and adolescents. *Muscle Nerve*, 24, 1339–1345.

Merskey, H. and Bogduk, N. (1994). *Classification of chronic pain: descriptions of chronic pain syndromes and definitions of pain terms* (2nd edn). Seattle, WA: IASP Press.

Moloney, N. A., Hall, T. M., O'Sullivan, T. C., and Doody, C. M. (2011). Reliability of thermal quantitative sensory testing of the hand in a cohort of young, healthy adults. *Muscle Nerve*, 44, 547–552.

Neziri, A. Y., Curatolo, M., Nuesch, E., Scaramozzino, P., Andersen, O. K., Arendt-Nielsen, L, *et al*. (2011a). Factor analysis of responses to thermal, electrical, and mechanical painful stimuli supports the importance of multi-modal pain assessment. *Pain*, 152, 1146–1155.

Neziri, A. Y., Scaramozzino, P., Andersen, O. K., Dickenson, A. H., Arendt-Nielsen, L, and Curatolo, M. (2011b). Reference values of mechanical and thermal pain tests in a pain-free population. *Eur J Pain*, 15, 376–383.

Nikolajsen, L., Kristensen, A. D., Pedersen, L. K., Rahbek, O., Jensen, T. S., and Moller-Madsen, B. (2011). Intra- and interrater agreement of pressure pain thresholds in children with orthopedic disorders. *J Child Orthop*, 5, 173–178.

Oelkers-Ax, R., Schmidt, K., Bender, S., Reimer, I., Mohler, E., Knauss, E., *et al*. (2008). Longitudinal assessment of response preparation and evaluation in migraine gives evidence for deviant maturation. *Cephalalgia*, 28, 237–249.

Pathirana, S., Champion, D., Jaaniste, T., Yee, A., and Chapman, C. (2011). Somatosensory test responses in children with growing pains. *J Pain Res*, 4, 393–400.

Peters, E. W., Bienfait, H. M., de Visser, M., and de Haan, R. J. (2003). The reliability of assessment of vibration sense. *Acta Neurol Scand*, 107, 293–298.

Pizzagalli, D. (2007). Electroencephalography and high-density electrophysiological source localization. In J. T. Cacciopo, L. G. Tassinary, and G. G. Bernston, (eds). *Handbook of psychophysiology*, pp. 56–85. New York: Cambridge University Press.

Racine, M., Tousignant-Laflamme, Y., Kloda, L. A., Dion, D., Dupuis, G., and Choiniere, M. (2012a). A systematic literature review of 10 years of research on sex/gender and experimental pain perception—part 1: are there really differences between women and men? *Pain*, 153, 602–618.

Racine, M., Tousignant-Laflamme, Y., Kloda, L. A., Dion, D., Dupuis, G., and Choiniere, M. (2012b). A systematic literature review of 10 years of research on sex/gender and pain perception—part 2: do biopsychosocial factors alter pain sensitivity differently in women and men? *Pain*, 153, 619–635.

Ranger, M., Johnston, C. C., Limperopoulos, C., Rennick, J. E., and du Plessis, A. J. (2011). Cerebral near-infrared spectroscopy as a measure of nociceptive evoked activity in critically ill infants. *Pain Res Manag*, 16, 331–336.

Riley, J. L. III, Robinson, M. E., Wise, E. A., Myers, C. D., and Fillingim, R. B. (1998). Sex differences in the perception of noxious experimental stimuli: a meta-analysis. *Pain*, 74, 181–187.

Rodriguez-Raecke, R., Niemeier, A., Ihle, K., Ruether, W., and May, A. (2009). Brain gray matter decrease in chronic pain is the consequence and not the cause of pain. *J Neurosci*, 29, 13746–13750.

Rolke, R., Baron, R., Maier, C., Tolle, T. R., Treede, R. D., Beyer, A., *et al.* (2006a). Quantitative sensory testing in the German Research Network on Neuropathic Pain (DFNS): standardized protocol and reference values. *Pain*, 123, 231–243.

Rolke, R., Magerl, W., Campbell, K. A., Schalber, C., Caspari, S., Birklein, F., *et al.* (2006b). Quantitative sensory testing: a comprehensive protocol for clinical trials. *Eur J Pain*, 10, 77–88.

Sand, T., Nilsen, K. B., Hagen, K., and Stovner, L. J. (2010). Repeatability of cold pain and heat pain thresholds: the application of sensory testing in migraine research. *Cephalalgia*, 30, 904–909.

Sava, S., Lebel, A. A., Leslie, D. S., Drosos, A., Berde, C., Becerra, L., *et al.* (2009). Challenges of functional imaging research of pain in children. *Mol Pain*, 5, 30.

Schmelzle-Lubiecki, B. M., Campbell, K. A., Howard, R. H., Franck, L., and Fitzgerald, M. (2007). Long-term consequences of early infant injury and trauma upon somatosensory processing. *Eur J Pain*, 11, 799–809.

Seminowicz, D. A., Wideman, T. H., Naso, L., Hatami-Khoroushahi, Z., Fallatah, S., Ware, M. A., *et al.* (2011). Effective treatment of chronic low back pain in humans reverses abnormal brain anatomy and function. *J Neurosci*, 31, 7540–7550.

Siao, P. and Cros, D. P. (2003). Quantitative sensory testing. *Phys Med Rehabil Clin North Am*, 14, 261–286.

Siniatchkin, M., Jonas, A., Baki, H., van, B. A, Gerber, W. D, and Stephani, U. (2010). Developmental changes of the contingent negative variation in migraine and healthy children. *J Headache Pain*, 11, 105–113.

Slater, R., Cantarella, A., Gallella, S., Worley, A., Boyd, S., Meek, J., *et al.* (2006). Cortical pain responses in human infants. *J Neurosci*, 26, 3662–3666.

Slater, R., Cornelissen, L., Fabrizi, L., Patten, D., Yoxen, J., Worley, A., *et al.* (2010a). Oral sucrose as an analgesic drug for procedural pain in newborn infants: a randomised controlled trial. *Lancet*, 376, 1225–1232.

Slater, R., Fabrizi, L., Worley, A., Meek, J., Boyd, S., and Fitzgerald, M. (2010b). Premature infants display increased noxious-evoked neuronal activity in the brain compared to healthy age-matched term-born infants. *Neuroimage*, 52, 583–589.

Slater, R., Worley, A., Fabrizi, L., Roberts, S., Meek, J., Boyd, S., *et al.* (2010). Evoked potentials generated by noxious stimulation in the human infant brain. *Eur J Pain*, 14, 321–326.

Strigo, I. A., Carli, F., and Bushnell, M. C. (2000). Effect of ambient temperature on human pain and temperature perception. *Anesthesiology*, 92, 699–707.

Thibault, A., Forget, R., and Lambert, J. (1994). Evaluation of cutaneous and proprioceptive sensation in children: a reliability study. *Dev Med Child Neurol*, 36, 796–812.

Tracey, I. and Bushnell, M. C. (2009). How neuroimaging studies have challenged us to rethink: is chronic pain a disease? *J Pain*, 10, 1113–1120.

Tracey, I. and Mantyh, P. W. (2007). The cerebral signature for pain perception and its modulation. *Neuron*, 55, 377–391.

Treede, R. D., Jensen, T. S., Campbell, J. N., Cruccu, G., Dostrovsky, J. O., Griffin, J. W., *et al.* (2008). Neuropathic pain: redefinition and a grading system for clinical and research purposes. *Neurology*, 70, 1630–1635.

Tsao, J. C., Myers, C. D., Craske, M. G., Bursch, B., Kim, S. C., and Zeltzer, L. K. (2004). Role of anticipatory anxiety and anxiety sensitivity in children's and adolescents' laboratory pain responses. *J Pediatr Psychol*, 29, 379–388.

Wager, T., Hernandez, L., Jonides, J., and Lindquist, M. (2007). Elements of functional neuroimaging. In J. T. Cacciopo, L. G. Tassinary, and G. G. Berntson, (eds) *Handbook of psychophysiology*, pp. 19–55. New York: Cambridge University Press.

Walco, G. A., Dampier, C. D., Hartstein, G., Djordjevic, D., and Miller, L. (1990). The relationship between recurrent clinical pain and pain threshold in children. In D. C. Tyler and E. J. Krane (eds) *Advances in pain research and therapy* (Vol. 15), pp. 333–340. New York: Raven Press, Ltd.

Walk, D., Sehgal, N., Moeller-Bertram, T., Edwards, R. R., Wasan, A., Wallace, M., *et al.* (2009). Quantitative sensory testing and mapping: a review of nonautomated quantitative methods for examination of the patient with neuropathic pain. *Clin J Pain*, 25, 632–640.

Walker, S. M., Franck, L. S., Fitzgerald, M., Myles, J., Stocks, J., and Marlow, N. (2009). Long-term impact of neonatal intensive care and surgery on somatosensory perception in children born extremely preterm. *Pain*, 141, 79–87.

Wiech, K., Ploner, M., and Tracey, I. (2018). Neurocognitive aspects of pain perception. *Trends Cogn Sci*, 12, 306–313.

Wiech, K. and Tracey, I. (2019). The influence of negative emotions on pain: behavioral effects and neural mechanisms. *Neuroimage*, 47, 987–994.

Woolf, C. J. (2011). Central sensitization: implications for the diagnosis and treatment of pain. *Pain*, 152, S2–15.

Wylde, V., Palmer, S., Learmonth, I. D., and Dieppe, P. (2011). Test-retest reliability of quantitative sensory testing in knee osteoarthritis and healthy participants. *Osteoarthritis Cartilage*, 19, 655–658.

Yarnitsky, D. (1997). Quantitative sensory testing. *Muscle Nerve*, 20, 198–204.

Yarnitsky, D. and Ochoa, J. L. (1990). Studies of heat pain sensation in man: perception thresholds, rate of stimulus rise and reaction time. *Pain*, 40, 85–91.

Zohsel, K., Hohmeister, J., Flor, H., and Hermann, C. (2008a). Altered pain processing in children with migraine: an evoked potential study. *Eur J Pain*, 12, 1090–1101.

Zohsel, K., Hohmeister, J., Flor, H., and Hermann, C. (2008b). Somatic pain sensitivity in children with recurrent abdominal pain. *Am J Gastroenterol*, 103, 1517–1523.

Zohsel, K., Hohmeister, J., Oelkers-Ax, R., Flor, H., and Hermann, C. (2006). Quantitative sensory testing in children with migraine: preliminary evidence for enhanced sensitivity to painful stimuli especially in girls. *Pain*, 123, 10–18.

CHAPTER 41

Measurement of health-related quality of life and physical function

See Wan Tham, Anna C. Wilson, and Tonya M. Palermo

Summary

This chapter reviews the measurement of health-related quality of life (HRQOL) and physical function in paediatric pain populations. We present available data on HRQOL and physical function in children with pain, methods of assessment, details about specific questionnaire and performance-based measures, and recommendations for the use of measures based on available evidence. Because many children and adolescents with pain report impairment in participation in physical activities such as walking, running, and sports, physical functioning is a core target and outcome for intervention, particularly for youth with chronic pain. However, the domain of physical functioning encompasses a number of constructs such as physical fitness, physical activity, and subjective disability, which are interrelated, but represent distinct aspects of functioning. Moreover, HRQOL is a broader concept that subsumes physical and psychosocial function. A wide variety of measurement tools are in use, but no guidelines for measurement have been established. A better understanding of measurement of HRQOL and physical function may enable researchers and clinicians to track children's functional impact and changes in function over time, and to improve the design and testing of potentially effective interventions for children with pain.

Introduction

It is well recognized that medical conditions and ill health may have significant impact across different areas of a child's life. Pain, particularly chronic pain, may impair school attendance, mobility, self-care, interpersonal interactions, life activities, and community activities (Palermo, 2000). Health-related quality of life (HRQOL) refers to an individual's perception of the impact of an illness, symptoms, and its consequent treatment on their physical, psychological, and social well-being, as well as perception of overall well-being in relation to their health (Eiser et al. 2001). Measurement of HRQOL incorporates assessment of three levels: (1) components of specific domains of functioning (e.g. difficulty walking up stairs), (2) individual domains of functioning (e.g. psychosocial, physical, school, and role functioning), and (3) an overall assessment of well-being (e.g. global health status). HRQOL scores are often summarized as broadband scores for physical health and psychosocial health. Integral to the assessment of HRQOL is the domain of physical functioning. Physical functioning refers to actual participation in physical activities and ability to perform physical tasks, as well as the individual's perception of difficulty or restriction in activity participation.

Physical function should be a primary treatment outcome for youth with pain and represents a specific domain requiring detailed assessment. The Pediatric Initiative on Methods, Measurement, and Pain Assessment in Clinical Trials (Ped-IMMPACT) recommended outcome measures for clinical trials investigating acute and chronic pain in children (McGrath et al., 2008) and identified physical and role functioning as two of the eight core outcome domains. In this chapter, we review approaches for assessment of HRQOL as a multidimensional construct that incorporates the domains of physical and role functioning, and we separately review specific approaches to the assessment of physical functioning. We further describe measures of HRQOL and physical functioning in paediatric pain populations.

Health-related quality of life and physical function in children with painful conditions

Several examinations of HRQOL in children and adolescents with pain conditions (e.g. headache, sickle cell disease, mixed pain conditions) have found that they report significantly poorer HRQOL in comparison to healthy children (Nodari et al., 2002; Palermo et al., 2002). Moreover, unexplained chronic pain in adolescents has been associated with poor quality of life for the adolescent and his or her family (Hunfeld et al., 2001). Predictors of poor HRQOL within pain populations include the presence of sleep problems (Palermo and Kiska, 2005), fatigue (Berrin et al., 2007), pain-related hospitalizations (Palermo et al., 2002), low socioeconomic conditions (Palermo et al., 2008c) and increasing child age. Little is known, however, about how HRQOL changes over time in youth with pain.

Similarly, physical function has also been fairly extensively studied in youth with various pain conditions primarily to identify how chronic pain can affect children's participation in developmentally appropriate physical and social activities. In one epidemiological study of chronic pain in a community sample of youth (Roth-Isigkeit, et al., 2005), impairments most commonly reported were: sleep problems (53.6%), inability to pursue hobbies (53.3%), eating problems (51.1%), school absence (48.8%), and inability to meet friends (46.7%). Huguet and Miro (2008) examined pain severity including impact from pain using validated measures in a population based sample. They found that 36.8% of youth had some disability, with 31.7% categorized as having a low level of disability and 5.1% having moderate to severe disability. These studies highlight that pain and disability can vary considerably among children with pain.

Prior reviews of HRQOL and function measures

Several recent reviews have provided summaries of measures that have been used to assess HRQOL and physical function in medical populations experiencing chronic pain or chronic illness. Eccleston et al. (2006) identified nine measures of the impact of pain on HRQOL and physical functioning in children with headache, arthritis, abdominal pain, and mixed pain conditions. They concluded that for the majority of the measures, the psychometric evaluations were limited in scope, and had only been used in a few studies.

Palermo et al. (2008b) reviewed 16 measures of HRQOL and functional impairment that have been used with paediatric populations including children with painful conditions. This review classified measures as being well established, approaching well established, or promising. Several well-established measures were found used in pain populations including the Pediatric Quality of Life Inventory (PedsQL; Varni et al., 1999), the Functional Disability Inventory (FDI; Walker and Greene, 1991), and the Child Activity Limitations Interview (CALI; Palermo, et al., 2004). Specific measures are discussed in more detail in later sections. This review called for further research, particularly regarding the validity of HRQOL and functional disability measures in response to interventions, and the clinical utility of changes in these measures (Palermo et al., 2008b).

There is little information available concerning measurement of HRQOL, physical or role functioning in children experiencing acute pain. This is in large part due to the way that measures have been developed in the field where the primary focus has been on the longer-term impact of illness on children. However, we recognize that HRQOL, physical, and role function may be important endpoints in the treatment of children with acute pain as well.

Methods of evaluation of HRQOL and physical function

Starting with the most commonly used method of evaluation, a clinical interview can be used to evaluate physical function. However, the evidence base reviewed here pertains to the use of standardized measures of HRQOL and physical function using validated questionnaires and objective/observational measures of performance. Examples of measurements within each of these methods are reviewed in the following sections; however, this is not intended to serve as an exhaustive review of the literature.

Clinical interview

The cornerstone of the clinical evaluation and assessment of the child in pain is the clinical interview. The clinician uses the interview to establish rapport, obtain a pain history, and to understand impact of pain on aspects of the child's daily life. Interview probes about school, daily activities, sports participation, recreational and peer activities, and self-care activities can uncover areas of significant limitation in physical function (see Table 41.1). See supplementary online materials for additional interview probes in multiple domains of assessment.

Functional goals are often developed with children and parents around specific areas of limitation tailored to each child's needs. Re-assessment of these allows for monitoring and tracking of patient outcomes. There are limitations to the use of clinical interviews to assess physical function, however, including that questions may be asked in different ways (i.e. lack of standardization), demand characteristics may influence responses, and there is a limited ability to make comparisons across children. Empirical support is not yet available to recommend a standardized clinical interview for assessing physical function in paediatric pain.

HRQOL questionnaires

HRQOL can be assessed on questionnaires that can be generic or condition-specific measures (Palermo et al., 2008b). Generic measures are not intended for a specific population, and allow for comparisons across children with different pain or medical conditions. Condition-specific HRQOL measures, on the other hand, are developed for examination of specific impairments experienced by children with the same health conditions. This may increase sensitivity in capturing the nuances of living with specific conditions. However, condition-specific instruments do not allow for comparative measurements across different illness groups, or between children with and without pain.

Two commonly used, well-established generic HRQOL measures that have been applied to pain populations are the Child Health Questionnaire (CHQ) and PedsQL. The CHQ is a widely used instrument, initially developed for use in healthy children

Table 41.1 Clinical interview questions to assess physical and role function

Domain	Sample question
Overall health status	How would you describe your overall health?
Daily living	Describe a typical day. What is your routine? What activities do you do during the day?
Self-care	What do you do to take care of yourself and your body?
School participation	How often do you attend school? When you go to school, how long do you stay? Do you have any difficulties completing schoolwork?
Community participation	Do you participate in hobbies, like clubs or after-school activities, or church?
Physical activities	Do you participate in sports or other athletic activities? What activities are difficult for you to do because of your pain? What would you like to be able to do that you can't do now?
Activities with peers	How often do you spend time with friends? What do you do with friends?
Activities with family	What activities do you do with your family (parents, siblings)?

(Landgraf et al., 1996). It incorporates 13 domains including psychosocial functioning, physical and role functioning, family cohesion, school and activity limitations, behaviour, self-esteem, and the emotional and time impact on the parent. Broad band measures of physical health and psychosocial health can be derived. This instrument has been used for HRQOL assessment in children with chronic pain conditions such as juvenile idiopathic arthritis and sickle cell disease (e.g. Panepinto et al., 2005; Selvaag et al., 2003). Notable strengths of the CHQ are the broad generalizability across different medical conditions (Bruijn et al., 2009; Krab et al., 2009), widespread international experience (Ruperto et al., 2001), and feasibility via Internet administration (Raat et al., 2007). Primary disadvantages of the CHQ are the excessive length of the scale in comparison to other HRQOL measures, the more limited range of child self-report (only available for age 10 and above), and that the parent and child versions are not parallel which prohibits direct comparison of parent and child reports.

Another commonly used instrument is PedsQL (Varni et al., 1999). Initially developed to assess HRQOL in children with cancer, it has undergone development and validation as both a core instrument and disease-specific modules within numerous paediatric medical populations. It assesses four core broad-band domains of physical, psychological, social and school functioning. The PedsQL 4.0 has been used for descriptive purposes in general pain populations and in specific pain conditions such as sickle cell disease and fibromyalgia (Dale et al., 2011; Gold et al., 2009; Varni et al., 2007a). It has been used in several intervention studies for outcome assessment (Hicks et al., 2006; Langley et al., 2011). Several disease-specific modules may be relevant for use with pain populations such as the Rheumatology Module (Varni et al., 2002) which includes subscales for pain and hurt, daily activities, treatment, worry, and communication. One unique feature of the PedsQL is the applicability across a wide age range; it has been validated for use from birth to 18 years old, with multiple versions for different ages (Varni et al., 2011). Research on the validity of this measure has been conducted internationally (Amiri et al., 2010; Tsuji et al., 2011) and across several ethnic and racial groups (Limbers et al., 2009). Construct validity was demonstrated by determining responsiveness following medical intervention over time (Varni et al., 1999). Several studies have found that the electronic (e-PedsQL) Internet mode of administration demonstrates equivalent properties to the paper and pencil mode of administration (Varni et al., 2008a; Young et al., 2009). The disadvantage of the PedsQL 4.0 is that the instrument provides a broad assessment of HRQOL and may not be responsive to changes in disease-specific symptoms. Additional details on psychometric evaluation of the generic measures of HRQOL can be found in Table 41.2.

Table 41.2 Psychometric characteristics of HRQOL and physical function measures

Name of measure	Number of items/ administration burden	Validity			Reliability					Population developed
		Construct	Criterion	Content	Temporal stability	Test–retest	Internal consistency	Sensitivity to change	Interrater reliability	
Child Health Questionnaire (CHQ)	Child: 87 Parent: 98, 50, and 28 (3 versions)	x		x		x	x			Healthy and medical paediatric populations
Pediatric Quality of Life Inventory (PedsQL)	Child: 23 Parent: 23 Short form: 15	x		x			x	x		Paediatric medical populations
Pain Experience Questionnaire (PEQ)	Child: 15 Parent: 12	x		x			x			Paediatric chronic pain
Bath Adolescent Pain questionnaire (BAPQ)	Child: 61 Parent: 61	x				x	x			Paediatric chronic pain
Functional Disability Inventory (FDI)	Child: 15 Parent: 15	x	x		x		x	x	x	Paediatric chronic pain
Child Activity Limitations Interview (CALI)	Child: 21 Parent: 21	x				x	x	x		Paediatric chronic pain
Timed walk task	Up to 10 min to administer	x						x		Healthy and medical paediatric populations
Sit-to-stand task	Approx. 1 min to administer	x						x		Healthy and medical paediatric populations

There are two newer multidimensional measures designed specifically for children with pain conditions: the Bath Adolescent Pain Questionnaire (BAPQ; (Eccleston et al., 2005) and the Pain Experience Questionnaire (Hermann et al., 2008). Although a HRQOL framework was not used to develop these instruments, they both cover a range of constructs important in HRQOL assessment and were designed specifically to assess pain-related interference and functioning. The BAPQ was designed for adolescent and parent report and focuses on assessment of psychosocial, activity limitations, social, and family functioning. The PEQ was based on the Multidimensional Pain Inventory, commonly used in adults with chronic pain, and is a multidimensional pain measure designed for ages 7 and up. Both instruments require additional psychometric evaluation. However, the strengths of both measures are that they were developed for children and adolescents with chronic pain and may capture unique limitations and impact experienced by this population.

There are also HRQOL measures designed for specific paediatric pain populations. For children and adolescents with chronic headaches or migraines, available instruments include The Quality of Life Headache in Youth (QLH-Y) and The Migraine Specific Quality of Life Questionnaire Version 2.1(MSQ). The QLH-Y assesses the domains of psychological and social functioning, functional status, physical status, and satisfaction with life and health (Langeveld et al., 1996). The MSQ assesses impact of pain on physical, emotional, and social functioning (Martin et al., 2000). Both measures have been validated in relatively small samples. For children with arthritis, the Arthritis Impact Measurement Scales 2 (AIMS 2) and Juvenile Arthritis Quality of Life Questionnaire (JAQQ) have been used as disease specific measures of physical and psychosocial function in children with juvenile idiopathic arthritis (Duffy et al., 1997; Meenan et al., 1992).

Questionnaires for assessment of physical function

Questionnaires designed to capture activity limitations, restriction, and functional impairment or disability related to pain fall under the domain of physical function. They may provide a more comprehensive examination of areas of impact or disability that may be overlooked by general measures of HRQOL. For the child with a pain condition, measures of physical function may identify specific areas of decreased activity performance secondary to pain that could serve as the goal of intervention. Two generic and five condition-specific instruments of physical function are discussed in the following paragraphs.

Measures of functional impairment that assess subjective perception of difficulty performing activities include the Functional Disability Inventory (FDI) and the Child Activity Limitations Interview (CALI). Both were developed for children and adolescents with chronic pain. The FDI (Walker and Greene, 1991) was initially developed for adolescents with abdominal pain; it has since been used in children with other chronic pain conditions (headaches, musculoskeletal pain; Claar et al., 2006), as a descriptive measure (Kashikar-Zuck et al., 2011), and as a treatment outcome measure (Kashikar-Zuck et al., 2005). The CALI (Palermo et al., 2004; Palermo et al., 2008a) was developed to assess activity limitations associated with chronic pain in broader populations, and to allow for both retrospective assessment and daily prospective assessment in a diary format. It has been factor analysed and has been shown to be responsive to change in treatment outcome research (Palermo et al., 2009). Details of the psychometric evaluation of these measures can be found in Table 41.2.

Condition-specific measures of functional impairment are also available. For example, two measures assessing function in arthritis are the Child Health Assessment Questionnaire (CHAQ; Stephens et al., 2007) and the Juvenile Arthritis Functional Assessment Report (JAFAR). The CHAQ is a valid and reliable measure used to guide clinical decisions for level of assistance for functional impairment and to evaluate functional improvement after intervention (Halbig et al., 2009). The JAFAR has demonstrated good construct validity, reliability and responsiveness (Howe et al., 1991), and has been widely used in juvenile idiopathic arthritis. In the migraine population, the PedMIDAS (Hershey et al., 2004) is a brief measure with promising initial validation, and includes items assessing school, physical, recreation and peer participation.

Objective and observational measures of physical function

Certain constructs within the domain of physical function, including physical fitness and activity, are traditionally measured with objective and performance-based tools. For example, physical fitness may be measured using oxygen exchange for aerobic or anaerobic capacity, isokinetic machines or force dynamometers that measure torque and strength, and body mass index or skinfold calipers for body composition. Objective measures of physical activity may include motion sensing devices such as pedometers and accelerometers.

Observational performance-based measures of function provide information about an individual's actual performance on tasks which are typically designed to mimic naturalistic tasks that would be encountered in daily life (e.g. lifting, walking). In rehabilitation settings, performance-based measures of function are routinely used in evaluation and re-evaluation of patients with chronic pain.

In adult pain research, a broad range of observational measurement systems have been developed to assess physical functioning, such as the Sorenson back extension test (Harding et al., 1994), the sit-to-stand (the number of times an individual can move from a seated to a standing position in a 1 min time period), and the timed walk (how long it takes an individual to walk a certain distance such as 10 metres, or how far a person walks in a certain time period such as 2 or 6 min). These measures are administered using standardized conditions (often in a gym).

Observational and performance measures have been used surprisingly little in paediatric pain populations. In juvenile arthritis, standardized measures of fitness such as grip strength have been shown to correlate with self-report measures of physical function (Wessel et al., 1999). Standardized back muscle endurance measures have also been used with youth who have chronic musculoskeletal pain (O'Sullivan et al., 2011). Only one study of which we are aware has utilized performance measures to assess intervention outcome. In this study, improvements were found in adolescents with chronic pain on sit-to-stand and timed walk measures following an intensive interdisciplinary physical therapy and psychological treatment day hospital programme (Eccleston et al., 2003). Observational measures have the advantage of reduced subjectivity compared to self-report. Disadvantages of these measures include some burden in terms of additional time needed to administer the tasks, as well as necessitating training research or clinical staff. At this time, however, the most significant limitation is the lack of available data on any particular performance-based measure of physical function in children with painful conditions.

Physical activity, a specific domain of overall physical function, can be measured via self-report, proxy-report, or via activity monitors that capture physical activity in daily life such as pedometers or actigraphic monitoring devices. This domain of physical function is relevant for acute and chronic pain conditions, as pain is often characterized by limitations in movement and withdrawal from physical activities (Sullivan et al., 2008). Additionally, low levels of physical activity have been associated with the development of pain in adolescents (Skoffer et al., 2008).

Several self- and proxy-report measurement systems, including diary and recall reports, have been developed for assessment of physical activity in healthy adolescents (see review by Sirard et al., 2001). Examples of available measures include the International Physical Activity Questionnaire (IPAQ), which shows adequate reliability and has been validated with objective measures of energy expenditure in adolescents (Arvidsson et al., 2005). Brief physical activity screening measures are also available for use with adolescents (e.g. Prochaska et al., 2001). These measures typically prompt the adolescent to recall a specific time period (e.g. the last 7 days) and estimate the amount of time spent in various levels of activity (e.g. vigorous enough to sweat).

Despite the availability of self-report measures of physical activity, there are few published studies examining these measures in youth with acute or chronic pain. Among youth with musculoskeletal pain, diary reports of physical activity demonstrate less time spent in physical activity compared to healthy controls (Kashikar-Zuck et al., 2010; Tarakci et al., 2011). Similarly, youth with nonspecific musculoskeletal pain reported lower levels of activity using the Youth Activity Questionnaire (Ainsworth et al., 1993), compared to healthy youth matched for age and sex (O'Sullivan et al., 2011). While there are limitations to self-report of physical activity in children and adolescents, particularly among those with chronic pain (Kashikar-Zuck et al., 2010), additional research in this area would provide more information about the impact of pain on physical activity and to understanding of how these measures perform in pain populations.

Activity monitoring or actigraphy typically uses wrist- or hip-mounted accelerometers to track an individual's movements in daily life activities, which may be converted to caloric expenditure. These measures of physical activity provide proxy data on actual movement patterns and have been used in a few studies of adolescents with chronic pain. Two studies have compared adolescents with mixed chronic pain problems (headaches, abdominal pain, and musculoskeletal pain) to matched healthy controls on actigraphic measures of daytime activity, and found lower activity levels and more time spent in sedentary activity among youth with chronic pain (Long et al., 2008; Wilson et al., 2012). In one study of adolescents with juvenile primary fibromyalgia syndrome, between-subject variability in physical activity levels were high; among these untreated youth, higher activity was associated with significantly lower levels of self-reported pain intensity, depressive symptoms, and functional disability (Kashikar-Zuck et al., 2010). Overall, actigraphic measures have been moderately correlated with self-reports of physical functioning among youth with chronic pain. There are various monitoring devices and computer programs that have been developed for research purposes and can be used to assess physical activity (see review of activity monitoring in children and adolescents by Bjornson et al. (2004)). To our knowledge, no published studies have examined physical activity in children experiencing acute or postoperative pain, or in association with acute or chronic

pain management or treatment. There has been too little empirical work performed to date to recommend specific objective measures of functional assessment in youth with pain.

Outcomes measurement

Enhancing children's functioning is often the primary treatment goal for youth with chronic pain. Re-assessment of HRQOL and function is important for understanding the impact of treatments, both on individuals and on groups. To date, the majority of studies have used HRQOL and function to describe paediatric medical and pain populations, however, there have been limited studies using these tools as outcome measurements after intervention. There are a few paediatric studies that utilized HRQOL as an outcome measure after pharmacologic intervention for rheumatologic conditions (Ruperto et al., 2010). With respect to psychological intervention, similarly, few randomized controlled trials of psychological treatments have measured change in children's physical or role functioning from pre- to post-treatment (Palermo et al., 2010). While psychological interventions are largely found to be effective in reducing pain intensity, a significant gap remains in our knowledge of the effects of psychological interventions on physical and role functioning, especially in randomized controlled trials.

Given the broad range of assessment measures and approaches available, clinicians must make choices to prioritize what information about HRQOL and functioning will be useful to collect when evaluating an individual child with chronic pain and his or her family. Interview and questionnaire reports of HRQOL and physical function should ideally be obtained from self-report if the child is cognitively and physically able to provide it. Parent or caregiver proxy reports can provide additional information on parent perception of the HRQOL and functioning of the child. As there is imperfect agreement between self and proxy report (Varni et al., 2007b), proxy report should be used to supplement assessment of the child, not to replace information provided by self-report. Parent report has some unique correlates; for example, parental perception of HRQOL (rather than child perception) and function has been shown to be associated with children's healthcare utilization (Campo et al., 2002; Janicke et al., 2001).

There are several new developments in measurement of physical function. Most notably, considerable work has been invested in the Patient Reported Outcomes Measurement Information System (PROMIS) funded by the National Institutes of Health. At present, preliminary validation has been conducted on a new measure of pain interference in children (Varni et al., 2010) that can be administered via self-report or computerized adaptive testing. Pain and function are areas identified by PROMIS where ongoing work will continue to advance assessment of health related outcomes in the paediatric pain population.

Best available evidence to guide current use of assessment tools

A wide variety of methods have been used to measure HRQOL, physical function, physical activity, and physical fitness. Clear guidelines are not presently available for measurement of physical function domains in the paediatric pain population. Further research on psychometric properties of measures and comparative analysis of measurement methods is needed in this area to establish

Table 41.3 Recommendations for assessment of HRQOL and physical function in children and adolescents with painful conditions

Assessment	Name of measure (acronym)	Reference	Primary scale content
HRQOL–generic measures	Child Health Questionnaire (CHQ)	Landgraf et al. (1996)	Physical functioning, role functioning: emotional/behavioural, role functioning: physical, bodily pain, general behaviour, mental health, self-esteem, general health perceptions, parental impact: emotional, parental impact: time, family activities, family cohesion, change in health
Multidimensional pain-specific measures	Pediatric Quality of Life Inventory 4.0 (PedsQL4.0)	Varni et al. (1999)	Physical, psychological, social, and school functioning
	Pain Experience Questionnaire (PEQ)	Hermann et al. (2008)	Pain severity, pain related interference, affective distress, perceived social support
	Bath Adolescent Pain Questionnaire (BAPQ)	Eccleston et al. (2005)	Physical functioning, social functioning, depression, general anxiety, pain-specific anxiety, family functioning, and developmental functioning
Functional Impairment	Functional Disability Inventory (FDI)	Walker and Greene (1991)	Physical and psychosocial limitations due to pain
	Child Activity Limitations Interview (CALI)	Palermo et al. (2004)	Activity restrictions in daily, personal, recreational, physical, and social activities due to pain

these guidelines. We have made recommendations to guide the use of instruments for measurement of HRQOL and physical function in paediatric pain populations in Table 41.3. We have chosen not to recommend measures within specific pain conditions given the small available evidence base within any one condition. In addition, due to the limited available data on objective and performance-based measures in children with pain, it is premature to recommend their routine use.

Conclusion

Collectively, information obtained from the clinical interview, questionnaires, and observational measures allow for global evaluation of HRQOL and physical function in the child with pain. Due to the availability of numerous measures, the choice of instrument(s) needs to be guided by measurement quality of the instruments and the goals set by and the clinician and/or the researcher. In examination of the wide range of available instruments, we have identified several research priorities:

◆ Validation of HRQOL and physical function measures for use in children with pain conditions requires further attention. At this time it is not clear whether currently available measures are appropriate in the context of acute pain or whether adaptations to existing measures or the development of new measures will be needed.

◆ To extend the clinical utility of measures, additional work is required to establish the clinical meaning of changes in scores for individuals. The development of cut-points to indicate clinical severity of the limitation in HRQOL or physical function may be useful for certain measures. For an example, see Kashikar-Zuck et al. (2011) concerning clinical utility of the FDI.

◆ There is limited information on any objective or performance-based measure of physical function or activity in children with pain. Additional work is needed with performance-based tasks (e.g. timed walk), activity devices (e.g. actigraphy), and with physical fitness measures (e.g. grip strength) to develop normative data in paediatric pain populations and understand relative

levels of impairment. Moreover, the relationship between subjective measures (questionnaires) and objective performance measures requires specific consideration.

In summary, HRQOL and physical functioning instruments may allow for objective assessment of the global functioning of the child, enable standardized comparison within and across painful medical populations, and provide longitudinal monitoring of outcomes over time and in response to intervention. Applications of HRQOL measurement reviewed by Varni et al. (2005) suggest that standardized measures may improve communication between the health care provider and the child and family as well as improve child and parent satisfaction by actively eliciting information about the child's functioning. Thus, in order to optimize the use of these measures, further research into the potential benefits are needed in paediatric pain populations.

Case example

Kristy is a 16-year-old female who began experiencing low back pain about 2 years ago. Prior to pain onset, she participated in softball and volleyball at her school, but has now given up these sports activities due to pain. Kristy has missed an increasing number of school days in the past year, which she attributes to worsening pain from sitting for long periods. Her parents report that she is more sedentary than she used to be, spending much time lying down at home. They also note that she often refuses to do household chores that involve lifting. Kristy has begun to avoid interactions with her friends because they often choose activities that involve walking long distances. Currently, Kristy reports that she can go on walks on days when her pain is less intense, but only walks for 20 to 30 min once or twice a week. She also experiences increased pain when walking up and down stairs, and when her pain is severe she will sleep on the couch at night to avoid walking upstairs to her bedroom. Her night-time sleep has been disrupted for the past several months and she is often fatigued during the day.

Assessment that includes a combination of interview questions, standardized measures of HRQOL and physical function in conjunction with performance measures may provide clinically relevant information. The clinical interview could be used to assess in detail Kristy's participation in physical and role activities (e.g. doing family chores at home, attending school, doing things with friends). Specific interview probes could be used with Kristy and her parent(s) to understand Kristy's expectations for activity and role participation and what her individual values are around functional activities. A measure of overall HRQOL, such as the PedsQL 4.0, would provide information about perception of overall health impact, while a measure of pain-related activity limitations or disability such as the FDI or the CALI-21 would provide information about pain impact on functioning that may identify specific intervention targets or goals. Because Kristy reports trouble walking, and a timed 10-metre walk would establish a baseline performance that could be used throughout treatment to assess progress. Additional measures of performance and fitness might be chosen by a physical or occupational therapist.

These measures can provide valuable information to assess Kristy on an individual basis, and to also compare the level of impairment secondary to pain in comparison to other adolescents with pain conditions. Furthermore, the measures can also allow the clinician to track Kristy's progress over time to objectively monitor her level of functioning and assess for changes in impairment if treatment is undertaken.

References

Ainsworth, B. E., Haskell, W. L., Leon, A. S., Jacobs, D. R.Jr., Montoye, H. J., Sallis, J. F., et al. (1993). Compendium of physical activities: classification of energy costs of human physical activities. Med Sci Sports Exerc, 25, 71–80.

Amiri, P., Ardekani, E. M., Jalali-Farahani, S., Hosseinpanah, F., Varni, J. W., Ghofranipour, F., et al. (2010). Reliability and validity of the Iranian version of the Pediatric Quality of Life Inventory 4.0 Generic Core Scales in adolescents. Qual Life Res, 19, 1501–1508.

Arvidsson, D., Slinde, F., and Hulthen, L. (2005). Physical activity questionnaire for adolescents validated against doubly labelled water. Eur J Clin Nutr, 59, 376–383.

Berrin, S. J., Malcarne, V. L., Varni, J. W., Burwinkle, T. M., Sherman, S. A., Artavia, K., et al. (2007). Pain, fatigue, and school functioning in children with cerebral palsy: a path-analytic model. J Pediatr Psychol 32(3), 330–337.

Bjornson, K. F., and Belza, B. (2004). Ambulatory activity monitoring in youth: state of the science. Pediatr Phys Ther, 16, 82–89.

Bruijn, J., Arts, W. F., Duivenvoorden, H., Dijkstra, N., Raat, H., and Passchier, J. (2009). Quality of life in children with primary headache in a general hospital. Cephalalgia, 29, 624–630.

Campo, J. V., Comer, D. M., Jansen-Mcwilliams, L., Gardner, W., and Kelleher, K. J. (2002). Recurrent pain, emotional distress, and health service use in childhood. J Pediatr, 141, 76–83.

Claar, R. L., and Walker, L. S. (2006). Functional assessment of pediatric pain patients: psychometric properties of the functional disability inventory. Pain, 121, 77–84.

Dale, J. C., Cochran, C. J., Roy, L., Jernigan, E., and Buchanan, G. R. (2011). Health-related quality of life in children and adolescents with sickle cell disease. J Pediatr Health Care, 25, 208–215.

Duffy, C. M., Arsenault, L., Duffy, K. N., Paquin, J. D., and Strawczynski, H. (1997). The Juvenile Arthritis Quality of Life Questionnaire—development of a new responsive index for juvenile rheumatoid arthritis and juvenile spondyloarthritides. J Rheumatol, 24, 738–746.

Eccleston, C., Jordan, A., McCracken, L. M., Sleed, M., Connell, H., and Clinch, J. (2005). The Bath Adolescent Pain Questionnaire (BAPQ): development and preliminary psychometric evaluation of an instrument to assess the impact of chronic pain on adolescents. Pain, 118, 263–270.

Eccleston, C., Jordan, A. L., and Crombez, G. (2006). The impact of chronic pain on adolescents: a review of previously used measures. J Pediatr Psychol, 31, 684–697.

Eccleston, C., Malleson, P. N., Clinch, J., Connell, H., and Sourbut, C. (2003). Chronic pain in adolescents: evaluation of a programme of interdisciplinary cognitive behaviour therapy. Arch Dis Child, 88, 881–885.

Eiser, C. and Morse, R. (2001). The measurement of quality of life in children: past and future perspectives. J Dev Behav Pediatr, 22, 248–256.

Gold, J. I., Mahrer, N. E., Yee, J., and Palermo, T. M. (2009). Pain, fatigue, and health-related quality of life in children and adolescents with chronic pain. Clin J Pain, 25, 407–412.

Halbig, M. and Horneff, G. (2009). Improvement of functional ability in children with juvenile idiopathic arthritis by treatment with etanercept. Rheumatol Int, 30, 229–238.

Harding, V. R., Williams, A. C., Richardson, P. H., Nicholas, M. K., Jackson, J. L., Richardson, I. H., et al. (1994). The development of a battery of measures for assessing physical functioning of chronic pain patients. Pain, 58, 367–375.

Hermann, C., Hohmeister, J., Zohsel, K., Tuttas, M. L., and Flor, H. (2008). The impact of chronic pain in children and adolescents: development and initial validation of a child and parent version of the Pain Experience Questionnaire. Pain, 135, 251–261.

Hershey, A. D., Powers, S. W., Vockell, A. L., LeCates, S. L., Segers, A., and Kabbouche, M. A. (2004). Development of a patient-based grading scale for PedMIDAS. Cephalalgia, 24, 844–849.

Hicks, C. L., von Baeyer, C. L., and McGrath, P. J. (2006). Online psychological treatment for pediatric recurrent pain: a randomized evaluation. J Pediatr Psychol, 31, 724–736.

Howe, S., Levinson, J., Shear, E., Hartner, S., McGirr, G., Schulte, M., et al. (1991). Development of a disability measurement tool for juvenile rheumatoid arthritis. The Juvenile Arthritis Functional Assessment Report for Children and their Parents. Arthritis Rheum, 34, 873–880.

Hunfeld, J. A., Perquin, C. W., Duivenvoorden, H. J., Hazebroek-Kampschreur, A. A., Passchier, J., van Suijlekom-Smit, L. W., et al. (2001). Chronic pain and its impact on quality of life in adolescents and their families. J Pediatr Psychol 26(3), 145–153.

Janicke, D. M., Finney, J. W., and Riley, A. W. (2001). Children's health care use: a prospective investigation of factors related to care-seeking. Med Care, 39, 990–1001.

Kashikar-Zuck, S., Flowers, S. R., Claar, R. L., Guite, J. W., Logan, D. E., Lynch-Jordan, A. M., et al. (2011). Clinical utility and validity of the Functional Disability Inventory among a multicenter sample of youth with chronic pain. Pain, 152, 1600–1607.

Kashikar-Zuck, S., Flowers, S. R., Verkamp, E., Ting, T. V., Lynch-Jordan, A. M., Graham, T. B., et al. (2010). Actigraphy-based physical activity monitoring in adolescents with juvenile primary fibromyalgia syndrome. J Pain, 11, 885–893.

Kashikar-Zuck, S., Goldschneider, K. R., Powers, S. W., Vaught, M. H., and Hershey, A. D. (2001). Depression and functional disability in chronic pediatric pain. Clin J Pain, 17, 341–349.

Kashikar-Zuck, S., Swain, N. F., Jones, B. A., and Graham, T. B. (2005). Efficacy of cognitive-behavioral intervention for juvenile primary fibromyalgia syndrome. J Rheumatol, 32, 1594–1602.

Krab, L. C., Oostenbrink, R. de Goede-Bolder, A., Aarsen, F. K., Elgersma, Y., and Moll, H. A. (2009). Health-related quality of life in children with neurofibromatosis type 1: contribution of demographic factors, disease-related factors, and behavior. J Pediatr, 154, 420–425, 425.e421.

Landgraf, J. M., Abetz, L., and Ware, J. E. (1996). The CHQ user's manual. Boston, MA: The Health Institute, New England Medical Center.

Langeveld, J. H., Koot, H. M., Loonen, M. C., Hazebroek-Kampschreur, A. A., and Passchier, J. (1996). A quality of life instrument for adolescents with chronic headache. *Cephalalgia*, 16, 183–196; discussion 137.

Langley, R. G., Paller, A. S., Hebert, A. A., Creamer, K., Weng, H. H., Jahreis, A., *et al.* (2011). Patient-reported outcomes in pediatric patients with psoriasis undergoing etanercept treatment: 12-week results from a phase III randomized controlled trial. *J Am Acad Dermatol*, 64, 64–70.

Limbers, C. A., Newman, D. A., and Varni, J. W. (2009). Factorial invariance of child self-report across race/ethnicity groups: a multigroup confirmatory factor analysis approach utilizing the PedsQL 4.0 Generic Core Scales. *Ann Epidemiol*, 19, 575–581.

Long, A. C., Palermo, T. M., and Manees, A. M. (2008). Brief report: using actigraphy to compare physical activity levels in adolescents with chronic pain and healthy adolescents. *J Pediatr Psychol*, 33, 660–665.

Martin, B. C., Pathak, D. S., Sharfman, M. I., Adelman, J. U., Taylor, F., Kwong, W. J., *et al.* (2000). Validity and reliability of the migraine-specific quality of life questionnaire (MSQ Version 2.1). *Headache*, 40, 204–215.

McGrath, P. J., Walco, G. A., Turk, D. C., Dworkin, R. H., Brown, M. T., Davidson, K., *et al.* (2008). Core outcome domains and measures for pediatric acute and chronic/recurrent pain clinical trials: PedIMMPACT recommendations. *J Pain*, 9, 771–783.

Meenan, R. F., Mason, J. H., Anderson, J. J., Guccione, A. A., and Kazis, L. E. (1992). AIMS2. The content and properties of a revised and expanded Arthritis Impact Measurement Scales Health Status Questionnaire. *Arthritis Rheum*, 35, 1–10.

Nodari, E., Battistella, P. A., Naccarella, C., and Vidi, M. (2002). Quality of life in young Italian patients with primary headache. *Headache* 42(4), 268–274.

O'Sullivan, P., Beales, D. Jensen, L. Murray, K., and Myers, T. (2011). Characteristics of chronic non-specific musculoskeletal pain in children and adolescents attending a rheumatology outpatients clinic: a cross-sectional study. *Pediatr Rheumatol Online J*, 9, 3.

Palermo, T. M. (2000). Impact of recurrent and chronic pain on child and family daily functioning: a critical review of the literature. *J Dev Behav Pediatr*, 21, 58–69.

Palermo, T. M. (2009). Assessment of chronic pain in children: current status and emerging topics. *Pain Res Manag*, 14, 21–26.

Palermo, T. M. (2012). *Cognitive-behavioral therapy for chronic pain in children and adolescents.* New York: Oxford University Press.

Palermo, T. M., Eccleston, C., Lewandowski, A. S., Williams, A. C., and Morley, S. (2010). Randomized controlled trials of psychological therapies for management of chronic pain in children and adolescents: an updated meta-analytic review. *Pain*, 148, 387–397.

Palermo, T. M., Lewandowski, A. S., Long, A. C., and Burant, C. J. (2008a). Validation of a self-report questionnaire version of the Child Activity Limitations Interview (CALI): the CALI-21. *Pain*, 139, 644–652.

Palermo, T. M., Long, A. C., Lewandowski, A. S., Drotar, D., Quittner, A. L., and Walker, L. S. (2008b). Evidence-based assessment of health-related quality of life and functional impairment in pediatric psychology. *J Pediatr Psychol*, 33, 983–996; discussion 997–988.

Palermo, T. M., and Kiska, R. (2005). Subjective sleep disturbances in adolescents with chronic pain: relationship to daily functioning and quality of life. *J Pain* 6(3), 201–207.

Palermo, T.M., Riley, C.A., and Mitchell, B. A. (2008c). Daily functioning and quality of life in children with sickle cell disease pain: relationship with family and neighborhood socioeconomic distress. *J Pain* 9(9), 833–40.

Palermo, T. M., Schwartz, L., Drotar, D., AND McGowan, K. (2002). Parental report of health-related quality of life in children with sickle cell disease. *J Behav Med* 25(3), 269–283.

Palermo, T. M., Wilson, A. C., Peters, M. Lewandowski, A., and Somhegyi, H. (2009). Randomized controlled trial of an Internet-delivered family cognitive-behavioral therapy intervention for children and adolescents with chronic pain. *Pain*, 146, 205–213.

Palermo, T. M., Witherspoon, D. Valenzuela, D., and Drotar, D. D. (2004). Development and validation of the Child Activity Limitations Interview: a measure of pain-related functional impairment in school-age children and adolescents. *Pain*, 109, 461–470.

Panepinto, J. A., O'Mahar, K. M., DeBaun, M. R., Loberiza, F. R., and Scott, J. P. (2005). Health-related quality of life in children with sickle cell disease: child and parent perception. *Br J Haematol*, 130, 437–444.

Prochaska, J. J., Sallis, J. F., and Long, B. (2001). A physical activity screening measure for use with adolescents in primary care. *Arch Pediatr Adolesc Med*, 155, 554–559.

Raat, H., Mangunkusumo, R. T., Landgraf, J. M. Kloek, G., and Brug, J. (2007). Feasibility, reliability, and validity of adolescent health status measurement by the Child Health Questionnaire Child Form (CHQ-CF): internet administration compared with the standard paper version. *Qual Life Res*, 16, 675–685.

Roth-Isigkeit, A., Thyen, U. Stoven, H. Schwarzenberger, J., and Schmucker, P. (2005). Pain among children and adolescents: restrictions in daily living and triggering factors. *Pediatrics*, 115, e152–162.

Ruperto, N., Lovell, D. J., Li, T. Sztajnbok, F. Goldenstein-Schainberg, C. Scheinberg, M., *et al.* (2010). Abatacept improves health-related quality of life, pain, sleep quality, and daily participation in subjects with juvenile idiopathic arthritis. *Arthritis Care Res (Hoboken)*, 62, 1542–1551.

Ruperto, N., Ravelli, A. Pistorio, A. Malattia, C. Cavuto, S. Gado-West, L., *et al.* (2001). Cross-cultural adaptation and psychometric evaluation of the Childhood Health Assessment Questionnaire (CHAQ) and the Child Health Questionnaire (CHQ) in 32 countries. Review of the general methodology. *Clin Exp Rheumatol*, 19, S1–9.

Selvaag, A. M., Flato, B. Lien, G. Sorskaar, D. Vinje and Forre, O. (2003). Measuring health status in early juvenile idiopathic arthritis: determinants and responsiveness of the child health questionnaire. *J Rheumatol*, 30, 1602–1610.

Sirard, J. R., and Pate, R. R. (2001). Physical activity assessment in children and adolescents. *Sports Med*, 31, 439–454.

Skoffer, B. and Foldspang, A. (2008). Physical activity and low-back pain in schoolchildren. *Eur Spine J*, 17, 373–379.

Stephens, S., Singh-Grewal, D., Bar-Or, O., Beyene, J., Cameron, B., Leblanc, C. M., *et al.* (2007). Reliability of exercise testing and functional activity questionnaires in children with juvenile arthritis. *Arthritis Rheum*, 57, 1446–1452.

Sullivan, M. J. (2008). Toward a biopsychomotor conceptualization of pain: implications for research and intervention. *Clin J Pain*, 24, 281–290.

Tarakci, E., Yeldan, I., Kaya Mutlu, E., Baydogan, S. N., and Kasapcopur, O. (2011). The relationship between physical activity level, anxiety, depression, and functional ability in children and adolescents with juvenile idiopathic arthritis. *Clin Rheumatol*, 30, 1415–1420.

Tsuji, N., Kakee, N., Ishida, Y., Asami, K., Tabuchi, K., Nakadate, H., *et al.* (2011). Validation of the Japanese version of the Pediatric Quality of Life Inventory (PedsQL) Cancer Module. *Health Qual Life Outcomes*, 9, 22.

Varni, J. W., Burwinkle, T. M., and Lane, M. M. (2005). Health-related quality of life measurement in pediatric clinical practice: an appraisal and precept for future research and application. *Health Qual Life Outcomes*, 3, 34.

Varni, J. W., Limbers, C. A., and Burwinkle, T. M. (2007a). Impaired health-related quality of life in children and adolescents with chronic conditions: a comparative analysis of 10 disease clusters and 33 disease categories/severities utilizing the PedsQL 4.0 Generic Core Scales. *Health Qual Life Outcomes* 5, 43.

Varni, J. W., Limbers, C. A., and Burwinkle, T. M. (2007b). Parent proxy-report of their children's health-related quality of life: an analysis of 13,878 parents' reliability and validity across age subgroups using the PedsQL 4.0 Generic Core Scales. *Health Qual Life Outcomes*, 5, 2.

Varni, J. W., Limbers, C. A., Burwinkle, T. M., Bryant, W. P., and Wilson, D. P. (2008a). The ePedsQL in type 1 and type 2 diabetes: feasibility, reliability, and validity of the Pediatric Quality of Life Inventory Internet administration. *Diabetes Care*, 31, 672–677.

Varni, J. W., Limbers, C. A., Neighbors, K., Schulz, K., Lieu, J. E., Heffer, R. W., et al. (2011). The PedsQL Infant Scales: feasibility, internal consistency reliability, and validity in healthy and ill infants. *Qual Life Res*, 20, 45–55.

Varni, J. W., Limbers, C. A., Newman, D. A., and Seid, M. (2008b). Longitudinal factorial invariance of the PedsQL 4.0 Generic Core Scales child self-report Version: one year prospective evidence from the California State Children's Health Insurance Program (SCHIP). *Qual Life Res*, 17, 1153–1162.

Varni, J. W., Seid, M., Smith Knight, T., Burwinkle, T., Brown, J., et al. (2002). The PedsQL in pediatric rheumatology: reliability, validity, and responsiveness of the Pediatric Quality of Life Inventory Generic Core Scales and Rheumatology Module. *Arthritis Rheum* 46(3), 714–725.

Varni, J. W., Seid, M. and Rode, C. A. (1999). The PedsQL: measurement model for the pediatric quality of life inventory. *Med Care*, 37, 126–139.

Varni, J. W., Stucky, B. D., Thissen, D., Dewitt, E. M., Irwin, D. E., Lai, J. S., et al. (2010). PROMIS Pediatric Pain Interference Scale: an item response theory analysis of the pediatric pain item bank. *J Pain* 11(11), 1109–1119.

Walker, L. S., and Greene, J. W. (1991). The functional disability inventory: measuring a neglected dimension of child health status. *J Pediatr Psychol*, 16, 39–58.

Wessel, J., Kaup, C., Fan, J., Ehalt, R., Ellsworth, J., Speer, C., et al. (1999). Isometric strength measurements in children with arthritis: reliability and relation to function. *Arthritis Care Res*, 12, 238–246.

Wilson, A. C., and Palermo, T. M. (2012). Physical activity and function in adolescents with chronic pain: a controlled study using actigraphy. *J Pain*, 13, 121–130.

Young, N. L., Varni, J. W., Snider, L., McCormick, A., Sawatzky, B., Scott, M., et al. (2009). The Internet is valid and reliable for child-report: an example using the Activities Scale for Kids (ASK) and the Pediatric Quality of Life Inventory (PedsQL). *J Clin Epidemiol*, 62, 314–320.

Online supplementary materials

Table 41.4 Interview probes for assessing physical functioning.
Reproduced from Tonya M. Palermo, *Cognitive-Behavioral Therapy for Chronic Pain in Children and Adolescents*, Table 4.4, p.50, Oxford University Press, Inc., New York, USA, Copyright © 2012, by permission of Oxford University Press.

Table 41.5 Interview probes for assessing sleep problems.
Reproduced from Tonya M. Palermo, *Cognitive-Behavioral Therapy for Chronic Pain in Children and Adolescents*, Table 4.6, p.52, Oxford University Press, Inc., New York, USA, Copyright © 2012, by permission of Oxford University Press.

Table 41.6 Interview probes for assessing family relationships.
Reproduced from Tonya M. Palermo, *Cognitive-Behavioral Therapy for Chronic Pain in Children and Adolescents*, Table 4.7, p.53, Oxford University Press, Inc., New York, USA, Copyright © 2012, by permission of Oxford University Press.

SECTION 6

Pharmacological interventions

Principles of pain pharmacology in paediatrics

Kim Chau and Gideon Koren

Summary

Changes during growth and development may profoundly alter the pharmacokinetic and pharmacodynamics profile of medications in children of different ages, and in comparison to adults. Genetic factors can also influence the disposition and action of a drug, and contribute to interindividual differences in clinical response. Safe and effective pharmacological management of pain in neonates, infants, and children requires a thorough understanding of the principles of analgesic pharmacology in paediatric patients. Analgesic dosing regimens should take into account the severity of pain, the age or developmental state of the infant, and the therapeutic window of the drug.

Introduction

Growth and development differences exist between children and adults and these may profoundly alter the pharmacokinetics and pharmacodynamics of medications in children (Anderson and Palmer, 2006; Kearns et al., 2003). In the past, formulaic approaches were used to determine paediatric drug doses, with some using discrete age points or principles that assume that infant growth is a predictable and linear process. For example, using Young's rule and Clark's rule, a child's dose is based on a mathematical fractionation of the adult dose. To calculate an approximate child's dose, these formulae divide the child's weight (in pounds) by the assumed average weight of an adult (150 lbs) and multiply the fractional result by the adult dose (Munzenberger and McKercher, 1980). With advances and integration of developmental pharmacology into clinical practice, it is now recognized that neonates and infants are not merely 'small adults' and thus, they do not respond to pharmacological therapy in a similar manner to adults (Kearns et al., 2003). When approaching pharmacological decisions in managing pain in paediatric patients, there needs to be an appreciation of the interaction between pharmacokinetics and pharmacodynamics of therapeutics. As a result, factors that must be considered when treating infants and children include:

- Rate of drug absorption via oral route of administration is slower in neonates than in infants and older children; thus, time to achieve maximal plasma levels is prolonged (Heimann, 1980).

- Neonates and infants have higher percentage of body weight as water and smaller fat and muscle stores compared to adults; therefore, water-soluble drugs may have larger volume of distribution (Echeverria et al., 1975).

- They have an anatomically developed liver at birth; however, functional maturation is delayed and as a result, neonates exhibit delayed maturation of hepatic drug metabolizing enzymes compared to older children, until around 6 months of age (Tateishi et al., 1997).

- The kidney exhibits slower glomerular filtration rate and tubular secretion.

- Plasma concentrations of albumin and alpha-1 acid glycoprotein are lower than in adults; for some drugs (e.g. sulphonamides) this may result in greater availability of unbound active drugs and thereby, greater drug effect or increased risk of drug toxicity (Heimann, 1980).

- Neonates have an immature blood–brain barrier (BBB), which may allow increased passage of certain drugs, such as morphine and merperidine, into the brain (Bouwmeester et al., 2003; Way et al., 1965).

Unfortunately, there are still gaps in our understanding of the impact of maturational changes on the clinical pharmacology of most drugs; however, it is abundantly clear that the continuous physiological development of neonates, infants, and children influences the disposition of most drugs (Holford, 1996; Kearns et al., 2003). Therefore, to safely and effectively manage pain in neonates, infants, and young children, a thorough understanding of the principals of pain pharmacology in paediatric patients is essential.

Developmental paediatric pharmacokinetics

The use of pharmacological agents for the treatment of pain in paediatric patients should be guided by the general principles of developmental pharmacology. Accordingly, paediatric analgesic dosing regimens should take into account the severity of pain and the age or developmental state of the infant (Helms and Barone, 2008), as well as the therapeutic window of the drug, to avoid dose-dependent toxicities. The traditional empirical approach to determining paediatric drug doses was based on the allometric size scaling principle, whereby pharmacokinetic parameters were based on relative body size and it was generally assumed there is a linear relationship between body mass and body surface area in infants, children, adolescents, and adults (Ritschel, 1980). However, infant growth and development are not always linear processes when growth and age-related changes in body composition and organ function are considered (Kearns, 2000). Therefore, simply scaling an adult dose for infants and children based on body weight or body surface area may result, at times, in either ineffective pain management or severe, unexpected toxicity (Holford, 1996). As such, using a non-linear relationship between weight and drug elimination capacity is more appropriate for determining drug dosing regimens of pain treatments in paediatric patients (Dawson, 1940). Of note, such guidelines are primarily applicable for initiating pain therapy, and long-term maintenance of pain therapy must be individualized and requires consideration of developmental variations in pharmacokinetics and pharmacodynamics. Thus, to safely and effectively manage and treat pain in paediatric patients, a fundamental understanding of the interplay between growth and development on the disposition and actions of drugs is necessary.

Absorption of drugs

The absorption of drugs administered to neonates and infants is significantly influenced by developmental changes in absorptive surfaces, such as the gastrointestinal tract, pulmonary bronchioles, and skin; these sites of absorption determine the rate and extent of the bioavailability of a drug (Kearns, 2000). Furthermore, the relative amount of drug available for absorption is affected by the intraluminal pH. For example, gastric pH is higher (greater than 4) in neonates compared to older children, affecting the stability and the degree of ionization of a drug, and thus influencing the amount of drug that can be absorbed (Agunod et al., 1969). Therefore, strong acidic drugs, such as penicillin, administered orally have a greater bioavailability in neonates than in older children; whereas, for neonates to achieve therapeutic plasma levels of orally administered drugs that are weak acids, such as phenobarbital, larger doses may be required due to the higher intraluminal pH (Kearns et al., 2003; Koren et al., 1993).

Following birth, neonates experience a marked increase in gastric emptying due to the improvement of the coordination of antral contractions (Gupta and Brans, 1978; Ittmann et al., 1992). This is clinically significant as the rate of drug exposure along the mucosal surface of the small intestine is determined by the transit time of the drug within the gastrointestinal tract. As a result of increased gastric emptying in neonates, orally administered drugs are less well absorbed and more time is required to achieve therapeutic plasma levels of drugs in neonates compared to older children and adults (Heimann, 1980). Although few bioavailability studies have examined the absorption of drugs in infants and older children, it has been suggested that both passive and active transport are fully mature in infants by approximately 4 months of age (Anderson and Holford, 2008; Heimann, 1980).

Delayed maturation or developmental differences in the activity of intestinal drug-metabolizing enzymes in neonates and infants may affect the bioavailability of drugs (Hines and McCarver, 2002), and can alter the systemic absorption of therapeutically active metabolites of certain drugs, such as theophylline. For example,

the intestinal activity of cytochrome P450 (CYP) 1A1 (CYP1A1) is lower during infancy compared to late childhood; however, it appears that the activity level increases with age (Stahlberg et al., 1988). At birth, glutathione-S-transferase (GST) activity is high compared to older children, but decreases during infancy through early adolescence (Gibbs et al., 1999).

Relative to adults, the stratum corneum is thinner and the epidermis is also more hydrated in neonates and throughout childhood, which may result in an increase in percutaneous absorption during infancy (Fluhr et al., 2000). As infants and young children have a greater total body surface area to body mass ratio than adults, topically applied drugs display greater systemic exposure in infants, which may result in toxic effects if the dose administered is not age-appropriately adjusted (Fluhr et al., 2000; West et al., 1981).

Rectal administration of drugs is increasingly being used in infants and young children, but may have greater bioavailability in neonates due to the delayed developmental maturity of hepatic drug-metabolizing enzymes. Conversely, neonates and infants may absorb less drug following rectal administration compared to adults (van Lingen et al., 1999) due to a greater number of high-amplitude pulsatile contractions resulting in greater expulsion of drugs (Di Lorenzo et al., 1995). As absorption and bioavailability of acetaminophen suppositories are unpredictable, and delayed peak plasma concentration is observed compared to oral administration, rectal administration may result in subtherapeutic plasma concentrations (Autret et al., 1993; Goldstein et al., 2008; Rumore and Blaiklock, 1992; see also Anderson, Chapter 43, this volume).

Distribution of drugs

Developmental changes in body composition are primarily responsible for the age-associated differences in drug distribution. As neonates and infants have relatively larger extracellular and total-body water, coupled with smaller fat and muscle stores compared to adults, when water-soluble drugs are administered, plasma levels in these compartments may be lower (i.e. larger volume of distribution; Echeverria et al., 1975; Siber et al., 1975). Additionally, neonates and young infants have lower amounts of total circulating plasma proteins, such as albumin and α_1-acid glycoprotein, resulting in an increase in the free fraction of drugs, which influences the availability of the active moiety of drugs (Ehrnebo et al., 1971). The free fraction of highly protein-bound drugs is higher in neonates compared to older children and adults, as foetal albumin has lower binding affinity for weak acids, and there is an increase in endogenous substances (e.g. free fatty acids) with a high affinity for displacing drugs from albumin binding sites (Ehrnebo et al., 1971; Windorfer et al., 1974). Other age-related physiological changes, such as differences in organ perfusion, regional blood flow, and permeability of cell membranes, can also dramatically influence drug binding and distribution.

Drug metabolism

Compared to older children and adults, neonates and infants exhibit distinct developmental immaturity of many phase I (oxidation; Hines and McCarver, 2002) and phase II (conjugation) drug-metabolizing enzymes (McCarver and Hines, 2002; Tateishi et al., 1997), which can contribute to observed drug toxicities in this age group (Weiss et al., 1960). During postnatal development, distinct patterns of change are observed in the isoform-specific expression and activity of phase I enzymes, such as the cytochrome P450 family of drug-metabolizing enzymes:

- The activity of CYP2E1 surges within hours after birth (Vieira et al., 1996).

- This is immediately followed by the detection of CYP2D6 (Treluyer et al., 1991).

- By the first week of life, the expression of CYP3A4 (Lacroix et al., 1997) and CYP2C (CYP2C9 and CYP2C19; Treluyer et al., 1997) become detectable.

- By 1 to 3 months of life, CYP1A2 begins to appear (Sonnier and Cresteil, 1998).

The cytochrome P450 superfamily of enzymes catalyses the oxidation of opioids, converting the parent opioid to a more polar metabolite to facilitate its excretion. Of importance in opioid metabolism are CYP3A4 and CYP2D6. Relatively low levels of P450s are expressed in the foetal liver; the level of CYP2D6 expression reaches only 3% to 5% of adult expression in the third trimester (Ladona et al., 1991). However, expression and activity level of CYP2D6 approaches 95% of adult capacity by 2 weeks of life (Blake et al., 2007). In comparison, the expression of CYP3A4/5 begins to increase at 1 week of life reaching 30% of adult levels by the age of 1 month.

Although the ontogeny of phase II drug-metabolizing enzymes is less well established than phase I drug-metabolizing enzymes, available data suggests that specific isoforms of uridine diphosphate (UDP)-glucuronosyltransferase (UGT) display distinct patterns of maturation, which can markedly affect the pharmacokinetics of drugs (Barrett et al., 1996):

- The expression and activity of the isoforms UGT1A6 and UGT1A9, are lower in neonates and infants, and the glucuronidation of acetaminophen by UGT1A6 and, to a lesser extent, UGT1A9, is markedly decreased relative to adolescents and adults (Miller et al., 1976)

- The isoform UGT2B7 can be detected from 24 weeks of gestational age, and glucuronidation of morphine can occur in premature infants (Barrett et al., 1996). As the expression and activity of UGT2B7 markedly increases between 27 and 40 weeks postconceptual age, increases in morphine dose are necessary to maintain therapeutic plasma levels of morphine (Scott et al., 1999).

Glucuronidation plays an important role in the metabolism of many opioids and their metabolites, as the enzyme, uridine 5-diphophoglucuronosyltransferase, attaches glucuronic acid onto a functional group on the parent opioid to form a highly polar metabolite, which is then eliminated by the kidneys. For example, codeine is converted into codeine-6-glucuronide via UGT2B7. Although the ontogeny of UGT expression is still incompletely understood, it is known that at 15 weeks of gestational age, glucuronidation activity is present. Immediately after birth, UGT activity increases to approximately 10% of adult levels and by 3 to 6 months of age, neonatal activity level of UGT reaches full adult capacity (Pacifici et al., 1982).

Glucuronidation of acetaminophen to produce its toxic metabolite, N-acetyl-p-benzoquinone-imine (NAPQI), is capable of depleting hepatic glutathione and results in hepatotoxicity (Rumore and Blaiklock, 1992). In contrast to sulphation processes, which are more developed in young children, glucuronidation activity increases with age explaining less hepatotoxicity observed in children under 6 years of age even when acetaminophen plasma levels are within the range that is toxic at older ages (Rumore and Blaiklock, 1992).

Elimination of drugs

Beginning at 9 weeks of age, there is a developmental increase in the glomerular filtration rate, a process that is dependent on normal nephrogenesis but is complete by 36 weeks of gestation, and then influenced by postnatal changes in renal and intrarenal blood flow (Robillard et al., 1988). During the first 2 weeks of life, there is a rapid and marked increase in the glomerular filtration rate, which reaches its peak adult values by 8 to 12 months of age (Arant, 1978; van den Anker et al., 1995). Correspondingly, delayed maturation of tubular secretion is observed following birth; however, it reaches adult capacity by the first year of life (Arant, 1978).

As developmental differences in the maturation of renal function can significantly influence the plasma clearance of drugs extensively eliminated by the kidneys (e.g. ceftazidime and famotidine; James et al., 1998), consideration of the ontogeny of renal function and age-appropriate dosing regimens for infants is necessary to avoid potential toxicity.

Developmental paediatric pharmacodynamics

It is well-established that physiological development plays an important role in the mechanism of action of, and the response to, a drug. However, the effect of ontogeny on the interactions between a drug within the human body and the consequence of these interactions are still incompletely understood. Certain drugs, such as cyclosporine (Marshall and Kearns, 1999) and warfarin (Takahashi et al., 2000), demonstrate developmental differences in the interaction between a drug and the targeted receptor. Whereas, drugs such as midazolam show a clearer relationship between plasma level and the pharmacological effect of the drug (e.g. sedative effect; Marshall et al., 2000).

Functionally and morphologically, the human brain is immature at birth, which contributes to the variability in opioid-related analgesia and respiratory depression. Moreover, the ontogeny of the BBB, drug metabolizing enzymes, and transporters also alter the pharmacodynamics of opioids in neonates. Opioids must travel across the BBB in order to elicit their therapeutic effect; therefore, the amount of opioid that an infant brain is exposed to is in part dependent on the maturity of the BBB. For example, neonates are more sensitive to the respiratory effects of morphine and merperidine compared to older children and adults (Way et al., 1965), and the greater permeability of neonatal brain to opioids (Koren et al., 1985) is one contributing factor. Additionally, human newborns display age-related differences in morphine requirement, and full-term neonates aged 7 days or younger require significantly less morphine to achieve an analgesic effect compared to older children (Bouwmeester et al., 2003; see also Hathway, Chapter 44; Strassels, Chapter 45, this volume).

Low expression and function of P-glycoprotein (P-gp), an efflux transporter, in neonates also contributes to heightened central nervous system (CNS) exposure to morphine. The localization of P-gp along the luminal plasma membrane of the brain capillary endothelium is important, as these transporters efflux xenobiotics to prevent entry and accumulation of neurotoxins or drugs in the brain (de Vries et al., 2007; Fellner et al., 2002). Although limited data is available regarding the developmental differences in the expression the P-gp transporter, it is known that neonates express P-gp as early as 22 weeks of gestational age, however, at relatively low levels compared to that of adults (Daood et al., 2008). Postmortem analysis of CNS tissue obtained from neonates at 23 to 42 weeks gestational age revealed significantly lower expression levels, but with a similar pattern of P-gp localization to that of adults (Tsai et al., 2002). As such, it is probable that delayed expression and function of P-gp may contribute to a heightened and sustained CNS exposure to morphine (Bouwmeester et al., 2004). Further studies examining the contribution of the ontogeny of P-gp in the analgesic effect of opioids, such as morphine, in neonates are required to fully understand the impact of age-related differences in opioid response.

Developmental paediatric pharmacogenomics and pharmacogenetics

There are a multitude of genetic factors that can influence the disposition and action of a drug, and these interindividual differences can also elicit very different clinical responses to the same dose of a drug. In addition to physiological developmental differences, genetic polymorphisms in drug metabolizing enzymes and drug transporters also significantly influence the pharmacokinetic and pharmacodynamic responses to certain drugs, such as opioids.

Polymorphisms in drug metabolizing enzymes

Codeine is an alkaloid of the opium poppy *Papaver somniferum* and its analgesic effects are derived from metabolic conversion to morphine by demethylase activity (International Narcotic Control Board, United Nations: Narcotic Drug, Estimated World Requirements for 2013- Statistics for 2011 and Chen Z.R, Somogyi A.A, Reynolds .G, Bochner .F., 1991). As codeine is considered a 'weak' opioid, it is understood that use was associated with a low incidence of adverse events when compared to 'stronger' opioids. As a result, codeine had been the most commonly prescribed opioid for treatment of mild-to-moderate pain in children (Conroy and Peden, 2001; de Lima et al., 1996). Codeine is available in an oral elixir form for oral administration to infants and young children, and is often used in combination with acetaminophen in a 10:1 ratio of acetaminophen (120 mg/5 ml) to codeine (12 mg/5 ml) (Reisine and Pasternak, 1996). Recent reports have recognized that genetic factors play a major role in the disposition and analgesic effect of codeine (Madadi and Koren, 2008; Madadi et al., 2009), as the primary enzyme cytochrome P450 2D6 (CYP2D6) that O-demethylates codeine to morphine is highly polymorphic (Madadi and Koren, 2008; Olkkola et al., 1995; Yaster and Deshpande, 1988). Functional polymorphisms in genes encoding for metabolic enzymes may lead to altered drug response with either a diminished, excessive, or absent metabolism. The enzymatic activity of CYP2D6 is determined by measuring the urinary metabolic ratio, which is the amount of unchanged drug in urine/amount of O-demethylated metabolite in urine, in comparison with a specified known probe substrate, such as dextromethorphan or desbrisoquinie. Four phenotypic classifications have been established: poor metabolizers (PM), intermediate (IM) or extensive metabolizers (EM) and ultrarapid metabolizers (UM) (Ito et al., 2010). Genetically, PM exhibit non-functional homozygotes CYP2D6 alleles, IM displays one functional allele and one decrease or null function allele, EM have two functional alleles and UM possess more

than two functional alleles (Ito et al., 2010). In relation to codeine analgesia, metabolism of codeine by CYP2D6 to the active metabolite, morphine, is necessary to achieve an analgesic effect. Therefore, phenotypes of clinical significance are:

+ PM which are associated with therapeutic failure, as deletion or inactive variants of CYP2D6 results in reduced formation of morphine and lack of analgesia. Approximately 5% to 10% of Caucasians are phenotypically classified as PM and thus, are unable to make the conversion of codeine to morphine and they fail to elicit analgesic effects with codeine (Caraco et al., 1999; Madadi and Koren, 2008; Madadi et al., 2009; Sistonen et al., 2007).

+ UM which are associated with severe opioid intoxication, as individuals carrying more than two functional CYP2D6 alleles may produce an excess amount of morphine from codeine (Ciszkowski et al., 2009). Approximately 1% to 2% of Caucasians are classified into the UM phenotype and therefore, these individuals very rapidly and readily convert codeine to morphine resulting in approximately 50% higher plasma concentrations of morphine corresponding to severe opioid intoxication, which may result in a high incidence of CNS depression (Dalen et al., 1997; Kirchheiner et al., 2007; Madadi and Koren, 2008).

In conjunction with genetic polymorphisms in the *CYP2D6* gene, ontogeny further contributes to the interindividual variability in CYP2D6 activity. Some studies have demonstrated very low levels of CYP2D6 expression in foetal liver, where only 3% to 5% of adult expression of CYP2D6 is present during the third trimester with a significant increase following the first week of life (Blake et al., 2007; Ladona et al., 1991; Neville et al., 2011). Furthermore, *in vitro* data of CYP2D6 ontogeny demonstrates that CYP2D6 protein expression and activity remain constant after 1 week of life up to 18 years (Neville et al., 2011; Stevens et al., 2008) and that the contribution of CYP2D6 phenotypes in children approaches adult levels at 10 years of age (Stevens et al., 2008). However, significant interindividual variability in CYP2D6 activity is observed during the first year of life (Blake et al., 2007) suggesting that both genetic variation in CYP2D6 expression and activity and developmental factors involving CYP2D6 maturity play important roles in the metabolism of drugs, such as codeine.

Of concern, very few studies have investigated the effects of phenotype, genotype, and adverse events associated with codeine use for infant pain (Williams et al., 2002, 2004). Furthermore, despite several guidelines suggesting a paediatric therapeutic safe dose of less than 2 mg/kg, a threshold that is unlikely to result in adverse drug reactions (ADRs; American Academy of Pediatrics, 1997), there have been reports of severe and life-threatening ADRs associated with the use of codeine at the recommended dose of less than 2 mg/kg in infants and children (Meyer and Tobias, 2005; Sachdeva and Stadnyk, 2005; von Muhlendahl et al., 1976). As such, it is evident that genetic variations, in addition to developmental factors, may amplify the risk of ADRs associated with codeine use in infants and young children and therefore, caution should be taken when prescribing codeine.

Polymorphisms in opioid transporters

The P-gp transporter, which is encoded by the *ATP-binding cassette B1* (*ABCB1*) gene, is expressed in the BBB at the luminal membrane of the brain endothelial cells where it effluxes opioids from the brain to the blood (Xie et al., 1999). P-gp is a major determinant of opioid bioavailability in the CNS, as it is capable of limiting entry of opioids into the brain (Wandel et al., 2002). Therefore, functional polymorphisms in *ABCB1* may affect opioid disposition into the CNS (Kharasch et al., 2003; Lee et al., 2005; Xie et al., 1999; Zwisler et al., 2010). There have been approximately 35 single nucleotide polymorphisms identified in the coding region of the *ABCB1* gene and it has been suggested that, of these, homozygous 3435T/T carriers undergoing chronic oral morphine exposure may experience greater pain relief than homozygous wild-type 3435C/C (Campa et al., 2008); however, the impact of this variant on P-gp expression in the brain remains unknown.

Analgesic therapy for paediatric patients

Most pain medications, which include peripheral (e.g. non-steroidal anti-inflammatory drugs (NSAIDs)) and centrally (e.g. morphine and related opioid compounds) acting analgesics, are metabolized by several hepatic enzyme systems, including sulphation, glucuronidation, oxidation, and cytochrome P450 subtypes (Tateishi et al., 1997). However, delayed functional maturation of these enzyme systems in neonates and infants significantly influences the pharmacokinetic properties of these agents with additional age-dependent changes in pharmacodynamic responses to analgesic drugs. The pharmacology of specific drug therapies are covered in more detail in other chapters, but are briefly mentioned here. Acetaminophen and NSAIDs, frequently used to treat mild to moderate pain, have antipyretic effects in infants and young children, and NSAIDs also have anti-inflammatory effects (Brooks and Day, 1991; Maunuksela and Olkkola, 1993; Savvas and Brooks, 1991). With the exception of the neonatal period, the pharmacokinetics and pharmacodynamics of NSAIDs in young children are similar to adults (Berde and Sethna, 2002; Mak et al., 2011) and although there is the potential for gastrointestinal and renal toxicities, the incidence in infants and older children is less frequent than observed in adults (Szer et al., 1991; see Anderson, Chapter 43, this volume).

Morphine is the most commonly used intravenous opioid in neonates, infants, and children, as it provides potent analgesia (Anand et al., 2008), but age-related differences in both pharmacokinetic and pharmacodynamic responses during development pose challenges for selection of an appropriate dose (Pasternak et al., 1980). As sensitivity to morphine's CNS effects is increased in neonates (Koren et al., 1993; Reisine and Pasternak, 1996), a lower initial dose of morphine is recommended (Olkkola et al., 1995), which is then titrated against individual response. In addition, the elimination half-life of morphine is more than twice as long as that observed in adults due to the immaturity of neonate's hepatic enzyme system (McRorie et al., 1992). Morphine clearance increases in accordance with the maturation of the glomerular filtration rate (Bouwmeester et al., 2004) and by 1 year of age, the ratio of plasma to cerebral spinal fluid morphine concentration is comparable to that of adults (Hain et al., 1999) (see also Hathway, Chapter44; Strassels, Chapter 45, this volume).

Conclusion

Many challenges arise when managing pain in paediatric patients, as pain is a complicated subjective experience and the physiological development of neonates, infants, and children has significant impact on the pharmacokinetic and pharmacodynamics profile of many analgesic agents. Although there has been significant progress, ongoing investigation and research is required to achieve a thorough understanding of the impact of developmental changes in drug disposition, metabolism and action, to enhance safe and effective pharmacological management of pain in neonates, infants and children.

References

Agunod, M., Yamaguchi, N., Lopez, R., Luhby, A. L., and Glass, G. B. (1969). Correlative study of hydrochloric acid, pepsin, and intrinsic factor secretion in newborns and infants. *Am J Dig Dis*, 14, 400–414.

American Academy of Pediatrics. (1997). Use of codeine- and dextromethorphan-containing cough remedies in children. American Academy of Pediatrics. Committee on Drugs. *Pediatrics*, 99, 918–920.

Anand, K. J., Anderson, B. J., Holford, N. H., Hall, R. W., Young, T., Shephard, B., *et al.* (2008). Morphine pharmacokinetics and pharmacodynamics in preterm and term neonates: secondary results from the NEOPAIN trial. *Br J Anaesth*, 101, 680–689.

Anderson, B. J., and Holford, N. H. (2008). Mechanism-based concepts of size and maturity in pharmacokinetics. *Annu Rev Pharmacol Toxicol*, 48, 303–332.

Anderson, B. J., and Palmer, G. M. (2006). Recent pharmacological advances in paediatric analgesics. *Biomed Pharmacother*, 60, 303–309.

Anonymous. (1999). Codeine for child pain: new preparation. Helpful in some cases. *Prescrire Int*, 8, 107–109.

Arant, B. S. Jr. (1978). Developmental patterns of renal functional maturation compared in the human neonate. *J Pediatr*, 92, 705–712.

Autret, E., Dutertre, J. P., Breteau, M., Jonville, A. P., Furet, Y., and Laugier, J. (1993). Pharmacokinetics of paracetamol in the neonate and infant after administration of propacetamol chlorhydrate. *Dev Pharmacol Ther*, 20, 129–134.

Barrett, D. A., Barker, D. P., Rutter, N., Pawula, M., and Shaw, P. N. (1996). Morphine, morphine-6-glucuronide and morphine-3-glucuronide pharmacokinetics in newborn infants receiving diamorphine infusions. *Br J Clin Pharmacol*, 41, 531–537.

Berde, C. B., and Sethna, N. F. (2002). Analgesics for the treatment of pain in children. *N Engl J Med*, 347, 1094–1103.

Blake, M. J., Gaedigk, A., Pearce, R. E., Bomgaars, L. R., Christensen, M. L., Stowe, C., *et al.* (2007). Ontogeny of dextromethorphan O- and N-demethylation in the first year of life. *Clin Pharmacol Ther*, 81, 510–516.

Bouwmeester, N. J., Anderson, B. J., Tibboel, D., and Holford, N. H. (2004). Developmental pharmacokinetics of morphine and its metabolites in neonates, infants and young children. *Br J Anaesth*, 92, 208–217.

Bouwmeester, N. J., Hop, W. C., van Dijk, M., Anand, K. J., van den Anker, J. N., and Tibboel, D. (2003). Postoperative pain in the neonate: age-related differences in morphine requirements and metabolism. *Intensive Care Med*, 29, 2009–2015.

Brooks, P. M., and Day, R. O. (1991). Nonsteroidal antiinflammatory drugs—differences and similarities. *N Engl J Med*, 324, 1716–1725.

Campa, D., Gioia, A., Tomei, A., Poli, P., and Barale, R. (2008). Association of ABCB1/MDR1 and OPRM1 gene polymorphisms with morphine pain relief. *Clin Pharmacol Ther*, 83, 559–566.

Caraco, Y., Sheller, J., and Wood, A. J. (1999). Impact of ethnic origin and quinidine coadministration on codeine's disposition and pharmacodynamic effects. *J Pharmacol Exp Ther*, 290, 413–422.

Chen, Z. R., Somogyi, A. A., Reynolds, G., Bochner, F., (1991). Disposition and metabolism of codeine after single and chronic doses in poor and seven extensive metabolizers. *Br J Clin Pharmacol*, 31(4), 381–390.

Ciszkowski, C., Madadi, P., Phillips, M. S., Lauwers, A. E., and Koren, G. (2009). Codeine, ultrarapid-metabolism genotype, and postoperative death. *N Engl J Med*, 361, 827–828.

Conroy, S. and Peden, V. (2001). Unlicensed and off label analgesic use in paediatric pain management. *Paediatr Anaesth*, 11, 431–436.

Dalen, P., Frengell, C., Dahl, M. L., and Sjoqvist, F. (1997). Quick onset of severe abdominal pain after codeine in an ultrarapid metabolizer of debrisoquine. *Ther Drug Monit*, 19, 543–544.

Daood, M., Tsai, C., Ahdab-Barmada, M., and Watchko, J. F. (2008). ABC transporter (P-gp/ABCB1, MRP1/ABCC1, BCRP/ABCG2) expression in the developing human CNS. *Neuropediatrics*, 39, 211–218.

Dawson, W. T. (1940). Relations between age and weight and dosage of drugs*. *Annals of Internal Med*, 13, 1594–1615.

de Lima, J., Lloyd-Thomas, A. R., Howard, R. F., Sumner, E., and Quinn, T. M. (1996). Infant and neonatal pain: anaesthetists' perceptions and prescribing patterns. *Br Med J*, 313, 787.

de Vries, N. A., Zhao, J., Kroon, E., Buckle, T., Beijnen, J. H., and van Tellingen, O. (2007). P-glycoprotein and breast cancer resistance protein: two dominant transporters working together in limiting the brain penetration of topotecan. *Clin Cancer Res*, 13, 6440–6449.

Di Lorenzo, C., Flores, A. F., and Hyman, P. E. (1995). Age-related changes in colon motility. *J Pediatr*, 127, 593–596.

Echeverria, P., Siber, G. R., Paisley, J., Smith, A. L., Smith, D. H., Jaffe, N., and Paed, D. (1975). Age-dependent dose response to gentamicin. *J Pediatr*, 87, 805–808.

Ehrnebo, M., Agurell, S., Jalling, B., and Boreus, L. O. (1971). Age differences in drug binding by plasma proteins: studies on human foetuses, neonates and adults. *Eur J Clin Pharmacol*, 3, 189–193.

Fellner, S., Bauer, B., Miller, D. S., Schaffrik, M., Fankhanel, M., Spruss, T., et al. (2002). Transport of paclitaxel (Taxol) across the blood-brain barrier in vitro and in vivo. *J Clin Invest*, 110, 1309–1318.

Fluhr, J. W., Pfisterer, S., and Gloor, M. (2000). Direct comparison of skin physiology in children and adults with bioengineering methods. *Pediatr Dermatol*, 17, 436–439.

Gibbs, J. P., Liacouras, C. A., Baldassano, R. N., and Slattery, J. T. (1999). Up-regulation of glutathione S-transferase activity in enterocytes of young children. *Drug Metab Dispos*, 27, 1466–1469.

Goldstein, L.H., Berlin, M., Berkovitch, M., and Kozer, E. (2008). Effectiveness of oral vs rectal acetaminophen: A meta-analysis. *Arch Pediatr Adolesc Med*, 162, 1042.

Gupta, M. and Brans, Y. W. (1978). Gastric retention in neonates. *Pediatrics*, 62, 26–29.

Hain, R. D. Hardcastle, A., Pinkerton, C. R., and Aherne, G. W. (1999). Morphine and morphine-6-glucuronide in the plasma and cerebrospinal fluid of children. *Br J Clin Pharmacol*, 48, 37–42.

Heimann, G. (1980). Enteral absorption and bioavailability in children in relation to age. *Eur J Clin Pharmacol*, 18, 43–50.

Helms, J.E. and Barone, C.P. (2008). Physiology and treatment of pain. *Critical Care Nurs*, 28, 38–49.

Hines, R. N., and McCarver, D. G. (2002). The ontogeny of human drug-metabolizing enzymes: phase I oxidative enzymes. *J Pharmacol Exp Ther*, 300, 355–360.

Holford, N. H. (1996). A size standard for pharmacokinetics. *Clin Pharmacokinet*, 30, 329–332.

International Narcotic Control Board, United Nations: Narcotic Drug, Estimated World Requirements for 2013- Statistics for 2011. 30–31 (2013).

Ito, T., Kato, M., Chiba, K., Okazaki, O., and Sugiyama, Y. (2010). Estimation of the interindividual variability of cytochrome 2D6 activity from urinary metabolic ratios in the literature. *Drug Metab Pharmacokinet*, 25, 243–253.

Ittmann, P. I., Amarnath, R., and Berseth, C. L. (1992). Maturation of antroduodenal motor activity in preterm and term infants. *Dig Dis Sci*, 37, 14–19.

James, L. P., Marotti, T., Stowe, C. D., Farrar, H. C., Taylor, B. J., and Kearns, G. L. (1998). Pharmacokinetics and pharmacodynamics of famotidine in infants. *J Clin Pharmacol*, 38, 1089–1095.

Kearns, G. L. (2000). Impact of developmental pharmacology on pediatric study design: overcoming the challenges. *J Allergy Clin Immunol*, 106 (Suppl.), S128–38.

Kearns, G. L., Abdel-Rahman, S. M., Alander, S. W., Blowey, D. L., Leeder, J. S., and Kauffman, R. E. (2003). Developmental pharmacology—drug disposition, action, and therapy in infants and children. *N Engl J Med*, 349, 1157–1167.

Kharasch, E.D., Hoffer, C., Whittington, D., and Sheffels, P. (2003). Role of P-glycoprotein in the intestinal absorption and clinical effects of morphine. *Clin Pharmacol Ther*, 74, 543–554.

Kirchheiner, J., Schmidt, H., Tzvetkov, M., Keulen, J. T., Lotsch, J., Roots, I., and Brockmoller, J. (2007). Pharmacokinetics of codeine and its metabolite morphine in ultra-rapid metabolizers due to CYP2D6 duplication. *Pharmacogenomics J*, 7, 257–265.

Koren, G., Butt, W., Chinyanga, H., Soldin, S., Tan, Y. K., and Pape, K. (1985). Postoperative morphine infusion in newborn infants: assessment of disposition characteristics and safety. *J Pediatr*, 107, 963–967.

Koren, G., Jacobson, S. Schester, N., Berde, C., and Yaster, M. (1993). Developmental considerations in the clinical pharmacology of analgesics. *Pain in infants, children, and adolescents. Baltimore: Williams and Wilkins* 33–38.

Lacroix, D., Sonnier, M., Moncion, A., Cheron, G., and Cresteil, T. (1997). Expression of CYP3A in the human liver—evidence that the shift between CYP3A7 and CYP3A4 occurs immediately after birth. *Eur J Biochem*, 247, 625–634.

Ladona, M. G., Lindstrom, B., Thyr, C., Dun-Ren, P., and Rane, A. (1991). Differential foetal development of the O- and N-demethylation of codeine and dextromethorphan in man. *Br J Clin Pharmacol*, 32, 295–302.

Madadi, P. and Koren, G. (2008). Pharmacogenetic insights into codeine analgesia: implications to pediatric codeine use. *Pharmacogenomics*, 9, 1267–1284.

Madadi, P., Ross, C. J., Hayden, M. R., Carleton, B. C., Gaedigk, A., Leeder, J. S., et al. (2009). Pharmacogenetics of neonatal opioid toxicity following maternal use of codeine during breastfeeding: a case-control study. *Clin Pharmacol Ther*, 85, 31–35.

Mak, W.Y., Yuen, V., Irwin, M., and Hui, T. (2011). Pharmacotherapy for acute pain in children: current practice and recent advances. *Expert Opin Pharmacother*, 12, 865–881.

Marshall, J., Rodarte, A., Blumer, J., Khoo, K. C., Akbari, B., and Kearns, G. (2000). Pediatric pharmacodynamics of midazolam oral syrup. Pediatric Pharmacology Research Unit Network. *J Clin Pharmacol*, 40, 578–589.

Marshall, J. D., and Kearns, G. L. (1999). Developmental pharmacodynamics of cyclosporine. *Clin Pharmacol Ther*, 66, 66–75.

Maunuksela, E.L. and Olkkola, K.T. (1993). Nonsteroidal anti-inflammatory drugs in pediatric pain management. In N. L. Shechter, C. B. Beroe, and M. Yaster, (eds) *Pain in infants, children, and adolescents*, pp. 135–143. Baltimore: Williams & Wilkins.

McCarver, D. G., and Hines, R. N. (2002). The ontogeny of human drug-metabolizing enzymes: phase II conjugation enzymes and regulatory mechanisms. *J Pharmacol Exp Ther*, 300, 361–366.

McRorie, T. I., Lynn, A. M., Nespeca, M. K., Opheim, K. E., and Slattery, J. T. (1992). The maturation of morphine clearance and metabolism. *Am J Dis Child*, 146, 972–976.

Meyer, D. and Tobias, J. D. (2005). Adverse effects following the inadvertent administration of opioids to infants and children. *Clin Pediatr (Phila)*, 44, 499–503.

Miller, R. P., Roberts, R. J., and Fischer, L. J. (1976). Acetaminophen elimination kinetics in neonates, children, and adults. *Clin Pharmacol Ther*, 19, 284–294.

Munzenberger, P. J., and McKercher, P. (1980). Pediatric dosing—the pharmacist's dilemma. *Contemp Pharm Pract*, 3, 11–14.

Neville, K. A., Becker, M. L., Goldman, J. L., and Kearns, G. L. (2011). Developmental pharmacogenomics. *Paediatr Anaesth*, 21, 255–265.

Olkkola, K. T., Hamunen, K., and Maunuksela, E. L. (1995). Clinical pharmacokinetics and pharmacodynamics of opioid analgesics in infants and children. *Clin Pharmacokinet*, 28, 385–404.

Pacifici, G.M., Sawe, J., Kager, L., and Rane, A. (1982). Morphine glucuronidation in human foetal and adult liver. *Eur J Clin Pharmacol*, 22, 553–558.

Reisine, T. and Pasternak, G. (1996). Opioid analgesics and antagonists. In J. G. Hardman, and L. E. Limbird (eds) *Goodman & Gilman's the pharmacological basis of therapeutics* (9th edn), pp. 521–555. New York: McGraw Hill.

Ritschel, W. A. (1980). Drug dosage in children. In W. A. Ritschel, (eds) *Handbook of basic pharmacokinetics* (2nd edn), pp. 296–310. Hamilton, IL: Drug Intelligence.

Robillard, J. E., Nakamura, K. T., Matherne, G. P., and Jose, P. A. (1988). Renal hemodynamics and functional adjustments to postnatal life. *Semin Perinatol*, 12, 143–150.

Rumore, M. M., and Blaiklock, R. G. (1992). Influence of age-dependent pharmacokinetics and metabolism on acetaminophen hepatotoxicity. *J Pharm Sci*, 81, 203–207.

Sachdeva, D. K., and Stadnyk, J. M. (2005). Are one or two dangerous? Opioid exposure in toddlers. *J Emerg Med*, 29, 77–84.

Savvas, P. and Brooks, P. M. (1991). Non steroidal anti-inflammatory drugs. Risk factors versus benefits. *Aust Fam Physician*, 20, 1726–9, 1732–3.

Scott, C. S., Riggs, K. W., Ling, E. W., Fitzgerald, C. E., Hill, M. L., Grunau, R. V., *et al.* (1999). Morphine pharmacokinetics and pain assessment in premature newborns. *J Pediatr*, 135, 423–429.

Siber, G. R., Echeverria, P., Smith, A. L., Paisley, J. W., and Smith, D. H. (1975). Pharmacokinetics of gentamicin in children and adults. *J Infect Dis*, 132, 637–651.

Simon, L. S., and Mills, J. A. (1980a). Drug therapy: nonsteroidal antiinflammatory drugs (first of two parts). *N Engl J Med*, 302, 1179–1185.

Simon, L. S., and Mills, J. A. (1980b). Nonsteroidal antiinflammatory drugs (second of two parts). *N Engl J Med*, 302, 1237–1243.

Sistonen, J., Sajantila, A., Lao, O., Corander, J., Barbujani, G., and Fuselli, S. (2007). CYP2D6 worldwide genetic variation shows high frequency of altered activity variants and no continental structure. *Pharmacogenet Genomics*, 17, 93–101.

Sonnier, M. and Cresteil, T. 1998. Delayed ontogenesis of CYP1A2 in the human liver. *Eur J Biochem*, 251, 893–898.

Stahlberg, M. R., Hietanen, E., and Maki, M. (1988). Mucosal biotransformation rates in the small intestine of children. *Gut*, 29, 1058–1063.

Stevens, J. C., Marsh, S. A., Zaya, M. J., Regina, K. J., Divakaran, K., Le, M., and Hines, R. N. (2008). Developmental changes in human liver CYP2D6 expression. *Drug Metab Dispos*, 36, 1587–1593.

Szer, I. S., Goldenstein-Schainberg, C., and Kurtin, P. S. (1991). Paucity of renal complications associated with nonsteroidal antiinflammatory drugs in children with chronic arthritis. *J Pediatr*, 119, 815–817.

Taiwo, Y. O., and Levine, J. D. (1988). Prostaglandins inhibit endogenous pain control mechanisms by blocking transmission at spinal noradrenergic synapses. *J Neurosci*, 8, 1346–1349.

Takahashi, H., Ishikawa, S., Nomoto, S., Nishigaki, Y., Ando, F., Kashima, T., *et al.* (2000). Developmental changes in pharmacokinetics and pharmacodynamics of warfarin enantiomers in Japanese children. *Clin Pharmacol Ther*, 68, 541–555.

Tateishi, T., Nakura, H., Asoh, M., Watanabe, M., Tanaka, M., Kumai, T., *et al.* (1997). A comparison of hepatic cytochrome P450 protein expression between infancy and postinfancy. *Life Sci*, 61, 2567–2574.

Treluyer, J. M., Gueret, G., Cheron, G., Sonnier, M., and Cresteil, T. (1997). Developmental expression of CYP2C and CYP2C-dependent activities in the human liver: in-vivo/in-vitro correlation and inducibility. *Pharmacogenetics*, 7, 441–452.

Treluyer, J. M., Jacqz-Aigrain, E., Alvarez, F., and Cresteil, T. (1991). Expression of CYP2D6 in developing human liver. *Eur J Biochem*, 202, 583–588.

Tsai, C. E., Daood, M. J., Lane, R. H., Hansen, T. W., Gruetzmacher, E. M., and Watchko, J. F. (2002). P-glycoprotein expression in mouse brain increases with maturation. *Biol Neonate*, 81, 58–64.

van den Anker, J. N., Schoemaker, R. C., Hop, W. C., van der Heijden, B. J., Weber, A., Sauer, P. J., *et al.* (1995). Ceftazidime pharmacokinetics in preterm infants: effects of renal function and gestational age. *Clin Pharmacol Ther*, 58, 650–659.

van Lingen, R. A., Deinum, J. T., Quak, J. M., Kuizenga, A. J., van Dam, J. G., Anand, K. J., *et al.* (1999). Pharmacokinetics and metabolism of rectally administered paracetamol in preterm neonates. *Arch Dis Child Fetal Neonatal Ed*, 80, F59–63.

Vieira, I., Sonnier, M., and Cresteil, T. (1996). Developmental expression of CYP2E1 in the human liver. Hypermethylation control of gene expression during the neonatal period. *Eur J Biochem*, 238, 476–483.

von Muhlendahl, K. E., Scherf-Rahne, B., Krienke, E. G., and Baukloh, G. (1976). Codeine intoxication in childhood. *Lancet*, 2, 303–305.

Wandel, C., Kim, R., Wood, M., and Wood, A. (2002). Interaction of morphine, fentanyl, sufentanil, alfentanil, and loperamide with the efflux drug transporter P-glycoprotein. *Anesthesiology*, 96, 913–920.

Way, W. L., Costley, E. C., and Leongway, E. (1965). Respiratory sensitivity of the newborn infant to meperidine and morphine. *Clin Pharmacol Ther*, 6, 454–461.

Weiss, C. F., Glazko, A. J., and Weston, J. K. (1960). Chloramphenicol in the newborn infant. A physiologic explanation of its toxicity when given in excessive doses. *N Engl J Med*, 262, 787–794.

West, D. P., Worobec, S., and Solomon, L. M. (1981). Pharmacology and toxicology of infant skin. *J Invest Dermatol*, 76, 147–150.

Williams, D. G., Dickenson, A., Fitzgerald, M, and Howard, R. F. (2004). Developmental regulation of codeine analgesia in the rat. *Anesthesiology*, 100, 92–97.

Williams, D. G., Patel, A., and Howard, R. F. (2002). Pharmacogenetics of codeine metabolism in an urban population of children and its implications for analgesic reliability. *Br J Anaesth*, 89, 839–45.

Windorfer, A, Kuenzer, W., and Urbanek, R. (1974). The influence of age on the activity of acetylsalicylic acid-esterase and protein-salicylate binding. *Eur J Clin Pharmacol*, 7, 227–231.

Xie, R., Hammarlund-Udenaes, M., de Boer, A. G., and de Lange, E. C. (1999). The role of P-glycoprotein in blood-brain barrier transport of morphine: transcortical microdialysis studies in mdr1a (-/-) and mdr1a (+/+) mice. *Br J Pharmacol*, 128, 563–568.

Yaster, M, and Deshpande, J. K. (1988). Management of pediatric pain with opioid analgesics. *J Pediatr*, 113, 421–429.

Zwisler, S. T., Enggaard, T. P., Noehr-Jensen, L., Mikkelsen, S., Verstuyft, C., Becquemont, L., *et al.* (2010). The antinociceptive effect and adverse drug reactions of oxycodone in human experimental pain in relation to genetic variations in the OPRM1 and ABCB1 genes. *Fundam Clin Pharmacol*, 24, 517–524.

CHAPTER 43

The non-steroidal anti-inflammatory drugs and acetaminophen

Brian J. Anderson

Summary

The non-steroidal anti-inflammatory drugs (NSAIDs) and acetaminophen (N-acetyl-p-aminophenol, APAP) are the commonest analgesic drugs used in childhood. Although both drugs act through inhibition of prostaglandin H_2 synthetase (PGHS), acetaminophen lacks the anti-inflammatory effects of the NSAIDs. Neonatal acetaminophen hepatic clearance is reduced in premature neonates (5–10% adult rates) and increases to 30% adult rates in neonates born at term; adult rates (approximately 16–20 L/h/70 kg) are reached within the first year of life. NSAID clearance maturation, mostly through cytochrome P450 mixed oxidases, is more rapid. Concentration–response relationships suggest a maximum pain reduction of 5 or 6 on a 10-point scale for both drugs. Combination therapy does not increase this maximum effect but does prolong duration of analgesia. While both drugs have good safety profiles, dosing of both drug groups is tempered by concerns about toxicity. Acetaminophen hepatotoxicity is associated with single doses (>250 mg/kg in preschool children, >150 mg/kg in adults) and therapy duration longer than 3 to 5 days (>90 mg/kg/day). The most common minor adverse events in NSAID recipients are nausea, dizziness, and headache. More concerning is the potential of NSAIDs to cause gastrointestinal irritation, blood clotting disorders, renal impairment, neutrophil dysfunction, and bronchoconstriction. These adverse effects are uncommon provided care is taken with drug dose, duration of therapy, and recognition of contraindications.

Acetaminophen

Mechanism of action

Acetaminophen (N-acetyl-p-aminophenol, APAP, paracetamol) has been used in clinical practice for more than 100 years and is the most commonly prescribed paediatric medicine. Acetanilid, the parent compound of acetaminophen, was introduced in 1886. Toxicity-related problems with acetanilid led to the introduction of acetaminophen in 1893. The popularity of acetaminophen over the non-steroidal anti-inflammatory drugs (NSAIDs) ascended after the reported association between Reye's syndrome and aspirin in the 1980s (Committee on Infectious Disease, 1982). Acetaminophen is widely used in the management of pain and fever, but is lacking anti-inflammatory effects.

Debate exists about the site of action. Prostaglandin H_2 synthetase (PGHS) is the enzyme responsible for metabolism of arachidonic acid to the unstable prostaglandin H_2. The two major forms of this enzyme are the constitutive PGHS-1 and the inducible PGHS-2. PGHS is comprised of two sites; a cyclo-oxygenase (COX) site and a peroxidise (POX) site (Figure 43.1). The conversion of arachidonic acid to prostaglandin G_2 is dependent on a tyrosine-385 radical at the COX site. Acetaminophen acts as a reducing cosubstrate on the POX site and lessens the amount of tyrosine-385 radical at the COX site. Alternatively, acetaminophen effects may be mediated by an active metabolite (p-aminophenol). P-aminophenol is conjugated with arachidonic acid by fatty acid amide hydrolase to form AM404. AM404 exerts effect through cannabinoid receptors (Anderson, 2008).

Pharmacodynamics

The relation between drug concentration and response may be described by the Hill equation or E_{max} model:

$$Effect = E0 + \frac{\left(E\max \cdot Ce^N\right)}{\left(EC_{50}^N + Ce^N\right)} \qquad \text{Equation 43.1}$$

where E_0 is the baseline response, E_{max} is the maximum effect change, Ce is the concentration in the effect compartment, EC_{50} is the concentration producing 50% E_{max} and N is the Hill coefficient defining the steepness of the concentration-response curve (Figure 43.2). Efficacy is the maximum response on a dose or concentration-response curve.

A delay often exists between plasma and effect site concentration. A single first-order parameter ($T_{1/2}$keo) describes the equilibration half-time between plasma and effect site. The concentration in the effect compartment is used to describe the concentration–effect relationship.

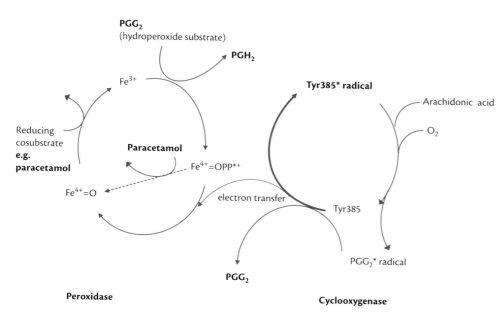

Figure 43.1 Prostaglandin H_2 synthetase (PGHS) is the enzyme responsible for metabolism of arachidonic acid to the unstable prostaglandin H_2. Formation of tyrosine-385 radical (Tye385*) at the COX site is dependent on the reduction of a ferrylprotoporphyrin IX radical cation ($Fe^{4+} = OPP^{*+}$) at the POX site. Acetaminophen is a reducing cosubstrate that partially reduces $Fe^{4+} = OPP^{*+}$, decreasing the amount available for regeneration of Tyr385*. Reproduced from Brian J. Anderson, Paracetamol (Acetaminophen): mechanisms of action, *Paediatric Anasthesia*, Volume 18, Issue 10, pp. 915–921, Copyright © 2008 The Author, by permission of John Wiley & Sons, Inc., http://onlinelibrary.wiley.com/journal/10.1111/%28ISSN%291460-9592.

Analgesia

Acetaminophen is an effective analgesic drug. Thirty seven per cent of patients (>13 years of age) given an intravenous (IV) acetaminophen formulation for postoperative pain experienced at least 50% pain relief over 4 h compared with 16% receiving placebo (number needed to treat (NNT) 4.0, 95% confidence interval (CI) 3.5–4.8; Inomata et al., 2003). Increased analgesia has been reported with increasing plasma concentration until a maximum effect (e.g. E_{max} 5.17/10; visual analogue pain score 0–10 after paediatric tonsillectomy). However, the analgesic effect of acetaminophen is not directly related to plasma concentration. Further time is required for the drug to move from the plasma into the effect site. There are time delays of approximately 1 h between peak concentration and peak effect (Figure 43.3); the equilibration half-time ($T_{1/2}$keo) was 53 min (Figure 43.4). A target effect compartment concentration of 10 mg/L is associated with a pain reduction of 2.6/10 (Anderson et al., 2001). Pain fluctuations, pain type, and placebo effects complicate interpretation of clinical studies.

Attempts to unravel these time relationships with studies using oral or rectal acetaminophen are difficult because there are further time delays associated with absorption from the gastrointestinal (GI) tract into the blood. The use of an IV acetaminophen formulation allows greater dosing accuracy, less pharmacokinetic variability attributable to absorption, and more rapid speed of effect onset (Gibb and Anderson, 2008). Infusions over 15 min of IV acetaminophen 15 mg/kg following inguinal hernia repair in children resulted in a steep reduction in pain between 15 and 30 min (Murat et al., 2005), consistent with a delay achieving effect site concentrations in the brain. Two European Centres have published dosing guidelines in neonates (Allegaert et al., 2007; Bartocci and Lundeberg, 2007). These regimens attempt to achieve a steady-state target concentration of 10 mg/L.

Acetaminophen is commonly used to supplement postoperative analgesia from morphine infusion, but this usually only reduces morphine consumption by 10% to 20% and is probably insufficient to decrease morphine-related adverse effects (Maund et al., 2011).

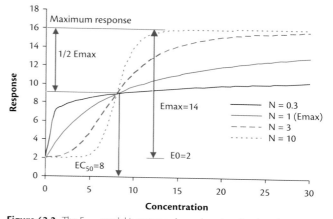

Figure 43.2 The E_{max} model is commonly used to describe the relationship between drug response and concentration. Changing the Hill coefficient dramatically alters the shape of the curve.

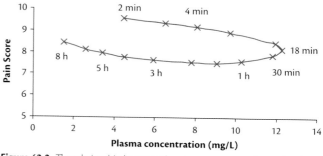

Figure 43.3 The relationship between the plasma concentration and analgesic effect demonstrates clockwise hysteresis. The equilibration half-time ($T_{1/2}$keo) of the analgesic effect compartment was 53 min. Reproduced with permission from I. A. Gibb and B. J. Anderson, Paracetamol (acetaminophen) pharmacodynamics: interpreting the plasma concentration, *Archives of Disease in Childhood*, Volume 93, Issue 3, pp. 241–247, Copyright © 2008 BMJ Publishing Group Ltd and Royal College of Paediatrics and Child Health, http://adc.bmj.com/.

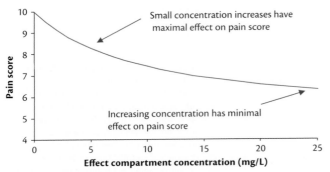

Figure 43.4 The effect compartment–response relationship for acetaminophen analgesia after tonsillectomy.
Reproduced with permission from I. A. Gibb and B. J. Anderson, Paracetamol (acetaminophen) pharmacodynamics: interpreting the plasma concentration, *Archives of Disease in Childhood*, Volume 93, Issue 3, pp. 241–247, Copyright © 2008 BMJ Publishing Group Ltd and Royal College of Paediatrics and Child Health, http://adc.bmj.com/.

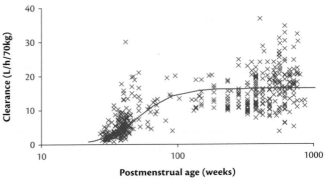

Figure 43.5 Clearance changes with age. Individual predicted clearances, standardized to a 70 kg person, from the NONMEM program's post hoc step are plotted against age. The thin line demonstrates the predicted non-linear relationship between clearance and age.
Reproduced from Brian J. Anderson and Karel Allegaert, Intravenous neonatal acetaminophen dosing; the magic of ten days, *Paediatric Anaesthesia*, Volume 19, Issue 4, pp. 289–295, Copyright © 2009 The Authors, by permission of John Wiley & Sons, Inc., http://onlinelibrary.wiley.com/journal/10.1111/%28ISSN%291460-9592.

Pharmacokinetics

Oral absorption

Acetaminophen has low first-pass metabolism, and the hepatic extraction ratio is 0.11 to 0.37. Acetaminophen is rapidly absorbed from the duodenum to the systemic circulation. There is usually a short interval before the drug enters the duodenum from the stomach (5 min) and then absorption is rapid; absorption half-life is 2 to 5 min (Anderson et al., 2000; Brown et al., 1992). Absorption in children under the age of 3 months is delayed because absorption depends on gastric emptying, and gastric emptying is slow and erratic in the neonate. Normal adult rates may not be reached until 6 to 8 months.

Rectal absorption

Rectal acetaminophen is widely used in children presenting for surgical procedures because of GI dysfunction or preoperative fasting guidelines that disallow food or fluids up to 6 h before surgery. It is also preferable in children with nausea and vomiting. The relative bioavailability of rectal compared with oral acetaminophen formulations ranges from 0.24 to 0.98. Absorption through the rectal route is slow and erratic (absorption half-life 0.65–1.34 h). The absorption half-life for rectal formulations is prolonged in infants younger than 3 months (1.51 times greater) compared to values in older children (Anderson et al., 2002).

Clearance

Acetaminophen is metabolized predominantly by uridine diphospho-glucuronosyltransferases (UGT1A6). This enzyme is immature in neonates, although some acetaminophen can be metabolized by sulphate conjugation, which is mature in term neonates. Maturation of clearance is completed in within the first few years of life and reflects the maturation of the UGT1A6 isoenzyme (Miyagi and Collier, 2011). Clearance increases from 27 weeks postmenstrual age (1.87 L/h/70 kg) to reach 84% of the mature value (c.16–20 L/h/70 kg) by 1 year of age (Figure 43.5) (Anderson et al., 2002, 2005). Clearance through sulphate conjugation is saturable and dependent on substrate availability (Reith et al., 2009). It is also possible that APAP may induce glucutonosyltransferase, leading to increased clearance after repeat therapeutic dosing (Gelotte et al., 2007). Total body clearance is first order after very high doses

(20 g/m^2) when used to augment alkylating drugs for melanoma treatment (Wolchok et al., 2003).

Volume of distribution

The volume of distribution in children is similar to those reported in adults (56–70 L; Prescott, 1996). Peripheral volume of distribution decreased from 27 weeks postmenstrual age (45.0 L/70 kg) to reach 110% of its mature value by 6 months of age (Figure 43.6) (Anderson et al., 2005), reflecting neonatal body composition and the rapid changes in body water distribution in early life.

Disease states

The effects of altered physiology such as fever, anaesthesia, or mildly impaired hepatic dysfunction on pharmacokinetic parameters have received little attention, but appear to have minimal impact in children. Similarly, chronic conditions such as diabetes and renal failure have minimal impact on pharmacokinetics. Clearance is reduced in disease states where we might expect reduced hepatic function; hypothyroidism, congestive heart failure, acute viral hepatitis. The impact of obesity is unknown. Bilirubin is also cleared by a glucuronosyltransferase (UGT1A1); increased unconjugated bilirubin concentration in neonates is an indicator of reduced hepatic function and consequently reduced clearance. However size (predicted by weight) is the major covariate of clearance variance in neonates (Allegaert et al., 2011).

Toxicity

Chronic use of acetaminophen

Hepatotoxicity is the principal adverse effect. The toxic metabolite of acetaminophen, *N*-acetyl-*p*-benzoquinone imine (NAPQI), is formed by the CYP2E1. Hepatotoxicity is dependent on the balance between the rate of NAPQI formation, capacity of the safe elimination pathways of sulphate and glucuronide production, and the initial content and maximal rate of synthesis of hepatic glutathione that mops up NAPQI. NAPQI binds to intracellular hepatic macromolecules to produce cell necrosis and damage. During hepatocyte lysis APAP-protein adducts are released into plasma and these can be used as specific biomarkers of APAP toxicity in patients with acute liver injury (Bond, 2009; James et al., 2009).

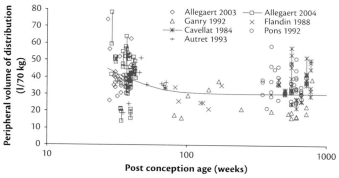

Figure 43.6 Peripheral volume of distribution changes with age. Individual predicted volumes, standardized to a 70 kg person, against age. The solid line demonstrates the non-linear relationship between volume of distribution and age. Those children given multiple doses have volume of distribution estimates linked by a fine line to demonstrate between occasion variability.
Reproduced from Brian J. Anderson et al., Paediatric intravenous acetaminophen (propacetamol) pharmacokinetics; a population analysis. *Paediatric Anaesthesia*, Volume 15, Issue 4, pp. 282–292, Copyright © 2005 The Authors, by permission of John Wiley & Sons, Inc., http://onlinelibrary.wiley.com/journal/10.1111/%28ISSN%291460-9592

Significant hepatic and renal disease, malnutrition, and dehydration may increase the propensity for toxicity. Medications that induce the NAPQI formation (e.g. phenobarbitone, phenytoin, and rifampicin) may also increase the risk of hepatotoxicity. The influence of disease on acetaminophen toxicity is unknown. Hepatotoxicity causing death or requiring liver transplantation has been reported with doses above 75 mg/kg/day in children and 90 mg/kg/day in infants. It is possible that even these traditional regimens may cause hepatotoxicity if used for longer than 2 to 3 days (Kearns et al., 1998).

Hepatic enzyme profiles have been used as a surrogate assessment in neonatal studies. Although no hepatic changes occurred during the treatment periods that extended over a median of 4 days, the value of hepatic changes is debated (Anderson and Allegaert, 2009). It is currently impossible to predict which individuals have an enhanced susceptibility to cellular injury from acetaminophen.

Single dose of acetaminophen

The Rumack and Matthew (Rumack and Matthew, 1975) acetaminophen toxicity nomogram is widely used to guide management of acetaminophen overdose in adults and children. Acetaminophen concentrations of more than 300 mg/L at 4 h were always associated with severe hepatic lesions, but none were observed in adults with concentrations less than 150 mg/L. The half-life was less than 4 h in all patients without liver damage.

Clearance, expressed as L/h/kg is greater in children than adults. The 4 h concentration is determined by clearance in preschool children following accidental ingestion of elixir where absorption is rapid. As a consequence, younger children (1–5 years) require larger doses than older children and adults to achieve similar concentrations at 4 h. Children (1–5 years) with reported accidental ingestion of greater than 250 mg/kg (compare to 150 mg/kg in adults) can have serum concentration measured at 2 h after ingestion rather than the 4 h time point recommended in adults (Anderson et al., 1999).

Neonates can produce NAPQI, but CYP2E1 in neonates is immature at birth. This may explain the low occurrence of acetaminophen-induced hepatotoxicity seen in neonates, despite reports of high serum concentrations in newborn neonates. Neonatal hepatotoxicity has been reported in an ex-term (41-week) neonate who presented encephalopathic at 5 days following 3 days of oral acetaminophen dosing—initially 156 mg/kg/day and then 78 mg/kg/day. The neonate had an unconjugated hyperbilirubinaemia (130 μmol/L) on admission with marked liver derangement and after receiving N-acetyl cysteine recovered fully over 7 days (Walls et al., 2007).

Dosing with formulation

Suggested acetaminophen dosing for different age groups is shown in Table 43.1. These dosing regimens achieve a target concentration of 10 mg/L, but may be considered too high as concerns about dose and hepatotoxicity increase. Children seek rapid relief from symptoms, be they pain or fever. In general, the smaller the child, the shorter the $T_{1/2}$keo, but absorption characteristics of enteral acetaminophen in neonates delays analgesia onset. Speed of onset may be shortened by giving a larger initial dose or improving absorption characteristics or changing the formulation (Gibb and Anderson, 2008). Target effect compartment concentrations (and effect) will be reached earlier as dose is increased. The administration of a large initial oral or rectal 'loading' dose will achieve the target concentration speedily, but such dosing may exceed the subsequent daily dose recommendation. Formulation has considerable impact. For example the slow absorption of rectal acetaminophen suppositories means peak concentrations are only reached after several hours. In contrast an IV formulation has rapid onset of analgesia (Figure 43.7).

Non-steroidal anti-inflammatory drugs

Mechanism of action

The NSAIDs are a heterogeneous group of compounds that share common antipyretic, analgesic, and anti-inflammatory effects (Table 43.2). Their major action is through inhibition of prostaglandin synthesis. NSAIDs act by reducing prostaglandin biosynthesis through inhibition at the COX site of PGHS (Figure 43.8). The two major forms of this enzyme are the constitutive PGHS-1 and the inducible PGHS-2 (COX-1 and COX-2). This enzyme converts arachidonic acid to cyclic endoperoxides. The prostinoids produced by COX-1 protect the gastric mucosa, regulate renal blood flow, and induce platelet aggregation. NSAID-induced GI toxicity, for example, is generally believed to occur through blockade of COX-1 activity, whereas the anti-inflammatory effects of NSAIDs are thought to occur primarily through inhibition of the inducible isoform, COX-2. Relative COX-1/COX-2 specificity ratios vary from greater than 1 (aspirin, indomethacin, ibuprofen), approximately 1 (diclofenac, naproxen), to less than 1 (celecoxib, etoricoxib).

Pharmacodynamics

The NSAIDs are commonly used in children for antipyresis and analgesia. The anti-inflammatory properties of the NSAIDs have, in addition, been used in such diverse disorders as juvenile idiopathic arthritis, renal and biliary colic, dysmenorrhoea, Kawasaki disease, and cystic fibrosis. The NSAIDs indomethacin and ibuprofen are also used to treat delayed closure of patent ductus arteriosis in premature neonates.

Pain relief attributable to NSAIDs has been compared to pain relief from other analgesics or analgesic modalities (e.g. caudal blockade, acetaminophen, and morphine). Studies comparing

Table 43.1 Suggested acetaminophen dosing

Age	Typical body weight (kg)	Acetaminophen clearance (L/h/kg)	Acetaminophen dose (oral)
Neonate	3.3	0.21	50 mg, 8 h
3 months	6	0.25	90 mg, 6 h
6 months	7.5	0.27	120 mg, 6 h
1 year	10	0.29	120 mg, 4 h
5 years	18	0.25	250 mg, 4 h
8 years	24	0.24	300 mg, 4 h
12 years	38	0.21	375 mg, 4 h
16 years	50	0.3	500 mg, 4 h
Adult	70	0.3	1000 mg, 6 h

The maintenance dose of acetaminophen for a patient is calculated as follows: acetaminophen maintenance dose = acetaminophen clearance × target concentration. Individual clearance values can be predicted from weight and age (Anderson et al., 2002). Most of the age-related changes in clearance are complete by 1 year of age. There are also size-related changes in clearance so that the value per kg continues to decrease as weight increases in children (Anderson and Meakin, 2002; Anderson et al., 1997). Clearance in adults is reported as higher than in children. The doses have been calculated to maintain a target serum acetaminophen concentration of 10 mg/L and a lower target may be preferred because of hepatotoxicity concerns

For patients more than 20% overweight, use ideal body weight. Children prefer elixir to capsules or tablets. It is important to note that elixir formulation is available in different formulation strengths when prescribing the dose by volume. Proprietary cough and cold medications containing acetaminophen are also available. Concurrent use of such medications can result in inadvertent acetaminophen toxicity. The relative bioavailability of rectal formulations is reduced out of the neonatal period and dose can be increased by 30%. Dose is reduced in premature neonates (e.g. 24 and 45 mg/kg/d at 30 and 34 weeks postmenstrual age, respectively.

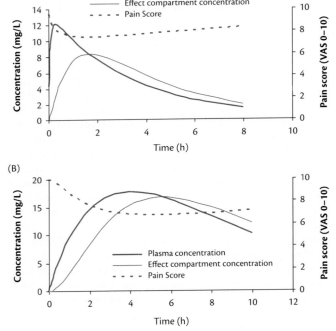

Figure 43.7 (A) The temporal relationships for plasma concentration, effect compartment concentration and analgesic effect after 12.5 mg/kg acetaminophen elixir in a child. The absorption half-time used was 4.5 min. (B) The temporal relationships for plasma concentration, effect compartment concentration and analgesic effect after 20 mg/kg acetaminophen suppository in an adult. Maximum effect lags an hour behind the 4 h peak concentration. Reproduced with permission from I. A. Gibb and B. J. Anderson, Paracetamol (acetaminophen) pharmacodynamics: interpreting the plasma concentration, *Archives of Disease in Childhood*, Volume 93, Issue 3, pp. 241–247, Copyright © 2008 BMJ Publishing Group Ltd and Royal College of Paediatrics and Child Health, http://adc.bmj.com/.

ketorolac (0.75–1 g/kg) to morphine (0.1 mg/kg) for analgesia after paediatric tonsillectomy, strabismus surgery, or general surgery have demonstrated similar degrees of analgesia with reduced emesis with some increased bleeding in children given ketorolac. Diclofenac and ketorolac reduce morphine use by up to 40% in children after a surgical insult.

Conflicting reports plague the literature as to whether NSAIDs or acetaminophen display greater analgesic effect when given alone. An early meta-analysis comparing single doses of acetaminophen 7 to 15 mg/kg with ibuprofen 4 to 10 mg/kg found similar analgesic effect in children (Perrott et al., 2004). A more recent meta-analysis identified 54 studies directly comparing the analgesic effect of acetaminophen with ibuprofen (Pierce and Voss, 2010). The authors concluded that ibuprofen is at least as effective as, if not more so than, acetaminophen in both adults and children. These comparisons are difficult to interpret because of differences in pain insult, timing of response, duration and nature of pain scores, patient ages, doses administered, and formulations used (Anderson, 2004).

NSAIDs appear to be equally effective at commonly used doses (Davies and Skjodt, 2000). It has been suggested (Maunuksela and Olkkola, 2003) that 1 mg/kg of rectal diclofenac = 10 mg/kg of oral ibuprofen = 40 mg/kg of rectal acetaminophen = 5 mg/kg of IV ketoprofen = 0.5 mg/kg of IV ketorolac. A single dose of ibuprofen 400 mg had a NNT of 2.5 for at least 50% pain relief compared with placebo (Collins et al., 2002; Kopacz and Bernards, 2001). This means that two of every five adults with pain of moderate to severe intensity will experience at least 50% pain relief with ibuprofen, which they would not have had with placebo. The equivalent NNTs for ibuprofen 200 and 600 mg were 3.3 and 2.4, respectively, and those for diclofenac 25, 50, and 100 mg were 2.6, 2.3, and 1.8, respectively (Table 43.3).

NSAID concentration–response relationships are rare in children, but have been described for adults. Data from adults given

Table 43.2 Classification of common NSAIDs

Sulphonanilides	Fenamic acid derivatives	Selective COX-2 inhibitors
Nimesulide	Mefenamic acid	Etoricoxib
	Meclofenamic acid	Paracoxib
Salicylic acid derivatives	Tofenamic acid	Celecoxib
Aspirin	Flufenamic acid	
Sodium salicylate		**Acetic acid derivatives**
Diflunisal	**Propionic acid derivatives**	Etodolac
	Fenoprofen	Indomethacin
Enolic acids	Ibuprofen	Sulindac
Meloxicam	Flurtiprofen	Ketorolac
Phenylbutazone	Ketoprofen	Diclofenac
Piroxicam	Naproxen	
Tenoxicam	Dexketoprofen	

Table 43.3 Number needed to treat (NNT) for ibuprofen and diclofenac in adults

Ibuprofen (mg)	NNT (95% CI)	Diclofenac (mg)	NNT (95% CI)
50	4.7 (3.3–8)	25	2.6 (2.2–3.3)
100	4.3 (3.2–6.4)	50	2.7 (2.4–3)
200	2.7 (2.5–3)	100	2.3 (2–2.5)
400	2.5 (2.4–2.6)		
600	2.7 (2.0–4.2)		
800	1.6 (1.3–2.2)		

Source: data from Derry, P., Derry, S., Moore, R. A., and McQuay, H.J., Single dose oral diclofenac for acute postoperative pain in adults, *Cochrane Database of Systematic Reviews* 2009, Issue 2, Copyright © 2009 The Cochrane Collaboration and Derry, C. J., Derry, S., Moore, R. A., and McQuay, H. J., Single dose oral ibuprofen for acute postoperative pain in adults, *Cochrane Database of Systematic Reviews* 2009, Issue 3, Copyright © 2009 The Cochrane Collaboration.

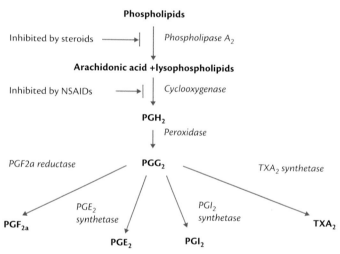

Figure 43.8 The conversion of arachidonic acid to PGG_2, the precursor of the prostaglandins is controlled by prostaglandin H_2 synthetase (PGHS). PGHS comprises of two sites; a cyclooxygenase (COX) site and a peroxidise (POX) site

ibuprofen after dental extraction suggest a similar E_{max} to that described for acetaminophen (1.54 of a scale 0–3; Li et al., 2012). The equilibration half-time ($T_{1/2}keo$) of 28 min was less than the 53 min reported for acetaminophen (Anderson et al., 2001). In addition, the slope of the concentration–response curve was steeper than that for acetaminophen (Hill = 2 for ibuprofen, Hill = 1 for acetaminophen) indicating a more rapid onset of analgesia. Data from adult patients given ketorolac for postoperative pain relief after orthopaedic surgery revealed an E_{max} of 8.5/10 (VAS 0–10) and $T_{1/2}keo$ 24 min (Mandema and Stanski, 1996).

Interpretation of analgesia is also complicated by active metabolites. Naproxcinod is an active metabolite of naproxen (Ingelmo and Fumagalli, 2005). Diclofenac's 4'-hydroxyl metabolite has 30% of the anti-inflammatory and antipyretic activity of the parent

compound. Approximately 20% of the parent drug is processed to this metabolite. Despite the impact of this metabolite, there are reasonable data to support the contention that diclofenac 50 mg is as effective as diclofenac 100 mg in adults (McQuay and Moore, 1998; Wong and Baker, 1988). Little or no information on developmental differences in arachidonic acid release, prostaglandin formation, or COX-2 expression is available for the paediatric population. It has been assumed that attaining similar adult exposure to 50 mg in children should give similar effectiveness. This argument has been used to support a single dose of diclofenac 0.3 mg/kg for IV, 0.5 mg/kg for suppositories, and 1 mg/kg for oral diclofenac in children aged 1 to 12 years (Standing et al., 2011).

Pharmacokinetics

Pharmacokinetic age-related changes and covariate effects are poorly documented for many of the NSAIDs. There are limited data in infants less than 6 months age (Litalien and Jacqz-Aigrain, 2001). NSAID formulations may be administered orally, topically, intraocularly, intra-articularly, intravenously, intramuscularly, and rectally. NSAIDs are rapidly absorbed in the GI tract after oral administration. Time to maximal concentration is generally 1 to 2 h, but depends on formulation and concomitant food intake. Absorption due to the dissolution time of diclofenac tablets is slower than that associated with effervescent or liquid formulations (Standing et al., 2011). An absorption lag time of 1 h has been reported in children given enteric-coated diclofenac tablets (Romsing et al., 2001). The relative bioavailability of oral preparations approaches 1 compared to IV administration. The rate and extent of rectal absorption of NSAIDs such as ibuprofen, diclofenac, flurbiprofen, indomethacin, and nimesulide is generally less than those by oral routes.

The apparent volume of distribution (V/F) is small in adults (less than 0.2 L/kg, suggesting minimal tissue binding) but is larger in children; for example, ketorolac V/F in children 4 to 8 years old is twice that of adults (Forrest et al., 1997; Olkkola and Maunuksela, 1991). Premature neonates (22 to 31 weeks gestational age) given IV ibuprofen had a V/F of 0.62 (SD 0.04) L/kg (Aranda et al., 1997). A dramatic reduction in ibuprofen central volume following closure of the PDA in premature neonates (0.244 versus 0.171 L/kg) is reported (Van Overmeire et al., 2001).

The NSAIDs, as a group, are weakly acidic, lipophilic, and highly protein bound. The bound fraction in children and premature neonates is slightly lower than in adults. The impact of this reduced protein binding is probably minimal with routine dosing because NSAIDs cleared by the liver have a low hepatic extraction ratio and they have a long equilibration time between plasma and effect compartments (Benet and Hoener, 2002). There is relatively little transfer from maternal to fetal blood. Excretion of NSAIDs into breast milk of lactating mothers is low.

NSAIDs undergo extensive phase I and phase II enzyme biotransformation in the liver, with subsequent excretion into urine or bile. Enterohepatic recirculation occurs when a significant amount of an NSAID or its conjugated metabolites are excreted into the bile and then reabsorbed in the distal intestine. Pharmacokinetic parameter estimate variability is large, partly attributable to covariate effects of age, size, and pharmacogenomics. Ibuprofen, for example, is metabolized by the CYP2C9 and CYP2C8 subfamily. It is known that considerable variation exists in the expression of CYP2C activities among individuals, and functional polymorphism of the gene coding for CYP2C9 has been described.

NSAID elimination is all too frequently described only in terms of half-life, which is therefore confounded by volume of distribution. The plasma half-lives of NSAIDs in adults range from 0.25 to greater than 70 h, indicating wide differences in clearance rates. Elimination half-lives are longer in neonates than in children. An elimination half-life of 30.5 h was reported in premature infants receiving ibuprofen within the first 12 h of life (Aranda et al., 1997), in contrast with 1.6 h in infants and children aged 3 months to 10 years (Kelley et al., 1992). Clearance increases from birth; ibuprofen clearance increases from 2.06 ml/h/kg at 22 to 31 weeks postmenstrual age (Aranda et al., 1997), 9.49 ml/h/kg at 28 weeks postmenstrual age (Van Overmeire et al., 2001), to 140 ml/h/kg at 5 years (Scott et al., 1999) (Table 43.4). Clearance (L/h/kg) is generally increased in childhood both for the established NSAIDs and for the newer COX-2 inhibitors. This increased clearance is common for most drugs in childhood. Age-related ketorolac pharmacokinetic parameter estimates after 0.5 mg per kg intravenously are shown in Table 43.5. Elimination clearance, corrected for size using an allometric $^3/_4$-power model (Anderson and Holford, 2008), is similar to adult estimates from 1 year of age. Data from infants under the age of 1 year suggest higher clearance estimates of 1.5 ml/min/kg (Cederholm et al., 1992; Demiraran et al., 2008).

Many NSAIDs are formulated as a racemic mixture where only one isomer is active, but where the other may influence pharmacokinetics (stereoselectivity). Ibuprofen stereoselectivity has been reported in premature neonates (<28 weeks of gestation). R- and S-ibuprofen half-lives were about 10 h and 25.5 h, respectively. The mean clearance of R-ibuprofen (12.7 ml/h) was about 2.5-fold higher than for S-ibuprofen (5.0 ml/h) (Gregoire et al., 2004). Similar data have been reported for ketorolac (Hansen et al., 2001; Kristensen et al., 1998). Single-isomer NSAIDs are appearing for the treatment of acute pain and may have fewer adverse effects than traditional NSAIDs.

Reports of the use of COX-2 selective inhibitors in children are appearing in the literature, but their future use is still uncertain following reports of atherothrombosis in adults. Future benefits may be derived from nitric oxide or hydrogen sulphide releasing NSAIDs

that have increased potency and reduced side effects (Fiorucci and Distrutti, 2011).

Drug interactions

High protein binding among the NSAIDs has been used to explain drug interactions with oral anticoagulant agents, oral hypoglycaemics, sulphonamides, bilirubin, and other protein-bound drugs. Warfarin administered with phenylbutazone increased plasma warfarin concentrations and prothrombin time in normal volunteers. Phenylbutazone displaces warfarin from its albumin-binding sites *in vitro*, but this observation cannot be extrapolated to an *in vivo* effect. The observed effect is due to changes in drug metabolic clearance and not from changes in protein binding.

The NSAIDs can reduce the antihypertensive effect of angiotensin-converting enzyme inhibitors and β-blockers with possible loss of blood pressure control and can attenuate the natriuretic effect of thiazide diuretics and furosemide. Concurrent administration of probenecid decreases NSAID renal clearance. Lithium and methotrexate concentrations may be increased due to decreased renal clearance. Significant drug interactions have also been demonstrated for aspirin, digoxin, cyclosporine, cholestyramine, and colestipol (Davies and Anderson, 1997).

Renal failure

Renally excreted NSAIDs such as azapropazone may accumulate in renal failure. Ketoprofen and naproxen are metabolized via the acyl glucuronidation pathway, and also may accumulate in renal failure. Renal impairment is a risk factor for NSAID-induced renal toxicity (Davies and Skjodt, 2000).

Hepatic disease

Hypoalbuminaemia will alter the volume of distribution of NSAIDs. NSAIDs that are mainly eliminated by hepatic oxidative metabolism may require dose reduction, or should be avoided in the presence of significant liver disease (Davies and Skjodt, 2000).

Safety issues

The most common adverse events in NSAID recipients are nausea, dizziness, and headache. NSAIDs have potential to cause GI irritation, blood clotting disorders, renal impairment, neutrophil dysfunction, and bronchoconstriction; effects postulated to be related to COX-1/COX-2 ratios, although this concept may be an oversimplification. COX-2, for example, is constitutively expressed in renal tissues of all species. It seems unlikely that these COX-2 inhibitors will offer renal safety benefits over non-selective NSAID therapies. It is reasonable to assume that all NSAIDs, including COX-2-selective inhibitors, share a similar risk for adverse renal effects (Brater et al., 2001).

One other concern is the sudden and profound bradycardia after rapid IV administration of ketorolac. Although the mechanism of this response is unclear, ketorolac should be administered slowly when given intravenously. Most children are asymptomatic after NSAID accidental overdose. Symptoms may comprise tinnitus, diarrhoea, nausea, blurred vision, drowsiness, vomiting, headache, agitation, confusion, rash, and sweating with increasing dose (e.g. >100 mg/kg ibuprofen). Severe overdose (e.g. ibuprofen >400 mg/kg) can be life threatening and present with respiratory depression, cardiovascular compromise, metabolic acidosis, renal failure, and altered neurological state.

Table 43.4 Pharmacokinetic parameter estimates for some commonly used NSAIDs

Age	No.	Formulation	CL/F (mL/h/kg)	V/F (L/kg)	$T_{1/2}$ (h)	Reference
Salicylic acid						
0.3–4 years	6	Suspension	ND	0.3 (0.1)	4 (2.1)	(Treluyer et al., 1991)
0.8–1.8 years	5	Suspension	ND	0.3 (0.06)	5.6 (6.4)	(Treluyer et al., 1991)
5.5 (0.8) years	10	Tablet	22.1 (1.8)	0.113 (0.005)	3.24	(Wilson et al., 1982)
Diclofenac						
4.3–6.8 years	10	IV	462 (90)	0.9 (0.25)	1.3 (0.3)	(Korpela and Olkkola, 1990)
4–8 years	26	Suppository	875	0.32	4.2	(van der Marel et al., 2004)
5–15 years	11	Tablet	754 (207)	0.71 (0.23)	0.65 (0.14)	(Romsing et al., 2001)
1–14 years	141[b]	IV (F = 1), dissolvable tablet F = 0.35, suppository F =0.63	291	0.21	–	(Standing et al., 2011)
Ibuprofen						
22–31 weeks	21[d]	IV	2.06 (0.33)	0.062 (0.004)	30.5	(Aranda et al., 1997)
28.6 (1.9) weeks	13[d]	IV	9.49 (6.82)	0.357 (0.121)	43.1 (26.1)	(Van Overmeire et al., 2001)
0.5–1.5 years	11	Suspension	110 (40)	0.20 (0.09)	1.6 (0.4)	(Rey et al., 1994)
11 months–11 years	18	Suspension	57.6	0.164	1.97	(Kelley et al., 1992)
3 months–12 years	28	Suspension	80 (SE 10)	0.16 (SE 0.02)	1.44 (SE 0.15)	(Brown et al., 1998)
3 months–12 years	39	Suspension	110 (SE 10)	0.22 (SE 0.02)	1.37 (SE 0.09)	(Brown et al., 1998)
5.2 (1.7) years	22	Suspension	140 (32)	0.27 (0.11)	1.4 (0.5)	(Scott et al., 1999)
5.2 (2.5) years	4	Tablet	114 (26)	0.26 (0.1)	1.6 (0.4)	(Scott et al., 1999)
4–16 years	103[b]	Suspension/ granules	71 (CV 24%) (4.05 L/h/70 kg)	V_c 0.06, V_p 0.1 (CV 65%)	—	(Troconiz et al., 2000)
4–11 years	24	suspension	77.5 (16.4)	0.147 (0.0037)	1.3	(Granfors et al., 2004)
Indomethacin						
28.8 (2.5) weeks[c]	83[e]	IV	2.63 × wt (kg) + 0.244PNA (d) mL/h (CV 77%)	0.28 × wt (kg) + 0.0041PNA (d) L (CV 28%)		(Wiest et al., 1991)
5.7 (4.7) days[d]						
1.2–4.6 years	14	IV	192 (102)	0.74 (0.75)	6.1 (4.9)	(Olkkola et al., 1989)
Ketoprofen						
7 months–16 years	18	IV	90 (60–130)	0.16 (0.12–0.21)	1.3 (0.8–1.7)	(Kokki et al., 2002)
Ketorolac						
0.4–33 weeks	12	IV	100	0. 18	–	(Cederholm et al., 1992)
2–11 months	17	IV	89.4 (69.2)	0.31 (0.11)	3.9 (2.8)	(Demiraran et al., 2008)
1–16 years	36	IV	34.2 (10.2)	0.113 (0.033)	–	(Dsida et al., 2002)
4–8 years	10	IV	42 (30–58)	0.26 (0.19–0.44)	6.1 (3.5–10)	(Olkkola and Maunuksela, 1991a)
3–18 years	50	IV	66 (30)	0.35 (0.2)	4.1 (2.3)	(Kauffman et al., 1999)
3.3–8 years	7	IV	80 (50)	0.26 (0.17)	2.26 (1.35)	(Gonzalez-Martin et al., 1997)
2.6–7.3 years	7	IV	70 (30)	0.21 (0.08)	2.09 (0.57)	(Gonzalez-Martin et al., 1997)

(Continued)

Table 43.4 *(Continued)*

Age	No.	Formulation	CL/F (mL/h/kg)	V/F (L/kg)	T$_{1/2}$ (h)	Reference
Naproxen						
8.1–14.1 years	12	Tablet	9.2 (2.6)	0.11 (0.02)	8.1 (2.1)	(Wells et al., 1994)
10.4–14.1 years	10	Suspension	9 (2.4)	0.13 (0.03)	9.6 (3.2)	(Wells et al., 1994)

[a]Variability is given in parentheses as SD, range, or SE. *CL/F* = apparent drug plasma clearance; IV = intravenous; *T$_{1/2}$* = elimination half-life; *V/F* = apparent volume of distribution; *V$_c$* = initial volume of distribution; *V$_p$*= apparent volume of distribution of peripheral compartment, ND = not determined, CV = coefficient of variation; PNA = postnatal age.

[b]Data reported using allometric model. Estimate presented for a 30 kg individual.

[c]Age is gestational age (weeks).

[d]Covariates age and weight included in parameter estimates.

Adapted from *Seminars in Fetal and Neonatal Medicine*, Volume 11, Issue 4, Jacqz-Aigrain E and Anderson BJ, Pain Control—Nonsteroidal anti-inflammatory agents, pp. 251–259, Copyright © 2006, with permission from Elsevier, http://www.sciencedirect.com/science/journal/1744165X.

Table 43.5 Ketorolac age-related pharmacokinetic changes

Age (years)	Weight (kg)	V$_{ss}$ (SD) (L/kg)	CL (SD) (mL/min/kg)	CL$_{std}$ (SD) (mL/min/70 kg)
1–3	12	0.111 (0.025)	0.6 (0.2)	27.0 (9.0)
4–7	20	0.128 (0.047)	0.61 (0.22)	31.2 (11.3)
8–12	30	0.099 (0.014)	0.54 (0.15)	30.6 (8.5)
12–16	50	0.116 (0.040)	0.51 (0.12)	32.8 (7.7)
Adult (Mandema and Stanski, 1996)	70	0.18	0.47	32.7

V$_{ss}$ = volume of distribution at steady state; *CL$_{std}$* = total body clearance standardized to a 70 kg person using an allometric $^3/_4$-power model; weight is estimated. Data are from Dsida et al. (2002).

Reprinted with permission from Caroline D. van der Marel et al., Diclofenac and metabolite pharmacokinetics in children, *Paediatric Anaesthesia*, Volume 14, Issue 6, pp. 443–451, Copyright © 2004 Blackwell Publishing Ltd, http://onlinelibrary.wiley.com/journal/10.1111/%28ISSN%291460-9592.

Renal effects

The effect of short-term treatment with NSAIDs on healthy kidneys is negligible. Ibuprofen reduced the glomerular filtration rate by 20% in premature neonates, affecting aminoglycoside clearance, and this effect appears independent of gestational age (Allegaert et al., 2005). Large studies involving ibuprofen (Lesko and Mitchell, 1997, 1999) and ketorolac (Houck et al., 1996) have shown little risk in children (e.g. upper 95% bound was 5.4 per 100 000 ibuprofen-treated children). Similar data are reported in children suffering juvenile rheumatoid arthritis (JIA) given NSAIDs as long-term treatment. However, renal compromise is described in children suffering dehydration, hypovolaemia, hypotension, or pre-existing renal disease. NSAIDs may also potentiate the toxicity of other drugs such as aminoglycosides and ciclosporin.

Gastrointestinal effects

Adverse GI effects are significant in adults, particularly in those with peptic ulcer disease, *Helicobacter pylori*, or advanced age. The risk of acute GI bleeding in children given short-term ibuprofen was estimated to be 7.2 in 100 000 (95% CI, 2–18 in 100 000) (Lesko and Mitchell, 1995, 1999) and was not different from those children given acetaminophen. Similar data are reported in children given ketorolac for acute pain (Forrest et al., 1997). The incidence of clinically significant gastropathy is comparable to adults in children given NSAIDs for JIA (Dowd et al., 1995; Keenan et al., 1995), but gastroduodenal injury may be very much higher depending on assessment criteria.

Bone healing

NSAIDs, but not acetaminophen, impair fracture healing in animal models. COX-2 activity plays an important role in bone healing and the use of NSAIDs decreases osteogenic activity that may increase the incidence of non-union after spinal surgery. The effect on osteogenic activity is dose-dependent and reversible. These effects are cause for concern after major orthopaedic surgery (Dodwell et al., 2010), but there was no risk of non-union with NSAID exposure when high-quality studies were assessed.

Bleeding propensity

The commonly used NSAIDs such as ketorolac, diclofenac, ibuprofen, and ketoprofen have reversible antiplatelet effects, which are attributable to the inhibition of thromboxane synthesis. Bleeding time is usually slightly increased in the perioperative period, but it remains within normal limits in children with normal coagulation systems. A Cochrane review has established that even after tonsillectomy, NSAIDs did not cause any increase in bleeding that required a return to theatre in children (Cardwell et al., 2005). There was significantly less nausea and vomiting with NSAIDs compared to alternative analgesics, suggesting their benefits outweigh their negative aspects.

The use of ketorolac analgesia for tonsillectomy, however, has been associated with increased bleeding. This was attributable to the dose used and whether it is given preoperatively or postoperatively and duration of therapy (Strom et al., 1996). The risk associated with the drug was larger and clinically important when ketorolac was used in higher doses, in older subjects, and for more than 5 days. It is reasonable to not administer this medication until the end of surgery after haemostasis is achieved. Forrest et al. have suggested an IV dose of ketorolac in children of 0.5 mg/kg, followed either by bolus injections of 1.0 mg/kg every 6 h or an IV infusion of 0.17 mg/kg/h (Forrest et al., 1997). The maximum daily dose is 90 mg, and the maximum duration of treatment is 48 h. The recommended oral dosage is 0.25 mg/kg to a maximum of 1.0 mg/kg/day, with a maximum duration of 7 days.

Asthma

Aspirin or NSAID exacerbated respiratory disease (ERD) is more a disorder of adults but exacerbations in children and teenagers have been reported. This adverse effect is countered by a beneficial reduction of asthma symptoms where ibuprofen was administered for antipyresis. Benefit is likely seen in younger children with mild episodic asthma and ERD is a concern in one in three teenagers with severe asthma and coexistent nasal disease. COX-2 inhibitors are reported as safe in NSAID-ERD (Palmer, 2005).

The acetaminophen–NSAID interaction

Acetaminophen and NSAIDs are often given together for the management of pain or fever. They can be safely combined without increases in their associated adverse effect profiles and combination therapy is popular. A review of randomized controlled studies comparing combined acetaminophen and ibuprofen therapy for postoperative pain management identified six studies (Ong et al., 2010). Of these, three were conducted in paediatric populations: oral premedication with acetaminophen and ibuprofen was supported over acetaminophen alone for tonsillectomy pain in children and following tooth extraction; while rectally administered acetaminophen and ibuprofen showed no benefit over acetaminophen alone for pain following adenoidectomy, although a reduction in rescue analgesia was seen in the combination group once home.

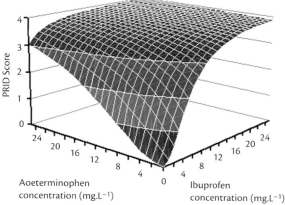

Disparities between results may stem from differences in the endpoint studied (particularly for assessments of analgesia) and dissimilar dosing regimens, as well as a plethora of other factors relating to study design, conduct and analysis. Dose–response curves published in adults (Mehlisch et al., 2010) for combination acetaminophen-ibuprofen therapy have been investigated for combination therapy response. Pain after dental surgery was measured using pain intensity differences (PRID, 0–8) from 0 to 8 h. Analysis of the response surface area (Figure 43.9) allowed dose interpretation in children (Hannam and Anderson, 2011). Simulation for a 20 kg child showed the addition of acetaminophen to ibuprofen doses of less than 5 mg/kg was effective; acetaminophen had minimal effect when given with ibuprofen at doses greater than 5 mg/kg in the immediate postoperative period. A more sustained analgesic effect was noted at 4 to 8 h after combination dosing (Figure 43.10).

Hepatotoxicity attributed to the therapeutic administration of acetaminophen

Case example

A 3-year-old boy suffered a depressed compound right-sided skull fracture with underlying brain contusion. He presented 1 h after injury with apnoea, hypovolaemia, and a Glasgow Coma Score of 6/15. Intubation, ventilation, volume resuscitation, and inotropes were instituted and the child went forward for emergency right fronto-temporal craniotomy and debridement of the fracture site. Postoperatively he remained stable. Prophylactic phenytoin was used for possible seizure activity and intermittent phenobarbital for sedation. Acetaminophen 100 mg/kg/day was administered through the nasogastric tube to control hyperpyrexia. Serum concentrations of acetaminophen were not measured. Serum aspartate aminotransferase (AST) was elevated to 610 IU/L on day 2. On day 3 he developed a metabolic acidosis with a base deficit of 9 mmol/L. There was a dramatic rise in AST (10 000 IU/L) and a moderate increase in gammaglutamyltransferase (GGT 113 IU/L) concentrations. The coagulation profile was disordered (APTT 79, PR 3.3, fibrinogen 1.6g/L).

Abdominal contrast-enhanced computed tomography (CT) revealed a large wedged-shaped area of non-enhancement in the right lobe of the liver with a large volume of free intraperitoneal fluid in the hepatorenal fossa, the right paracolic gutter, and the lesser sac of the pelvis. The lesion was assumed to represent a laceration and was managed conservatively; however, over the subsequent 48 h the child developed fulminant hepatic failure with multiple system organ involvement. Treatment was withdrawn on day 5.

Postmortem liver sections showed coagulative necrosis involving zone 3 which, in some areas, extended into zone 2 of the liver acinus. There was sparing of periportal areas. The portal triads were unremarkable. There was a mild acute inflammatory response associated with the coagulative necrosis. There was no evidence of centrilobular congestion or sinusoidal engorgement. There was no evidence of a laceration in the right lobe.

Figure 43.9 Theoretical response surface of effect between acetaminophen and ibuprofen. Concentrations are those in the effect compartment. The concentration response for acetaminophen is plotted on the x–y axis, while that for ibuprofen is on the z–y axis. The 'surface' is that plotted between these axes. Reproduced with permission from Jacqueline Hannam and Brian J. Anderson, Explaining the acetaminophen–ibuprofen analgesic interaction using a response surface model, *Paediatric Anaesthesia*, Volume 21, Issue 12, pp. 1234–1240, Copyright © 2011 Blackwell Publishing Ltd, http://onlinelibrary.wiley.com/journal/10.1111/%28ISSN%291460-9592.

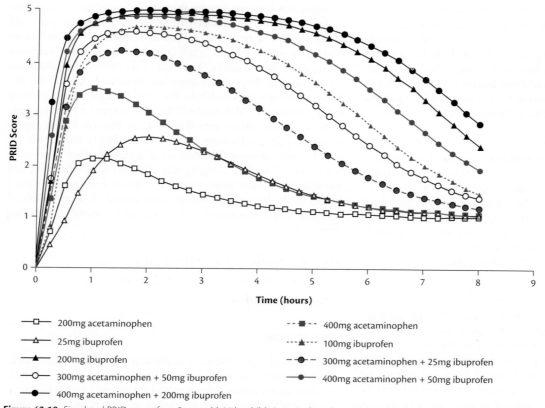

Figure 43.10 Simulated PRID scores for a 5-year-old, 20 kg child given single and combination acetaminophen-ibuprofen therapy. Reproduced with permission from Jacqueline Hannam and Brian J. Anderson, Explaining the acetaminophen–ibuprofen analgesic interaction using a response surface model, *Paediatric Anaesthesia*, Volume 21, Issue 12, pp. 1234–1240, Copyright © 2011 Blackwell Publishing Ltd, http://onlinelibrary.wiley.com/journal/10.1111/%28ISSN%291460-9592.

Discussion

In the case example, acetaminophen was implicated as a cause of hepatic necrosis in the child. Diagnosis was delayed because CT abdominal findings, performed 3 days after the presenting injury, were misinterpreted as hepatic trauma. The pattern of necrosis described in this child's liver is consistent with damage related to acetaminophen where zone 3 is the main area of concentration of the enzyme system responsible for the conversion of acetaminophen into hepatotoxic metabolites. None of the other drugs used in his management are commonly implicated in hepatoxicity, although co-administration of anticonvulsants may induce hepatic microsomal enzymes resulting in increased NAPQI after subsequent acetaminophen administration. While some anticonvulsant drugs may induce CYP2E1, phenytoin and phenobarbital are not metabolized through CYP2E1 and have not been considered to be CYP2E1 inducers, although there are reports that suggest phenobarbital induces a modest increase (1.7-fold) in CYP2E1 (Madan et al., 2003).

Acetaminophen has recognized hepatotoxicity after doses above 150 mg/kg in children (Penna and Buchanan, 1991), although data subsequent to this report has implicated lower threshold doses (75–90 mg/kg/day) used for 3 days or more (Kearns et al., 1998). Children may have raised serum concentrations after 2–3 days of repeated therapeutic doses, resulting in hepatic damage. Liver function is further reduced in the presence of ischaemic hepatitis, which occurs in association with severe shock and is due to a reduction in liver blood flow. The condition is manifested by elevation of plasma hepatic transaminase concentrations with peak concentrations occurring within 24 h of the ischaemic episode. It is likely that the combination of therapeutic acetaminophen doses in the presence of a liver compromised by ischaemic hepatitis, contributed to this boy's death.

Consideration should be given to both the indication for acetaminophen and the dose in children with hepatic pathology. Acetaminophen has poor effect on temperature changes due to cerebral pathology. Temperature reduction in this child would have been better achieved by external cooling and neuromuscular blockade to prevent shivering. Acetaminophen contributes little additional analgesia and does not reduce opioid adverse effects when used to supplement morphine (Maund et al., 2011). The use of acetaminophen to control fever continues to be debated. It has not been established conclusively that the benefits of antipyretic therapy outweigh its risks (Plaisance and Mackowiak, 2000).

References

Allegaert, K., Cossey, V., Debeer, A., Langhendries, J. P., Van Overmeire, B., De Hoon, J., *et al.* (2005). The impact of ibuprofen on renal clearance in preterm infants is independent of the gestational age. *Pediatr Nephrol*, 20, 740–743.

Allegaert, K., Murat, I., and Anderson, B. J. (2007). Not all intravenous paracetamol formulations are created equal. *Paediatr Anaesth*, 17, 811–812.

Allegaert, K., Palmer, G. M., and Anderson, B. J. (2011). The pharmacokinetics of intravenous paracetamol in neonates: size matters most. *Arch Dis Child*, 96, 575–580.

Anderson, B. J. (2004). Comparing the efficacy of NSAIDs and paracetamol in children. *Paediatr Anaesth*, 14, 201–217.

Anderson, B. J. (2008). Paracetamol (acetaminophen): mechanisms of action. *Paediatr Anaesth*, 18, 915–921.

Anderson, B. J., and Allegaert, K. (2009). Intravenous neonatal paracetamol dosing: the magic of 10 days. *Paediatr Anaesth*, 19, 289–295.

Anderson, B. J., and Holford, N. H. (2008). Mechanism-based concepts of size and maturity in pharmacokinetics. *Annu Rev Pharmacol Toxicol*, 48, 303–332.

Anderson, B. J., Holford, N. H. G., Armishaw, J. C., and Aicken, R. (1999). Predicting concentrations in children presenting with acetaminophen overdose. *J Pediatrics*, 135, 290–295.

Anderson, B. J., Mckee, A. D., and Holford, N. H. (1997). Size, myths and the clinical pharmacokinetics of analgesia in paediatric patients. *Clin Pharmacokinet*, 33, 313–327.

Anderson, B. J., and Meakin, G. H. (2002). Scaling for size: some implications for paediatric anaesthesia dosing. *Paediatr Anaesth*, 12, 205–219.

Anderson, B. J., Pons, G., Autret-Leca, E., Allegaert, K., and Boccard, E. (2005). Pediatric intravenous paracetamol (propacetamol) pharmacokinetics: a population analysis. *Paediatr Anaesth*, 15, 282–292.

Anderson, B. J., Van Lingen, R. A., Hansen, T. G., Lin, Y. C., and Holford, N. H. (2002). Acetaminophen developmental pharmacokinetics in premature neonates and infants: a pooled population analysis. *Anesthesiology*, 96, 1336–1345.

Anderson, B. J., Woollard, G. A., and Holford, N. H. (2000). A model for size and age changes in the pharmacokinetics of paracetamol in neonates, infants and children. *Br J Clin Pharmacol*, 50, 125–134.

Anderson, B. J., Woollard, G. A., and Holford, N. H. (2001). Acetaminophen analgesia in children: placebo effect and pain resolution after tonsillectomy. *Eur J Clin Pharmacol*, 57, 559–569.

Aranda, J. V., Varvarigou, A., Beharry, K., Bansal, R., Bardin, C., Modanlou, H., *et al.* (1997). Pharmacokinetics and protein binding of intravenous ibuprofen in the premature newborn infant. *Acta Paediatr*, 86, 289–293.

Bartocci, M., and Lundeberg, S. (2007). Intravenous paracetamol: the 'Stockholm protocol' for postoperative analgesia of term and preterm neonates. *Paediatric Anaesthesia*, 17, 1120–1121.

Benet, L. Z., and Hoener, B.-A. (2002). Changes in plasma protein binding have little clinical consequence. *Clin Pharm Ther*, 71, 115–121.

Bond, G. R. 2009. Acetaminophen protein adducts: a review. *Clin Toxicol (Phila)*, 47, 2–7.

Brater, D. C., Harris, C., Redfern, J. S., and Gertz, B. J. (2001). Renal effects of COX-2-selective inhibitors. *Am J Nephrol*, 21, 1–15.

Brown, R. D., Kearns, G. L., and Wilson, J. T. (1998). Integrated pharmacokinetic-pharmacodynamic model for acetaminophen, ibuprofen, and placebo antipyresis in children. *J Pharmacokinet Biopharm*, 26, 559–579.

Brown, R. D., Wilson, J. T., Kearns, G. L., Eichler, V. F., Johnson, V. A., and Bertrand, K. M. (1992). Single-dose pharmacokinetics of ibuprofen and acetaminophen in febrile children. *J Clin Pharmacol*, 32, 231–241.

Cardwell, M., Siviter, G., and Smith, A. (2005). Non-steroidal anti-inflammatory drugs and perioperative bleeding in paediatric tonsillectomy. *Cochrane Database Syst Rev*, 2, CD003591.

Cederholm, I., Evers, H., and Lofstrom, J. B. (1992). Skin blood flow after intradermal injection of ropivacaine in various concentrations with and without epinephrine evaluated by laser Doppler flowmetry. *Reg Anesth*, 17, 322–328.

Collins, S. L., Moore, R. A., Mcquay, H. J., Wiffen, P. J., and Edwards, J. E. (2002). Single dose oral ibuprofen and diclofenac for postoperative pain. *Cochrane Database Syst Rev*, 2, CD001548.

Committee On Infectious Disease. (1982). Aspirin and Reye's syndrome. *Pediatrics*, 69, 810.

Davies, N. M., and Anderson, K. E. (1997). Clinical pharmacokinetics of diclofenac. Therapeutic insights and pitfalls. *Clin Pharmacokinet*, 33, 184–213.

Davies, N. M., and Skjodt, N. M. (2000). Choosing the right nonsteroidal anti-inflammatory drug for the right patient: a pharmacokinetic approach. *Clin Pharmacokinet*, 38, 377–392.

Demiraran, Y., Ozturk, O., Guclu, E., Iskender, A., Ergin, M. H., and Tokmak, A. (2008). Vasoconstriction and analgesic efficacy of locally infiltrated levobupivacaine for nasal surgery. *Anesth Analg*, 106, 1008–1011.

Dodwell, E. R., Latorre, J. G., Parisini, E., Zwettler, E., Chandra, D., Mulpuri, K., *et al.* (2010). NSAID exposure and risk of nonunion: a meta-analysis of case-control and cohort studies. *Calcif Tissue Int*, 87, 193–202.

Dowd, J. E., Cimaz, R., and Fink, C. W. (1995). Nonsteroidal antiinflammatory drug-induced gastroduodenal injury in children. *Arthritis Rheum*, 38, 1225–1231.

Dsida, R. M., Wheeler, M., Birmingham, P. K., Wang, Z., Heffner, C. L., Cote, C. J., *et al.* (2002). Age-stratified pharmacokinetics of ketorolac tromethamine in pediatric surgical patients. *Anesth Analg*, 94, 266–720.

Fiorucci, S., and Distrutti, E. (2011). COXIBs, CINODs and HS-releasing NSAIDs: current perspectives in the development of safer non steroidal anti-inflammatory drugs. *Curr Med Chem*, 18, 3494–3505.

Forrest, J. B., Heitlinger, E. L., and Revell, S. (1997). Ketorolac for postoperative pain management in children. *Drug Saf*, 16, 309–329.

Gelotte, C. K., Auiler, J. F., Lynch, J. M., Temple, A. R., and Slattery, J. T. (2007). Disposition of acetaminophen at 4, 6, and 8 g/day for 3 days in healthy young adults. *Clin Pharmacol Ther*, 81, 840–848.

Gibb, I. A., and Anderson, B. J. (2008). Paracetamol (acetaminophen) pharmacodynamics; interpreting the plasma concentration. *Arch Dis Child*, 93, 241–247.

Gonzalez-Martin, G., Maggio, L., Gonzalez-Sotomayor, J., and Zuniga, S. (1997). Pharmacokinetics of ketorolac in children after abdominal surgery. *Int J Clin Pharmacol Ther*, 35, 160–163.

Granfors, M. T., Backman, J. T., Laitila, J., and Neuvonen, P. J. (2004). Tizanidine is mainly metabolized by cytochrome p450 1A2 in vitro. *Br J Clin Pharmacol*, 57, 349–353.

Gregoire, N., Gualano, V., Geneteau, A., Millerioux, L., Brault, M., Mignot, A., and Roze, J. C. (2004). Population pharmacokinetics of ibuprofen enantiomers in very premature neonates. *J Clin Pharmacol*, 44, 1114–1124.

Hannam, J., and Anderson, B. J. (2011). Explaining the acetaminophen-ibuprofen analgesic interaction using a response surface model. *Paediatr Anaesth*, 21, 1234–1240.

Hansen, T. G., Morton, N. S., Cullen, P. M., and Watson, D. G. (2001). Plasma concentrations and pharmacokinetics of bupivacaine with and without adrenaline following caudal anaesthesia in infants. *Acta Anaesthesiol Scand*, 45, 42–47.

Houck, C. S., Wilder, R. T., McDermott, J. S., Sethna, N. F., and Berde, C. B. (1996). Safety of intravenous ketorolac therapy in children and cost savings with a unit dosing system. *J Pediatr*, 129, 292–296.

Ingelmo, P. M., and Fumagalli, R. (2005). Central blocks with levobupivacaina in children. *Minerva Anestesiol*, 71, 339–345.

Inomata, S., Nagashima, A., Osaka, Y., Tanaka, E., and Toyooka, H. (2003). Effects of clonidine on lidocaine metabolism in human or rat liver microsomes. *J Anesth*, 17, 281–283.

James, L. P., Letzig, L., Simpson, P. M., Capparelli, E., Roberts, D. W., Hinson, J. A., *et al.* (2009). Pharmacokinetics of acetaminophen-protein adducts in adults with acetaminophen overdose and acute liver failure. *Drug Metab Dispos*, 37, 1779–1784.

Kauffman, R. E., Lieh-Lai, M. W., Uy, H. G., and Aravind, M. K. (1999). Enantiomer-selective pharmacokinetics and metabolism of ketorolac in children. *Clin Pharmacol Ther*, 65, 382–388.

Kearns, G. L., Leeder, J. S., and Wasserman, G. S. (1998). Acetaminophen overdose with therapeutic intent. *J Pediatr*, 132, 5–8.

Keenan, G. F., Giannini, E. H., and Athreya, B. H. (1995). Clinically significant gastropathy associated with nonsteroidal antiinflammatory drug use in children with juvenile rheumatoid arthritis. *J Rheumatol*, 22, 1149–1151.

Kelley, M. T., Walson, P. D., Edge, J. H., Cox, S., and Mortensen, M. E. (1992). Pharmacokinetics and pharmacodynamics of ibuprofen isomers and acetaminophen in febrile children. *Clin Pharmacol Ther*, 52, 181–189.

Kokki, H., Karvinen, M., and Jekunen, A. (2002). Pharmacokinetics of a 24-hour intravenous ketoprofen infusion in children. *Acta Anaesthesiol Scand*, 46, 194–198.

Kopacz, D. J., and Bernards, C. M. (2001). Effect of clonidine on lidocaine clearance in vivo: a microdialysis study in humans. *Anesthesiology*, 95, 1371–1376.

Korpela, R. and Olkkola, K. T. (1990). Pharmacokinetics of intravenous diclofenac sodium in children. *Eur J Clin Pharmacol*, 38, 293–295.

Kristensen, J. D., Karlsten, R., and Gordh, T. (1998). Spinal cord blood flow after intrathecal injection of ropivacaine and bupivacaine with or without epinephrine in rats. *Acta Anaesthesiol Scand*, 42, 685–690.

Lesko, S. M., and Mitchell, A. A. (1995). An assessment of the safety of pediatric ibuprofen. A practitioner-based randomized clinical trial. *JAMA*, 273, 929–933.

Lesko, S. M., and Mitchell, A. A. (1997). Renal function after short-term ibuprofen use in infants and children. *Pediatrics*, 100, 954–957.

Lesko, S. M., and Mitchell, A. A. (1999). The safety of acetaminophen and ibuprofen among children younger than two years old. *Pediatrics*, 104, e39.

Li, H., Mandema, J., Wada, R., Jayawardena, S., Desjardins, P., Doyle, G., *et al.* (2012). Modeling the onset and offset of dental pain relief by ibuprofen. *J Clin Pharmacol*, 52(1), 89–101.

Litalien, C. and Jacqz-Aigrain, E. (2001). Risks and benefits of nonsteroidal anti-inflammatory drugs in children: a comparison with paracetamol. *Paediatr Drugs*, 3, 817–858.

Madan, A., Graham, R. A., Carroll, K. M., Mudra, D. R., Burton, L. A., Krueger, L. A., *et al.* (2003). Effects of prototypical microsomal enzyme inducers on cytochrome P450 expression in cultured human hepatocytes. *Drug Metab Dispos*, 31, 421–431.

Mandema, J. W., and Stanski, D. R. (1996). Population pharmacodynamic model for ketorolac analgesia. *Clin Pharmacol Ther*, 60, 619–635.

Maund, E., McDaid, C., Rice, S., Wright, K., Jenkins, B., and Woolacott, N. (2011). Paracetamol and selective and non-selective non-steroidal anti-inflammatory drugs for the reduction in morphine-related side-effects after major surgery: a systematic review. *Br J Anaesth*, 106, 292–297.

Maunuksela, E.-L., and Olkkola, K. T. (2003). Nonsteroidal anti-inflammatory drugs in pediatric pain management. In Schechter, N. L., Berde, C. B., and Yaster, M. (eds.) *Pain in infants, children, and adolescents* (2nd edn), pp. 171–180. Philadelphia, PA: Lippincott Williams & Wilkins.

McQuay, H. J., and Moore, R. A. (1998). Postoperative analgesia and vomiting, with special reference to day-case surgery: a systematic review. *Health Technol Assess*, 2, 1–236.

Mehlisch, D. R., Aspley, S., Daniels, S. E., Southerden, K. A., and Christensen, K. S. (2010). A single-tablet fixed-dose combination of racemic ibuprofen/paracetamol in the management of moderate to severe postoperative dental pain in adult and adolescent patients: a multicenter, two-stage, randomized, double-blind, parallel-group, placebo-controlled, factorial study. *Clin Ther*, 32, 1033–1049.

Miyagi, S. J., and Collier, A. C. (2011). The development of UDP-glucuronosyltransferases 1A1 and 1A6 in the pediatric liver. *Drug Metab Dispos*, 39, 912–919.

Murat, I., Baujard, C., Foussat, C., Guyot, E., Petel, H., Rod, B., *et al.* (2005). Tolerance and analgesic efficacy of a new i.v. paracetamol solution in children after inguinal hernia repair. *Paediatr Anaesth*, 15, 663–670.

Olkkola, K. T., and Maunuksela, E. L. (1991). The pharmacokinetics of postoperative intravenous ketorolac trimethamine in children. *Br J Clin Pharmacol*, 31, 182–184.

Olkkola, K. T., Maunuksela, E. L., and Korpela, R. (1989). Pharmacokinetics of postoperative intravenous indomethacin in children. *Pharmacol Toxicol*, 65, 157–160.

Ong, C. K., Seymour, R. A., Lirk, P., and Merry, A. F. (2010). Combining paracetamol (acetaminophen) with nonsteroidal antiinflammatory drugs: a qualitative systematic review of analgesic efficacy for acute postoperative pain. *Anesthes Analg*, 110, 1170–1179.

Palmer, G. M. (2005). A teenager with severe asthma exacerbation following ibuprofen. *Anaesth Intensive Care*, 33, 261–265.

Penna, A., and Buchanan, N. (1991). Paracetamol poisoning in children and hepatotoxicity. *Br J Clin Pharmacol*, 32, 143–149.

Perrott, D. A., Piira, T., Goodenough, B., and Champion, G. D. (2004). Efficacy and safety of acetaminophen vs ibuprofen for treating children's pain or fever: a meta-analysis. *Arch Pediatr Adolesc Med*, 158, 521–526.

Pierce, C. A., and Voss, B. (2010). Efficacy and safety of ibuprofen and acetaminophen in children and adults: a meta-analysis and qualitative review. *Ann Pharmacother*, 44, 489–506.

Plaisance, K. I., and Mackowiak, P. A. (2000). Antipyretic therapy: physiologic rationale, diagnostic implications, and clinical consequences. *Arch Intern Med*, 160, 449–456.

Prescott, L. F. (1996). *Paracetamol (acetaminophen). A critical bibliographic review*, London: Taylor and Francis Publishers.

Reith, D., Medlicott, N. J., Kumara De Silva, R., Yang, L., Hickling, J., and Zacharias, M. (2009). Simultaneous modelling of the Michaelis-Menten kinetics of paracetamol sulphation and glucuronidation. *Clin Exp Pharmacol Physiol*, 36, 35–42.

Rey, E., Pariente-Khayat, A., Gouyet, L., Vauzelle-Kervroedan, F., Pons, G., D'athis, P., *et al.* (1994). Stereoselective disposition of ibuprofen enantiomers in infants. *Br J Clin Pharmacol*, 38, 373–375.

Romsing, J., Ostergaard, D., Senderovitz, T., Drozdziewicz, D., Sonne, J., and Ravn, G. (2001). Pharmacokinetics of oral diclofenac and acetaminophen in children after surgery. *Paediatr Anaesth*, 11, 205–213.

Rumack, B. H., and Matthew, H. (1975). Acetaminophen poisoning and toxicity. *Pediatrics*, 55, 871–876.

Scott, C. S., Retsch-Bogart, G. Z., Kustra, R. P., Graham, K. M., Glasscock, B. J., and Smith, P. C. (1999). The pharmacokinetics of ibuprofen suspension, chewable tablets, and tablets in children with cystic fibrosis. *J Pediatr*, 134, 58–63.

Standing, J. F., Tibboel, D., Korpela, R., and Olkkola, K. T. (2011). Diclofenac pharmacokinetic meta-analysis and dose recommendations for surgical pain in children aged 1–12 years. *Paediatr Anaesth*, 21, 316–324.

Strom, B. L., Berlin, J. A., Kinman, J. L., Spitz, P. W., Hennessy, S., Feldman, H., *et al.* (1996). Parenteral ketorolac and risk of gastrointestinal and operative site bleeding. A postmarketing surveillance study. *JAMA*, 275, 376–382.

Treluyer, J. M., Sultan, E., Alexandre, J. A., Roux, A., Flouvat, B., and Lagardere, B. (1991). [Pharmacokinetics of aspirin in African children with normal nutrition and malnutrition]. *Arch Fr Pediatr*, 48, 337–341.

Troconiz, I. F., Armenteros, S., Planelles, M. V., Benitez, J., Calvo, R., and Dominguez, R. (2000). Pharmacokinetic-pharmacodynamic modelling of the antipyretic effect of two oral formulations of ibuprofen. *Clin Pharmacokinet*, 38, 505–518.

Van Der Marel, C. D., Anderson, B. J., Romsing, J., Jacqz-Aigrain, E., and Tibboel, D. (2004). Diclofenac and metabolite pharmacokinetics in children. *Paediatr Anaesth*, 14, 443–451.

Van Overmeire, B., Touw, D., Schepens, P. J., Kearns, G. L., and Van Den Anker, J. N. (2001). Ibuprofen pharmacokinetics in preterm infants with patent ductus arteriosus. *Clin Pharmacol Ther*, 70, 336–343.

Walls, L., Baker, C. F., and Sarkar, S. (2007). Acetaminophen-induced hepatic failure with encephalopathy in a newborn. *J Perinatol*, 27, 133–135.

Wells, T. G., Mortensen, M. E., Dietrich, A., Walson, P. D., Blasier, D., and Kearns, G. L. (1994). Comparison of the pharmacokinetics of naproxen tablets and suspension in children. *J Clin Pharmacol*, 34, 30–33.

Wiest, D. B., Pinson, J. B., Gal, P. S., Brundage, R. C., Schall, S., Ransom, J. L., *et al.* (1991). Population pharmacokinetics of intravenous indomethacin in neonates with symptomatic patent ductus arteriosus. *Clin Pharmacol Ther*, 49, 550–557.

Wilson, J. T., Brown, R. D., Bocchini, J. A., Jr., and Kearns, G. L. (1982). Efficacy, disposition and pharmacodynamics of aspirin, acetaminophen and choline salicylate in young febrile children. *Ther Drug Monit*, 4, 147–180.

Wolchok, J. D., Williams, L., Pinto, J. T., Fleisher, M., Krown, S. E., Hwu, W. J., *et al.* (2003). Phase I trial of high dose paracetamol and carmustine in patients with metastatic melanoma. *Melanoma Res*, 13, 189–196.

Wong, D. L., and Baker, C. M. (1988). Pain in children: comparison of assessment scales. *Pediatr Nurs*, 14, 9–17.

CHAPTER 44

Developmental pharmacology of opioids

Gareth J. Hathway

Summary

Recognition of the need for alternative analgesic regimens for managing neonatal and childhood pain has led to a rich literature concerning the ways in which early life pain differs from that at older ages. As in adults, opiates are often considered the gold standard analgesic class of drugs, of which morphine is the prototypical agent. There is a wealth of data detailing clinical observations, measurements, and interventions with regard to the use of opioids in treating pain in children. Studies in the early part of this century have highlighted that, in humans, age is an important factor that influences the morphine requirement of neonates following surgery; and dose requirements are influenced by both pharmacokinetic and pharmacodynamic factors. Laboratory studies have extended our understanding of changes within the peripheral and central nervous systems that underlie alterations in nociception in early life. This chapter will review what is currently known about the actions of opioids upon nociceptive and nociresponsive elements of the nervous system in early life, how they differ from adult responses, and ask whether manipulating endogenous opioid systems in early life may have consequences on neurodevelopment.

Introduction

The response of neonatal and young animals to pain can be generally considered to be hyperexcitable; and characterized by poorly coordinated, inappropriately organized reflexes and reduced thermal and mechanical pain thresholds (Fitzgerald, 2005). The dorsal horn (DH) of the spinal cord is important for the primary integration of somatosensory and nociceptive information in the central nervous system (CNS). Delayed maturation of inhibitory neurotransmission in the spinal cord contributes to the alterations in nociceptive responses exhibited in early life. At a cellular level this is manifested as an increased cutaneous receptive field of nociresponsive neurons in the spinal DH (Fitzgerald and Jennings, 1999). These immature physiological responses are underpinned by a lack of synaptic inhibition in the DH through the first 2 to 3 postnatal weeks in the rat (a time period which correlates with infancy through to late childhood in human development). Intrinsic spinal neurotransmitters such as GABA and glycine fail to evoke measurable mIPSCs (inhibitory currents) in the neonatal and infant spinal

cord (Baccei and Fitzgerald, 2004, 2006; Baccei et al., 2003; see also Walker and Baccei, Chapter 6, this volume).

Further sources of inhibitory drive to the adult spinal cord are descending projections from the ventral brainstem. In the adult, these projections that emanate from the rostroventral medulla (RVM) are able to powerfully facilitate and inhibit spinal excitability, increasing and decreasing spinal reflexes (Fields and Anderson, 1978; Fields et al., 1983). Furthermore, there is considerable evidence that these brainstem centres are important for the maintenance of chronic pain states in adults (Porreca et al., 2002; Zhang et al., 2009). The RVM receives a dense afferent input from the periaqueductal grey (PAG) which in turn acts as a common target for numerous more rostral structures such as the amygdala, hypothalamus, hippocampus, and anterior cingulate cortex (Fields et al., 2006; see Fitzgerald, Chapter 8, this volume). As this brief summary demonstrates, pain is a complex phenomenon involving numerous parts of the peripheral and central nervous systems. When considering the analgesic action of opioids, it is therefore necessary to consider the expression and actions of both endogenous and exogenous ligands, at multiple sites within the nervous system.

Opioid peptides

History

Opium has been used as a recreational and analgesic drug for centuries, yet it was Stertürner's isolation of the active ingredient morphine in 1806 that began the pharmacological evaluation of how this drug and other similar drugs act. Some considerable time passed before the first description of specific opiate receptors (see later) (Pert and Snyder, 1973; Simon et al., 1973; Terenius, 1973). The ability of opiates to mediate analgesia in a dose-dependent manner when administered into the midbrain of rats and humans, and the observation that electrical stimulation of the same brain regions resulted in similar inhibition of pain, led to the hypothesis that an endogenous opiate-like neurotransmission system existed in the mammalian CNS (Mayer and Liebeskind, 1974; Reynolds, 1969; Tsou and Jang, 1964).

The pioneering work of many groups in the late 1960s and 1970s led to the final identification of a family of endogenous opioid-like peptides in the forebrain that were intrinsically linked with nociception (Goldstein et al., 1979; Hughes et al., 1975; Li et al., 1976; Loh et al., 1976). The endogenous opioids include β-endorphin, the endomorphins 1 and 2, the enkephalins and dynorphins. Each of these are synthesized from precursor peptides: pre-opiomelano-cortin (POMC), pro-enkephalin, and pro-dynorphin respectively. Work on the ontogeny of these systems was largely carried out in the 1980s and is expertly reviewed by McDowell and Kitchen (1987). Although predating developments within the field of molecular neurobiology, this is a valuable review of the subject.

Specific peptides

β-endorphin can be detected prenatally in the rat from embryonic day 13 (E13), levels increase within several brain areas with age (Ng et al., 1984) until E18 (just prior to birth at E20–21 in the rat), when adult levels have been reached (Bayon et al., 1979; Bloom et al., 1980). Analysis of the literature from this time shows general agreement that β-endorphin levels change postnatally, including in the pons, which has direct relevance to the descending control of pain processing. However, there is significant disagreement as to the temporal profile of these changes and the absolute levels of β-endorphin that can be measured in specific brain regions (McDowell and Kitchen, 1987), but marked regional differences in the development of β-endorphin expression in the CNS are apparent. The mechanisms for β-endorphin release in the brain are not fully developed at birth; both the spontaneous and potassium-stimulated release of the peptide from hypothalamic slices appear to be immature until at least postnatal day 20 (P20) in the rat (Hompes et al., 1982).

Enkephalin (both Met and Leu) can also be detected prenatally. Within the brainstem levels are thought to peak around the second postnatal week in the rat (McDowell and Kitchen, 1987; Ng et al., 1984) with levels then diminishing to those found in the adult. It has been proposed that the development of the enkephalinergic system proceeds in a rostrocaudal manner (Tsang et al., 1982).

Pro-dynoprhin is the pro-peptide responsible for the synthesis of dynorphin. Studies detailing the developmental expression profile of either the pro-peptide or the actual peptide in pain related areas of the CNS are very sparse and no clear consensus or opinion has been reached (McDowell and Kitchen, 1987).

Developmental expression

It is apparent from the current literature that investigations into the normal development of the endogenous opioid system have slowed considerably from the late 1980s and early 1990s. There is little data regarding the presence of endogenous opioid peptides in the primary afferent fibres through postnatal development. There is limited evidence for the presence of opioid peptides in some afferent fibres in the prenatal environment (Haynes et al., 1982), but this weak immunoreactivity disappeared postnatally and was restricted to white matter tracts. Fibre staining within the spinal DH was absent. This study pre-dated a full description of the composition of the family of opioid peptides and concentrated only on the expression of β-endorphin. More recent studies regarding the distribution of these peptides in the peripheral nervous system has focussed on the adult rat. In these studies (Marvizón et al., 2009), although enkephalin was never observed to be co-localized with primary afferent terminals in the spinal DH, there was some co-localization of dynorphin with calcitonin gene-related peptide (CGRP), a marker of peptidergic C fibres. A thorough study through postnatal development has not yet been performed.

Impact of developmental interventions on opioid systems

Stress and maternal separation

Subsequent research has focussed on pre- or perinatal manipulations to either the rat pups or their mothers, and the impact this has upon the development of opioidergic systems, particularly in the forebrain (Belcheva et al., 1998; Lin et al., 2009; McLaughlin et al., 2002). Most of these manipulations take the form of stress such as maternal separation in the early postnatal period, or of pharmacological manipulations such as exposure to opiates whilst *in utero*. The overriding hypotheses of these studies are that the ontogeny of the opioidergic system in the CNS will be altered, and there is considerable supporting data. In one example (Gustafsson et al., 2008), rats were either collectively or individually separated from their mothers for 15 or 360 min over the first three postnatal weeks. This resulted in altered met-enkephalin and dynorphin levels in a number of forebrain regions in 3-week and 10-week old offspring, and this was particularly pronounced if pups were individually separated. Whilst many areas of the brain were assayed, focusing on the PAG which is directly involved in pain processing, it can be seen that the normal increase in met-enkephalin levels seen in control rats is blunted in rats that underwent separation, with inconclusive changes in dynorphin levels. This study, which is one of many, demonstrates that early life interventions can radically change the expression and therefore the functional role of endogenous opioid systems through to adulthood.

Opioid exposure

Clinically it is important to determine whether exposure to opiate analgesics early in life has any effect on subsequent response to the same compounds later in life. In rats, administration of opioids either prenatally to the mother, or in the first 10 postnatal days, can significantly shift the morphine dose–response relationship later in life. Single morphine administration on postnatal days 1 or 2 (1 mg/kg) produced 'tolerance' to subsequent morphine analgesia at postnatal day 29 (Bardo and Hughes, 1981). Repeated administration of morphine over the first 9 postnatal days (3 mg/kg subcutaneously) resulted in significantly lower basal thermal and mechanical thresholds in the juvenile period (P29). Additionally, there was a significant rightward-shift in the cumulative dose–response curves at both postnatal days 20 and 49 (Zhang and Sweitzer, 2008). Prenatal exposure (twice daily from E5 to E12) altered morphine dose–response in offspring at postnatal day 35 (O'Callaghan and Holtzman, 1976). These data suggest that opiate exposure early in life can alter the development of components of the nervous system necessary for mediating the analgesic effects of exogenous opioids; and also that early life opiate exposure can alter other elements of the 'pain pathway' development as indexed by alterations in basal sensory thresholds in some studies (Zhang and Sweitzer, 2008).

Role of opioid peptides in normal development

Do opioid peptides have a role in normal development? Reviewing the available literature suggests that opioid peptides act as inhibitory growth factors at a cellular level, with antagonism of opioid receptors *in vivo* resulting in increased dendritic length and spine formation in neurons in the cerebellum (Hauser et al., 1987, 1989). However, alterations in the anatomical development of the nervous system by opioids are not restricted to neurons. Astrocyte numbers have decreased in mouse cortical cultures exposed to met-enkephalin by a receptor-dependent mechanism (Stiene-Martin and Hauser, 1990). More recently this effect of opioids on the development of non-neuronal cells in the nervous system has been confirmed. To model effects of prolonged opiate exposure of offspring of opiate-dependent mothers, Sanchez et al. (2008) implanted pregnant rat dams with osmotic mini-pumps that continuously delivered buprenorphine from day 7 of gestation until postnatal day 21, ensuring that pups were exposed prenatally to the drug via the placenta and postnatally via maternal milk. In these pups it was shown that lower doses of buprenorphine increased the expression of myelin basic protein whilst higher doses significantly decreased levels of this protein, particularly when animals were examined at postnatal day 12. Anatomical examination of the corpus callosum showed that in rats exposed to buprenorphine there were significantly more large calibre myelinated fibres but the same distributions of non-myelinated fibres compared to controls. This increase in calibre was also associated with a thinner myelin sheath surrounding these axons suggesting an altered balance between axon growth and myelin thickness. Thus, exposure to high levels of opioid for relatively prolonged periods during prenatal development can alter CNS structure. Further studies are required to evaluate the impact of different doses and durations of exposure during postnatal development.

More recently data from our laboratory has demonstrated a specific trophic role for endogenous opioids in the maturation of supraspinal centres responsible for the descending control of spinal pain processing (Hathway et al., 2012). In this study we implanted subcutaneous mini-pumps containing naloxone HCl at P14, P21, or P28, and continuously delivered the drug for 7-day periods. Animals were then allowed to mature to P40. In the group that had drug delivered between P21 to P28, the RVM failed to mature properly, and descending inhibition of spinal pain processing could not be evoked in adulthood. These data showed that the action of endogenous opioids are central to the normal maturation of supraspinal pain control systems, but even more interestingly that this occurs relatively late in postnatal development, at a period when rats would be judged to be adolescent. This is a true 'critical period' as the same manipulation one week before or after this does not prevent or effect normal maturation. In an extension of this study we implanted neonatal, 7-day-old, rats with mini-pumps that delivered morphine for 7 days and showed that at developmental stages where the RVM is normally immature and unable to provide descending inhibitory control of spinal processing, that neonatal morphine treatment had accelerated the maturation of the RVM. In these animals adult like stimulus response profiles from the RVM were evoked. This work demonstrates the importance of the opioidergic system for the normal postnatal development of pain processing in the nervous system.

It is intriguing to speculate on the results of studies using more recent quantitative and non-quantitative methods to further evaluate the changing expression of opioid peptides in the developing nervous system. The majority of studies listed above utilized the most sensitive assays available at the time, such as radioimmunoassay and *in situ* hybridization. The value of these studies remains high and they are still our best source of information regarding the ontogeny of adult endogenous opioid networks in the CNS, however the application of quantitative genomic and post-genomic techniques would significantly add to this work. Equally, utilizing immunohistochemical techniques to uncover the distribution of these peptides and the co-transmitters utilized in different neuronal populations through the postnatal period would be valuable. Many of the supraspinal structures involved in pain modulation are anatomically small and the analyses detailed earlier were too crude to detect subtle variations in expression levels within refined brain nuclei. Even with today's state-of-the art RNA amplification methods accurately and repeatedly dissecting these areas from postmortem tissue is technically challenging.

Opioid receptors

Opioid peptides mediate their effects via interactions with a family of opioid receptors, which are metabotropic, membrane-expressed receptors that act through second messengers (i.e. in contrast to ionotropic receptors that form an ion channel pore). There are three main subclasses of opioid receptor named mu (μ), delta (δ), and kappa (κ), as well as a less well recognized and investigated receptor, ORL-1 (opioid-like receptor). Receptors are composed of seven hydrophobic membrane-spanning domains, with extracellular components that are involved in specifying interactions with ligands, and intracellular domains that interact with intracellular signalling mediators. Opioid receptors mediate their actions via second messenger G-proteins (see later). In the adult nervous systems activation of opioid receptors engage intracellular signalling systems that are in large part inhibitory, and act to decrease neuronal excitability by increasing inwardly rectifying potassium (K^+) conductances, decreasing voltage-dependent calcium (Ca^{2+}) channels, and by decreasing the production of cyclic adenosine monophosphate (cAMP).

Peripheral nervous system

The peripheral nervous system detects stimuli and conveys sensory information to the CNS. Peripheral sensory afferent neurons are subdivided into three broad categories according to their physiological and anatomical properties:

- Aβ fibres are large, myelinated fibres that usually convey non-noxious information to the CNS.

- Aδ fibres are small myelinated fibres and convey both noxious and non-noxious information.

- C fibres are small unmyelinated fibres that convey noxious information to the CNS, that are further subdivided into peptidergic or non-peptidergic, depending on their neurotransmitter phenotype.

All of these primary afferent fibres innervate target tissues such as skin, muscle, and viscera and their cell bodies are to be found in the dorsal root ganglia (DRG) which run parallel to the spinal cord. These neurons then have spinal projections which enter the DH of the spinal cord. Each primary afferent subtype has different central termination patterns within the DH. These terminations are immature at birth and refine to their adult state via activity dependent processes (see Walker and Baccei, Chapter 6, this volume).

A detailed study of the expression pattern of μ-opioid receptors in the DRG over postnatal development has shown considerable changes in early life (Nandi et al., 2004). Receptor expression in adulthood was confined to mainly small and medium sized neurons (presumably C and Aδ fibres). However, in the neonatal rat, there were significantly more μ-opioid receptors expressed on large-diameter myelinated fibres (Beland and Fitzgerald, 2001). This increased expression was mirrored when Ca^{2+} imaging demonstrated increased fluorescence in response to activation of the μ-opioid receptor with the receptor agonist DAMGO, in a greater proportion of DRG neurons than in the adult (Nandi et al., 2004). This suggests that not only are more receptors present, but they are also functional and can be activated by agonists, as confirmed by an enhanced response or leftward shift in the dose–response relationship for systemic morphine in younger rats. The mechanisms that regulate the expression of the μ-opioid receptor in primary afferent neurons are not known. Although age-dependent alterations in the central terminals of primary afferent neurons in the DH are related to changes in levels of neural activity (Beggs et al., 2002; Bremner and Fitzgerald, 2008), it is not known if opioid receptor expression is similarly regulated. Both the κ and δ subtypes are expressed on the terminals of adult primary afferent neurons, but developmental changes have not been evaluated.

The presence of opioid receptors on the terminals of primary afferent neurons suggests a role in inhibiting primary afferent firing in response to noxious stimuli. In postnatal rats, electrical stimulation of incoming fibres in the dorsal root produces excitatory postsynaptic potentials in the DH; but these were reduced by the μ-opioid receptor agonist DAMGO via inhibition of both Aδ and C fibres. DAMGO was also more efficacious and potent at inhibiting C fibres than Aδ fibres, but identical intracellular processes mediated the inhibition in both fibre types. Tissue from 17- to 25-day-old rat pups, which is toward the limit of technical feasibility of the techniques employed were used, but these are not fully mature animals (Heinke et al., 2011). It was not reported whether stimulating the dorsal root at Aβ strengths was also sensitive to DAMGO application in young animals, as would be predicted on the basis of developmental studies (Nandi et al., 2004).

Spinal cord

The spinal cord is the first site of integration of sensory information within the CNS. Primary afferent sensory neurons enter the spinal cord via the dorsal root and synapse with second-order neurons. These second-order neurons are central to the perception of pain; being intrinsically involved in both the transmission of nociception-related information to supraspinal centres, and also in receiving converging descending information from other supraspinal sites that can act to increase or decrease their excitability. Autoradiographic and immunohistochemical studies have shown that the majority of opioid receptors are located either in laminae I and II of the DH and to a lesser extent in deeper layers (Besse et al., 1990; Rahman et al., 1998). This reflects termination of primary afferents (see earlier), but approximately 30% (Besse et al., 1990) of receptors are located postsynaptically and may relate to descending projections.

Studies in the 1990s using *in situ* hybridization illustrated that mRNA for at least the μ- and κ-opioid receptors can be found within the DH (Maekawa et al., 1994). The highest density of mRNA for the μ-opioid receptor could be found in laminae I, II, and VIII whilst κ was densest in laminae I and II. Recent immunohistochemical studies examined the anatomical distribution of

μ-, δ-, and κ-opioid receptor expression in the spinal cord, with intense staining to all three seen in the superficial layers in adult rats (Gray et al., 2006). Positive cells were generally ovoid in shape and aligned to follow the rostrocaudal axis of the spinal cord itself. μ staining was most intense in lamina II and was localized to the cell membrane of cell bodies and dendrites, whereas δ immunoreactivity was restricted to cell bodies. κ staining was particularly intense in lamina I due to the presence of heavily stained fibres, but cell body staining was also prominent here. Immunohistochemistry uses antibodies to selectively label different proteins and provides increased spatial resolution, as protein expression can be directly detected at a subcellular level. This is a distinct advantage over other techniques, such as radioligand binding, which requires tissue to be exposed to irradiated drug and resultant images on X-ray or similar films to then be analysed. Improvements in immunohistochemical technologies, from antibody design and production, through to signal amplification and advances in microscopy, have meant that immunohistochemistry is now more routinely employed in laboratory studies, but to date there has been limited immunohistochemical investigation of the postnatal expression of opioid receptors in the spinal cord.

Autoradiography has been used to map postnatal changes in opioid receptor biding in the spinal cord (Rahman et al., 1998). At birth, μ binding is relatively diffuse, increases over the first postnatal week, and then decreases until P21. A progressive pattern and refinement of μ binding could be seen with increasing age, so that binding sites became progressively more restricted to the superficial laminae of the DH as seen in the adult. κ binding followed a similar pattern to μ in that diffuse binding was present at birth. Total κ binding increased over the first postnatal week and then decreased so that at P14 there was approximately 50% of the binding seen at P7. At P21 and P56 (adult) greater preference for κ binding in the superficial DH was observed. δ opioid receptor binding was not present at birth, was first observed at P7, but was diffuse and remained like this until at least P56.

Brainstem

Analysis of the published literature shows that, as with other areas of the nervous system, a detailed account of the postnatal development of opioid receptors is elusive. For the purposes of this chapter, changes in opioid receptor expression that take place in areas of the brain that are recognized as being central to the modulation of spinal cord excitability, namely the PAG and the RVM, have been highlighted (Figure 44.1). Immunohistochemical studies (Gray et al., 2006) have shown intense immunoreactivity for all three opioid receptors within the PAG; with considerable co-localization of μ and δ receptors in the medial and lateral parts of this midbrain structure. Light to moderate κ staining was seen and κ positive cells were closely apposed to those that expressed μ opioid receptors. κ immunoreactivity was also most noticeable within the caudal and venterolateral parts; the latter is of particular interest as it is this part of the PAG that projects to the RVM. Within the nucleus raphe magnus of the RVM strong μ staining was seen in dense cell bodies whereas δ immunoreactivity was associated with fibres and was more diffuse. As in the PAG there was some co-localization of both μ and δ receptors. Small round cells which were positive for κ immunoreactivity were noted to be 'intermingled' with μ positive cell bodies. The locus coeruleus (LC) is the source of noradrenaline

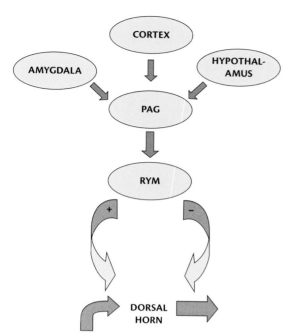

Figure 44.1 Supraspinal modulation of dorsal horn excitability. The ability of supraspinal sites to control the excitability of neurons within the dorsal horn of the spinal cord is one of the major mechanisms that underpin opioid analgesia. Forebrain regions commonly innervate the periaqueductal grey (PAG) which in turns innervates the rostroventral medical medulla (RVM). Via spinally projecting neurons this structure directly controls pain processing in the spinal cord. The RVM bi-directionally controls spinal excitability it is able to both facilitate (+) or inhibit (−) the spinal cord depending on the nature of the input to the RVM itself. The RVM is therefore central to opioid analgesia mediating these effects via descending inhibitory pathways and in the maintenance of chronic pain states via facilitatory pathways.

for the entire central nervous system and also has descending projections which powerfully control spinal excitability. Intense μ staining was found within cell bodies of the LC in adult rats; δ staining although above background levels was weak; and a few κ-positive cells were present (Gray et al., 2006).

Multiple radioligand binding studies have quantified opioid receptor binding at different postnatal ages in brain tissue. In general, it appears that the expression of opioid receptor binding sites within the brain alters with age and that the different opioid receptors follow different trajectories (Kitchen et al., 1990; McDowell and Kitchen, 1986, 1987; Spain et al., 1985; Volterra et al., 1986,). Despite the difficulty in making comparisons between studies it appears that μ receptors are present at birth and are able to bind ligands with the same affinity (dissociation constant, Kd) as in the adult. Binding of μ selective ligands increase from birth and reach adult levels around the third postnatal week. δ receptors seem to be absent at birth, but reliable binding is detectable from the second postnatal week, and then increases with age. κ binding is detectable at P5, increases to high levels by P10, then decreases to adult levels by P25. Binding characteristics of the δ and κ receptor are the same in neonates as they are in adults. Whilst informative, these studies provide no data regarding the expression of opioid receptors in specific brain nuclei. Most use whole brain homogenates which have limited sensitivity, and Spain et al. (1985) use rostral and caudal brain portions. It is not unreasonable to hypothesize that as well as following different paths between subtypes, the maturation of opioid

receptors may follow different trajectories in different regions of the brain. Again the application of modern post-genomic approaches to the study of the development of opioid receptor expression and their pharmacology is required.

Idiosyncrasies of age and receptor function

It is tempting to think of neonates, children, or young animals as smaller versions of adults. Compensations are clearly made in terms of the dosing requirements based on weight and pharmacokinetic data, but what of the fundamental action of the drug at its receptor? Previously we have shown that the action of midazolam at the GABA$_A$ receptor is significantly altered in neonatal rats as it is pronociceptive and fails to produce sedation (Koch et al., 2008). Could the result of opioid receptor agonism also undergo age-dependent changes? As discussed previously, there seem to be no major differences in the basic receptor-agonist interaction with postnatal age as assessed by radio-ligand binding in whole brain homogenates. It must be stressed that the available literature confirms that opioid mediated analgesia can be evoked at all ages. This is true via whichever route the drugs are administered; be that systemic (Abbott and Guy, 1995; Nandi et al., 2004; Thornton et al., 1998), epidural (Marsh et al., 1999a, 1999b), intrathecal (Barr et al., 1992; Westin et al., 2010) or peripherally (Barr, 1999).

Assumptions seem to have been made in the literature that μ-opioid receptor activity–function relationships in one part of the CNS reflect the situation in the entire CNS. Recently we have shown that this is not the case. Microinjection of the μ-opioid receptor agonist DAMGO into the RVM of juvenile (P21) rats is able to dose-dependently facilitate spinal nociception, that is it increases pain, which is in contrast to adult (>P40) rats where the same intervention results in dose-dependent analgesia (Hathway et al., 2012). This alteration in response to receptor agonism is not associated with an age-related alteration in the level or pattern of expression of μ-opioid receptors within the RVM, but seems to be a fundamental shift in the signalling pathways activated by the receptor following its activation. It is therefore apparent that although the same receptor can be expressed within the same animal in multiple tissues at any point during postnatal development there can be subtle, tissue specific alterations in the receptor that radically alter the consequences of its activation.

Analysis of the literature reveals some interesting developmental changes. There are age-related *increases* in the total μ-opioid expression within the brainstem of the developing rat whilst there is a concomitant *decrease* in δ expression (Kivell et al., 2004). It was also been noted that MOR in brainstem tissue existed as two different isoforms, both a 50 kD protein and a 70 kD protein, and that levels of the heavier isoform increased with postnatal age whilst the lighter isoform decreased. No alteration in the expression pattern of μ-opioid receptor was seen, in agreement with our later study (Hathway et al., 2012). This age-related alteration in receptor mass may represent alterations in: the splicing of mRNA for the receptor; post-translational glycosylation; use of alternative promoters for the *OPRM1* gene that encodes the receptor; or oligomerization of the receptor. Several studies have noted region specific distribution of μ-opioid receptor splice variants across the adult rodent CNS (Abbadie et al., 2000a, 2000b; Pan et al., 1999; Schulz et al., 1998), yet this study was the first to detail an apparent change in receptor isoform expression that correlated with postnatal age.

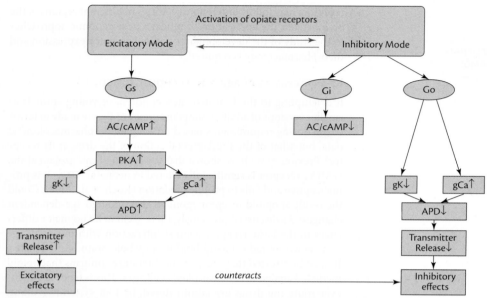

Figure 44.2 Bi-modal actions of opioid receptors. Classical opioid receptors act in an inhibitory mode mediating their actions via Gi and Go pathways, decreasing production of cAMP, reducing calcium currents and increasing potassium currents which ultimately leads to decreased neurotransmitter release. Alternatively opioid receptors can operate in an excitatory mode (at certain times in postnatal development or in states of opiate tolerance). In this mode receptors operate Gs (stimulatory) pathways increasing calcium currents and cAMP levels with increase neurotransmitter release.

Adapted with permission from *Trends in Pharmacological Sciences*, Volume 19, Issue 9, Stanley M. Crain and Ke-Fei Shen, Modulation of opioid analgesia, tolerance and dependence by Gs-coupled, GM1 ganglioside-regulated opioid receptor functions, pp. 358–365, Copyright © 1998, with permission from Elsevier, http://www.sciencedirect.com/science/journal/01656147.

Another age-related alteration in opioid receptor pharmacology is the propensity of neonatal opioid receptors to weakly couple to their effector mechanisms. This is thought to be due to modifications in the way that the receptor interacts with G-proteins (Figure 44.2). All opioid receptors couple to Gi G-proteins and therefore have inhibitory effects on cellular excitability. The classic view of the intracellular events that take place following activation of the receptor is that K^+ currents are increased and Ca^{2+} currents are decreased, leading to a decrease in neurotransmitter release from the neuron (Crain and Shen, 1998). However, what if this is too simple an explanation? Evidence for altered μ-opioid receptor G-protein coupling was first observed in 2003 (Nitsche and Pintar, 2003), when this group demonstrated radioligand binding to the receptor prior to agonist stimulated [^{35}S]GTPγS production in embryonic brain. Within the striatum of the postnatal rat, there is an age-dependent increase in Gi μ-opioid receptor coupling with postnatal age (Talbot et al., 2005); with levels of Gi coupling at P15 approximately 50% of those in the adult, and maximum levels of Gi coupling not being achieved until greater than P40 (approximately 250 g body weight). Further work is required to establish the functional consequences of this, but it implies that if the μ-opioid receptor is not coupled to Gi then it must either be coupled to some other G-protein, or is functionally inert and has no physiological role. However, this previous study concentrated on opioid signalling within the basal ganglia, and this may not be the case in areas more pertinent to pain. We, and others, have clearly shown functional responses to opioid in the RVM (Hathway et al., 2012), but further work in different brain regions is required.

Conclusion

Developmental alterations in opioid pharmacology from the laboratory experimental perspective are complex, and based on a solid but dated literature that has not applied modern post-genomic methodologies, and without a full appreciation that neonatal and young animals are not just smaller versions of adults. Behavioural studies clearly demonstrate analgesic responses to opioids from early development, but changes in opioid receptor expression and signalling mature at different rates in different parts of the nervous system, and this contributes to age-related differences in the degree and nature of response. In the coming years it is hoped that fresh approaches to evaluating postnatal alterations in opioid systems may shed new light on the role that endogenous and exogenous opioids may play in neurodevelopment, and potentially allow for the development of new therapies that take into account the ontogeny of the opioidergic system.

References

Abbadie, C., Pan, Y., Drake, C. T., and Pasternak, G. W. (2000a). Comparative immunohistochemical distributions of carboxy terminus epitopes from the mu-opioid receptor splice variants MOR-1D, MOR-1 and MOR-1C in the mouse and rat CNS. *Neuroscience*, 100, 141–153.

Abbadie, C., Pan, Y. X., and Pasternak, G. W. (2000b). Differential distribution in rat brain of mu opioid receptor carboxy terminal splice variants MOR-1C-like and MOR-1-like immunoreactivity: evidence for region-specific processing. *J Comp Neurol*, 419, 244–256.

Abbott, F. V., and Guy, E. R. (1995). Effects of morphine, pentobarbital and amphetamine on formalin-induced behaviours in infant rats: sedation versus specific suppression of pain. *Pain*, 62, 303–312.

Baccei, M. and Fitzgerald, M. (2006). Development of pain pathways and mechanisms. In S. B. McMahon, and M. Koltzenburg (eds) *The textbook of pain*, pp. 143–158. London: Elsevier.

Baccei, M. L., Bardoni, R., and Fitzgerald, M. (2003). Development of nociceptive synaptic inputs to the neonatal rat dorsal horn: glutamate release by capsaicin and menthol. *J Physiol*, 549, 231–242.

Baccei, M. L., and Fitzgerald, M. (2004). Development of GABAergic and glycinergic transmission in the neonatal rat dorsal horn 5. *J Neurosci*, 24, 4749–4757.

Bardo, M. T., and Hughes, R. A. (1981). Single-dose tolerance to morphine-induced analgesic and hypoactive effects in infant rats. *Dev Psychobiol*, 14, 415–423.

Barr, G. A. (1999). Antinociceptive effects of locally administered morphine in infant rats. *Pain*, 81, 155–161.

Barr, G. A., Miya, D. Y., and Paredes, W. (1992). Analgesic effects of intraventricular and intrathecal injection of morphine and ketocyclazocine in the infant rat. *Brain Res*, 584, 83–91.

Bayon, A., Shoemaker, W. J., Bloom, F. E., Mauss, A., and Guillemin, R. (1979). Perinatal development of the endorphin- and enkephalin-containing systems in the rat brain. *Brain Res*, 179, 93–101.

Beggs, S., Torsney, C., Drew, L. J., and Fitzgerald, M. (2002). The postnatal reorganization of primary afferent input and dorsal horn cell receptive fields in the rat spinal cord is an activity-dependent process. *Eur J Neurosci*, 16, 1249–1258.

Beland, B. and Fitzgerald, M. (2001). Mu- and delta-opioid receptors are downregulated in the largest diameter primary sensory neurons during postnatal development in rats 474. *Pain*, 90, 143–150.

Belcheva, M. M., Bohn, L. M., Ho, M. T., Johnson, F. E., Yanai, J., Barron, S., *et al.* (1998). Brain opioid receptor adaptation and expression after prenatal exposure to buprenorphine. *Dev Brain Res*, 111, 35–42.

Besse, D., Lombard, M. C., Zajac, J. M., Roques, B. P., and Besson, J. M. (1990). Pre- and postsynaptic distribution of mu, delta and kappa opioid receptors in the superficial layers of the cervical dorsal horn of the rat spinal cord. *Brain Res*, 521, 15–22.

Bloom, F., Bayon, A., Battenberg, E., French, E., Koda, L., Koob, G., *et al.* (1980). Endorphins: developmental, cellular, and behavioral aspects. *Adv Biochem Psychopharmacol*, 22, 619–632.

Bremner, L. R., and Fitzgerald, M. (2008). Postnatal tuning of cutaneous inhibitory receptive fields in the rat. *J Physiol*, 586, 1529–1537.

Coggeshall, R. E., Jennings, E. A., and Fitzgerald, M. (1996). Evidence that large myelinated primary afferent fibers make synaptic contacts in lamina II of neonatal rats. *Brain Res Dev Brain Res*, 92, 81–90.

Crain, S. M and Shen, K. F. (1998). Modulation of opioid analgesia, tolerance and dependence by Gs-coupled, GM1 ganglioside-regulated opioid receptor functions. *Trends Pharmacol Sci*, 19, 358–365.

Fields, H. L., and Anderson, S. D. (1978). Evidence that raphe-spinal neurons mediate opiate and midbrain stimulation-produced analgesias. *Pain*, 5, 333–349.

Fields, H. L., Basbaum, A. I., and Heinricher, M. M. (2006) Central nervous system mechanisms of pain modulation. In S. B. McMahon, and M. Koltzenburg (eds) *The textbook of pain* (vol. 5), pp. 125–142 London: Elsevier Churchill Linvingstone.

Fields, H. L., Bry, J., Hentall, I., and Zorman, G. (1983). The activity of neurons in the rostral medulla of the rat during withdrawal from noxious heat. *J Neurosci*, 3, 2545–2552.

Fitzgerald, M. (2005). The development of nociceptive circuits. *Nat Rev Neurosci*, 6, 507–520.

Fitzgerald, M. and Jennings, E. (1999). The postnatal development of spinal sensory processing. *Proc Natl Acad Sci U S A*, 96, 7719–7722.

Goldstein, A., Tachibana, S., Lowney, L. I., Hunkapiller, M., and Hood, L. (1979). Dynorphin-(1-13), an extraordinarily potent opioid peptide. *Proc Natl Acad Sci U S A*, 76, 6666–6670.

Gray, A. C., Coupar, I. M., and White, P. J. (2006). Comparison of opioid receptor distributions in the rat central nervous system. *Life Sci*, 79, 674–685.

Gustafsson, L., Oreland, S., Hoffmann, P., and Nylander, I. (2008). The impact of postnatal environment on opioid peptides in young and adult male Wistar rats. *Neuropeptides*, 42, 177–191.

Hathway, G. J., Vega-Avelaira, D., and Fitzgerald, M. (2012). A critical period in the supraspinal control of pain: opioid-dependent changes in brainstem rostroventral medulla function in preadolescence. *Pain*, 153, 775–783.

Hauser, K. F., McLaughlin, P. J., and Zagon, I. S. (1987). Endogenous opioids regulate dendritic growth and spine formation in developing rat brain. *Brain Res*, 416, 157–161.

Hauser, K. F., McLaughlin, P. J., and Zagon, I. S. (1989). Endogenous opioid systems and the regulation of dendritic growth and spine formation. *J Comp Neurol*, 281, 13–22.

Haynes, L. W., Smyth, D. G., and Zakarian, S. (1982). Immunocytochemical localization of beta-endorphin (lipotropin C-fragment) in the developing rat spinal cord and hypothalamus. *Brain Res*, 232, 115–128.

Heinke, B., Gingl, E., and Sandkühler, J. (2011). Multiple targets of mu-opioid receptor-mediated presynaptic inhibition at primary afferent Adelta- and C-fibers. *J Neurosci*, 31, 1313–1322.

Hompes, P. G., Vermes, I., Tilders, F. J., and Schoemaker, J. (1982). Immunoreactive beta-endorphin in the hypothalamus of female rats: changes in content and release during prepubertal development. *Brain Res*, 281, 281–286.

Hughes, J., Smith, T. W., Kosterlitz, H. W., Fothergill, L. A., Morgan, B. A., and Morris, H. R. (1975). Identification of two related pentapeptides from the brain with potent opiate agonist activity. *Nature*, 258, 577–580.

Kitchen, I., Kelly, M., and Viveros, M. P. (1990). Ontogenesis of Îº-opioid receptors in rat brain using [3H]U-69593 as a binding ligand. *Eur J Pharmacol*, 175, 93–96.

Kivell, B. M., Day, D. J., McDonald, F. J., and Miller, J. H. (2004). Developmental expression of [mu] and [delta] opioid receptors in the rat brainstem: evidence for a postnatal switch in [mu] isoform expression. *Dev Brain Res*, 148, 185–196.

Koch, S. C., Fitzgerald, M., and Hathway, G. J. (2008). Midazolam potentiates nociceptive behavior, sensitizes cutaneous reflexes, and is devoid of sedative action in neonatal rats. *Anesthesiology*, 108, 122–129.

Li, C. H., Lemaire, S., Yamashiro, D., and Doneen, B. A. (1976). The synthesis and opiate activity of beta-endorphin. *Biochem Biophys Res Commun*, 71, 19–25.

Lin, C. S., Tao, P. L., Jong, Y. J., Chen, W. F., Yang, C. H., Huang, L. T., *et al.* (2009). Prenatal morphine alters the synaptic complex of postsynaptic density 95 with N-methyl-d-aspartate receptor subunit in hippocampal CA1 subregion of rat offspring leading to long-term cognitive deficits. *Neuroscience*, 158, 1326–1337.

Loh, H. H., Tseng, L. F., Wei, E., and Li, C. H. (1976). beta-endorphin is a potent analgesic agent. *Proc Natl Acad Sci U S A*, 73, 2895–2898.

Maekawa, K., Minami, M., Yabuuchi, K., Toya, T., Katao, Y., Hosoi, Y., *et al.* (1994). In situ hybridization study of mu- and kappa-opioid receptor mRNAs in the rat spinal cord and dorsal root ganglia. *Neurosci Lett*, 168, 97–100.

Marsh, D., Dickenson, A., Hatch, D., and Fitzgerald, M. (1999a). Epidural opioid analgesia in infant rats I: mechanical and heat responses. *Pain*, 82, 23–32.

Marsh, D., Dickenson, A., Hatch, D., and Fitzgerald, M. (1999b). Epidural opioid analgesia in infant rats II: responses to carrageenan and capsaicin. *Pain*, 82, 33–38.

Marvizón, J. C. G., Chen, W., and Murphy, N. (2009). Enkephalins, dynorphins, and β-endorphin in the rat dorsal horn: an immunofluorescence colocalization study. *J Comp Neurol*, 517, 51–68.

Mayer, D. J., and Liebeskind, J. C. (1974). Pain reduction by focal electrical stimulation of the brain: an anatomical and behavioral analysis. *Brain Res*, 68, 73–93.

McDowell, J. and Kitchen, I. (1986). Ontogenesis of delta-opioid receptors in rat brain using [3H][D-Pen2, D-Pen5]enkephalin as a binding ligand. *Eur J Pharmacol*, 128, 287–289.

McDowell, J. and Kitchen, I. (1987). Development of opioid systems: peptides, receptors and pharmacology. *Brain Res Rev*, 12, 397–421.

McLaughlin, P. J., Wylie, J. D., Bloom, G., Griffith, J. W., and Zagon, I. S. (2002). Chronic exposure to the opioid growth factor, [Met5]-enkephalin, during pregnancy: maternal and preweaning effects. *Pharmacol Biochem Behav*, 71, 171–181.

Nandi, R., Beacham, D., Middleton, J., Koltzenburg, M., Howard, R. F., and Fitzgerald, M. (2004). The functional expression of mu opioid receptors on sensory neurons is developmentally regulated; morphine analgesia is less selective in the neonate 2. *Pain*, 111, 38–50.

Ng, T. B., Ho, W. K., and Tam, P. P. (1984). Brain and pituitary beta-endorphin levels at different developmental stages of the rat. *Int J Pept Protein Res*, 24, 141–146.

Nitsche, J. F., and Pintar, J. E. (2003). Opioid receptor-induced GTPgamma35S binding during mouse development. *Dev Biol*, 253, 99–108.

O'Callaghan, J. P., and Holtzman, S. G. (1976). Prenatal administration of morphine to the rat: tolerance to the analgesic effect of morphine in the offspring. *J Pharmacol Exp Ther*, 197, 533–544.

Pan, Y. X., Xu, J., Bolan, E., Abbadie, C., Chang, A., Zuckerman, A., *et al.* (1999). Identification and characterization of three new alternatively spliced mu-opioid receptor isoforms. *Mol Pharmacol*, 56, 396–403.

Pert, C. B., and Snyder, S. H. (1973). Opiate receptor: demonstration in nervous tissue. *Science*, 179, 1011–1014.

Porreca, F., Ossipov, M. H., and Gebhart, G. F. (2002). Chronic pain and medullary descending facilitation. *Trends Neurosci*, 25, 319–325.

Rahman, W., Dashwood, M. R., Fitzgerald, M., Aynsley-Green, A., and Dickenson, A. H. (1998). Postnatal development of multiple opioid receptors in the spinal cord and development of spinal morphine analgesia 658. *Brain Res Dev Brain Res*, 108, 239–254.

Reynolds, D. V. (1969). Surgery in the rat during electrical analgesia induced by focal brain stimulation. *Science*, 164, 444–445.

Sanchez, E. S., Bigbee, J. W., Fobbs, W., Robinson, S. E., and Sato-Bigbee, C. (2008). Opioid addiction and pregnancy: perinatal exposure to buprenorphine affects myelination in the developing brain. *Glia*, 56, 1017–1027.

Schulz, S., Schreff, M., Koch, T., Zimprich, A., Gramsch, C., Elde, R., *et al.* (1998). Immunolocalization of two mu-opioid receptor isoforms (MOR1 and MOR1B) in the rat central nervous system. *Neuroscience*, 82, 613–622.

Simon, E. J., Hiller, J. M., and Edelman, I. (1973). Stereospecific binding of the potent narcotic analgesic (3H) Etorphine to rat-brain homogenate. *Proc Natl Acad Sci U S A*, 70, 1947–1949.

Spain, J., Roth, B., and Coscia, C. (1985). Differential ontogeny of multiple opioid receptors (mu, delta, and kappa). *J Neurosci*, 5, 584–588.

Stiene-Martin, A., and Hauser, K. F. (1990). Opioid-dependent growth of glial cultures: suppression of astrocyte DNA synthesis by met-enkephalin. *Life Sci*, 46, 91–98.

Talbot, J. N., Happe, H. K., and Murrin, L. C. (2005). Mu opioid receptor coupling to Gi/o proteins increases during postnatal development in rat brain. *J Pharmacol Exp Ther*, 314, 596–602.

Terenius, L. (1973). Characteristics of the 'receptor' for narcotic analgesics in synaptic plasma membrane fraction from rat brain. *Acta Pharmacol Toxicol (Copenh)*, 33, 377–384.

Thornton, S. R., Compton, D. R., and Smith, F. L. (1998). Ontogeny of mu opioid agonist anti-nociception in postnatal rats. *Brain Res Dev Brain Res*, 105, 269–276.

Tsang, D., Ng, S. C., Ho, K. P., and Ho, W. K. (1982). Ontogenesis of opiate binding sites and radioimmunoassayable beta-endorphin and enkephalin in regions of rat brain. *Brain Res*, 281, 257–261.

Tsou, K. and Jang, C. S. (1964). Studies on the site of analgesic action of morphine by intracerebral micro-injection. *Sci Sin*, 13, 1099–1109.

Volterra, A., Brunello, N., Restani, P., Galli, C. L., and Racagni, G. (1986). Ontogenetic studies on mu, delta and kappa opioid receptors in rat brain. *Pharmacol Res Commun*, 18, 979–990.

Westin, B. D., Walker, S. M., Deumens, R., Grafe, M., and Yaksh, T. L. (2010). Validation of a preclinical spinal safety model: effects of intrathecal morphine in the neonatal rat. *Anesthesiology*, 113, 183–199.

Zhang, G. H., and Sweitzer, S. M. (2008). Neonatal morphine enhances nociception and decreases analgesia in young rats. *Brain Res*, 1199, 82–90.

Zhang, W., Gardell, S., Zhang, D., Xie, J. Y., Agnes, R. S., Badghisi, H, *et al.* (2009). Neuropathic pain is maintained by brainstem neurons co-expressing opioid and cholecystokinin receptors. *Brain*, 132, 778–787.

CHAPTER 45

Opioids in clinical practice

Scott A. Strassels

Introduction

Opioid analgesics occupy a unique position in modern medicine. They are indispensable tools for the treatment of many types of moderate to severe pain, but are also the focus of intense attention and criticism in the biomedical literature, lay press, and media (Meldrum, 2003; Whelan et al., 2011).

The epidemiology of painful conditions and diseases, as well as other common sources of pain, including invasive procedures to diagnose and monitor diseases, help provide insight into the need at the population level for opioids to provide safe and effective prevention and management of moderate to severe pain. At the patient level, the importance of these medications is illustrated by tools such as the World Health Organization (WHO) pain ladder (Ventafridda et al., 1985), in which opioids are central to steps two and three, and by the inclusion of morphine in the WHO essential medicines list of priority medicines for mothers and children (World Health Organization, 2011a), the WHO *Model List of Essential Medicines for Children*, *3rd list*, published in March 2011 (WHO, 2011b), and the WHO guidelines on the pharmacological treatment of persisting pain in children with medical illnesses (WHO, 2012).

Nonetheless, there is mixed consensus about the roles opioids play in society and medical practice, particularly as part of the care of persons with chronic, non-cancer pain. In part, this state of affairs is due to our evolving understanding of opioids and their effects at the individual and population levels, to limited time spent educating clinicians on the appropriate use of these and other analgesics, and to substantial gaps in the evidence base, overall and particularly within children (Chou et al., 2009a, 2009b; Chapman et al., 2010). Despite this uncertainty, the view of morphine, and by extension, other opioids, as not just important, but absolutely essential contributors to clinical practice underscores the belief that these are among the most useful medications of any sort. Yet, while the medications in this class have numerous advantages, including a high degree of effectiveness and safety when they are used appropriately, there are important patient and population issues and concerns regarding the use of these medications. As a result, it is critically important that all medical practitioners, as well as other clinical decision-makers be familiar with the pharmacological and pharmacodynamic characteristics and effects of these agents, as well as related issues that are of interest, such as opioid-induced hyperalgesia (OIH) and efforts to address inappropriate opioid use at the population level.

Clinical outcomes associated with use of opioids

Evidence-based medicine plays an important part of clinical practice in many countries, from reimbursement decisions through pay for performance incentives. Yet, the evidence base for the use of opioids in children with painful conditions is uneven. The result of this situation is that there are few clinical practice guidelines (CPGs) focused on specific treatments for pain in children and adolescents. In the absence of high-quality evidence, clinicians are often left to practise according to habit, which may or may not result in optimal outcomes. Furthermore, there is a lack of consensus on the outcomes that are best to assess. For example, it is generally easy to assess a patient's pain (and, indirectly, the quality of care) using a numeric analogue 0 to 10 or verbal rating scale, but pain intensity is just one of many facets of a complex multidimensional experience (Gordon et al., 2005). Other dimensions of the pain experience, such as the ability to function in ways that are important to the patient, family, and caregivers, are also likely to be important.

To illustrate the current state of the biomedical literature on this topic, a literature search using the strategy [(pediatric OR paediatric) AND pain AND clinical practice guideline AND opioid] identified ten English-language, Pubmed-indexed papers published between 2007 and 2012. Of these, two were guidelines based on a systematic review of the literature. In one, the authors reviewed papers and abstracts published between 1996 and 2006 to provide recommendations for treatment of chronic and procedural pain in paediatric patients with rheumatic disease (Kimura and Walco, 2007). The other guideline provides recommendations from the Canadian Pain Society for drug treatment of neuropathic pain, and while none of the contents are specific to paediatric patients, it makes sense that the insights may be used in caring for children as well as adults (Moulin et al., 2007). Other topics identified in this search included the use of intravenous (IV) bolus morphine in a paediatric setting (Ellis et al., 2011), regulatory aspects of paediatric pain management in Europe (Fortinguerra et al., 2010), use of the WHO analgesic ladder to provide pain management to 39 children with leukaemia in a teaching hospital in India (Geeta et al., 2010), the results of a survey on the effect of guidelines on pain management in Austrian, German, and Swiss neonatal intensive care units (Gharavi et al., 2007), and the results of a survey of paediatric anaesthesiologists in the US, published in 2010, which was undertaken to describe patient demographics, as well as whether

IV patient-controlled (or proxy-controlled) analgesia was available and used, and the degree to which serious and life-threatening opioid-related adverse events occurred (Nelson et al., 2010). Among other findings, these authors reported that facilities with more paediatric beds were more likely to have a paediatric pain service, that IV patient-controlled analgesia was available at nearly all of the 252 institutions surveyed, and that only 38% of these institutions offered IV proxy-controlled analgesia.

Other CPGs have also been published. In 2012, an updated practice guideline was published by the American Society of Anesthesiologists for acute pain management in the perioperative setting (American Society of Anesthesiologists, 2012). While not specific to children, this document includes general recommendations for assessing, preventing, and treating pain in paediatric patients. The National Comprehensive Cancer Network (NCCN) has also published guidelines for the treatment of paediatric cancer pain in the past, most recently in 2007 (National Comprehensive Cancer Network, 2007). While the recommendations in this CPG are primarily based on lower-level evidence, including consensus, the authors recommend that treatment be titrated to pain intensity and the patient's clinical condition, reflecting the understanding that pain affects and is affected by many other dimensions of the pain experience besides just intensity. The Association of Paediatric Anaesthetists of Great Britain and Ireland published the second edition of *Good Practice in Postoperative and Procedural Pain Management* in 2012. This document is useful not only because it provides recommendations by age (i.e. procedural pain in the neonate versus older children), it also addresses assessment systematically, using explicit criteria for the evaluation of evidence. Thus, while pain intensity is clearly important, other issues, such as distress, consolability, and parental report are also discussed.

The 2012 WHO guidelines on the pharmacological treatment of persisting pain in children with medical illnesses is important for three main contributions (World Health Organization, 2012).

First, this guideline focuses on chronic pain and excludes pain due to trauma, surgery, or invasive procedures, although the recommendations are likely to apply to other patient populations, in other settings, and with other types and sources of pain. It also includes strength of recommendation and quality of evidence ratings. For example, one such guideline is that 'the use of strong opioids is recommended for the relief of moderate to severe persisting pain in children with medical illnesses' (recommendation 4, World Health Organization, 2012). Although this statement is rated as a strong recommendation, the quality of evidence supporting this suggestion is low. Notably, it is unlikely that the strength of evidence for this and similar statements will be addressed. In order to strengthen the quality of evidence, it would be necessary to conduct well-designed clinical and epidemiological research to compare the ability of strong opioids to other drugs and non-pharmacological approaches to treat moderate to severe pain in medically ill children with persisting pain—an effort that would bring up questions of appropriate and ethical resource use.

The second contribution made by the 2012 WHO guidelines is explicit discussion of codeine and tramadol—drugs that were excluded from these recommendations. Codeine, a prodrug with analgesic activity due to its conversion to morphine via cytochrome P450 (CYP) 2D6, was excluded because of problems with safety and efficacy due to the variability caused by genetic polymorphism in that metabolic pathway. Further, fetal CYP2D6 activity is extremely low compared to adult levels, and rises to no more than 25% of the adult level in children under 5 years of age. The result has been no analgesia from codeine (in poor or low metabolizers) and potential toxicity due to increased morphine production at the other end of the spectrum of activity. Tramadol was excluded due to a lack of evidence for its use in this patient population, and lack of regulatory approval for paediatric use in some countries.

The third major contribution in the new WHO guidelines is a two-step approach to the choice of medications, as opposed to the three-step ladder used in previous WHO publications. In this new method, the first step consists of treatment for mild pain using acetaminophen (paracetamol) and ibuprofen. In contrast to the three-step WHO ladder, the second step now consists of adding a strong opioid to non-opioid therapy for moderate to severe pain.

Underlying these CPGs, there is also a small group of clinical trials that assess opioid use perioperatively or in specific painful conditions. Using the strategy [(child* OR pediatric OR paediatric) AND outcome AND opioid AND pain], 207 articles published between 2007 to 2012 were identified. Of these, 30 papers remained after a review of the titles and abstracts. One paper assessed the use of all opioids in US emergency departments for any diagnosis (Pletcher et al., 2008). Several papers were reviews: one of opioid pharmacogenomics in the perioperative setting, one of analgesia in neonates (Allegaert et al., 2009), and one of the pharmacotherapy for acute pain in children (Mak et al., 2011). Additionally, one paper was a systematic review of the effect of a continuous infusion with IV patient-controlled analgesia on respiratory depression, and one was a report from a Food and Drug Administration workshop on the design of paediatric analgesic clinical trials (Berde et al., 2012).

When considered as a group, the outcomes assessed in these papers typically emphasized pain relief, whether a drug or route of administration was used, or an adverse event occurred, rather than the result of care for the patient. For example, outcomes reported included the occurrence of adverse events (Ou et al., 2008), whether opioids were used in children with abdominal pain who presented to an emergency department (Goldman et al., 2008), the use of patient-controlled analgesia in children at the end of life (Schiessl et al., 2008), and the use of ketamine as a way to decrease morphine use in children who underwent tonsillectomy (Abu-Shahwan, 2008). In one trial, changes in pain intensity were compared between children who received ibuprofen and those who received acetaminophen with codeine for extremity injuries (Friday et al., 2009). Other outcomes studied included quality of sleep, play and level of activity, eating, speech, and cry (Ruggiero et al., 2013), assessment of pain compared to hospital standards (Vijenthira et al., 2012), and emergence delirium, emesis, hypoxaemia, and the need for airway intervention in a group of children who underwent bilateral myringotomy and placement of ventilating tubes (Hippard et al., 2012). Notably, in this last paper, although administering drugs by intramuscular injection is not recommended due to pain and unpredictable absorption from tissue, the authors of this study concluded that the intramuscular route would be preferred due to the lack of a difference in the efficacy of intranasal fentanyl, intramuscular, or intravenous morphine, and the utility from the clinician's perspective of avoiding having to establish vascular access and the potential for laryngospasm from intranasal medications.

Pharmacokinetics

Pharmacokinetics refers to how physiological processes affect the absorption, distribution, metabolism, and excretion of drugs—in short, these processes are often referred to as what the body does to the drug, as opposed to pharmacology or pharmacodynamics, which are what the drug does to the body (Benet, 1984). The aspects of pharmacokinetics are absorption, distribution, metabolism, and elimination. Each of these phases includes issues that may affect use of the opioids in paediatrics.

Absorption

The stratum corneum is structurally complete by 34 weeks of gestation, and in a term infant, continues to thicken until about 4 months of age (Maples et al., 2006). Since younger infants have greater water loss than older infants as a function of body surface area: body weight, preterm infants and term infants early in life have greater absorption of drugs through the skin than older children and adults, potentially making the transdermal route more efficient in younger infants, although the changing nature of the skin also presents important challenges (Maples et al., 2006, p. 214).

Prodrugs are inactive, and require transformation to become active. As a result, activity of these medications may be decreased if enzymatic activity is insufficient to produce the active drug (as in preterm infants); lipophilic drugs may be absorbed erratically secondary to evolving lipolytic capacity; bile acids may be diminished, resulting in changes in enterohepatic recirculation of glucuronidated metabolites (morphine, hydromorphone), absorption may be increased, as a function of delayed gastric emptying and gastrointestinal transit time, which can be affected by diet.

Rectal administration may be useful when administration of meds orally or by other routes is not available, but absorption may be unpredictable (Birmingham et al., 1997; Nolke 1956). One study of 48 persons after minor surgery found that the amount of oxycodone was absorbed from a rectal suppository was similar to that from the oral route, but was about 42% of the IV dose (Leow et al., 1992). In healthy, young men, approximately bioavailability of rectal hydromorphone was approximately 33% (Parab et al., 1988).

The nasal and transmucosal routes of administration have also become popular. For example, in the US, fentanyl is available as a buccal tablet, a transmucosal lozenge, which is rubbed on inside of the cheek, a nasal solution, and a sublingual spray. It is critically important to note that these products are not bioequivalent and cannot be used interchangeably without careful titration.

Distribution

Total body water accounts for approximately 75% of total body weight in a newborn infant and about 92% in premature infants, gradually decreasing to 60% at 6 months of life (Friis-Hansen 1971, 1983). Similarly, extracellular fluid accounts for a greater percentage of total body weight than in adults (45% at birth (50% in premature infants), 28% at year 1, 20% for adults). The result is that water-soluble drugs, such as morphine, have a larger volume of distribution. In contrast, the amount of body fat increases over the first year of life before decreasing over time to adult levels. Fat levels as a percentage of body weight are higher in girls than boys during adolescence. The implication here is that fat-soluble drugs (among the opioids, diamorphine, fentanyl, alfentanil, and sufentanil are more lipophilic than morphine) may have a longer duration of action for infants compared to older children and adults, as well as in adolescent girls compared to adolescent boys.

In general, once absorbed into the bloodstream, a given drug must be free (unbound) in order to be pharmacologically active. As a result, the degree to which drugs are bound to plasma proteins has the potential to influence medications; this fraction can be affected by the concentration of the protein, the affinity of the drug for the protein, and the ability of the protein to interact with the drug (Maples et al., 2006, p. 217). As a result, in persons with hypoalbuminaemia or in persons with conditions in which the binding sites on albumin for a drug are altered and binding is decreased, pharmacological activity of a drug is likely to be increased. Acidic drugs are generally bound to albumin, while basic drugs are bound to alpha-1 acid glycoprotein. For example, albumin levels are lower in premature than in term babies, and there are fewer binding sites. In neonates, alpha-1-acid glycoprotein is present, but at about one-third of adult levels, which occur at approximately 1 year of age.

The opioids thought to be most likely to be affected by changes in plasma proteins are those that are at least 80% protein bound (Maples et al., 2006, p. 217). Among the opioids, these include alfentanil (92%), buprenorphine (96%), fentanyl (84%), methadone (90%), and sufentanil (79% in neonates, 91–93% otherwise). Morphine is approximately 30% bound. The extent to which hydrocodone is bound to plasma proteins is not completely understood, although it is thought to be in the same range as other semisynthetic opioids, such as hydromorphone and oxycodone, approximately 19% to 45% (Vintage Pharmaceuticals, 2012). The clinical implications of these phenomena are not well understood, however, preterm infants and neonates may require lower doses of these drugs.

Metabolism

Generally speaking, fetal drug metabolism is lower than in infants, and then increases in early childhood. The hepatic enzymes most commonly discussed in the context of opioid metabolism are CYP2D6 and CYP3A4, and the drugs most commonly affected are codeine, fentanyl, and hydrocodone. CYP2D6 is particularly important because it is known to show genetic polymorphism, with poor and extensive metabolizer groups (Leeder and Kearns 1997; May 1994). The drug most affected by variations in 2D6 activity is codeine, although about 4% of hydrocodone is metabolized to hydromorphone via this route. About 10% of a codeine dose is metabolized to morphine, however since poor metabolizers are not expected to generate any morphine and codeine is a prodrug, these individuals will not receive any analgesia from codeine (Yaksh and Wallace 2011). Extensive metabolizers, on the other hand, will produce more morphine from the same amount of codeine, which may result in significant toxicity. Codeine use by a nursing extensive-metabolizer mother has also resulted in death of the infant, and several children after tonsillectomy. A similar case in which a child who was a CYP2D6 poor metabolizer and was also receiving other drugs that interfered with metabolism of hydrocodone and its metabolites died has also been published.

The CYP3A4 isozyme is important in this context mainly in the biotransformation of alfentanil, fentanyl, sufentanil, and methadone (Yaksh and Wallace 2011). Persons with diminished enzyme activity or who are taking drugs that are themselves metabolized by this route or that inhibit this enzyme (e.g. macrolide antibiotics (erythromycin, clarithromycin, telithromycin)), azole antifungals (ketoconazole, itraconazole), or protease inhibitors, among others, are at risk for toxicity due to increased levels of these opioids (see Table 45.1).

Elimination

With the exception of methadone, the kidney is the primary route of elimination for the opioids. Methadone is eliminated via the gastrointestinal tract in bile, as well as in urine (Yaksh and Wallace, 2011). For children with decreased renal function, the doses of renally eliminated drugs are decreased (Nahata and Taketomo, 2011). In general, however, conditions and diseases that reduce blood flow to the liver (e.g. cirrhosis, congestive heart failure) reduce the clearance and increase oral bioavailability of drugs with high hepatic extraction. Among the opioids, the drugs that are highly hepatically extracted in adults include morphine, meperidine, fentanyl, sufentanil, but not alfentanil or remifentanil (Davis 2007; Tegeder et al., 1999).

Nursing and lactation

As shown in Table 45.2, data on opioid use by nursing mothers is limited. In general, clinical decision-making rests on a foundation of assessing risk-to benefit ratio, and the expected duration of therapy.

One clinical scenario involving use of codeine by a nursing mother bears mention here. Although use by nursing mothers for short periods has been considered safe, use over a 2-week period by an ultrarapid metabolizer of has resulted in the death of a nursing infant (Koren et al., 2006).

Language

Among the many challenges to providing high-quality pain management is making sure that patients, clinicians, and other caregivers, families, and regulatory officials are all speaking the same language. This is particularly important because the words and concepts involved are not only emotionally powerful, they have implications for clinicians' willingness to prescribe, and pharmacies' ability and willingness to fill prescriptions.

One of the challenges that complicates the treatment of pain and, particularly, the use of opioids is that the definitions (and consequently, understanding) of commonly used terms differ between medicine and psychology. For example, in the 2003 consensus definitions published by the American Society of Addiction Medicine, the American Pain Society, and the American Academy of Pain Medicine, addiction is defined as a primary, chronic, multifactorial,

Table 45.1 Opioid metabolism

Opioid	Metabolic pathway	Major metabolites	Comments
Alfentanil	CYP3A4	NA	NA
Codeine	CYP2D6	Morphine	Approximately 10% of codeine dose is converted to morphine, however pharmacogenetic variation may result in varying clinical effects, from no production of morphine to higher conversion to morphine (resulting in toxicity or death)
Fentanyl	CYP3A4	NA	Fentanyl is available in various dosage forms (transdermal, transmucosal, buccal, sublingual, nasal), which are NOT bioequivalent.
Hydrocodone	CYP2D6	Hydromorphone	About 4% of dose is converted to hydromorphone
Hydromorphone	Glucuronidation	Hydromorphone-3-glucuronide	NA
Levorphanol	Glucuronidation	NA	NA
Meperidine	Hepatic	Normeperidine	Normeperidine is toxic, and may cause seizures. Accumulation may occur in persons with decreased renal function
Methadone	CYP3A4, CYP2D6	2-ethylidene-1, 5-dimethyl-3, 3-diphenylpyrrolidine (EDDP)	EDDP is inactive; Higher doses of methadone are associated with QT prolongation and potential for torsades de pointes
Morphine	Conjugation	Morphine-3-glucuronide, morphine-6-glucuronide	Metabolites accumulate with decreased renal function. M6G is analgesic, M3G may be proalgesic
Oxycodone	CYP2D6	Oxymorphone	Present only in small amounts
	Glucuronidation	Noroxycodone	Weaker than parent drug
Oxymorphone	Glucuronidation	Oxymorphone-6-glucuronide, 6-OH-oxymorphone	
Remifentanil	Ester hydrolysis	NA	NA
Sufentanil	N-dealkylation, O-demethylation via CYP3A4	NA	NA
Tapentadol	Conjugation, CYP2C9, CYP2C19, CYP2D6	Tapentadol-O-glucuronide	No active metabolites
Tramadol	CYP2D6, CYP3A4, conjugation	O-desmethyltramadol (M1)	M1 contributes to analgesic activity

Source: data from Yaksh and Wallace, 2011; Tegeder et al., 1999; Lundeberg and Roelofse, 2011; Tateishi et al., 1996; Sullivan and Due, 1973 and Eap et al., 2002. NA = not applicable.

Table 45.2 Opioids in breast milk

Drug	Excreted into breast milk?	Clinically important?
Alfentanil	Yes	Limited human data—probably compatible
Codeine	Yes	Limited human data—potential toxicity
Fentanyl	Yes	Compatible
Hydrocodone	Not known	No human data—probably compatible
Hydromorphone	Yes	Limited human data - probably compatible
Levorphanol	Not known	No human data – probably compatible
Meperidine	Yes	Compatible
Methadone	Yes	Limited human data – probably compatible
Morphine	Yes	Limited human data—probably compatible
Oxycodone	Yes	Limited human data—probably compatible
Oxymorphone	Not known	No human data—probably compatible
Remifentanil	Not known	No human data—probably compatible
Sufentanil	Not known	No human data—probably compatible
Tapentadol	Not known	Manufacturer does not recommend use during breastfeeding
Tramadol	Yes	Limited human data—probably compatible

Compatible: either the drug is not excreted in clinically significant amounts into human breast milk or its use during lactation does not, or is not expected to, cause toxicity in a nursing infant.

No (limited) human data—probably compatible: there may or may not be human pregnancy experience, but the characteristics of the drug suggest that it does not represent a significant risk to the embryo/fetus. For example, other drugs in the same class or with similar mechanisms are compatible or the drug does not obtain significant systemic concentrations. Any animal reproduction data are not relevant.

Reproduced with permission from Briggs et al. (ed.) *Drugs in Pregnancy and Lactation: A Reference Guide to Fetal and Neonatal Risk* (8th edn), Lippincott Williams & Wilkins, Philadelphia, USA, Copyright ©2008.

neurobiological disease, characterized by impaired control over drug use, compulsive use, continued use despite harm, and craving. In the *Diagnostic and Statistical Manual of Mental Disorders, fourth edition, text revision* the term 'dependence' is used (American Psychiatric Association, 2000; Savage et al., 2003).

Drugs are often referred to as being addictive. Yet, while it is generally true that the reward experienced from a given drug is an important component of the decision to repeat use, there are also patient-specific factors that are important patient contributors to the development of addiction (Savage et al., 2003). In general, then, rather than blaming a drug or class of drugs for addiction, it is the combination of a physiologically and psychologically vulnerable person (and the degree of vulnerability is not constant), with a substance that produces reward that requires our attention. This idea also seems to help explain why some people prefer a class of drugs over others (alcohol versus nicotine versus opioids, and so on), as well as drugs within a class (codeine versus fentanyl, and so on).

Physical dependence is defined as a state of physiological adaptation in which a class-specific withdrawal syndrome occurs upon suddenly stopping use of a drug, quickly reducing the dose, use of an antagonist, or otherwise decreasing the blood level of drug (Savage et al., 2003). In other words, when sudden discontinuation of a drug is not recommended (for whatever reason), it can be viewed as dependence. Many drug classes fall into this category, not just opioids, including corticosteroids, anticonvulsants, and antihypertensives, among others.

Tolerance occurs when a specific effect of a drug decreases over time (Savage et al., 2003). Like physical dependence, tolerance is currently understood to be a state of physiological adaptation, and can be a measure of safety. The heart of this definition is centred on the diminution of a specific effect. Thus, in referring to tolerance to an opioid, the assumption may be that the drug's analgesic effect has decreased, even if it is another effect of that drug. For example, in the opioids, tolerance to respiratory depression typically occurs fairly quickly, while tolerance to the constipating effects generally occurs slowly, if at all.

Opioid analgesics

In general, opioids can be organized by the main type of opioid receptor the drug interacts with (Table 45.3), and by the drugs' general chemical structure (Table 45.4). The three main types of opioid receptor are mu, kappa, and delta (Yaksh and Wallace, 2011). While agonism at each of these receptors produces analgesia, most opioids currently available are mu agonists, and none of the opioids used in the US are delta agonists. Although the partial agonists and kappa agonists/mu antagonists were originally developed to be safer alternatives to the mu agonist drugs, the difference between these groups when given in equianalgesic doses is small and not thought to be clinically meaningful.

Opioids are categorized chemically as phenanthrenes, phenylpiperidines, or diphenylpropylamines (Yaksh and Wallace, 2011). The clinical implication of these differences is that, generally speaking, if a person cannot take a drug in one chemical group, such as morphine, it may be possible to cautiously use a drug from one of the other groups, such as methadone or fentanyl.

Table 45.3 Opioids by receptor activity

Mu agonists		Kappa agonist/Mu antagonists	Mu antagonists
Alfentanil	Opium	Buprenorphine (partial agonist)	Nalmefene
Codeine	Oxycodone	Butorphanol	Naloxone
Diamorphine (Heroin; not used clinically in the US)	Oxymorphone	Nalbuphine	Naltrexone
Fentanyl	Propoxyphene (withdrawn from the US market in 2010)	Pentazocine	
Hydrocodone	Remifentanil		
Hydromorphone	Sufentanil		
Levorphanol	Tapentadol		
Meperidine (Pethidine)	Tramadol		
Methadone			
Morphine			

Table 45.4 Opioid analgesics by chemical structure

Phenanthrenes	Phenylpiperidines	Diphenylpropylamines
Codeine	Alfentanil	Methadone
Hydrocodone	Fentanyl	Propoxyphene (withdrawn from the US market in 2010)
Levorphanol (a morphinan)	Meperidine	
Morphine	Remifentanil	
Oxycodone	Sufentanil	
Oxymorphone		

Since the focus of this chapter is to provide general clinical insight into opioid use for the treatment of pain, the discussion in this section will emphasize those opioids that are most commonly used in that setting (see Table 45.5). Alfentanil, remifentanil, and sufentanil are primarily used in surgical settings, and while nalmefene and naltrexone are opioid antagonists, they are used mainly in the treatment of alcohol dependence. As a result, the use of these drugs is beyond the scope of this effort.

Buprenorphine

Buprenorphine is a partial agonist at the mu opioid receptor, as well as an antagonist at the kappa and delta opioid receptors (Yaksh and Wallace, 2011). Its half-life in premature neonates after IV use is approximately 20 h (standard deviation 8), and it is metabolized to norbuprenorphine and other compounds. The role of buprenorphine in caring for children with pain is unclear, in part because of limited research on this topic, and in part because use of the agonist-antagonist drugs (buprenorphine, butorphanol, nalbuphine, and pentazocine) may precipitate withdrawal in persons who have been receiving mu agonist opioids. In two studies of children with postoperative pain after orthopaedic surgery, morphine and buprenorphine were each considered good or very good analgesics, with similar side effect profiles, despite the studies being considered to be low quality (World Health Organization, 2012). Transdermal buprenorphine has also

been studied in a small group of children with cancer-related pain (Ruggiero et al., 2013).

Codeine

Codeine is not recommended for use in children with persistent pain, due to well-documented problems with efficacy and safety (World Health Organization, 2012). This recommendation makes sense for children with other types of pain, as well. Specifically, codeine is a prodrug, and its analgesic activity is dependent on its conversion to morphine via CYP2D6. Persons with an absolute or functional lack of this will not experience analgesia from codeine or they may experience diminished analgesia relative to a given dose. Conversely, persons who are considered rapid or extensive metabolizers will experience more analgesia than would otherwise be expected. Toxicity and deaths have occurred in rapid metabolizers, as well as in children of nursing mothers who were taking codeine. Approximately 10% of a codeine dose is converted to morphine, and bioavailability is estimated as 30% to 60%. Thus, a 10 mg oral dose of codeine would be expected to provide approximately 0.3 to 0.6 mg of morphine. Given that genetic polymorphism with codeine has been well documented, there have been serious adverse events due to the use of therapeutic codeine doses, and morphine is readily available, the continued need to use codeine for analgesia is questionable at best (Ciszkowski et al., 2009; Kelly et al., 2012; Koren et al., 2006).

Table 45.5 Dosing for commonly used opioids

Drug	Neonates	Infants	Children	Adolescents
Buprenorphine: slow IV			2–6 mcg/kg every 4–8 h (2–12 years of age)	3 mcg/kg every 6–8 h (≥13 years of age)
Fentanyl[a]				
Oral transmucosal			0.01 mg/kg/dose or 10–15 mcg/kg (oralet)	
Intranasal			1–2 mcg/kg	
IV bolus			0.001 mg/kg/dose or 0.5–1 mcg/kg every 1–2 h	
IV infusion			0.5 mcg/kg/h	
Hydrocodone			0.1–0.2 mg/kg every 4 h	
Hydromorphone				
Oral		40–80 mcg/kg every 4 h		
IV bolus		10–20 mcg/kg every 3–4 h		
IV infusion		3–5 mcg/kg/h		
Methadone				
Initial intravenous			0.05–0.1 mg/kg (up to 10 mg) every 3–4 h for 2–3 doses, then every 6–12 h	
Oral and subcutaneous			0.1 mg/kg (up to 10 mg) every 4 h for 2–3 doses, then every 6–12 h. Alternately, 0.7 mg/kg/day (up to 10 mg/dose) divided every 4–6 h	
Morphine				
Oral, immediate release		0.2–0.5 mg/kg every 3–4 h		
Oral, sustained release (older children & adolescents)			0.25–0.5 mg/kg every 8–12 h	
IV bolus	Preterm: 10–25 mcg/kg every 2–4 h	50–100 mcg/kg every 3 h		
	Full-term: 25–50 mcg/kg every 3–4 h			
IV infusion	Preterm: 0.01–0.03 mg/kg/h or 2–10 mcg/kg/h	15–30 mcg/kg/h		
	Full-term: 5–20 mcg/kg/h			
Oxycodone			0.05–0.2 mg/kg every 4–6 h	

[a]Fentanyl: transdermal, transmucosal, intranasal use is not for use in outpatient or unobserved settings, or in opioid-naïve patients.

Source: dosing data from Johns Hopkins Hospital, Kristin Arcara and Megan Tschudy, *The Harriet Lane Handbook*, 19th Edition, Mosby, Inc., an affiliate of Elsevier Inc., Copyright © 2012; Lexicomp® and Facts & Comparisons®, Copyright © Wolters Kluwer Health, Inc. and John Barnes Rose, Analgesic Medications for Acute Pain Management in Children, in Gary A. Walco and Kenneth R. Goldschneider (eds), *Pain in Children: A Practical Guide for Primary Care*, Humana Press, Totowa, New Jersey, USA, pp. 73–85, Copyright © 2008.

Diamorphine (diacetylmorphine, heroin)

Although not available for clinical use in the US, diamorphine is used in the UK in children for a variety of painful conditions and for pain at the end of life (Hewitt et al., 2008), intranasal use in emergency settings (Finn and Harris, 2010; Hadley et al., 2010), and sickle cell pain (Telfer et al., 2009).

Metabolism to 3- and 6-monoacetylmorphine and then to morphine occurs quickly when diamorphine is given by mouth. In contrast, administration by injection or other routes that avoid the first-pass effect allows the drug to cross the blood–brain barrier more rapidly than morphine or other, less fat-soluble opioids. It is not known if diamorphine offers any clinical advantage in terms of

its ability to produce analgesia over drugs that are even more lipid-soluble, such as methadone or fentanyl, when given by the same route.

Fentanyl

Fentanyl is approximately 100 times more potent than morphine on a milligram-to-milligram basis (Yaksh and Wallace, 2011). It is also lipophilic, which results in relatively rapid onset of action (except when used transdermally). Although fentanyl is metabolized to inactive products via CYP3A4, this process is decreased by a wide variety of drugs. These drugs include, but are not limited to amiodarone, aprepitant, the azole antifungals (i.e. fluconazole, itraconazole, ketoconazole), calcium channel blockers (e.g. diltiazem, verapamil), macrolide antibiotics (clarithromycin, erythromycin, telithromycin), nefazodone, and protease inhibitors (e.g. fosamprenavir, ritonavir, indinavir, nelfinavir, saquinavir). The result of this interaction has included fatalities due to respiratory depression. As a result, close monitoring (including dose reduction of fentanyl as indicated) is absolutely required, particularly when using fentanyl with drugs that inhibit the CYP3A4 pathway.

Fentanyl is also of interest because it is one of the only opioids that is available for transdermal use, along with buprenorphine, or intranasal use (diamorphine is used intranasally in the UK) and fentanyl is the only opioid available for transmucosal use. Transdermal fentanyl should not be used in people who are opioid-naïve. Additionally, although there are several transmucosal and one intranasal fentanyl products available, they are not bioequivalent to each other, and cannot be interchanged without titrating. Further, using these products in children is a challenge because the doses are chosen based on adult opioid dosing, although Borland et al. (2011) assessed the use of intranasal fentanyl in 50 mcg/ml or 300 mcg/ml concentrations using a calibrated delivery device to provide 1.5 mcg/kg (up to 0.2 ml per nostril) in 189 children aged 3 to 15 years who presented to an Australian emergency department with clinically deformed closed long bone fractures. These authors concluded that these concentrations were clinically equivalent in their provision of analgesia, and that the lower concentration was reasonable for children weighing less than 50 kg.

Hydrocodone

Most hydrocodone is used in the US, although it is also available (to a much smaller degree) in other countries, including Argentina, Belgium, Canada, Columbia, Germany, Guatemala, and Switzerland (International Narcotics Control Board, 2013). Bioavailability information is not available, and limited data suggest that hydrocodone is roughly equipotent to morphine on a milligram to milligram basis. Approximately 4% of a hydrocodone dose is transformed to hydromorphone via CYP2D6. Since CYP2D6 is the same pathway that biotransforms codeine, similar safety and efficacy problems are possible.

In the US, hydrocodone is not available for parenteral use, and it is always used in combination with other drugs, most typically acetaminophen (paracetamol). While the usual initial dose in opioid-naïve children who weigh less than 50 kg is 0.1 to 0.2 mg/kg every 3 to 4 h, and 5 to 10 mg every 3 to 4 h in children who weight at least 50 kg, maximum dosing is a function of other drugs (i.e. acetaminophen) present (Lexicomp, 2013a).

Hydromorphone

Hydromorphone is approximately five times as potent than morphine on a milligram to milligram basis (Yaksh and Wallace, 2011). Its oral bioavailability is approximately 20% to 60% (Lexicomp, 2013b) by mouth and approximately 51% intranasally, although, in one study, the interindividual variability was 59%. Metabolism is via glucuronidation to inactive products, which are eliminated in the urine. Usual initial doses for infants older than 6 months of age who weigh more than 10 kg are 0.03 to 0.06 mg/kg given by mouth every 3 to 4 h as needed, 0.01 mg/kg intravenously, given every 3 to 6 h, or 0.003 to 0.005 mg/kg/h by continuous IV infusion (Friedrichsdorf and Kang 2007; Lexicomp 2013b; Zernikow et al.,

2009). In older children and adolescents who weigh less than 50 kg, oral doses of 0.03 to 0.08 mg/kg every 3 to 4 h, 0.015 mg/kg intravenously every 3 to 6 h, or 0.003 to 0.005 mg/kg/h up to a maximum of 0.2 mg/h by continuous IV infusion.

Meperidine (British approved name: pethidine)

Meperidine is not recommended for use as an analgesic, due to its active and toxic metabolite, normeperidine, which can accumulate (elimination half-life in neonates is 30–85 h) and cause seizures. Because of its poor risk:benefit profile, meperidine has been removed from many formularies in the US. Meperidine is about one-tenth as potent as morphine and it is about 30% bioavailable when given by mouth (Lexicomp, 2013c). If alternatives to meperidine are not available or are contraindicated, usual meperidine dosing in children is 1 to 1.5 mg/kg every 3 to 4 h by mouth or parenterally. By continuous IV infusion, a loading dose of 0.5 to 1 mg/kg can be given, followed by 0.3 mg/kg/h initially, with titration to effect up to 0.5 to 0.7 mg/kg/h.

Methadone

Methadone is a potent opioid that is challenging to use, due to its long elimination half-life of approximately 19 h (range 4–62), and because the elimination half-life is substantially longer than the duration of analgesia, which is 6 to 8 h initially (Lexicomp, 2013d). Methadone is approximately 80% bioavailable and is metabolized to an inactive product via CYP3A4 and CYP2D6, and eliminated in the urine (approximately 10% of unchanged drug) and faeces. It also has the potential to cause cardiac arrhythmias. Choice of a dose must be done carefully, and is best viewed as a process, rather than a single event, since the dose and dosing interval will likely change over the first few days of therapy due to accumulation (Weschules and Bain, 2008). It is also critically important to recognize that equianalgesic conversion involving methadone is not a linear calculation. For example, in contrast to the idea that hydromorphone is about five times as potent as morphine or that fentanyl is about 100 times as potent as morphine, the ratio of methadone to morphine varies based in part on how much morphine the person was receiving. There are several methods available to estimate methadone doses, and while each differs slightly from each other, the hallmark is that the expected dose of methadone decreases as the dose of morphine increases.

Morphine

Morphine is the prototypical opioid and is generally the opioid of first choice, due to its effectiveness, extensive clinical experience using it, and low cost. When given by mouth, it is approximately 30% bioavailable, and is metabolized to morphine-3- and morphine-6-glucuronides (Lexicomp, 2013e; Yaksh and Wallace, 2011). While morphine-3-glucuronide is not an analgesic, some evidence suggests that it may be proalgesic. In contrast, morphine-6-glucuronide has analgesic activity. Both compounds can accumulate in people with decreased renal function. The elimination half-life of morphine generally decreases from 10 to 20 h in preterm infants to 1 to 2 h in preschool-aged children.

Opium

Although used primarily as an antidiarrheal, opium can also be used as an analgesic. It contains several alkaloids, including morphine (10% of opium) and codeine (0.5% of opium) (Yaksh and

Wallace, 2011). It is important to note that opium is available as a tincture (10 mg morphine/ml), as well as in paregoric (2 mg morphine/5 ml). The difference between these products is critical, since opium tincture contains 25 times more morphine than paregoric. Paediatric dosing of paregoric is 0.25–0.50 ml/kg one to four times a day (Lexicomp, 2013f).

Oxycodone

The main differences between oxycodone and morphine have to do with metabolism and bioavailability. Oxycodone is metabolized via CYP2D6 to oxymorphone (which is present only in small amounts) and is glucuronidated to noroxycodone (Yaksh and Wallace, 2011). The relative lack of clinically important active metabolites makes oxycodone a reasonable choice for patients with diminished renal function. Oxycodone is approximately 80% bioavailable.

Tapentadol

Metabolism of tapentadol is via conjugation, as well as CYP2C9, CYP2C19, and CYP2D6 to inactive products. In terms of efficacy, tapentadol is broadly considered to be similar to tramadol, although tapentadol has less effect on serotonin reuptake inhibition than tramadol (Yaksh and Wallace, 2011). No articles on tapentadol and children were identified in a literature search of PubMed-indexed journals. According to the professional prescribing information, the safety and effectiveness of tapentadol has not been established in patients less than 18 years of age (Janssen Pharmaceuticals, 2012).

Tramadol

Tramadol is not recommended for treatment of persistent pain in medically ill children, due to lack of evidence and lack of regulatory approval in this population (World Health Organization, 2012). This recommendation likely applies to children with other kinds of pain as well. Although tramadol is considered a codeine analogue, it is structurally dissimilar from the other phenanthrene opioids, thus, it may be a reasonable choice in people who cannot take other opioids (Yaksh and Wallace, 2011).

Side effects and adverse events

While respiratory depression is commonly considered the most concerning potential side effect of the opioids, other side effects closely associated with the opioids include nausea and vomiting, itching, urinary retention, dizziness, and sedation (see Table 45.6). Since adverse events considered broadly are simply things that are undesirable at the time and from the perspective being considered, it also makes sense to think about these occurrences more broadly. One example of this is a commentary by Chorney et al. (2010), in which the authors consider the implications of viewing pain as an adverse event itself.

Pain management aside for a moment, the general approach to addressing adverse events and side effects consists of prevention when possible, followed by decreasing the dose (or administration frequency), using a different drug in place of the implicated medication, or as a last resort, continuing with the medication associated with the adverse event and adding another drug to treat the unwanted event or symptom. An example of the latter situation is to use low doses of a central nervous system stimulant in a person whose pain is well controlled, but who is sedated. A variety of treatment methods have been used, including opioid rotation, use of different routes of administration, and use of drugs with different mechanisms of action to help decrease the patient's opioid requirement. Although we are moving into a time in which comparative effectiveness studies are considered increasingly important, much of the published biomedical literature relies heavily on placebo-controlled trials. As a result, although randomized, controlled trials comparing opioids are not very common, clinical practice often includes trying another drug in a class if the patient doesn't tolerate the first drug chosen.

Nausea and vomiting

Nausea and vomiting are among the most undesirable adverse effects of clinical anaesthesia, from the points of view of patients as well as clinicians (Macario et al., 1999a, 1999b). Despite the importance of avoiding these adverse effects, prevention and treatment have remained challenging, in part due to varying mechanisms of action. While opioids are often implicated as causes due to their effects on the central nervous system, gastrointestinal tract, and other physiological systems, other drugs and pain also cause nausea. Depending on the underlying cause, treatment typically consists of a variety of drugs, including phenothiazines, haloperidol, and the 5-HT$_3$ receptor antagonists, of which dolasetron, ondansetron, and palonosetron have been approved by the US Food & Drug Administration for prevention of postoperative nausea and vomiting (Hardy et al., 2002; Schug et al., 1992; Sussman et al., 1999). Antihistamines, transdermal scopolamine, and metoclopramide have also been used.

Itching

Although commonly attributed to histamine release (and treated that way), the pathophysiological mechanisms underlying opioid-related itching are hypothesized multiple pathways to involve spinal opioid receptors, disinhibition of specific neurons, or central serotonin (5-HT-3) receptors (McNicol, 2007; Schmelz, 2002; Schug et al., 1992). It is also important to recognize that itching may be caused or aggravated by other diseases and conditions, including cholestatic liver disease, as well as skin conditions, like dry skin or eczema, although the latter are typically localized versus generalized.

Treatment of itching is often focused on H$_1$-receptor antagonists, although itching also occurs with fentanyl and sufentanil, which do not cause histamine release (Schug et al., 1992). If antihistamines are used, there is potential for drug interactions to enhance sedation. In these individuals, more frequent monitoring for respiratory function will be important. Nalbuphine has also been used, but this drug is an antagonist at the mu opioid receptor, so there is the potential for analgesia to be reversed or withdrawal to be induced (Yaksh and Wallace, 2011). In one recent review, Miller and Hagemann (2011) evaluated the published biomedical literature on the use of naloxone, naltrexone, or methylnaltrexone for management of opioid-induced itching. These authors concluded that IV doses of 0.25 to 1 mcg/kg/h of naloxone is optimal for reversal of itching without also affecting analgesia. Yet, since most people in an ambulatory setting don't have percutaneous access, optimal treatment of itching in community-based patients will likely centre on opioid rotation.

Respiratory depression/sedation

Opioids produce a dose-related decrease on all phases of respiration (Yaksh and Wallace, 2011). It is a more common occurrence in individuals who are opioid-naïve or -inexperienced, as well as persons

Table 45.6 Selected drugs and dosing for opioid-related side effects

Side effect and drugs	Neonates	Infants	Children	Adolescents
Nausea				
Diphenhydramine, by mouth or intravenously			0.5–1 mg/kg every 4–6 h as needed	
Lorazepam, by mouth or intravenously			0.02–0.04 mg/kg (up to 2 mg) every 6 h	
Ondansetron, by mouth or intravenously			0.15 mg/kg (up to 8 mg) 1–4 times a day	
Prochlorperazine, by mouth or rectally			0.1–0.15 mg/kg every 6–8 h	
Promethazine, by mouth or intravenously			0.25–0.5 mg/kg every 4–6 h as needed	
Respiratory depression/sedation				
Naloxone			0.02 mg every 30–60 secs until improvement (may need to repeat)	
Itching: diphenhydramine, by mouth or intravenously			0.5–1 mg/kg every 6–8 h	
Nalbuphine, intravenously[a]			0.01–0.02 mg/kg every 6–8 h as needed	
Naloxone, by infusion			0.25–1 mcg/kg/h	
Constipation: docusate (1–4 divided doses by mouth per day)				
<3 years of age			10–40 mg	
3–6 years of age			20–60 mg	
6–12 years of age			40–150 mg	
>12 years of age			50–400 mg	
Senna, by mouth			10–20 mg/kg/dose 1–2 times a day	
Bisacodyl tablets, by mouth			5–10 mg (must be able to swallow a tablet whole)	
Suppository, rectally			5 mg (<2 years of age), 10 mg (>2 years of age)	
Magnesium citrate, by mouth: <6 years of age			2–4 ml/kg a day (in single or divided doses)	
6–12 years of age			100–150 ml once a day	
12 years of age or older				150–300 ml by mouth once a day
Magnesium hydroxide, by mouth: <2 years of age			0.5 ml once a day	
2–5 years of age			5–15 ml once a day	
6–12 years of age			5–30 ml once a day	
12 years of age or older				30–60 ml once a day
Mineral oil: 5–11 years of age, by mouth			5–15 ml once a day	
12 years of age or older, by mouth				15–45 ml once a day
2–11 years of age, rectally			30–60 ml	
12 years of age or older, rectally				60–150 ml retention enema
Glycerine: under 6 years of age, rectal or enema			1 infant suppository, one or two times, or 2–5 ml as an enema	
6 years of age or older, rectal or enema			1 adult suppository, one or two times, or 5–15 ml as an enema	
Lactulose, by mouth			7.5 ml once a day after breakfast	
Polyethylene glycol, by mouth (in 4–8 ounces of fluid)			8.5–17 grams (0.5–1 capful or packet) one to three times a day	

(Continued)

Table 45.6 *(Continued)*

Side effect and drugs	Neonates	Infants	Children	Adolescents
Polyethylene glycol–electrolyte solution, by mouth			25–40 ml/kg/h until constipation is relieved	
Methylnaltrexone,[b] subcutaneously or enterally			0.15 mg/kg once every other day to every day	
Naloxone, by mouth[a]			2–12 mg three times a day	

Prevention of constipation should be with a stool softener/laxative combination, such as senna with docusate.

[a]Naloxone and nalbuphine must be titrated carefully to avoid reversing opioid analgesia and precipitating withdrawal symptoms.

[b]Methylnaltrexone dosing is based on a case report of one 4-year-old patient with epidemolysis bullosa (Lee and Mooney, 2012; Facts & Comparisons). Safety and efficacy have not been evaluated for labelling purposes in children. The dose of 0.15 mg/kg is the usual adult dose for persons weighing less than 38 kg. For adults who weigh 38–less than 62 kg, the dose is 8 mg, and for persons who weigh 62–114 kg, the dose is 12 mg.

Source: data from Lexicomp® and Facts & Comparisons®, Copyright © Wolters Kluwer Health, Inc.; Johns Hopkins Hospital, Kristin Arcara and Megan T Schudy, *The Harriet Lane Handbook*, 19th Edition, Mosby, Inc., an affiliate of Elsevier Inc., Copyright © 2012; Bruce P. Himelstein et al., Pediatric Palliative Care, *New England Journal of Medicine*, Volume 350, Number 17, pp. 1752–1763, Copyright © 2004 Massachusetts Medical Society and NCCN 2007 Pediatric Cancer Pain (pp. 23, PEDP-E 2 of 3, 3 of 3).

who have limited respiratory function, or conditions like asthma. Tolerance to this effect generally happens reasonably quickly.

Sedation is a more useful measure of the risk of respiratory depression than respiratory rate alone, since sedation occurs before the person's breathing is depressed. A variety of sedation scales are used in clinical practice; these typically include a measure of how sedated the person is, as well as how easily the person is aroused. The level of sedation may be useful, along with the trend. Treatment for respiratory depression focuses on use of naloxone and, if needed, oxygen. If naloxone is used, however, it should be given slowly to avoid antagonizing analgesia. Additionally, since the half-life of naloxone is short, the dose will likely need to be repeated (Yaksh and Wallace, 2011).

Constipation

Although constipation is common in persons who are treated with opioids, tolerance to this effect develops only slowly, if at all. As a result, prophylactic use of laxatives—typically a stimulant such as senna with a stool softener—is considered first-line therapy. In practice, however, as well as in persons at the end of life, either no treatment or prevention, or use of only a stool softener remains relatively common. In one study of paediatric and adult hospice patients, for example, approximately 26% of persons were not prescribed any laxatives, and 4% were prescribed only a stool softener (Strassels et al., 2010). The problem with using just a stool softener is that it doesn't address the decreased gastrointestinal motion that occurs with opioid use. Additionally, as gastrointestinal transit time is increased, there is more time for water to be absorbed, in addition to drying effects of the opioids. Other options include drugs such as methylnaltrexone, alvimopan, nalbuphine, and naloxone. Alvimopan and methylnaltrexone are peripheral mu-opioid receptor antagonists. The concept underlying these drugs is that antagonism of peripheral opioid receptors is useful to treat opioid-induced side effects, like constipation, without affecting centrally-mediated analgesia. Although no English-language reports of the use of alvimopan in children with opioid-induced constipation have been published in PubMed-indexed journals as of this writing (January 2013), two case reports of the use of methylnaltrexone in children with opioid-induced constipation have been published (Kissling et al., 2012; Lee and Mooney, 2012) In each of these reports, 0.15 mg/kg was used. It is worth noting that, in a 2008 Cochrane review conducted on the use of mu-opioid antagonists for opioid-induced bowel dysfunction, the authors concluded that the evidence at the time supported neither a class effect of the opioid antagonists, nor was there evidence of superiority of one drug over another (McNicol et al., 2008). Similarly, they found that neither safety nor efficacy of naloxone or nalbuphine was supported for use in patients with postoperative ileus or opioid-induced constipation.

Hyperalgesia

Hyperalgesia refers to an increased response to a painful stimulus at either a normal or increased threshold (IASP 2011). In contrast, the term opioid-induced hyperalgesia (OIH) is broadly defined as patients becoming more sensitive to pain due specifically to the use of opioids (Compton et al., 2001; Mao, 2008; McNicol, 2007; Werner, 2012). There are significant gaps in understanding the mechanisms underlying OIH, as well as the clinical relevance of this phenomenon (Chapman et al., 2010; Werner, 2012).

The pathophysiology of OIH is incompletely understood, and it remains important to emphasize that decreased analgesia from opioids may reflect hyperalgesia, tolerance, worsening disease, or a combination of these phenomena which remains a puzzle that has not yet been solved (Ballantyne and Shin, 2008).

Having said that, the science underlying increases in pain sensitivity is growing rapidly. Specifically, hyperalgesia appears to occur in a wide variety of clinical settings and patient populations, including persons on maintenance opioid use and in withdrawal of opioid, as well as persons receiving methadone for opioid maintenance and surgical patients (Angst and Clark, 2006). There also appears to be variation in the type of increased painful response to different stimulation. For example, in persons being maintained on methadone, hyperalgesia was found to occur to cold, but to a lesser degree for electrical stimuli and not to mechanical pain. In persons who underwent surgery, the development of hyperalgesia appeared to be associated with receiving higher opioid doses, although this finding has not been consistent, nor is it necessarily easy to separate hyperalgesia from tolerance.

Remifentanil, a potent opioid that is used primarily in surgical settings, is known to produce a post-infusion hyperalgesia. In a recent study of ten patients, persons who received remifentanil and propranolol did not experience mechanical hyperalgesia, while individuals who received remifentanil and placebo did have hyperalgesia (Chu et al., 2012a). Although the sample size for this study was very small, these authors concluded that propranolol may be useful to prevent hyperalgesia in persons treated with opioids.

In a separate publication, in a study of adults with chronic non-radicular low back pain who used sustained-release morphine, these authors have also demonstrated that tolerance can occur independently from OIH (Chu et al., 2012b).

Another recent study provides some insight into the molecular link between increased pain and opioids. In the *OPRM1* gene (which codes for the mu opioid receptor) higher levels of DNA methylation was associated with chronic opioid use in former opioid addicts being treated with methadone as replacement compared with matched healthy controls, (Doehring et al., 2013; Stone and Szyf, 2013). Although this change was not associated with coding for the mu opioid receptor, it was associated with increased chronic pain.

Risk factors for development of OIH are not yet well understood. In the 2010 research guideline on future research pertaining to the use of opioids for chronic non-cancer pain, the authors note that several critical topics have yet to be addressed, including the epidemiology of OIH, the likelihood of developing OIH as a function of clinical and demographic characteristics, the interaction between hyperalgesia and acute pain, and, notably, dose and duration of therapy. While facets of a patient's clinical presentation such as dose, duration of therapy, and quantitative sensory testing may be helpful to identify patients at increased risk for altered pain sensitivity, these factors are neither sensitive nor specific.

Treatment regimens for suspected OIH generally include options such as dose increase (to rule out tolerance), dose decrease, adding (or changing to) drugs that are antagonists at the N-methyl D-aspartate receptor (ketamine and methadone, respectively), clonidine, and dexmedetomidine. Buprenorphine may be useful, and multimodal analgesia also has potential, as a function of the opioid-sparing effect of these regimens. There are not many studies of treatment for hyperalgesia in children, thus dosing information is similarly limited.

In one case report of suspected OIH in a medically complex infant with gastroschisis, morphine and fentanyl were used for postoperative pain initially. In the face of increasing pain and irritability, a variety of pharmacological approaches were tried with success after 46 days, including addition of IV clonidine at 0.33–0.45 mcg/kg/h, switching the opioid to hydromorphone, introduction of IV ketamine at 0.1 mg/kg/h, and IV dexmedetomidine at 0.7 mcg/kg/h in place of clonidine (Hallett and Chalkiadis, 2012). Use of dexmedetomidine (dose range 0.2–0.7 mcg/kg/h) in a case series of 11 patients, including a 9-year-old male and two adolescents, has also been reported (Belgrade and Hall, 2010). More than half of the individuals reported in this series experienced substantial decreases in their opioid requirements after use of dexmedetomidine, none had clinically significant withdrawal symptoms, and pain intensity was stable or decreased for most patients.

Efforts to improve safe access to opioids

There is ample evidence in the biomedical literature documenting the need for improved care for people with pain. At the same time, there is significant concern about the potential for opioids to be misused, abused, or diverted, resulting in adverse events and deaths. In 2011, the US Centers for Disease Control and Prevention estimated that the rate of deaths related to prescription analgesic overdose had increased by more than threefold since 1990, that the number of these events was greater than that of motor vehicle deaths and larger than deaths attributed to cocaine and heroin overdoses. (Alexander et al., 2012; Centers for Disease Control and Prevention, 2011). While these data do not tell us important information such as where the drugs were obtained, whether the overdose was intentional or accidental, and if the event was due to use of one drug or multiple medications, it is clear that there is a serious problem. As a result, there are a variety of efforts underway to better educate healthcare providers, and to monitor use of controlled medications.

Prescription monitoring programmes (PMP)

As of October, 2012, 41 US states have an operational PMP in place and an additional ten (including the District of Columbia and Guam) have enacted legislation, but the programme has not yet begun operating (Alliance of States with Prescription Monitoring Programs, 2012). These programmes generally collect information about the patient, the drug and amount being prescribed, the date the prescription was written and the date it was filled, and the pharmacy that filled the prescription. States differ in terms of what data are collected, what time lag between filling the prescription and submitting the information is allowed, and who is responsible for maintaining the dataset (In Texas, it is the Department of Public Safety, in other states, the Board of Pharmacy or other groups are responsible.) Yet, despite the prevalence of PMPs, it remains unclear how to best use this information to achieve optimally safe and effective pain management. Here are a few challenges and opportunities that remain for healthcare providers and health policy decision-makers before the promise of these data can be fully realized.

Much of the PMP-related literature and discussions focus on drug abuse, often using prescriber- or pharmacy-shopping as markers of inappropriate use of controlled substances. Yet, we don't know the right number of prescribers or pharmacies, the right time period to consider, or whether there is even a right number. For example, in a literature search of 'prescription monitoring program' AND 'opioid', time intervals used to define either doctor- or pharmacy shopping included zero (concurrent use of opioids or controlled substances from different prescribers; Ives et al., 2006), 6 months (Pradel et al., 2009), 30 days (prescription for the same medication from at least two practitioners filled by at least two pharmacies; Gilson et al., 2012; Wilsey et al., 2010), and 1 year (Baehren et al., 2010; Hall et al., 2008; Wilsey et al., 2011), although one consensus statement published in 2004 defined use of multiple prescribers as at least six prescribers over a 1-year period (Parente et al., 2004). In a recent analysis, Wilsey and colleagues used California PMP data to assess differences between people who used only one prescriber compared to individuals who used two to five prescribers over a 1-year period (Wilsey et al., 2010). These investigators found that people who used two to five prescribers were not different in terms of male sex, younger age, or location in larger geographic areas—factors thought to be associated with drug abuse.

To make things more complex, the allure of considering data in isolation is powerful, even though looking at a broader picture often provides insight that a simple view cannot. As H. L. Mencken (1917) said, 'There is always an easy solution to every human problem—neat, plausible, and wrong'. One example of this idea is that the period of time in which the prescriptions were filled may help explain the observed numbers of prescribers and pharmacies. The longer that period, the more likely it is that multiple explanations for a patient's behaviour are important in understanding their medication use.

Along these lines, it is worth looking beyond the absolute number of prescribers and pharmacies from multiple prescribers or pharmacies to ask why people might get prescriptions, aside from potential abuse, misuse, or diversion. A single medical practice may include several people writing prescriptions, individuals may see other prescribers when their usual caregiver is not available, and people who are medically complex may have good reasons for obtaining controlled substances from multiple prescribers. Similarly, there may be important differences between groups of people who use prescription opioids non-medically, but for pain only as opposed to persons who obtain these drugs for nonmedical and non-pain use (Zacny and Lichtor, 2008). The count of pharmacies is also suspect. People may choose to go to different pharmacies for any number of reasons, and this is not necessarily a problem. It is common for pharmacies to offer financial incentives to people who transfer prescriptions, convenience of location is often important, and pharmacies don't always carry (or can't get) the specific medication the patient is looking for in the needed timeframe. Despite the potential to limit legitimate access to pain management services, in November 2011, the pharmacy chain CVS/Caremark (2011) announced a new policy to refuse to fill prescriptions for Schedule II controlled medications from some prescribers in Florida. Pharmacies' decisions to not carry certain medications or blanket refusals to fill prescriptions are likely to result in unnecessary suffering among the vast majority of pain patients who use their medications appropriately and to increase the barriers to needed health care these people must face.

Data quality is another issue that needs close attention (Strassels, 2012). The information that comes out of PMPs is only as good as the data that are put in. These data are generally input at busy pharmacies, patient names and birthdates may be the same, and prescribers often have multiple offices. Data may also be missing, misspelled, or otherwise incorrect. Furthermore, as a result, interpretation of these data may be challenging, and prescribers and pharmacists must not jump to conclusions and inadvertently contribute to difficulties in access to appropriate pain management services.

Assessment and identification of prescription drug abuse or misuse in paediatric populations presents challenges in addition to those that apply to adults. For example, while many discussions of PMPs and prescription drug abuse, misuse, and diversion focus on opioids, we must recognize that these drugs and prescribing rates do not tell the whole story. Individuals being treated for chronic pain are often on multiple psychoactive medications, such as muscle relaxants, benzodiazepines, and antidepressants, and that these combinations may have their own problems. For example, in a 2006 editorial on whether being on chronic opioid therapy should be a contraindication to driving, Zacny (2006) counsels caution, since we don't know to what extent different combinations of drugs result in what outcomes.

Although much of the discussion surrounding PMPs emphasizes their use as tools for drug enforcement, they can also be used to better understand patient outcomes, including estimating the present and future needs for pain management services based on incidence and prevalence trajectories, and use of geospatial tools to better understand access issues. PMP data are also useful to better understand and improve the safety of opioid use, whether these drugs are used alone or in combination with other analgesics. Last, it may be possible to link these data to other population-level resources to better understand the results and consequences of using pain management resources, including unintended consequences of public policy.

PMPs and other data collection efforts are used elsewhere as well. While systems that are used to collect information about prescribed drugs are common in many countries, allowing surveillance of opioid prescribing and dispensing, the literature on this topic published in the last 5 years pertains primarily to Australia, Canada, and France.

In one examples of PMP use in New South Wales, Australia, with other large datasets to establish drug source and reason for use, the mortality associated with overdoses of methadone or buprenorphine was estimated (Bell et al., 2009). In this analysis, investigators found that approximately five times as many people were treated with methadone than with buprenorphine for opioid dependence. Of the individuals who died, 60 were on methadone and seven were using buprenorphine. Half of the methadone patients and none of the buprenorphine patients who died were in treatment. The authors concluded that the risk of overdose death was lower in buprenorphine patients than in methadone patients, although the confidence interval for the relative rate was wide (relative risk 4.25, 95% confidence interval 1.03–17.54). The authors also noted that use of more than one drug was common among the persons treated with methadone, particularly of heroin, benzodiazepine, and antidepressants.

Among the analyses exploring opioid use in Canada, one study found that interprovincial disparities in the numbers and types of opioids prescribed were common during 2005 to 2010 (Fischer et al., 2011). The authors also found that increases in the use of strong opioids was an important driver of this result, although this paper focused on the drug dispensing and not specific outcomes as a result of dispensing.

Building on these results, an analysis was carried out to estimate the relation between use of prescription opioids and mortality in British Columbia and Ontario from 2005 to 2009 (Fischer et al., 2013). These authors found strong correlations between the use of fentanyl, hydromorphone, morphine, and oxycodone and drug-related mortality, although they also noted that non-retail dispensing was not included here, nor were they able to assess concomitant use of drugs that may have contributed to death, such as non-opioid medications or alcohol.

In France, analyses were conducted to estimate the diversion of opioids relative to benzodiazepines and to quantify the effect of a PMP on doctor-shopping for high-dose buprenorphine therapy from 2000 to 2004. In the first paper, the authors found that, although benzodiazepines were dispensed more frequently than opioids, abuse, and diversion were observed mainly in association with opioid maintenance therapy, morphine, and benzodiazepines, and less so to non-morphine opioids (Pauly et al., 2012). In the second analyses, the authors estimated that, from 2004 to 2005, the prescription drug database contributed to a decrease in doctor-shopping, without adversely affecting the number of patients treated or the total prescribed doses (Pradel et al., 2009).

Case example

Jackson is a 13-year-old, 50 kg boy with sickle cell disease. He usually manages his pain at home with oxycodone 5 mg as needed. He has not been hospitalized in 2 years. Over the last 2 days Jackson has had persistent pain in his abdomen and legs which has not improved despite taking oxycodone every 3 to 4 h. His mother brings him to the emergency department.

At triage in the emergency department Jackson reports his pain score as 10 out of 10 on a visual analogue scale. He is given fentanyl 50 mcg intranasally and brought immediately back to a patient care room.

He is then evaluated by the physician and 30 min after the fentanyl his pain score is a 9. An IV line is started and he is given 5 mg of morphine IV as well as 30 mg of ketorolac and IV fluids. His pain score remains a 9 and 40 min later he is given another 5 mg dose of morphine. This does not result in improvement and he is transferred to the inpatient unit.

On the inpatient floor he reports a pain score of 9. He also complains of itching and requests that he be switched to hydromorphone as that did not cause him as much itching during his last hospitalization.

He is placed on a hydromorphone via patient-controlled analgesia with a 0.2 mg per hour continuous infusion and a 0.1 mg bolus every 6 min as needed. He is also placed on IV fluids and senna. He is encouraged to use an incentive spirometer.

Over the next 24 h Jackson continues to have severe pain. His continuous infusion is increased to 0.3 mg per hour.

By day 3 of hospitalization he reports his pain is now a 5. On this day his continuous infusion is stopped and he is placed on extended release oxycodone (10 mg every 12 h). He remains on a bolus only PCA for 24 more hours and then this is discontinued. He is sent home on the extended release oxycodone as well as 5 mg of immediate-release oxycodone to be used as needed. He is told to remain on the senna as long as he is taking the oxycodone. A follow-up appointment is made for 5 days after discharge.

References

Abu-Shahwan, I. (2008). Ketamine does not reduce postoperative morphine consumption after tonsillectomy in children. *Clin J Pain*, 24(5), 395–398.

Alexander, G. C., Kruszewski, S. P., and Webster, D. W. (2012). Rethinking opioid prescribing to protect patient safety and public health. *JAMA*, 308(18), 1865–1866.

Allegaert, K., Veyckemans, F., and Tibboel, D. (2009). Clinical practice: analgesia in neonates. *Eur J Pediatr*, 168, 765–770.

Alliance of States with Prescription Monitoring Programs. (2012). *Status of prescription drug monitoring programs (PDMPs)*. Available at: <http://www.pmpalliance.org/> (accessed 19 November 2012).

American Psychiatric Association. (2000). Opioid use disorders. Opioid dependence. In *Diagnostic and statistical manual of mental disorders, fourth edition, text revision*, p. 270. Washington, DC: American Psychiatric Association.

American Society of Anesthesiologists Task Force on Acute Pain Management. (2012). Practice guidelines for acute pain management in the perioperative setting. *Anesthesiology*, 116, 248–273.

Angst, M. S., and Clark, J. D. (2006). Opioid-induced hyperalgesia. A qualitative systematic review. *Anesthesiology*, 104, 570–587.

Association of Paediatric Anaesthetists of Great Britain and Ireland. (2012). Good practice in postoperative and procedural pain management (2nd edn). *Pediatr Anesth*, 22(Supplement 1), 1–79.

Baehren, D. F., Marco, C. A., Droz, D. E., Sinha, S., Callan, E. M., and Akpunonu, P (2010). A statewide prescription monitoring program affects emergency department prescribing behaviors. *Ann Emerg Med*, 56, 19–23.

Ballantyne, J. C., and Shin, N. S. (2008). Efficacy of opioids for chronic pain: a review of the evidence. *Clin J Pain*, 24(6), 469–478.

Benet, L. Z. (1984). Pharmacokinetics: basic principles and its use as a tool in drug metabolism. In J. R. Mitchell, and M. G. Horning (eds) *Drug metabolism and drug toxicity*, pp. 199–211. New York: Raven Press.

Belgrade, M. and Hall, S. (2010). Dexmedetomidine infusion for the management of opioid-induced hyperalgesia. *Pain Med*, 11, 1819–1826.

Bell, J. R., Butler, B., Lawrance, A., Batey, R., and Salmelainen, P. (2009). Comparing overdose mortality associated with methadone and buprenorphine treatment. *Drug Alcohol Depend*, 104(1–2), 73–77.

Berde, C. B., Walco, G. A., Krane, E. J., Anand, K. J., Aranda, J. V., Craig, K. D., *et al.* (2012). Pediatric analgesic clinical trial designs, measures, and extrapolation: report of an FDA scientific workshop. *Pediatrics*, 129(2), 354–364.

Borland, M., Milson, S., and Esson, A. (2011). Equivalency of two concentrations of fentanyl administered by the intranasal route for acute analgesia in children in a paediatric emergency department: a randomized controlled trial. *Emerg Med Australas*, 23(2), 202–208.

Birmingham, P. K., Tobin, M. J., Henthorn, T. K., Fisher, D. M., Berkelhammer, M. C., Smith, F. A., *et al.* (1997). Twenty-four-hour pharmacokinetics of rectal acetaminophen in children. An old drug with new recommendations. *Anesthesiology*, 87, 244–252.

Briggs, G. C., Freeman, R. K., and Yaffe, S. J (2008). *Drugs in pregnancy and lactation: a reference guide to fetal and neonatal risk* (8th edn). Philadelphia, PA: Lippincott Williams & Wilkins.

Centers for Disease Control and Prevention. (2011). *Policy impact: prescription painkiller overdoses*. Available at: <http://www.cdc.gov/homeandrecreationalsafety/rxbrief/> (accessed 16 January 2013).

Chapman, C. R., Lipschitz, D. L., Angst, M. S., Chou, R., Denisco, R. C., Donaldson, G. W., *et al.* (2010). Opioid pharmacotherapy for chronic non-cancer pain in the United States: a research guideline for developing an evidence-base. *J Pain*, 11(9), 807–829.

Chorney, J. M., McGrath, P., and Finley, G. A. (2010). Pain as the neglected adverse event. *CMAJ*, 182(7), 732.

Chou, R., Fanciullo, G. J., Fine, P. G., Adler, J. A., Ballantyne, J. C., Davies, P., *et al.* (2009a). Clinical guidelines for the use of chronic opioid therapy in chronic noncancer pain. *J Pain*, 10(2), 113–130.

Chou, R., Ballantyne, J. C., Fanciullo, G. J., Fine, P. G., and Miaskowski, C. (2009b). Research gaps on use of opioids for chronic noncancer pain: findings from a review of the evidence for an American Pain Society and American Academy of Pain Medicine clinical practice guideline. *J Pain*, 10(2), 147–159.

Chu, L. F., Cun, T., Ngai, L. K., Kim, J. E., Zamora, A. K., Young, C. A., *et al.* (2012a). Modulation of remifentanil-induced postinfusion hyperalgesia by the β-blocker propranolol in humans. *Pain*, 153(5), 974–981.

Chu, L. F., D'Arcy, N., Brady, C., Zamora, A. K., Young, C. A., Kim, J. E., *et al.* (2012b). Analgesic tolerance without demonstrable opioid-induced hyperalgesia: a double-blinded, randomized, placebo-controlled trial of sustained-release morphine for treatment of chronic nonradicular low-back pain. *Pain*, 153(8), 1583–1592.

Ciszkowski, C., Madadi, P., Phillips, M. S., Lauwers, A. E., and Koren, G. (2009). Codeine, ultrarapid-metabolism genotype, and postoperative death. *N Engl J Med*, 361(8), 827–827.

Compton, P., Charuvastra, V. C., and Ling, W. (2001). Pain intolerance in opioid-maintained former opiate addicts: effect of long-acting maintenance agent. *Drug Alcohol Depend*, 63, 139–146.

CVS/Caremark. (2011). *Letter to Florida prescribers*. Available at: <http://www.cfnews13.com/article/news/2011/december/351997/CVS-to-Florida-doctors:-No-more-oxycodone-prescriptions> (accessed 12 December 2011).

Davis, M. (2007). Cholestasis and endogenous opioids: liver disease and exogenous opioid pharmacokinetics. *Clin Pharmacokinet*, 46, 825–850.

Doehring, A., Oertel, B. G., Sittl, R., and Lotsch, J. (2013). Chronic opioid use is associated with increased DMA methylation correlating with increased clinical pain. *Pain*, 154(1), 15–23.

Eap, C. B., Buclin, T., and Baumann, P. (2002). Interindividual variability of the clinical pharmacokinetics of methadone. Implications for the treatment of opioid dependence. *Clin Pharmacokinet*, 41(14), 1153–1193.

Ellis, J., Martelli, B., Lamontagne, C., Pasquet, E., Taillefer, L., Gaboury, I., et al. (2011). Improved practices for safe administration of intravenous bolus morphine in a pediatric setting. *Pain Manag Nurs*, 12(3), 146–153.

Finn, M. and Harris, D. (2010). Intranasal fentanyl for analgesia in the paediatric emergency department. *Emerg Med J*, 27(4), 300–301.

Fischer, B., Jones, W., and Rehm, J. (2013). High correlations between levels of consumption and mortality related to strong prescription opioid analgesics in British Columbia and Ontario, 2005–2009. *Pharmacoepidemiol Drug Saf*, 22(4), 438–442.

Fischer, B., Jones, W., Krahn, M., and Rehm, J. (2011). Differences and over-time changes in levels of prescription opioid analgesic dispensing from retail pharmacies in Canada, 2005–2010. *Pharmacoepidemiol Drug Saf*, 20(12), 1269–1277.

Friedrichsdorf, S. J., and Kang, T. I. (2007). The management of pain in children with life-limiting illnesses. *Pediatr Clin North Am*, 54(5), 645–672.

Fortinguerra, F., Maschi, S., Clavenna, A., and Bonati, M. (2010). Pain management in the paediatric population: the regulatory situation in Europe. *Arch Dis Child*, 95(9), 749–753.

Friday, J. H., Kanegaye, J. T., McCaslin, I., Zheng, A., and Harley, J. R. (2009). Ibuprofen provides analgesia equivalent to acetaminophen-codeine in the treatment of acute pain in children with extremity injuries: a randomized clinical trial. *Acad Emerg Med*, 16, 711–716.

Friis-Hansen, B. (1971). Body composition during growth: in vivo measurements and biochemical data correlated to differential anatomical growth. *Pediatrics*, 47, 264–274.

Friis-Hansen, B. (1983). Water distribution in the fetus and newborn infant. *Acta Pediatr Scand*, 305(Suppl 1), 7–11.

Geeta, M. G., Geetha, P., Ajithkumar, V. T., Krishnakumar, P., Kumar, K. S., and Mathews, L. (2010). Management of pain in leukemic children using the WHO analgesic ladder. *Ind J Pediatr*, 77(6), 665–8.

Gharavi, B., Schott, C., Nelle, M., Reiter, G., and Linderkamp, O. (2007). Pain management and the effect of guidelines in neonatal units in Austria, Germany, and Switzerland. *Pediatr Int*, 49(5), 652–658.

Gilson, A. M., Fishman, S. M., Wilsey, B. L., Casamalhuapa, C., and Baxi, H. (2012). Time series analysis of California's prescription monitoring program: impact on prescribing and multiple provider episodes. *J Pain*, 13(2), 103–111.

Goldman, R. D., Narula, N., Klein-Kremer, A., Finkelstein, Y., and Rogovik, A. L. (2008). Predictors for opioid analgesia administration in children with abdominal pain presenting to the emergency department. *Clin J Pain*, 24(1), 11–15.

Gordon, D. B., Dahl, J. L., Miaskowski, C., McCarberg, B., Todd, K. H., Paice, J. A., et al. (2005). American pain society recommendations for improving the quality of acute and cancer pain management: American Pain Society Quality of Care Task Force. *Arch Intern Med*,165(14), 1574–15780.

Hadley, G., Maconochie, I., and Jackson, A. (2010). A survey of intranasal medication use in the paediatric emergency setting in England and Wales. *Emerg Med J*, 27(7), 553–554.

Hall, A. J., Logan, J. E., Toblin, R. L., Kaplan, J. A., Kraner, J. C., Bixler, D., et al. (2008). Patterns of abuse among unintentional pharmaceutical overdose fatalities. *JAMA*, 300, 2613–2620.

Hallett, B. R., and Chalkiadis, G. A. (2012). Suspected opioid-induced hyperalgesia in an infant. *Br J Anaesth*, 108(1), 116–118.

Hardy, J., Daly, S., McQuade, B., Albertsson, M., Chimontsi-Kypriou, V., Stathopoulos, G. P., et al. (2002). A double-blind, randomised, parallel group, multinational, multicentre study comparing a single dose of ondansetron 24 mg p.o. with placebo and metoclopramide 10 mg t.d.s. p.o. in the treatment of opioid-induced nausea and emesis in cancer patients. *Support Care Cancer*, 10(3), 231–236.

Hewitt, M., Goldman, A., Collins, G. S., Childs, M., and Hain, R. (2008). Opioid use in palliative care of children and young people with cancer. *J Pediatr*, 152(1), 39–44.

Hippard, H. K., Govindan, K., Friedman, E. M., Sulek, M., Giannoni, C., Larrier, D., et al. (2012). Postoperative analgesic and behavioral effects of intranasal fentanyl, intravenous morphine, and intramuscular morphine in pediatric patients undergoing bilateral myringotomy and placement of ventilating tubes. *Anesth Analg*, 115(2), 356–363.

International Association for the Study of Pain (IASP). (2011). *IASP taxonomy*. Available at: <http://www.iasp-pain.org/Content/NavigationMenu/GeneralResourceLinks/PainDefinitions/default.htm#Hyperalgesia> (accessed 11 January 2013).

International Narcotics Control Board. (2013). Available at: <http://www.incb.org> (accessed 18 January 2013).

Ives, T. J., Chelminski, P. R., Hammett-Stabler, C. A., Malone, R. M., Perhac, J. S., Potisek, N. M., et al. (2006). Predictors of opioid misuse in patients with chronic pain: a prospective cohort study. *BMC Heath Serv Res*, 6(46). doi: 10.1186/1472-6963-6-46.

Kelly, L. E., Rieder, M., van den Anker, J., Malkin, B., Ross, C., Neely, M. N., et al. (2012). More codeine fatalities after tonsillectomy in North American children. *Pediatrics*, 129(5), e1343-1347.

Kissling, K. T., Mohassel, L. R., and Heintz, J. (2012). Methylnaltrexone for opioid-induced constipation in a pediatric oncology patient. *J Pain Symptom Manage*, 44(1), e1–e3.

Kimura, Y. and Walco, G. A. (2007). Treatment of chronic pain in pediatric rheumatic disease. *Nat Clin Pract Rheumatol*, 3, 210–218.

Koren, G., Cairns, J., Chitayat, D., Gaedigk, A., and Leeder, S. J. (2006). Pharmacogenetics of morphine poisoning in a breastfed neonate of a codeine-prescribed mother. *Lancet*, 368(9536), 704.

Lee, J. M., and Mooney, J. (2012). Methylnaltrexone in treatment of opioid-induced constipation in a pediatric patient. *Clin J Pain*, 28, 338–341.

Leeder, J. S., and Kearns, G. L. (1997). Pharmacogenetics in practice: implications for practice. *Pediatr Clin North Am*, 44, 55–77.

Leow, K. P., Smith, M. T., Watt, J. A., Williams, B. E., and Cramond, T. (1992). Comparative oxycodone pharmacokinetics in humans after intravenous, oral, and rectal administration. *Ther Drug Monitor*, 14(6), 479–484.

Lexicomp. (2013a). *Hydrocodone*. Available at: <http://online.lexi.com/lco/action/doc/retrieve/docid/pdh_f/129885> (accessed 18 January 2013).

Lexicomp. (2013b). *Hydromorphone*. Available at: <http://online.lexi.com/lco/action/doc/retrieve/docid/pdh_f/129887> (accessed 18 January 2013).

Lexicomp. (2013c). *Meperidine*. Available at: <http://online.lexi.com/lco/action/doc/retrieve/docid/pdh_f/129907> (accessed 18 January 2013).

Lexicomp. (2013d). *Methadone*. Available at: <http://online.lexi.com/lco/action/doc/retrieve/docid/pdh_f/129909> (accessed 18 January 2013).

Lexicomp. (2013e). *Morphine*. Available at: <http://online.lexi.com/lco/action/doc/retrieve/docid/pdh_f/2853079> (accessed 18 January 2013).

Lexicomp. (2013f). *Paregoric*. Available at: <http://online.lexi.com/lco/action/doc/retrieve/docid/pdh_f/129941> (accessed 18 January 2013).

Lundeberg, S. and Roelofse, J. A. (2011). Aspects of pharmacokinetics and pharmacodynamics of sufentanil in pediatric practice. *Pediatr Anesth*, 21, 274–279.

Macario, A., Weinger, M., Carney, S., and Kim, A. (1999a). Which clinical anesthesia outcomes are important to avoid. The perspective of patients. *Anesth Analg*, 89(3), 652–658.

Macario, A., Weinger, M., Truong, P., and Lee, M. (1999b). Which clinical anesthesia outcomes are both common and important to avoid? The perspective of a panel of expert anesthesiologists. *Anesth Analg*, 88(5), 1085–1091.

Mak, W. Y., Tuen, V., Irwin, M., and Hui, T. (2011). Pharmacotherapy for acute pain in children: current practice and recent advances. *Expert Opin Pharmacother*, 12(6), 865–881.

Mao J (2008). Opioid-induced hyperalgesia. *Pain: Clinical Updates*, XVI(2).

Maples, H. D., James, L. P., and Stowe, C. D. (2006). Special pharmacokinetic and pharmacodynamic considerations in children. In M. E. Burton, L. M. Shaw, J. J. Schentag, and W. E. Evans (eds) *Applied pharmacokinetics*

& *pharmacodynamics. Principles of therapeutic drug monitoring*, pp. 213–230. Philadelphia, PA: Lippincott Williams & Wilkins.

May, D. G. (1994). Genetic differences in drug disposition. *J Clin Pharmacol*, 34, 881–897.

McNicol, E. (2007). Opioid side effects. *Pain: Clin Update*, XV(2).

McNicol, E. D., Boyce, D., Schumann, R., and Carr, D. B. (2008). Mu-opioid antagonists for opioid-induced bowel dysfunction. *Cochrane Database Syst Rev*, 2, CD006332.

Meldrum, M. L. (2003). Preface. In M. L. Meldrum, (ed.) *Opioids and pain relief: a historical perspective*, pp. ix–x. Seattle, WA: IASP Press.

Mencken, H. L. (1917, 16 November). The divine afflatus. *New York Evening Mail*.

Miller, J. L., and Hagemann, T. M. (2011). Use of pure opioid antagonists for management of opioid-induced pruritus. *Am J Health Syst Pharm*, 68, 1419–1425.

Moulin, D. E., Clark, A. J., Gilron, I., Ware, M. A., Watson, C. P. N., Sessle, B. J., *et al.* (2007). Pharmacologic management of chronic neuropathic pain—consensus statement and guidelines from the Canadian Pain Society. *Pain Res Manag*, 12(1), 13–21.

Nahata, M. C., and Taketomo, C. (2011). Pediatrics. In J. T. DiPiro, R. L. Talbert, G. C. Yee, G. R. Matzke, B. G. Wells, L. M. Posey (eds) *Pharmacotherapy: a pathophysiologic approach* (8th edn), pp. 47–56. New York: McGraw Hill. Available at: <http://www.accesspharmacy.com/content.aspx?aid=7967211> (accessed 19 November 2012).

Nolke, A. C. (1956). Severe toxic effects from aminophylline and theophylline suppositories in children. *JAMA*, 161, 693–697.

Janssen Pharmaceuticals. (2012). Nucynta prescribing information. Available at: <http://www.nucynta.com/> (accessed 17 January 2013).

National Comprehensive Cancer Network. (2007). *Pediatric cancer pain*. Fort Washington, PA: National Comprehensive Cancer Network.

Nelson, K. L., Yaster, M., Kost-Byerly, S., and Monitto, C. L. (2010). A national survey of American Pediatric Anesthesiologists: patient-controlled analgesia and other intravenous opioid therapies in pediatric acute pain management. *Anesth Analg*, 110(3), 754–760.

Ou, C. H., Kent, S. K., Hammond, A. M., Bowen-Roberts, T., Steinbok, P., and Warren, D. T. (2008). Morphine infusions after pediatric cranial surgery: a retrospective analysis of safety and efficacy. *Can J Neurosci Nurs*, 30(3), 21–30.

Parab, P. V., Ritschel, W. A., Coyle, D. E., Gregg, R. V., and Denson, D. D. (1988). Pharmacokinetics of hydromorphone after intravenous, peroral and rectal administration to human subjects. *Biopharm Drug Dispos*, 9(2), 187–199.

Parente, S. T., Kim, S. S., Finch, M. D., Schloff, L. A., Rector, T. S., Seifeldin, R., *et al.* (2004). Identifying controlled substance patterns of utilization requiring evaluation using administrative claims data. *Am J Manag Care*, 10, 783–790.

Pauly, V., Pradel, V., Pource, L., Nordmann, S., Frauger, E., Lapeyre-Mestre, M., *et al.* (2012). Estimated magnitude of diversion and abuse of opioids relative to benzodiazepines in France. *Drug Alcohol Depend*, 126(1–2), 13–20.

Pletcher, M. J., Kertesz, S. G., Kohn, M. A., and Gonzales, R. (2008). Trends in opioid prescribing by race/ethnicity for patients seeking care in US emergency departments. *JAMA*, 299(1), 70–78.

Pradel, V., Frauger, E., Thirion, X., Ronfle, E., Lapierre, V., Masut, A., *et al.* (2009). Impact of a prescription monitoring program on doctor-shopping for high dosage buprenorphine. *Pharmacoepidemiol Drug Saf*, 18, 36–43.

Ruggiero, A., Coccia, P., Arena, R., Maurizi, P., Battista, A., Ridola, V., *et al.* (2013). Efficacy and safety of transdermal buprenorphine in the management of children with cancer-related pain. *Pediatr Blood Cancer*, 60(3), 433–437.

Sadhasivam, S. and Chidambaran, V. (2012). Pharmacogenomics of opioids and perioperative pain management. *Pharmacogenomics*, 13(15), 1719–1740.

Savage, S. R., Joranson, D. E., Covington, E. C., Schnoll, S. H., Heit, H. A., and Gilson, A. M. (2003). Definitions related to the medical use of opioids: evolution toward universal agreement. *J Pain Symptom Manage*, 26(1), 655–667.

Schiessl, C., Gravou, C., Zernikow, B., Sittl, R., and Griessinger, N. (2008). Use of patient-controlled analgesia for pain control in dying children. *Support Care Cancer*, 16(5), 531–536.

Schug, S. A., Zech, D., and Grond, S. (1992). Adverse effects of systemic opioid analgesics. *Drug Saf*, 7(3), 200–213.

Stone, L. S., and Szyf, M. (2013). The emerging field of pain epigenetics. *Pain*, 154(1), 1–2.

Strassels, S. A., Maxwell, T. L., and Iyer, S. (2010). Constipation in persons receiving hospice care. *J Pain Symptom Manage*, 40(6), 810–820.

Strassels, S. A. (2012). Prescription monitoring programs: pitfalls and opportunities. *J Pain Palliat Care Pharmacother*, 26, 48–50.

Sullivan, H. R., and Due, S. L. (1973). Urinary metabolites of dl-methadone in maintenance subjects. *J Med Chem*, 16, 909–913.

Sussman, G., Shurman, J., Creed, M. R., Larsen, L. S., Ferrer-Brechner, T., Noll, D., *et al.* (1999). Intravenous ondansetron for the control of opioid-induced nausea and vomiting. International S3AA3013 Study Group. *Clin Ther*, 21(7), 1216–1227.

Tateishi, T., Krivoruk, Y., Ueng, Y. F., Wood, A. J., Guengerich, F. P., and Wood, M. (1996). Identification of human liver cytochrome P-450 3A4 as the enzyme responsible for fentanyl and sufentanil N-dealkylation. *Anesth Analg*, 82, 167–172.

Tegeder, I., Lötsch, J., and Geisslinger, G. (1999). Pharmacokinetics of opioids in liver disease. *Clin Pharmacokinet*, 37, 17–40.

Telfer, P., Criddle, J., Sandell, J., Davies, F., Morrison, I., and Challands, J. (2009). Intranasal diamorphine for acute sickle cell pain. *Arch Dis Child*, 94(12), 979–980.

Ventafridda, V., Saita, L., Ripamonti, C., and De Conno, F. (1985). WHO guidelines for the use of analgesics in cancer pain. *Int J Tissue React*, 7(1), 93–96.

Vijenthira, A., Stinson, J., Friedman, J., Palozzi, L., Taddio, A., Scolnik, D., *et al.* (2012). Benchmarking pain outcomes for children with sickle cell disease hospitalized in a tertiary referral pediatric hospital. *Pain Res Manag*, 17(4), 291–296.

Vintage Pharmaceuticals, LLC. (2012). *Hydrocodone bitartrate and ibuprofen tablet, film coated* [Vintage Pharmaceuticals, LLC]. Available at: <http://nccs-dailymed-1.nlm.nih.gov/dailymed/archives/fdaDrugInfo.cfm?archiveid=3898> (accessed 13 November 2012).

Werner, M. U. (2012). Vanguard research in opioid-induced hyperalgesia—but guard the basics. *Pain*, 153, 943–944.

Weschules, D. J., and Bain, K. T. (2008). A systematic review of opioid conversion ratios used with methadone for the treatment of pain. *Pain Med*, 9(5), 595–612.

Whelan, E., Asbridge, M., and Haydt, S. (2011). Representations of OxyContin in North American newspapers and medical journals. *Pain Res Manag*, 16(4), 252–258.

Wilsey, B. L., Fishman, S. M., Gilson, A. M., Casamalhuapa, C., Baxi, H., Lin, T. C., *et al.* (2011). An analysis of the number of multiple prescribers for opioids utilizing data from the California Prescription Monitoring Program. *Pharmacoepidemiol Drug Saf*, 20, 1262–1268.

Wilsey, B. L., Fishman, S. M., Gilson, A. M., Casamalhuapa, C., Baxi, H., Zhang, H., *et al.* (2010). Profiling multiple provider prescribing of opioids, benzodiazepines, stimulants, and anorectics. *Drug Alcohol Depend*, 112, 99–106.

World Health Organization. (2011a). *Priority medicines for mothers and children*. Geneva: World Health Organization.

World Health Organization. (2011b). *Model list of essential medicines for children, 3rd list*. Geneva: World Health Organization.

World Health Organization. (2012). *Guidelines on the pharmacological treatment of persisting pain in children with medical illnesses*. Geneva: World Health Organization.

Yaksh, T. L., and Wallace, M. S. (2011). Opioids, analgesia, and pain management. In L. L. Brunton, D. K. Blumenthal, N. Murri, R. Hilal-Dandan, and B. C. Knollmann (eds) *Goodman & Gilman's the pharmacological basis of therapeutics* (12th edn), pp. 481–526. New York: McGraw-Hill. Available at: <http://www.accesspharmacy.com/content.aspx?aID=16664296> (accessed 19 November 2012).

Zacny, J. P. (2006). Chronic pain and driving: proceed with caution. *Pain*, 122, 6–7.

Zacny, J. P., and Lichtor, S. A. (2008). Nonmedical use of prescription opioids: motive and ubiquity issues. *J Pain*, 9, 473–486.

Zernikow, B., Michel, E., Craig, F., and Anderson, B. J. (2009). Pediatric palliative care: use of opioids for the management of pain. *Paediatr Drugs*, 11(2), 129–125

CHAPTER 46

Interventional pain management techniques for chronic pain

Navil F. Sethna, Pradeep Dinakar, and Karen R. Boretsky

Summary

As part of multidisciplinary management of paediatric chronic pain, interventional pain management techniques can play an important role when pain is unrelieved by conventional treatment modalities. Many procedures and indications are extrapolated from adult studies, and evidence for long-term efficacy in paediatric populations is limited. Interventions range from injection techniques with local anaesthetic and/or corticosteroids to neuraxial blockade with implanted catheters. Paediatric case series have reported benefit in selected patients with complex regional pain syndrome and cancer-related pain.

Introduction

Significant improvement in our understanding of paediatric pain neurobiology and its adverse effects has increased awareness for the need for early analgesic intervention to mitigate the acute and long-term consequences of pain. As part of multidisciplinary management of paediatric chronic pain, interventional pain management (IPM) techniques play an important role when pain is unrelieved by conventional treatment modalities. Although these techniques have long been the mainstay of adult chronic pain management, the lack of outcome data in paediatric populations has limited its utility. As with adults, paediatric chronic pain requires multidisciplinary management, combining psychosocial support and pharmacotherapy, and including IPM when required to provide the best possible options for managing pain and improving quality of life.

Several textbooks and manuals have been published describing detailed applied anatomy and approaches and techniques of IPM in adults (Peng and Tumber, 2008) but only a few case reports and case series are described in children. The experience with application of these blockades in paediatric population is very limited and citation of references in this chapter refers to adult literature unless specified for children. It is not the intention of this chapter to duplicate these technical details and readers are referred to adult standard textbooks for detailed technical information (Cousins et al., 2009; Fishman et al., 2010; Prithvi Raj, 2008). This chapter focuses on commonly useful procedures that are increasingly used in paediatric patients with chronic pain syndromes. Physicians who perform IPM techniques in children should be familiar with differences in developmental anatomy and pharmacology and trained and experienced in regional nerve blocks in adults and children. As a general principle all IPM procedures for chronic pain disorders must be performed as adjunct to multimodal therapies in the setting of interdisciplinary programme.

General patient considerations

Interventional pain management techniques are widely used in the paediatric population in acute postoperative pain, but also have a role in chronic paediatric pain management. Patients and families should be fully informed about the benefit and risks of the IPM procedure, how a particular procedure is conducted, potential rare but serious complications, and alternative options should be reviewed. The patients and guardians should be informed that IPM techniques have limitations, and responses may vary for different patients and different chronic pain conditions. The details of procedures, setting appropriate expectations, long-term benefits and risks must be explained in days or weeks before the scheduled procedure rather than on the day of the planned procedure. Depending on his/her age, the procedure should be discussed with the child, who is encouraged to express concerns and ask questions. The guardians must provide a written informed consent for the procedure and when appropriate (usually over age of 7 years) the child should provide assent, not only to protect the patient's right to autonomy but also to protect the physician from medical malpractice. The analgesic effect of a single intervention is typically temporary and may offer little to no long-term pain relief. These IPM techniques are often performed in a series to achieve longer duration of analgesia or discontinued if no benefit obtained. Younger children and anxious adolescents may require intravenous sedation or general anaesthesia, which will require additional preparation. The absolute contraindications for IPM technique are same as in adults including presence of infections at the site of the procedure, intake of anticoagulants, a history of coagulopathy, and hyperglycaemia.

Pharmacology of agents

The most common medications used in paediatric interventional pain management include local anaesthetics and corticosteroids.

Local anaesthetics

Local anaesthetics are reversible voltage-gated sodium channel blockers, and blockade of (Na^+) ion influx leads to inhibition of nociceptive impulse propagation. The success and safety of a nerve blockade depends on delivery of the optimal dose and volume of a local anaesthetic, preferably at the precise site of the suspected pain generator foci of a nerve or plexus. Adding 1 ml of sodium bicarbonate 8.4% to each 10 ml of a local anaesthetic (e.g. lidocaine or mepivacaine) or 0.1 ml to 10 ml of bupivacaine can hasten the onset of the nerve blockade and lessen the discomfort associated with the local anaesthetic injection. Amide local anaesthetics, such as lidocaine, bupivacaine, and ropivacaine have delayed hepatic clearance in infants less than 2 months and variable clearance between 3 and 6 months. Reduced plasma proteins (albumin and alpha-1 glycoproteins) in this age group increase the unbound and free local anaesthetic concentration that is potentially available to cause central nervous system (CNS) and cardiac toxicity. Similarly, ester local anaesthetics such as chloroprocaine are metabolized at a lower rate in infants under the age of 6 months due to decreased plasma cholinesterase activity (Mazoit and Dalens, 2004)

Steroids

Glucocorticoids are commonly used anti-inflammatory drugs and suppress inflammatory process through many routes despite its limited efficacy. It is most frequently used via lumbar and caudal epidural routes for targeting the radicular pain of L5, S1, and other nerve roots. They exert their action by blocking the synthesis of prostaglandins, leukotrienes, and platelet activating factor. Steroids also stabilize the neuronal membrane and so are used to reduce pain from neural irritability and diminish perineural inflammation and oedema. There is no supporting scientific evidence in children, but a maximum series of three nerve blocks are proposed, to achieve longer-term relief. There is no consensus on the type or optimal dose of steroids that should be used for various central and peripheral nerve blocks in adults and no data in children. The most common steroid preparations used include triamcinolone, methylprednisolone acetate, and dexamethasone. Even though the first two are particulate steroids with better efficacy, the potential risk of vascular injury and infarction makes their use undesirable. The main risks of repeat injections of steroids are systemic absorption and Cushing's syndrome, skin atrophy, and poor healing. The use of steroid for interventional chronic pain in children is not approved by Federal Drug Administration in US (Eckel and Bartynski, 2009).

Correct needle placement technique

Although many axial and peripheral nerve blockades have traditionally been performed without aids to correct placement a number of options may now be utilized to improve accuracy and safety of the procedures:

+ Nerve stimulation aims to stimulate the motor component of a mixed peripheral nerve to elicit painless muscle contraction. A current of usually between 0.4 and 0.5 mA is the threshold current at lowest twitch response. Higher current intensity should not be used to avoid stimulating the sensory component and causing painful paraesthesia. Responses at lower currents may indicate contact with the neural tissue and potential for inadvertent intraneural injection (Abrahams et al., 2009).

+ Fluoroscopic guidance (i.e. X-ray image intensifier or a C-arm X-ray system with injection of radiopaque contrast to confirm needle tip position) for epidural steroid injections and other IPM techniques enhances accuracy of locating the target tissue and reduces the potential injury to the surrounding structures. Safe and efficient use of these modalities requires formal training, skills and experience, with attention to minimizing radiation exposure to patients' vital organs and clinicians (Eckel and Bartynski, 2009; Hodge, 2005).

+ Ultrasound imaging allows visualization of soft tissue, bony, vascular, and neural structures, and can differentiate various tissue planes and spaces (e.g. epidural, intrathecal, pleural and peritoneal). The operator can confirm desirable spread of the injectate in real time. Ultrasound imaging avoids radiation and is virtually without side effects (Peng and Narouze, 2009).

Interventional pain management for CRPS

Sympathetic ganglion blockade

Sympathetic ganglia blockade with local anaesthetics may be used as a diagnostic test, and a positive response is interpreted as sympathetically mediated pain (SMP), however, this view is not shared by all researchers and is not supported by rigorous investigation. Although favourable responses to sympathetic blockade has been used to predict pain relief from implanted spinal cord stimulators in adult patients with CRPS, the evidence is weak (Bogduk, 2002; Sharma et al., 2006). Response to sympathetic ganglion blockade success could not be predicted from any of the presenting signs or symptoms (Sethna and Berde, 2012; van Eijs et al., 2012).

Sympathetic ganglia blockade and/or epidural analgesia must be offered in the context of multidisciplinary management of chronic pain disorders. Preliminary experience in rehabilitation of children and adolescents with intractable CRPS reported significant improvement in many domains of the child's quality of life including pain reduction, functional improvement to remission, return to normal activities, and improvement of school attendance after a 3-week outpatient intensive interdisciplinary rehabilitative programme, consisting of physical and occupational therapies, cognitive-behavioural therapy, and child and family education (Logan et al., 2012).

Stellate ganglion blockade

The stellate ganglion is located on the anterior surface of C7 transverse process. Sympathetic innervation to the head and neck arises from T1/T2 and passes through the stellate ganglion; and the sympathetic innervation to the upper extremity arises from T2 to T8, but some fibres synapse at the second thoracic ganglion and may not be fully interrupted by a stellate ganglion blockade (Tong and

Nelson, 2000). Blockade is achieved by injection of 3 to 5 ml of local anaesthetic; larger volumes may spread to the somatic nerve via epidural sleeves, or cause serious systemic toxicity if inadvertently injected in a vessel (particularly the nearby vertebral artery). Signs of successful sympathetic blockade include: ipsilateral Horner's syndrome, nasal congestion, cutaneous vasodilation, and increased cutaneous temperature in the arm. Stellate ganglion blockade is infrequently performed in children because CRPS affects predominantly the lower extremity. Recent cases report use for post-traumatic headache, and pain management of acute herpes zoster ophthalmicus using an indwelling catheter for injection of a series stellate ganglion blockade (Agarwal and Joseph, 2006; Chan and Chalkiadis, 2010; Elias and Chakerian, 1994).

Lumbar sympathetic blockade

This procedure is the more commonly performed in children for management of CRPS-I which predominantly affects the lower extremity (80–90%). It is typically performed at L2 to L3 level, and the technique is similar to that described in adults (Meier et al., 2009, Sethna and Wilder, 1993). Successful sympathetic blockade is indicated by interruption of sympathetic innervation to the skin manifested by vasodilation, increased blood flow and rise in skin temperature of the ipsilateral limb (Irazuzta et al., 1992; Krumova et al., 2011). Despite widespread use of sympathetic blockade in pain management clinics, only a few controlled trials have shown significant differences between sympathetic blockade and control. Systematic reviews have concluded that the overall evidence for therapeutic benefit for temporary or neuroablative sympathetic interruption for CRPS is weak (Sethna and Berde, 2012).

The precise mechanism(s) of CRPS is complex and remains a research challenge, as it involves somatosensory, motor, and sympathetic nervous systems. Potential mechanisms include: disordered regulation of sympathetic system with sympathetically maintained pain, peripheral and central sensitization, somatosensory and body perception changes (Krumova et al., 2011; Price et al., 1998). In a few CRPS patients, a series of temporary blockade with local anaesthetics leads to long-lasting pain relief (Krumova et al., 2011; Meier et al., 2009; Price et al., 1998), but the long-term benefit of sympathetic blockade in children and adults has not been investigated or demonstrated (Perez et al., 2010; Wilder et al., 1992). As an alternative technique, epidural and peripheral nerve blockade with indwelling catheters has been used for continuous infusion of local anaesthetic to alleviate CRPS pain and facilitate physical therapy for mobilization of the affected limb (Dadure et al., 2005; Sethna and Wilder, 1993).

A recent controlled trial in children with CRPS, ages 7 to 17 years, demonstrated thermal and mechanical quantitative sensory abnormalities suggestive of central sensitization (Sethna et al., 2007). A second double-blind, placebo-controlled crossover trial by the same investigators compared intravenous versus lumbar sympathetic blockade with lidocaine in a small number of children (ages 10–18 years) and found that a single lumbar sympathetic blockade produced significant reduction in pain intensity in response to evoked tactile and mechanical stimulation, mechanical temporal summation and spontaneous pain scores in approximately 40% of the patients. The findings of this study support the concept that in some patients a component of pain involves a sympathetic efferent and somatic afferent cycle of activities, and suggest that selective sympathetic ganglia blockade can alleviate pain (Meier et al., 2009).

Complications

Potential serious infectious complications can occur with temporary epidural catheters and SCS, particularly in immune suppressed children due to malignancy, chronic steroid therapy, chronic pain disorders or those with coexisting infection (Aram et al., 2001; Olsson et al., 2008; Sethna et al., 2010; Strafford et al., 1995). In a large paediatric population the incidence of externalized (through a short subcutaneous tunnel) tunnelled epidural catheter-associated cellulitis, paravertebral muscle, and epidural space infections was evaluated and significantly higher rate of infection was found in children with CRPS when compared to postoperative children: 3.2% versus 0.06% (Sethna et al., 2010). The median duration of epidural infusion was similar in the two groups of patients (3 versus 4 days, ranging 1–12 days). The diagnosis of the infection in CRPS children (10–16 years) was made between 3 and 5 days after insertion of the catheters. All CRPS children were otherwise healthy whereas the children who developed postoperative epidural catheter-associated infection were immunosuppressed due to malignancy and/or chronic steroid therapy. The most common pathogen was *Staphylococcus aureus*. The reasons for the higher incidence of infection in otherwise healthy CRPS children are not entirely understood, but are attributed to impaired immune response caused by chronic pain and stress.

Spinal cord stimulation (SCS) for intractable CRPS

Adult controlled trials of intractable CRPS reported that SCS significantly reduced pain (more than 50%) with SCS, but did not alleviate sensory abnormalities of allodynia or improve function (Kemler et al., 2004). Regrettably, the long-term benefit at 3-year follow-up waned and was not statistically different compared to control group. The benefit of SCS for management of challenging cases of CRPS-I in children has been reported in one retrospective review of 7 children ages 11 to 14 years who benefited transiently from sympathetic blockade with local anaesthetic (Olsson et al., 2008). The duration of SCS ranged from 3 weeks to 4 years. The pain alleviation onset occurred after 1 to 2 weeks and complete relief at 2 to 6 weeks in five patients, which persisted for 1 to 8 years; but in two patients the there was only partial relief. In one patient after a few-day trial, the SCS was removed due to local infection, but the pain reduction persisted, and a recurrence some months later resolved spontaneously. Follow-up data were collected via telephone interviews and only three out of seven patients responded favourably to the question 'Would you have SCS again?'. In view of the limitations of this retrospective review and invasiveness of the procedure, prospective placebo-control trials are needed before application of this intervention can be justified (Olsson et al., 2008; van Eijs et al., 2012).

Neuraxial blockade for intractable cancer-related pain

Many of the principles and fundamental tenets of adult palliative care are applied to refractory paediatric cancer and chronic non-malignant pain conditions, but bearing in mind the differences in child development, pharmacology, and the spectrum of malignancies.

For the majority of children (90–95%) with cancer, pain is effectively managed with conventional analgesics (opioids, non-opioids, adjuvants) via parenteral, enteral, subcutaneous, and transdermal routes (Collins, 2002). Analgesia requires optimization as parents reported only 27% of children with end-stage cancer pain received adequate conventional analgesia (Wolfe et al., 2000). Pain complaints, other than headache, were reported more commonly in children with solid tumours including brain and nervous system, compared to other types (leukaemia, lymphoma, etc.). In last days of life 92% of children with all types of childhood malignancy reported pain and in approximately two-thirds of these patients the pain constituted a difficult problem to manage (Goldman et al., 2006).

In a small number of children even large doses of opioids do not adequately control pain, because of development of opioid tolerance and/or opioid-induced hyperalgesia; or because severe diffuse pain, involving somatic, neuropathic, and visceral components, develops. During the terminal stages of childhood malignancy, the opioid requirement may escalate exponentially to massive doses. Approximately 3% to 6% of these patients can benefit from interventional pain therapies for management of the refractory pain unresponsive to standard cancer and conventional analgesic therapies, or because opioid dose escalation is limited by intolerable side effects such as nausea, vomiting, sedation, and obtunded mentation (Collins et al., 1995, 1996).

Interventional therapies are offered when the overall benefits outweigh the risks. Such therapies include epidural, intrathecal, plexus, and peripheral nerve analgesic infusions or ablative therapies. The published experience in children is very limited but includes (Table 46.1):

+ Neuraxial blockade via an epidural (caudal, lumbar, thoracic, cervical) or intrathecal catheter.

+ Externalized catheter and infusion for peripheral nerve blockade.

+ Neurolytic nerve and plexus blockade.

Efficacy and safety of continuous infusion of neuraxial analgesics

Several paediatric cancer case reports and small series of have reported effective analgesia with short-term (weeks to months) use of externalized and internalized epidural and intrathecal catheters for infusion of various combinations of opioids, local anaesthetics, and clonidine (Tables 46.1 and 46.2). The spread, absorption, and pharmacodynamics of analgesics administered via epidural and intrathecal routes in children are influenced by multiple factors such as the age, weight, height, presence of increased intra-abdominal and intrathoracic pressure, cerebrospinal fluid (CSF) flow characteristics, and patency of the epidural space. There is no clear standardization or consensus for the use of various analgesics, either given alone or in combination, in children. Most approaches are derived from paediatric acute pain management studies and clinical experience. The published experience (and our own) would suggest starting with a single analgesic for patients who are on systemic opioid and other adjuvants such as a local anaesthetic for epidural administration, and opioids for intrathecal administration for the first 24 h. Combinations of analgesics are used when pain is not adequately controlled (e.g. an opioid plus local anaesthetic and/or clonidine) to enhance analgesia and/or reduce dose requirements of an individual analgesic agent and minimize the side effects. As the need for systemic opioids reduces a second agent may be added (e.g. opioid to epidural solution, or local anaesthetic to intrathecal solution). Morphine and hydromorphone are the most commonly used opioids. The initial dose is estimated by conversion of the total daily dose of enteral and parenteral opioids. The average ratio of opioid conversion between routes, for instance, for morphine oral:intravenous:epidural:intrathecal is 3:1:0.1:0.01 mg respectively (Krames, 1996). Initially, frequent dose adjustment is required to titrate analgesic dose, concentrations and volume against individual response. Additional small doses may be necessary for breakthrough pain.

Regular monitoring for side effects is required, with close nursing observation, continuous electrocardiogram, chest wall impedance plethysmography, and pulse oximetry. In addition, systemic opioids should be gradually reduced as neuraxial analgesia is titrated up, to avoid opioid withdrawal symptoms. In terminally ill children the analgesic requirement by all routes of administration may escalate to massive doses (Queinnec et al., 1999; Whyte and Lauder, 2012).

Inadequate analgesia with neuraxial delivery has been reported in a few children with advanced and extensive malignancy, particularly with the epidural route, and which necessitated conversion to intrathecal analgesia (Collins et al., 1996; Portas et al., 1998; Queinnec et al., 1999; Tobias, 2000). Children with extensive visceral and pelvic malignancy refractory to intrathecal analgesia may require neurolytic intrathecal or coeliac blockade (Galloway et al., 2000; Patt et al., 1995; Shimazaki et al., 2003), and one rare case of cordotomy has been reported in a 10-year-old child (Queinnec et al., 1999).

Contraindications

Many of the absolute contraindications for placement of epidural, intrathecal, and peripheral nerve blockade in healthy patients are considered to be relative contraindications in children with uncontrolled cancer pain. Advanced malignancy is associated with immune suppression and possible coagulopathy, but complications and particularly infections are surprisingly low (Anghelescu et al., 2010). Benefits should outweigh the potential side effects, and patients and their families must be fully informed of the potential serious side effects.

Neuraxial delivery systems

A percutaneous tunnelled epidural or intrathecal catheter connected to a regular syringe pump may be used when life expectancy is limited to days or a few weeks. For children with longer life expectance (weeks to a few months), an implanted delivery system is a better therapeutic option to reduce catheter displacement and the risk of infection. Intrathecal delivery circumvents incomplete epidural absorption kinetics, irregular spread of analgesic solution, and formation of catheter tip granulomas. Smaller volumes of analgesic are required, which is more convenient for children being cared for in the community (Galloway et al., 2000; Queinnec et al., 1999; Tobias, 2000).

Before proceeding with implantation of the drug delivery system, all patients must undergo a screening trial of intrathecal or epidural analgesia for at least 24 h to ensure pain reduction of 50% or greater and/or reduction in opioid requirement, as well as observing for potential drug reactions. It is advisable to use fluoroscopic guidance and inject contrast to ensure correct catheter placement, and epidural catheter tips should be placed at the optimal spinal dermatome to cover the location of maximum pain (Collins et al., 1996;

Table 46.1 Continuous externalized neuraxial and peripheral nerve blockade management of intractable malignant pain in children

Reference	Age (years)	n	Intervention	Site	Infusion	Duration
(Berde et al., 1989)	0.4	1	Epidural	Caudal	Intermittent morphine	1 week
(Berde et al., 1990)	19	1	Intrathecal	Lumbar to thoracic	Bupivacaine	7 months
(Plancarte and Patt 1991)	3.8	1	Epidural	Thoracic	Meperidine	1 month
					Droperidol	
(Meignier et al., 1992)	1.4–12	5	Intrathecal	Lumbar	Bupivacaine	20 days–3 months
					Morphine	
					Fentanyl	
(Veyckemans et al., 1994)	1.9	1	Epidural	Cervical	Morphine and	35 days
					Bupivacaine	
					Intermittent	
(Patt et al., 1995)	3	5	Intrathecal	Lumbar	Phenol 10%	8 days until demise
(Collins, 1996)	0.4–16	4	Intrathecal	Lumbar	Bupivacaine	3 days–7 weeks
		6	Epidural	Caudal/lumbar	Morphine	
					Fentanyl Hydromorphone	
(Portas et al., 1998)	1–15	7	Epidural	Lumbar	Bupivacaine	2 days–6 months
					Sufentanil	
					Clonidine	
(Queinnec et al., 1999)	10	1	Epidural	Lumbar	Bupivacaine	4.8 months
					Morphine	
					Clonidine	
(Tobias, 2000)	16	1	Intrathecal	Lumbar	Bupivacaine	4 weeks
					Sufentanil	
(Galloway et al., 2000)	15	1	Intrathecal	Lumbar	Bupivacaine	5 months
					Sufentanil	
(Aram et al., 2001)	6	7–21	Epidural	Lumbar thoracic	Bupivacaine, Morphine	5–54 days
					Fentanyl Hydromorphone	
(Bozkurt et al., 2005)	2.5	1	Epidural	Thoracic	Bupivacaine	2 weeks
					Fentanyl	
(Anghelescu et al., 2010)	4.4–21	10	Epidural	Lumbar	Local anaesthetic	4–85 days
				Thoracic	Opioids clonidine	
(Cooper et al., 1994)	6	1		Brachial plexus	Bupivacaine intermittent	5 days
(Anghelescu et al., 2010)	2, 3, 18	3	Femoral		Ropivacaine	3–81 days
			Axillary			
			Interscalene			
(Burgoyne et al., 2012)	14, 13, 8	3	Femoral		Ropivacaine	22–41 days
			Brachial plexus			

Queinnec et al., 1999). In addition to meticulous attention to aseptic handling of externalized and internalized catheters, catheters should be clearly labelled to avoid inadvertent administration of drugs not intended for epidural or intrathecal therapy. All drugs used for epidural and intrathecal administration should be preservative free to minimize the risk of neurotoxicity.

In adults, the subcutaneous Port-A-Cath™ device has been used for delivery of opioids via epidural and intrathecal routes for long-term management of cancer and non-malignant intractable chronic pain syndromes (Dahm et al., 1998; Plummer et al., 1991). A special Port-A-Cath system™ is designed specifically for analgesic drug delivery and repeated access to the epidural or

Table 46.2 Clinical data on neuraxial and peripheral nerve blockade infusion reported in the literature

Site of administration and analgesic agent[a]	Dose
Epidural opioid and clonidine (mcg/kg/h)	
Lumbar morphine	1–4
Lumbar hydromorphone	0.6
Lumbar fentanyl	0.4–0.5
Lumbar sufentanil	5–30
Lumbar clonidine	5–10
Cervical meperidine	5 mg three times a day
Epidural local anaesthetic (mg/kg/h)	
Lumbar bupivacaine	0.2
Thoracic bupivacaine/ropivacaine	0.2–0.3
Lumbar/thoracic lidocaine	1.5 (maximum 2)
Intrathecal opioid (mcg/kg/h)	
Lumbar morphine	2.5–252
Thoracic and lumbar fentanyl	0.2–0.4
Intrathecal local anaesthetic (mg/kg/h)	
Thoracic bupivacaine 0.5%	2–4 ml/h
Lumbar bupivacaine	0.04–0.25
Thoracic bupivacaine	0.01–0.12
Intrathecal clonidine	0.04–0.9
Peripheral nerve blockade	
Femoral nerve ropivacaine 0.2–0.4%	10–12 ml/h for 81 days
Interscalene ropivacaine 0.2%	8–12 ml/h for 35 days

[a]The lower rates of infusion are for initial dosing. The higher rates of infusion of opioids and/or local anaesthetics were administered to children tolerant to opioids.

intrathecal space. A subarachnoid or epidural silicon catheter is tunnelled subcutaneously to a small reservoir that has a self-sealing silicone septum for needle insertion and connection to an external infusion device. Successful use of epidural or intrathecal Port-A-Cath system™ has been reported in paediatric case reports for delivery of opioid, local anaesthetic and clonidine (Table 46.1) (Galloway et al., 2000; Queinnec et al., 1999; Tobias, 2000). In one case the Port-A-Cath system™ was used for epidural analgesia on four occasions with effective analgesia over 143 days. Complications occurred on two occasions: a catheter dysfunction, and abscess that necessitated removal of the system (Queinnec et al., 1999).

In the past decade fully implanted intrathecal pumps have been used for infusion of baclofen to manage intractable spasticity. The drawbacks of this system are potential technical problems, it requires a surgical procedure and a special percutaneous needle and kit for accessing and refilling the pump reservoir, and the high cost makes it impractical for children with cancer-related pain and limited life expectancy.

Although the use of subcutaneous implanted systems in children is appealing, in reality the full potential for delivery of various combinations of analgesic agents is yet to be realized with respect to efficacy, failure rates, and technical complications.

Complications of neuraxial infusions

In children, estimation of the incidence of adverse events with neuraxial infusion is not possible due to the small number of retrospective cases reported, and because many side effects either did not occur or were not documented. Systemic toxicity has occurred with large doses of epidural bupivacaine (3–4 mg/kg/h) in three patients (Portas et al., 1998). Cases of tolerance or tachyphylaxis to opioid and/or local anaesthetics were treated by converting to another analgesic with a different mechanism of action, or adding clonidine to enhance analgesia (Anghelescu et al., 2010; Berde et al., 1990a; Whyte and Lauder, 2012). Drug-related side effects have included: urinary retention, which usually improved with time (Collins et al., 1996; Queinnec et al., 1999); constipation (Queinnec et al., 1999); mild reversible somnolence and respiratory depression (Berde et al., 1990a; Collins et al., 1996). Other potential side effects and complications such as nausea, vomiting, pruritus, opioid-induced myoclonus and hyperalgesia, CSF-hygroma, implantation pocket seroma, meningitis, and cardiovascular instability and death were not reported in these paediatric case reports. Reported catheter-related or technical complications include: catheter leakage and fracture (Anghelescu et al., 2010); epidural catheter occlusion by tumour or kinking (Anghelescu et al., 2010; Collins et al., 1996); catheter dislodgement (Anghelescu et al., 2010; Aram et al., 2001), and Port-A-Cath system malfunction (Queinnec et al., 1999); post-dural puncture headache (Collins et al., 1996); and infection at the skin entry port or catheter tip (Aram et al., 2001; Berde et al., 1990a; Queinnec et al., 1999)

Plexus blockade for intractable malignant and chronic non-malignant pain

The coeliac plexus is located at the T12/L1 vertebral level, anterior to the aorta and crus of the diaphragm, and supplies sympathetic innervation to the upper abdominal viscera (liver, gall bladder, spleen, stomach, pancreas, kidneys, small bowel, and proximal two-thirds of the large bowel). The preganglionic sympathetic innervation consists of T5 to T12 spinal segments. It supplies sympathetic supply to greater splanchnic nerve (T5–10), lesser splanchnic nerve (T10–11) and least splanchnic nerve (T11–12) (Loukas et al., 2010; Kambadakone et al., 2011; Puli et al., 2009). The standard coeliac plexus blockade is performed in adults with the aid of imaging or under direct vision during surgery (Arcidiacono et al., 2011; Kambadakone et al., 2011; Levy et al., 2012, Sharma et al., 2011).

Coeliac plexus blockade is primarily indicated for cancer and life limiting/terminating conditions. The principles of pain management and palliative care in adults are incorporated in the care of children with cancer, including use of neurolytic blockade. Drugs (e.g. alcohol, phenol) and dosing regimens in paediatric case reports have been based on the age of the child and extrapolation from adult experience. Neoplastic diseases such as pancreatic and hepatic malignancies can produce intense pain from stretch, compression, invasion, or distension of the visceral structures. Neurolysis of the coeliac plexus is an important adjunct for relief of intractable pain, aiming to optimizing analgesia and reduce the need for, and adverse effects of, opioid and non-opioid analgesics. As neurolytic blockade is associated with potential serious side effects, this modality of intervention is offered when the benefits clearly outweigh the potential risks.

In children, CT-guided coeliac blockade has safely achieved effective pain management in a small number of patients aged 3 to 7 years. Reported cases include:

- Neurolytic block for management of refractory upper abdomen visceral pain from cancer (Berde et al., 1990b; Staats and Kost-Byerly, 1995).
- Neurolytic splanchnic nerve blockade in an 18-year-old with mitochondrial neurogastrointenstinal encephalopathy and superior mesenteric artery syndrome for management of intractable abdominal pain, which resulted in pain relief at one-year follow-up (Celebi et al., 2006).
- Diagnostic and temporary treatment of acute on chronic pancreatitis with local anaesthetic and steroid (Attila et al., 2009; Goldschneider et al., 2007).
- Chronic abdominal pain due to inflammatory bowel disorder (Tanelian and Cousins, 1989) or due to neurodegenerative disorders (Goldschneider et al., 2007; Teitelbaum et al., 2002).

Superior hypogastric plexus blockade (anterior to lower third of L5 and upper two-thirds of S1 vertebral bodies) has been used in adults for management of intractable pain of the pelvic organs and descending colon and rectum as well as perineal hyperhidrosis (Schmidt et al., 2005; Nabil and Eissa, 2010).

Ganglion impar, a small ganglion formed by convergence of the two pelvic sympathetic trunks in front of the sacro-coccygeal junction, supplying perineum, distal rectum, anus, distal urethra, vulva and distal third of the vagina. A trans-sacrococcygeal block with local anaesthetic successfully managed chronic post-traumatic coccydynia in an adolescent (Ellinas and Sethna, 2009). Neurolytic blockade, with appropriate imaging and confirmation of a successful diagnostic local anaesthetic block, has been used for adult malignant pain conditions unresponsive to conventional treatment (Lin et al., 2010).

Interventional pain management for intractable acute and chronic pain

Neuraxial blockade

Safe and effective (defined as decrease in mean dose of opioid requirement) use of short-term caudal, lumbar and thoracic epidural infusions via tunnelled catheters are also reported in a small number of 14 children and adolescents, a mean age 4.4 years, and a mean duration of 16 days (range 5–14 days) for management of pain following trauma, extensive surgery and CRPS type I (Aram et al., 2001). Long-term continuous peripheral nerve block has also been used for management of severe pain from pathological fracture of the femur in 3 children, aged 8, 13, and 14 years, with osteosarcoma while awaiting chemotherapy and surgical treatment. The duration of the externalized catheters was 22 to 41 days with significant reduction in pain and opioid use, and without complications related to the catheter, infection or local anaesthetic toxicity (Burgoyne et al., 2012b).

Phantom limb pain (PLP)

In children, the clinical characteristics, preventive measures and treatment of PLP have not been investigated rigorously, with only a few retrospective reviews and one prospective study in small numbers of paediatric patients (Krane and Heller, 1995; McGrath and Hillier, 1992; Melzack et al., 1997; Simmel, 1962; Smith and Thompson, 1995; Thomas et al., 2003; Wilkins et al., 1998). The current pharmacotherapy is inadequate to completely prevent or alleviate the pain after limb amputation in children and adults. The development of PLP is best conceptualized as multifactorial and treatment requires a multimodal approach. See elsewhere in this volume for further description of PLP (Walker, Chapter 21), and for pharmacological management options (Rastogi and Campbell, Chapter 48). While PLP cannot be entirely prevented after surgery, growing anecdotal data suggests that perioperative neuraxial and peripheral nerve blocks in addition to systemic analgesics may minimize the immediate and short-term post-amputation PLP. A recent review of cancer amputee children and young adults reported a very lower incidence of only 10% of PLP at 1 year after amputation (Burgoyne et al., 2012a). In this review 17 out of 25 patients had pain prior to amputation and the low incidence post-surgical PLP was partly ascribed to the preoperative pain management. This included administration of gabapentin in all patients and continuous epidural or continuous peripheral nerve blockade in 21 out of 26 cases.

Epidural steroid injection (ESI)

The indication for ESI is local alleviation of perineural inflammation of the spinal nerve roots that are irritated or compressed by herniated nucleus pulposus, annular tear, spinal stenosis and post-laminectomy syndrome. Fluoroscopic-guidance is used to place steroid in the vicinity of the affected nerve roots. Evidence for ESI is restricted to adult practice, predominantly for radicular pain that radiates along the distribution of a specific spinal nerve distally below the knee. Radicular pain is neuropathic pain in the distribution of specific spinal nerve roots, and can arise from mechanical or chemical irritation due to a herniated nucleus pulposus or spondylosis with stenosis of nerve pathways (Manchikanti et al., 2012).

Interlaminar epidural steroid injections may be performed in the cervical and lumbar spine using the traditional loss of resistance technique. For accurate placement of the needle, within the epidural space and close to the affected nerve fluoroscopic guidance is recommended to avoid misplacement of the needle and confirm spread of contrast medium in proximity to the target spinal nerve. In adults, typical injectate is 80 mg (2ml) of triamcinolone. In the lumbar region a small amount of local anaesthetic is added to produce pain relief. In the cervical spine local anaesthetics are avoided to minimize excessive cephalad spread of the injectate (Manchikanti et al., 2012).

Transforaminal epidural steroid injections is intended to deposit the medication around the nerve root sleeve for more accurate targeting of the affected nerve in the anterior epidural space where disc herniation occurs. It is primarily performed in the lumbar spine under fluoroscopic guidance. In adults, typical dose is 40 mg (1ml) of triamcinolone, with or without a small amount of local anaesthetic (Manchikanti et al., 2012, Quraishi, 2012).

Selective spinal nerve blockade (SNRB) is a diagnostic technique to determine if a specific nerve root is the source of pain prior to surgical removal of the offending ruptured intervertebral disc. The needle tip is placed just outside of the neural foramen, lateral to the position for transforaminal ESI site but outside the foramina.

Caudal epidural steroid injection is performed by a technique similar to that performed for caudal anaesthesia, with lateral fluoroscopy to visualize the spread of contrast medium (Parr et al., 2012).

Facet joint pain

The facet joint is formed by articulation of processes of two adjacent vertebrae and the joint capsule is innervated by a medial nerve branch. The joint is susceptible to chondral damage (e.g. whiplash injury, repetitive strain, sports injury), inflammation and degeneration (e.g. congenital, post-surgical spinal fusion, old age). Estimation of the true incidence of facet joint pain is difficult because the diagnosis cannot be made by history, physical examination or imaging, and the most reliable diagnostic test is response to intra-articular or medial nerve branch blockade (Schwarzer et al., 1994a, 1994b). Although some studies report pain relief up to one year, the lack of RCT crossover studies precludes drawing definitive conclusions about specificity of this blockade.

Intra-articular facet blockade is performed with local anaesthetic and steroid, and repeat injections may be required to relief flare-ups. If the pain recurs some practitioners consider positive response to steroid injection a criterion to perform radiofrequency lesioning for providing prolonged pain relief (Atluri et al., 2008; Boswell et al., 2007).

Medial branch nerve blockade (MBB) interrupt pain conduction by nerves that innervate the facet joints. MBB is performed using a local anaesthetic alone or in combination with steroids, potentially followed by a series of blocks, or radiofrequency lesioning to provide prolonged pain relief.

Radiofrequency nerve lesioning (RFNL) (thermo-coagulation or thermal injury) is utilized to interrupt nerve conduction for 6 to 9 months. Although RFNL is used for interruption of various nerves, e.g. peripheral (e.g. occipital neuralgia), visceral (e.g. splanchnic) and sympathetic (e.g. CRPS), presently it is primarily used for the treatment of axial back pain produced by facet and sacroiliac joint arthropathy, and therefore is most often used in adults (van Boxem et al., 2008). Pulsed RFNL was introduced recently because of a wider margin of safety, and to expand the application of this therapy to various peripheral neuropathies, joints arthropathy and painful trigger points as well as treatment of facet joints, sacroiliac joints, dorsal root ganglion, stellate ganglion, Gasserian ganglion and intervertebral discs (van Boxem et al., 2008).

Sacroiliac joint injection

The sacroiliac joint connects the pelvis to spine, has limited mobility and is a major source of low back pain in aged adults secondary to degenerative processes of the intra-articular cartilage. In adolescents, sacroiliac joint pain may follow trauma, particularly sports injury. There is no one clinical test that reliably confirms that the pain emanates specifically from the sacroiliac joint and diagnosis is based on a combination of clinical tests of the sacroiliac joint and radiographic imaging. Most patients benefit from anti-inflammatory drugs and physical therapy. Some support performance of diagnostic/therapeutic blockade with a local anaesthetic alone or in combination with steroid. If repeated treatment is required radiofrequency nerve lesioning has been utilized in adults (Hansen et al., 2012; Simopoulos et al., 2012).

Peripheral nerve blockade

Many different types of peripheral nerve blockade have been utilized for either diagnosis or management of various chronic pain syndromes. Local anaesthetic blockade can provide several hours of pain relief, and may aid in diagnosis or predict responses to sustained pain relief following prolonged nerve blockade techniques. Steroid provides lasting relief in cases of perineural inflammation from entrapment syndromes. Common peripheral nerve blockade used in management of adult chronic pain are described below, but for the majority evidence is limited. For many, paediatric use is predominantly for acute or perioperative pain, and the role for chronic pain management is unclear.

Trigeminal nerve blockade

The sensory afferent inputs from the orofacial structures that sense mechanical, thermal and pain stimuli are served by the fifth (trigeminal) cranial nerve, and divided into:

* Ophthalmic branch innervates nasal and frontal sinuses mucosa.

* Maxillary branch innervates the nares, upper teeth and gums, nasal mucosa, palate and roof of the pharynx, maxillary, ethmoid, and sphenoid sinuses.

* Mandibular branch innervates the lower teeth and gums. The trigeminal system is the main source of sensory innervations to the supra-tentorial dura, venous sinuses and meningeal arteries.

The sensory afferent input projects to the trigeminal (Gasserian) ganglion. The trigeminal brainstem sensory neuron complex receives descending inhibitory modulation from higher centres (periaqueductal grey, reticular formation and sensory-motor cortex) mediated through release of neuropeptides including endogenous opioids, noradrenaline, 5-HT, and GABA through synaptic connections (Sessle, 2000).

The classic presentation of trigeminal neuralgia (TN) is paroxysms of lancinating pain, which occur in the territory of one or more trigeminal nerve branches, associated with muscle spasms in the absence of sensory and motor deficit. The pain is easily triggered by non-noxious stimuli such as minor mechanical stimulation or light touch. Trigeminal neuralgia is rare in the paediatric age group, with case reports of typical (at ages 1.5, 6, 9, and 12 years) and atypical (at 9 years) TN described. The youngest child in whom TN was retrospectively suspected was 13 months of age; the child suffered pain attacks for years before TN was finally diagnosed at age 7 years (Bender et al., 2011).

As in adults, children in whom the medical treatment of TN is ineffective or the side effects prove unacceptable, microvascular decompression of the trigeminal nerves in the posterior cranial fossa may be indicated (Kalkanis et al., 2003; Resnick et al., 1998). There is no satisfactory long-term medical or ablative treatment for TN. In 18 children, percutaneous retro-Gasserian glycerol injection resulted in complete pain relief in 72%, good in 11%, poor 11%, and recurrence in 22%. None of the children experienced a permanent facial sensory deficit. Although this procedure is less invasive than a microvascular decompression craniotomy, its performance requires the full cooperation of an awake and non-sedated child and the long-term benefit is not known (Yue, 2004).

Greater occipital nerve

Occipital nerve irritation or inflammation can produce localized pain or ipsilateral tension-type headache or intractable neuropathic headache. Perineural injection of a combination of local anaesthetic and steroid can relieve pain. Best results are reported for occipital nerve neuralgia presenting with shooting, stinging or burning pain and the symptoms are reproducible by pressure palpation of the occipital nerve at its exist from the skull. Some degree of temporary success is also reported for patients with unilateral migraines, cluster headaches and cervical facet arthropathy. Blockade is usually performed using surface landmarks in children and adolescents (Suresh and Voronov, 2012). Care is needed to avoid direct needle trauma of the nerve or puncturing the occipital artery, which runs lateral and parallel to the nerve. To improve safety occipital nerve block can be performed with use of ultrasound guide as described for adults (Shim et al., 2011).

Suprascapular nerve blockade

The suprascapular nerve arises from C5 and C6 and innervates the supraspinatus and infraspinatus muscles and gives of twigs to shoulder joint. In a randomized control trial of adults with chronic shoulder pain this blockade has improved pain, range of motion and disability (Shanahan et al., 2003). This nerve blockade has been performed in adults with aid of anatomical landmarks, electromyography, computed tomography scan, ultrasound guide, or with fluoroscopy (Fernandes et al., 2012).

Intercostal nerve blockade

Intercostal nerve blockade is performed for management of intercostal neuralgia following nerve injury or inflammation. It is also performed for diagnosis of painful conditions such as post-thoracotomy pain syndrome, and slipping rib syndrome. This procedure is commonly performed in children with the use of anatomical landmarks but ultrasound imaging may improve safety (Bhalla et al., 2012) as pneumothorax can occur if the needle is advanced deep beyond the internal intercostal muscles.

Rectus abdominis sheath blockade

The rectus sheath consists of anterior and posterior layers that envelop the rectus abdominis muscle, which is innervated by T7 to T12. The intercostal nerves enter the rectus sheath through the posterior rectus sheath, and pierce the rectus muscles and the anterior sheath to innervate the anterior abdominal wall. In one-third of the population the intercostal nerve bypasses the rectus sheath compartment and innervates the overlying skin directly (Skinner and Lauder, 2007) and subcutaneous infiltration should be used to supplement the posterior rectus sheath blockade.

Entrapment of the nerves may occur after trauma, repetitive and excessive abdominal crunches in athletes, rectus sheath hematoma, postsurgical entrapment in a scar or suture ligation. This presents with intermittent pain at the edge of the rectus muscle sheath (entry site of the intercostal nerves), which is aggravated with contraction of the rectus muscles and alleviated by lying down and flexion of the ipsilateral hip. Differential diagnoses include hernia, irritation of intercostal nerve roots, rib-tip syndrome, myofascial pain and trigger points of the recuts muscles.

Block with local anaesthetic with or without steroid can be performed with loss of resistance technique and feel of posterior rectus sheath as an end point, ultrasound imaging clearly defines the end-point and reduces the risk of perforating the posterior rectus sheath

and bowel injury (Bhalla et al., 2012; Gurnaney et al., 2011; Skinner and Lauder, 2007).

Ilioinguinal and iliohypogastric nerve blockade

The ilioinguinal and iliohypogastric nerves are branches of the first L1 root, occasionally with contribution from T12. The ilioinguinal nerve exits from the abdomen through the obliquus internus and accompanies the spermatic cord through superficial inguinal ring. The iliohypogastric anterior branch perforates the external oblique muscle just medial to the anterior superior iliac spine and provides cutaneous sensory innervation to the abdominal skin above the pubis. Ilioinguinal neuralgia can cause lower abdominal and pelvic pain in adults (often following direct blunt trauma, inguinal herniorrhaphy or pelvic surgery), and has been reported in adolescent athletes. The nerve is compressed as it exits the transverse abdominis muscle just lateral to anterior superior iliac spine, presenting as burning pain, paraesthesia, and infrequent numbness over the nerve's lower abdominal distribution, with radiation to the scrotum or labia and sometimes the inner upper thigh. Slouching forward may improve, and extension of the spine worsens the pain.

In children both these nerves are in close proximity between transversus abdominis and internal oblique muscle and are amenable to blockade with a single injection medial and cephalad to anterior superior iliac spine. Possible complications are perforation of the bowel if the needle further posteriorly and femoral nerve blockade if the local anaesthetic tracks down caudad. This blockade can be easily and safely performed with ultrasound guidance (Ecoffey et al., 2010; Jansen et al., 2008; Peng and Tumber, 2008; Stark et al., 1999).

Lateral femoral cutaneous neuropathy (LFCN)

LFCN neuropathy, also known as meralgia paraesthetica, presents with paraesthesia (tingling, pins and needles), burning, cutaneous hypersensitivity to warm shower, groin pain or numbness over the distribution of the nerve on the anterolateral area of the thigh. The symptoms are aggravated by prolonged walking, standing or biking. Compression of the nerve may be due to tight clothing or belt, obesity or fast weight gain, pregnancy, pelvic pathology, local injury from direct trauma or after inguinal hernia repair. Conservative therapy includes elimination of the offending compression cause. Neuropathic pain pharmacotherapy is effective in most patients with mild pain (see Rastogi and Campbell, Chapter 48, this volume). In some patients nerve blockade at the inguinal ligament with a combination of a local anaesthetic and corticosteroid may provide pain relief for days to weeks (Fernandez-Mayoralas et al., 2010).

Pudendal nerve blockade

The pudendal nerve arises from S2 to S4 nerve roots, passes out the pelvis through lesser sciatic foramen and crosses the ischial spine to innervate the rectum, perineum and the penis or clitoris and posterior aspect of the penis or labia majora. Injury to these nerves occurs following trauma, injury during surgery, inflammation, compression/entrapment, or due to invasion by malignancy. Pain is aggravated by sitting and alleviated by standing, sitting on toilet seat or lying on the painful side. Pudendal nerve blockade has been described in children using percutaneous transperineal approach and nerve stimulator for management of postoperative pain management (Kfoury et al., 2008; Naja et al., 2011).

Conclusion

In adults and now in paediatric patients there have been concerns about efficacy and acceptability of the various interventional techniques for management of chronic pain disorders due to the lack of well-designed randomized control trials. Interventional techniques for management of chronic pain in children and adolescents are still being developed and there are no controlled trials on their long-term effectiveness. The best available evidence synthesized here is primarily extrapolation from adult interventional procedures for chronic pain management literature, paediatric case reports and case series, and the authors' experience. The authors of this chapter are of the view that the practitioners of paediatric interventional techniques must have a basic understanding of paediatric development, pharmacology, resuscitation skills, and competency in performing paediatric regional anaesthesia techniques as well as experience with specific adult interventional techniques for chronic pain management before applying these techniques in young patients. The readers are also advised to review the adult controlled trials and evidence-based data before integrating these techniques into paediatric practice. However, as part of multidisciplinary management of paediatric cancer and chronic pain, well-selected IPM techniques can play an important role when pain is unrelieved by conventional treatment modalities.

References

Abrahams, M. S., Aziz, M. F., Fu, R. F., and Horn, J. L. (2009). Ultrasound guidance compared with electrical neurostimulation for peripheral nerve block: a systematic review and meta-analysis of randomized controlled trials. *Br J Anaesth*, 102, 408–417.

Agarwal, V. and Joseph, B. (2006). Recurrent migratory sympathetically maintained pain syndrome in a child: a case report. *J Pediatr Orthop B*, 15, 73–74.

Anghelescu, D. L., Faughnan, L. G., Baker, J. N., Yang, J., and Kane, J. R. (2010). Use of epidural and peripheral nerve blocks at the end of life in children and young adults with cancer: the collaboration between a pain service and a palliative care service. *Paediatr Anaesth*, 20, 1070–1077.

Aram, L., Krane, E. J., Kozloski, L. J., and Yaster, M. (2001). Tunneled epidural catheters for prolonged analgesia in pediatric patients. *Anesth Analg*, 92, 1432–1438.

Arcidiacono, P. G., Calori, G., Carrara, S., Mcnicol, E. D., and Testoni, P. A. (2011). Celiac plexus block for pancreatic cancer pain in adults. *Cochrane Database Syst Rev*, 3, CD007519.

Atluri, S., Datta, S., Falco, F. J., and Lee, M. (2008). Systematic review of diagnostic utility and therapeutic effectiveness of thoracic facet joint interventions. *Pain Physician*, 11, 611–629.

Attila, T., Adler, D. G., Hilden, K., and Faigel, D. O. (2009). EUS in pediatric patients. *Gastrointest Endosc*, 70, 892–898.

Bender, M. T., Pradilla, G., James, C., Raza, S., Lim, M., and Carson, B. S. (2011). Surgical treatment of pediatric trigeminal neuralgia: case series and review of the literature. *Childs Nerv Syst*, 27, 2123–2129.

Berde, C. B., Fischel, N., Filardi, J. P., Coe, C. S., Grier, H. E., and Bernstein, S. C. (1989). Caudal epidural morphine analgesia for an infant with advanced neuroblastoma: report of a case. *Pain*, 36, 219–223.

Berde, C. B., Sethna, N. F., Conrad, L. S., Hershenson, M. B., and Shillito, J.Jr. (1990a). Subarachnoid bupivacaine analgesia for seven months for a patient with a spinal cord tumor. *Anesthesiology*, 72, 1094–1096.

Berde, C. B., Sethna, N. F., Fisher, D. E., Kahn, C. H., Chandler, P., and Grier, H. E. (1990b). Celiac plexus blockade for a 3-year-old boy with hepatoblastoma and refractory pain. *Pediatrics*, 86, 779–781.

Bhalla, T., Sawardekar, A., Dewhirst, E., Jagannathan, N., and Tobias, J. D. (2012). Ultrasound-guided trunk and core blocks in infants and children. *J Anesth*, 27(1), 109–123.

Bogduk, N. (2002). Diagnostic nerve blocks in chronic pain. *Best Pract Res Clin Anaesthesiol*, 16, 565–578.

Boswell, M. V., Colson, J. D., Sehgal, N., Dunbar, E. E., and Epter, R. (2007). A systematic review of therapeutic facet joint interventions in chronic spinal pain. *Pain Physician*, 10, 229–253.

Bozkurt, P., Bakan, M., and Kilinc, L. T. (2005). [Challenges in the treatment of pain in children with cancer and tunneling of epidural catheter for long term infusion]. *Agri*, 17, 28–32.

Burgoyne, L. L., Billups, C. A., Jiron, J. L.Jr., Kaddoum, R. N., Wright, B. B., Bikhazi, G. B., et al. (2012a). Phantom limb pain in young cancer-related amputees: recent experience at St Jude children's research hospital. *Clin J Pain*, 28, 222–225.

Burgoyne, L. L., Pereiras, L. A., Bertani, L. A., Kaddoum, R. N., Neel, M., Faughnan, L. G., et al. (2012b). Long-term use of nerve block catheters in paediatric patients with cancer related pathologic fractures. *Anaesth Intensive Care*, 40, 710–713.

Celebi, N., Sahin, A., Canbay, O., Uzumcugil, F., and Aypar, U. (2006). Abdominal pain related to mitochondrial neurogastrointestinal encephalomyopathy syndrome may benefit from splanchnic nerve blockade. *Paediatr Anaesth*, 16, 1073–1076.

Chan, C. W., and Chalkiadis, G. A. (2010). A case of sympathetically mediated headache treated with stellate ganglion blockade. *Pain Med*, 11, 1294–1298.

Collins, J. J. (1996). Intractable pain in children with terminal cancer. *J Palliat Care*, 12, 29–34.

Collins, J. J. (2002). Palliative care and the child with cancer. *Hematol Oncol Clin North Am*, 16, 657–670.

Collins, J. J., Grier, H. E., Kinney, H. C., and Berde, C. B. (1995). Control of severe pain in children with terminal malignancy. *J Pediatr*, 126, 653–657.

Collins, J. J., Grier, H. E., Sethna, N. F., Wilder, R. T., and Berde, C. B. (1996). Regional anesthesia for pain associated with terminal pediatric malignancy. *Pain*, 65, 63–69.

Cooper, M. G., Keneally, J. P., and Kinchington, D. (1994). Continuous brachial plexus neural blockade in a child with intractable cancer pain. *J Pain Symptom Manage*, 9, 277–281.

Cousins, M. J., Carr, D. B., Horlocker, T. T., and Bridenbaugh, P. O. (2009). *Cousins & Bridenbaugh's neural blockade in clinical anesthesia and pain medicine* (4th edn). Philadelphia, PA: Wolters Kluwer Health, Lippincott. Williams & Wilkins.

Dadure, C., Motais, F., Ricard, C., Raux, O., Troncin, R., and Capdevila, X. (2005). Continuous peripheral nerve blocks at home for treatment of recurrent complex regional pain syndrome I in children. *Anesthesiology*, 102, 387–391.

Dahm, P., Nitescu, P., Appelgren, L., and Curelaru, I. (1998). Efficacy and technical complications of long-term continuous intraspinal infusions of opioid and/or bupivacaine in refractory nonmalignant pain: a comparison between the epidural and the intrathecal approach with externalized or implanted catheters and infusion pumps. *Clin J Pain*, 14, 4–16.

Eckel, T. S., and Bartynski, W. S. (2009). Epidural steroid injections and selective nerve root blocks. *Tech Vasc Interv Radiol*, 12, 11–21.

Ecoffey, C., Lacroix, F., Giaufre, E., Orliaguet, G., and Courreges, P. (2010). Epidemiology and morbidity of regional anesthesia in children: a follow-up one-year prospective survey of the French-Language Society of Paediatric Anaesthesiologists (ADARPEF). *Paediatr Anaesth*, 20, 1061–1069.

Elias, M. and Chakerian, M. U. (1994). Repeated stellate ganglion blockade using a catheter for pediatric herpes zoster ophthalmicus. *Anesthesiology*, 80, 950–952.

Ellinas, H. and Sethna, N. F. (2009). Ganglion impar block for management of chronic coccydynia in an adolescent. *Paediatr Anaesth*, 19, 1137–1138.

Fernandes, M. R., Barbosa, M. A., Sousa, A. L., and Ramos, G. C. (2012). Suprascapular nerve block: important procedure in clinical practice. Part II. *Rev Bras Reumatol*, 52, 616–622.

Fernandez-Mayoralas, D. M., Fernandez-Jaen, A., Jareno, N. M., Perez, B. C., Fernandez, P. M., and Sola, A. G. (2010). Meralgia paresthetica in the pediatric population: a propos of 2 cases. *J Child Neurol*, 25, 110–113.

Fishman, S. C., Ballantyne, J. C., Rathmell, J. P. (eds) (2010). *Bonica's Management of Pain. Fourth Edition.* Philadelphia, PA: Lippincott Williams & Wilkins Wolters Kluwer,

Galloway, K., Staats, P. S., and Bowers, D. C. (2000). Intrathecal analgesia for children with cancer via implanted infusion pumps. *Med Pediatr Oncol,* 34, 265–267.

Goldman, A., Hewitt, M., Collins, G. S., Childs, M., and Hain, R. (2006). Symptoms in children/young people with progressive malignant disease: United Kingdom Children's Cancer Study Group/Paediatric Oncology Nurses Forum survey. *Pediatrics,* 117, e1179–1186.

Goldschneider, K. R., Racadio, J. M., and Weidner, N. J. (2007). Celiac plexus blockade in children using a three-dimensional fluoroscopic reconstruction technique: case reports. *Reg Anesth Pain Med,* 32, 510–515.

Gurnaney, H. G., Maxwell, L. G., Kraemer, F. W., Goebel, T., Nance, M. L., and Ganesh, A. (2011). Prospective randomized observer-blinded study comparing the analgesic efficacy of ultrasound-guided rectus sheath block and local anaesthetic infiltration for umbilical hernia repair. *Br J Anaesth,* 107, 790–795.

Hansen, H., Manchikanti, L., Simopoulos, T. T., Christo, P. J., Gupta, S., Smith, H. S., *et al.* (2012). A systematic evaluation of the therapeutic effectiveness of sacroiliac joint interventions. *Pain Physician,* 15, E247–278.

Hodge, J. (2005). Facet, nerve root, and epidural block. *Semin Ultrasound CT MR,* 26, 98–102.

Irazuzta, J. E., Berde, C. B., and Sethna, N. F. (1992). Laser Doppler measurements of skin blood flow before, during, and after lumbar sympathetic blockade in children and young adults with reflex sympathetic dystrophy syndrome. *J Clin Monit,* 8, 16–19.

Jansen, J. A., Mens, J. M., Backx, F. J., Kolfschoten, N., and Stam, H. J. (2008). Treatment of longstanding groin pain in athletes: a systematic review. *Scand J Med Sci Sports,* 18, 263–274.

Kalkanis, S. N., Eskandar, E. N., Carter, B. S., and Barker, F. G. 2nd. (2003). Microvascular decompression surgery in the United States, 1996 to 2000: mortality rates, morbidity rates, and the effects of hospital and surgeon volumes. *Neurosurgery,* 52, 1251–1261; discussion 1261–1262.

Kambadakone, A., Thabet, A., Gervais, D. A., Mueller, P. R., and Arellano, R. S. (2011). CT-guided celiac plexus neurolysis: a review of anatomy, indications, technique, and tips for successful treatment. *Radiographics,* 31, 1599–1621.

Kemler, M. A., De Vet, H. C., Barendse, G. A., Van Den Wildenberg, F. A., and Van Kleef, M. (2004). The effect of spinal cord stimulation in patients with chronic reflex sympathetic dystrophy: two years' follow-up of the randomized controlled trial. *Ann Neurol,* 55, 13–18.

Kfoury, T., Staiti, G., Baujard, C., and Benhamou, D. (2008). Pudendal nerve block by nerve stimulation in a child with Waardenburg disease. *Paediatr Anaesth,* 18, 1267–1268.

Krames, E. S. (1996). Intraspinal opioid therapy for chronic nonmalignant pain: current practice and clinical guidelines. *J Pain Symptom Manage,* 11, 333–352.

Krane, E. J., and Heller, L. B. (1995). The prevalence of phantom sensation and pain in pediatric amputees. *J Pain Symptom Manage,* 10, 21–29.

Krumova, E. K., Gussone, C., Regeniter, S., Westermann, A., Zenz, M., and Maier, C. (2011). Are sympathetic blocks useful for diagnostic purposes? *Reg Anesth Pain Med,* 36, 560–567.

Levy, M. J., Chari, S. T., and Wiersema, M. J. (2012). Endoscopic ultrasound-guided celiac neurolysis. *Gastrointest Endosc Clin N Am,* 22, 231–247, viii.

Lin, C. S., Cheng, J. K., Hsu, Y. W., Chen, C. C., Lao, H. C., Huang, C. J., *et al.* (2010). Ultrasound-guided ganglion impar block: a technical report. *Pain Med,* 11, 390–394.

Logan, D.E., Carpino, E.A., Chiang, G., Condon, M., Firn, E., Gaughan, V.J., *et al.* (2012). *A day-hospital approach to treatment of pediatric complex regional pain syndrome: initial functional outcomes. Clin J Pain,* 28, 766–774.

Loukas, M., Klaassen, Z., Merbs, W., Tubbs, R. S., Gielecki, J., and Zurada, A. (2010). A review of the thoracic splanchnic nerves and celiac ganglia. *Clin Anat,* 23, 512–522.

Manchikanti, L., Buenaventura, R. M., Manchikanti, K. N., Ruan, X., Gupta, S., Smith, H. S., *et al.* (2012). Effectiveness of therapeutic lumbar transforaminal epidural steroid injections in managing lumbar spinal pain. *Pain Physician,* 15, E199–245.

Mazoit, J. X., and Dalens, B. J. (2004). Pharmacokinetics of local anaesthetics in infants and children. *Clin Pharmacokinet,* 43, 17–32.

Mcgrath, P. A., and Hillier, L. M. (1992). Phantom limb sensations in adolescents: a case study to illustrate the utility of sensation and pain logs in pediatric clinical practice. *J Pain Symptom Manage,* 7, 46–53.

Meier, P. M., Zurakowski, D., Berde, C. B., and Sethna, N. F. (2009). Lumbar sympathetic blockade in children with complex regional pain syndromes: a double blind placebo-controlled crossover trial. *Anesthesiology,* 111, 372–380.

Meignier, M., Ganansia, M. F., Lejus, C., and Testa, S. (1992). [Intrathecal morphine therapy in children with cancer]. *Cah Anesthesiol,* 40, 487–490.

Melzack, R., Israel, R., Lacroix, R., and Schultz, G. (1997). Phantom limbs in people with congenital limb deficiency or amputation in early childhood. *Brain,* 120 (Pt 9), 1603–1620.

Nabil, D. and Eissa, A. A. (2010). Evaluation of posteromedial transdiscal superior hypogastric block after failure of the classic approach. *Clin J Pain,* 26, 694–697.

Naja, Z., Al-Tannir, M. A., Faysal, W., Daoud, N., Ziade, F., and El-Rajab, M. (2011). A comparison of pudendal block vs dorsal penile nerve block for circumcision in children: a randomised controlled trial. *Anaesthesia,* 66, 802–807.

Olsson, G. L., Meyerson, B. A., and Linderoth, B. (2008). Spinal cord stimulation in adolescents with complex regional pain syndrome type I (CRPS-I). *Eur J Pain,* 12, 53–59.

Parr, A. T., Manchikanti, L., Hameed, H., Conn, A., Manchikanti, K. N., Benyamin, R. M., *et al.* (2012). Caudal epidural injections in the management of chronic low back pain: a systematic appraisal of the literature. *Pain Physician,* 15, E159–198.

Patt, R. B., Payne, R., Farhat, G. A., and Reddy, S. K. (1995). Subarachnoid neurolytic block under general anesthesia in a 3-year-old with neuroblastoma. *Clin J Pain,* 11, 143–146.

Peng, P. W., and Narouze, S. (2009). Ultrasound-guided interventional procedures in pain medicine: a review of anatomy, sonoanatomy, and procedures: part I: nonaxial structures. *Reg Anesth Pain Med,* 34, 458–474.

Peng, P. W., and Tumber, P. S. (2008). Ultrasound-guided interventional procedures for patients with chronic pelvic pain—a description of techniques and review of literature. *Pain Physician,* 11, 215–224.

Perez, R. S., Zollinger, P. E., Dijkstra, P. U., Thomassen-Hilgersom, I. L., Zuurmond, W. W., Rosenbrand, K. C., *et al.* (2010). Evidence based guidelines for complex regional pain syndrome type 1. *BMC Neurol,* 10, 20.

Plancarte, R. and Patt, R. (1991). Intractable upper body pain in a pediatric patient relieved with cervical epidural opioid administration. *J Pain Symptom Manage,* 6, 98–99.

Plummer, J. L., Cherry, D. A., Cousins, M. J., Gourlay, G. K., Onley, M. M., and Evans, K. H. (1991). Long-term spinal administration of morphine in cancer and non-cancer pain: a retrospective study. *Pain,* 44, 215–220.

Portas, M., Marty, J. Y., Buttin, C., Gentet, J. C., Coze, C., Fallouh, K., *et al.* (1998). [Refractory pain in children with cancer: role of peridural analgesia]. *Arch Pediatr,* 5, 851–860.

Price, D. D., Long, S., Wilsey, B., and Rafii, A. (1998). Analysis of peak magnitude and duration of analgesia produced by local anesthetics injected into sympathetic ganglia of complex regional pain syndrome patients. *Clinical Journal of Pain,* 14, 216–226.

Prithvi Raj, P. (2008). *Interventional pain management: image-guided procedures* (2nd edn). Philadelphia, PA: Saunders Elsevier.

Puli, S. R., Reddy, J. B., Bechtold, M. L., Antillon, M. R., and Brugge, W. R. (2009). EUS-guided celiac plexus neurolysis for pain due to chronic pancreatitis or pancreatic cancer pain: a meta-analysis and systematic review. *Dig Dis Sci,* 54, 2330–2337.

Queinnec, M. C., Esteve, M., and Vedrenne, J. (1999). Positive effect of regional analgesia (RA) in terminal stage paediatric chondrosarcoma: a case report and the review of the literature. *Pain*, 83, 383–385.

Quraishi, N. A. (2012). Transforaminal injection of corticosteroids for lumbar radiculopathy: systematic review and meta-analysis. *Eur Spine J*, 21, 214–219.

Resnick, D. K., Levy, E. I., and Jannetta, P. J. (1998). Microvascular decompression for pediatric onset trigeminal neuralgia. *Neurosurgery*, 43, 804–807; discussion 807–808.

Schmidt, A. P., Schmidt, S. R., and Ribeiro, S. M. (2005). Is superior hypogastric plexus block effective for treatment of chronic pelvic pain? *Rev Bras Anestesiol*, 55, 669–679.

Schwarzer, A. C., Aprill, C. N., Derby, R., Fortin, J., Kine, G., and Bogduk, N. (1994a). Clinical features of patients with pain stemming from the lumbar zygapophysial joints. Is the lumbar facet syndrome a clinical entity? *Spine (Phila Pa 1976)*, 19, 1132–1137.

Schwarzer, A. C., Derby, R., Aprill, C. N., Fortin, J., Kine, G., and Bogduk, N. (1994b). Pain from the lumbar zygapophysial joints: a test of two models. *J Spinal Disord*, 7, 331–336.

Sessle, B. J. (2000). Acute and chronic craniofacial pain: brainstem mechanisms of nociceptive transmission and neuroplasticity, and their clinical correlates. *Crit Rev Oral Biol Med*, 11, 57–91.

Sethna, N. F., and Berde, C. B. (2012). Sympathetic nerve blocks, pragmatic trials, and responder analysis. *Anesthesiology*, 116, 12–14.

Sethna, N. F., Clendenin, D., Athiraman, U., Solodiuk, J., Rodriguez, D. P., and Zurakowski, D. (2010). Incidence of epidural catheter-associated infections after continuous epidural analgesia in children. *Anesthesiology*, 113, 224–232.

Sethna, N. F., Meier, P. M., Zurakowski, D., and Berde, C. B. (2007). Cutaneous sensory abnormalities in children and adolescents with complex regional pain syndromes. *Pain*, 131, 153–161.

Sethna, N. F., and Wilder, R. T. (1993). Regional anesthetic techniques for chronic pain. In N. L. Schechter, C. B. Berde, and M. Yasters, (eds) *Pain in infants, children, and adolescents*, pp. 281–293. Baltimore, MD: Williams & Wilkins.

Shanahan, E. M., Ahern, M., Smith, M., Wetherall, M., Bresnihan, B., and Fitzgerald, O. (2003). Suprascapular nerve block (using bupivacaine and methylprednisolone acetate) in chronic shoulder pain. *Ann Rheum Dis*, 62, 400–406.

Sharma, A., Williams, K., and Raja, S. N. (2006). Advances in treatment of complex regional pain syndrome: recent insights on a perplexing disease. *Curr Opin Anaesthesiol*, 19, 566–572.

Sharma, C., Eltawil, K. M., Renfrew, P. D., Walsh, M. J., and Molinari, M. (2011). Advances in diagnosis, treatment and palliation of pancreatic carcinoma: 1990–2010. *World J Gastroenterol*, 17, 867–897.

Shim, J. H., Ko, S. Y., Bang, M. R., Jeon, W. J., Cho, S. Y., Yeom, J. H., *et al.* (2011). Ultrasound-guided greater occipital nerve block for patients with occipital headache and short term follow up. *Korean J Anesthesiol*, 61, 50–4.

Shimazaki, M., Egawa, H., Motojima, F., Fujimaki, K., Hamaguchi, S., Okuda, Y., *et al.* (2003). [Intrathecal phenol block in a child with cancer pain—a case report]. *Masui*, 52, 756–758.

Simmel, M. L. (1962). Phantom experiences following amputation in childhood. *J Neurol Neurosurg Psychiatry*, 25, 69–78.

Simopoulos, T. T., Manchikanti, L., Singh, V., Gupta, S., Hameed, H., Diwan, S., *et al.* (2012). A systematic evaluation of prevalence and diagnostic accuracy of sacroiliac joint interventions. *Pain Physician*, 15(3), E305–344.

Skinner, A. V., and Lauder, G. R. (2007). Rectus sheath block: successful use in the chronic pain management of pediatric abdominal wall pain. *Paediatr Anaesth*, 17, 1203–1211.

Smith, J. and Thompson, J. M. (1995). Phantom limb pain and chemotherapy in pediatric amputees. *Mayo Clin Proc*, 70, 357–364.

Staats, P. S., and Kost-Byerly, S. (1995). Celiac plexus blockade in a 7-year-old child with neuroblastoma. *J Pain Symptom Manage*, 10, 321–324.

Stark, E., Oestreich, K., Wendl, K., Rumstadt, B., and Hagmuller, E. (1999). Nerve irritation after laparoscopic hernia repair. *Surg Endosc*, 13, 878–881.

Strafford, M. A., Wilder, R. T., and Berde, C. B. (1995). The risk of infection from epidural analgesia in children: a review of 1620 cases. *Anesth Analg*, 80, 234–238.

Suresh, S. and Voronov, P. (2012). Head and neck blocks in infants, children, and adolescents. *Paediatr Anaesth*, 22, 81–87.

Tanelian, D. and Cousins, M.J. (1989). Celiac plexus block following high-dose opiates for chronic noncancer pain in a four-year-old child. *J Pain Symptom Manage*, 4, 82–85.

Teitelbaum, J. E., Berde, C. B., Nurko, S., Buonomo, C., Perez-Atayde, A. R., and Fox, V.L. (2002). Diagnosis and management of MNGIE syndrome in children: case report and review of the literature. *J Pediatr Gastroenterol Nutr*, 35, 377–383.

Thomas, C. R., Brazeal, B. A., Rosenberg, L., Robert, R. S., Blakeney, P. E., and Meyer, W. J. (2003). Phantom limb pain in pediatric burn survivors. *Burns*, 29, 139–1342.

Tobias, J. D. (2000). Applications of intrathecal catheters in children. *Paediatr Anaesth*, 10, 367–375.

Tong, H. C., and Nelson, V. S. (2000). Recurrent and migratory reflex sympathetic dystrophy in children. *Pediatr Rehabil*, 4, 87–89.

Van Boxem, K., Van Eerd, M., Brinkhuizen, T., Patijn, J., Van Kleef, M., and Van Zundert, J. (2008). Radiofrequency and pulsed radiofrequency treatment of chronic pain syndromes: the available evidence. *Pain Pract*, 8, 385–393.

Van Eijs, F., Geurts, J., Van Kleef, M., Faber, C. G., Perez, R. S., Kessels, A. G., *et al.* (2012). Predictors of pain relieving response to sympathetic blockade in complex regional pain syndrome type 1. *Anesthesiology*, 116, 113–121.

Veyckemans, F., Scholtes, J. L., and Ninane, J. (1994). Cervical epidural analgesia for a cancer child at home. *Med Pediatr Oncol*, 22, 58–60.

Whyte, E. and Lauder, G. (2012). Intrathecal infusion of bupivacaine and clonidine provides effective analgesia in a terminally ill child. *Paediatr Anaesth*, 22, 173–175.

Wilder, R. T., Berde, C. B., Wolohan, M., Vieyra, M. A., Masek, B. J., and Micheli, L. J. (1992). Reflex sympathetic dystrophy in children. Clinical characteristics and follow-up of seventy patients. *J Bone Joint Surg*, A-74, 910–919.

Wilkins, K. L., Mcgrath, P. J., Finley, G. A., and Katz, J. (1998). Phantom limb sensations and phantom limb pain in child and adolescent amputees. *Pain*, 78, 7–12.

Wolfe, J., Klar, N., Grier, H. E., Duncan, J., Salem-Schatz, S., Emanuel, E. J., and Weeks, J. C. (2000). Understanding of prognosis among parents of children who died of cancer: impact on treatment goals and integration of palliative care. *JAMA*, 284, 2469–2475.

Yue, W. L. (2004). Peripheral glycerol injection for the relief of facial neuralgia in children. *Int J Pediatr Otorhinolaryngol*, 68, 37–41.

CHAPTER 47

Topical anaesthetics and analgesics

William T. Zempsky

Summary

Topical administration of anaesthetics and analgesics can allow for the efficient, painless delivery of medications which may reduce systemic side effects associated with the medication while providing clinical advantages over injected or oral administration for the same clinical situation. Topical anaesthetics have become widely used prior to a variety of painful procedures in children including venous access, laceration repair, and injections. Topical administration of non-steroidal anti-inflammatory drugs, lidocaine, capsaicin, and other agents also are useful for a range of conditions including acute and chronic musculoskeletal pain, and neuropathic pain.

Background

It is important to differentiate between topical and transdermal medications. Topical medications target the site of application and ideally produce effective drug concentrations locally with minimal systemic absorption. Topical anaesthetics and analgesics target the peripheral nerves and soft tissue at that site (Galer, 2001). In contrast, transdermal medications do not have to be applied over an involved site and attempt to reach systemic drug concentrations to achieve therapeutic results (Argoff, 2004). This chapter will focus on topical medications (Table 47.1).

Benefits of topical drug delivery in general may include the potential for local therapeutic drug levels with reduced side effects, painless drug delivery, improved patient adherence (which is especially important in children) and acceptance, ease of dose termination, avoidance of first-pass metabolism, and direct access to the target site.

The skin is an effective barrier to drug delivery, its primary role being to prevent the ingress or egress of compounds across it (Tadicherla, 2006). The stratum corneum, the uppermost layer of the skin consists of a thin layer of cornified non-viable keratinocytes interconnected by highly ordered lipid bilayers, and has evolved to be a highly effective barrier to water-soluble substances, which typically include anaesthetics (Houck and Sethna, 2005). Topical medications must transverse the stratum corneum to reach their site of action which may be the peripheral transducing terminals of cutaneous sensory fibres located in the dermis and epidermis (Lumpkin and Caterina, 2007), or the local soft tissues including synovial fluid, synovial tissue and cartilaginous structures (Bandolier extra, 2005) (Figure 47.1).

Three delivery methods have been utilized to bypass the stratum corneum barrier (Zempsky, 2008):

- Injection of local anaesthetics or other medications, usually via a small-gauge hypodermic syringe, is the oldest of the methodologies.

- Passive diffusion from creams, gels, or patches comprises the second general class of methodologies. Passive diffusion of topical agents require that they have a molecular weight under 500 Daltons, with a hydrophobic component to allow it to transverse the stratum corneum but also some hydrophilic features to penetrate the epidermis (Stamos, 2007).

- Active drug delivery methods which enhance the rate of drug passage through the skin and shorten the time to onset of action. There are a diverse group of technologies which facilitate the drug delivery process. These include heat-enhanced diffusion, iontophoresis, sonophoresis, laser-assisted transdermal passage, or pressurized gas delivery of powdered drug particles (Zempsky, 2008). Microporation, a newer technology, uses tiny microneedles to penetrate the stratum corneum and directly place the drug within the epidermis (Yadav, 2011).

Topical as well as transdermal drug delivery is a rapidly expanding field. Most of the drugs and technologies used for topical anaesthesia have been well studied in children; however, this is not the case for topical medications used for musculoskeletal and neuropathic pain which will be discussed in this chapter. The extrapolation of use of the these agents in children seem reasonable given several factors: the pharmacodynamic response to most medications including local anaesthetics, opioids, and non-steroidal anti-inflammatories (NSAIDs) are substantially mature by age 2 years, the degree of systemic absorption of these topical medications is low, and the local skin effects are for the most part minimal and short lived (Berde, 2012).

Topical anaesthetics for procedural pain

The ideal topical anaesthetic should have good efficacy, an excellent safety profile, convenient application, enduring effect, and reasonable cost. Specific properties important for topical anaesthesia prior to a procedure include rapid onset of analgesia to minimize disruption and delay of needed medical procedures, minimal systemic

Table 47.1 Common topical anaesthetics and analgesics

Drug	Brand or other names	Use
Lidocaine prilocaine cream	EMLA® and others	Procedural pain
Tetracaine	Amethocaine®, Ametop®	Procedural pain
Liposomal lidocaine	LMX⁴®, Maxilene®	Procedural pain
Vapocoolant spray	Painease® and others	Procedural pain
5% lidocaine patch	Lidoderm®	Neuropathic and musculoskeletal pain
Topical NSAIDs	Flector®, Voltaren®, Pennsaid®, and others	Musculoskeletal pain
Capsaicin	Zostrix®, Qutenza®, and others	Neuropathic pain
Menthol and methylsalicylates	Many	Musculoskeletal pain
Ketamine and amitriptyline	Compounding pharmacist	Neuropathic pain

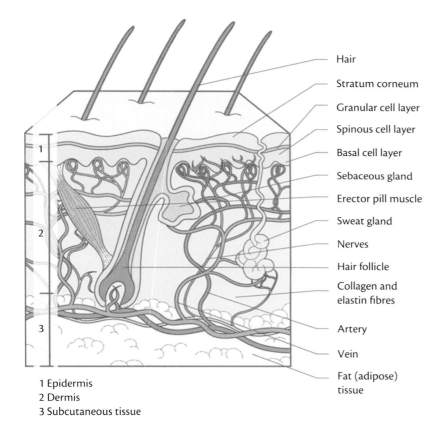

Hair

Stratum corneum

Granular cell layer

Spinous cell layer

Basal cell layer

Sebaceous gland

Erector pill muscle

Sweat gland

Nerves

Hair follicle

Collagen and elastin fibres

Artery

Vein

Fat (adipose) tissue

1 Epidermis
2 Dermis
3 Subcutaneous tissue

Figure 47.1 Reproduced from Mark Gardiner et al, Training in Paediatrics: *The Essential Curriculum*, Figure 9.1, p.194, Oxford University Press, Oxford, UK, Copyright © 2009, by permission of Oxford University Press.

absorption, no untoward dermal effects, and no adverse effect on the success rate of the procedure (Zempsky, 2008). No commercially available agent is likely to have all of these properties.

Topical anaesthetics for procedural pain differ from one another primarily in their drug delivery mechanisms, rather than in their underlying pharmacological modes of action. Most available agents utilize lidocaine, prilocaine, and/or tetracaine (also known as amethocaine) and produce their analgesia through similar mechanisms involving inhibition of sodium ion channels in sensory neurons.

Lidocaine and prilocaine cream, 2.5%/2.5% (EMLA® Cream (eutectic mixture of local anaesthetics), AstraZeneca LP, Wilmington, DE) is the most well studied topical anaesthetic and has been used in clinical practice for approximately 25 years. When mixed in a 1:1 ratio, crystals of lidocaine and prilocaine produce a 'eutectic mixture', a mixture that has a lower melting point than either component alone. Within the cream, the local anaesthetics exist as a liquid oil rather than as crystals; this leads to higher concentration of anaesthetic within the oil thus an increase in the rate of diffusion into the epidermal and dermal layers. In some countries a eutectic mixture of lidocaine and prilocaine is also available in a patch formulation.

A large number of clinical trials in both children and adults have analysed its efficacy for venepuncture pain and intravenous cannulation pain (Ehrenstrom-Reiz, 1983; Hallen and Uppfeldt, 1982; D. L. Halperin et al., 1989; Lander et al., 1996; Maunuksela and Korpela, 1986; Moller, 1985). A meta-analysis of these trials concluded that lidocaine and prilocaine cream provided significant analgesia for both venepuncture and cannulation procedures, with similar and consistent effects across both procedures, with 85% of patients receiving exhibiting significant analgesic benefit from its application prior to the procedure (Fetzer, 2002). The analgesia appears to be independent of age, location of the procedure, and intravenous insertion technique (Fetzer, 2002). Lidocaine and prilocaine cream also reduces pain associated with vaccination and has not been shown to impact immunogenicity (S. A. Halperin, 2000).

The efficacy of lidocaine and prilocaine cream is dependent upon dosage and application time. A thick layer (2.0 ml) is more effective than a thin layer (0.5 ml) in reducing pain (Sims, 1991). The minimum recommended treatment time is 60 min, but longer durations (>90 min) are known to produce greater pain relief (Houck and Sethna, 2005). Protocols (such as application in triage in the emergency department) can overcome the practical challenge of delayed onset of anaesthesia for use in clinical settings.

Lidocaine and prilocaine cream is efficacious and safe for use in neonates and prematures down to 26 weeks for blood drawing (Taddio, 1998), lumbar puncture (Kaur, 2003), suprapubic aspiration (Nahum, 2007) and circumcision (Taddio, 1997, 1998). Efficacy for heel lancing has not been demonstrated (Taddio, 1998). For neonates 0 to 3 months of age or in any child less than 5 kg, maximum total dose of lidocaine and prilocaine cream should be 1 g, the maximum application area should be 10 cm^2, and the maximum application time should be 1 h (Taddio et al., 1998) (Table 47.2).

Lidocaine and prilocaine cream causes vasoconstriction, which leads to blanching of the skin. Allergic and anaphylactoid reactions associated with lidocaine or prilocaine can rarely occur. In young infants who do not have adult levels of methaemoglobin reductase, in patients who are on medications which put them at increased risk, or have prolonged application times use of lidocaine and prilocaine cream may be associated with methaemoglobinaemia. However methaemoglobinaemia was not demonstrated with appropriate use of this agent in neonates (Taddio, 1998).

Tetracaine or amethocaine gel (Ametop Gel™, Smith & Nephew, London, UK), currently available in Australia, Canada, New Zealand, and the UK, consists of 4% tetracaine base in an aqueous gel (Obrien et al., 2005). When applied to skin, solid tetracaine particles liquefy to form an oil emulsion that better penetrates the stratum corneum (Obrien et al., 2005). Like lidocaine and prilocaine cream, tetracaine gel is usually applied with an occlusive dressing.

Tetracaine gel has been demonstrated to provide comparable anaesthesia to lidocaine and prilocaine for venous access and other dermal procedures (Bishai et al., 1999; Lawson et al., 1995; Rømsing et al., 1999). For intravenous cannulation a tetracaine gel is preferred over lidocaine- prilocaine cream (Lander, 2006). In neonates, tetracaine is effective for pain of venepuncture and injection but not heel lance (Jain and Ruttner, 2000; Jain et al., 2001; Shah et al., 2008). Tetracaine gel produces analgesia in 30 to 45 min, and has a longer duration of anaesthesia (4–6 h) than lidocaine and prilocaine cream (2 h) (Houck and Sethna, 2005; Lander, 2006). Tetracaine gels' prolonged duration of action may be due to a depot effect in the stratum corneum and an affinity of tetracaine for proteins, which may prolong its binding to sodium channels on sensory neurons (Obrien, 2005).

No significant systemic adverse events with tetracaine gel have been reported. Transient erythema followed by oedema and pruritus are the most common side effects (Obrien et al., 2005). Tetracaine causes vasodilation which has been theorized to facilitate vascular access (Houck and Sethna, 2005); however, in a comparative study first attempt success rates between 4% tetracaine and lidocaine-prilocaine cream were not different (75.8% versus 73.9%) (Newbury and Herd, 2009).

Liposomes are vesicles consisting of concentric lipid bilayers (phospholipids and cholesterol) that enclose an aqueous compartment (Kshirsagar, 2005). By encapsulating a drug in liposomes the surrounding bilayer protects it from *in vivo* degradation enzymes and allows fusion with other bilayers (Kshirsagar, 2005). Liposomal lidocaine 4% is available in the US (LMX4®, Ferndale Laboratories, Detroit, MI) and Canada (Maxilene®, Ferndale Laboratories, Detroit, MI) and can be used with or without an occlusive dressing.

Liposomal lidocaine 4% is efficacious in children undergoing venous access procedures (Eichenfield et al., 2002; Koh et al., 2004; Taddio et al., 2005). Procedural success rate was higher in a liposomal lidocaine 4% group compared to the placebo group in patients undergoing venous access (Taddio et al., 2005). A systematic review found liposomal lidocaine to be as efficacious as lidocaine prilocaine cream and tetracaine gel (Eidelman et al., 2005).

Safety of liposomal lidocaine is similar to other creams and gels. Adverse events are usually limited to pallor, redness, and mild itching at the application site (Eichenfield et al., 2005). Liposomal lidocaine 4% has not been investigated in great detail in children younger than 2 years of age (Zempsky, 2008).

Table 47.2 Lidocaine and prilocaine cream maximum recommended dose, application area, and application time by age and weight (EMLA® package insert, n.d.)

Age and body weight	Maximum total dose	Maximum application area	Maximum application time
0–3 months or <5 kg	1 g	10 cm^2	1 h
3–12 months and >5 kg	2 g	20 cm^2	4 h
1–6 years and >10 kg	10 g	100 cm^2	4 h
7–12 years and >20 kg	20 g	200 cm^2	4 h

Please note: if a patient greater than 3 months old does not meet the minimum weight requirement, the maximum total dose of lidocaine and prilocaine cream should be restricted to that which corresponds to the patient's weight.

These are broad guidelines for avoiding systemic toxicity in applying lidocaine and prilocaine cream to patients with normal intact skin and with normal renal and hepatic function.

For more individualized calculation of how much lidocaine and prilocaine may be absorbed, physicians can use the following estimates of lidocaine and prilocaine absorption for children and adults: the estimated mean (±SD) absorption of lidocaine is 0.045 (±0.016) mg/cm^2/h; the estimated mean (±SD) absorption of prilocaine is 0.077 (±0.036) mg/cm^2/h.

Unlike the other topical anaesthetic options, vapocoolant sprays do not rely on a chemical anaesthetic. Instead, they rapidly cool the skin, which slows initiation and conduction of impulses in cutaneous sensory nerves and increases their refractoriness (Burke et al., 1999). Composed of volatile liquid refrigerants, vapocoolant sprays are applied to the skin and their rapid evaporation produces a short-lived (<1 min) anaesthetic effect. These agents can be directly sprayed onto the skin or applied via saturated cotton balls.

Studies of vapocoolant sprays for prevention of procedural pain have reported mixed results. In a review of trials for venous access pain four out of eight trials could not demonstrate increased efficacy over placebo or no treatment while the other four demonstrated significant benefit (Bandolier extra, n.d.).

Studies are also inconsistent for injection pain. A vapocoolant spray provided significantly more analgesia than cold saline spray in adults (Mawhorter et al., 2004) and, when combined with distraction, provided significantly more pain relief than distraction alone in children and the analgesic effect was similar to lidocaine and prilocaine cream plus distraction (Reis and Holubkuv, 1997.) However, a meta-analysis of five studies evaluating vapocoolants for immunization did not demonstrate benefit (Shah, 2009).

The heterogeneous results provided by vapocoolants may be due to the short-lived nature of the anaesthesia, small sample sizes of the study, differences in the length of anaesthesia needed for the procedure, and varied administration technique of the vapocoolant itself (Bandolier extra, n.d.). Studies that demonstrated benefit for immunization pain applied the vapocoolant using a cotton ball held in place for 10 to 15 sec (Shah, 2009).

Use of vapocoolant sprays has been associated with some rare cases of allergic contact dermatitis, and prolonged spraying can cause hypo-pigmentation and atrophic scarring, especially in patients with poor circulation. Most vapocoolant sprays contain chemicals that are eye irritants (Bircher, 1994).

Penetration of local anaesthetics through the stratum corneum is accelerated by heat (Hull, 2002). The lidocaine/tetracaine topical patch (Synera™, Nuvo Research Inc. Mississauga, Ontario; Rapydan™, EUSA, England), has a heating component that generates a mild warming when exposed to air, and an adhesive to fix the patch to the skin (Sethna et al., 2005). The lidocaine/tetracaine patch provided superior analgesia to placebo in a paediatric venous access study of children aged 3 to 17 who received treatment for 20 min prior to venous access (Sethna et al., 2005). In an adult study the lidocaine/tetracaine patch provided superior analgesia for 10-, 20-, and 30-minute application times prior to venous access than lidocaine/prilocaine cream but at 60 min the two anaesthetics were equivalent (Sawyer 2004). The lidocaine/tetracaine patch was also equivalent to 4% tetracaine in a study of 100 adults requiring venous cannulation for day surgery. The warmth has the potential to ease venous access by dilating veins but this has not been evaluated. Adverse events with the lidocaine/tetracaine patch are limited to local irritation and erythema.

There are several other active drug delivery technologies which have been demonstrated to be effective for speeding lidocaine delivery allowing for more rapid skin anaesthesia prior to dermal procedures. The following technologies described are not currently in clinical use.

Lidocaine iontophoresis is the process where positively charged lidocaine is accelerated into the skin under the influence of a low-voltage direct electrical current (Figure 47.2). The quantity and distribution of delivered drug is dependent on the ion charge, molecular weight, intensity of the electric current, concentration of the drug, contact surface area of the delivery electrode, and duration of current (Zempsky and Ashburn, 1998). Lidocaine iontophoresis provides better anaesthesia with a 10 min application than iontophoresis of placebo, and at least equivalent anaesthesia to a 60 min application of lidocaine and prilocaine cream, and lidocaine infiltration (Galinkin et al., 2002; Miller 2001; Zempsky et al., 1998, 2004). However, tingling, itching, burning sensation, and discomfort have been documented in trials, and burns, which have been reported to occur at incidences of 1 per 15 000 to 20 000 treatments, remain a concern clinical acceptability of this technology for topical anaesthesia (Rattenbury and Worthy, 1996; Zempsky et al., 1998).

The Epiture Easytouch™ System (Norwood Abbey Ltd, Frankston, Australia), is a single-pulse laser device that can be used before dermal procedures to ablate a patch of stratum corneum 6 mm in diameter which allows for a topical anaesthetic such as liposomal lidocaine to provide anaesthesia in about 5 min (Shapiro, 2002). This system has been shown to be effective in reducing pain associated with needle procedures in healthy adults (Baron, 2003; Shapiro 2002). Mild pain, itching, and erythema of the skin may be apparent at the ablation site following treatment. Patients treated with dermatological lasers are known to experience temporary hyper-pigmentation or hypopigmentation at the treatment site (Zempsky, 2008).

Low-frequency ultrasound produces gaseous cavities in a liquid medium, a process known as acoustic cavitation which can disrupt lipid bilayers in the stratum corneum to accelerate transdermal passage of drugs (Mitragotri and Kost, 2004). This technology can be used in conjunction with anaesthetic creams with shorter application times. Sonophoresis followed by a 5 min application of liposomal lidocaine has been evaluated in both adults and children for venous access pain and is superior to no treatment or placebo and equivalent to a 30 min treatment of liposomal lidocaine (Becker et al., 2005; Skarbek-Borowska et al., 2006; Zempsky et al., 2008). Adverse events immediately after ultrasound are limited to redness and mild discomfort.

Lidocaine particles can be delivered painlessly into the skin under pressure. Helium gas when released accelerates lidocaine particles to velocities that are sufficient to penetrate the epidermis and produce local analgesia. Onset of action for venous access procedures is within 1 to 3 min with superiority over placebo in large randomized controlled trials in children. Skin reactions such as erythema, petechiae are short-lived and self-limited (Zempsky, 2008a, 2008b).

Topical anaesthetics can also be used to provide either complete or partial anaesthesia prior to wound repair (Eidelman et al., 2011). The most well studied of these solutions are tetracaine adrenaline and cocaine (TAC) and lidocaine, epinephrine (adrenaline), and tetracaine (LET). Due to the disruption of the epidermis these solutions are easily absorbed into the wound with the vasoconstrictor minimizing diffusion. LET has essentially replaced TAC in the US due to the expense of cocaine as well as drug control and safety issues. LET which can be made by the in-hospital pharmacy as a liquid or gel preparation, provides excellent wound anaesthesia for facial lacerations in 20 to 30 min (Ernst et al., 1995; Schilling et al., 1995). TAC and LET are less effective for extremity wounds and repair of these lacerations often requires supplemental anaesthesia (Singer and Stark, 2001; Zempsky and Karasic, 1997). A Cochrane

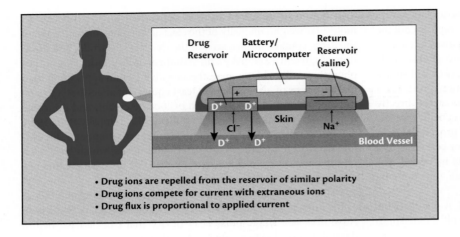

Figure 47.2 Schematic of iontophoretic drug delivery. Reprinted from *Advanced Drug Delivery Reviews*, Volume 54S, H. E Junginger, Iontophoretic delivery of apomorphine: from in-vitro modelling to the Parkinson patient, pp. S57–75, Copyright © 2002, with permission from Elsevier, http://www.sciencedirect.com/science/journal/0169409X. Figure includes data from *Journal of Controlled Release*, Volume 41, Issues 1–2, Philip G. Green, Iontophoretic delivery of peptide drugs, pp. 33–48, Copyright © 1996, with permission from Elsevier, http://www.sciencedirect.com/science/journal/01683659.

review of topical anaesthetics for wound repair recommended future trials comparing LET to other cocaine-free compounds, as well as further study of in pre-verbal and non-verbal children. Application on or near mucous membranes should be avoided with these compounds to minimize the potential for systemic absorption.

Topical medications for the treatment of musculoskeletal and neuropathic pain

While indicated for the treatment of postherpetic neuralgia in the US, lidocaine 5% topical anaesthetic patch (Lidoderm®, Endo Pharmaceuticals, Chadds Ford, PA) has gained usage in a variety of clinical conditions both neuropathic and musculoskeletal. A 5% lidocaine patch is composed of an adhesive material containing that is applied to a non-woven polyester felt backing which allows for slow release of lidocaine. The patch provides analgesic action, reducing pain with some decrease in sensory function but without the complete loss of sensation thus it is not effective for procedural pain (Krumova et al., 2012; Wehrfritz et al., 2011). The size of the patch is 10 cm × 14 cm (Galer, 1999).

In addition to treatment of postherpetic neuralgia, the 5% lidocaine patch has been used with efficacy in a variety of neuropathic pain conditions such as post-thoracotomy pain, complex regional pain syndrome, and post amputation pain (Devers and Galer, 2000). The lidocaine patch is also effective for musculoskeletal conditions. The 5% lidocaine patch has been shown to be effective in adults with osteoarthritis (Galer, 2004a; Gammaaitoni, 2004) and with lower back pain (Galer et al., 2004b; Gimbel et al., 2005). The lack of significant side effects makes topical 5% lidocaine an appropriate option in adults for any focal neuropathic pain with allodynia or hyperalgesia (Jensen et al., 2009). The patch must be placed at the site of pain in order to be effective.

While it has not been studied specifically in children we have used it successfully in many of the conditions described previously, especially lower back pain and focal neuropathic pains. Lidocaine absorption in adult usage amounts to only 3% to 5% of the total dose available in the patch and systemic levels do not increase with daily use, and systemic toxicity in adults is felt not to be a significant risk (Campbell et al., 2002; Lidoderm Package Insert, n.d.). For children under 50 kg we limit the treatment to one to two patches for 12 h per day to insure safety. Children over 50 kg can use the adult dose of three patches for 12 h per day. Often 7 to 10 days of

treatment is necessary before efficacy is noted. Side effects are usually limited to redness or other signs of skin irritation.

Topical NSAIDS can provide local relief without the risks of an orally or parenterally delivered NSAID. They have primarily been evaluated for osteoarthritis and acute musculoskeletal injury. These drugs are applied over the injured or painful body part and penetrate into the subcutaneous tissues, musculature, and tendons where they exert their therapeutic action (Esparza et al., 2007).

After administration of topical NSAIDs peak plasma concentrations are 0.2% to 8% of concentrations achieved with appropriate oral dosing (Heyneman et al., 2000). However, levels of NSAID in the meniscus and cartilaginous structures as well as in muscular tissues are four to seven times greater after topical administration than oral administration (Bandolier extra, 2005; Tegeder et al., 1995). Concentrations in the tendon sheath are several hundred times greater than plasma concentration after topical administration. Length of time to Cmax is about ten times longer in topically rather than orally administered NSAIDs with Cmax for topical preparations ranging from 2.2 to 23 h (Heyneman et al., 2000).

Unlike orally administered NSAIDs, topical NSAIDs have not been associated with increased risk of bleeding, and the risk of any gastrointestinal side effects for topical administration is considerably lower (Bandolier extra, 2005). Adverse events with topical NSAIDs are predominately local cutaneous reactions. Photosensitivity is a rare adverse reaction to topical NSAIDs (Bandolier extra, 2005).

There are a variety of preparations of topical NSAIDs including creams, gels, patches, and plasters. NSAIDS delivered topically include diclofenac, ketoprofen, and ibuprofen. Superiority of topical NSAIDs compared with placebo has been demonstrated for both diclofenac and ketoprofen patches for acute musculoskeletal conditions (Haroutiunian et al., 2010). Based on a large meta-analysis ketoprofen may be the most effective of the topical NSAIDs for acute pain (Mason et al., 2004). Though there are fewer comparative trials, in general, topical NSAIDs appear as effective and have a better safety profile in adults than oral NSAIDs, though onset of action is slower (Heyneman et al., 2000; Underwood et al., 2008).

Unfortunately there are no randomized trials of topical NSAIDs in the paediatric age group. Given the excellent safety profile and low systemic absorption of topical NSAIDs, utilization of these agents in children and adolescents with acute or chronic musculoskeletal pain is a reasonable option.

Capsaicin, the active compound in chilli peppers, is a counter irritant (a substance applied to the skin which, by acting as an irritant on a painful zone, attenuates the sensation of pain) which provides some relief in neuropathic pain conditions. Capsaicin is a TRPV1 agonist that first activates nociceptive nerve fibres in the skin and causes the release of substance P which results in neurogenic inflammation. This is followed by reversible defunctionalization of nerve endings resulting in the inhibition of pain transmission (Derry et al., 2009; Irving et al., 2011; Knoktova et al., 2008).

Low-concentration (0.025% and 0.075%) capsaicin creams have shown mild efficacy in a variety of neuropathic conditions including postherpetic neuralgia, diabetic neuropathy, polyneuropathy, and postsurgical neuropathic pain. These creams must be applied several times a day and can take several weeks of application to have effect (Knotkova et al., 2008). More recently an 8% capsaicin patch has been developed for one-time use and shown efficacy in postherpetic neuralgia and HIV neuropathic pain (Irving et al., 2011). Oral capsaicin has shown some efficacy in reducing mucositis pain in adult cancer patients (Berger et al., 1995).

Local skin irritation with capsaicin cream use is common with burning and erythema and itching are predominant side effects. These effects usually diminish after 1 to 2 weeks of use. Pretreatment of the skin with topical anaesthetic is necessary prior to use of the capsaicin 8% patch to improve tolerability.

Use of capsaicin in paediatrics is limited to case reports. This includes the use of a compounded form of 10% capsaicin in a 9-year-old with erythromelalgia (McElhiney, 2011). Given the rare incidence of systemic side effects, use of capsaicin for neuropathic pain in children and adolescents could be considered and will be limited by tolerance to the application.

Other counter irritants such as methyl salicylates and menthol have also been used for musculoskeletal pain. Methyl salicylate may have direct analgesic effects but also provides tissue warming by its vasodilatory effects (Higashi et al., 2010). Menthol's mode of action is likely the cooling effect it has on the skin. There is limited evidence for the efficacy of these compounds however a recent study of a 10% methyl salicylate 3% menthol patch demonstrated greater pain relief than placebo in 208 adults with muscle strains (Higashi et al., 2010).

The identification of peripheral opioid receptors and the adverse systemic effects of opioids have led to the use of topical opioids primarily in the palliative care setting for ulcers and mucositis (Coggeshell and Carlton, 1997; Lebon et al., 2009). Morphine is the most common opioid reported in the literature although diamorphine, methadone, oxycodone, and meperidine have also been studied. A review of 19 studies (six randomized controlled trials and 13 case reports) found support for efficacy but recommended further larger trials (Lebon et al., 2009). Morphine is used either mixed with intrasite gel to apply to ulcers, or swished and spit as a 1% or 2% mouthwash for mucositis (Cerchietti et al., 2003; Zeppetella et al., 2003). A case report on the use of topical morphine gel in two adolescents with epidermolysis bullosa reported good efficacy with no side effects despite prolonged use for 4 weeks and 5 months (Watterson et al., 2004).

Ketamine and amitriptyline either alone or in various combinations have been used to provide pain relief in neuropathic pain conditions. The evidence supporting their use is mixed although negative studies may reflect lower concentrations of the agents used. A study of 4% amitriptyline and 2% ketamine demonstrated reduced pain in adults with postherpetic neuralgia compared with a lower concentration cream or placebo and a randomized controlled trial of 10% ketamine reduced allodynia in adults with complex regional pain syndrome (Finch et al., 2009; Lockhart 2004). In the second trial no systemic ketamine was detected 1 h after application in ten patients (Fisch et al., 2009). For clinical use these preparations may require the expertise of a compounding pharmacist.

Dexamethasone, a steroid, can be delivered iontophoretically for a variety of inflammatory conditions such as medical and lateral epicondylitis, Achilles tendonitis, and plantar fasciitis (Gudeman, 1997; Neeter, 2003; Nirschl, 2003). In the US this procedure is primarily performed by physiotherapists. Unlike lidocaine iontophoresis described earlier, dexamethasone is negatively charged so it must be placed on the negatively charged electrode to facilitate drug delivery. The data supported the efficacy of dexamethasone iontophoresis is variable. The largest study which evaluated dexamethasone iontophoresis for epicondylitis demonstrated reduced pain in the active drug group versus placebo iontophoresis, however the results of several other smaller trials including one for epicondylitis were mixed. It is likely that dexamethasone iontophoresis provides short-term benefits including pain relief in acute musculoskeletal injuries (Torro, 2011).

One paediatric study of dexamethasone iontophoresis demonstrated efficacy in a case series of 28 patients with juvenile idiopathic arthritis treated for temporomandibular joint involvement (Mina, 2011). Side effects in this study and others are similar to those mentioned previously with iontophoresis.

Conclusion

There are a variety of effective topical medications for both procedural pain as well as musculoskeletal and neuropathic pain. For procedural pain these medications have been well studied in children and their use should be encouraged. There is limited data to support the efficacy of topical medications in the paediatric population for musculoskeletal and neuropathic pain conditions. However, given the excellent safety profile including lack of systemic absorption and minimal local side effects the use of these medications in the paediatric age group should be considered.

Case example

A 15-year-old girl presents to the chronic pain clinic with a 4-month history of back pain. Her pain is usually a 4 to 6 out of 10 at rest but increases to an 8 to 9 out of 10 with activity. She continues to attend school, has no trouble sleeping, and her mood as reported by her both herself and her mother is good. She does say it is hard to concentrate at school because she has to shift positions multiple times during class to stay comfortable. She is frustrated because she has not been able to participate in dance since her pain started. She has had an extensive workup that includes orthopaedic evaluation, plain films and a magnetic resonance imaging scan of the lumbosacral spine. The radiological studies were normal. She took ibuprofen for several weeks after the onset of pain; however, this was not helpful. She has had eight sessions of physiotherapy focused on core strengthening. She says the physiotherapy has not reduced her pain but that the electrical stimulation they do during therapy does reduce her pain temporarily.

On physical exam she is a comfortable appearing, pleasant, non-obese female. Notable findings on her exam include paraspinal muscular tenderness and tightening in the lumbar region. She has increased pain with forwards and especially backwards flexion. She has no evidence of hypermobility and her neurological exam is normal.

Recommendations: you recommend a lidocaine 5% patch. She should apply it for 12 h daily (usually at night). She should cut the patch in half and place the halves over the areas of maximal tenderness. The patches should be placed in the same location every night. You tell her to give it at least 2 weeks of regular use to expect results (the manufacturer recommends 7 to 10 days for pain reduction from postherpetic neuralgia but our experience for back pain is that it takes a longer period of time).

You also recommend that she obtain a TENS (transcutaneous electric nerve stimulation) unit from her physiotherapist. She can wear this at times during the day when her pain becomes severe. It is also helpful during school classes to help reduce pain and enable her to concentrate.

Follow-up: she returns to the clinic 6 weeks later with her pain essentially resolved. She experienced no local irritation or other side effects from the patch. She continues to use the lidocaine patches and has now transitioned from physiotherapy and is doing some low-intensity dancing. You tell her to use the patches for another 2 weeks and return to see you again if her pain returns.

References

Argoff, C. E. (2004). Topical treatments for pain. *Curr Pain Headache Rep*, 8, 261–267.

Bandolier extra. (2005). *Topical analgesics: a review of reviews and a bit of perspective.* Available at: <http://www.medicine.ox.ac.uk/bandolier/Extraforbando/Topextra3.pdf> (accessed 1 February 2012).

Bandolier extra. (n.d.). *Vapocollant sprays for cannulation pain.* Available at: <http://www.medicine.ox.ac.uk/bandolier/booth/painpag/Acutrev/Analgesics/Vapocoolant.html> (accessed 3 February 2012).

Baron, E. D., Harris, L., Redpath, W. S., Shapiro, H., Hetzel, F., Morley, G., et al. (2003). Laser-assisted penetration of topical anesthetic in adults. *Arch Dermatol*, 139(10), 1288–1290.

Becker, B. M., Helfrich, S., Baker, E., Lovgren, K., Minugh, P. A., and Machan, J. T. (2005). Ultrasound with topical anesthetic rapidly decreases pain of intravenous cannulation. *Acad Emerg Med*, 12(4), 289–295.

Berde C. B., Walco G. A., Krane E. J., Anand, K. J., Aranda, J. V., Craig, K. D., et al. (2012). Pediatric analgesic clinical trial designs, measures, and extrapolation: report of an FDA scientific workshop. *Pediatrics*, 129, 354–364.

Berger, A., Henderson, M., Nadoolman, W., Duffy, V., Cooper, D., Saberski, L. et al. (1995). Oral capsaicin provides temporary relief for oral mucositis pain secondary to chemotherapy/radiation therapy. *J Pain Symptom Manage*, 10, 243–248.

Bircher, A. J., Hampl, K., Hirsbrunner, P., Buechner, S. A., and Schneider, M. (1994). Allergic contact dermatitis from ethyl chloride and sensitization to dichlorodifluoromethane (CFC 12). *Contact Dermatitis*, 31(1), 41–44.

Bishai, R., Taddio, A., Bar-Oz, B., Freedman, M. H., and Koren, G. (1995). Relative efficacy of amethocaine gel and lidocaine-prilocaine cream for Port-a-Cath puncture in children. *Pediatrics*, 104(3), e31.

Campbell, B. J., Rowbotham, M., Davies, P. S., Jacob, P., and Benowitz, N. J. (2002). Systemic absorption of topical lidocaine in normal volunteers,

patients with post-herpetic neuralgia, and patients with acute herpes zoster. *J Pharm Sci*, 91, 1343–1350.

Cerchietti, L. C., Navigante, A. H., Korte, M. W., Cohen, A. M., Quiroga, P. N., Villaamil, E. C., et al. (2003). Potential utility of the peripheral analgesic properties of morphine in stomatitis related pain: a pilot study. *Pain*, 105, 265–273.

Coggeshell, R. E., and Carlton, S. M. (1997). Receptor localization in mammalian dorsal horn d primary afferent neurons. *Brain Res Rev*, 24, 28–66.

Derry, S., Lloyd, R., Moore, R. A., and McQuay, H. J. (2009). Topical capsaicin for chronic neuropathic pain in adults. *Cochrane Database Syst Rev*, 7(4), CD007393.

Devers, A. and Galer, B. S. (2000). Topical lidocaine patch relieves a variety of neuropathic pain conditions: an open label study. *Clin J Pain*, 16, 205–208.

Ehrenstrom-Reiz, G., Reiz, S., and Stockman, O. (1983). Topical anaesthesia with EMLA, a new lidocaine-prilocaine cream and the Cusum technique for detection of minimal application time. *Acta Anaesthesiol Scand*, 27(6), 510–512.

Eichenfield, L. F., Funk, A., Fallon-Friedlander, S., and Cunningham, B. B. (2002). A clinical study to evaluate the efficacy of ELA-Max (4% liposomal lidocaine) as compared with eutectic mixture of local anesthetics cream for pain reduction of venipuncture in children. *Pediatrics*, 109(6), 1093–1099.

Eidelman, A., Weiss, J. M., Baldwin, C. L., Enu, I. K., McNicol, E. D., and Carr, D. B. (2011). Topical anaesthetics for repair of dermal laceration. *Cochrane Database Syst Rev*, 6, CD005364.

EMLA® Package Insert. (n.d.). Astra Zeneca.

Epiture EasyTouch™ System User Manual. (2003). Frankston, Australia: Norwood Abbey Ltd.

Ernst, A. A., Marvez, E., Nick, T. G., Chin, E., Wood, E., and Gonzaba, W. T. (1995). Lidocaine adrenaline tetracaine gel versus tetracaine adrenaline cocaine gel for topical anesthesia in linear scalp and facial lacerations in children aged 5 to 17 years. *Pediatrics*, 95, 255–258.

Esparza, F. Cobian, C., Jiminez, J. F., García-Cota, J. J., Sánchez, C., Maestro, A., et al. (2007). Topical ketoprofen TDS patch versus diclofenac gel: efficacy and tolerability in benign sport related soft-tissue injuries. *Br J Sports Med*, 41, 134–139.

Fetzer, S. J. (2002). Reducing venipuncture and intravenous insertion pain with eutectic mixture of local anesthetic: a meta-analysis. *Nurs Res*, 51(2), 119–124.

Finch, P. M., Knudsen, L., and Drummond, P. D. (2009). Reduction of allodynia in patients with complex regional pain syndrome: a double-blind placebo-controlled trial of topical ketamine. *Pain*, 146, 18–25.

Galer, B. S. (2001). Topical medications. In J. D. Loeser, (ed.) *Bonica's Management of Pain*, pp. 1736–1741. Philadelphia, PA: Lippincott Williams & Wilkins.

Galer, B. S., Gammaitoni, A. R., Oleka, N., Jensen, M. P., Argoff, C. E. (2004b). Use of the lidocaine 5% patch in reducing intensity of various pain qualities reported by patients with low-back pain. *Curr Res Med Opin*, 20, S5–S12.

Galer, B. S., Rowbotham, M. C., Perander, J., and Friedman, E. (1999). Topical lidocaine patch relieves postherpetic neuralgia more effectively than a vehicle topical patch: results of an enriched enrollment study. *Pain*, 80(3), 533–538.

Galer, B. S., Sahaler, E., and Patel, N. (2004a). Topical lidocaine patch 5% may target a novel underlying pain mechanism in osteoarthritis. *Curr Med Res Opin*, 20, 1455–1458.

Galinkin, J. L., Rose, J. B., Harris, K., and Watcha, M. F. (2002). Lidocaine iontophoresis versus eutectic mixture of local anesthetics (EMLA) for IV placement in children. *Anesth Analg*, 94(6), 1484–1488.

Gammaaitoni, A. R., Galer, B. S., Onwala, R. Jensen, M. P., and Argoff, C. E. (2004). Lidocaine patch 5% and its positive impact on pain qualities in osteoarthritis: results of a pilot 2-week, open label study using the neuropathic pain scale. *Curr Res Med Opin*, 20, S13–S19.

Gimbel, J., Linn, R., Hale, M., and Nicholson, B. (2005). Lidocaine patch treatment in patients with low back pain: results of an open-label, non-randomized pilot study. *Am J Ther*, 12, 311–319.

Gudeman S. D., Eisele S. A., Heidt R. S. Jr, Colosimo, A. J., and Stroupe, A. L. (1997). Treatment of plantar fasciitis by iontophoresis of 0.4% dexamethasone. A randomized, double-blind, placebo-controlled study. *Am J Sports Med*, 25, 312–316.

Hallen, B. and Uppfeldt, A. (1982). Does lidocaine-prilocaine cream permit painfree insertion of IV catheters in children? *Anesthesiology*, 57(4), 340–342.

Halperin, D. L., Koren, G., Attias, D., Pellegrini, E., Greenberg, M. L., and Wyss, M. (1989). Topical skin anesthesia for venous, subcutaneous drug reservoir and lumbar punctures in children. *Pediatrics*, 84(2), 281–284.

Halperin, S. A., McGrath, P., Smith, B., and Houston, T. (2000). Lidocaine-prilocaine patch decreases the pain associated with the subcutaneous administration of measles-mumps-rubella vaccine but does not adversely affect the antibody response. *J Pediatr*, 136(6)789–794.

Haroutiunian, S., Drennan, D. A., and Lipman, A. G. (2010). Topical NSAID therapy for musculoskeletal pain. *Pain Med*, 11, 535–549.

Heyneman, C. A., Lawless-Liday, C., and Wall, G. C. (2000). Oral versus topical NSAIDs in rheumatic disease: a comparison. *Drugs*, 60, 555–574.

Higashi, Y., Kiuchi, T., and Furuta, K. (2009). Efficacy and safety profile of a topical methyl salicylate and menthol patch in adult patients with mild to moderate muscle strain: a randomized double-blind, parallel-group, placebo-controlled, multicenter study. *Clinical Therapeutics*, 32, 34–43.

Houck, C. S., and Sethna, N. F. (2005). Transdermal analgesia with local anesthetics in children: review, update and future directions. *Expert Rev Neurother*, 5(5), 625–634.

Hull, W. (2002). Heat-enhanced transdermal drug delivery: a survey paper. *J App Res*, 2, 69–75.

Irving, G. A., Backonja, M. M., Dunteman, E., Blonsky, R., Vanhove, G. F., Lu, S., *et al*. (2011). A multicenter, randomized, double-blind controlled study of NGX-4010, a high-concentration capsaicin patch, for the treatment of post herpetic neuralgia. *Pain Medicine*, 12, 99–109.

Jain, A. and Rutter, N. (2000). Does topical amethocaine gel reduce the pain of venepuncture in newborn infants? A randomised double blind controlled trial. *Arch Dis Child Fetal Neonatal* Ed, 83(3), F207–10.

Jain, A., Rutter, N., and Ratnayaka, M. (2001). Topical amethocaine gel for pain relief of heel prick blood sampling: a randomised double blind controlled trial. *Arch Dis Child Fetal Neonatal Ed*, 84(1), F56–9

Jensen, T. S., Madesen, C. S., and Finnerup, N. B. (2009). Pharmacology and treatment of neuropathic pains. *Curr Opin Neurol*, 22, 467–474

Kaur, G., Gupta, P., and Kumar, A. (2003). A randomized trial of eutectic mixture of local anesthetics during lumbar puncture in newborns. *Arch Pediatr Adolesc Med*, 157(11), 1065–1070.

Knoktova, H., Pappagallo, M., and Szallasi, A. (2008). Capsaicin (TRPV1 agonist) the pay for pain relief. Farwell or revival? *Clin J Pain*, 24, 142–154

Koh, J. L., Harrison, D., Myers, R., Dembinski, R., Turner, H., and McGraw, T. (2004). A randomized, double-blind comparison study of EMLA and ELA-Max for topical anesthesia in children undergoing intravenous insertion. *Paediatr Anaesth*, 14(12), 977–982

Krumova, E. K., Zeller, M., Westermann, A., and Maier, C. (2012). Lidocaine patch (5%) produces a selective, but incomplete block of Aδ and C fibers. *Pain*, 153(2), 273–280.

Kshirsagar, N. A., Pandya, S. K., Kirodian, G. B., Sanath, S. (2005). Liposomal drug delivery system from laboratory to clinic. *J Postgrad Med*, 51(Suppl 1), S5–15.

Lander, J., Hodgins, M., Nazarali, S., McTavish, J., Ouellette, J., and Friesen, E. (1996). Determinants of success and failure of EMLA. *Pain*, 64(1), 89–97.

Lander, J. A., Weltman, B. J., and So, S. S. (2006). EMLA and amethocaine for reduction of children's pain associated with needle insertion. *Cochrane Database Syst Rev*, 3, CD004236.

Lawson, R. A., Smart, N. G., Gudgeon, A. C., and Morton, N. S. (1995). Evaluation of an amethocaine gel preparation for percutaneous analgesia before venous cannulation in children. *Br J Anaesth*, 75(3), 282–285.

Lidoderm Package Insert. (n.d.). Endo pharmaceuticals.

Lockhart, E. (2004). Topical combination of amytriptyline and ketamine for post herpetic neuralgia. *J Pain*, 5, 82.

Lebon, B., Zeppetella, G., and Higginson, I. J. (2009). Effectiveness of topical administration of opioids in palliative care: a systematic review. *J Pain Symptom Manage*, 37, 913–917.

Lumpkin, E. A., and Caterina, M. J. (2007). Mechanisms of sensory transduction in the skin. *Nature*, 445(7130), 858–865.

Mason, L., Moore, R. A., Edwards, J. E., Derry, S., and Mcquay H. J. (2004). Topical NSAIDs for chronic musculoskeletal pain: systematic review and meta-analysis. *BMC Musculoskelet Disord*, 5, 28.

Maunuksela, E. L., and Korpela, R. (1986). Double-blind evaluation of a lignocaine-prilocaine cream (EMLA) in children. Effect on the pain associated with venous cannulation. *Br J Anaesth*, 58(11), 1242–1245.

Mawhorter, S., Daugherty, L., Ford, A., Hughes, R., Metzger, D., and Easley, K. (2004). Topical vapocoolant quickly and effectively reduces vaccine-associated pain: results of a randomized, single-blinded, placebo-controlled study. *J Travel Med*, 11(5), 267–272.

McElhiney, L. (2011). Case report: the use of topical concentrated capsaicin cream to treat erythromelalgia in a pediatric patient. *Int J Pharm Compounding*, 15(3), 386–387.

Miller, K. A., Balakrishnan, G., Eichbauer, G., and Betley, K. (2001). 1% lidocaine injection, EMLA cream, or 'Numby Stuff' for topical analgesia associated with peripheral intravenous cannulation. *AANA J*, 69(3), 185–187.

Mina, R., Melson, P., Powell, S., Rao, M., Hinze, C., Passo, M., *et al*. (2011). Effectiveness of dexamethsone iontophoresis for temporomandibular joint involvement in juvenile idiopathic arthritis. *Arthritis Care Res*, 63, 1511–1516.

Mitragotri, S. and Kost, J. (2004). Low-frequency sonophoresis: a review. *Adv Drug Deliv Rev*, 56(5), 589–601.

Moller, C. (1985). A lignocaine-prilocaine cream reduces venipuncture pain. *Ups J Med Sci*, 90(3), 293–298.

Nahum, Y., Tenenbaum, A., Isaiah, W., Levy-Khademi, F. (2007). Effect of eutectic mixture of local anesthetics (EMLA) for pain relief during suprapubic aspiration in young infants: a randomized, controlled trial. *Clin J Pain*, 23(9), 756–759.

Neeter, C., Thomee, R., Silbernagel, K. G., Thomeé, P., and Karlsson, J. (2003). Iontophoresis with or without dexamethasone in the treatment of acute Achilles tendon pain. *Scand J Med Sci Sports*, 13, 376–382.

Newbury, C. and Herd, D. W. (2009). Amethocaine versus EMLA for successful intravenous cannulation in a children's emergency department: a randomised controlled study. *Emerg Med J*, 26(7), 487–491.

Nirschl, R. P., Rodin, D. M., Ochiai, D. H., Maartmann-Moe, C.; DEX-AHE-01–99 Study Group. (2003). Iontophoretic administration of dexamethasone sodium phosphate for acute epicondylitis. A randomized, double-blinded, placebo-controlled study. *Am J Sports Med*, 31,189–195.

O'Brien, L., Taddio, A., Lyszkiewicz, D. A., and Koren, G. (2005). A critical review of the topical local anesthetic amethocaine (Ametop) for pediatric pain. *Paediatr Drugs*, 7(1), 41–54.

Rattenbury, J. M., and Worthy, E. (1993). Is the sweat test safe? Some instances of burns received during pilocarpine iontophoresis. *Ann Clin Biochem*, 33(5), 456–458.

Reis, E. and Holubkov, R. (1997). Vapocoolant spray is equally effective as EMLA cream in reducing immunization pain in school-aged children. *Pediatrics*, 100(6), E5.

Rømsing, J., Henneberg, S. W., Walther-Larsen, S., and Kjeldsen, C. (1999). Tetracaine gel vs EMLA cream for percutaneous anaesthesia in children. *Br J Anaesth*, 82(4), 637–638.

Sawyer, J., Febbraro, S., Masud, S., Ashburn, M. A., Campbell, J. C. (2009). Heated lidocaine/tetracaine patch (Synera, Rapydan) compared with lidocaine/prilocaine cream (EMLA) for topical anaesthesia before vascular access. *Br J Anaesth*, 102(2), 210–215.

Schilling, C. G., Bank, D. E., Borchert, B. A., Klatzko, M. D., and Uden, D. L. (1995). Tetracaine, epinephrine and cocaine (TAC) versus lidocaine, epinephrine, and tetracaine (LET) for anesthesia of lacerations in children. *Ann Emerg Med*, 25, 203–220.

Sethna, N. F., Verghese, S. T., Hannallah, R. S., Solodiuk, J. C., Zurakowski, D., and Berde, C. B. (2005). A randomized controlled trial to evaluate S-Caine patch for reducing pain associated with vascular access in children. *Anesthesiology*, 102(2), 403–408.

Shah, V. S., Taddio, A., Hancock, R., Shah, P., and Ohlsson, A. (2008). Topical amethocaine gel 4% for intramuscular injection in term neonates: a double-blind, placebo-controlled, randomized trial. *Clin Ther*, 30(1), 166–174.

Shah, V., Taddio, A., Rieder, M. J.; HELPinKIDS Team. (2009). Effectiveness and tolerability of pharmacologic and combined interventions for reducing injection pain during routine childhood immunizations: systematic review and meta-analyses. *Clin Ther*, 31(Suppl 2), S104–151.

Shapiro, H., Harris, L., Hetzel, F.W., and Bar-Or, D. (2002). Laser assisted delivery of topical anesthesia for intramuscular needle insertion in adults. *Lasers Surg Med*, 31(4), 252–256.

Sims, C. (1991). Thickly and thinly applied lignocaine-prilocaine cream prior to venepuncture in children. *Anaesth Intensive Care*, 19(3), 343–345.

Singer, A. J., and Stark, M. J. (2001). LET versus EMLA for pretreating lacerations: a randomized trial. *Acad Emerg Med*, 8, 223–230.

Skarbek-Borowska, S., Becker, B. M., Lovgren, K., Bates, A., and Minugh, P.A. (2006). Brief focal ultrasound with topical anesthetic decreases the pain of intravenous placement in children. *Pediatr Emerg Care*, 22(5), 339–345.

Stamos, S. P. (2007). Topical agents for the management of musculoskeletal pain. *J Pain Symptom Manage*, 33, 342–355.

Taddio, A., Ohlsson, A., Einarson, T.R., Stevens, B., and Koren, G. (1998). A systematic review of lidocaine-prilocaine cream (EMLA) in the treatment of acute pain in neonates. *Pediatrics*, 101(2), E1.

Taddio, A., Soin, H.K., Schuh, S., Koren, G., and Scolnik, D. (2005). Liposomal lidocaine to improve procedural success rates and reduce procedural pain among children: a randomized controlled trial. *CMAJ*, 172(13), 1691–1695.

Taddio, A., Stevens, B., Craig, K., Rastogi, P., Ben-David, S., Shennan, A., *et al.* (1997). Efficacy and safety of lidocaine prilocaine cream for pain during circumcision. *N Engl J Med*, 336, 1197–1201.

Tadicherla, S. and Berman, B. (2006). Percutaneous dermal drug delivery for local pain control. *Ther Clin Risk Manage*, 2, 99–113.

Tegeder, I., Muth-Selbach, U., Lotsch, J., Rüsing, G., Oelkers, R., Brune, K., *et al.* (1999). Application of microdialysis for the determination of muscle and subcutaneous tissue concentrations after oral and topical ibupfofen administration. *Clin Pharmacol Ther*, 65, 357–368.

Torro, J., Bruneti, L., and Patel, M. (2011). Ionotphoretic administration of dexamethasone for musculoskeletal pain. *J Musculoskel Med*, 28, 410–421.

Underwood, M., Ashby, D., Carnes, D., Castelnuovo, E., Cross, P., Harding, G., *et al.* (2008). Topical or oral iburpofen for chronic knee pain in older people. The TOIB study. *Health Technol Assess*, 12, ix–155.

Watterson, G., Howard, R., and Goldman, A. (2004). Peripheral opioids in inflammatory pain. *Arch Dis Child*, 89, 679–681.

Wehrfritz, A., Namer, B., Ihmsen, H., Mueller, C., Filitz, J., Koppert, W., *et al.* (2011). Differential effects on sensory functions and measures of epidermal nerve fiber density after application of a lidocaine patch (5%) on healthy human skin. *Eur J Pain*, 15(9), 907–912.

Yadav, J. D., Vaidya, K. A., Kulkarni, P. R., and Raut, R. A. (2011). Microneedles: promising technique for transdermal drug delivery. *Int J Pharma Biosciences*, 2, 684–708.

Zempsky, W. T. (2008a). Pharmacologic approaches for reducing venous access pain. *Pediatrics*, 122, S140–153.

Zempsky, W. T., Anand, K. J., Sullivan, K. M., Fraser, D., and Cucina, K. (1998). Lidocaine iontophoresis for topical anesthesia before intravenous line placement in children. *J Pediatr*, 132(6), 1061–1063.

Zempsky, W. T., and Ashburn, M. A. (1998). Iontophoresis: noninvasive drug delivery. *Am J Anesthesiol.*, 25(4), 158–162.

Zempsky, W. T., Bean-Lejewski, J., Kaufman, R. E., Koh, J. L., Malviya, S. V., Rose, J. B., *et al.* (2008c). Needle free powder lidocaine delivery system provides rapid and effective analgesia for venipuncture or cannulation pain in children: The randomized double-blind COMFORT-003 trial. *Pediatrics*, 121, 979–987.

Zempsky, W. T., and Karasic, R. B. (1997). EMLA versus TAC for topical anesthesia of extremity wounds in children. *Ann Emerg Med*, 30, 163–166.

Zeppetella, G., Paul, J., and Ribeiro, M. D. (2003). Analgesic efficacy of morphine applied topically to painful ulcers. *J Pain Symptom Manage*, 25, 555–558.

Zempsky, W. T., Robbins. B., and McKay, L. (2008b). Reduction of topical anesthetic onset time using ultrasound: A randomized controlled trial prior to venipuncture in young children. *Pain Med*, 9, 795–802.

Zempsky, W. T., Robbins, B., Richards, P. T., Leong, M. S., and Schechter, N. L. (2008d). A study evaluating venipuncture pain in children receiving a novel needlefree powder lidocaine delivery system for rapid local analgesia. *J Pediatr*, 152, 405–411.

Zempsky, W. T., Sullivan, J., Paulson, D. M., and Hoath, S. B. (2004). Evaluation of a low-dose lidocaine iontophoresis system for topical anesthesia in adults and children: a randomized, controlled trial. *Clin Ther*, 26(7), 1110–1119.

CHAPTER 48

Drugs for neuropathic pain

Sachin Rastogi and Fiona Campbell

Summary

Neuropathic pain is defined as 'pain arising as a direct consequence of a lesion or disease affecting the somatosensory system'. It is often contrasted with nociceptive pain which is associated with tissue injury or inflammation. Neuropathic pain exhibits certain clinical features that differentiate it from nociceptive pain. Neuropathic pain conditions in children are different from those in adults and include complex regional pain syndrome (CRPS), phantom limb pain, postoperative and post-traumatic neuropathic pain, and autoimmune and degenerative neuropathies, e.g. Guillain–Barré syndrome, Charcot–Marie–Tooth disease. However, a lack of randomized controlled trials in children means that evidence from adult studies guides pharmacological management of neuropathic pain in children, which is problematic as the aetiologies and mechanisms are different.

In this chapter we propose an algorithm for drug therapy for neuropathic pain in children based on best available evidence, our clinical experience, and the safety of these drugs in paediatric practice. We suggest a step-wise approach incorporating first-, second-, third-, and fourth-line therapies that should be tried methodically according to effectiveness and side effects. Neuropathic pain in children, if identified and treated in a timely manner as part of an interdisciplinary framework, using multimodal strategies can be managed effectively.

Introduction

Neuropathic pain

The International Association for the Study of Pain (IASP) defines pain as 'an unpleasant sensory and emotional experience associated with actual or potential tissue damage, or described in terms of such damage' (Merskey and Bogduk, 1994, p. 210). Pain can be categorized in various ways; by (1) its temporal profile (i.e. acute, chronic, recurrent), (2) disease type (e.g. sickle cell pain, cancer pain), or (3) pain mechanism (nociceptive, neuropathic). Neuropathic pain has recently been defined as 'pain arising as a direct consequence of a lesion or disease affecting the somatosensory system' (Treede et al., 2008). Traditionally, pain type is broadly classified into nociceptive and neuropathic. Nociceptive pain is initiated by normal activation of pain pathways by noxious stimuli, whereas neuropathic pain is associated with abnormal activation of pain pathways involving both the peripheral and central nervous system. It is a complex,

partially understood phenomenon with characteristic clinical features, which have predominantly been described in adults. For the purposes of this chapter the term 'children' will refer to all children and adolescents unless indicated otherwise. Though it is well known that children suffer from neuropathic pain, there have been few paediatric studies. Moreover, it is likely that given the differences in nervous system anatomy and physiology between adults and children, as well as different aetiologies of neuropathic pain, there are significant differences in mechanisms and prognoses.

Though basic mechanisms underlying pain transmission are reasonably well understood, neuropathic pain is a complex, interdependent dynamic state, which is likely influenced by multiple factors including aetiology, previous pain experience, and genetic factors. Interindividual variability in chronic pain expression and response to analgesics are known to have a genetic basis, which may guide future treatments (Sorge et al., 2012), including those for neuropathic pain. Translation of these mechanisms into drug therapy has not been simple, further complicated by the fact that underlying mechanisms in children are different from those in adults. Examples include the increased plasticity of the developing nervous system and altered response to injury, and the reduced spinal microglial response to nerve injury during earlier stages of development (Moss et al., 2007; Vega-Avelaira et al., 2007; see also Vega-Avelaira and Beggs, Chapter 7, this volume). One could postulate that these differences might improve the prognosis of neuropathic pain in children.

Clinical features

Neuropathic pain is characterized by positive symptoms and negative symptoms (sensory loss, numbness). Positive symptoms are either spontaneous pains that can be (1) continuous (e.g. burning, throbbing) or intermittent (e.g. shooting, stabbing) or (2) evoked (e.g. hyperalgesia and allodynia). Hyperalgesia is defined as 'increased pain from a stimulus that usually provokes pain' and allodynia as 'pain due to a stimulus that does not normally provoke pain' (Merskey and Bogduk, 1994). Positive symptoms may be understood in terms of pathological changes in the peripheral nerves, as a way in which the nervous system attempts to compensate for sensory loss. A high index of suspicion is required to make a diagnosis of neuropathic pain, and an early clue is the poor response to simple analgesics such as acetaminophen and non-steroidal anti-inflammatory drugs. Diagnosis is presently based upon the history comprising qualitative pain descriptors and basic neurological examination. Common pain descriptors include burning, throbbing, electrical, stabbing, shooting, pricking, and pins and needles. In addition to positive and negative symptoms, autonomic dysfunction can sometimes be seen (e.g. vasomotor, sudomotor, and trophic changes), particularly in the context of complex regional pain syndrome (CRPS) (see Clinch, Chapter 24; Vega-Avelaira and Beggs, Chapter 21; Walker, Chapter 7, this volume).

Neuropathic pain: children versus adult

Neuropathic pain in adults affects up to 8% of the population with significant impact on quality of life (Torrance et al., 2006); no epidemiological data exists regarding prevalence in children (Walker, 2008). This might in part be due to a lack of an agreed definition and diagnostic criteria for paediatric neuropathic pain. In addition, compared to adults, the common causes of neuropathic pain in adults are rare in children. Diabetic neuropathy, trigeminal neuralgia, postherpetic neuralgia (PHN) (Hempenstall et al., 2005) and central post-stroke pain are conditions that seldom affect children, but are major causes of neuropathic pain in adults. Moreover, most of the adult literature from which paediatric neuropathic pain management is extrapolated is based on common adult aetiologies. Causes of neuropathic pain in children are heterogeneous (Walco et al., 2010) (Table 48.1). According to the latest definition of neuropathic pain for adults (Treede et al., 2008)—CRPS type 1 would not fit into the classification as there is no evidence of direct nerve disease or injury. However, given its frequency and response to anti-neuropathic pain medications, CRPS type 1 in children will be considered in this chapter.

With clearer diagnostic instruments for paediatric neuropathic pain, and improved recognition and understanding, it is likely that the prevalence in children is more than we would like to think. Neuropathic pain is often part of a mixed picture alongside nociceptive pain, for example, vaso-occlusive pain in sickle cell disease (Niscola et al., 2009).

A paucity of randomized controlled trials (RCTs) in children, a lack of validated neuropathic pain scales in children, uncertainty over definitions of neuropathic pain and diagnosis has led to a lack of data and over-reliance on extrapolation of adult studies, case reports and expert opinion (Level 4). For these reasons many of the drugs described are used off-licence.

Drugs

The drugs used in the symptomatic management of neuropathic pain in children are presented in a step-wise, practical manner, based on our clinical experience in paediatric practice, the implications of committing children to certain therapies, and best quality evidence (Levels 1 and 2). The evidence comes from adult studies as very few clinical trials have been conducted in children with neuropathic pain, and the literature is predominantly case series or isolated case reports. With inadequate or partial pain relief, additional drugs can be added in combination (with exceptions noted in the text—see Table 48.2 for detailed dosing and side effect information for first-, second-, and third-line medications).

First-line agents

Tricyclic antidepressants

Tricyclic antidepressants (TCAs) such as amitriptyline and nortriptyline are commonly used to treat neuropathic pain, with

Table 48.1 Causes of neuropathic pain in children

Causes of neuropathic pain in children	Specific examples
Peripheral causes	
Postsurgical pain	Pain after amputation
	Postoperative neuropathic pain
Complex regional pain syndrome	Type 1 (without nerve injury)
	Type 2 (with nerve injury)
Plexus injuries	Congenital
	Traumatic
Childhood cancer	Tumour related
	Treatment related
Autoimmune neuropathy	Guillain–Barré syndrome
Hereditary neurodegenerative disorders	Fabry disease
	Charcot–Marie–Tooth disease
Toxic and metabolic neuropathies	Lead, mercury, alcohol
Infection	(HIV)
Mitochondrial disorders	
Erythromelalgia	Primary
	Secondary
Burns	
Haematological	Sickle cell disease
Central causes	
Spinal cord injury	Congenital
	Traumatic
Brain	Traumatic
	Tumour

a proven track record over time (Finnerup et al., 2005; Saarto and Wiffen, 2005). The mechanism of action of TCAs in neuropathic pain is separate from its mode of action in depression (Max et al., 1987). This is reflected in the lower doses required for neuropathic pain. The multimodal mechanism of action comprises blockade of serotonin and noradrenaline reuptake, interaction with sodium and calcium ion channels, as well as some antihistamine and anticholinergic antagonism. The onset of pain relief is generally quicker (1–2 weeks) than its antidepressant effect. The metabolism of TCAs is dependent upon cytochrome P450 (CYP) metabolism (CYP2D6) and susceptible to genetic polymorphism. Therefore, in 'poor metabolizers' (up to 25% of the population) an increase in plasma levels can be seen (Lotsch and Geisslinger, 2006).

There are no published RCTs in children. In adults, the NNT (number needed to treat) for TCAs in neuropathic pain is just over 2. This equates to roughly one in every two patients receiving a 50% reduction in pain with a TCA (Finnerup et al., 2005, 2010). Studies looking at the efficacy of TCAs in neuropathic pain have looked at adults with a range of 'classic' neuropathic pain conditions such as PHN, painful neuropathies, traumatic nerve injury, and trigeminal neuralgia (Saarto and Wiffen, 2005).

Table 48.2 Commonly used first-, second-, and third-line drugs; dosages and side effects

Drug group	Drug name	Dose	Side effects
First line			
TCA	Amitriptyline	*<50 kg*: 0.1 mg/kg PO QHS, increase as tolerated every 4–6 days by 0.25 mg/kg increments until good analgesia occurs, limiting side effects or to a max of 0.5–2 mg/kg. Decrease by same rate if unhelpful. *>50 kg*: start at 10 mg, increase as tolerated by 10 mg increments every 4–6 days until a maximum of 75 mg Decrease by same rate if unhelpful	Sedation, dry mouth, blurred vision, urinary retention, tachycardia, constipation, prolongation of QTc interval, orthostatic hypotension
	Nortriptyline	See above	See above
α_2-δ ligand	Gabapentin	*<50kg*: Day 1: 3–5 mg/kg PO QHS Day 2: 3–5 mg/kg BID Day 3: 3–5 mg/kg TID Escalate more slowly if required Maintenance 20–30 mg/kg/day TID	Sedation, dizziness, caution in renal failure
		>50kg and adolescents: Day 1: 300 mg PO QHS Day 2: 300 mg BID Day 3: 300 mg TID Escalate dose as tolerated until good analgesia, limiting side effects or a maximum dose of 3600 mg/day. Additional benefit may not be seen beyond 2400 mg/day	
		Decrease by same rate if unhelpful.	
	Pregabalin	*<50kg*: 1–2 mg/kg/day PO BID. Titrate upwards weekly to effect *>50kg*: start at 75 mg PO BID.	See above
		Titrate upwards weekly to effect, to a maximum dose of 600 mg BID	
		Decrease by same rate if unhelpful.	
Topical	Lidocaine 5% patch	Each plaster or patch is applied over intact, dry and non-irritated skin for a period of 12 h on and 12 h off. A maximum of 3 plasters is recommended at any one time	Skin irritation
Second line			
SSNRI	Duloxetine	*>50 kg*: starting dose 30 mg PO daily for 1 week before increasing to 60 mg	Dry mouth, sedation, dizziness, loss of appetite, nausea, constipation
	Venlafaxine	1–2 mg/kg per day divided BID or TID increased weekly to a maximum of 225 mg/day	See above, prolongation of QTc interval
Topical	Capsaicin	Can be administered in the form of creams, lotions and patches in a range of 0.025–8% by weight. 8% capsaicin patch involves a single 60 min application with up to 12 weeks of effective subsequent analgesia in adults	Initial local burning discomfort
Third line			
Weak mu opioid receptor agonist	Tramadol	1–3 mg/kg PO every 6 h Also available in extended-release 12 h formulation, and in combination with acetaminophen (Tramacet™)	Nausea, vomiting, pruritus, constipation, hallucinations, sedation
Opioid	Morphine	Initial 0.2–0.5 mg/kg PO every 4 h PRN. After 2 weeks convert total daily dose to long-acting preparation and keep short-acting preparation for breakthrough. No ceiling effect; dose escalation can proceed with careful titration, but at high daily doses (180 mg), efficacy should be re-assessed and opioid switch or alternative options considered. An adequate trial should last between 4–6 weeks; and discontinued if there is no improvement in pain or function	Nausea, vomiting, pruritus, constipation, hallucinations, sedation, dry mouth, respiratory depression, urinary retention, caution in hepatic and renal failure, tolerance, dependence, addiction, opioid-induced hyperalgesia, immunosuppression, endocrine dysfunction (infertility)
	Oxycodone	Initial 0.1–0.2 mg/kg PO every 4–6 h as needed. After 2 weeks convert to long-acting preparation, and keep short acting dose for breakthrough	See above
Cannabinoid	Nabilone	<50 kg: 10 mcg/kg PO BID >50 kg: 1 mg BID	Sedation, dizziness, nausea, vomiting

BID = twice daily; PO = orally; QHS = every night at bedtime; TID = three times daily.

TCAs confer additional advantages in that they are inexpensive, have once-daily dosing, and can be helpful for patients in whom sleep is a problem. Side effects of TCAs are predominantly anticholinergic and antihistaminic (Table 48.2). Cardiac toxicity is a concern due to the risk of prolongation of the QTc interval, and there have been case reports of sudden death in children with arrhythmias (Varley, 2001). While there is currently no published evidence-based guideline, it is our practice for every child to have a baseline electrocardiogram (ECG) to rule out conduction abnormalities before commencing a TCA. Adverse effects can be minimized by starting the TCA at a low dose at night (see Table 48.2).

Most experience of TCAs in children is with nocturnal amitriptyline since sedation is common and this can be capitalized upon to aid sleep. Nortriptyline is similar to amitriptyline but is a secondary amine so exhibits fewer side effects.

Desiprimine, another TCA, is no longer used in children following several reports of sudden death (Biederman et al., 1995). Should TCAs not be helpful, they should be weaned slowly and not stopped abruptly. Children should be advised that vivid dreams may occur as the drug is tapered.

Alpha-2-delta ligands

The alpha-2-delta (α_2-δ) ligands, sometimes referred to as gabapentinoids (gabapentin and pregabalin), are effective treatments in many forms of neuropathic pain (Backonja et al., 1998; Freynhagen et al., 2005; Rowbotham et al., 1998; Serpell, 2002). Gabapentin binds to voltage-gated calcium channels at the α_2-δ subunit (Gee et al., 1996), as well as modulating gamma-aminobutyric acid (GABA) synthesis, release, and metabolism. Gabapentin and pregabalin are lipophilic analogues of GABA which interact with the α_2-δ subunit common to all voltage-gated calcium channels, which explains their therapeutic effect in neuropathic pain. There is evidence to suggest that these drugs selectively target those calcium channels that display abnormal activity (Li et al., 2006), as well as evidence of α_2-δ upregulation with nerve injury (Boroujerdi et al., 2011; Luo et al., 2002).

Gabapentin has been used extensively in paediatric practice (Golden et al., 2006). Though it has been superseded by other anticonvulsants in the treatment of epilepsy, its use in paediatric neuropathic pain is now established. There have been numerous case reports and series in paediatric neuropathic pain and CRPS (McGraw and Kosek, 1997; Rusy et al., 2001; Wheeler et al., 2000), as well as strong evidence from the adult literature to support its use. Gabapentin has also been successfully used in neurologically-impaired children with unexplained (neuro) irritability, improving behaviour and pain scores, which has contributed to the familiarity of the drug in paediatrics (Haney et al., 2009; Hauer et al., 2007).

There is less experience with pregabalin than gabapentin in the treatment of paediatric neuropathic pain. Pregabalin is effective in adults (Freynhagen et al., 2005), but there is no strong evidence that it is any better than gabapentin. There is limited evidence to support its used in children (Vondracek et al., 2009). Pregabalin demonstrates a similar efficacy and side effect profile to gabapentin; however, it has the advantage of twice daily (BID) dosing. In adults, pregabalin has been licensed for generalized anxiety disorder, painful diabetic neuropathy, and been shown to be effective in fibromyalgia. The increased cost of pregabalin in some countries might make it prohibitive and favour gabapentin as a first-line treatment.

Topical lidocaine 5% plasters (patches) (see also Zempsky, Chapter 47, this volume)

The purported mode of action is due to the local anaesthetic action of lidocaine, which stabilizes neuronal membranes causing downregulation of sodium channels (Rosielle, 2008).

Topical lidocaine 5% medicated plasters provide an alternative pharmacological non-systemic option in the treatment of neuropathic pain with good evidence in adults supporting its use in herpetic neuralgia (Binder et al., 2009) and focal peripheral neuropathy (Meier et al., 2003). Lidocaine plasters are also effective in combination with other antineuropathic analgesics and reduction in co-analgesic consumption was demonstrated in a retrospective observational study in adults. Their efficacy in children for neuropathic pain is supported by case series (Nayak and Cunliffe, 2008).

Systemic absorption of lidocaine is very low so side effects are minimal and therefore advantageous for children. Additional benefit comes from the patch providing a physical barrier to painful touch and a cool sensation from the patch itself. It is applied for 12 h followed by 12 h off over the focal painful area. Cost can be prohibitive in some countries, and it is not licensed for use in many countries, e.g. Canada. A less expensive 5% lidocaine gel is also available and is effective in PHN (Rowbotham et al., 1995).

Second-line agents

Selective serotonin and noradrenaline reuptake inhibitors

Balanced selective serotonin and noradrenaline reuptake inhibitors (SSNRIs) such as duloxetine and venlafaxine cause an increase in serotonin and noradrenaline, which work either presynaptically to reduce nociceptive transmission or postsynaptically to increase endogenous spinal inhibition (Smith, 2006). SSNRIs are predominantly used as antidepressants, although the analgesic mode of action is independent of the antidepressant effect.

Duloxetine has proven efficacy in painful diabetic polyneuropathy (Wernicke et al., 2006), depression, generalized anxiety, and fibromyalgia (Hauser et al., 2009) in adults. However, the role of duloxetine in paediatric neuropathic pain is not clear. Venlafaxine also has well-documented efficacy in painful diabetic polyneuropathy (Rowbotham et al., 2004), but not PHN in adults (Grothe et al., 2004). SSNRIs cannot currently be recommended as first-line treatments in paediatrics, and should only be used as a second-line agent if there is a contraindication to or failure of TCAs. According to the adult literature, selective serotonin reuptake inhibitors (SSRIs) such as fluoxetine and citalopram are poorly effective in neuropathic pain which may partially be explained by a predilection for facilitatory serotonin (5-HT)-3 receptors by SSRIs rather than inhibitory 5-HT1 receptors (Mattia et al., 2002); however, more good quality trials are needed. As it stands, there is little to suggest that they are more effective than TCAs, so their use in neuropathic pain is currently not recommended.

SSNRIs do not have anticholinergic effects so have an improved side effect profile compared to TCAs in adults. Duloxetine appears to be safe from an adverse cardiac conduction effect in adults (Wernicke et al., 2007). Venlafaxine has been linked with cardiac conduction abnormalities and increases in blood pressure, so a baseline ECG and blood pressure monitoring is recommended (Rowbotham et al., 2004). SSNRIs should not be used in conjunction with a TCA, given the risk of precipitating serotonin syndrome. When discontinuing SSNRIs the dose should be tapered to avoid a withdrawal response.

Topical capsaicin cream (see also Zempsky, Chapter 47, this volume)

Capsaicin is derived from chilli pepper and has been used for its medicinal properties for over 150 years. Its mechanism of action was originally thought to be due to depletion of substance P at peripheral nerve endings, though this does not fully explain its analgesic action. Capsaicin has a complex mechanism of action; it activates the transient receptor potential vanilloid 1 (TRPV1) receptor which initially results in sensory neuronal depolarization causing burning and itching, but over time leads to localized 'defunctionalization' of cutaneous nociceptors and analgesia (Anand and Bley, 2011).

Low-concentration formulations of capsaicin are supported by modest evidence but require daily application which may limit its use in children (Derry et al., 2009). The newer high concentration preparation 8% capsaicin patch (Qutenza™) has been used with success in adults with focal peripheral neuropathic pain (Backonja et al., 2008). It should be considered as a second-line topical intervention in children with focal neuropathic pain where lidocaine patches are either unavailable or have failed to show improvement in symptoms after an adequate trial.

Topical capsaicin is available in a variety of strengths and formulations to manage pain (Table 48.2). Although it is generally safe in terms of toxicity, the initial burning discomfort with application can result in problems with compliance, especially in children. These problems usually diminish with time, but the drug can take up to 4 weeks to produce benefit, requiring considerable patience in young patients. The newer stronger 8% capsaicin patch involves a single 60 min application with up to 12 weeks of effective subsequent analgesia. Pretreatment with a topical anaesthetic agent (e.g. EMLA®) may help with compliance, but its efficacy in children is not yet known.

Third-line agents

Tramadol

Tramadol has a unique dual mode of action whereby it inhibits the reuptake of central serotonin and noradrenaline as well as being a weak mu receptor agonist (five to eight times weaker than morphine). This unique mechanism of action may explain its efficacy in neuropathic pain.

Tramadol is effective in adults with PHN (Boureau et al., 2003) and painful diabetic neuropathy (Harati et al., 1998; Sindrup et al., 1999). A Cochrane review demonstrated its usefulness in neuropathic pain with a NNT of 3.5 (Hollingshead et al., 2006).

Tramadol is often seen as occupying a middle ground before starting a pure opioid agonist. The abuse potential of tramadol is thought to be less than that of opioids in adults (Cicero et al., 2005). Caution is required when combining tramadol with a TCA, SSNRI, or SSRI, given the risk of precipitating serotonin syndrome. This may not be an issue when tramadol is combined with low-dose TCA (e.g. amitriptyline 10 mg). Tramadol is metabolized by the CYP enzyme system (CYP2D6) and is therefore susceptible to genetic polymorphism and variable pharmacokinetics (e.g. poor metabolizers). Such variation in response to tramadol may be reduced by the introduction of the new similar compound tapentadol, which neither requires metabolic activation nor is dependent on isomer-related pharmacodynamics. However, RCTs in neuropathic pain are lacking and as such the use of tapentadol in children cannot currently be recommended.

Opioids

The term opioid refers to any compound synthetic or natural that activates the mu receptor; opiates specifically refer to drugs which derive directly from *Papaver somniferum*. Central inhibitory systems are the site of action of opioids which are agonists at inhibitory opioid receptors found in the brain, spinal cord, and periphery (see Hathway, Chapter 44, this volume); the action of endogenous opioid peptides is much less than that seen with opioid drugs.

The historical dogmatic view that opioids do not demonstrate efficacy in neuropathic pain has long been refuted. Opioids have shown consistent analgesic efficacy in treatment of neuropathic pain (Eisenberg et al., 2006), especially supporting the use of morphine, oxycodone (and tramadol), and have considerably faster onset of action compared to other agents. Little evidence exists to favour the use of fentanyl, buprenorphine, or meperidine in neuropathic pain ahead of other opioids, so will not be discussed further. We do not use codeine in children at our institutions due to unpredictable analgesic effects and significant adverse effects caused by its genetic polymorphism (Ciszkowski et al., 2009; Madadi and Koren, 2008). Problems surrounding the use of opioids relate not to their efficacy but to both their short- and long-term side effects, especially when used in children (Table 48.2). Long-term effects on sexual hormone production (Katz and Mazer, 2009) and immune function (Vallejo et al., 2004) have significant implications for children. For this reason opioids are not considered first- or second-line treatments for neuropathic pain in children, unless the pain is acutely severe or in neuropathic cancer pain. Before committing a child to opioid therapy, risk factors for abuse should be screened including previous substance abuse, history of psychiatric disease, and family history of drug abuse (National Opioid Use Guideline Group (NOUGG), 2010; Zacny et al., 2003). Particular care is required when treating adolescents. We advocate using an opioid contract system when initiating therapy; we include a generic example of a contract for children and adolescents (see Figure 48.1) based on NOUGG recommendations (NOUGG, 2010).

Morphine

Morphine is the gold standard opioid and the one with which most practitioners treating children have most experience. It is a natural derivative of *Papaver somniferum* (opium poppy).

Morphine is the prototypical mu receptor agonist, given orally its bioavailability is low (30%) and duration of action is 3 to 5 h, or 12 h if using a sustained-release preparation. It is metabolized in the liver to morphine 3-glucoronide (M3G) and morphine 6-glucuronide (M6G); the latter is a more potent analgesic than morphine itself. Both M3G and M6G are renally excreted and morphine should be used with caution in patients with any degree of renal insufficiency (see Strassels, Chapter 45, this volume).

Morphine is effective in peripheral neuropathic pain and mixed neuropathic pain in adults (Eisenberg et al., 2006), with particular evidence in painful diabetic neuropathy, PHN, and phantom limb pain (Dworkin et al., 2007). It has been shown to be as effective as gabapentin in one trial (Gilron et al., 2005).

Morphine is a versatile drug which can be administered via a number of routes. For chronic neuropathic pain, the oral route is typically used. Both short-acting and long-acting oral preparations are available, in addition to injectable forms. If the decision is made to discontinue opioid therapy, it should be carefully tapered under medical supervision to avoid withdrawal.

Patient/Family/Health Care Team Agreement for Opioid Therapy

History

1. Family history of substance use (alcohol, illicit drugs, prescription drugs)   yes   no
   If yes, please describe:

   _____

2. Personal history of substance use (alcohol, illicit drugs, prescription drugs):   yes   no

   If yes, please describe:

   _____

3. Age of first alcoholic drink? _____

4. Have you ever passed out/blacked out?   yes   no

5. Psychiatric History:

   a. Self harm   yes   no

   b. Intentional overdose   yes   no

   c. Suicide attempts   yes   no

   d. Trauma/abuse   yes   no

6. Have you ever been diagnosed with:

   a. Depression   yes   no

   b. Anxiety   yes   no

7. Education History:

   a. Learning disability   yes   no

   b. ADD/ADHD   yes   no

8. History of sleep apnea

   a. Snoring   yes   no

   b. Sleep study positive   yes   no

9. Using sedating medications   yes   no

   If yes, please list: _____

Side Effects:

Opioids can help pain but they can also have side effects. These may include:

- Sleepiness, confusion, dizziness
- Decreased breathing
- Constipation
- Nausea and/or vomiting
- Itchiness
- Difficulty urinating

I understand to let my team know if I experience any of these side effects.

Goals of Opioid Therapy:

I understand that the goals of opioid therapy are:

1. Improve function (such as school attendance, physical activity, seeing friends).
2. Decrease pain scores by at least 30% (eg. from 10/10 to 7/10)
3. Personal goal(s):

   _____

   _____

   _____

I further understand that if the above goals are not achieved within 4 weeks of starting therapy this therapy will be considered unhelpful and adjusted or discontinued. Our team will work together with you to wean this medication gradually to avoid negative effects/withdrawal.

Opioid therapy will be reviewed at least once a month and adjustments made as needed.

Figure 48.1 An example of an opioid contract for children and adolescents.

Agreement:

I understand that I am receiving opioid medication from Dr. _____ to treat my chronic pain condition. I agree to the following:

1. I/my child will not seek opioid medications from another physician. Only

   Dr. _____ will prescribe opioids for me/my child. In exceptional circumstances (such as my doctor's absence) other anesthesiologists in the Sick Kids pain clinic may prescribe.

2. I/my child will not take opioid medications in larger amounts or more frequently than is prescribed by Dr. _____.

3. I/my child will not give or sell my medication to anyone else, including family members; nor will I/my child accept any opioid medication from anyone else.

4. I/my child will not use over-the-counter opioid medications such as 222's and Tylenol® No. 1.

5. I understand that if my/my child's prescription runs out early for any reason (for example, if I lose the medication, or take more than prescribed), Dr. _____ may not prescribe extra medications for me; I will have to wait until the next prescription is due.

6. I/my child will not stop the opioid medication suddenly, as this may cause withdrawal.

7. I will fill my/my child's prescriptions at one pharmacy of my choice; pharmacy name:

8. I will store my medication in a secured location.

9. I agree to monitor for side effects of opioids (such as itchiness, nausea/vomiting, constipation, sleepiness/lethargy) and notify the chronic pain team if they are present.

10. I will not drive when starting or increasing the dose of opioids, and will discuss my ability to drive with Dr._____ prior to driving.

11. I/my child agree(s) to provide a urine sample upon request for opioid screening purposes.

12. I understand that if I break these conditions, Dr. _____ may choose to cease to write opioid prescriptions for me.

Patient's signature:

Parent/Guardian signature:

Physician/Advanced Practice Nurse signature:

Figure 48.1 (Continued)

Oxycodone

Oxycodone is a semisynthetic opioid which is 1.5 to 2 times the potency of morphine. It exerts its analgesic effect through both mu and kappa agonism, which has been suggested for its efficacy in neuropathic pain (Nielsen et al., 2007). It has a higher oral bioavailability than morphine at 75% due to minimal first-pass metabolism. It is demethylated to noroxycodone and oxymorphone by hepatic CYP2D6, both of which are less active than oxycodone, and then conjugated to inactive glucoronides. Oxycodone has a comparable effect to morphine in neuropathic pain in adults. It has an NNT of 2.6, which means that 1 in every 2.6 patients with neuropathic pain will get a 50% reduction in neuropathic pain with oxycodone (Finnerup et al., 2005). It is available orally as immediate release (4–6 h) and modified release (OxyContin™ 12 h), in addition to preparations combined with acetaminophen (Percocet™) and naloxone (Targin™). Generally speaking we do not support the use of combination analgesics, as the presence of acetaminophen can prevent the upward titration of the opioid analgesic. Parenteral preparations are also available. Unfortunately, oxycodone is one of the most abused opioids in North America, and carries a stigma which may limit its use amongst children (Sproule et al., 2009). When switching from another opioid, it is important to be cognizant of the phenomenon of *incomplete cross-tolerance* whereby a less than equianalgesic dose is required of the second opioid. We recommend converting to a dose of two-thirds of an equianalgesic dose of the second opioid with generous breakthrough analgesia until steady state is reached.

Methadone

Methadone is a synthetic opioid with multiple mechanisms of action making it unique amongst opioids. Originally used for opioid addiction and dependence, methadone is now used for neuropathic pain, particularly for palliative cancer pain management in adults. It comes as a racemic mixture which consists of S- and D-methadone. It has more affinity than morphine for delta receptors and less for mu receptors. It is also a N-methyl-D-aspartate (NMDA) receptor antagonist as well as noradrenaline and serotonin reuptake inhibitor, which may explain its effectiveness in the treatment of neuropathic pain. Methadone is metabolized in the liver by the CYP enzyme family (CYP3A4, CYP1A2, and CYP2D6) to inactive metabolites. Individual pharmacogenetics may therefore go some way to explain the variation in response to the drug. It is excreted via the faecal route and does not accumulate in renal failure (Layson-Wolf et al., 2002).

In adults, methadone has significantly better efficacy than placebo in mixed neuropathic and nociceptive pain (Morley et al., 2003); however, whether it is better than other opioids is not certain. Theoretically, the additional NMDA antagonism of methadone suggests that neuropathic pain should respond better than other opioids but a Cochrane review has not demonstrated additional efficacy of methadone over other opioids in either cancer pain or neuropathic pain within that population (Nicholson, 2007). More trials are needed as anecdotally methadone is perceived to have additional benefit than other opioids in recalcitrant neuropathic pain.

Methadone is usually taken orally once a day, has a high bio-availability (80%), and accumulates with chronic use. The half-life is unpredictable: 12 to 18 h after a single oral dose, and 10 to 75 h after chronic use. In general, the half-life of methadone increases with patient age. Methadone is approximately five to ten times more potent than morphine; however, conversion ratios depend on the pre-switch opioid dose. The general principle of conversion is that the higher the opioid dose, the lower the conversion ratio, and when commencing methadone to 'start low and go slow'. Care should be taken when combining methadone with a TCA, SSNRI, or SSRI due to its effect on serotonin and noradrenaline reuptake. SSRIs also decrease methadone metabolism and increase plasma levels. Carbamazepine and phenytoin interact with methadone by lowering plasma levels by up to 50%. High doses (>200 mg) can result in torsades de pointes, and methadone should only be pre-scribed by an experienced specialist physician.

Cannabinoids

Cannabinoids represent a relatively new pharmacological option as part of a multimodal treatment plan for the management of neuropathic pain (Lynch and Campbell, 2011). With the increasing knowledge of the endocannabinoid system and compelling preclinical work indicating that cannabinoid agonists are analgesic there is increasing attention on their potential role in the management of neuropathic pain. There are no studies in children, but a systematic review of randomized trials of cannabinoids for the treatment of adults with chronic non-cancer pain concluded that cannabinoids are safe and modestly effective in neuropathic pain (Lynch and Campbell, 2011). There were no serious adverse effects reported. Adverse effects that were reported were generally well tolerated, mild to moderate in severity and led to withdrawal from the studies in only a few cases. Cannabinoids studied included smoked cannabis, oromucosal extracts of cannabis-based medicine, nabilone, dronabinol, and a novel tetrahydrocannabinol (THC) analogue. Given that safety and effectiveness have not been established in patients younger than 18 years of age, caution is recommended in prescribing cannabinoids to children predominantly because of psychoactive effects. In practice we recommend the use of nabilone titrated from a very low dose at night (0.005 mg/kg)—and increased to 0.025 mg/kg BID. Nabilone can be compounded—we have used it in very young children through to adolescents. Empirically about one-third of the children obtain some benefit, one-third obtain benefit but limited by side effects, and one-third do not obtain benefit.

Fourth-line agents

Ketamine

Ketamine, an anaesthetic agent and analgesic, is a phencyclidine derivative that can be administered orally, parenterally, topically, intranasally and via the intrathecal or epidural route for neuropathic pain. As an analgesic, ketamine has been used extensively in cancer pain and refractory neuropathic pain, usually as an adjuvant with opioids. Side effects include unpleasant psychomimetic effects, confusion, dysphoria, hallucinations, tachycardia, and hypertension. These adverse effects are usually dose dependent and less pronounced in the lower doses required for analgesia. There is considerable experience with the use of ketamine in children, and the psychomimetic effects appear to be reasonably

well tolerated. Ketamine is usually presented as a racemic mixture of two enantiomers: S(+)-ketamine and R(−)-ketamine. The S(+) enantiomer alone formulation is available in some countries. Ketamine mediates analgesia primarily through non-competitive antagonism at the NMDA receptor at the spinal cord and within the CNS. Reduction in presynaptic release of glutamate may also explain some of the analgesic effect. The S(+) enantiomer has three to four times greater affinity for the NMDA receptor and therefore provides greater analgesia than the R(−) enantiomer at equipotent doses. Ketamine also has a weak effect on opioid receptors, not antagonized by naloxone, as well as antagonistic effects on muscarinic, nicotinic, and monoaminergic receptors. It also exhibits local anaesthetic properties possibly by blocking neuronal sodium ion channels (Bergman, 1999).

Ketamine is metabolized in the liver to norketamine which has a lower anaesthetic potency but greater analgesic potency than ketamine. Oral ketamine therefore is a more potent analgesic than parenteral. Norketamine is then hydroxylated and conjugated by CYP enzyme system in the liver before being excreted via the kidneys.

Systematic reviews of intravenous (IV) ketamine as an adjuvant to opioid analgesia have failed to show a clear benefit in acute perioperative pain (Bell et al., 2005; Elia and Tramer, 2005). IV ketamine infusions may relieve neuropathic pains of different origins, including PHN (Sang, 2000), peripheral neuropathy, and refractory neuropathic pain syndromes, including CRPS in adults (Schwartzman et al., 2009; Sigtermans et al., 2009). Topical ketamine (see also Zempsky, Chapter 47, this volume) can be effective for allodynia in CRPS type 1 (Finch et al., 2009). Studies in children with neuropathic pain are limited to case reports (Takahashi et al., 1998), with successful use in opioid-refractory cancer pain (Klepstad et al., 2001). Ketamine is not currently recommended as a frontline treatment for neuropathic pain in children as the racemic preparation is hampered by problematic side effects and more trials are needed.

Dosage (for analgesia): 0.1 to 0.5 mg/kg PO every 6 h, can be titrated upwards by 0.1 mg/kg per dose. For weight greater than 50 kg the usual oral dose range is 10 to 100 mg every 6 h, and by IV infusion is: 0 to 0.25 mg/kg/h.

Intravenous lidocaine infusion

Lidocaine works by blocking conduction of sodium ion channels to reduce spontaneous action potentials in nerve cells. The analgesic properties of IV lidocaine outlast its pharmacokinetic predicted half-life, and analgesia can last for many weeks after a single infusion (Carroll, 2007).

IV lidocaine has been used with success to treat not only neuropathic pain in adults but also CRPS types 1 and 2, cancer pain, and fibromyalgia (McCleane, 2007). An infusion should be administered in a hospital setting with ECG monitoring, but the treatment is generally safe and well tolerated. There is no consensus on infusion dosages or duration but the pharmacokinetic profiles of lidocaine in adults and children are similar; an infusion rate of 1 mg/kg/h has been used with success in children (Wallace et al., 1997). IV lidocaine represents a useful option in the treatment of neuropathic pain in cases refractory to conventional therapy or cases limited by side effects of oral medications. While plasma levels of lidocaine can be measured (levels between 2 and 5 mcg/ml are thought to be therapeutic); we are not aware that this is done in routine clinical practice. Doses should be adjusted in cases of hepatic and renal insufficiency to avoid toxicity.

Mexiletine

Mexiletine is an oral type 1b antiarrhythmic agent that is analogous to lidocaine in its mechanism of action. It also acts by blocking sodium channels and has been shown to be of some benefit in adults with painful diabetic neuropathy, though not much superior to placebo (Duby et al., 2004). Its oral preparation is an advantage as opposed to IV lidocaine, however its use in children is limited (Wallace et al., 2000) although there are paediatric case reports of its efficacy in erythromelalgia (Jang et al., 2004; Nathan et al., 2005).

Other anticonvulsants

Older anticonvulsant drugs such as carbamazepine and phenytoin, typically used in adults with trigeminal neuralgia, have been superseded by newer drugs which are generally safer more effective (e.g. gabapentin). In addition the need for monitoring of liver function with these drugs makes them less appealing in children (Dworkin et al., 2007). The evidence in adults for the use of lamotrigine, oxcarbazepine, valproate, topiramate, lacosamide, and levetiracetam in neuropathic pain has not been convincing, so their place in paediatric neuropathic pain management is uncertain at this time and should only be considered in recalcitrant cases (Finnerup et al., 2010).

Miscellaneous

Other oral NMDA receptor antagonists such as dextromethorphan, memantine, and riluzide have showed only minor or no improvement in neuropathic pain in adults (Finnerup et al., 2005, 2007), with little experience in children. Magnesium is also an NMDA receptor antagonist that has been shown to be of benefit in neuropathic pain in animal models (Rondon et al., 2010). Its obvious benefit over ketamine is the improved side effect profile, but the drug needs to be given as an IV infusion and further work is required before its role can be fully clarified.

Botulinum toxin A has been used extensively in the treatment of spasticity in children with cerebral palsy (Lukban et al., 2009), and there is emerging data that it may also be effective in neuropathic pain (Francisco et al., 2012). Trials have not shown consistent benefit yet (Dworkin et al., 2010), but familiarity with the drug in children suggests it might have a role.

Combination strategies

Frequently a single first-line drug is insufficient in alleviating pain to an acceptable level, or side effects become limiting at the higher dose range. In these situations adding in a second agent can provide an additive or synergistic effect to improve analgesia and reduce side effects. The combination of nortriptyline and gabapentin has been demonstrated in an RCT to be superior in neuropathic pain than either drug alone (Gilron et al., 2009). Many RCTs that provide good evidence for combination strategies in adults with neuropathic pain involve opioids as the co-analgesic. The combination of an α_2-δ ligand with an opioid has been studied for painful diabetic neuropathy and PHN in adults (Gilron et al., 2005). In fact, morphine was slightly more effective than gabapentin but

the combination provided better analgesia than either drug alone. Combinations of oxycodone and gabapentin have also demonstrated combined improved efficacy at lower dosages than either drug alone (Hanna et al., 2008), however a trial with oxycodone and pregabalin showed no enhanced dual effect (Zin et al., 2010). If based solely on efficacy then opioids would deserve to be second-line treatments for neuropathic pain, however the choice of medication needs to be considered also in terms of potential risks and tolerability, especially in the paediatric population. The relatively improved side effect profile and long-term superior health-related quality of life indices of α_2-δ ligands as compared to opioids makes them the better first-line choice.

Key recommendations

The algorithm in Figure 48.2 is based upon the current literature and our clinical experience in treating neuropathic pain cognizant of risks and long-term effects in children, and extrapolating the best quality evidence from controlled trials in adults with neuropathic pain. This algorithm should be followed in the context of an interdisciplinary approach also incorporating physical and psychological strategies.

After a reasonable trial of 4 to 6 weeks of the selected first-line medication, and only partial analgesia (NRS ≥4/10) or troublesome side effects, an additional co-analgesic should be commenced. In acute severe neuropathic pain scenarios (e.g. Guillain–Barré syndrome or cancer pain), one may escalate more quickly and have a lower threshold for combination strategies

Third-line medications can be added if there is some pre-existing benefit of first or second line, or alone *de novo* if not.

The decision to use fourth-line medications with limited evidence, such as ketamine or IV lidocaine, should only be made at specialist paediatric centres

Conclusion

Neuropathic pain in children can be debilitating with significant impact on mood, sleep, and function, whilst posing a difficult challenge to health care practitioners. The challenge is made more problematic with an over reliance on evidence extrapolated from studies in adults, whose neuropathic pain conditions are uncommon in children and may be quite separate phenomena. Clearly, specific screening and diagnostic tools for neuropathic pain in children are required, in addition to good quality multicentre drug trials. In our experience, the early identification and treatment of neuropathic pain in children can often result in effective sustained reversal of symptoms in many cases, likely due in part to the plasticity of the developing nervous system.

Future directions for pharmacological management will include pharmacogenomics, with a view to tailoring specific drug regimens for individual patients, and stem cell research which also carries promise (Braz et al., 2012). However, it must be reiterated that the pharmacological management alone of neuropathic pain is very unlikely to fully alleviate symptoms. Drugs must form part of an interdisciplinary approach incorporating physical, psychological, and occasionally interventional techniques to achieve successful outcomes in children with neuropathic pain.

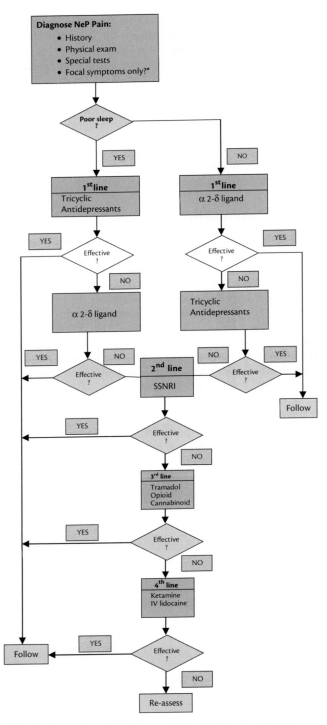

*for focal neuropathic pain, topical agents could be used either along with or in lieu of systemic neuropathic medication. In this case 5% lidocaine patch would be the first line followed by capsaicin.

Figure 48.2 Drug treatment for neuropathic pain (NeP); an algorithm.

Case example

A 13-year-old girl diagnosed with Charcot–Marie–Tooth disease (CMT) type 1A (confirmed by genetic testing—*PMP22* gene duplication) was referred to the chronic pain clinic with a 2-month history of neuropathic pain in the hands and feet. CMT disease is a hereditary polyneuropathy condition presenting with distal weakness and muscular atrophy (myopathy). It is a slowly progressing, demyelinating disease of peripheral nerves, and is also known as hereditary motor and sensory neuropathy (HMSN) of which there are several subtypes. Clinical features include loss of reflexes, pes cavus foot deformity, and hammertoes. It is an increasingly recognized cause of neuropathic pain in children.

The pain was described as a constant burning, tingling and itchy 'deep' sensation. There was intermittent stabbing pain in her toes. There were no autonomic symptoms such as changes in colour, sweating, temperature or hair or nail growth, suggestive of CRPS. She rated the pain intensity as 7/10 on the numeric pain scale (NRS) at the clinic appointment. The range of pain intensity scores varied between 6 to 10/10. The average pain score was 7/10. She reported that the pain needed to be 4/10 or less to find it manageable. When asked to score how unpleasant she found her pain she rated it as 8/10. Her sleep was disturbed by pain; taking at least 1 h to fall asleep, and waking her two to three times per night due to allodynia from the bed sheets. She was frustrated rather than depressed; she reported lethargy, reduced energy and difficulty concentrating at school. She was missing 1 day of school per week because of pain. Her physical activities were significantly affected in that she had stopped participating in gym and swimming. There was some evidence of fear-avoidance to her pain behaviours on a background of mild anxiety. Previous pharmacological interventions had not been helpful at either reducing pain or improving function; these included acetaminophen and ibuprofen, and a topical compound of ketamine, ketoprofen, and lidocaine. Neither physical nor psychological interventions had been tried. She lived with her parents and two younger brothers, all of whom were healthy.

Physical examination revealed an age-appropriate, somewhat shy 13-year-old girl in no acute distress (150 cm tall, weight 48 kg). Pain was outlined on the palmer aspect of both hands and feet with reduced sensation. Allodynia and hyperalgesia were present over the toes. Wrist and ankle deep tendon reflexes were reduced.

Neuropathic pain secondary to CMT disease affecting the hands and feet was diagnosed; with significant pain related disability. Education was provided regarding the nature of neuropathic pain and a pain management plan comprising pharmacological, physical, and psychological strategies was developed in collaboration with the patient and her parents. She was started on gabapentin 100 mg PO once daily to be slowly increased in a step-wise manner to 300 mg PO three times daily as tolerated.

Physical strategies comprised education around promoting normal function, desensitization, and a graded exercise programme. A psychological evaluation was scheduled to evaluate to what extent cognitive and emotional factors were contributing to pain and pain related disability; with a view to teaching some relaxation and distraction strategies.

The patient was reviewed in the pain clinic 6 weeks later. The gabapentin had been increased to 100 mg PO three times daily resulting in excessive daytime somnolence, with marginal benefit in pain relief. Furthermore, she had difficulty swallowing the pills given their relatively large size. Given that pain was worse at night with subsequent sleep disturbance, she was switched to amitriptyline 10 mg PO every night at bedtime after an ECG was reported as normal. She was advised that the dose could be doubled if well-tolerated and additional analgesia was required. The next time she was seen in clinic, her pain was better controlled, with an average pain intensity score of 1/10 using the NRS. She had stabilized on a 20 mg dose of amitriptyline, which was well tolerated. She also found physical strategies (ice packs, massage) and psychological strategies (distraction, relaxation) helpful. She reported improved sleep, mood (less frustration), and function (participating in school, hobbies, and seeing friends).

References

Anand, P. and Bley, K. (2011). Topical capsaicin for pain management: therapeutic potential and mechanisms of action of the new high-concentration capsaicin 8% patch. *Br J Anaesth*, 107, 490–502.

Backonja, M., Beydoun, A., Edwards, K. R., Schwartz, S. L., Fonseca, V., Hes, M., *et al.* (1998). Gabapentin for the symptomatic treatment of painful neuropathy in patients with diabetes mellitus: a randomized controlled trial. *JAMA*, 280, 1831–1836.

Backonja, M., Wallace, M. S., Blonsky, E. R., Cutler, B. J., Malan, P., Jr., Rauck, R., *et al.* (2008). NGX-4010, a high-concentration capsaicin patch, for the treatment of postherpetic neuralgia: a randomised, double-blind study. *Lancet Neurol*, 7, 1106–1112.

Bell, R. F., Dahl, J. B., Moore, R. A., and Kalso, E. (2005). Peri-operative ketamine for acute post-operative pain: a quantitative and qualitative systematic review (Cochrane review). *Acta Anaesthesiol Scand*, 49, 1405–1428.

Bergman, S. A. (1999). Ketamine: review of its pharmacology and its use in pediatric anesthesia. *Anesth Prog*, 46, 10–20.

Biederman, J., Thisted, R. A., Greenhill, L. L., and Ryan, N. D. (1995). Estimation of the association between desipramine and the risk for sudden death in 5- to 14-year-old children. *J Clin Psychiatry*, 56, 87–93.

Binder, A., Bruxelle, J., Rogers, P., Hans, G., Bosl, I., and Baron, R. (2009). Topical 5% lidocaine (lignocaine) medicated plaster treatment for post-herpetic neuralgia: results of a double-blind, placebo-controlled, multinational efficacy and safety trial. *Clin Drug Investig*, 29, 393–408.

Boroujerdi, A., Zeng, J., Sharp, K., Kim, D., Steward, O., and Luo, Z. D. (2011). Calcium channel alpha-2-delta-1 protein upregulation in dorsal spinal cord mediates spinal cord injury-induced neuropathic pain states. *Pain*, 152, 649–655.

Boureau, F., Legallicier, P., and Kabir-Ahmadi, M. (2003). Tramadol in post-herpetic neuralgia: a randomized, double-blind, placebo-controlled trial. *Pain*, 104, 323–331.

Braz, J. M., Sharif-Naeini, R., Vogt, D., Kriegstein, A., Alvarez-Buylla, A., Rubenstein, J. L., *et al.* (2012). Forebrain GABAergic neuron precursors integrate into adult spinal cord and reduce injury-induced neuropathic pain. *Neuron*, 74(4), 663–675.

Carroll, I. (2007). Intravenous lidocaine for neuropathic pain: diagnostic utility and therapeutic efficacy. *Curr Pain Headache Rep*, 11, 20–24.

Cicero, T. J., Inciardi, J. A., Adams, E. H., Geller, A., Senay, E. C., Woody, G. E., *et al.* (2005). Rates of abuse of tramadol remain unchanged with the introduction of new branded and generic products: results of an abuse monitoring system, 1994–2004. *Pharmacoepidemiol Drug Saf*, 14, 851–859.

Ciszkowski, C., Madadi, P., Phillips, M. S., Lauwers, A. E., and Koren, G. (2009). Codeine, ultrarapid-metabolism genotype, and postoperative death. *N Engl J Med*, 361, 827–828.

Derry, S., Lloyd, R., Moore, R. A., and McQuay, H. J. (2009). Topical capsaicin for chronic neuropathic pain in adults. *Cochrane Database Syst Rev*, 4, CD007393.

Duby, J. J., Campbell, R. K., Setter, S. M., White, J. R., and Rasmussen, K. A. (2004). Diabetic neuropathy: an intensive review. *Am J Health Syst Pharm*, 61, 160–173.

Dworkin, R. H., O'Connor, A. B., Audette, J., Baron, R., Gourlay, G. K., Haanpaa, M. L., *et al.* (2010). Recommendations for the pharmacological management of neuropathic pain: an overview and literature update. *Mayo Clin Proc*, 85, S3–14.

Dworkin, R. H., O'Connor, A. B., Backonja, M., Farrar, J. T., Finnerup, N. B., Jensen, T. S., *et al.* (2007). Pharmacologic management of neuropathic pain: evidence-based recommendations. *Pain*, 132, 237–251.

Eisenberg, E., McNicol, E., and Carr, D. B. (2006). Opioids for neuropathic pain. *Cochrane Database Syst Rev*, 3, CD006146.

Elia, N. and Tramer, M. R. (2005). Ketamine and postoperative pain—a quantitative systematic review of randomised trials. *Pain*, 113, 61–70.

Finch, P. M., Knudsen, L., and Drummond, P. D. (2009). Reduction of allodynia in patients with complex regional pain syndrome: A double-blind placebo-controlled trial of topical ketamine. *Pain*, 146, 18–25.

Finnerup, N. B., Otto, M., Jensen, T. S., and Sindrup, S. H. (2007). An evidence-based algorithm for the treatment of neuropathic pain. *MedGenMed*, 9, 36.

Finnerup, N. B., Otto, M., Mcquay, H. J., Jensen, T. S., and Sindrup, S. H. (2005). Algorithm for neuropathic pain treatment: an evidence based proposal. *Pain*, 118, 289–305.

Finnerup, N. B., Sindrup, S. H., and Jensen, T. S. (2010). The evidence for pharmacological treatment of neuropathic pain. *Pain*, 150, 573–581.

Francisco, G. E., Tan, H., and Green, M. (2012). Do botulinum toxins have a role in the management of neuropathic pain?: A focused review. *Am J Phys Med Rehabil*, 91(10), 899–909.

Freynhagen, R., Strojek, K., Griesing, T., Whalen, E., and Balkenohl, M. (2005). Efficacy of pregabalin in neuropathic pain evaluated in a 12-week, randomised, double-blind, multicentre, placebo-controlled trial of flexible- and fixed-dose regimens. *Pain*, 115, 254–263.

Gee, N. S., Brown, J. P., Dissanayake, V. U., Offord, J., Thurlow, R., and Woodruff, G. N. (1996). The novel anticonvulsant drug, gabapentin (Neurontin), binds to the alpha2delta subunit of a calcium channel. *J Biol Chem*, 271, 5768–5776.

Gilron, I., Bailey, J. M., Tu, D., Holden, R. R., Jackson, A. C., and Houlden, R. L. (2009). Nortriptyline and gabapentin, alone and in combination for neuropathic pain: a double-blind, randomised controlled crossover trial. *Lancet*, 374, 1252–1261.

Gilron, I., Bailey, J. M., Tu, D., Holden, R. R., Weaver, D. F., and Houlden, R. L. (2005). Morphine, gabapentin, or their combination for neuropathic pain. *N Engl J Med*, 352, 1324–1334.

Golden, A. S., Haut, S. R., and Moshe, S. L. (2006). Nonepileptic uses of antiepileptic drugs in children and adolescents. *Pediatr Neurol*, 34, 421–432.

Grothe, D. R., Scheckner, B., and Albano, D. (2004). Treatment of pain syndromes with venlafaxine. *Pharmacotherapy*, 24, 621–629.

Haney, A. L., Garner, S. S., and Cox, T. H. (2009). Gabapentin therapy for pain and irritability in a neurologically impaired infant. *Pharmacotherapy*, 29, 997–1001.

Hanna, M., O'Brien, C., and Wilson, M. C. (2008). Prolonged-release oxycodone enhances the effects of existing gabapentin therapy in painful diabetic neuropathy patients. *Eur J Pain*, 12, 804–813.

Harati, Y., Gooch, C., Swenson, M., Edelman, S., Greene, D., Raskin, P., *et al.* (1998). Double-blind randomized trial of tramadol for the treatment of the pain of diabetic neuropathy. *Neurology*, 50, 1842–1846.

Hauer, J. M., Wical, B. S., and Charnas, L. (2007). Gabapentin successfully manages chronic unexplained irritability in children with severe neurologic impairment. *Pediatrics*, 119, e519–522.

Hauser, W., Bernardy, K., Uceyler, N., and Sommer, C. (2009). Treatment of fibromyalgia syndrome with antidepressants: a meta-analysis. *JAMA*, 301, 198–209.

Hempenstall, K., Nurmikko, T. J., Johnson, R. W., A'Hern, R. P., and Rice, A. S. (2005). Analgesic therapy in postherpetic neuralgia: a quantitative systematic review. *PLoS Med*, 2, e164.

Hollingshead, J., Duhmke, R. M., and Cornblath, D. R. (2006). Tramadol for neuropathic pain. *Cochrane Database Syst Rev*, 3, CD003726.

Jang, H. S., Jung, D., Kim, S., Jo, J., Lee, J., Kim, M., Oh, C., and Kwon, K. (2004). A case of primary erythromelalgia improved by mexiletine. *Br J Dermatol*, 151, 708–710.

Katz, N., and Mazer, N. A. (2009). The impact of opioids on the endocrine system. *Clin J Pain*, 25, 170–175.

Klepstad, P., Borchgrevink, P., Hval, B., Flaat, S., and Kaasa, S. (2001). Long-term treatment with ketamine in a 12-year-old girl with severe neuropathic pain caused by a cervical spinal tumor. *J Pediatr Hematol Oncol*, 23, 616–619.

Layson-Wolf, C., Goode, J. V., and Small, R. E. (2002). Clinical use of methadone. *J Pain Palliat Care Pharmacother*, 16, 29–59.

Li, C. Y., Zhang, X. L., Matthews, E. A., Li, K. W., Kurwa, A., Boroujerdi, A., *et al.* (2006). Calcium channel alpha2delta1 subunit mediates spinal hyperexcitability in pain modulation. *Pain*, 125, 20–34.

Lotsch, J., and Geisslinger, G. (2006). Current evidence for a genetic modulation of the response to analgesics. *Pain*, 121, 1–5.

Lukban, M. B., Rosales, R. L., and Dressler, D. (2009). Effectiveness of botulinum toxin A for upper and lower limb spasticity in children with cerebral palsy: a summary of evidence. *J Neural Transm*, 116, 319–331.

Luo, Z. D., Calcutt, N. A., Higuera, E. S., Valder, C. R., Song, Y. H., Svensson, C. I., *et al.* (2002). Injury type-specific calcium channel alpha 2 delta-1 subunit up-regulation in rat neuropathic pain models correlates with antiallodynic effects of gabapentin. *J Pharmacol Exp Ther*, 303, 1199–1205.

Lynch, M. E., and Campbell, F. (2011). Cannabinoids for treatment of chronic non-cancer pain; a systematic review of randomized trials. *Br J Clin Pharmacol*, 72, 735–744.

Madadi, P. and Koren, G. (2008). Pharmacogenetic insights into codeine analgesia: implications to pediatric codeine use. *Pharmacogenomics*, 9, 1267–1284.

Mattia, C., Paoletti, F., Coluzzi, F., and Boanelli, A. (2002). New antidepressants in the treatment of neuropathic pain. A review. *Minerva Anestesiol*, 68, 105–114.

Max, M. B., Culnane, M., Schafer, S. C., Gracely, R. H., Walther, D. J., Smoller, B., *et al.* (1987). Amitriptyline relieves diabetic neuropathy pain in patients with normal or depressed mood. *Neurology*, 37, 589–596.

McCleane, G. (2007). Intravenous lidocaine: an outdated or underutilized treatment for pain? *J Palliat Med*, 10, 798–805.

McGraw, T. and Kosek, P. (1997). Erythromelalgia pain managed with gabapentin. *Anesthesiology*, 86, 988–990.

Meier, T., Wasner, G., Faust, M., Kuntzer, T., Ochsner, F., Hueppe, M., *et al.* (2003). Efficacy of lidocaine patch 5% in the treatment of focal peripheral neuropathic pain syndromes: a randomized, double-blind, placebo-controlled study. *Pain*, 106, 151–158.

Merskey, H. and Bogduk, N. (1994). *Classification of chronic pain* (2nd edn). Seattle, WA: IASP Press.

Morley, J. S., Bridson, J., Nash, T. P., Miles, J. B., White, S., and Makin, M. K. (2003). Low-dose methadone has an analgesic effect in neuropathic pain: a double-blind randomized controlled crossover trial. *Palliat Med*, 17, 576–587.

Moss, A., Beggs, S., Vega-Avelaira, D., Costigan, M., Hathway, G. J., Salter, M. W., *et al.* (2007). Spinal microglia and neuropathic pain in young rats. *Pain*, 128, 215–224.

Nathan, A., Rose, J. B., Guite, J. W., Hehir, D., and Milovcich, K. (2005). Primary erythromelalgia in a child responding to intravenous lidocaine and oral mexiletine treatment. *Pediatrics*, 115, e504–507.

National Opioid Use Guideline Group (NOUGG). (2010). *Canadian guideline for safe and effective use of opioids for chronic non-cancer pain*. Available at: <http://nationalpaincentre.mcmaster.ca/opioid/>.

Nayak, S. and Cunliffe, M. (2008). Lidocaine 5% patch for localized chronic neuropathic pain in adolescents: report of five cases. *Paediatr Anaesth*, 18, 554–558.

Nicholson, A. B. (2007). Methadone for cancer pain. *Cochrane Database Syst Rev*, 1, CD003971.

Nielsen, C. K., Ross, F. B., Lotfipour, S., Saini, K. S., Edwards, S. R., and Smith, M. T. (2007). Oxycodone and morphine have distinctly different pharmacological profiles: radioligand binding and behavioural studies in two rat models of neuropathic pain. *Pain*, 132, 289–300.

Niscola, P., Sorrentino, F., Scaramucci, L., De Fabritiis, P., and Cianciulli, P. (2009). Pain syndromes in sickle cell disease: an update. *Pain Med*, 10, 470–480.

Rondon, L. J., Privat, A. M., Daulhac, L., Davin, N., Mazur, A., Fialip, J., *et al.* (2010). Magnesium attenuates chronic hypersensitivity and spinal cord NMDA receptor phosphorylation in a rat model of diabetic neuropathic pain. *J Physiol*, 588, 4205–4215.

Rosielle, D. A. (2008). The lidocaine patch #148. *J Palliat Med*, 11, 502–503.

Rowbotham, M., Harden, N., Stacey, B., Bernstein, P., and Magnus-Miller, L. (1998). Gabapentin for the treatment of postherpetic neuralgia: a randomized controlled trial. *JAMA*, 280, 1837–1842.

Rowbotham, M. C., Davies, P. S., and Fields, H. L. (1995). Topical lidocaine gel relieves postherpetic neuralgia. *Ann Neurol*, 37, 246–253.

Rowbotham, M. C., Goli, V., Kunz, N. R., and Lei, D. (2004). Venlafaxine extended release in the treatment of painful diabetic neuropathy: a double-blind, placebo-controlled study. *Pain*, 110, 697–706.

Rusy, L. M., Troshynski, T. J., and Weisman, S. J. (2001). Gabapentin in phantom limb pain management in children and young adults: report of seven cases. *J Pain Symptom Manage*, 21, 78–82.

Saarto, T. and Wiffen, P. J. (2005). Antidepressants for neuropathic pain. *Cochrane Database Syst Rev*, 3, CD005454.

Sang, C. N. (2000). NMDA-receptor antagonists in neuropathic pain: experimental methods to clinical trials. *J Pain Symptom Manage*, 19, S21–25.

Schwartzman, R. J., Alexander, G. M., Grothusen, J. R., Paylor, T., Reichenberger, E., and Perreault, M. (2009). Outpatient intravenous ketamine for the treatment of complex regional pain syndrome: a double-blind placebo controlled study. *Pain*, 147, 107–115.

Serpell, M. G. (2002). Gabapentin in neuropathic pain syndromes: a randomised, double-blind, placebo-controlled trial. *Pain*, 99, 557–566.

Sigtermans, M. J., Van Hilten, J. J., Bauer, M. C., Arbous, M. S., Marinus, J., Sarton, E. Y., *et al.* (2009). Ketamine produces effective and long-term pain relief in patients with complex regional pain syndrome type 1. *Pain*, 145, 304–311.

Sindrup, S. H., Andersen, G., Madsen, C., Smith, T., Brosen, K., and Jensen, T. S. (1999). Tramadol relieves pain and allodynia in polyneuropathy: a randomised, double-blind, controlled trial. *Pain*, 83, 85–90.

Smith, T. R. (2006). Duloxetine in diabetic neuropathy. *Expert Opin Pharmacother*, 7, 215–223.

Sorge, R. E., Trang, T., Dorfman, R., Smith, S. B., Beggs, S., Ritchie, J., *et al.* (2012). Genetically determined P2X7 receptor pore formation regulates variability in chronic pain sensitivity. *Nat Med*, 18, 595–599.

Sproule, B., Brands, B., Li, S., and Catz-Biro, L. (2009). Changing patterns in opioid addiction: characterizing users of oxycodone and other opioids. *Can Fam Physician*, 55, 68–9, 69 e1–5.

Takahashi, H., Miyazaki, M., Nanbu, T., Yanagida, H., and Morita, S. (1998). The NMDA-receptor antagonist ketamine abolishes neuropathic pain after epidural administration in a clinical case. *Pain*, 75, 391–394.

Torrance, N., Smith, B. H., Bennett, M. I., and Lee, A. J. (2006). The epidemiology of chronic pain of predominantly neuropathic origin. Results from a general population survey. *J Pain*, 7, 281–289.

Treede, R., Jensen, T., Campbell, J., Cruccu, G., and Dostrovsky, J. (2008). Neuropathic pain—redefinition and grading system. *Neurology*, 70, 1630–1635.

Vallejo, R., De Leon-Casasola, O., and Benyamin, R. (2004). Opioid therapy and immunosuppression: a review. *Am J Ther*, 11, 354–365.

Varley, C. K. (2001). Sudden death related to selected tricyclic antidepressants in children: epidemiology, mechanisms and clinical implications. *Paediatr Drugs*, 3, 613–627.

Vega-Avelaira, D., Moss, A., and Fitzgerald, M. (2007). Age-related changes in the spinal cord microglial and astrocytic response profile to nerve injury. *Brain Behav Immun*, 21, 617–623.

Vondracek, P., Oslejskova, H., Kepak, T., Mazanek, P., Sterba, J., Rysava, M., *et al.* (2009). Efficacy of pregabalin in neuropathic pain in paediatric oncological patients. *Eur J Paediatr Neurol*, 13, 332–336.

Walco, G. A., Dworkin, R. H., Krane, E. J., Lebel, A. A., and Treede, R. D. (2010). Neuropathic pain in children: Special considerations. *Mayo Clin Proc*, 85, S33–41.

Walker, S. M. (2008). Pain in children: recent advances and ongoing challenges. *Br J Anaesth*, 101, 101–110.

Wallace, M. S., Lee, J., Sorkin, L., Dunn, J. S., Yaksh, T., and Yu, A. (1997). Intravenous lidocaine: effects on controlling pain after anti-GD2 antibody therapy in children with neuroblastoma—a report of a series. *Anesth Analg*, 85, 794–796.

Wallace, M. S., Magnuson, S., and Ridgeway, B. (2000). Efficacy of oral mexiletine for neuropathic pain with allodynia: a double-blind, placebo-controlled, crossover study. *Reg Anesth Pain Med*, 25, 459–467.

Wernicke, J., Lledo, A., Raskin, J., Kajdasz, D. K., and Wang, F. (2007). An evaluation of the cardiovascular safety profile of duloxetine: findings from 42 placebo-controlled studies. *Drug Saf*, 30, 437–455.

Wernicke, J. F., Pritchett, Y. L., D'souza, D. N., Waninger, A., Tran, P., Iyengar, S., *et al.* (2006). A randomized controlled trial of duloxetine in diabetic peripheral neuropathic pain. *Neurology*, 67, 1411–1420.

Wheeler, D. S., Vaux, K. K., and Tam, D. A. (2000). Use of gabapentin in the treatment of childhood reflex sympathetic dystrophy. *Pediatr Neurol*, 22, 220–221.

Zacny, J., Bigelow, G., Compton, P., Foley, K., Iguchi, M., and Sannerud, C. (2003). College on Problems of Drug Dependence taskforce on prescription opioid non-medical use and abuse: position statement. *Drug Alcohol Depend*, 69, 215–232.

Zin, C. S., Nissen, L. M., O'Callaghan, J. P., Duffull, S. B., Smith, M. T., and Moore, B. J. (2010). A randomized, controlled trial of oxycodone versus placebo in patients with postherpetic neuralgia and painful diabetic neuropathy treated with pregabalin. *J Pain*, 11, 462–471.

CHAPTER 49

Sucrose and sweet taste

Denise Harrison, Vanessa C. Z. Anseloni,
Janet Yamada, and Mariana Bueno

Summary

Abundant evidence demonstrates pain-reducing effects of sweet solutions in human infants and animals. Analgesic effects persist up to around 1 year of age in human infants, although the effects are more moderate than seen in the neonatal period. Effects are considered to be due to the relationship between sweet taste and the endogenous opiate system. Yet, despite extensive research, knowledge gaps remain relating to the exact mechanisms, the effectiveness and safety of sweet solutions when given over prolonged periods to preterm and sick infants, the effectiveness in sick infants receiving concomitant analgesics, and the effectiveness in children older than 12 months of age. Based on the extensive evidence to support sweet solutions, their use can be recommended prior to commonly performed short lasting minor painful procedures in newborn and young infants.

Introduction

Calming and pain-reducing effects of sweet-tasting solutions in infants have been demonstrated in more than 150 published studies, and are one of the most extensively studied interventions in infant care (Harrison and Bueno, 2012; Harrison et al., 2010a). With few exceptions, findings of trials, systematic reviews, and meta-analyses have consistently shown that sucrose and glucose reduce behavioural responses during commonly performed painful procedures in diverse populations of preterm and term newborn infants, and infants up to 12 months of age (Table 49.1) (Harrison et al., 2010a, 2010b; Stevens et al., 2010; Tsao et al., 2007). Based on this evidence, sweet solutions are recommended by national and international organizations (American Academy of Pediatrics Committee on Fetus and Newborn et al., 2006; Anand and International Evidence-Based Group for Neonatal Pain, 2001; Harrison and Australian College of Neonatal Nurses, 2006; Henderson-Smart and Australian & New Zealand Neonatal Network, 2007; Royal Australasian College of Physicians, 2005). Yet, despite such compelling evidence and recommendations, use of sucrose or glucose during painful procedures has not been translated into widespread consistent utilization in clinical practice in hospitals (Carbajal et al., 2008; Johnston et al., 2011; Losacco et al., 2011; Stevens et al., 2011) or ambulatory care settings (Harrison et al., 2013; Taddio et al., 2009). Reasons for this

knowledge/evidence practice gap are in all likelihood multifactorial, but may be related to remaining knowledge and research gaps or prevailing myths or controversies concerning analgesic effects of sweet solutions. This chapter will review (1) the mechanisms of sweet taste induced analgesia and (2) the evidence obtained from bench to bedside studies in animals, human infants, toddlers, pre-school children, and school-aged children. Uncertainties, knowledge gaps, and current controversies will be highlighted and translation of knowledge concerning effectiveness of sweet solutions in diverse patient populations and settings will be discussed. Finally, this chapter will provide implications for practice and directions for future research.

Sweet taste-induced analgesic mechanisms: the animal studies

Analgesic, calming, and distress-reducing effects of sweet taste were first demonstrated in rodent pups in 1987 (Blass et al., 1987). Effects of sweet solutions were demonstrated to occur rapidly, last for several minutes, and were blocked by systemic opioid receptor antagonists.

The effects were reported to be age dependent with a decline in effectiveness as the rodents aged. Analgesic and calming effects of oral sucrose were demonstrated as early as postnatal day 2 to 3, peaked at postnatal day 10, then declined by postnatal day 14, and were ineffective by postnatal day 21; the weaning time of rodents. In the presence of inflammation, the analgesic effects of sucrose (7.5%) are initially present on postnatal day 3 for inflamed forepaw and postnatal day 13 for inflamed hindpaw. By postnatal day 17, the analgesic effects of sucrose were no longer present for both inflamed fore- and hindpaws. These findings support that sucrose is age dependent and also has differential maturational effects that work in parallel to the changes in the endogenous analgesic mechanisms and the developmental features between gustatory and pain pathways in neonatal rats (Anseloni et al., 2002).

Reports from studies of rodents also showed that amongst sweet-tasting solutions there is a rank-order of potency in which sucrose is more analgesic and calming than glucose, and the latter is more effective than fructose and lactose had no analgesic effects (Blass and Shide, 1994). Studies also investigated a possible dose–response function of sugar concentrations; however, increasing the

Table 49.1 Systematic reviews of sweet solutions for analgesia in infants and children

Reference	Population and details	Summary of findings/recommendations
Stevens, B., Yamada, J., Lee, G. Y., and Ohlsson, A. (2013). Sucrose for analgesia in newborn infants undergoing painful procedures. *Cochrane Database Syst Rev*, 1, CD001069	N = 57 RCTs, 4,730 infants Population: term (29), preterm (27), both preterm and term (1) neonates Procedures: HL (30); eye examination (6); VP (9); circumcision (3); subcutaneous injection (2); combination of procedures (2); all procedures (2); NGT insertion (2), urethral catheterization (1)	◆ Sucrose is effective and safe for reducing procedural pain in neonates from single events ◆ NNS and other non-pharmacological methods of pain relief should be considered in combination with sucrose ◆ Further research on sucrose in combination with other behavioural (e.g. facilitated tucking, kangaroo care) and pharmacological (e.g. morphine, fentanyl) interventions for more invasive procedures is warranted ◆ The use of repeated dosing of sucrose and its impact on clinical development is required
Bueno, M., Yamada, J., Harrison, D., Kahn, S., Adams-Webber, T., Beyene, J., *et al.* (2013). A systematic review and meta-analyses of non-sucrose sweet solutions sucrose for pain relief in neonates. *Pain Res Manage*	N = 38 RCTs, 3785 infants Population: term (23), preterm (10), both preterm and term (5) neonates Procedures: HL (19); VP (10); IM injections (3); eye examination (1); circumcision (1); subcutaneous injection (1); PICC (1); combination of procedures (2)	◆ Glucose is effective and safe for reducing procedural pain in neonates from single events ◆ Concentrations from 20–30% and higher were effective ◆ Small volumes were required ◆ Glucose can be incorporated into clinical settings as an alternative when sucrose is not readily available.
Harrison, D., Stevens, B., Bueno, M., Yamada, J., Adams-Webber, T., Beyene, J., *et al.* (2010). Efficacy of sweet solutions for analgesia in infants between one and 12 months of age: A systematic review. *Arch Dis Child*, 95(6), 406–413	N = 14 RCTs, 1674 injections in 1618 infants Population: infants 1–12 months during immunization Discussion included 3 other RCTS: HL, VP and urethral catheterization	◆ Sucrose or glucose is effective for reducing immunization pain. ◆ Other recommended pain reduction strategies, such as NNS, breastfeeding, and distraction should be consistently utilized for immunization, and considered for other painful procedures ◆ Total dose of sweet solution should be given in aliquots commencing 1–2 min prior to painful procedure, immediately prior to procedure, and at intervals throughout procedure to ensure sustained analgesic effects
Harrison, D., Yamada, J., Adams-Webber, T., Ohlsson, A., Beyene, J., and Stevens, B., *et al.* (2011). Sweet tasting solutions for reduction of needle-related procedural pain in children aged 1 to 16 years. *Cochrane Database Syst Rev*, 10, CD008408	N = 4 RCTs, 330 children Population: children 12 months–16 years during IM injection (3), venepuncture (1)	◆ Conflicting evidence in toddlers aged 12–18 months. Insufficient evidence to recommend use ◆ No evidence of efficacy in school aged children

concentration of sucrose did not result in increased analgesic and calming effects (Blass and Shide, 1994).

Opioid basis of effects

The neurochemical basis of the sweet-taste analgesia has been investigated both in human and animal newborns. Studies reported that the effects of orally administered sugars and fats are mediated by endogenous opioids (Anseloni et al., 2002; Blass et al., 1987, 1991). Analgesic and calming effects of sweet solutions and milk were reversed by injections of naloxone and naltrexone, non-selective opioid receptor antagonists (Anseloni et al., 2002; Blass and Fitzgerald, 1988; Blass et al., 1987, 1991; Shide and Blass, 1989). Several studies reported the mechanisms underlying sweet-taste analgesia. The stimulation of the taste buds in the oral cavity remains the main mechanistic explanation due to the rapid onset of the effects of sweet solutions given orally. It is clear that oral infusion of sweet solutions do not happen due to somatosensory stimulation in the oral cavity or gustatory stimulation in general,

since distilled water, saline, or other salty solutions do not produce analgesia (Anseloni et al., 2002, 2005; Blass, 1997; Blass et al., 1987; Ren et al., 1997; Shide and Blass, 1989).

Further evidence is needed to describe the mechanisms in which sweet-taste stimulation of the taste buds involve specific nerve branches. One study showed that, in rodents, sweet-taste receptors are located mainly on the palate, which is consistent with reports on the greater involvement of the greater petrosal nerve fibres instead of the chorda tympani fibres (Travers, 1993). The question of the possible contribution of post-ingestional mechanism remains unclear since there has been only one study in human infants and none in animal models. Ramenghi and colleagues (Ramenghi et al., 1999) reported that direct administration of sucrose to the stomach via a nasogastric tube (NGT) had no analgesic effects during heel lance.

Another remarkable finding relating to the basic neurobiology of sucrose analgesia was that oral sucrose did not require involvement of the forebrain, but was dependent on brainstem activity

(Anseloni et al., 2005). Sucrose was seen to activate neurons in the two main brainstem structures involved in descending modulation of pain; the caudal periaqueductal grey matter and the raphe magnus. These findings contribute significantly to the knowledge concerning mechanisms of sweet taste analgesia.

Sweet taste-induced analgesic mechanisms: the human infant studies

The early animal laboratory studies discussed in the preceding section set the scene for more than 150 studies of sweet taste-induced analgesia in human infants conducted over two decades (Harrison and Bueno, 2012; Harrison et al., 2010a). The first published study identified showing calming effects of sweet solutions in human infants was published in 1989 by Blass and colleagues (Blass et al., 1989), the same authors responsible for many of the early investigations into the stress moderating and analgesic effects of sweet taste in rodents. In this earliest study, 0.2 ml 12% sucrose solution given in two aliquots 2 min apart, to healthy crying, term newborn infants, resulted in immediate calming, immediate cessation of crying, and vigorous mouthing and hand to mouth activity. Sustained calming persisted for up to 5 min. Successive trials continued to demonstrate calming effects of small volumes of oral sucrose on healthy crying infants (Barr et al., 1994, 1999a, 1999b; Blass and Smith, 1992; Graillon et al., 1997; Smith and Blass, 1996; Smith et al., 1992). Such profound calming effects were considered to be non-sedating, with most of the infants remaining alert following sucrose administration (Blass and Ciaramitaro, 1994).

Further research established that calming effects were dependent on sweet *taste* rather than volume. A step-wise sweetness effect on calming was clearly demonstrated, with the sweetest solutions of sucrose and fructose resulting in more rapid and sustained calming compared to the less sweet sugars of glucose and lactose (Blass and Smith, 1992). Lactose was no more effective than water and in fact, led to some infants to cry more. As volumes of 0.2 ml sucrose were equally as effective in soothing infants as larger volumes of 0.6 ml and 1.0 ml, calming effects were considered to be independent of volume (Blass and Smith, 1992).

To further explore the endogenous opioid basis of sweet taste-induced calming, the effects of sucrose on infants with chronic antenatal exposure to opiates were evaluated (Blass and Ciaramitaro, 1994). Sucrose was hypothesized to be ineffective in infants with antenatal methadone exposure and suffering from withdrawal symptoms, due to low circulating endogenous opioid levels precluding an increase in response to sweet taste. Findings were that sucrose was less effective in this population compared to infants with no antenatal methadone exposure, further confirming the association between sweet taste, an intact endogenous opioid system, and analgesia.

Following these studies demonstrating calming effects of sweet taste, the questions turned to whether sweet solutions, if given prior to painful procedures could in fact be analgesic. In the first published placebo controlled trial of sucrose for reducing procedural pain in human newborn infants, Blass and Hoffmeyer demonstrated that 2 ml of a 12% sucrose solution significantly reduced crying duration during capillary sampling via heel lance (HL), compared to water, and 24% sucrose solution combined with non-nutritive sucking (NNS) significantly reduced crying duration during circumcision, compared to water with NNS (Blass and Hoffmeyer, 1991).

These first studies conducted over two decades ago, clearly demonstrating profound and sustained calming and analgesic effects of sweet solutions, set the scene for the conduct and subsequent publication of large numbers of studies, reviews, systematic reviews, commentaries, and guidelines concerning effects of sweet taste in diverse populations of human infants (Harrison et al., 2010a). In the next section, systematic reviews of randomized controlled trials (RCTs) evaluating sweet solutions for reducing procedural pain in the neonatal period will be reviewed.

Effectiveness of sweet taste in newborn infants

Sucrose has been the most commonly investigated strategy for reduction of procedural pain in infants. As already mentioned, the first study evaluating sucrose during a painful procedure was published in 1991 (Blass and Hoffmeyer, 1991) and was the forerunner for extensive evaluation of sweet solutions for procedural pain management in infants and children over the next two decades. Six years after this first trial, the first systematic review and meta-analysis of studies of sucrose included 13 trials and 982 neonates (Stevens et al., 1997). Procedures investigated were HL (11 studies) and one study each evaluated venepuncture (VP), immunization, and circumcision. Findings were that sucrose reduced cry duration, facial expressions, pain intensity scores, and heart rate compared to water or no intervention, with the exception of one study in which an 18% sucrose solution was used. Fifteen years later, this systematic review has been substantially updated a number of times, with the most recent update in 2013 including 57 studies with 4730 term or preterm infants (Stevens et al., 2013). Predominantly, HL was studied (29) while other painful procedures included VP (nine), eye examination for retinopathy of prematurity (six), combination of procedures (four), circumcision (three), subcutaneous injection (two), NGT insertion (two), bladder catheterization (one), and heel stroke (one). Sucrose consistently and statistically significantly decreased individual behavioural pain indicators, unidimensional, multidimensional and composite pain scores compared to water or no treatment. A meta-analysis including four studies (264 neonates) showed that a range of doses ranging from the pacifier dipped in 24% sucrose up to administering 0.5 ml 24% sucrose significantly reduced Premature Infant Pain Profile (PIPP) scores compared to control or no treatment (1) at 30 sec following HL (weighted mean difference (WMD) −1.76 (95% confidence interval (CI) −2.54 to −0.97; p <0.001)), and (2) at 60 sec following HL (WMD −2.05 (95% CI −3.08 to −1.02; p <0.001)). Another meta-analysis including only two trials and 88 neonates showed that sucrose also reduced total crying time following HL. Based on the meta-analyses of four studies, the authors recommended the routine use of sucrose 0.012 to 0.12 g (0.05 ml of 24% sucrose to 0.5 ml of 24% sucrose) be administered approximately 2 min prior to single painful procedures. However, given the broad range of effectiveness of sucrose doses and the heterogeneity of studies in this review, further research is needed to identify a more precise dose for the different gestational ages. The authors also recommended further research in extremely preterm, sick ventilated infants, and relationships between validated pain assessment tools and indicators that measure nociceptive brain activity.

Sweet-tasting solutions other than sucrose have also been investigated. A systematic review and meta-analysis exploring the effects of solutions other than sucrose included 38 studies, 3785 infants, and eight different procedures (Bueno et al., in press). Glucose was the most frequently investigated solution (35, 92% of trials) with one study each including artificial sweetener, fructose, glycine, honey, and maltitol. Nineteen studies evaluated non-sucrose solutions during HL; ten studies during VP, and three during intramuscular (IM) injections (Table 49.1). Results were analogous to the sucrose systematic review; glucose of sufficient concentrations consistently reduced individual behavioural responses and unidimensional, multidimensional and composite pain scores compared to water or no treatment in preterm and term newborn infants during single episodes of painful procedures. A meta-analysis showed that glucose (20–50%) given prior to HL resulted in a 36 sec reduction in duration of cry (two studies, 90 infants, 95% CI −43.3, −29.5; p <0.001), and a 3.6-point reduction in mean PIPP scores (two studies, 124 infants, 95% CI −4.6, −2.6; p <0.001) compared to water or no treatment.

Both systematic reviews highlighted that analgesic effects were independent of volume of sweet solutions; as small volumes were as effective as larger volumes, yet the effects were reported to be sweet-taste dependent. Sweeter, more concentrated solutions more effectively reduced pain responses compared to less sweet solutions (Bueno et al., in press; Stevens et al.,2013). Although sucrose and glucose consistently reduced behavioural indicators, both reviews reported inconsistent effects of sweet solutions on reducing physiological responses. Inconsistency between behavioural, physiological, and even cortical responses (Norman et al., 2008; Slater et al., 2010) highlights the different mechanisms and actions of sweet solutions as well as the loose correlation in infants between physiological and behavioural responses to pain (Barr, 1998).

The large majority of studies included in the systematic reviews were single episodes of short lasting painful procedures, with fewer studies evaluating sucrose or glucose during procedures of more prolonged duration such as eye examination for retinopathy of prematurity. In addition, very few studies investigated repeated use of sucrose over days, weeks, or months of use. Only three studies to date have examined repeated use of sucrose and showed that sucrose was effective and safe over time (Harrison et al., 2009; Mucignat et al., 2004; Stevens et al., 2005). However, one study of consistent use of sucrose for preterm infants during the first 7 days of life showed that more than ten doses of sucrose in a 24 h period was associated with poorer neurodevelopmental outcomes compared to ten or less doses for infants less than 31 weeks gestational age (Johnston et al., 2002, 2007). In contrast, there were no differences in neurodevelopmental outcomes in preterm infants who received multiple doses of sucrose compared to water over a 4-week period (Stevens et al., 2005). To date, these are the only two studies examining neurodevelopmental outcomes following repeated use of sweet solutions for procedural pain management in infants.

The most important limitation of the systematic reviews was that inconsistencies across studies in outcome measures and metrics used to report results meant that the number of outcomes that could be pooled for meta-analysis was severely restricted. In fact, despite the inclusion of 57 individual studies of sucrose in the 2013 review, the largest number of studies included in any meta-analysis was only four, highlighting the large variability in study outcomes and reporting of statistics. Based on the results of the meta-analyses only, the use of 24% sucrose within a range of 0.05–0.5 ml was recommended prior to single episodes of painful procedures.

However, this recommendation needs to be viewed with caution given the large number of studies demonstrating effectiveness of a broad range of sucrose doses (e.g. 0.02–2.0 ml) that were excluded from these analyses.

In conclusion, systematic reviews and meta-analyses of large numbers of trials show that sucrose and glucose consistently and significantly reduce behavioural responses and unidimensional, multidimensional and composite pain scores in newborn preterm and term infants compared to water or no treatment, during single episodes of commonly performed short lasting painful procedures. Evidence to support use of sucrose or glucose during procedures of longer duration is less clear. As analgesic effects of sucrose persist for around 2 to 5 min in newborn infants (Barr et al., 1994; Blass et al., 1989; Smith et al., 1990), and for a shorter period of around 1min in 6-week old infants (Barr et al., 1994), administering solutions in divided doses throughout procedures that are prolonged for more than a few minutes may be more effective than single doses. Further research is warranted to confirm this hypothesis. Further knowledge gaps include safety and efficacy of repeated doses of sweet solutions for extremely preterm infants and term infants requiring prolonged hospitalization.

Effectiveness of sweet taste in infants beyond the newborn period

Does the same sweet taste-induced analgesic effect persist beyond the neonatal period? As highlighted in the first section of this chapter, analgesic effects of sweet taste in rodents declined as the rodents aged. However, this same age-related decline of effectiveness is not as clear cut in human infants. As highlighted in a systematic review and meta-analysis of 14 trials of sweet solutions during immunization in infants aged 1 to 12 months of age (Table 49.1), sweet solutions at sufficient concentrations (at least 30% glucose or 24% sucrose) consistently reduced pain scores and individual behavioural indicators during or following immunization (Harrison et al., 2010b). Effect sizes were however smaller than reported in neonatal studies (Stevens et al., 2013). Conflicting results were also reported concerning; (1) effectiveness of a weak 12% sucrose concentration, and (2) effectiveness of single doses of sucrose for prolonged procedures.

A single dose of 12% sucrose, given 2 min prior to immunization, was no more effective than water in reducing pain in infants beyond the newborn period in two trials (Allen et al., 1996; Poulsen, 2009), yet the same dose was effective in a third study (Dilli et al., 2009). Dilli et al. reported that 12% sucrose not only substantially reduced immunization pain in infants, but also in children up to 4 years of age. These conflicting results may be attributed to possible cultural differences, or maternal interventions, including holding, comforting, and distraction techniques which may have potentiated the sucrose effects (Harrison et al., 2010b). As there are no other published studies of analgesic effects of sucrose in pre-school children during medically related painful procedures, comparison with other findings is not possible at this time.

Whether the analgesic effects of a single dose of sucrose given prior to procedures can be sustained throughout the duration of painful procedures, especially in infants beyond the newborn period, is questionable. Single doses of sucrose given 2 min prior to venepuncture (Curtis et al., 2007) and urethral catheterization (Rogers et al., 2006) were ineffective in reducing pain in infants beyond the newborn period (Curtis et al., 2007; Rogers et al., 2006). Although neither study reported the duration of the procedures, it is well known that these procedures can take a long time to successfully complete. Single doses of sucrose given 2 min prior to these more prolonged procedures may not result in sustained analgesic effects in older infants. In fact, a key important difference in effectiveness of sweet solutions in infants beyond the neonatal period compared to newborn infants, is the shorter peak effect time and duration of effect, reported to be 1 min only in 6-week-old infants, compared to around 5 min for newborn infants (Barr et al., 1994). This difference has important implications as, based on previous studies showing the peak onset of analgesic effects following sucrose administration is 2 min (Blass and Shah, 1995; Blass et al., 1987); the large majority of study protocols use this timing, regardless of the age of the infants. For infants beyond the newborn period, dividing the dose of sucrose and administering throughout the duration of painful and distressing procedures is recommended to ensure sustained analgesic effects (Harrison et al., 2010b).

Effectiveness of sweet taste throughout childhood

There are few studies of sweet taste for pain reduction in children beyond 1 year of age, and results of these studies are conflicting. Seven published studies investigating sweet taste during painful procedures in toddlers and children aged from 1 to 16 years have been identified (Allen et al., 1996; Dilli et al., 2009; Lewkowski et al., 2003; Mennella et al., 2010; Miller et al., 1994; Pepino and Mennella, 2005). Four trials involved needle-related procedures (Allen et al., 1996; Dilli et al., 2009, Lewkowski et al., 2003) and were included in a recent Cochrane systematic review of sweet-tasting solutions for needle-related pain in children (Table 49.1) (Harrison et al., 2011). Three further trials involved experimental pain invoked by cold pressor testing (CPT) (Mennella et al., 2010; Miller et al., 1994; Pepino and Mennella, 2005).

Effectiveness of sweet taste in toddlers and pre-school children

Only two studies have included toddlers, both of which investigated 12% sucrose during immunization (Allen et al., 1996; Dilli et al., 2009). Both studies included children aged 15 and 18 months of age, but Dilli et al., 2009 also included children up to 4 years of age. Dilli et al. reported that sucrose significantly reduced crying duration and pain scores across all ages of children, while Allen et al. reported a lack of analgesic effects of sucrose compared to water, in infants beyond the newborn period. Possible reasons for the conflicting findings were proposed, including cultural differences and differences in comfort strategies used by parents during the immunization procedure (Harrison et al., 2011). Valid conclusions from these two trials, both of which used 12% sucrose which is considerably less concentrated and less sweet than the 24% recommended for effective pain reduction in newborn infants (Stevens et al., 2013), and both of which included small numbers of children in this age bracket, are unable to be drawn. Children in this age group often become exceedingly distressed during procedures and effective pain management is problematic. Further research determining effective interventions, including use of sucrose, is strongly recommended in this age group.

Effectiveness of sweet taste in school-aged children

Five published studies have evaluated whether sweet taste reduces pain in school-aged children (Lewkowski et al., 2003; Miller et al., 1994; Mennella et al., 2010; Pepino and Mennella, 2005). Lewkowski and colleagues compared sweetened and unsweetened chewing gum during immunization and VP or finger prick (Lewkowski et al., 2003). Results showed no differences in self-report of pain for children who chewed sweet gum either prior to, or during the procedures compared to children chewing non-sweet gum. Three studies were conducted during CPT and results were conflicting (Mennella et al., 2010; Miller et al., 1994; Pepino and Mennella, 2005). Miller et al (1994) reported that pain threshold (time until pain/discomfort was reported) was reduced, but neither pain tolerance (removal of arm from the water), or self-report of pain were effected by 24% sucrose (Miller et al., 1994). Limitations to the study included incomplete data collection with over half the children having no pain tolerance or self-report data. Similar problems with incomplete data collection were also reported in the two other studies of sucrose during CPT in children (Mennella et al., 2010; Pepino and Mennella, 2005). In addition to examining analgesic effects of sucrose, the two more recently published studies also reported that preference for sweet taste influenced whether sucrose exerted analgesic effects. Based on the findings from these five published studies including school aged children, sucrose or other sweet substances are not sufficiently effective as a pain management strategy in this population and their use cannot be recommended.

Uncertainties, knowledge gaps, and current controversies

Despite over 150 studies, predominately including neonates, the use of sweet solutions for painful procedures has not been translated into consistent clinical practice (Carbajal et al., 2008; Harrison et al., 2013, Johnston et al., 2011; Losacco et al., 2011; Stevens et al., 2011). Additionally, there are a number of key knowledge gaps concerning mechanisms of action and effectiveness and safety of sucrose in specific populations of infants. These gaps include:

1. Physiological mechanisms of sucrose.

2. Effectiveness and safety of sucrose given repeatedly over prolonged periods to preterm and sick infants.

3. Effectiveness and utilization of sucrose for managing non-procedural pain and distress in sick infants.

4. Effectiveness of sucrose in sick infants receiving concurrent opioid or equivalent analgesics.

5. Effectiveness of consistent use of sucrose in addition to non-pharmacological pain management interventions in reducing or preventing long-term adverse outcomes of repeated painful procedures in sick hospitalized infants.

6. Effectiveness of sucrose in children older than 12 months of age.

Physiological mechanisms of sucrose

Despite the current understanding of a sweet taste, orally-induced endogenous opioid effect, considered to be due to a beta-endorphin response (Anseloni et al., 2002; Blass et al., 1987; Dum et al., 1983; McKay et al., 1981), the exact mechanism has not been definitively confirmed in human infants (Taddio et al., 2003). Further research aimed to elucidate the calming and analgesic mechanism of oral sucrose in infants is warranted.

Effectiveness and safety of sucrose given repeatedly over prolonged periods to preterm and sick infants

Only three disparate studies, two trials and one longitudinal study, have evaluated the use of sucrose for prolonged periods (Harrison et al., 2009; Mucignat et al., 2004; Stevens et al., 2005). All three studies showed that sucrose remained effective and safe when used for 4 weeks or longer, however further research is warranted to corroborate these findings.

Effectiveness and utilization of sucrose for managing non-procedural pain and distress in sick infants

This is a key unexplored question which has not been addressed in any published reports to date. Although, anecdotally sucrose is used to calm crying, distressed, agitated hospitalized infants, the effectiveness of sucrose, in this context, as well as the extent of this practice is unknown. As effects of sweet solutions are short lasting, consistent use for ongoing pain and distress could potentially lead to excessive volumes being given over the course of the hospitalization. Setting maximum daily doses may reduce this risk. Tracking the utilization of sweet solutions in hospitalized infants is imperative for furthering our understanding of the degree of sucrose exposure which can in turn, inform if there are any long-term effects based on degree of exposure. Currently there is little evidence to inform the question 'How much is too much?'. When tracking sucrose use, it is important to be cognizant that sucrose is also present in commonly administered proprietary syrups, including antibiotics, vitamins, and antipyretics (Harrison, 2008).

Effectiveness of sucrose in sick infants receiving concurrent opioid or equivalent analgesics

As the proposed mechanism of oral sweet taste in infants is the invoking of an endogenous opioid response, whether this response can occur in the context of exogenous opioid delivery is an important question. As maintenance doses of continuous opioid analgesics, given for postoperative pain management or for sedation, do not sufficiently reduce pain during acute painful procedures (Carbajal et al., 2005), it important that the effectiveness of sucrose in this context is evaluated.

Effectiveness of consistent use of sucrose in addition to non-pharmacological pain management interventions in reducing or preventing long-term adverse outcomes of repeated painful procedures in sick hospitalized infant

Adverse long-term effects of repeated painful procedures have been reported. The question whether consistent use of effective pain management strategies including sucrose with NNS and breastfeeding or skin-to-skin care, can ameliorate such effects is not known. The design of such a study is challenging, as a control group would be considered to be unethical, given what is currently known. Furthermore, using historical controls is problematic as rapid changes have been made in many NICU care practices; thus attributing differences in outcomes to pain management practices

could be flawed reasoning. Nevertheless, close follow-up of preterm and sick infants following discharge from hospital, which includes all relevant behavioural and developmental outcomes including pain responses to future procedures such as immunization, and pain sensitivity, will contribute to the knowledge gap regarding long-term effects of effective early pain management.

Effectiveness of sucrose in children older than 12 months of age

Young children often become extremely distressed during medical procedures. Effective management of procedural pain and distress in this age-group is challenging. Whether sucrose can be of benefit beyond 1 year of age is an important question warranting further investigation.

Due to the abundant research consistently showing effectiveness of oral sucrose or glucose in newborns and infants up to 1 year of age during single episodes of short-lasting painful procedures, there is no longer uncertainty regarding benefits of using sweet solutions. It is therefore no longer ethical to conduct further no treatment or placebo-controlled trials of sweet solutions during commonly performed painful procedures in this population (Harrison et al., 2010a). Sweet solutions, with NNS if possible, should be considered a standard of care, along with breastfeeding and skin-to-skin care when feasible. Further research needs to focus on addressing existing knowledge gaps.

Clinical practice implications

Practice pointers—guidelines for use

- Sweet solutions only work if given orally. Administer in small doses on the top of the tongue, with a pacifier if the infant is able to suck.

- Solutions need to be sufficiently sweet for endogenous opioid effect (24% sucrose or 25–30% glucose).

- Suggested doses range from 0.05 to 2 ml in total for single painful procedures.

- Delivery: only small volumes are required. For newborn infants, a single dose given 2 min before a painful procedure reduces pain during procedures. For infants beyond the newborn period—administer about one-quarter of the dose on the anterior part of the infant's tongue, one min before the procedure and give remaining dose immediately prior to, and throughout the procedure.

- For more painful or prolonged procedures, such as eye examination, use additional pain-relieving strategies as recommended.

- Sucrose or glucose should be considered as adjuvant pain management strategies for procedures associated with moderate to severe pain intensity (e.g. circumcision) and used in conjunction with topical and regional anaesthetics such as dorsal penile block.

- Document the administration and effectiveness of sucrose.

- Use additional strategies as feasible such as skin-to-skin care, facilitated tucking, and NNS if part of infant's care.

- Support parents to provide pain management and advise of additional ways they can help reduce their baby's pain (e.g. breastfeeding or skin-to-skin care during non-urgent blood draws, newborn screening, and immunization) (see Johnston and Campbell-Yeo, Chapter 58, this volume on mothercare).

◆ Parent education may need to include recommendations to avoid using sucrose for crying in the home.

Availability and accessibility of sweet solutions in all settings where infants undergo painful procedures is necessary to enable their use. Sucrose may be purchased pre-manufactured or made by hospital pharmacy departments or independent pharmacists. Sucrose recipes are available from most large paediatric hospital pharmacy departments. Glucose for intravenous use is readily available in hospitals and can be used orally, as an alternative to sucrose when sucrose is not available. Clearly written, user-friendly clinical practice guidelines which have been approved by relevant stakeholders are necessary to promote consistent best pain

management practices. Guidelines should highlight how to achieve optimal effectiveness of sweet solutions over the course of painful procedures. Examples of mini pocket clinical practice guideline cards developed during the course of a Canadian Institutes of Health Research knowledge synthesis and dissemination project are shown in Figures 49.1 and 49.2.

Infants no longer need to suffer unnecessarily during painful procedures. Sucrose or glucose, alongside other effective pain management strategies including pacifier, breastfeeding, and skin-to-skin care cost little to use, are effective, and can easily be incorporated into infants' care during painful procedures. Health professionals have an ethical responsibility to consistently use best pain management practices and to support parents to do the same. Researchers have an ethical responsibility to work at effectively disseminating their research and to address existing research gaps.

(a)

(b)

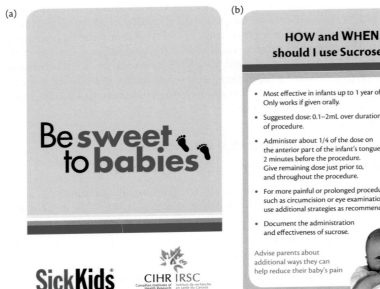
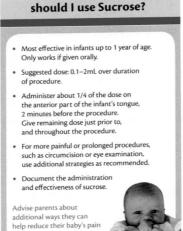

Figure 49.1 Clinical practice guideline (CPG) care in English.
Republished with kind permission of the author Denise Harrison, Copyright © 2013. Guidelines designed by Hospital for SickKids Toronto.

(a)

(b)

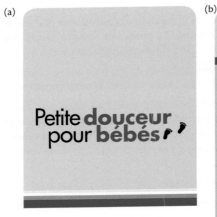

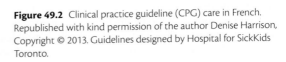

Figure 49.2 Clinical practice guideline (CPG) care in French.
Republished with kind permission of the author Denise Harrison, Copyright © 2013. Guidelines designed by Hospital for SickKids Toronto.

References

Allen, K. D., White, D. D., and Walburn, J. N. (1996). Sucrose as an analgesic agent for infants during immunization injections. *Arch Pediatr Adolesc Med*, 150, 270–274.

American Academy of Pediatrics Committee on Fetus and Newborn, American Academy of Pediatrics Section on Surgery, Canadian Paediatric Society Fetus and Newborn Committee, Batton, D. G., Barrington, K. J., Wallman, C., *et al.* (2006). Prevention and management of pain in the neonate: an update. *Pediatrics*, 118, 2231–2241.

Anand, K. J. and International Evidence-Based Group for Neonatal Pain.(2001). Consensus statement for the prevention and management of pain in the newborn. *Arch Pediatr Adolesc Med*, 155, 173–180.

Anseloni, V. C., Weng, H. R., Terayama, R., Letizia, D., Davis, B. J., Ren, K., *et al.* (2002). Age-dependency of analgesia elicited by intraoral sucrose in acute and persistent pain models. *Pain*, 97, 93–103.

Anseloni, V. C. Z., Ren, K., Dubner, R., and Ennis, M. (2005). A brainstem substrate for analgesia elicited by intraoral sucrose. *Neuroscience*, 133, 231–243.

Barr, R. G. (1998). Reflections on measuring pain in infants: dissociation in responsive systems and 'honest signalling'. *Arch Pediatr Adolesc Med Fetal Neonatal Ed*, 79, F152–156.

Barr, R. G., Pantel, M. S., Young, S. N., Wright, J. H., Hendricks, L. A., and Gravel, R. (1999a). The response of crying newborns to sucrose: is it a 'sweetness' effect? *Physiol Behav*, 66, 409–417.

Barr, R. G., Quek, V. S. H., Cousineau, D., Oberlander, T. F., Brian, J. A., and Young, S. N. (1994). Effects of intra-oral sucrose on crying, mouthing, and hand-mouth contact in newborn and six-week old infants. *Dev Med Child Neurol*, 36, 608–618.

Barr, R. G., Young, S. N., Wright, J. H., Gravel, R., and Alkawaf, R. (1999b). Differential calming responses to sucrose taste in crying infants with and without colic. *Pediatrics*, 103, e68.

Blass, E. and Ciaramitaro, V. (1994). A new look at some old mechanisms in human newborns. *Monogr Soc Res Child Dev*, 59.

Blass, E., Fitzgerald, E., and Kehoe, P. (1987). Interactions between sucrose, pain and isolation distress. *Pharmacol Biochem Behav*, 26, 483–489.

Blass, E. M. (1997). Interactions between contact and chemosensory mechanisms in pain modulation in 10-day-old rats. *Behavioral Neurosci*, 111, 147–154.

Blass, E. M., Fillion, T. J., Rochat, P., Hoffmeyer, L. B., Rochat, P., and Metzger, M. A. (1989). Sensorimotor and motivational determinants of hand-mouth coordination in 1–3-day-old human infants. *Dev Psychol*, 25, 963–975.

Blass, E. M., and Fitzgerald, E. (1988). Milk-induced analgesia and comforting in 10-day-old rats: opioid mediation. *Pharmacol Biochem Behav*, 29, 9–13.

Blass, E. M., and Hoffmeyer, L. B. (1991). Sucrose as an analgesic for newborn infants. *Pediatrics*, 87, 215–218.

Blass, E. M., Jackson, A. M., and Smotherman, W. P. (1991). Milk-induced, opioid-mediated antinociception in rats at the time of cesarean delivery. *Behav Neurosci*, 105, 677–686.

Blass, E. M., and Shah, A. (1995). Pain-reducing properties of sucrose in human newborns. *Chem Senses*, 20, 29–35.

Blass, E. M., and Shide, D. J. (1994). Some comparisons among the calming and pain-relieving effects of sucrose, glucose, fructose and lactose in infant rats. *Chem Senses*, 19, 239–249.

Blass, E. M., and Smith, B. A. (1992). Differential effects of sucrose, fructose, glucose, and lactose on crying in 1- to 3-day-old human infants: qualitative and quantitative considerations. *Dev Psychol*, 28, 804–810.

Bueno, M., Yamada, J., Harrison, D., Kahn, S., Adams-Webber, T., Beyene, J., *et al.* (2013). A systematic review and meta-analyses of non-sucrose sweet solutions sucrose for pain relief in neonates. *Pain Res Manage*, 18, 153–161.

Carbajal, R., Lenclen, R., Jugie, M., Paupe, A., Barton, B. A., and Anand, K. J. S. (2005). Morphine does not provide adequate analgesia for acute procedural pain among preterm neonates. *Pediatrics*, 115, 1494–1500.

Carbajal, R., Rousset, A., Danan, C., Coquery, S., Nolent, P., Ducrocq, S., *et al.* (2008). Epidemiology and treatment of painful procedures in neonates in intensive care units. *JAMA*, 300, 60–70.

Curtis, S. J., Jou, H., Ali, S., Vandermeer, B., and Klassen, T. (2007). A randomized controlled trial of sucrose and/or pacifier as analgesia for infants receiving venipuncture in a pediatric emergency department. *BMC Pediatr*, 7, 27.

Dilli, D., Küçük, I., and Dallar, Y. (2009). Interventions to reduce pain during vaccination in infancy. *J Pediatr*, 154, 385–390.

Dum, J., Gramsch, C., and Herz, A. (1983). Activation of hypothalamic beta-endorphin pools by reward induced by highly palatable food. *Pharmacol Biochem Behav*, 18, 443–7.

Graillon, A., Barr, R. G., Young, S. N., Wright, J. H., and Hendricks, L. A. (1997). Differential response to intraoral sucrose, quinine and corn oil in crying human newborns. *Physiol Behav*, 62, 317–25.

Guyatt, G. H., Oxman, A. D., Vist, G. E., Kunz, R., Falck-Ytter, Y., Alonso-Coello, P., *et al.* (2008). GRADE: an emerging consensus on rating quality of evidence and strength of recommendations. *Br Med J*, 336, 924–6.

Harrison, D. (2008). Oral sucrose for pain management in infants: myths and misconceptions. *J Neonatal Nurs*, 14, 39–46.

Harrison, D. and Australian College of Neonatal Nurses (2006). Management of pain in sick hospitalised infants. *Neonatal Paediatr Child Health Nurs*, 9, 27–29.

Harrison, D. and Bueno, M. (2012). Sweet solutions for pain in infants—how many studies are too many studies? *Pain Res Manage*, 17(3), 211, P134

Harrison, D., Bueno, M., Yamada, J., Adams-Webber, T., and Stevens, B. (2010a). Analgesic effects of sweet tasting solutions in infants: Do we have equipoise yet? *Pediatrics*, 126, 894–902.

Harrison, D., Elia, S., Royle, J., and Manias, E. (2013). Pain management strategies used during early childhood immunisations. *J Paediatr Child Health*, 49, 313–318

Harrison, D., Loughnan, P., Manias, E., Gordon, I., and Johnston, L. (2009). Repeated doses of sucrose in infants continue to reduce procedural pain during prolonged hospitalizations. *Nursing Res*, 58, 427–434.

Harrison, D., Stevens, B., Bueno, M., Yamada, J., Adams-Webber, T., Beyene, J., *et al.* (2010b). Efficacy of sweet solutions for analgesia in infants between 1 and 12 months of age: a systematic review. *Arch Dis Child*, 95, 406–413.

Harrison, D., Yamada, J., Adams-Webber, T., Ohlsson, A., Beyene, J., and Stevens, B. (2011). Sweet tasting solutions for reduction of needle-related procedural pain in children aged 1 to 16 years. *Cochrane Database Syst Rev*, 10, CD008408.

Henderson-Smart, D. and Australian & New Zealand Neonatal Network. (2007). *Evidence uptake using networks—Newborn Pain project*. Sydney: National Institute of Clinical Studies, National Health & Medical Research Council.

Johnston, C., Barrington, K. J., Taddio, A., Carbajal, R., and Filion, F. (2011). Pain in Canadian NICUs: have we improved over the past 12 years? *Clin J Pain*, 27, 225–232.

Johnston, C. C., Filion, F., Snider, L., Limperopoulos, C., Majnemer, A., Pelausa, E., *et al.* (2007). How much sucrose is too much sucrose? *Pediatrics*, 119(1), 226.

Johnston, C. C., Filion, F., Snider, L., Majnemer, A., Limperopoulos, C., Walker, C. D., *et al.* (2002). Routine sucrose analgesia during the first week of life in neonates younger than 31 weeks' postconceptional age. *Pediatrics*, 110, 523–528.

Lewkowski, M. D., Barr, R. G., Sherrard, A., Lessard, J., Harris, A. R., and Young, S. N. (2003). Effects of chewing gum on responses to routine painful procedures in children. *Physiol Behav*, 79, 257–265.

Losacco, V., Cuttini, M., Greisen, G., Haumont, D., Pallas-Alonso, C. R., Pierrat, V., *et al.* (2011). Heel blood sampling in European neonatal intensive care units: compliance with pain management guidelines. *Arch Dis Child Fetal Neonatal Ed*, 96, F65–68.

McKay, L. D., Kenney, N. J., Edens, N. K., Williams, R. H., and Woods, S. C. (1981). Intracerebroventricular beta-endorphin increases food intake of rats. *Life Sci*, 29, 1429–1434.

Mennella, J. A., Pepino, M. Y., Lehmann-Castor, S. M., and Yourshaw, L. M. (2010). Sweet preferences and analgesia during childhood:effects of family history of alcoholism and depression. *Addiction*, 105, 666–675.

Miller, A., Barr, R. G., and Young, S. N. (1994). The cold pressor test in children: methodological aspects and the analgesic effect of intraoral sucrose. *Pain*, 56, 175–183.

Mucignat, V., Ducrocq, S., Lebas, F., Mochel, F., Baudon, J. J., and Gold, F. (2004). Analgesic effects of EMLA cream and saccharose solution for subcutaneous injections in preterm newborns: a prospective study of 265 injections. *Arch Pediatr*, 11, 921–925.

Norman, E., Rosen, I., Vanhatalo, S., Stjernqvist, K., Okland, O., Fellman, V., and Hellstrom-Westas, L. (2008). Electroencephalographic response to procedural pain in healthy term newborn infants. *Pediatric Res*, 64, 429–434.

Pepino, M. Y., and Mennella, J. A. (2005). Sucrose-induced analgesia is related to sweet preferences in children but not adults. *Pain*, 119, 210–218.

Poulsen, M. (2009). Cane sugar unsuitable for use as analgesic in paediatric vaccination. *Sygeplejersken/Dan J Nurs*, 106, 54–57.

Ramenghi, L. A., Evans, D. J., and Levene, M. I. (1999). 'Sucrose analgesia': absorptive mechanism or taste perception? *Arch Dis Child Fetal Neonatal Ed*, 80, F146–1467.

Ren, K., Blass, E. M., Zhou, Q., and Dubner, R. (1997). Suckling and sucrose ingestion suppress persistent hyperalgesia and spinal Fos expression after forepaw inflammation in infant rats. *Proc Natl Acad Sci U S A*, 94, 1471–1475.

Rogers, A. J., Greenwald, M. H., Deguzman, M. A., Kelley, M. E., and Simon, H. K. (2006). A randomized, controlled trial of sucrose analgesia in infants younger than 90 days of age who require bladder catheterization in the pediatric emergency department. *Acad Emerg Med*, 13, 617–622.

Royal Australasian College of Physicians. (2005). *Guideline statement: management of procedure-related pain in neonates*. Sydney: Paediatrics & Child Health Division, The Royal Australasian College of Physicians.

Shide, D. J., and Blass, E. M. (1989). Opioidlike effects of intraoral infusions of corn oil and polycose on stress reactions in 10-day-old rats. *Behav Neurosci*, 103, 1168–1175.

Slater, R., Cornelissen, L., Fabrizi, L., Patten, D., Yoxen, J., Worley, A., et al. (2010). Oral sucrose as an analgesic drug for procedural pain in newborn infants: a randomised controlled trial. *Lancet*, 376(9748), 1225–1232.

Smith, B. A., and Blass, E. (1996). Taste-mediated calming in premature, preterm, and full-term infants. *Dev Psychol*, 32, 1084–1089.

Smith, B. A., Fillion, T. J., and Blass, E. M. (1990). Orally mediated sources of calming in 1- to 3-day-old human infants. *Dev Psychol*, 26, 731–737.

Smith, B. A., Stevens, K., Torgerson, W. S., and Kim, J. H. (1992). Diminished reactivity of postmature human infants to sucrose compared with term infants. *Dev Psychol*, 28, 811–820.

Stevens, B., Abbott, L., Yamada, J., Harrison, D., Stinson, J., Taddio, A., et al. (2011). Epidemiology and management of painful procedures in hospitalized children across Canada. *CMAJ*, 183, E403–E410.

Stevens, B., Taddio, A., Ohlsson, A., and Einarson, T. (1997). The efficacy of sucrose for relieving procedural pain in neonates-a systematic review and meta-analysis. *Acta Pædiatr*, 86, 837–842.

Stevens, B., Yamada, J., Beyene, J., Gibbins, S., Petryshen, P., Stinson, J., and Narciso, J. (2005). Consistent management of repeated procedural pain with sucrose in preterm neonates: Is it effective and safe for repeated use over time? *Clin J Pain*, 21, 543–548.

Stevens, B., Yamada, J., and Ohlsson, A. (2010). Sucrose for analgesia in newborn infants undergoing painful procedures. *Cochrane Database Syst Rev*, 1, CD001069.

Stevens, B., Yamada, J., and Ohlsson, A. (2013). Sucrose for analgesia in newborn infants undergoing painful procedures. *Cochrane Database Syst Rev*, 1, CD001069.

Taddio, A., Chambers, C. T., Halperin, S. A., Ipp, M., Lockett, D., Rieder, M. J., and Shah, V. (2009). Inadequate pain management during routine childhood immunizations: the nerve of it. *Clin Ther*, 31(Suppl 2), S152–167.

Taddio, A., Shah, V., Shah, P., and Katz, J. (2003). Beta-endorphin concentration after administration of sucrose in preterm infants. *Arch Pediatr Adolesc Med*, 157, 1071–1074.

Travers, S. (1993). Orosensory processing in neural systems of the nucleus of the solitary tract. In S. Simon, and S. Roper (eds) *Mechanisms of taste transduction*, pp. 339–394. Boca Raton, FL: CRC Press.

Tsao, J. C. I., Evans, S., Meldrum, M., Altman, T., and Zeltzer, L. K. (2007). A review of CAM for procedural pain in infancy: part I. sucrose and non-nutritive sucking. *Evid Based Complement Alternat Med*, 371–381.

SECTION 7

Psychosocial interventions

CHAPTER 50

Cognitive-behavioural interventions

Deirdre E. Logan, Rachael M. Coakley, and Brittany N. Barber Garcia

Cognitive-behavioural therapy (CBT) is the most commonly researched and empirically supported psychological treatment for the management of paediatric pain. CBT is a brief, goal-oriented psychotherapy treatment using a hands-on, practical problem-solving approach (Kendall, 2012). It is based on the concept that thoughts, feelings, and behaviours are causally interrelated. This chapter offers an overview of CBT and its application to pain management, describes specific cognitive-behavioural strategies commonly used for paediatric acute and chronic pain problems, presents the empirical evidence supporting these approaches, and highlights key considerations and emerging directions in the use of CBT and related treatments for paediatric pain.Cognitive-behavioural theory

Cognitive-behavioural theory

Cognitive-behavioural theory, which underlies CBT, represents a convergence of two psychological theories; *cognitive theory* (Beck, 1979), which focuses on mental interpretations of experiences, and *behavioural learning theory* (Thorndike, 1913), which emphasizes the shaping of behaviours through reinforcement. Cognitive-behavioural theory merges these concepts into a model of treatment that targets cognitive appraisals and their influence on emotional and behavioural responses. In practice, CBT relies heavily on the modification of thoughts and behaviours using the principles of reinforcement (Turk and Rudy, 1989; see Slifer et al., Chapter 51, this volume).

CBT in practice

CBT first emerged in the early 1970s and quickly gained recognition due to both its effectiveness for a wide array of mood and behavioural disturbances and its time-limited model of care. There are many components of CBT that distinguish it from other types of psychotherapy. CBT is usually provided by psychologists, though some skilled licensed social workers and masters-level counsellors also practise CBT. CBT is present-focused and time-limited. It is typically delivered individually in weekly therapy sessions, though it can also be effectively administered in a group format (Barakat et al., 2007; Hayutin et al., 2009; Logan and Simons, 2010). CBT is highly instructive in nature, often incorporating the use of manuals and workbooks in session, and homework assignments to solidify skills. Within a CBT framework, the therapist and patient work collaboratively to identify problems and design learning experiences that will help to modify negative cognitions and dysfunctional behavioural patterns (Kendall, 2012).

In practice today, CBT is an amalgam of cognitive and behavioural approaches that can be applied in various combinations. Cognitive interventions include the use of skills such as reframing, cognitive distraction, and positive self-talk statements. Behavioural strategies include skills such as relaxation, exposure and desensitization, and modelling. Overarching elements of CBT include education, goal-setting (establishing desired outcomes and incorporating incentives to help achieve these outcomes), self-monitoring (increasing awareness of symptoms and responses through tracking in a diary-like fashion), and problem-solving (identifying obstacles to one's goals and working collaboratively with the therapist to overcome these obstacles). Importantly, a CBT model also attends to the relationship of cognition and behaviour in the context of a child's environment (Kendall, 2012).

CBT for pain

The use of CBT for pain problems is based on the understanding that pain is a complex biopsychosocial experience shaped not only by underlying pathophysiology but also by individuals' thoughts, feelings, and behaviours (e.g. Keefe and Gil, 1986). Within a CBT framework for paediatric pain, children are taught *cognitive strategies* to identify and restructure illogical or maladaptive thoughts related to pain. Children are also taught *behavioural strategies* to relieve physiological discomfort and relearn adaptive functioning patterns. CBT for pain specifically targets the common distorted thought that pain cannot be controlled (Rogers, 2008). Treatment focuses on modifying this negative belief, enhancing ability to solve pain-related problems, and providing a set of skills for managing pain in an adaptive way. Goals of CBT for pain include gaining a sense of control over pain, reducing fear of pain, enhancing function, increasing feelings of hopefulness and resourcefulness, and improving mood.

Within the literature on paediatric pain, CBT interventions have demonstrated promising improvements in self-efficacy, self-management, family functioning, psychosocial well-being, pain severity, school attendance, and feelings of hopefulness (Barlow and Ellard, 2004). Although the literature has not yet clearly identified which constellation of cognitive or behavioural interventions are most effective for specific groups based on characteristics such as age, gender, or type of pain, there is strong evidence that taken as a whole, these strategies are highly effective for treatment of acute and chronic pain for children as well as adults (Eccleston et al., 2002; Turk et al., 2008).

CBT for pain management typically focuses *initially* on the provision of developmentally targeted education about a child's condition (Rogers, 2008), but *most importantly* on the relationship between thoughts, physiological changes in the body, and behaviours or actions. For example, a child with a chronic pain condition such as complex regional pain syndrome would be taught that she would not cause harm to herself by using her affected limb. A child preparing for a painful procedure would be taught that pain sensations are diminished when attention is allocated away from painful stimuli. Treatment addresses the negative or fearful thoughts (e.g. 'it's going to hurt too much', 'I can't do this') that produce physiological changes (e.g. racing heart, shortness of breath, increased discomfort) and resultant behavioural changes (e.g. poor adherence, withdrawal from activity). CBT also directly addresses maladaptive behavioural responses with the use of strategies such as graded exposure to anxiety producing stimuli and reinforcement for adaptive behaviours.

Specific CBT techniques for paediatric pain

Many cognitive-behavioural techniques are useful both in the acute context of procedural pain (e.g. injections, blood draws, laceration repairs) and for chronic pain conditions (e.g. headache, abdominal pain, disease-related pain, musculoskeletal pain). Each technique reviewed here (see Table 50.1) aims to achieve one or more of the following CBT goals: (1) to direct the child's attention away from pain, (2) to enhance the child's sense of control over pain, and (3) to diminish negative thoughts and feelings related to pain. Although operant strategies (i.e. providing reinforcement or incentives for coping adaptively with pain) are sometimes included within the scope of cognitive-behavioural pain management, those strategies are detailed elsewhere by Slifer et al. (Chapter 51, this volume).

Preparation and psychoeducation

Education is a fundamental component of all CBT interventions. Educational interventions provide a rationale for how and why other cognitive-behavioural strategies can effectively reduce pain and distress.

Preparation for procedural pain

Preparation is a specific educational intervention that entails explaining to the child in advance exactly what the procedure will involve. Typically this includes breaking down the procedure into detailed steps to reduce anxiety and uncertainty. Incorporating sensory information is useful (e.g. 'The nurse will tie a rubber band around your arm; this will feel tight'). Preparation can include showing the child where the procedure will occur and specific equipment that will be used. There are also child-friendly procedure preparation kits available for purchase. It is important to note

Table 50.1 CBT techniques and their typical uses

CBT technique	Used for procedural pain?	Used for chronic pain?
Cognitive reframing	✓	✓
Desensitization	✓	✓
Distraction	✓	✓
Modelling	✓	
Multicomponent packages	✓	✓
Positive self-statements (aka coping statements)	✓	✓
Preparation	✓	
Psychoeducation		✓
Rehearsal	✓	
Relaxation	✓	✓

that detailed preparation prior to a medical procedure may reduce anxiety in some children but may create more anticipatory attention to the procedure than is helpful for others. Both developmental level and individual child coping style may influence utility of these techniques.

Psychoeducation for chronic pain

For chronic pain, psychoeducation entails providing the child and family with a clear explanation of what chronic pain is (e.g. the non-protective nature of chronic pain), how pain signals are transmitted in the body, the role of the brain in processing pain information, and an explanation of the biopsychosocial model of pain (see Pillai Riddell et al., Chapter 9, this volume) and the transactional relationship between stress and pain. Psychoeducation should include a rationale for how and why cognitive-behavioural strategies can effectively reduce pain and restore function. It is helpful to incorporate written educational materials so that children and families can refer back to them as needed.

Evidence base for preparation and psychoeducation

A few randomized controlled trials (RCTs) have examined the effects of preparation on children's response to procedure pain (Harrison, 1991; Tak and van Bon, 2006). A meta-analysis of this evidence shows positive effects of preparation on observer reports of pain during needle procedures but insufficient evidence of effects on self-report of pain or behavioural measures of distress (Uman et al., 2008). Results from one early study (Dahlquist et al., 1985) suggest that individual factors such as the quality (but not quantity) of a child's previous medical experience can affect whether preparation helps the child to cope more adaptively with procedural pain, but more research is needed in this area.

Psychoeducation for paediatric chronic pain is rarely delivered as a stand-alone intervention; thus, there is little literature examining its effectiveness in isolation. One RCT of adult chronic pain patients (Moseley et al., 2004) showed that education about pain neurophysiology resulted in changes in pain cognitions and physical task performance, although the education intervention did not result in changes in reported disability.

Distraction

The primary goal of distraction is to shift the child's attention away from pain toward more enjoyable, engaging stimuli. Recent theories, backed by empirical support, hold that distraction can exert a powerful analgesic effect that alters the activity on pain processing pathways in the brain (Bantick et al., 2002). Distraction is addressed by Cohen et al. (Chapter 53, this volume). It is briefly discussed here due to its central role in CBT package treatments. Distraction can include both behaviourally oriented strategies such as blowing bubbles or playing a videogame, and cognitively oriented strategies such as non-procedure focused conversation or tasks (e.g. discussing a favourite movie or counting objects). Reading stories or watching videos are also effective distractions for many children. Recently, virtual reality (VR) technology has been employed to create interactive and highly engaging distractions from pain (Lange et al., 2006; Mahrer and Gold, 2009).

Distraction for procedural pain

Distraction is perhaps the most commonly employed cognitive-behavioural technique for coping with procedural pain. It is easily employed in this setting and can work well across a variety of ages and temperaments. Distraction techniques are generally not time intensive, require little advance preparation, and can be implemented by a variety of clinicians. Parents can also be recruited to employ these strategies.

Distraction for chronic pain

Distraction works similarly in chronic pain, but the chronicity of the pain requires distractions that remain effective over time. Children and adolescents can identify activities that they enjoy and find absorbing and can be encouraged to use those activities in attempts to cope with pain. Distractions may be social or solitary. School can also be framed as an adaptive distraction from pain, since children are more likely able to distract themselves from pain in school than when home in bed, for example. It is important to work with the individual child to identify the distractions that work best.

Evidence base for distraction

Among all the specific cognitive behavioural tools for managing procedural pain, distraction has the largest base of empirical support (Cohen et al., 1997; Kleiber and Harper, 1999) Several systematic and critical reviews (Chambers et al., 2009; DeMore and Cohen, 2005; Powers, 1999; Uman et al., 2008) show large effect sizes for distraction as an intervention for paediatric procedural pain, with several recent studies specifically supporting VR-based distraction approaches in comparison to other distraction techniques (Mahrer and Gold, 2009). For further information see Cohen et al. (Chapter 53, this volume).

Modelling and rehearsal

Modelling and rehearsal techniques are aimed at reducing anticipatory anxiety by helping the child to develop more realistic expectations of a potentially painful situation and increasing comfort and familiarity with the situation. They are therefore most well-suited to the procedural pain context.

Modelling and rehearsal for procedural pain

For young children who are anxious about anticipated painful procedures, it is often helpful to provide a demonstration (i.e. modelling) of an adult or another child undertaking the procedure and using positive coping strategies. Videotaped demonstrations can be used for such purposes, or this can be done with a clinician (e.g. child life specialist) or through coaching a parent to demonstrate appropriate coping techniques. Often, children benefit most from education strategies that require them to assume a more active role. Therefore, rehearsal, in which the child him/herself acts out the procedure, such as through medical play, can reduce anxiety and foster positive coping. Often, assuming the role of the doctor or nurse and performing the procedure on a stuffed animal or parent helps children acquire a sense of mastery of an anxiety-provoking situation that may otherwise feel uncontrollable.

In general, studies support preparation and modelling/rehearsal strategies as effective tools for reducing anxiety and distress about medical procedures (Harbeck-Weber and McKee, 1995) with some indication that they may help reduce pain as well. Only one small RCT specifically focused on modelling was reported in a meta-analysis (Zabin, 1982), cited in Uman et al. (2008), and its results were not found to provide sufficient evidence of benefits from this technique alone.

Cognitive reframing/positive self-statements

Cognitive reframing refers to modifying one's thoughts about a distressing situation so that they are less focused on negative aspects of the situation. Typically, children are taught first to *identify* their negative thoughts or 'self-talk' about pain, then to *challenge* these thoughts, for example, by listing out evidence in support of the thought and evidence against it, and finally to *modify* these thoughts to produce less negative emotional responses. A related technique, positive self-statements, focuses on developing a set of statements that emphasize one's ability to cope positively with a challenging situation. Statements should be brief, such as 'I can do it!' or 'This will be over soon!'

Cognitive reframing and positive self-statements in procedural pain

A child facing a painful procedure might say, 'I don't want to do this, it will hurt too much!'. Reframing this statement might entail highlighting how quickly the procedure will be over and reminding the child that s/he has strategies for coping with pain, so that the statement can be reframed as, 'This might be uncomfortable, but it will be over soon and I can listen to my favourite song so I don't notice it as much'. Cognitive reframing can take place prior to, during, and after a painful procedure. Using cognitive reframing after a procedure, sometimes referred to as memory alteration, is aimed at reducing the negative memories of a painful experience so they are not as distressing and do not predispose the child toward greater anxiety in subsequent painful procedures (Chen et al., 1999).

Cognitive reframing and positive self-statements in chronic pain

A child with chronic pain might say, 'This pain is never going to get better'. This negative thinking, referred to as 'catastrophizing', is commonly associated with chronic pain (Sullivan et al., 2001; Turner and Aaron, 2001) The first step in reframing negative or catastrophic thinking is to help a child gain awareness of his/her negative thinking patterns using questionnaire assessments or thought monitoring procedures. Once recurrent negative thoughts are identified, the therapist and child examine evidence supporting the thought (e.g. 'I've seen a lot of doctors but haven't gotten better yet') and evidence against the thought (e.g. 'there are treatments available that help with this kind of pain'). If the evidence fails to fully support the negative thought, the child is taught to reframe this thought into a new, more adaptive thought such as 'This pain has been with me for a long time, but now I'm working on ways to feel better'. Positive self-statements (e.g. 'I know I can do this!', 'My pain WILL get better') can be used to foster adaptive coping and help challenge negative thought patterns.

Evidence base for cognitive reframing

There are few published studies of interventions that test cognitive reframing or positive self-statement approaches in isolation; typically they are incorporated into multicomponent CBT packages. One study (Chen et al., 1999) of memory alteration following lumbar puncture found that the group of children who participated in the memory alteration intervention reported less distress and pain than a control group, both immediately after the procedure and at follow-up. However, this small study has not been replicated, so results should be interpreted cautiously. The overall pattern of findings did not meet criteria to be considered efficacious in a meta-analysis (Uman et al., 2008).

Exposure and psychological desensitization

Exposure and psychological desensitization techniques, widely used in CBT for anxiety problems, involve gradually increasing exposure to a feared stimulus over time while minimizing associated anxiety. The roots of this approach lie in classical conditioning theory, which holds that the association between the stimulus (e.g. needle) and the response (fear, anxiety) is conditioned (learned) and can be progressively weakened. Typically, systematic desensitization entails developing a hierarchy of anxiety-provoking situations ordered from least- to most-feared. Through a process called graded *in vivo* exposure, the child is then exposed to the fearful situations beginning with those identified as least feared and gradually working up the hierarchy. The goal is to encounter the situations safely, without the previously experienced distress, to unlink them from associated anxiety. The clinician may teach the child to engage in positive coping strategies (e.g. relaxation) during this desensitization process.

Desensitization in procedural pain

Desensitization is a time-intensive strategy that requires a number of sessions with a trained clinician prior to the procedure. Therefore, in the procedural pain context it is typically used with children who are known to have high levels of pain-related anxiety in response to medical procedures such as injections. Prior to a procedure, children can work with a CBT therapist to develop and undergo a systematic process of pairing successive exposures to the feared stimulus (e.g. needle) with relaxation and use of other adaptive coping skills. Over time, the previously feared situation (e.g. the needle stick) ceases to produce significant pain-related anxiety.

Desensitization in chronic pain

Expectancy effects have a strong influence on pain perception (e.g. Logan and Rose, 2005). Many children with chronic pain develop a pattern of avoiding activities they believe will trigger or increase pain (Martin et al., 2007). Desensitization can be used to reduce this pain-avoidance pattern, unlink the association between activities and fear of pain, and help children to re-engage in activities, which can in turn help to reduce pain.

Evidence base for exposure/desensitization

A recent systematic review of exposure and desensitization treatments for adults with chronic pain (Bailey et al., 2010) included several RCTs (Leeuw et al., 2008; Woods and Asmundson, 2008) as well as many single case design studies. Current evidence suggests that graded *in vivo* exposure effectively reduces pain and fear-avoidance beliefs and behaviours. Few trials have examined exposure-based treatments in paediatric pain, but this is an emerging area of inquiry given the role of exposure in newer treatment approaches such as acceptance and commitment therapy (ACT). Wicksell and colleagues (2009) conducted a RCT of a ten-session ACT-based treatment with exposure as the primary intervention. The intervention led to greater reductions in pain, disability, pain-related discomfort, and fear of pain compared to standard multidisciplinary treatment (including medication) for children with chronic pain.

Relaxation techniques: breathing, guided imagery, muscle relaxation

Relaxation strategies focus on acquiring specific skills that can be used to decrease pain perception by promoting a general sense of physical and psychological well-being. This relaxed state is incongruent with intense pain perceptions. Relaxation approaches include deep (diaphragmatic) breathing, progressive muscle relaxation (PMR), and guided imagery techniques. Hypnosis also relies heavily on relaxation. See Liossi et al. (Chapter 54, this volume) for detailed explanations of these specific techniques.

Relaxation techniques in procedural pain

In the brief context of procedural pain experiences, deep breathing is perhaps the most commonly used relaxation tool. Often props such as bubbles or party blowers are employed, particularly with younger children; these tools incorporate a component of distraction that can augment the benefits of deep breathing. Recorded instructions for progressive muscle relaxation and guided imagery procedures are available and can be used in procedural settings when there is less preparation time available.

Relaxation techniques for chronic pain

Relaxation is widely used in chronic pain (e.g. Palermo et al., 2010). Learning to employ relaxation strategies in a self-directed manner provides children a greater sense of control over their physiological processes, which may help counteract feelings of helplessness induced by chronic pain. Sometimes these techniques are taught using computer-based biofeedback (see Zeltzer, Chapter 60, this volume), providing concrete visual and/or audio feedback to help the child gain increased awareness over previously involuntary physiological processes. Many therapists provide children with audio-recordings to practise techniques between sessions.

In addition to using guided imagery to develop relaxing images, this technique can also focus on pain-reducing imagery. For example, a child might be guided to imagine the 'pain control centre' in the brain and then locate specific controls that can help to turn down pain messages travelling to a specific body area. These techniques are typically more effective when the child has been guided into a general state of relaxation prior to engaging in imagery exercises (Kuttner, 1991).

Evidence base for relaxation strategies

Relaxation strategies have a good base of evidence supporting their use with paediatric patients in procedural pain contexts (Dahlquist, et al., 1985; French et al., 1994). Breathing exercises have been shown to be effective in reducing children's self-reported pain, observer rated distress, and nurse reported distress during routine immunization procedures (Chambers et al., 2009). In a meta-analysis published in 2010, Palermo and colleagues (Palermo et al., 2010) concluded that relaxation as a stand-alone cognitive-behavioural treatment was effective in reducing pain across studies of children and adolescents with a variety of chronic pain conditions including headache, abdominal pain, and fibromyalgia. Typically, however, these strategies along with most others described earlier, are incorporated into multicomponent CBT packages.

Biofeedback/biofeedback-assisted relaxation training

Biofeedback is a therapeutic procedure that measures and 'feeds back' information about an individual's physiological activity (typically indicators of autonomic arousal) to increase awareness of and voluntary control over those physiological processes (Arena and Blanchard, 1996; Olson and Schwartz, 2003). In the treatment of paediatric pain, biofeedback is often taught in conjunction with other relaxation strategies. As biofeedback is only one component of this approach, it is often referred to as biofeedback-assisted relaxation therapy. Because of the need for trained practitioners (most often psychologists), specialized equipment, and the need for practice to become skilled with these techniques, biofeedback is most commonly used for chronic and recurrent pain conditions.

Biofeedback for chronic pain

Biofeedback uses electrical sensors to measure and receive information (feedback) about a patient's body. The biofeedback sensors are connected to a computer interface and provide real-time information about physiological processes such as muscle tension. This information provides concrete evidence to patients, demonstrating when they are successful in making positive changes in their body, such as relaxing certain muscles, to achieve pain reduction. Biofeedback for pain management typically incorporates a focus on one or more of the following physiological processes: respiration (pace and depth of breathing), muscle electromyography, peripheral skin temperature, and blood flow or heart rate variability. The 'feedback' can be visual and/or auditory. Visual information can be displayed in graphic or numeric form, such as readout of skin temperature, or it can be transformed into other interactive displays. For example, a child engaging in thermal biofeedback might watch an image of a hot air balloon that gradually rises as the child increases their peripheral skin temperature, or sinks back down if the child's temperature drops. Similarly, relaxing music and images might play as long as the child maintains muscle relaxation below a specified surface electromyograph (EMG) level, but stop if the child surpasses the muscle tension threshold.

Each biofeedback modality has a different mechanism that accounts for its benefits for pain management; for example, EMG biofeedback promotes muscle relaxation, whereas skin-temperature biofeedback produces changes in peripheral and cranial blood flow. These physical changes can be directly beneficial to certain pain conditions, particularly migraine and tension headaches. Biofeedback can also help to foster mind–body connections, decrease overall sympathetic arousal, promote general relaxation, and enhance a child's sense of self control. Children often find

biofeedback engaging and benefit from the concrete, visual aspects of this technique. In fact, studies have shown that children with headaches derive greater benefit from biofeedback compared to adults (Sarafino and Goehring, 2000).

Evidence base for biofeedback

The most established evidence exists for the use of thermal biofeedback to treat migraine headache and for surface EMG biofeedback in the treatment of tension-type headaches (Herman and Blanchard, 2002). Several studies have demonstrated support for combining biofeedback training with interventions targeting parental responses to pain (Allen and Shriver, 1998; Kroner-Herwig et al., 1998), with results suggesting that this combined approach yields modestly better long-term outcomes than biofeedback treatment alone. In a meta-analytic review, Hermann et al. (1995) found evidence showing greater effectiveness of biofeedback compared to placebo or prophylactic drugs for the treatment of headache.

Studies have also begun to demonstrate the efficacy of biofeedback with paediatric patients with chronic abdominal pain (Schurman et al., 2010; Weidert et al., 2003). Several studies provide support for the use of biofeedback in the treatment of fibromyalgia symptoms (Buckelew et al., 1998; van Santen et al., 2002), although none of these studies is specific to the paediatric population. In their recent meta-analysis of psychological therapies for paediatric chronic pain, Palermo and colleagues (2010) concluded that biofeedback was effective in reducing pain, with an odds ratio of 23.34. However, additional well-designed studies of specific biofeedback modalities and biofeedback assisted relaxation approaches are needed, particularly studies that examine pain conditions other than headache and that include outcomes beyond pain reduction, such as improvements in physical and psychological functioning. Additionally, research is needed to compare biofeedback training to placebo conditions to elucidate its specific and non-specific effects. This is an important design consideration given the potential influence of the novelty of this treatment approach. Patients and families may have a negative bias towards psychological therapy for chronic pain, but may have a positive bias towards expectations for improvement when relaxation or pain management is taught via biofeedback. Teasing apart whether biofeedback-assisted relaxation is more beneficial for chronic pain management as compared to relaxation taught without biofeedback is an ongoing effort in the study of psychological interventions for chronic pain.

Multicomponent approaches

The techniques described earlier in this chapter are frequently combined into multicomponent cognitive-behavioural treatment packages. Such packages typically combine one or more behaviourally-oriented strategies, such as distraction, breathing, muscle relaxation, modelling/rehearsal, or desensitization, with one or more cognitively-focused strategies, such as imagery/hypnosis, education, cognitive reframing, or positive coping statements (Uman et al., 2008).

Multicomponent CBT for procedural pain

When using multicomponent CBT in the context of a painful procedure, techniques can be delivered all at once during the procedure itself, or in stages (e.g. with some pre-procedural preparation, some intervention during the procedure, and some post-procedural intervention). Parent or staff coaching in the use of the strategies is also a common component of these treatment packages in the procedural pain context, particularly for younger children (e.g. under age 8). Although combined approaches may be more time intensive to deliver, which is sometimes a challenge in the procedural setting, children are likely to benefit more from this comprehensive approach.

Multicomponent CBT for chronic pain

For children with chronic pain conditions, psychologists typically teach a broad complement of CBT strategies, often in the context of multidisciplinary treatments that might also incorporate physical therapy and medication use. Patients are encouraged to develop a 'toolbox' of diverse strategies for coping with pain and to adopt a self-management approach to their use outside of therapy sessions. The literature includes many reports of effective multicomponent CBT for treatment of paediatric chronic pain. For example, Sanders and colleagues (1994) developed a comprehensive cognitive-behavioural family intervention for children with recurrent abdominal pain that included psychoeducation, muscle relaxation, breathing, positive self-talk, distraction and imagery techniques along with some operant strategies. Biofeedback and relaxation strategies have frequently been delivered in combination in the treatment of paediatric headache (Holden et al., 1999). Logan and Simons (2010) developed a CBT package consisting of psychoeducation, relaxation, and cognitive reframing skills for children with a range of chronic pain conditions and associated school impairment.

Evidence base for multicomponent CBT

A number of well-validated CBT treatment packages have been created for paediatric procedural pain. Table 50.2 provides examples of empirically tested intervention packages. Many of these packages have been found effective in reducing emotional/behavioural distress both by self-report and observation. Some studies have combined CBT with medications and found the combined approach to improve upon benefits from medication alone (Jay et al., 1991; Kazak et al., 1996). Reviewing empirically supported treatments for procedure-related pain, Powers (1999) concluded that CBT treatment packages were a 'well-established treatment' for procedural pain in children and adolescents. In a Cochrane review, Uman and colleagues (2008) studied psychosocial interventions for 2-to 19-year-olds undergoing needle procedures. They found strong effects on observer reports of pain and behavioural measures of distress for multicomponent CBT interventions. The review by Chambers and colleagues (Chambers, et al., 2009) on interventions to reduce pain during immunization also found combined cognitive-behavioural interventions to be effective for reducing children's self-reported pain and observer-rated distress.

In a series of reviews of cognitive-behavioural treatment for various paediatric chronic pain conditions published in 1999, CBT was found beneficial for children with headaches (Holden et al., 1999), recurrent abdominal pain (Janicke and Finney, 1999), and disease-related pain (Walco et al., 1999). Most evidence was in support of combined treatment packages, although some evidence existed to support relaxation alone and thermal biofeedback alone (Holden et al., 1999; Palermo et al. 2010). In a systematic Cochrane review, Eccleston and colleagues (2009) concluded that cognitive-behavioural treatments were effective in reducing pain in children with headache, with benefits lasting into follow-up assessment points. The authors concluded that these treatments may also benefit

children with other pain conditions including musculoskeletal pain and recurrent abdominal pain, but the number of RCTs for these pain conditions was low.

In a meta-analysis, Palermo and colleagues (Palermo, et al., 2010) addressed some of the limitations of previous reviews by including more recently published trials (focused on headache, abdominal pain, and fibromyalgia) and examining outcomes of functional disability and emotional distress in addition to pain. They analysed 25 RCTs of psychological treatments for paediatric chronic pain, with a total of 1247 participants. The meta-analysis found that multicomponent CBT (along with relaxation therapy and biofeedback training as stand-alone approaches) led to significant reductions in pain, but data were inconclusive regarding effects on functional disability and emotional functioning. Comparing studies on different pain populations, the greatest effects of CBT on reducing functional disability emerged for children with abdominal pain, although it is not clear whether findings related to the type of pain condition or differences among specific interventions. Overall, the evidence in support of CBT for paediatric chronic pain is strong, with the growing body of RCTs demonstrating generally positive effects for a variety of cognitive and behavioural treatment strategies for children with a range of pain conditions. See Table 50.3 for descriptions of sample multicomponent CBT packages for chronic pain.

Key considerations in the application of CBT to paediatric pain

Preparing patients for CBT

It is important for families to have accurate expectations for CBT prior to commencing treatment. For example, it is crucial to dispel the myth that psychological pain management strategies are only effective if there is a psychological cause for the pain. McGrath and colleagues (2003) suggest offering the analogy that morphine is often useful in reducing postoperative pain, but this does not mean that postoperative pain is *caused* by a lack of morphine. CBT is effective for pain management for several reasons. First, children with chronic or acute pain often find direct symptom relief from behavioural pain management strategies. Second, chronic or recurrent pain is often associated with functional impairment (e.g. poor adherence to medical procedures, inability to attend school, activity limitations), and CBT strategies can be effective in improving function even if there is not a reduction in pain. Third, pain and suffering are often linked to feelings of hopelessness, helplessness, frustration, fear, and anxiety. These feelings can exacerbate pain, interfere with medical care, increase disability, and contribute to long-standing mental health difficulties. Thus, CBT has tremendous value for the management of paediatric pain because it has demonstrated effectiveness for: (1) the direct modification of pain sensation, (2) improving maladaptive behavioural responses to pain (e.g. emotional distress, avoidance of activity), and (3) modification of the negative thoughts that can lead to feelings of depression and anxiety (Turk et al., 2008).

It is helpful to explain to children and families that even an empirically effective treatment such as CBT may not eliminate pain immediately or entirely. Over time and with adherence to treatment, however, CBT can often alter a child's experience of pain and thus change their long-term trajectory (Kendall, 2012). After treatment with CBT, it is common for children with chronic pain

Table 50.2 Sample CBT interventions for paediatric procedural pain

Study	Pain condition(s)	Sample	Study aims	CBT components and Tx dose	Outcomes (pain, function, distress)
Boivin et al. (2008).	Scheduled vaccination	N = 239, healthy 4–12-year-olds	Compare pharmacological + psychological approaches during vaccination to standard medical care (SMC), including pharmacological pain management	Treatment group received: parent + child education, anaesthetic medication, parents providing reassuring statements, and child distraction by blowing bubbles	Compared to SMC, those in the multifactorial treatment group self-reported less pain on a visual analogue scale and facial pain scale. Parents' reports of child's pain were also less for children in the treatment condition vs SMC
Cohen et al. (2002)	Routine immunization	N = 61, 3–6-year-olds	To examine the efficacy of children's use of coping skills training without trained parent/nurse coaches	Treatment included: video instruction in deep breathing; positive self-statements; video modelling; practice	Treatment group did not report using skills during the procedure, perhaps due to lack of parental/nurse coaching. More child training and/or coach involvement might be necessary for effective child coping. Nurses encouraged child coping, whereas parents tended to respond to child distress
Schiff et al. (2001).	Repeated blood draws	N = 43, 4–12-year-olds with HIV	Single group, repeated measures design to evaluate multicomponent pain management intervention for children with HIV under-going repeated venepuncture.	Treatment included: preparation, relaxation, distraction, reinforcement, parent involvement, local anaesthetic cream; no CBT or anaesthetic cream used at baseline	Children reported significant reductions in distress and pain by the second post-intervention procedure and maintained them at the third; parent anxiety was significantly reduced by the second post-intervention procedure
Blount et al. (1992).	Routine immunization	N = 60, healthy 3–7-year-olds	To determine if combined CBT package result in less pain and distress by patient and parent report vs. no-treatment control group	Treatment group received distraction, coping skills training, + use of a party blower for deep breathing; Control group received standard care	Trained parents prompted their child to use the blower more than untrained parents. Trained children engaged in more blower usage than untrained children. Child and parent reported distress lower than both comparison groups

to report that some pain persists, but that the pain is less noticeable and doesn't interfere with everyday life (Rogers, 2008). Children who use CBT strategies to manage procedural pain might report that the procedure was not pain-free, but that it hurt less and they did not feel as anxious or distressed about it.

Parent involvement

Parents play an integral role in CBT for children with chronic or acute pain, and there are multiple ways to incorporate parents into treatment. Kendall (2012) suggests that parents can be 'consultants, collaborators, or co-clients' in treatment. Parents serve as 'consultants' when they provide information about the social, developmental, or cultural contextual factors that may contribute to their child's pain. This information is crucial for establishing treatment goals and identifying barriers to treatment. Parents are 'collaborators' when they help to oversee the implementation of their child's newly learned cognitive behavioural skills (Kendall, 2012). For example, parents can be taught how to use distraction techniques during their child's painful procedure or taught how to effectively help implement long-term behavioural goals for a child with chronic pain. Lastly, parents can be directly incorporated into CBT treatment with children as 'co-clients' if they are viewed as contributing to the child's presenting problem. For example, many parents become highly focused on their

child's discomfort. This high level of concern may inadvertently reinforce poor adaptation in children with acute or chronic pain presentations. One important CBT goal for parents is to learn to emphasize their child's use of coping skills rather than focusing on the pain itself; decreasing parents' focus on the pain and has been shown to lead to reduced child pain and distress for both procedural and chronic pain (Chambers et al., 2002; McMurtry et al., 2006; Walker et al., 2006). Additionally, research suggests that the association between pain and depression in children is significantly reduced when parents use active pain coping strategies (Williamson et al., 2002).

Developmental considerations

CBT interventions are most effective when they conceptualize presenting problems within the context of the child's current developmental tasks and milestones. Over the past 10 years there has been a significant increase in research that examines developmental factors as moderators of treatment outcomes, with the goal of improving our understanding of the relationship between the developmental level of a child and specific components of CBT (Holmbeck, 2012).

Because CBT necessitates the acquisition of new or modified behavioural and cognitive skills, attention to a child's development is an important consideration in treatment planning. Although

Table 50.3 Sample CBT interventions for paediatric chronic pain

Study	Pain conditions	Sample	Study aims	CBT components and Tx dose	Outcomes (pain, function, distress)
Kashikar-Zuck et al. (2012).	Juvenile fibro-myalgia syndrome (FMS)	N = 114, 11–18-year-olds	RCT to compare CBT vs education in reducing functional disability, pain, and symptoms of depression in juvenile FMS	Ten individual sessions in both conditions; CBT included: psychoeducation, muscle relaxation, activity pacing, distraction, problem solving, calming statements, relapse prevention strategies; FM education condition included: education and discussion about FM, pain medications, diet, sleep, exercise, and lifestyle	CBT superior to FM education in reducing functional disability; both groups had decreases in pain and depressive symptoms. Reduction in pain statistically but not clinically significant
Palermo et al. (2009).	Chronic headache, abdominal, or musculoskeletal pain	N = 48, 11–17-year-olds	RCT to compare internet-delivered CBT vs. no treatment on reducing pain intensity and activity limitations	Treatment group vs. waitlist control. Internet treatment consisted of 8 weeks of online modules including relaxation training, cognitive strategies, parent operant techniques, communication strategies, sleep, and activity interventions	Internet treatment group had less activity limitations and pain intensity at post-treatment and 3-month follow-up vs. waitlist group. No differences in parental protectiveness or child depression
Connelly et al. (2006).	Recurrent headaches	N = 37, 7–12-year-olds	RCT to compare CBT via a CD-ROM (+ some therapist contact) vs wait-list control on headache management	Six 1-h CD modules included relaxation, guided imagery, deep breathing, muscle relaxation, coping thoughts, and behaviour management	CD-ROM group had significantly greater improvements in self-reported headache frequency, duration, and intensity vs wait-list controls. Gains maintained at 3-month follow-up
Robins et al. (2005).	Recurrent abdominal pain (RAP)	N = 69, 6–16-year-olds	RCT to compare combination of standard medical care (SMC) + CBT family groups vs SMC alone	Five child–parent CBT sessions included breathing, imagery, relaxation techniques; positive self-talk strategies; minimizing catastrophizing; distraction; parent reframing (i.e. encouraging coping, limiting secondary gains)	Treatment group had significantly less child- and parent-reported pain vs SMC group immediately post-intervention. Group differences maintained at 1 year. Treatment group had significantly fewer school absences vs SMC. No differences in functional disability or somatization

some behavioural strategies such as simple distraction techniques can be effective even among infants undergoing routine immunizations (Cohen et al., 2006), other skills may be less appropriate for younger children (e.g. understanding how changes in thinking impact future experiences). In general, behavioural strategies may be best suited to younger children and more verbal or cognitive strategies may work best for older children. However, given that age is only a proxy for development and that cognitive development impacts the rate and processing of information, executive functioning, meta-cognition, and self-regulation, a thorough understanding of a child's cognitive development is a critical factor in establishing CBT goals and tailoring interventions.

Relapse prevention

For children with chronic pain or those who undergo repeated painful procedures, CBT interventions should incorporate strategies for relapse prevention. While empirical studies support the

effectiveness of CBT across a wide array of pain-related difficulties, long-term maintenance of treatment gains is less well demonstrated. Symptom relapse is most likely to occur when: (1) pain symptoms change or intensify, (2) a patient's perceived ability to manage the symptoms declines, and (3) there is an increase in psychological distress (Keefe and Van Horn, 1993). Relapse prevention strategies typically include anticipation of minor setbacks, identification of the early signs that distress is increasing, rehearsal of cognitive and behavioural coping skills, and self-reinforcement for adaptive responses to relapse (Keefe and Van Horn, 1993). Additionally, some patients may benefit from intermittent 'tune-ups' with a therapist. This has been conceptualized as the 'dental model' of care (Kazdin, 1997). Meeting every 3 to 6 months after treatment may help to reinforce newly learned skills, identify new onset symptoms before they become problematic, and help children develop more advanced skills to meet their evolving psychological, psychosocial, and environmental demands (Kazdin, 1997).

Alternative delivery approaches and emerging directions in CBT for paediatric pain

Group therapy for chronic pain

Group-based CBT interventions have been shown to be cost- and time-efficient and as effective as individual treatment in numerous studies (Morrison, 2001; Sears et al., 2007). The group format also promotes psychosocial support, a particularly salient important factor for children with chronic pain who often feel alienated by their condition. Group therapy programmes can also incorporate other family members in treatment sessions to help modify pain responses within the family environment (e.g. Coakley and Barber 2012; Logan and Simons 2010). In the paediatric literature, group CBT has already demonstrated effectiveness for a variety of pain-related problems such as irritable bowel syndrome (Hayutin et al., 2009), headache (Kroener-Herwig and Denecke, 2002) and pain-related school absenteeism (Logan and Simons, 2010).

Web-based treatment

There has been a recent emergence of Internet-based CBT interventions for paediatric pain. Internet-delivered CBT for chronic pain has a number of advantages to traditional treatment delivery models. It reduces waiting lists and scheduling conflicts, can be self-paced, and minimizes stigma (Baer et al., 2007; Cuijpers et al., 2008). Both therapist-guided and unguided models exist. Limitations to this delivery method include the automated aspects of this approach, requirement of access to and comfort with appropriate technology, and in the case of unguided approaches, a lack of immediate response to individual needs (Baer et al., 2007; Cuijpers et al., 2008). One meta-analysis (Cuijpers et al., 2008) found that since 2000, six randomized studies have examined interventions delivered over the Internet for paediatric pain. Effect sizes for Internet-delivered CBT for pain were promising (ranging from 0.19 to 0.79), but overall below those found for Internet-delivered CBT for anxiety and depression in children (Cuijpers et al., 2008; Spek et al., 2007). At present, Web-based interventions for pain appear promising but require additional research to determine efficacy (Bender et al., 2011; Cuijpers et al., 2008; Macea et al., 2010).

Palermo and colleagues developed one such programme to deliver Web-based family CBT to adolescents with chronic pain (Long and Palermo, 2009). Adolescents received pain education, relaxation training, and other CBT skills and parents receive training on reinforcement of positive coping, reward systems, communication, and modelling positive coping (Long et al. 2009). Findings of a small RCT found significant reductions in pain and activity limitations post-treatment for the Internet CBT group compared to wait-list control group, with gains maintained at a 3-month follow-up (Palermo et al., 2009). Several Internet-based CBT interventions for children with headaches have also demonstrated reductions in pain and in pain-related negative thinking (Hicks et al., 2006; Trautmann and Kroner-Herwig, 2010).

Variations on CBT for chronic pain: acceptance and commitment therapy and contextual cognitive behavioural therapy

Acceptance and commitment therapy (ACT) and contextual cognitive-behavioural therapy (CCBT) are relatively new models of psychotherapy commonly referred to as 'third wave' CBT approaches (Hayes 2004). ACT and CCBT both blend many of the major tents of CBT with a functional, contextual philosophy of science or rational frame theory (Hayes and Smith, 2005; Hayes et al., 1999). Rather than focusing on controlling or changing unpleasant experiences (e.g. pain), these approaches incorporate acceptance and mindfulness techniques and promote the patient identifying their core values and findings ways to live consistently with these values in spite of pain. These treatments often include exposure-based therapy aimed at increasing psychological flexibility and restoring functioning.

ACT and CCBT for chronic pain management have gained attention in the clinical and research literature given that some individuals with chronic pain need to learn to function in the context of ongoing pain. As opposed to traditional CBT approaches where the goal is to change unwanted phenomena (e.g. reduce or eliminate pain), ACT and CCBT focus on reducing the distressing and disabling influences of pain, pain-related thoughts, and avoidance of potentially painful activities. These approaches assist patients in identifying how to increase functioning and quality of life in accordance with their personal values by shifting away from recurrent struggles with pain (Hayes and Smith, 2005; Hayes et al., 1999; McCracken et al., 2007).

Research on ACT and CCBT demonstrates their effectiveness in adult chronic pain populations (McCracken and Eccleston, 2003; Ruiz, 2010; Vowles and McCracken, 2008). At this time, there is a limited but growing body of literature supporting the application of CCBT and ACT in children with chronic pain (Gauntlett-Gilbert and Eccleston 2007; Wicksell et al. 2009). There is also modest emerging evidence that acceptance and values-based parenting behaviours are associated with improved adolescent functioning in the context of chronic pain (McCracken and Gauntlett-Gilbert, 2011). One RCT comparing CBT to ACT for adult chronic pain found similar outcomes across the two treatments; both approaches led to reductions in pain interference and emotional distress (Wetherell et al., 2011). ACT and CCBT offer promising evidence that the acceptance of pain may be an important component of cognitive-behavioural psychotherapeutic treatment for patients with chronic pain.

Case example: The Comfort Ability programme—a brief multicomponent CBT group intervention

Megan is a 14-year-old girl with complex regional pain syndrome in her right lower extremity. Her pain led to significant functional limitations; she struggled to attend school and withdrew from peer and extracurricular activities, spending most of her day at home on the couch. She was referred to physical therapy, but was so fearful of using her foot she was unable to fully engage in treatment. Megan was referred for CBT, but she and her parents were resistant because they felt that Megan did not have a psychological problem. They argued that because her pain was 'real', there would be no benefit in 'just talking about the problem'.

Megan and her parents attended 'The Comfort Ability', a 1-day pain management workshop designed to provide children and parents with a non-stigmatizing, cost-, and time-effective introduction to the principles of CBT (Coakley and Barber, 2012). By addressing the stigma and resource barriers that often prevent families from engaging in psychological services for pain management, an intervention such as this can provide the three important components of CBT including: (1) psychoeducation to help elicit motivation for pain self-management, (2) cognitive and behavioural skill acquisition, and (3) brief skill rehearsal. Other advantages of a group treatment include the benefit of peer-based psychosocial support.

Within the adolescent group, Megan expressed anxiety about whether her pain would get better, frustration over missed activities, social isolation, school absences, and friction at home. Megan engaged in a goal-setting activity to identify her individual goals for improved functioning, developmentally targeted psychoeducation about how pain functions in the body, interactive discussions and worksheets to learn how to identify and modify negative thoughts and maladaptive behaviours, problem solving skills, and an art activity that promoted self-efficacy. Additionally, she practised behavioural skills such as diaphragmatic breathing, guided imagery, and progressive muscle relaxation. She learned how to use these strategies to manage the discomfort and stress associated with physical therapy and returning to school. Finally, she created a personalized pain management plan, highlighting the individual cognitive and behavioural strategies she thought would work best for her. She left with a manual and a pain management tool kit inclusive of a relaxation CD.

Megan's mother and father attended the parent workshop. They expressed feeling sad, anxious, and overwhelmed by Megan's situation. They shared openly with other parents who had similar experiences. With guidance, Megan's parents were able to identify that Megan's chronic pain was exacerbated by factors such as her transition to a new school, the recent loss of her grandmother, her sensitive temperament, and her perfectionistic personality. They were taught how to minimize their responses to her pain (e.g. refraining from asking her to 'rate' her pain, encouraging her to be functional) and how to support her in using her coping skills. Importantly, they were also provided with guidance for how to advocate for Megan at school so that Megan would be well supported with a school re-entry plan.

Three weeks after attending the workshop Megan's parents reported significant changes in their approach to Megan's care, with observable benefits. They noted that Megan was regularly attending shortened days at school. She was participating in physical therapy and had set a motivating goal of getting her ears pierced when she 'graduated' from her treatment. Her parents noted that she still struggled with 'bad days' but that her mood and function were steadily improving. Megan's parents observed a shift in Megan's thinking and in her approach to pain management. They planned to initiate treatment with a local psychologist to provide ongoing CBT to Megan in order to further her initial gains.

References

Allen, K. D., and Shriver, M. D. (1998). Role of parent-mediated pain behavior management strategies in biofeedback treatment of childhood migraines. *Behav Ther*, 29(3), 477–490.

Arena, J. G., and Blanchard, E. B. (1996). Biofeedback and relaxation therapy for chronic pain disorders. In R. J. Gatchel, D. C. Turk, (eds) *Psychological approaches to pain management: a practitioner's handbook*, pp. 179–230. New York: Guilford Press.

Baer, L., Greist, J., and Marks, I. M. (2007). Computer-aided cognitive behaviour therapy. *Psychother Psychosom*, 76(4), 193–195.

Bailey, K. M., Carleton, R. N., Vlaeyen, J. W., and Asmundson, G. J. (2010). Treatments addressing pain-related fear and anxiety in patients with chronic musculoskeletal pain: a preliminary review. *Cogn Behav Ther*, 39(1), 46–63.

Bantick, S. J., Wise, R. G., Ploghaus, A., Clare, S., Smith, S. M., and Tracey, I. (2002). Imaging how attention modulates pain in humans using functional MRI. *Brain*, 125(Pt 2), 310–319.

Barakat, L. P., Gonzalez, E. R., and Weinberger, B. S. (2007). Using cognitive-behavior group therapy with chronic medical illness. In R. W. Christner, J. L. Stewart, and A. Freeman, (eds) *Handbook of cognitive-behavior group therapy with children and adolescents: specific settings and presenting problems*, pp. 427–446. New York: Routledge/Taylor & Francis Group.

Barlow, J. H., and Ellard, D. R. (2004). Psycho-educational interventions for children with chronic disease, parents and siblings: an overview of the research evidence base. *Child Care Health Dev*, 30(6), 637–645.

Beck, A. T. (1979). *Cognitive therapy and the emotional disorders*. New York: Meridian.

Bender, J. L., Radhakrishnan, A., Diorio, C., Englesakis, M., and Jadad, A. R. (2011). Can pain be managed through the Internet? A systematic review of randomized controlled trials. *Pain*, 152(8), 1740–1750.

Blount, R. L., Landolf-Fritsche, B., Powers, S. W., and Sturges, J. W. (1991). Differences between high and low coping children and between parent and staff behaviors during painful medical procedures. *J Pediatr Psychol*, 16(6), 795–809.

Boivin, J. M., Poupon-Lemarquis, L., Iraqi, W., Fay, R., Schmitt, C., and Rossignol, P. (2008). A multifactorial strategy of pain management is associated with less pain in scheduled vaccination of children. A study realized by family practitioners in 239 children aged 4–12 years old. *Fam Pract*, 25(6), 423–429.

Buckelew, S. P., Conway, R., Parker, J., Deuser, W. E., Read, J., Witty, T. E., et al. (1998). Biofeedback/relaxation training and exercise interventions for fibromyalgia: a prospective trial. *Arthritis Care Res*, 11, 196–209.

Chambers, C. T., Kenneth, D., and Bennett, S. M. (2002). The impact of maternal behavior on children's pain experiences: an experimental analysis. *J Pediatr Psychol*, 27(3), 293–301.

Chambers, C. T., Taddio, A., Uman, L. S., and McMurtry, C. M. (2009). Psychological interventions for reducing pain and distress during routine childhood immunizations: a systematic review. *Clin Ther*, 31(Suppl 2), S77–S103.

Chen, E., Zeltzer, L. K., Craske, M. G., and Katz, E. R. (1999). Alteration of memory in the reduction of children's distress during repeated aversive medical procedures. *J Consult Clin Psychol*, 67(4), 481–490.

Coakley, R. M., and Barber, B. N. (2012). Overcoming common barriers to engagement in psychological services for chronic pain: a one-day pediatric pain management workshop for youth and parents. *Pediatr Pain Lett*, 14(1), 10–15.

Cohen, L. L., Bernard, R. S., Greco, L. A., and McClellan, C. B. (2002). A child-focused intervention for coping with procedural pain: are parent and nurse coaches necessary? *J Pediatr Psychol*, 27(8), 749–757.

Cohen, L. L., Blount, R. L., and Panopoulos, G. (1997). Nurse coaching and cartoon distraction: an effective and practical intervention to reduce child, parent, and nurse distress during immunizations. *J Pediatr Psychol*, 22(3), 355–370.

Cohen, L. L., MacLaren, J. E., Fortson, B. L., Friedman, A., DeMore, M., Lim, C. S., et al. (2006). Randomized clinical trial of distraction for infant immunization pain. *Pain*, 125(1–2), 165–171.

Connelly, M., Rapoff, M. A., Thompson, N., and Connelly, W. (2006). Headstrong: a pilot study of a CD-ROM intervention for recurrent pediatric headache. *J Pediatr Psychol*, 31(7), 737–747.

Cuijpers, P., van Straten, A., and Andersson, G. (2008). Internet-administered cognitive behavior therapy for health problems: a systematic review. *J Behav Med*, 31(2), 169–177.

Dahlquist, L. M., Gil, K. M., Armstrong, F. D., Ginsberg, A., and Jones, B. (1985). Behavioral management of children's distress during chemotherapy. *J Behav Ther Exp Psychiatry*, 16(4), 325–329.

DeMore, M. and Cohen, L. L. (2005). Distraction for pediatric immunization pain: a critical review. *J Clin Psychol Med Sett*, 12(4), 281–291.

Eccleston, C., Morley, S., Williams, A., Yorke, L., and Mastroyannopoulou, K. (2002). Systematic review of randomised controlled trials of psychological therapy for chronic pain in children and adolescents, with a subset meta-analysis of pain relief. *Pain*, 99(1–2), 157–165.

Eccleston, C., Palermo, T. M., Williams, A. C., Lewandowski, A., and Morley, S. (2009). Psychological therapies for the management of chronic and recurrent pain in children and adolescents. *Cochrane Database Syst Rev*, 2, CD003968.

French, G. M., Painter, E. C., and Coury, D. L. (1994). Blowing away shot pain: a technique for pain management during immunization. *Pediatrics*, 93(3), 384–388.

Gauntlett-Gilbert J. and Eccleston, C. (2007). Disability in adolescents with chronic pain: patterns and predictors across different domains of functioning. *Pain*, 131(1–2), 132–141.

Harbeck-Weber, C. and McKee, D. (1995). Prevention of emotional and behavioral distress in children experiencing hospitalization and chronic pain. In M. Roberts, (ed.) *Handbook of pediatric psychology*, pp. 167–184. New York: Guilford.

Harrison, A. (1991). Preparing children for venous blood sampling. *Pain*, 45(3), 299–306.

Hayes, S. C., and Smith, S. (2005). *Get out of your mind and into your life: The new acceptance and commitment therapy*. Oakland, CA: New Barbinger Publications, Inc.

Hayes, S. C., Strosahl, K. D., and Wilson, K. G. (1999). *Acceptance and commitment therapy: an experiential approach to behavior change*. New York: Guilford Press.

Hayutin, L. G., Blount, R. L., Lewis, J. D., Simons, L. E., and McCormick, M. L. (2009). Skills-based group intervention for adolescent girls with inflammatory bowel disease. *Clin Case Stud*, 8(5), 355–365.

Hermann, C. and Blanchard, H. B. (2002). Biofeedback in the treatment of headache and other childhood pain. *Appl Psychophysiol Biofeedback*, 27(2), 143–162.

Hicks, C. L., von Baeyer, C. L., and McGrath, P. J. (2006). Online psychological treatment for pediatric recurrent pain: a randomized evaluation. *J Pediatr Psychol*, 31(7), 724–736.

Holden, E., Deichmann, M., and Levy, J. (1999). Empirically supported treatments in pediatric psychology: recurrent pediatric headache. *J Pediatr Psychol*, 24(2), 91–109.

Holmbeck, G. N. (2012). Guides from developmental psychology for therapy with adolescents. In P. C. Kendall, (ed.) *Child and adolescent therapy: cognitive-behavioral procedures* (4th edn), pp. 429–470. New York: Guilford Press.

Janicke, D. and Finney, J. (1999). Empirically supported treatments in pediatric psychology: recurrent abdominal pain. *J Pediatr Psychol*, 24(2), 115–127.

Jay, S. M., Elliott, C. H., Woody, P. D., and Siegel, S. (1991). An investigation of cognitive-behavior therapy combined with oral valium for children undergoing painful medical procedures. *Health Psychol*, 10(5), 317–322.

Kashikar-Zuck, S., Ting, T. V., Arnold, L. M., Bean, J., Powers, S. W., Graham, T. B., *et al.* (2012). Cognitive behavioral therapy for the treatment of juvenile fibromyalgia: a multisite, single-blind, randomized, controlled clinical trial. *Arthritis Rheum*, 64(1), 297–305.

Kazak, A. E., Penati, B., Boyer, B. A., Himelstein, B., Brophy, P., Waibel, M. K., *et al.* (1996). A randomized controlled prospective outcome study of a psychological and pharmacological intervention protocol for procedural distress in pediatric leukemia. *J Pediatr Psychol*, 21(5), 615–631.

Kazdin, A. E. (1997). A model for developing effective treatments: progression and interplay of theory, research, and practice. *J Clin Child Psychol*, 26, 114–129.

Keefe, F. J., and Gil, K. M. (1986). Behavioral concepts in the analysis of chronic pain syndromes. *J Consult Clin Psychol*, 54(6), 776–783.

Keefe, F. J., and Van Horn, Y. (1993). Cognitive-behavioral treatment of rheumatoid arthritis pain: maintaining treatment gains. *Arthritis Care Res*, 6, 213–222.

Kendall, P. C. (2012). Guiding theory for therapy with children and adolescents. In P. C. Kendall, (ed.) *Child and adolescent therapy: cognitive-behavioral procedures* (4th edn), pp. 3–24. New York: Guilford Press.

Kleiber, C. and Harper, D. C. (1999). Effects of distraction on children's pain and distress during medical procedures: a meta-analysis. *Nurs Res*, 48(1), 44–49.

Kroener-Herwig, B. and Denecke, H. (2002). Cognitive-behavioral therapy of pediatric headache: are there differences in efficacy between a therapist-administered group training and a self- help format? *J Psychosom Res*, 53(6), 1107–1114.

Kroener-Herwig, B., Mohn, U., and Pothmann, R. (1998). Comparison of biofeedback and relaxation in the treatment of pediatric headache and the influence of parent involvement on outcome. *Appl Psychophysiol Biofeedback*, 23(3), 143–157.

Kuttner, L. (1991). Helpful strategies in working with preschool children in pediatric practice. *Pediatr Ann*, 20(3), 120–122, 124–127.

Lange, B., Williams, M., and Fulton, I. (2006). Virtual reality distraction during pediatric medical procedures. *Pediatr Pain Lett*, 8(1), 6–10.

Leeuw, M., Goossens, M. E., van Breukelen, G. J., de Jong, J. R., Heuts, P. H., Smeets, R. J., *et al.* (2008). Exposure in vivo versus operant graded activity in chronic low back pain patients: results of a randomized controlled trial. *Pain*, 138(1), 192–207.

Logan, D. E., and Rose, J. B. (2005). Is postoperative pain a self-fulfilling prophecy? Expectancy effects on postoperative pain and patient-controlled analgesia use among adolescent surgical patients. *J Pediatr Psychol*, 30(2), 187–196.

Logan, D. E., and Simons, L. E. (2010). Development of a group intervention to improve school functioning in adolescents with chronic pain and depressive symptoms: a study of feasibility and preliminary efficacy. *J Pediatr Psychol*, 35(8), 823–836.

Long, A. C., and Palermo, T. M. (2009). Brief report: web-based management of adolescent chronic pain: development and usability testing of an online family cognitive behavioral therapy program. *J Pediatr Psychol*, 34(5), 511–516.

Macea, D. D., Gajos, K., Daglia Calil, Y. A., and Fregni, F. (2010). The efficacy of web-based cognitive behavioral interventions for chronic pain: a systematic review and meta-analysis. *J Pain*, 11(10), 917–929.

Mahrer, N. E., and Gold, J. I. (2009). The use of virtual reality for pain control: a review. *Curr Pain Headache Rep*, 13(2), 100–109.

Martin, A. L., McGrath, P. A., Brown, S. C., and Katz, J. (2007). Anxiety sensitivity, fear of pain and pain-related disability in children and adolescents with chronic pain. *Pain Res Manag*, 12(4), 267–272.

McCracken, L. M., and Eccleston, C. (2003). Coping or acceptance: what to do about chronic pain? *Pain*, 105(1), 197–204.

McCracken, L. M., and Gauntlett-Gilbert, J. (2011). Role of psychological flexibility in parents of adolescents with chronic pain: development of a measure and preliminary correlation analyses. *Pain*, 152(4), 780–785.

McCracken, L. M., MacKichan, F., and Eccleston, C. (2007). Contextual cognitive-behavioral therapy for severely disabled chronic pain sufferers: effectiveness and clinically significant change. *Eur J Pain*, 11(3), 314–322.

McMurtry, C. M., McGrath, P. J., and Chambers, C. T. (2006). Reassurance can hurt: Parental behavior and painful medical procedures. *J Pediatrics*, 148, 560–561.

Morrison, N. (2001). Group cognitive therapy: Treatment of choice or sub-optimal option? *Behav Cogn Psychother*, 29(3), 311–332.

Moseley, G. L., Nicholas, M. K., and Hodges, P. W. (2004). A randomized controlled trial of intensive neurophysiology education in chronic low back pain. *Clin J Pain*, 20(5), 324–330.

Olson, R. P., and Schwartz, M. S. (2003). A historical perspective on the field of biofeedback and applied physiology. In M. S. Schwartz and F. Andrasik (eds) *Biofeedback: a practitioner's guide* (2nd edn), pp. 3–19. New York: Guilford Press,

Palermo, T. M., Eccleston, C., Lewandowski, A. S., Williams, A. C., and Morley, S. (2010). Randomized controlled trials of psychological therapies for management of chronic pain in children and adolescents: an updated meta-analytic review. *Pain*, 148(3), 387–397.

Palermo, T. M., Wilson, A. C., Peters, M., Lewandowski, A., and Somhegyi, H. (2009). Randomized controlled trial of an Internet-delivered family cognitive-behavioral therapy intervention for children and adolescents with chronic pain. *Pain*, 146(1–2), 205–213.

Powers, S. W. (1999). Empirically supported treatments in pediatric psychology: procedure-related pain. *J Pediatr Psychol*, 24(2), 131–145.

Robins, P. M., Smith, S. M., Glutting, J. J., and Bishop, C. T. (2005). A randomized controlled trial of a cognitive-behavioral family intervention for pediatric recurrent abdominal pain. *J Pediatr Psychol*, 30(5), 397–408.

Rogers, R. (2008). *Managing persistent pain in adolescents*. Oxford: Radcliffe Publishing.

Ruiz, F. J. (2010). A review of acceptance and commitment therapy (ACT) empirical evidence: correlational, experimental psychopathology, component and outcome studies. *Int J Psychol Psychol Ther*, 10(1), 125–162.

Sanders, M., Shepherd, R., Cleghorn, G., and Woolford, H. (1994). The treatment of recurrent abdominal pain in children: a controlled comparison of cognitive-behavioral family intervention and standard pediatric care. *J Consult Clin Psychol*, 62(2), 306–314.

Sarafino, E. P., and Goehring, P. (2000). Age comparisons in acquiring biofeedback control and success in reducing headache pain. *Ann Behav Med*, 22(1), 10–16.

Schiff, W. B., Holtz, K. D., Peterson, N., and Rakusan, T. (2001). Effect of an intervention to reduce procedural pain and distress for children with HIV infection. *J Pediatr Psychol*, 26(7), 417–427.

Schurman, J. V., Wu, Y. P., Grayson, P., and Friesen, C. A. (2010). A pilot study to assess the efficacy of biofeedback-assisted relaxation training as an adjunct treatment for pediatric functional dyspepsia associated with duodenal eosinophilia. *J Pediatr Psychol*, 35(8), 837–847.

Sears, S. F., Sowell, L. D., Kuhl, E. A., Kovacs, A. H., Serber, E. R., Handberg, E., *et al.* (2007). The ICD shock and stress management program: a randomized trial of psychosocial treatment to optimize quality of life in ICD patients. *Pacing Clin Electrophysiol*, 30(7), 858–864.

Spek, V., Cuijpers, P., Nyklicek, I., Riper, H., Keyzer, J., and Pop, V. (2007). Internet-based cognitive behaviour therapy for symptoms of depression and anxiety: a meta-analysis. *Psychol Med*, 37(3), 319–328.

Sullivan, M. J., Thorn, B., Haythornthwaite, J. A., Keefe, F., Martin, M., Bradley, L. A., *et al.* (2001). Theoretical perspectives on the relation between catastrophizing and pain. *Clin J Pain*, 17(1), 52–64.

Tak, J. H., and van Bon, W. H. (2006). Pain- and distress-reducing interventions for venepuncture in children. *Child Care Health Dev*, 32(3), 257–268.

Thorndike, E. L. (1913). *The psychology of learning*. New York: Teachers College Press.

Trautmann, E. and Kroner-Herwig, B. (2010). A randomized controlled trial of Internet-based self-help training for recurrent headache in childhood and adolescence. *Behav Res Ther*, 48(1), 28–37.

Turk, D. C., and Rudy, T. E. (1989). A cognitive-behavioral perspective on chronic pain: beyond the scalpel and syringe. In C. D. Tollison, (ed.) *Handbook of chronic pain management*, pp. 222–236. Baltimore, MD: Williams & Wilkins.

Turk, D. C., Swanson, K. S., and Tunks, E. R. (2008). Psychological approaches in the treatment of chronic pain patients—when pills, scalpels, and needles are not enough. *Can J Psychiatry*, 53(4), 213–223.

Turner, J. A., and Aaron, L. A. (2001). Pain-related catastrophizing: what is it? *Clin J Pain*, 17(1), 65–71.

Uman, L. S., Chambers, C. T., McGrath, P. J., and Kisely, S. (2008). A systematic review of randomized controlled trials examining psychological interventions for needle-related procedural pain and distress in children and adolescents: an abbreviated Cochrane review. *J Pediatr Psychol*, 33(8), 842–854.

van Santen, M., Bolwijn, P., Verstappen, F., Bakker, C., Hidding, A., Houben, H., *et al.* (2002). A randomized clinical trial comparing fitness and biofeedback training versus basic treatment in patients with fibromyalgia. *J Rheumatol*, 29, 575–581.

Vowles, K. E., and McCracken, L. M. (2008). Acceptance and value-based action in chronic pain: A study of treatment effectiveness and process. *J Consult Clin Psychol*, 76(3), 397–407.

Walco, G. A., Sterling, C. M., Conte, P. M., and Engel, R. G. (1999). Empirically supported treatments in pediatric psychology: disease-related pain. *J Pediatr Psychol*, 24(2), 155–167.

Walker, L. S., Williams, S. E., Smith, C. A., Garber, J., Van Slyke, D. A., and Lipani, T. A. (2006). Parent attention versus distraction: impact on symptom complaints by children with and without chronic functional abdominal pain. *Pain*, 122(1–2), 43–52.

Weidert, J. A., Ball, T. M., and Davis, M. F. (2003). Systematic review of treatment for recurrent abdominal pain. *Pediatrics*, 111(1), e1–e11.

Wetherell, J. L., Afari, N., Rutledge, T., Sorrell, J. T., Stoddard, J. A., Petkus, A. J., *et al.* (2011). A randomized, controlled trial of acceptance and commitment therapy and cognitive-behavioral therapy for chronic pain. *Pain*, 152(9), 2098–20107.

Wicksell, R. K., Melin, L., Lekander, M., and Olsson, G. L. (2009). Evaluating the effectiveness of exposure and acceptance strategies to improve functioning and quality of life in longstanding pediatric pain—a randomized controlled trial. *Pain*, 141(3), 248–257.

Williamson, G. M., Walters, A. S., and Shaffer, D. R. (2002). Caregiver models of self and others, coping, and depression: predictors of depression in children with chronic pain. *Health Psychol*, 21(4), 405–410.

Woods, M. P., and Asmundson, G. J. (2008). Evaluating the efficacy of graded in vivo exposure for the treatment of fear in patients with chronic back pain: a randomized controlled clinical trial. *Pain*, 136(3), 271–280.

Zabin, A. M. (1982). The modification of children's behavior during blood work procedures. Doctoral dissertation, West Virginia University, WV.

CHAPTER 51

Operant treatment

Keith J. Slifer, Adrianna Amari and
Cynthia Maynard Ward

Introduction

Operant conditioning interventions for clinical pain involve the modification of environmental and social stimuli that are (1) antecedents (discriminative stimuli or setting events) to maladaptive pain behaviour or (2) consequent stimuli that maintain the maladaptive pain behaviour through positive reinforcement (social attention or assistance from others) or negative reinforcement (escape or avoidance of uncomfortable, effortful activity, or of social, academic, or work responsibilities). While aspects of operant conditioning theory have been included in the design of interventions to manage acute paediatric medical procedure-related pain (see Slifer et al., 1995, 2002, 2011), this chapter will not include these studies but will focus on operant conditioning based interventions for illness- and injury-related chronic or recurrent pain.

Before reviewing the history and empirical support for operant conditioning based interventions for pain, in general, and paediatric pain, in particular, it will be useful to note that much of the work in this area has been conducted by psychologists and behaviour analysts who have been trained in the research methods and conventions of the Experimental Analysis of Behaviour and Applied Behaviour Analysis (see Iversen, 2013; Cooper et al., 1987 for more background on these disciplines). These fields employ single-subject experimental designs in which each subject serves as his or her own control and careful, repeated observations are conducted on the same individual across time (referred to as a time series). The individual's behaviour is measured during these observations by recording the occurrence or not of operationally defined behavioural responses, features of the physical and social environment, and sometimes physiological responses of the participant (e.g. blood pressure, heart rate, body temperature, etc.). The preference for single-subject methods and research designs arose from the philosophical perspective that information about what controls behaviour can be learned from studying its variability across environmental conditions within a single participant. Observations of the antecedents and consequences of target behaviour lead to hypotheses about controlling variables. Single-subject research involves systematic control and manipulation of antecedent or consequent variables in order to demonstrate and confirm the hypothesized functional control over the behaviour being studied. The investigator's aim is to show that when hypothesized controlling variables are manipulated the occurrence of target behaviour can be reliably increased or decreased. In this type of research, rather than obtaining a single or a few observations of a large sample of participants, the investigator obtains many observations of only one or a few participants. One important advantage of this type of research is that variability within subjects is considered important information to be studied rather than error variance to be controlled by averaging across a large group of subjects or by other statistical methods. In single-subject experimental design research an emphasis is placed on replication of demonstrated functional control both within a given subject on different occasions and across settings and replication of the same or similar results for a given intervention across repeated applications with a relatively small series of participants. This is particularly useful when developing and testing new intervention approaches based on cumulative individual subject evidence. This approach is also preferred by behaviour analysts because it allows for more individualization of intervention procedures while basing them on a consistent rationale and set of learning and conditioning principles. This is especially important for working with children whose behaviour patterns are developing based on their ongoing learning experiences. This individualized approach to intervention is a hallmark of Applied Behaviour Analysis, and it is especially useful for demonstrating the effectiveness of novel interventions. These interventions may later become the focus of more conventional randomized clinical trials that assess for generalizability of effects across larger samples of participants. In light of this research philosophy many of the studies discussed in this chapter employed single-subject experimental design and the strength of the evidence derives from replication across studies demonstrating the same or similar behavioural phenomena. This evidence base is supplemented by the few relevant group design studies and systematic reviews across studies that are available in the literature.

Origins of operant treatment for chronic pain

Although the focus of this book and, therefore, this chapter is on methods for understanding and treating pain in infants, children, and youth, it will be helpful to consider the origins of the operant conceptualization of pain behaviour in the adult clinical pain management literature. Wilbert Fordyce and colleagues conducted some of the earliest work applying operant behavioural concepts to understanding and treating patients' pain (Fordyce, 1976). He and his colleagues proposed that a significant part of clinical pain is the patient's overt behaviour that can be influenced by myriad social and environmental factors in addition to being influenced by actual tissue damage or irritation (see Fordyce and colleagues' work summarized in Sanders, 2003).

The operant conceptual framework for understanding chronic pain is that consequences that immediately follow pain behaviours may have a powerful influence on the probability of the pain behaviours occurring again in the future. As a result of this behaviour-consequence association, pain behaviours that originated because of body damage or tissue irritation may come under control of consequences and conditioning that occur in the patient's social environment. According to Fordyce, the two general processes that are responsible for this operant conditioning are positive reinforcement and avoidance learning. Positive reinforcement suggests that the occurrence of pain behaviours will increase in frequency if followed by positive consequences. By definition, if a behaviour increases in frequency after a specific consequence consistently follows it, then whatever the consequence was is hypothesized to be a positive reinforcer. Positive reinforcers of pain behaviour may include contingent social attention in the form of attempts to comfort and console, efforts by others to soothe the pain, and providing contingent pain medication (pro re nata, prn, or 'take when needed' medication). Avoidance learning of pain behaviour occurs when the frequency of a behaviour increases after that behaviour allowed the patient to escape or avoid aversive stimulation.

In this process, pain behaviours such as limping, bracing, or activity avoidance become associated with decreased or no pain sensation, and as a result these behaviours are negatively reinforced and are maintained or increase in frequency. In chronic pain patients this process may become elaborated to the point that the anticipation of suffering becomes a conditioned aversive stimulus. Thus, in the context of anticipated pain, if the patient displays protective pain behaviours and pain perception or its exacerbation does not occur, then the same protective behaviours are more likely to be emitted in the future.

Furthermore, Fordyce noted that once such avoidance learning occurs, it requires little ongoing reinforcement to maintain it. In this context reinforcement refers to the avoidance of nociception. If a behaviour occurs due to anticipation of pain and motivation to avoid both the aversive experience of the anticipation (anxiety, physiological arousal) and the nociceptive stimulus, the patient will maintain the avoidance behaviour even if the nociceptive stimulation is never again experienced. In this situation the goal of operant treatment is to prompt and reinforce normative physical activity and arrange the environment such that the patient attempts typical physical activity without the self-protective pain behaviours, and does not experience pain or experiences it at much lower intensity or magnitude.

Fordyce et al. (1968) first applied operant conditioning methods to modify environmental contingencies in order to change chronic pain in an adult patient. These investigators hypothesized that responses by others to overt pain behaviour accompanying the patient's subjective pain experience may reinforce some aspects of the pain behaviour. If this occurs for a protracted period of time,

the environment may come to sustain the pain behaviour even after the condition that caused the pain has resolved. 'Environment' in this context refers primarily to the social environment. That is, overt expressions or demonstrations of pain behaviour may frequently be followed by attention and attempts by family members and/or medical personnel to provide comfort (Fordyce et al., 1968).

The patient in this case had complained of low back pain for 18 years and had decreased ability to function in the physical activities of daily living. She could maintain a maximum of 20 min of continuous activity without reclining to rest. When a pain episode occurred, she ceased all activity, laid down, took pain medication, and cried until the pain subsided. At these times she received a lot of solicitous and ministering attention from her husband and son. She had undergone surgical interventions to remove a herniated disk (the source of nerve root irritation) and a lumbosacral spine fusion to stabilize her spine. After a careful medical evaluation revealed no evidence of remaining neurological disorder, the investigators reasoned that this patient's behaviour was maintained by contingent attention, medication, and rest. Therefore, the first intervention based on operant conditioning theory was to remove the contingent relationships between pain complaints and medication administration. Instead of being provided on an 'as needed' basis in response to pain complaints, the medication was provided according to a standard medication schedule and gradually faded in dosage until completely discontinued. At the same time, the medical and rehabilitation staff were instructed to be as neutral and socially unresponsive as possible to the patient's complaints of pain or discomfort. Instead, whenever the patient was engaged in an out of bed activity and not speaking of her pain the staff provided positive social attention including praise for any observed increase in physical activity. In this way, pain behaviour was placed on operant extinction and physical functioning was differentially positively reinforced. Using these modified contingencies, a programme of occupational and physical therapy was developed that used rest and attention as the positive reinforcer for increasing participation in activities (e.g. weaving) and walking. As a result, the patient showed a marked increase in her activity level and her pain complaints nearly disappeared in a period of about 8 weeks.

During the 1970s and 1980s, a few similar case studies of children were published using the same type of operant behavioural contingencies as those first described by Fordyce and colleagues (1968). For example, Sank and Biglan (1974) used operant procedures within a controlled case study to treat a 10-year-old boy with severe stomach pains. The investigators developed a token economy in which tokens were awarded to positively reinforce non-pain behaviours while attention was withheld from the boy's pain complaints. This treatment was reported to decrease the frequency of pain attacks, the magnitude of the boy's pain ratings, and to increase his school attendance.

Miller and Kratochwill (1979) published another controlled case study in which time out was used to treat a 10-year-old girl with complaints of severe stomach pain that were hypothesized to be maintained by parental attention. The behavioural treatment in this case involved removing adult attention and social activities contingent on pain complaints. With this intervention, pain complaints in the home decreased from two per day during baseline observation to approximately one per week after treatment, and this improvement was maintained at 1-year follow-up. A similar decrease in pain complaints was reported to occur at school when the same treatment contingencies were introduced.

Varni et al. (1980) also published an early case demonstration that the overt pain behaviour of a child being treated for severe burns could be impacted by modifying environmental contingencies. These authors used a combination of multiple baseline and reversal single-subject experimental designs to document a reduction in the verbal and motor pain behaviour of a 3-year-old child across hospital bedroom, clinic, and physical therapy settings. Behavioural treatment consisted of rearranging reinforcement contingencies to minimize reinforcement of pain behaviour and maximize reinforcement of observed 'well' behaviours; including wearing required splints and participating in exercises in physical therapy.

The role of aversive conditioning and escape-avoidance learning in the development and maintenance of chronic pain behaviour

As already discussed, early operant conceptualizations by Fordyce and colleagues focused primarily on operant extinction of positively reinforced pain behaviour (eliminating pain behaviour-contingent positive reinforcement). However, these investigators subsequently conceptualized some pain behaviour in terms of escape-avoidance learning. For example when pain behaviour occurs in the context of physical exertion, the patient will discontinue the exertion and thereby escape the pain associated with the exertion. With experience, the patient may learn not only to stop physical activity that produces pain or discomfort, but may also learn to avoid the situations in which physical activity might be required. Thus, an adult may begin to avoid going to work, leaving the house or even getting out of bed. Children and adolescents may learn to avoid going to school, participating in athletics, or even having social interactions with peers.

Fordyce et al. (1982) published a description of the escape-avoidance conceptualization along with the case study of a 21-year-old-male with a 15-year history of hospitalizations for 'abnormal abdominal pain'. This publication described a procedural innovation specifically designed to modify chronic pain behaviours that were hypothesized to have been acquired through avoidance learning. In their article, Fordyce and colleagues presented the basic premises underlying the behaviour analysis and treatment of chronic pain, which are paraphrased in the following list (Fordyce et al., 1982):

1. Pain behaviour, defined as indicators of pain and suffering, may become chronic for reasons other than its original aetiology. That is, chronic pain behaviours may have little or no remaining link to nociception from the body site where the pain problem began.

2. A chronic pain problem may persist for reasons other than the originating aetiology, and a parsimonious explanation with empirical support is that chronic pain may be understood in terms of learning and conditioning factors occurring in the interactions between the patient and the social environment.

3. Given that pain behaviours may not be linked directly to nociception in individuals with chronic pain, but instead may be due to conditioning effects, strategies for treatment can be based on counterconditioning or behaviour-change principles.

4. Multiple behaviour change methods exist that can be focused on modifying pain behaviour directly, rather than attempting to directly change subjective pain perception.

This conceptualization does not suggest that nociception should not be changed directly, if possible, through medication or other medical intervention, but is based on the assumption that in chronic pain cases traditional medical approaches have not been effective in eliminating the patient's pain. In their 1982 case study Fordyce and colleagues demonstrated the effectiveness of behavioural intervention based on this avoidance–conditioning conceptualization. In that case the 21-year-old male with a 15-year history of pain, dizziness, and abnormal gait was treated with behavioural intervention because of his inactivity and severely impaired ability to walk. Treatment was introduced in two phases. First, improved walking was established by reintroducing walking between parallel bars and positively reinforcing patient participation and achievement of increasing distances. In the second phase reinforcement was provided for walking at increasing speeds that were incompatible with the patient's initially abnormal gait. In addition, a therapist met weekly with the patient and on three occasions with the patient's mother. These sessions focused on altering the social consequences of 'sick' and 'well' behaviour displayed by the patient. The therapist practised and taught the mother to withdraw social support for the patient's inactivity and to provide encouragement and social support for his progress with walking. After the provision of this multimodal intervention, the patient became normally active, ambulated normally, and returned to productive activity. After completing treatment he enrolled in and began attending college, and at 21 months post-treatment was maintaining his treatment gains. To demonstrate the effectiveness of this treatment, the authors employed a changing criterion single-subject experimental design. Using this design they showed that each time the criterion for reinforcement was changed, the patient's behaviour changed accordingly to meet the criterion set (e.g. increased walking speed requirement).

Application of operant conditioning principles to the management of children's pain behaviour during burn wound care

Following upon the conceptual and case study publications described earlier, Kelly et al. (1984) conducted a single-subject experimental study using a reversal design with two girls aged 4 and 6 years with severe burns who required daily hydrotherapy, wound debridement, and application of a topical antibiotic medication. In this study, the investigators noted that the child with burns encounters frequent pairings of environmental stimuli (sights, sounds, and smells in the hospital) with pain (nociceptive stimulation from burn wound care). As a result the child likely learns that in the presence of these stimuli he or she experiences pain. The children in this study responded to the pain with crying, thrashing, and other verbal and motor pain behaviours and these behaviours resulted in intermittent escape from or delay of the painful procedures as well as increased attention from adults attempting to soothe the distressed child.

Therefore, the authors employed an operant conceptualization that assumed burn treatment-related pain behaviour is both positively and negatively reinforced over time. They designed their behavioural intervention with this conceptualization in mind. They used a multicomponent behavioural treatment approach to reducing pain behaviour during these painful procedures. The intervention included cartoon viewing as a form of distraction during the procedures and implementation of a star feedback chart. The star feedback chart was used as an incentive for the children to use the TV cartoon viewing for distraction and for crying less than they had during the same procedure on the previous day. Direct observations were conducted and the occurrence of target behaviours was recorded during each 30-sec interval of the procedures. The target behaviours included the child's verbal and motor pain behaviours and parent or physical therapist interactions with the child. Following each treatment session the parent, physical therapist, and child also completed behaviour rating scales of the child's fear, cooperation, and pain using a 9-point scale. The star chart included a colourful graph showing the percentage of intervals during which the child displayed verbal or motor pain behaviour during each medical treatment session.

This intervention that combined distraction and positive reinforcement of decreased pain behaviour resulted in an approximately 40% reduction in the children's pain behaviour. In addition, both children indicated enjoying the TV cartoons (approximately 4 on a 5-point scale, with 5 = 'I enjoyed the TV very much'). Based on the study design and data it was not possible for the authors to determine the relative contribution of the distraction and reinforcement components of the intervention, but they speculated that the star chart positive reinforcement was critical because they had collected preliminary pilot data with three other children receiving the TV distraction only, and these children showed only slight reductions in pain behaviours.

Two caveats about this study should be noted. First, the most painful of these burn procedures are conducted under sedation, but prolonged periods of sedation and sleep are avoided because the child with burns needs to maintain high levels of caloric and fluid intake to prevent dehydration and ensure adequate nutrition for healing. Therefore, the child can benefit from being able to tolerate these treatments with reduced or no sedation as healing progresses. The second caveat stated by the authors is that the goal of this behavioural treatment is not to completely suppress the child's pain behaviour, but to distract the child to decrease pain perception during treatment and to teach the child to control their pain behaviour to some degree (Kelly et al., 1984).

From this pioneering work of Kelly et al. (1984) until the present day, principles of conditioning and learning have been applied to the management of children's pain and distress during burn wound care. A pair of informative review and discussion articles has been published that present a theoretical framework and associated treatment applications for burn wound care in children (Martin-Herz et al., 2000; Thurber et al., 2000). Three psychological principles are presented to help explain the association between burn care, pain and anxiety. The principles include: classical conditioning, operant conditioning, and control coping. Using these principles, the authors describe the developmentally normal emergence of avoidance behaviours that disrupt required wound care for burns. Using case examples, the authors present their conceptualization of how classical conditioning converts neutral environmental stimuli into anxiety-provoking, aversive stimuli, and nearly simultaneously operant delay, avoidance, and escape behaviours are both intentionally and unintentionally reinforced by medical and family caregivers. These authors also emphasize how the loss of ability to predict and control the environment with respect to aversive stimulation interferes with the ability of children undergoing burn wound care to cope in the hospital environment and likely promotes learned helplessness (Thurber et al., 2000). Following this conceptualization, Thurber and colleagues (2000) point out how behaviours of burn patients that are often labelled as 'manipulative' are, in fact, quite logical from the patient's perspective of trying to learn what will result in reinforcing outcomes or events in the context of burn wound care. Indeed, despite best pharmacological practices complete elimination of pain and distress may be impossible, and escape behaviour shaped through avoidance conditioning is expected and developmentally typical. The authors hypothesize that in the context of burn wound care, pauses and completion of painful procedures are the most salient reinforcers.

Based on this theoretical framework, a number of intervention strategies have been developed and applied. First, one way to reduce the occurrence of repeated undesirable pain behaviours, such as whining, complaining and constantly requesting pain medication, is to give the analgesic medication on a fixed, time-based schedule rather than giving it on an 'as needed' basis in response to increased pain behaviour. Another strategy based on operant conditioning theory that has been recommended is to place excessive pain behaviours 'on extinction' by withholding all unnecessary social attention (consoling, coaxing, apologizing, etc.) while, alternatively, positively reinforcing cooperation and coping behaviours such as participating in safe and distracting activities. Additional treatment strategies are based on the rationale of increasing the child's ability to predict and control at least some important aspects of his or her environment. This can be accomplished by providing the child with a limited quantity of 'passes' or 'break cards' that the child can use to request a brief break from the painful wound care. A case example on the application of this technique to another kind of wound care will be presented at the end of the present chapter. An alternative strategy is to allow the child to take planned or scheduled breaks that are established and explained to the child in advance. Making the temporary termination of painful stimulation contingent on the passing of a preset time interval (using a timer visible to the child) or contingent on the child presenting a break card helps to reduce the development of escape behaviour in the context of burn wound care (Martin-Herz et al., 2000).

Recent research on the use of behaviour analysis in clinical dentistry supports the beneficial effects of providing breaks from uncomfortable dental procedures according to a fixed time schedule. O'Callaghan et al. (2006) demonstrated that when five children (4–7 years of age) were undergoing tooth preparation and restoration procedures, providing them with intermittent, 10 sec breaks regardless of their level of disruptive behaviour resulted in clinically significant reductions in disruptive behaviour. Consequently, the need for physical restraint during treatment was reduced to near zero.

Pain behaviours as a class of operant responses

Pain behaviours can vary considerably in terms of modality of expression (vocal, verbal, motor), frequency, intensity, and duration. Yet, as Kalsher et al. (1985) pointed out, a variety of pain behaviours may have a similar effect on the patient's environment (e.g. attention from others, medication administration, avoidance of effortful physical demands). Given their common effect on the environment, these pain behaviours may be conceptualized as an operant response class. Kalsher and colleagues (1985) argued that examination of pain behaviours as a response class may identify behaviours that are most responsive to modification and might facilitate efficient treatment. The treatment efficiency may result from the phenomenon known as response covariation in which a change in the probability of one response in a response class results in corresponding changes in the probability of other members of the same response class. If screaming, crying and facial contortions are all members of the same response class, then an intervention that decreases the occurrence of screaming might also result in decreased crying and grimacing.

Based on this conceptualization, Kalsher et al. (1985) studied behavioural covariation in a patient exhibiting a variety of pain behaviours. These investigators studied the effects of reinforcement and contingent removal of reinforcement on one pain behaviour (screaming) and also measured the effects of these interventions on other pain behaviours that were not targeted directly for treatment. The participant in this study was a 24-year-old male with borderline intelligence and a medical diagnosis of dystonia musculorum deformans, a genetic neuromuscular disorder that is characterized by strong, sustained twisting and writhing motions of the somatic muscles, adduction of the thigh, and continuous torsion spasms with associated severe, chronic muscular pain. A variety of pharmacological treatments had resulted in little improvement and the patient was at risk of residential placement outside of the family home because of the severity of his screaming. In this study, screaming and five other pain behaviours including self-reports of pain were measured while varying behavioural contingencies for screaming. Pain behaviours that were measured in addition to screaming included facial contortions, muscle contractions, help-seeking, and sharp expulsion of breath. The experimental conditions involved non-contingent reinforcement compared to the removal of reinforcement contingent on screaming.

As hypothesized, the pain behaviours did co-vary during behavioural and drug conditions even though the intervention only directly targeted screaming. The untargeted pain behaviours covaried most during observations that followed rather than preceded pain drug administration. Furthermore, in contrast to the behavioural observation measures, physiological measures (electromyography) did not differ across conditions. Overall, the results of this study demonstrated that pain behaviour such as screaming can be brought under operant control via manipulation of environmental contingencies. Furthermore, because the other pain behaviours co-varied with screaming, together they appeared to form a response class that shared a similar reinforcement history. While this response covariation can be beneficial to the efficiency of behavioural intervention for pain behaviour, the authors caution that behaviour therapy for pain should be conducted in a manner that will assure the maintenance of at least one appropriate but non-disruptive method of pain expression to allow for successful medical management. That is, even though pain behaviours can be manipulated by modifying environmental contingencies, the goal is not to make the patient completely stoic. Having a consistent, reliable measure of pain behaviour is necessary to be able to monitor

the patient's biological status for evidence of illness, tissue damage, or irritation (Kalsher et al., 1985).

Systematic reviews of empirical support for the operant conditioning model of pain behaviour; the interactional mixed model of learning and associated intervention strategies

As can be seen from the case studies and single-subject design experiments discussed earlier, the literature supporting the operant behavioural conceptualization and treatment of chronic pain in children and adults, and of medical procedure-related pain in children, grew steadily during the 1970s and 1980s. Fordyce et al. (1985) published a comprehensive review article on the use of operant conditioning with adult chronic pain patients. These authors reviewed ten studies that supported the efficacy of behavioural interventions to systematically change the behaviour of patients and sustain these changes over follow-up intervals of up to several years. Based on these studies, they concluded that operant behavioural techniques typically applied in the context of interdisciplinary pain programmes have clinically significant effects on overt pain behaviours such as activity level, medication usage for pain, and verbal expression and self-ratings of pain.

Unfortunately, because of the interdisciplinary context in which the interventions were applied, it was not possible to conclude that operant conditioning-based behavioural interventions were solely responsible for the observed changes. Therefore, continued research was encouraged and needed to determine the specific effects of the operant techniques on immediate and long-term pain behaviour changes. Shortly thereafter, Linton (1986b) published a follow-up review that included five additional, somewhat more methodologically sound studies, resulting in similar conclusions that operant based interventions were effective at increasing activity level, reducing medication usage, and to a lesser degree improving subjective pain reports.

Since the pioneering work of Fordyce and colleagues, the operant conditioning conceptualization and strategies based on it have played a predominant role in understanding and treating adult chronic pain patients (Sanders, 1985, 2003). Sanders (2003) discussed, at length, the behavioural conceptualization of pain and the research supporting this model. In this conceptualization clinical pain is defined as 'an interacting cluster of individualized overt, covert and neurophysiological responses capable of being produced by relevant tissue damage or irritation, but also produced and maintained by other antecedent and consequent stimulus conditions'. Sanders' operant conditioning model is based on six decades of behavioural science, which has produced extensive empirical evidence that essentially all voluntary and most emotional behaviours are influenced by their environmental context and consequences. When applied to pain, the operant conditioning model emphasizes the equality of overt gross motor components of pain behaviour with the cognitive/subjective and neurophysiological components. Furthermore, evidence indicates that these three types of pain responses do not always co-vary consistently (are not reliably positively correlated).

Sander's model of pain is based on a larger Interactional Mixed Model of Learning that includes operant and respondent conditioning and observational learning effects. Fordyce et al. (1982) and Sanders (1985, 2003) argue that most gross motor and many cognitive/subjective responses can be characterized as escape-avoidance behaviours. For example crying, grimacing, avoiding activity and lying down all may allow the individual to remove, escape, or avoid unpleasant stimulation such as painful tissue damage or irritation, or anxiety from anticipation of this aversive stimulation. This, as introduced earlier, is consistent with a negative reinforcement paradigm, in which the termination of an unpleasant or non-preferred stimulus results in an increased probability of the behaviour that brought about its termination. Sanders (2003) elaborates that behaviours strengthened or maintained by negative reinforcement have been shown to be extremely resistant to change without direct intervention to modify their occurrence. This is especially true for avoidance behaviour because the behaviour functions to avoid the aversive consequence. Without direct intervention there is no opportunity for the individual to ever experience the avoided stimulus conditions in the absence of the aversive stimulus (pain perception), and to associate it with other positive consequences. Thus, with behaviour maintained by avoidance learning there is no spontaneous remedial learning mechanism for establishing new responses unless specific alterations are made in the controlling stimulus conditions associated with the avoidance response. Sanders (2003) cites multiple, well-controlled studies demonstrating that pain responses across response categories (cognitive/subjective, gross motor, neurophysiologic) can be influenced significantly by antecedent and consequent stimulus condition changes in both analogue and clinical environments.

Sander's (1985, 2003) conceptual model distinguishes between acute and chronic pain states. In acute pain, neurophysiological and gross motor pain responses are dominant and the most prevalent controlling consequent stimuli are those associated with the reduction of pain perception arising directly from tissue damage or irritation. When pain becomes chronic, pain responses may become more predominantly cognitive and subjective (anticipation, fear and avoidance of pain sensation). In chronic pain conditions, the most prevalent consequent stimuli maintaining pain behaviours involve escape or avoidance of anticipated pain. Indeed, the patient now may be avoiding aversive environmental stressors associated with pain (e.g. physical contact or exertion, social interactions) or confused with subjective pain perception (e.g. symptoms of anxiety, depression perceived as pain). In chronic pain states, this avoidance of physical activity and social interaction is maintained even after the original tissue damage or irritation is greatly diminished or no longer present. In addition, positive consequences such as social attention may play a greater role in chronic pain.

Given that the antecedent and consequent stimuli that maintain pain behaviour may have shifted when pain has become chronic, it is necessary to consider, and when possible, to modify these maintaining variables. As indicated by Sanders (2003), the effectiveness of any pain intervention is a function of the extent to which it significantly alters the primary antecedent and consequent stimuli initiating and maintaining the pain responses. For example, if a patient is actually experiencing tissue damage or irritation (an antecedent condition) then interventions that do not change the perception of this stimulus will not be effective. Rather, escape-avoidance motivated pain behaviour (e.g. avoiding physical activity) will be maintained to the extent that the behaviour reduces or eliminates perception of pain resulting directly from the tissue

damage or irritation. Interventions that may reduce pain perception include medication, nerve blocks, cognitive-behavioural coping strategies (distraction, hypnosis, controlled deep breathing, progressive muscle relaxation, visual imagery), acceptance and commitment interventions, and other physical interventions (heat, cold, massage, acupuncture, electrodermal stimulation). In situations in which environmental and psychosocial stressors are the antecedent events that set the occasion for pain behaviours, and these behaviours are positively reinforced by special social attention or ministering behaviour from others, and/or are negatively reinforced by physical, social, educational or work activity avoidance, these maintaining variables must be addressed or pain treatment will not be effective.

Following the logic and model just presented, Flor et al. (2002) conducted a study of the role of operant conditioning in the development and maintenance of chronic pain. The study compared 30 adult patients with chronic back pain to 30 healthy matched control participants on their verbal and neurophysiological responding to an operant conditioning paradigm. The results showed that both groups' verbal reports were able to be conditioned, but the patients with chronic low back pain showed different cortical and electromyographic responses. Specifically, the patients with chronic pain were more easily affected by operant conditioning factors at both the verbal and neurophysiological level. Flor and colleagues hypothesized that individuals with greater susceptibility to conditioning effects may be more likely to develop chronic pain conditions. In support of this hypothesis, there is recent evidence that after experiencing painful stimulation in an experiment, chronic pain patients evidenced decreased diffuse noxious inhibitory control (DNIC) in the brain when exposed to subsequent painful stimulation, while healthy control participants (Meeus et al., 2008) and individuals with major depressive disorder did not show this diminution of DNIC (Normand et al., 2011).

Positive reinforcement of wellness behaviour and the combination of operant and cognitive-behavioural interventions for clinical pain

It is important to note that operant interventions for pain also include modification of antecedent and consequent stimuli in order to strengthen wellness-oriented behaviours that are alternatives to, or incompatible with, maladaptive pain behaviour. Examples of positive alternative behaviours include participation in therapy, use of pain coping strategies (distraction, muscle relaxation, positive self-statements), increased physical and social activity, reduced use of narcotic pain medications, and return to role functioning (i.e. school or work).

In his excellent review article on operant therapy with patients with chronic pain, Sanders (2003) discussed the evidence base supporting the effectiveness of these operant interventions, and emphasized that although operant conditioning can play a major role in modifying pain behaviour, it is not considered a complete or comprehensive treatment for clinical pain. That is, medical, physical and cognitive-behavioural interventions also should be used, when appropriate, in addition to operant behavioural treatment strategies. In clinical practice, operant procedures are rarely, if ever, used in isolation, and research evidence supports the benefits of combining these strategies with cognitive-behavioural techniques such as distraction, relaxation training and cognitive coping skills training. The evidence indicates that the addition of cognitive-behavioural techniques to operant conditioning may significantly enhance the treatment effects accomplished with operant conditioning alone (Compas et al., 1998; Keefe et al., 1992; Lindstrom et al., 1992; Moraley et al., 1999; Sanders, 2003; Van Tulder et al., 2000). Based on his literature review and similar previous reviews by others, Sanders (2003) concluded that there is strong and substantial evidence for the effectiveness of operant conditioning interventions demonstrated primarily with adult patients with low back pain. The evidence supports that operant conditioning alone or in combination with other treatment (e.g. cognitive-behavioural) strategies can produce significant and sustained improvements in general activity level, work behaviour, use of pain medication, and to a lesser degree subjective pain intensity ratings of patients with chronic pain when applied in either inpatient or outpatient settings. The evidence base is strong for adults with low back pain, but there are fewer methodologically rigorous data on the efficacy of operant conditioning-based interventions on other pain conditions such as complex regional pain syndrome (CRPS), fibromyalgia, and headache. The research evidence on operant conditioning intervention effects with children, adolescents, and geriatric populations with diagnoses other than low back pain (either acute or chronic) were found to be less well developed when Sanders conducted his 2003 review.

Empirically supported psychological treatments for recurrent abdominal pain

Functional abdominal pain is one of the more frequently researched types of chronic pain. In these studies a number of factors associated with the exacerbation and regulation of pain behaviour have been identified (e.g. regulation of afferent input by the CNS, the patient's capacity for sustained attention to bodily sensations and painful stimuli, the amount of caregiver attention paid to pain behaviour, the child's emotional responding to pain, and the amount of effort devoted to using active coping strategies) (Hyams and Hyman, 1998; Lipani and Walker, 2006; Zeltzer et al., 1997, 2006).

With respect to operant behavioural conceptualizations of chronic functional pain in children, operant principles have been hypothesized to be a possible factor in the development of recurrent abdominal pain (RAP). The specific reasoning is that caregivers or others in the child's social environment may inadvertently reinforce illness behaviour and maladaptive coping strategies in the child. Children may receive increased parental attention and experience other reinforcing consequences for their pain complaints (e.g. being excused from school or household chores, or being allowed to avoid stressful social situations with peers; Janicke and Finney, 1999).

Other investigators have adopted a social learning (aka. observational learning or modelling) theory to explain the development of RAP (see Oster, 1972; Robinson et al., 1990; Stone and Barbero, 1970; Walker et al., 1991, 1993, 1994, 1995; Walker & Zeman, 1992; as cited in Janicke and Finney, 1999). According to social learning theory the child observes the pain complaints and corresponding reinforcement contingencies experienced by another person in his or her environment (usually a close family member) and adopts the same behaviour to deal with personal stressors. In support of

this theory are studies indicating a significant relationship between a family history of chronic pain and the occurrence of RAP. This relationship may be due to greater emphasis on bodily sensations throughout the family or modelling of illness behaviour by family members.

A few intervention studies based on operant and social learning theories have been conducted, and this literature was reviewed by Janicke and Finney (1999) to search for empirical support for treatments for RAP. Janicke and Finney (1999) found that based on the available studies and their methodological quality, operant procedures alone did not meet even the more lenient criteria for a 'promising' intervention. Dietary fibre treatments for RAP associated with constipation meet the criteria for a 'promising' intervention, and cognitive-behavioural interventions for RAP meet the criteria for a 'probably efficacious' intervention. While the two case studies using operant treatment alone reviewed by Janicke and Finney (1999) did not meet even the least stringent criteria for empirically supported 'promising' interventions, these early preliminary studies demonstrated preliminary evidence that operant conditioning principles have some influence on the symptoms that are reported by children with RAP, and they set the stage for pursuing alternatives to medical treatment for RAP, including cognitive-behavioural interventions that utilize operant procedures as part of their treatment strategies. From the time of Janicke and Finney's (1999) review to the present day, operant interventions alone rarely have been recommended for RAP or other chronic pain conditions, but have been frequently combined with cognitive-behavioural techniques (Banez and Gallagher, 2006; Blanchard and Scharf, 2002; Finney et al., 1989; Humphreys and Gevirtz, 2000; Linton, 1986a, 1986b; Sanders et al., 1989, 1994; Vervoort et al., 2011).

Robins et al. (2005) conducted a randomized controlled trial of a cognitive-behavioural family intervention for paediatric RAP. The intervention employed a social learning theory conceptualization of RAP, emphasizing the interactive effects of skill deficits in the child and maintenance of symptoms within the context of family interactions. Intervention strategies included presenting this conceptual model to both child and parents, instructing children on active pain management techniques (deep breathing, imagery, relaxation, positive self-statements) using modelling and behavioural rehearsal, and teaching parents more appropriate ways to respond to their child's pain behaviour (reinforcement of behaviour incompatible with pain behaviour, minimizing discussion of pain, refraining from allowing the child to gain special privileges or avoid age-appropriate responsibilities due to pain behaviour). Children and parents receiving the cognitive-behavioural intervention reported less abdominal pain and fewer school absences (Robins et al., 2005).

Hicks et al. (2006) conducted an intervention study with 47 children and youth (ages 9–16 years) with recurrent headache or abdominal pain. The 47 participating youth were randomly assigned to an Internet-based intervention group (n = 25) or a standard medical care waitlist control group (n = 22). The main components of the cognitive-behavioural intervention were relaxation skills training (deep breathing, visualization/imagery) and cognitive strategies (self-talk). Clinically significant improvement was defined a priori as a 50% or greater reduction in pain diary scores. Using this definition, 71% of the treatment group improved compared to 19% of the control group at 1-month follow-up, and 72% compared to 14% improved at 3-month follow-up.

Parent–child interactions

As can be discerned from the various operant and cognitive-behavioural and social learning-based studies described earlier, conducting parent training to change the ways in which parents respond to their children's pain versus wellness and coping behaviour is a common component of many of these intervention studies. The associated hypotheses are that parents or caregivers of children with chronic pain place too few demands on their children, attend excessively to pain symptoms, allow their children to escape or avoid activities and responsibilities because of pain behaviour, and allow their children to assume a developmentally inappropriate level of dependence on the parent or caregiver. They may try to protect the child from symptoms by decreasing activities and demands. They may increase the child's distress by overt expression of their own distress, and poor regulation of their own anxiety and frustration (Garber et al., 1990; Liakopoulou-Kairis et al., 2002).

In support of this conceptualization, Walker et al. (1995) studied parents' reactions to somatic complaints associated with unexplained illness and documented that parents often modify their interactions with their children in the presence of pain complaints or illness behaviour. Other studies by Walker and colleagues have reported similar findings that parents tend to encourage children to adopt the sick role for gastrointestinal symptoms (Walker and Zeman, 1992), and children with RAP often have families in which there is greater parental attention to abdominal pain (Walker et al., 1993). Furthermore, a laboratory study by Walker and colleagues (2006), experimentally induced visceral discomfort as an analogue of abdominal pain, and demonstrated that when social attention is provided contingent on gastrointestinal symptom complaints, these complaints nearly doubled in both children with a history of abdominal pain and controls without a history of abdominal pain.

Parents also may model pain behaviour (Schanberg et al., 2001). Parents' expressions of sympathy, attention to symptoms, emotional reactions, modelling of symptoms, and reinforcement of pain behaviour by allowing escape/avoidance of responsibilities, all have been associated with greater pain and disability in their children (Fordyce, 1976; Payne and Norfleet, 1986; Philips, 1987). A number of studies support that in at least some families, the child's pain symptoms play a functional role within family interaction patterns and relationships. In these families, functional disability may be more a function of these interaction patterns than of the subjective experience of pain (Covelman et al., 1990; Kopp et al., 1995; Logan and Scharff, 2005; Naidoo and Pillay, 1994; Palermo, 2000; Scharff et al., 2005). Other studies have examined the social consequences of chronic pain in children (Van Slyke and Walker, 2006; Walker and Zeman, 1992; Walker et al., 1993, 2002). Parental responses studied have included minimizing (shifting focus away from pain behaviours, or reacting in a negative or punishing manner), solicitous responses (encouragement, reinforcement, frequent attending to pain), and protecting (excusing child from regular activities, allowing child to miss school and to stay in bed, etc.) (Van Slyke and Walker, 2006; Walker et al., 1993). More solicitous parental responses have been associated with greater sick role behaviour and greater functional disability independent of stress level or pain intensity (Gidron et al., 1995; Walker et al., 2002; Whitehead et al., 1994).

Peterson and Palermo (2004) studied 215 children between 8 and 16 years of age with chronic or recurrent pain conditions (headache,

juvenile idiopathic arthritis, sickle cell disease) and their parents in order to examine how children's distress, parent indulgence and child functional disability are interrelated. Hierarchical linear regression analyses indicated that solicitous parental responding to child pain behaviour significantly predicted functional disability after controlling statistically for pain intensity. Furthermore, for children with greater distress (depression or anxiety symptoms), parental solicitous responses to the child's pain reports were more strongly associated with increased functional disability than for children with fewer symptoms of anxiety or depression (Peterson and Palermo, 2004).

The interdisciplinary behavioural rehabilitation model for treating chronic paediatric pain

Some clinicians and investigators have advocated using an interdisciplinary rehabilitation approach to the treatment of pain-associated disability syndrome (PADS) in children and adolescents (Bursch et al., 1998, 2003; Hyman et al., 2002). PADS is characterized by severe disability that continues for 2 months or greater (Bursch et al., 2003). PADS describes a chronic pain condition with frequent and severe difficulties in functioning, regardless of the location or cause of the pain (Bursch et al., 1998; Zeltzer et al., 1997). In PADS the actual tissue damage sustained by the patient, the perceived severity of the condition, and the degree of disability exhibited are often widely discrepant. PADS occurs with many variations in the aetiology and source of the original pain. It may begin with illness, injury, viral infection, or developmental or psychological challenge. In many cases the original trigger may not be identified. There also is wide variation in the time course of the development of the disability. Bursch and colleagues hypothesized that PADS develops when a physical trauma, illness, or other life circumstance becomes overwhelming to a vulnerable child who has poor coping skills and cannot regulate his/her own distress. The physical symptoms may allow the child to avoid or escape the stressor, associated discomfort, and negative emotions. Consequently, the child may fail to develop positive coping strategies and a behaviour pattern in which avoidance of stressful or painful stimulation occurs along with increasing dependence on others, social withdrawal, avoidance of school and physical activity, and progression of functional disability.

In the interdisciplinary behavioural rehabilitation model, children and families are encouraged to accept pain as a symptom that may or may not go away. They are encouraged to move their focus away from total elimination of pain as their sole objective. When underlying pain mechanisms can be identified, they are treated medically to the extent possible. However, central emphasis is placed on reinforcing more independent child functioning in activities of daily living, academics, social and physical activities. Interdisciplinary rehabilitation therapies are provided to treat specific symptoms of anxiety, depression, avoidance behaviour, diminished muscle strength, limited range of motion, and academic deficits, and to teach active coping skills to the child and family. Finally, adaptive functioning instead of pain severity is used to measure progress.

An inpatient interdisciplinary rehabilitation setting may be ideal for implementing systematic behavioural interventions to shape functional behaviour and reinforce its generalization across settings and situations (Amari et al., 1998; Palermo and Scher, 2001). However, there are few published data on inpatient interdisciplinary rehabilitation programmes that employ behavioural and cognitive-behavioural interventions in a comprehensive and systematic manner to treat chronic pain associated disability. In one case example, Palermo and Scher (2001) described improvements in the physical and psychosocial functioning of an adolescent with a severe pain disorder following an inpatient rehabilitation admission. Eccleston et al. (2003) studied the effects of a 3-week interdisciplinary residential programme that emphasized cognitive-behavioural and physical therapy interventions on 57 adolescents with chronic pain and their caregivers. Their results showed that the intervention effectively decreased distress and improved overall functioning and school attendance. Hechler et al. (2009) studied the effectiveness of a 3-week multimodal inpatient pain treatment for 167 adolescents with various pain disorders. Patients were evaluated at baseline and 3 months post-treatment. Results suggest that 72% and 45% of the patients demonstrated clinically significant changes in pain-related disability and pain intensity respectively.

More recently Maynard et al. (2010) conducted a study to assess the outcome of an inpatient interdisciplinary behavioural rehabilitation protocol to treat children and adolescents with pain-associated disability and distress. The conceptualization and the intervention approach were based on the prior work of Zeltzer et al. (2006). Maynard et al. (2010) conducted a retrospective review of the clinical outcomes from a sample of children and adolescents admitted to an inpatient rehabilitation programme for treatment of

PADS. The investigators hypothesized that the group would exhibit significant improvement across measures of functioning after completing the inpatient intervention protocol as compared to their pre-admission functioning. As a group, the participating patients showed clinically and statistically significant improvements in daily functioning and physical mobility after receiving the interdisciplinary behavioural rehabilitation intervention. Clinical significance was determined by comparing patient's admission and discharge functioning and physical mobility scores. Upon admission patients typically had significant difficulties with self-care, cognition and mobility. At discharge, the patients functioned more autonomously. The patients also showed improvement in school participation, sleep, and medication use. The patients were responsive to differential positive reinforcement of coping behaviour and compliance with task demands of gradually increasing difficulty within the rehabilitation context.

For those with available follow-up information, physical functioning was maintained or continued to improve after discharge. The investigators speculated that the protocol was feasible across development because of individualized shaping procedures and cognitive-behavioural interventions that could be modified for different ages. The use of shaping allowed the children to experience their first successes in small steps, which may have helped to promote coping, motivation and perception of self-efficacy. The rehabilitation hospital setting provided an environment in which multiple staff members prompted and differentially reinforced functional gains and coping behaviour while not reinforcing pain or illness behaviour. This

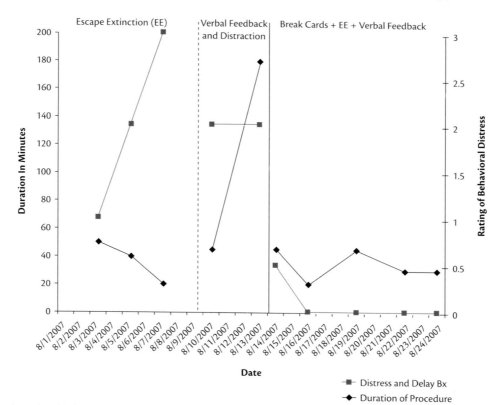

Figure 51.1 Observer ratings of Mark's distress and delay behaviour (squares) and the duration of the procedure in minutes (diamonds) across escape extinction, verbal feedback and distraction, and verbal feedback + distraction + escape extinction + break cards conditions.
Reproduced with permission of the author from Kim, F., Slifer, K., Amari, A., Herman, L., and DeMore, M., *The Utility of Operant Choice Using Patient-Controlled Break Cards during an Invasive Medical Procedure*, May, 2009 which was previously presented as a poster at the Annual Convention of the Association for Behavior Analysis International, Phoenix, AZ.

approach involving both fading of activity demands and shaping of increased effort and duration of physical functioning is consistent with the results of a randomized prospective clinical trial conducted with adults with low back pain, which combined graded activity goals and operant conditioning to significantly increase the patients' probability of returning to work and reducing their long-term use of sick leave (Lindstrom et al., 1992).

The emphasis on functional measures rather than subjective pain ratings was an important part of the behavioural rehabilitation approach in this study. Patients often showed little variability in their pain ratings during inpatient rehabilitation, continuing to give high ratings despite showing positive affect during participation in therapy and leisure activities. The Maynard et al. (2010) study was not a controlled experiment, and therefore could not claim a causal relationship or dismantle the relative contributions of the multiple therapeutic components included in the rehabilitation protocol. Therefore, the authors recommended that prospective randomized controlled clinical trials are needed involving multiple centres implementing the same protocol.

Case example

'Mark' was a 12-year-old African American male with obesity and spinal muscular dystrophy admitted to an inpatient rehabilitation unit following orthopaedic surgery. Postoperative complications included wound dehiscence (premature rupture of a wound along surgical suture) which required use of a wound vacuum-assisted closure (VAC) procedure to expedite healing. This case study was previously presented as a poster at the Annual Convention of the Association for Behavior Analysis (Kim et al., 2009). Mark was referred for behavioural psychology services secondary to his extreme anxiety and distress behaviour (e.g. screaming, crying, and pain verbalizations) related to this procedure early in admission.

Wound VAC procedures were completed by a physician and/or nurse every 2 to 3 days, with an additional staff member present to assist. Steps for the procedure included: removal of adhesive plastic sealant from wound site; removal of foam and drain tube; measurement of wound; lavage and removal of contamination and devitalized tissue; cutting foam dressing to approximate size of wound; insertion of dressing; application of adhesive plastic sealant; incision to sealant and insertion of suction tube, and activation of VAC system. Typical procedures last approximately 20 to 45 min.

Nursing staff completing the procedure recorded duration of procedure as well as Mark's behavioural responses on nursing flow sheets. Distress and/or delay behaviour (e.g. saying 'I'm not ready', asking questions unrelated to procedure, extending counting, e.g. 'two, two and a half …') were rated as follows: (0) no observed distress or attempts to delay procedure; (1) minimal distress behaviour (e.g. some pain verbalizations during more difficult steps); easily consolable; few attempts to delay; (2) moderate distress behaviour (e.g. crying, verbalizing pain) and some attempts to delay throughout the procedure; able to recover upon procedure completion; and (3) severe distress (screaming, inconsolable crying) and frequent attempts to delay procedure.

Prior to psychology consultation, when nursing staff implemented an escape extinction protocol (i.e. simply proceeded with the necessary task) and Mark's distress and delay behaviours did not result in a break, high levels of distress were observed (Figure 51.1; Phase 1). During initial treatment (Figure 51.1; Phase 2), the introduction of verbal feedback and distraction (conversation and access to a TV show) were provided by behavioural psychology and child life staff. This intervention decreased distress behaviours; however, delay behaviours, in the form of asking for frequent breaks and attempting to extend counting during each step increased. Therefore, the next phase of treatment involved use of a patient-controlled break card in combination with verbal feedback and escape extinction. Specifically, Mark was provided with a card before beginning the procedure, and was informed that he could exchange this card to request a 1 min break. Apart from natural breaks (e.g. between steps, while staff cut the foam), Mark was only provided breaks when he appropriately used his break card. He was prompted to use his break card (if still available) if he verbally requested a break or exhibited anxious behaviours (e.g. 'stop' or 'I'm scared').

Providing Mark with a choice of when to exercise limited control over aversive stimulation and extinguishing delay behaviours resulted in markedly decreased distress and enabled staff to complete the change in a timely manner (Phase 3, Figure 51.1).

References

Amari, A., Slifer, K. J., Sevier, R. C., Spezio, J., and Tucker, C. L. (1998). Using differential reinforcement to treat functional hypophonia in a paediatric rehabilitation patient. *Pediatr Rehabil*, 2(2), 89–94.

Banez, G. A., and Gallagher, H. M. (2006). Recurrent abdominal pain. *Behav Modif*, 30(1), 50–71.

Blanchard, E. B., and Scharff, L. (2002). Psychosocial aspects of assessment and treatment of irritable bowel syndrome in adults and recurrent abdominal pain in children. *J Consult Clin Psychol*, 70(3), 725–738.

Bursch, B., Joseph, M. H., and Zeltzer, L. K. (2003). Pain associated disability syndrome. In N. L. Schechter, C. B. Berde and M. Yaster (eds) *Pain in infants, children, and adolescents*, pp. 841–848. Philadelphia, PA: Lippincott, Williams, & Williams,

Bursch, B., Walco, G. A., and Zeltzer, L. (1998). Clinical assessment and management of chronic pain and pain associated disability syndrome. *Dev Behav Pediatr*, 19(1), 45–53.

Compas, B. E., Haaga, D. A., Keefe, F. J., Leitenberg, H., and Williams, D. A. (1998). Sampling of empirically supportive psychological treatments for health psychology: smoking, chronic pain, cancer, and bulimia nervosa. *J Consult Clin Psychol*, 66, 89–112.

Cooper, J. O., Heron, T. F., and Heward, W. L. (1987). *Applied behavior analysis*, pp. 2–34. Upper Saddle River, NJ: Prentice Hall, Inc.

Covelman, K., Scott, S., Buchanan, B., and Rossman, F. (1990). Pediatric pain control: a family systems model. In D. C. Tyler, and E. J. Krane (eds) *Advances in pain research and therapy* (Vol. 15), pp. 225–236. New York: Raven Press.

Eccleston, C., Malleson, P. N., Clinch, J., Connell, H., and Sourbut, C. (2003). Chronic pain in adolescents: evaluation of a programme of inter-disciplinary cognitive behaviour therapy. *Arch Dis Child*, 88, 881–885.

Finney, J. W. Lemaneka, K. L., Cataldoa, M. F., Katza, H. P., and Fuquaa, R. W. (1989). Pediatric psychology in primary care health care: brief targeted therapy for recurrent abdominal pain. *Behav Ther*, 20, 283–291.

Flor, H., Knost, B., and Birbaumer, N. (2002). The role of operant conditioning in chronic pain: an experimental investigation. *Pain*, 95, 111–118.

Fordyce, W. E. (1976). *Behavioral methods for chronic pain and illness*. St. Louis, MO: Mosby.

Fordyce, W. E., Fowler, R. S., and DeLateur, B. (1968). Case histories and shorter communications: an application of behavior modification technique to a problem of chronic pain. *Behav Res Ther*, 6, 105–107.

Fordyce, W. E., Roberts, A. H., and Sternbach, R. A. (1985). The behavioral management of chronic pain: a response to critics. *Pain*, 22, 113–125.

Fordyce, W. E., Shelton, J. L., and Dundore, D. E. (1982). The modification of avoidance learning pain behaviors. *J Behav Med*, 5, 405–414.

Garber, J., Zeman, J., and Walker, L. S. (1990). Recurrent abdominal pain in children: Psychiatric diagnoses and parental psychopathology. *J Am Acad Child Adolesc Psychiatry*, 29, 648–656.

Gidron, Y., McGrath, P. J., and Goodday, R. (1995). The physical and psychosocial predictors of adolescents' recovery from oral surgery. *J Behav Med*, 18, 385–399.

Hicks, C. L., von Baeyer, C. L., and McGrath, P. J. (2006). Online psychological treatment for pediatric recurrent pain: a randomized evaluation. *J Pediatr Psychol*, 31(7), 724–736.

Humphreys, P. A., and Gevirtz, R. (2000). Treatment of recurrent abdominal pain: components analysis of four treatment protocols. *J Pediatr Gastroenterol Nutr*, 31(1), 47–51.

Hyams, J. S., and Hyman, P. E. (1998). Recurrent abdominal pain and the biopsychosocial model of medical practice. *J Pediatr*, 133(4), 473–478.

Hyman, P. E., Bursch, B., Sood, M., Schwankovsky, L., Cocjin, J., and Zeltzer, L. K. (2002). Visceral pain-associated disability syndrome: a descriptive analysis. *J Pediatr Gastroenterol Nutr*, 35, 663–668.

Iversen, I. H. (2013). Single-case research methods: an overview. In G. J. Madden, (ed.) *APA handbook of behavior analysis (vol. 1): methods and principles*, pp. 3–32. Washington, DC: American Psychological Association.

Janicke, D. M., and Finney, J. W. (1999). Empirically supported treatments in pediatric psychology: recurrent abdominal pain. *J Pediatr Psychol*, 24(2), 115–127.

Kalsher, M. J., Cataldo, M. F., Deal, R. M., Traughber, B., and Jankel, W. R. (1985). Behavioral covariation in the treatment of chronic pain. *J Behav Ther Exper Psychiatry*, 16, 331–339.

Keefe, F. J., Dunsmore, J., and Burnett, R. (1992). Behavioral and cognitive-behavioral approaches to chronic pain: recent advances and future directions. *J Consult Clin Psychol*, 60, 528–536.

Kelly, M. L., Jarvie, G. J., Middlebrook, J. L., McNeer, M.F., and Drabman, R. S. (1984). Decreasing burned children's pain behavior: impacting the trauma of hydrotherapy. *J Appl Behav Anal*, 17, 147–158.

Kim, F., Slifer, K., Amari, A., Herman, L., and DeMore, M. (2009). The utility of operant choice using patient-controlled break cards during an invasive medical procedure. Poster presented at the Annual Convention of the Association for Behavior Analysis International, May, Phoenix, AZ.

Kopp, M., Richter, R., Rainer, J., Kopp-Wilfling, P., Rumpold, G., and Walter, M. H. (1995). Differences in family functioning between patients with chronic headache and patients with chronic low back pain. *Pain*, 63, 219–224.

Liakopoulou-Kairis, M., Alifieraki, T., Protagora, D., Korpa, T., Kondyli, K., Dimosthenous, E., *et al.* (2002). Recurrent abdominal pain and headache: psychopathology, life events and family functioning. *Eur Child Adolesc Psychiatry*, 11, 115–122.

Lindstrom, I., Ohlund, C., Eek, C., Wallin, L., Peterson, L. E., and Fordyce, W. E. (1992). The effect of graded activity on patients with subacute low back pain: a randomized prospective clinical study with an operant-conditioning behavioral approach. *Phys Ther*, 72, 279–293.

Linton, S. J. (1986a). A case study of the behavioural treatment of chronic stomach pain in a child. *Behav Change*, 3, 70–73.

Linton, S. J. (1986b). Behavioral remediation of chronic pain: a status report. *Pain*, 24, p.125.

Lipani, T. A., and Walker, L. S. (2006). Children's appraisal and coping with pain: relations to maternal ratings of worry and restriction in family activities. *J Pediatr Psychol*, 31(7), 667–673.

Logan, D. E., and Scharff, L. (2005). Relationships between family and parent characteristics and functional abilities in children with recurrent pain syndromes: an investigation of moderating effects on the pathway form pain to disability. *J Pediatr Psychol*, 30(8), 698–707.

Martin-Herz, S. P., Thurber, C. A., and Patterson, D. R. (2000). Psychological principles of burn wound pain in children. II: Treatment applications. *J Wound Care Rehabil*, 21, 458–472.

Maynard, C., Amari, A., Wieczorek, B., Christensen, J. R., and Slifer, K. J. (2010). Interdisciplinary behavioral rehabilitation of pediatric pain-associated disability: retrospective review of an inpatient treatment protocol. *J Pediatr Psychol*, 35(2), 128–137.

Meeus, M., Nijs, J., Van de Wauwer, N., Toeback, L., and Truijen, S. (2008). Diffuse noxious inhibitory control is delayed in chronic fatigue syndrome: an experimental study. *Pain*, 139, 439–448.

Miller, A. J., and Kratochwill, T. R. (1979). Reduction in frequent stomachache complaints by time out. *Behav Ther*, 10, 211–218.

Moraley, S., Eccleston, C., and Williams, A. (1999). Systematic review and meta-analysis of randomized control trials of cognitive behavioral therapy and behavior therapy for chronic pain in adults, excluding headache. *Pain*, 80, 1113.

Naidoo, P. and Pillay, Y. G. (1994). Correlations among general stress, family environment, psychological distress, and pain experience. *Percept Motor Skills*, 78, 1291–1296.

Normand, E., Potvin, S., Gaumond, I., Cloutier, G., Corbin, J. F., and Marchand, S. (2011). Pain inhibition is deficient in chronic widespread pain but normal in major depressive disorder. *J Clin Psychiatry*, 72, 219–224.

O'Callaghan, P. M., Allen, K. D., Powell, S., and Salama, F. (2006). The efficacy of noncontingent escape for decreasing children's disruptive behavior during restorative dental treatment. *J Appl Behav Anal*, 39, 161–171.

Oster, J. (1972). Recurrent abdominal pain, headache, and limb pains in children and adolescents. *Pediatrics*, 50, 429–436.

Palermo, T. M. (2000). Impact of recurrent and chronic pain on child and family daily functioning: a critical review of the literature. *J Dev Behav Pediatr*, 21, 58–69.

Palermo, T. M., and Scher, M. S. (2001). Treatment of functional impairment in somatoform pain disorder: a case example. *J Pediatr Psychol*, 26, 429–434.

Payne, B. and Norfleet, M. A. (1986). Chronic pain and the family: a review. *Pain*, 26(1), 1–22.

Peterson, C. C., and Palermo, T. M. (2004). Parental reinforcement of recurrent pain: the moderating impact of child depression and anxiety on functional disability. *J Pediatr Psychol*, 29(5), 331–341.

Philips, H. C. (1987). Avoidance behavior and its role in sustaining chronic pain. *Behav Res Ther*, 25, 273–279.

Robins, P. M., Smith, S. M., Glutting, J. J., and Bishop, C. T. (2005). A randomized controlled trial by a cognitive-behavioral family intervention for pediatric recurrent abdominal pain. *J Pediatr Psychol*, 30(5), 397–408.

Robinson, J. O., Alverez, J. H., and Dodge, J. A. (1990). Life events and family history in children with recurrent abdominal pain. *J Psychosomat Res*, 34, 171–181.

Sanders, M. R., Rebgetz, M., Morrison, M., Bor, W., Gordon, A., Dadds, M., *et al.* (1989). Cognitive-behavioral treatment of recurrent nonspecific abdominal pain in children: an analysis of generalization, maintenance, and side effects. *J Consult Clin Psychol*, 57, 294–300.

Sanders, M. R., Shepherd, R. W., Cleghorn, G., and Woolford, H. (1994). The treatment of recurrent abdominal pain in children: a controlled comparison of cognitive-behavioral family intervention and standard pediatric care. *J Consult Clin Psychol*, 62(2), 306–314.

Sanders, S. H. (1985). The role of learning and chronic pain states. In S. F. Brena, and S. L. Chapman (eds) *Clinics in anesthesiology: chronic pain: management principles*, pp. 41–55. Philadelphia, PA: Saunders.

Sanders, S. H. (2003). Operant therapy with pain patients: evidence for its effectiveness. *Semin Pain Med*, 1, 90–98.

Sank, L. I., and Biglan, A. (1974). Operant treatment of a case of recurrent abdominal pain in a 10-year-old boy. *Behav Ther*, 5, 677–681.

Schanberg, L. E., Anthony, K. K., Gil, K. M., Lefebvre, J. C., Kredich, D. W., and Macharoni, L. M. (2001). Family pain history predicts child health status in children with chronic rheumatic disease. *Pediatrics*, 108, p.E47.

Scharff, L., Langan, N., Rotter, N., Scott-Sutherland, J., Schenck, C., Tayor, N., *et al.* (2005). Psychological, behavioral, and family characteristics of pediatric patient with chronic pain. *Clin J Pain*, 21(5), 432–438.

Slifer, K. J., Babbitt, R. L., and Cataldo, M. D. (1995). Simulation and counterconditioning as an adjunct to pharmacotherapy for invasive pediatric procedures. *J Dev Behav Pediatr*, 16(3), 133–141.

Slifer, K. J., Hankinson, J. C., Zettler, M. A., Frutchey, R. A., Hendricks, M. C., Ward, C. M., *et al.* (2011). Distraction, exposure therapy, counterconditioning, and topical anesthetic for acute pain management during needle sticks in children with intellectual and developmental disabilities. *Clin Pediatr*, 50(8), 688–97.

Slifer, K. J., Tucker, C. L., and Dahlquist, L. M. (2002). Helping children and caregivers cope with repeated invasive procedures: how are we doing? *J Clin Psychol Med Sett* 9(2), 131–152.

Stone, R. T., and Barbero, G. J. (1970). Recurrent abdominal pain in childhood. *Pediatrics*, 45, 732–738.

Thurber, C. A., Martin-Herz, S. P., and Patterson, D. R. (2000). Psychological principles of burn wound pain in children. I: Theoretical framework. *J Wound Care Rehabil*, 21, 376–387.

Van Slyke, D. A. and Walker, L. S. (2006). Mothers' responses to adolescent's pain. *Clin J Pain*, 22(4), 387–391.

Van Tulder, M. W., Ostelo, R., Vlaeyen, J. W., Linton, S. J., Morley, S. J., and Assendelft, W. J. (2000). Behavioral treatment for chronic low back pain. *Spine*, 25, 2688–2699.

Varni, J. W., Bessman, C. A., Russo, D. C., and Cataldo, M. F. (1980). Behavioral management of chronic pain in children: a case study. *Arch Phys Med Rehabil*, 61, 375–379.

Vervoort, T., Caes, L., Trost, Z., Sullivan, M., Vangronsveld, K., and Goubert, L. (2011). Social modulation of facial pain display in high-catastrophizing children: an observational study in schoolchildren and their parents. *Pain*, 152, 1591–1599.

Walker, L. S., Claar, R. L., and Garber, J. (2002). Social consequences of children's pain: when do they encourage symptom maintenance? *J Pediatr Psychol*, 27, 689–698.

Walker, L. S., Garber, J., and Greene, J. W. (1993). Psychosocial correlates of recurrent childhood pain: a comparison of pediatric patients with recurrent abdominal pain, organic illness, and psychiatric disorders. *J Abnormal Psychol*, 102, 248–258.

Walker, L.S., Garber, J., and Greene, J.W. (1994). Somatic complaints in pediatric patients: a prospective study of the role of negative life events, child social and academic competence, and parental somatic symptoms. *J Consult Clin Psychol*, 62, 1213–1221.

Walker, L. S., Garber, J., and Greene, J.W. (1991). Somatization symptoms in pediatric abdominal pain patients: relation to chronicity of abdominal pain and parent somatization. *J Abnormal Child Psychol*, 19, 379–394.

Walker, L.S., Garber, J., and Van Slyke, D.A. (1995). Do parents excuse the misbehavior of children with physical or emotional symptoms? An investigation of the pediatric sick role. *J Pediatr Psychol*, 20, 329–345.

Walker, L. S., Williams, S. E., Smith, C. A., Garber, J., Van Slyke, D. A., and Lipani, T. A. (2006). Parent attention versus distraction: Impact on symptom complaints by children with and without chronic functional abdominal pain. *Pain*, 122(12), 43–52.

Walker, L. S., and Zeman, J. L. (1992). Parental response to child illness behavior. *J Pediatr Psychol*, 17, 49–71.

Whitehead, W.E., Crowell, M. D., Heller, B. R., Robinson, J. C., Schuster, M. M., and Horn, S. (1994). Modeling and reinforcement of the sick role during childhood predicts adult illness behavior. *Psychosomat Med*, 56, 541–550.

Zeltzer, L., Bursch, B., and Walco, G. (1997). Pain responsiveness and chronic pain: a psychobiological perspective. *J Dev Behav Pediatr*, 18(6), 413–422.

Zeltzer, L. K., Tsao, J. C., Bursch, B., and Myers, C. D. (2006). Introduction to the special issue on pain: From pain to pain-associated disability syndrome. *J Pediatr Psychol*, 31, 661–666.

CHAPTER 52

Child life interventions in paediatric pain

Chantal K. LeBlanc and Christine T. Chambers

Introduction

Child life specialists, as members of the health care team, are frequently involved in the assessment and management of pain in hospitalized children and children in emergency settings. Child life refers to a non-medical therapeutic service designed to address the developmental, educational, and psychosocial needs of paediatric patients. Child life specialists are professionals who 'promote effective coping through play, preparation, education, and self-expression activities. They provide emotional support for families, and encourage optimum development of children facing a broad range of challenging experiences, particularly those related to healthcare and hospitalization' (Child Life Council, 2012a), including painful procedures and coping with other types of pain (e.g. postoperative pain). This chapter provides an overview of the role of a child life specialist, including a historical perspective on the evolution of the field and current child life practices. The chapter then provides a summary of the specific contributions of child life specialists to pain assessment and management, including innovative uses of technology often facilitated by child life specialists.

Historical context

The child life profession originates from a time when children were left at the hospital to be cared for by doctors, nurses, nuns, psychiatric personnel, and volunteers. Many hospitals severely restricted visits, even by parents, limiting these familiar, and often comforting, interactions to only a few hours per week (Thompson, 1989). There was often no contact with siblings. Recovery included long stays, immobilization, lack of stimulation, sterile environments, and no play space or educational support. Little information was shared with children about the reason for their hospital admission, diagnosis, or treatments, let alone preparation for procedures, surgeries or support for painful experiences (Jun-Tai, 2008; McCue and Hicks, 2007; Thompson, 1989). The lack of family visits and information shared was thought to protect patients and families. It was believed children would not be able to understand complex information and would become more upset if family members stayed for long periods of time and then left.

The negative impact of this vacuous psychosocial environment on children's health became evident including the link between lack of stimulation and infant deaths (Spitz, 1945) and long-term psychological effects of hospitalization (Prugh et al., 1953). Hospitalized children were frequently withdrawn, quiet, and disengaged, coining the term 'hospitalism' (Spitz, 1945). Society at large began to develop a more sophisticated appreciation of the importance of cognitive, social, and emotional development during childhood. The effects of minimal stimulation, separation from family, and the potential trauma of hospitalization led to an appreciation that the experience of hospitalization put children at risk for significant emotional distress thereby impacting their overall health (Bowlby, 1952; Prugh et al., 1953; Spitz, 1945). This work prompted changes in health care (Thompson, 1989; Wojtasik and White, 2009), including the utilization of volunteers and staff, mostly women, to spend time with the children to engage them in play and learning. These individuals became known as 'play ladies', 'play teachers', or 'play leaders' (Rubin, 1992; Thompson, 1989). The Platt report, released in the UK in 1959 provided specific recommendations regarding the need for parents to be with their children while in hospital, the importance of specialized education and training of staff working with children, and the need for play and education during paediatric hospitalization (Anonymous, 1959). Changes in hospital visitation policies and programming and the realization of the need to meet the developmental and emotional needs of children during the provision of medical care (Barnes, 1995; Thompson, 1989; Wojtasik and White, 2009) provided the foundation for the child life profession.

Play programmes were noted as early as 1922 in the US and in 1936 in Canada, with nine identified programmes in North America by 1949. The 1960s and 1970s saw the coming together of professionals to organize associations such as the Association for the Wellbeing of Hospitalized Children and their Families in the US (later to be renamed the Association for the Care of Children's Health) and the Hospital Liaison Committee in the UK to lobby for stimulation and play for hospitalized children and specialized training to do this work. There are now over 480 programmes listed in the 2012 Child Life Council's Directory (Child Life Council, 2012b), in 18 countries around the world.

Child life today

The child life profession is a new profession, stemming from the need for personnel with specific training to acknowledge and address the developmental and psychosocial needs of hospitalized children. Child life has its roots in child development, psychology, recreation/leisure, education, sociology, and social science. Although there may be some overlap in professional roles with other psychosocial care providers, Thompson (1989) stresses the primary duty of the child life specialist is focusing on the developmental and psychosocial needs of the hospitalized child. In Canada, the US, and Kuwait, the title of 'child life specialist' is well recognized. In other parts of the world, this role is known as a 'hospital play specialist', 'hospital play staff', 'play leader', or 'child life therapist', however the philosophy, goals, and interventions are similar.

Child life specialists have specialized training, which in North America typically involves a minimum of a bachelor's degree in child life, child development, psychology or closely related field that incorporates a variety of coursework, including but not limited to child growth and development, function and development of play behaviours, family systems, behaviour management, child coping, psychology, and courses in child life methods. Additionally, successful completion of a child life internship, supervised by a certified child life specialist provides the minimum requirements to write the certification exam, offered through the Child Life Certifying Committee. Several countries (including Canada, the US, the UK, and New Zealand) offer credentialing processes for child life specialists to ensure specific and continued competencies in working with children in this field (Child Life Council, 2002; Hospital Play Specialist Association of Aotearoal/New Zealand, 2012).

Family centred care is a philosophy and way of interacting with families that is ingrained and intuitive to the child life specialist. As a result, child life specialists employ a collaborative approach to care, believing parents know their children best, should be true partners in care, and deserve to have information provided in a way they can understand. Cultural diversity is respected, focusing on the strengths of the family and its individuals, recognizing and respecting different coping styles, and being aware families require the appropriate supports to meet their needs (Shelton and Stepanek, 1994). Child life specialists work closely with all the members of the child's health care team to provide the best overall experience and outcomes for the child.

The role of child life specialists first originated in hospital-based paediatric inpatient units. However, many children outside of inpatient units experience repeated frightening or invasive procedures. As a result, child life specialists are involved in paediatric care in a number of settings, including: ambulatory clinics, diagnostic imaging (McGee, 2003), emergency department (Cavender et al., 2004; Gursky et al., 2010; Stevenson et al., 2005), sedation programme, day surgery (Brewer et al., 2006), mental health programmes (Breiner, 2003), neonatal intensive care, paediatric intensive care unit, critical care unit, laboratory medicine, children of adult inpatients (Thompson and Snow, 2009). A surgical event in day surgery or an urgent medical event in the emergency department can be painful and frightening for children and have profound effects on future encounters with health care providers. There are inequities in child life service delivery for different populations within and among hospitals and this continues to be a challenge.

Child life specialists provide valuable information about the child's perception and experience of medical events to the medical team. They are in a unique position because their role is typically viewed by the child and family as being non-threatening, non-invasive, and often 'fun'. They are able to quickly build rapport through

play and/or therapeutic dialogue, learn from the child/youth how they perceive and understand what is happening, clarify misconceptions and provide opportunities for questions, fears, or worries to be addressed. Strategies are then developed to assist with coping and adjustment to the situation, while ensuring a sense of mastery and control throughout the interventions. The child life specialist explores previous coping strategies and focuses on each family member's strengths, assessing the needs within the family (e.g. informational needs, emotional, parenting and/or sibling support needs) and partnering with them and other members of the team. When children and family members feel respected, engaged, and understood, they share their stories, their fears, worries, and needs, and become partners to make things better.

Child life assessment and interventions

Child life specialists first assess the key variables which are known to impact coping and adjustment to health care experiences in order to develop a child life plan of care and goals for the interprofessional plan of care. There are many variables that can impact coping responses to hospitalization and health care interventions. This information is gathered from the health record, the child and family, those involved in the care, as well as through observation. The assessment is an ongoing process; it is dynamic, and changes as the information and needs change. This in turn influences the child life interventions to be provided. The assessment variables associated with a child and family's ability to cope with hospitalization include (Blount and Loiselle, 2009; Gaynard et al., 1990; Koller, 2008a):

1. Child variables: age/developmental level, temperament and coping responses.

2. Family variables: parental anxiety, parental involvement, marital status and education.

3. Medical experiences: number of invasive procedures and memory of these experiences.

There are a range of interventions child life specialists will provide. At the core of the interventions is the use of developmentally appropriate toys/activities and conversation to assist the child and family. Some of the interventions described are provided predominantly by child life specialists such as medical play while others are also commonly utilized by a variety of health professionals, for example cognitive and behavioural distraction. A child life plan of care is developed including one or more of the following interventions (Skinner and LeBlanc, 2002):

1. *Play*: child life specialists use play/activities as their primary tool in assessing and intervening with children and youth regardless of the reason for involvement. There are many functions of play for the child life specialist including assessment, teaching, and expression of feelings, modelling, preparation, distraction and sheer enjoyment. Play for children is universal, how they learn about the world, make sense of the world, develop skills to socialize, make decisions, and learn how their actions have an impact on themselves and others. Play provides freedom and a sense of mastery and control. Play helps children gain the developmental and psychosocial skills they need for life. It can also be a way to work through stressful experiences and is known to reduce a child's anxiety (Thompson, 1989). The child's ability to engage in their environment, their understanding of concepts

and experiences, their social skills, their communication and language skills, their perception of the world, their hope for a better day, and their ability to control aspects of their world (Jessee and Gaynard, 2009) is revealed through their play.

2. *Play programming:* child life specialists ensure the child has developmentally appropriate play materials and supplies to encourage active participation in play, in the room, in play areas or a teen lounge, as appropriate (could be another child life specialist or an assistant or volunteer).

3. *Health care/medical play:* health care play encompasses the use of medical supplies and equipment, toy medical kits, body outline dolls or demonstration dolls in directive or non-directive play and even the use of music, photography, or technology applications to express oneself in regard to the health care experience. This play may include expressive or creative arts using medical supplies; use of expressive arts to allow children to share their experience, express their feelings through art, puppetry, dramatic play, writing/journaling, photography, video, etc. Medical play typically specifies the use of medical supplies and equipment to re-enact medical experiences on a 'patient' such as a body outline doll, puppet, or favourite toy. This form of play allows for the expression of feelings, clarification of misconceptions; exploration of coping strategies and working through feelings associated with painful or frightening experiences (Ostrenga, 1980). Very young children, even under the age of 2 years, can participate in medical play. The type of medical supplies used and the decision to use real needles in the play is dependent upon the age/developmental level of the child, the child's emotional response to needles and the ability to maintain a safe play area.

4. *Developmental support:* child life specialists implement individualized play programme to support the maintenance or progression of developmental and psychosocial skills.

5. *Teaching:* child life specialists provide simple clear and developmentally appropriate explanations about the reason for admission, the machinery, the diagnosis, the treatment to be undertaken, or a forthcoming surgery.

6. *Preparation:* child life specialists provide the child and family with developmentally appropriate information through play and/or discussion; based on anticipated sensory experiences; exploration of stress points, exploration of coping strategies to be used; opportunity for rehearsal and development of a coping plan with the team as needed. By its very nature, this should occur prior to interventions and surgery, be based on the developmental and coping needs, and responses of the child/family.

7. *Procedural support:* child life specialists support the child and family during a stressful encounter/examination, medical intervention or procedure. This might include behavioural or cognitive distraction, breathing exercises, coaching parents, advocating for positions of comfort, relaxation techniques, positive reinforcement, providing information, visualization, or guided imagery.

8. *Therapeutic dialogue:* child life specialists encourage the expression of feelings, clarification of misconceptions; determine coping strategies and work through feelings associated with painful or frightening experiences.

9. *Family support:* child life specialists provide information to navigate the system of care, general emotional support; translate medical jargon, liaise with the health care team, support brothers and sisters to cope effectively and help parents to recognize their child's coping style and support parenting roles.

These various interventions are adapted to fit the context of the work as the role of the child life specialist now extends beyond the hospital walls. Expertise and skills are utilized in rehabilitation centres (Davitt and Munn, 2008), dental offices (Glasrud and Feigal, 1984), community programmes (Chernoff et al., 2002), hospice programmes, funeral homes, specialized camps, the court system as well as consultation and support services for children of adult patients (American Academy of Pediatrics Child Life Council and Committee on Hospital Care, 2006; Hicks, 2008).

The role of child life specialists in paediatric pain

During the early years of the child life profession, it was recognized that children's pain responses were greatly influenced by distress and anxiety while developmentally appropriate information could influence coping responses and recovery (Plank, 1962). As is summarized throughout this volume, research regarding children's experience of pain and the contributions of various pharmacological and non-pharmacological interventions to improve pain has advanced our knowledge significantly since the 1960s. However, there is considerable evidence supporting the fact hospitalized children experience significant pain and still do not receive optimal pain management (Stevens et al., 2011).

The following two case examples illustrate some of the varied interventions child life specialists provide in the management of children's pain, followed by a description of some of the most commonly employed child life interventions when pain is an issue.

Case example: Jacob

Jacob is a 13-year-old admitted on the weekend with dehydration, 5 days post day surgery for tonsillectomy, articulating he was in a lot of pain and could not eat. Jacob was described by staff as a 'young' adolescent who was dramatic in his descriptions of his pain, was not eating or drinking well, and was likely going to need to stay for an additional night. Nurses reported that his mother was repeatedly voicing her concerns about her son's level of pain and was frustrated with the lack of pain control and intervention from staff.

Upon arrival, the child life specialist noted Jacob's affect was blunted; he reluctantly permitted her to enter the room, made fleeting eye contact, and initially answered questions quickly and hesitantly. His mother's posture was rigid and affect was neither welcoming nor engaging. When asked if he understood the reason for his admission, he stated his throat was bleeding, he couldn't drink, and the pain was unbearable. He repeatedly stated that the 'rotting flesh' in his throat gave his mouth an awful taste and he did not want to eat/drink because he did not want it to bleed again or to hurt more. His mother placed herself beside him on the bed, stroking his back, as he was curling into a fetal position.

Assessment

The child life specialist gathered further information from Jacob in a non-threatening confidant manner while indicating there were things that can be done to help with his pain. She explored his understanding of the surgery; the healing process post tonsillectomy; his typical coping style and previous successful strategies during stressful situations; his informational needs; his pain experience and what aspects of his experience were distressing; his personal interests and hobbies as well as expectation for improvement.

Child life interventions

The child life specialist clarified misconceptions and explained the medical equipment in the room, IV and medication being infused, and the importance of fluid intake to help the tissue heal. The use of thought stopping and cognitive reframing strategies (positive self-talk) were modelled and practised by Jacob ('my throat tissue is healing and will keep getting better') while his mother's negative statements were also reframed and more positive comments were reinforced.

Jacob stated he was an actor and loved to perform in plays. He often utilized deep breathing strategies to support voice projection and also as a calming strategy before he performed. His knowledge about deep breathing to assist with his pain and anxiety was encouraged. Rehearsal of breathing in slowly through the nose and out through the mouth several times to permitted his body to develop a rhythm and allow the sensation of relaxation to begin. His mother was eager and willing to be his coach and prompt him to stop his negative thinking and to use the deep breathing method. By the end of the session both mother and child were more friendly, physically more relaxed, exuded confidence that things would improve, and decided to physically leave the room to explore the unit and the teen lounge which the child life specialist had encouraged.

Case example: Carrie

Carrie is a 5-year-old girl referred to child life in anticipation of her upcoming bilateral ureter re-implantation surgery. The nurse recognized that Carrie would benefit from a child life preparation session and tour of the environment given that this was her first surgical experience.

Assessment

The child life specialist contacted the family 2 weeks in advance to plan a preparation session prior to the surgery and to screen for potential stressors that might impact on child/family coping. She was a typically developing child, with a generally easy-going temperament and who generally likes to know what will happen with enough detail to help her predict the situation. Mother reported Carrie's only experience with medical interventions, other than vaccines, was a cystogram 3 months previously for which she was not provided advance preparation. Parents reported this procedure was anxiety provoking for her and her parents; Carrie cried with pain during the catheter insertion, was able to settle during the procedure but was distressed when it was time to release the contrast material from her bladder. When she learned of her upcoming surgery, she was upset and did not want to go back to the hospital for the operation. Mother reported Carrie typically copes well when provided with information and a plan of action.

Mother had been reading stories about going to the hospital and answering Carrie's questions, as they arose. Parents were planning to be in attendance throughout the admission and reported no other significant stressors.

Interventions

Carrie and her mother met with the child life specialist and the pre-op nurse 1 week in advance of the surgery to learn what she would see, hear, smell, and experience in developmentally friendly language. The child life specialist offered Carrie a body outline doll for her to colour, as she wished, and offered to explain the medical equipment she would see. Carrie was interested in learning more. The child life specialist used Carrie's new hospital doll to demonstrate anaesthetic induction, explain the surgery in simple terms and 'perform' surgery, made a small opening, inserted external catheters to demonstrate what she would see upon waking, along with an IV and how the medicine goes through the IV to help her body get water and medicine to help with the 'ouch'. Carrie's body language and facial expressions were monitored closely to ensure the information was appropriate and to clarify any concerns, questions or misconceptions. Photographs of the surgical area, the hallways leading to the operating room (OR), the OR space and staff dressed in OR greens were shown after she indicated interest in seeing them. The family toured the surgical area and the inpatient unit, including the play areas and learned of the fun activities she would be able to do after the surgery.

After surgery, the child life specialist followed Carrie's progress. The first day post surgery, Carrie was playing contentedly in the bed, enjoying a craft left for her by the child life specialist. When asked, Carrie had no questions and stated the hardest part was 'it hurts when I move'. Strategies to cope with pain, such as the use of a pillow over the belly when moving, a warm blanket, slow breathing, counting, or using hand-held squeeze toys were discussed and she chose strategies she wanted to try. Daily visits occurred to assess her overall coping with the experience, monitoring for pain management issues, and promoting positive and fun activities in the playroom which motivated her to get up and walk. The child life specialist also provided procedural support for the removal of her catheters, once again preparing Carrie for what she would see, hear and feel as well as choosing distractions that would redirect her attention from the pain, this time by using applications on the iPad. Carrie's response post procedure was that 'it wasn't so bad'. Parents reported she slept well, and adjusted far better than anticipated; they felt confident and trusting of all members of the team given the coordinated approach to their daughter's care and pain management.

These two cases demonstrate the diverse nature of the interventions a child life specialist will provide. Building a strong rapport, conveying confidence and a belief that something can and will be done to decrease the pain are critical (Kuttner, 2010). Some of the most common interventions child life specialists provide for pain are summarized as follows.

Preparing children for procedures

Children report pain and discomfort most frequently as one of the worst aspects of hospitalization (Lindeke et al., 2006). Providing clear and accurate information to children results in fewer negative behaviours, reduces fear and anxiety, and leads to faster recovery postoperatively (Jaaniste et al., 2007; Koller, 2007). The key elements of effective preparation include: providing developmentally appropriate information, the opportunity to express emotions (fear, anxiety, and concerns), and the need for a trusting relationship (Koller, 2007). Early studies of preparatory programmes for parents (mothers) of children undergoing surgery using these same general principles showed significant decreases in parental anxiety and child coping as well (Mahaffy, 1965; Visintainer and Wolfer, 1975). The information should be child friendly, developmentally appropriate while using soft language versus words that provoke anxiety, for example, using the 'the doctor will make a small opening' versus a 'cut or incision'. Do not assume or insinuate something will hurt, but rather be honest about managing pain or discomfort should it occur. Balance the need to be honest while avoiding assumptions about how it will be experienced. Be aware of language and its double meaning, for example, for many children being 'put to sleep' reminds them of a pet that has been euthanized and may cause fear they may not awaken from the surgery, instead state 'the doctor will give you sleeping medicine'. Be prepared to address questions and misconceptions. Include not only specific and accurate information about the sequence of events (Jaaniste et al., 2007; Tak and van Bon, 2006), but also the rationale for the procedure (Campbell et al., 1995; Koller, 2007; Patterson and Ware, 1988) and the sensory information they will see, hear, taste, or smell (Koller, 2007; Suls and Wan, 1989). The preparation literature also consistently promotes the preparation for and modelling of coping strategies to cope with painful experiences (Jaaniste et al., 2007; LaMontagne et al., 2003a, 2003b; Patterson and Ware, 1988; Spafford et al., 2002).

In Carrie's case example, notice the key preparatory elements are present. Carrie was provided specific information through play and visual aids, in language she could understand. She was offered opportunities for questions; affective responses were monitored and the amount of information provided was guided by her throughout the session. Given her developmental level, information regarding anticipated pain was minimal; however, this was addressed postoperatively, with concrete strategies to rehearse and implement postoperatively as well as during procedures.

Distraction

The use of distraction during painful procedures is an effective strategy in reducing anxiety, distress, and paediatric pain (Uman et al., 2006). Distraction is the shifting of attention away from the painful or anxiety provoking stimuli to something more pleasant, interactive, or interesting. Distraction can be used with children as young as 10 months of age, can be cognitive in nature, and/or behaviourally focused (Kuttner, 2010). Some examples include non-procedural conversation, counting, bubble blowing, playing 'I Spy With my Little Eye', using pop-up books, the use of stress balls or hand held manipulative, and applications on an iPad. Providing a child with choices about the kind of distraction toys or activities provides a sense of control. Often children will use multiple distraction activities during a procedure or stressful experience. The distraction item(s) or activity(ies) must be highly engaging, be easy to use, and match the child's interest, developmental level, and ability (see Table 52.1 for examples). Younger children tend to need more active distracters and coach involvement whereas older children will often choose more passive distracters such as

music or videogame systems (Cavender et al., 2004; Sinha et al., 2006). Distraction is often used in conjunction with preparation and information sharing. Distraction is more effective with mild to moderate pain and can be particularly effective for children with chronic conditions (Kuttner, 2010).

Parent/staff coaching in the use of distraction

A distraction coach (parent or health professional) is an important role during any painful procedure. Child life specialists are trained in this type of intervention, are recommended in the emergency department (ED) literature on pain management (Madhok et al., 2011; Zempsky and Cravero 2004) and can be helpful in training others in these strategies (Cregin et al., 2008; Zempsky and Cravero 2004). A child's attention may direct itself to the painful procedure at intensely painful moments or with new sensory experiences. With support and education, parents or other health professionals can become effective distraction coaches (Kleiber et al., 2007). Engaging parents of children with long-term or chronic illness in this skill development is important in order to minimize dependency on health professionals, instil confidence and decrease parental anxiety caused by feelings of helplessness and guilt. Parents must be provided with information and positive feedback about their skills (Cavender et al., 2004; Kleiber et al., 2007).

In Jacob's case example, Jacob's mother did not initially engage with the child life specialist, but once she recognized Jacob was receiving concrete and practical information and strategies she recognized were useful for both of them, she was able to engage and accept a role of coach.

Breathing

Teaching children and parents slow, rhythmic breathing from the diaphragm rather than the chest is a simple and effective strategy. Children can be engaged in pretending to blow out candles, or blowing like the wind to move clouds in the sky, using party blowers, blowing bubbles, pretending to inflate or deflate a tyre or a balloon through inhaling/exhaling. Breathing in through the nose and out through the mouth, imagining the breath going down to the belly also give the child a visual image. One can also ask the child to imagine all their worries are collected in their belly and to blow them away, until they get smaller and smaller.

Jacob's case example demonstrates how using multiple strategies, thought stopping, positive self-statements, cognitive reframing with the addition of deep breathing can be very effective. Many children require a 'tool box' of skills and strategies.

Positive reinforcement

Positive reinforcement can come in the form of praise or in the form of a tangible reward (sticker/toy). Providing clear and specific positive statements is necessary. Making a statement 'Good job' will not likely encourage the reoccurrence of the specific behaviour desired, whereas 'You did a great job sitting still like a statue ... that really helped a lot' provides a clear understanding of the behaviour which was helpful.

The use of tangible rewards must be clearly defined by staff and family. For example, does the child receive a sticker for a specific, previously determined behaviour and does not receive it if the behaviour does not occur, or does the child receive the sticker because the procedure is complete or alternatively as a distracter

Table 52.1 Common distraction strategies used by child life specialists:—developmentally based distraction strategies

Age	Developmental issues	Behavioural/distraction techniques
Infant Birth to 2 years	1. Caregiver attachment 2. Basic needs need to be met in a consistent manner 3. Create calm environment, low lighting, low voice tone 4. Encourage touch and parental participation to decrease separation and detachment	Create a calm environment Magic Wand Toy Light up toys Singing Music Favourite object Use positions of comfort for procedures
Toddler 2–3 years	1. Motor skills and language are developing, understand more than can be expressed verbally 2. Increasing independence 3. Need for routines, consistent caregivers, parental involvement and security objects 4. Give positive reinforcement for specific behaviours 4. Need for mastery and control through play	Create a calm environment Magic Wand Toy Light up toys Pop-up picture books Video/DVD Bubbles Blowing (balloons/imaginary candles) Music, singing, counting Use positions of comfort Favourite object
Preschool 4–5 years	1. Communication skills are more developed. Important to provide information in a simple, concrete manner and check for misconceptions 2. Magical thinking and fear of bodily injury are common 3. Encourage parental participation, verbalization, and social interaction 4. Give positive reinforcement for specific behaviours 5. Clear limits and expectations are important to provide consistent structure	Create a calm environment Magic Wand toy Light up toys Pop-up picture books/books I Spy games/distraction walls Humour/jokes/joke books Video/DVD Bubbles Blowing (balloons/imaginary candles) Music, singing, counting Use positions of comfort Stress/squeeze balls Favourite object Guided imagery Wet noodle strategy 'Magic Glove' technique
School age 6–11 years	1. Need to understand why things are happening. Important to provide explanations and preparation for upcoming interventions, address misconceptions 2. There is often a fear of body mutilation 3. Encourage parental participation, verbalization, and social interaction 4. Give positive reinforcement for specific behaviours 5. Self-image and peer interactions are important at this stage 6. Clear limits and expectations are important to provide consistent structure 7. More aware and involved in health	Create a calm environment Magic Wand toy 'Search and find' books Distraction walls Humour/jokes/joke books Video/DVD Bubbles Blowing (balloons/imaginary candles) Deep breathing Music Use positions of comfort Stress/squeeze balls Favourite object Guided imagery Wet noodle strategy 'Magic Glove' technique 'Pain Switch' technique

Table 52.1 (*Continued*)

Age	Developmental issues	Behavioural/distraction techniques
Adolescence 12–18 years	1. Respect individual as separate from parents/caregivers 2. Body image, privacy, and peers are critically important 3. Often more active in own health care issues and active in decision-making re: treatment 4. Chronic health issues: need for independence conflicts with dependence eon parents/family for support	Humour/jokes/joke books Video/DVD Deep breathing Music Use positions of comfort Stress/squeeze balls Guided imagery 'Magic Glove' technique 'Pain Switch' technique

Developmentally Appropriate Behavioral Distraction Techniques. Adapted and used with permission from Boston Children's Hospital Interdisciplinary Pain Committee, Copyright © Boston Children's Hospital 2013.

near the end of procedure? It is important to be clear since one does not wish to reward unwanted behaviour.

Positioning for comfort

Children, especially preschool children, feel more vulnerable and fearful when lying in a supine position and this can be an immediate trigger that evokes a combative and/or uncooperative response (Cavender et al., 2004). Different positions can be utilized which allow the child to remain seated on the chair, stretcher, parent's lap or between the parent's legs (Stephens et al., 1999) while providing access for procedures and a comforting hold from parents. With the use of positions of comfort, children were observed by health professionals and parents alike to be less fearful (Cavender et al., 2004) and parents reported greater satisfaction (Sparks et al., 2007).

Modelling and rehearsal

Modelling is the demonstration of positive coping behaviours during a mock procedure by someone else. Child life specialists will often model breathing strategies or a desired behaviour for a procedure, such as 'keeping your arm still like a statue' or the use of physical strategies such as squeezing a stress toy. Once modelled, practice and positive reinforcement for the desired behaviour will increase its use.

In Jacob's case example, Jacob was shown how to breathe slowly and deeply (modelling) then was rehearsed with his mother. His mother agreed to be his coach and prompted him to use this breathing technique if she noted escalating anxiety or pain.

Therapeutic play

Koller's (2008b) review of therapeutic play in paediatric health care states 'therapeutic play refers to specialized activities that are developmentally supportive and facilitate the emotional well-being of a pediatric patient' and its focus is on the 'promotion of continuing 'normal development' while enabling children to respond more effectively to difficult situations such as medical experiences' (p. 3). This form of play can take many forms—puppet shows, dramatic play, creative or expressive art or medically focused play. Given that it is an integral part of a child life specialist's practice, more research evidence is needed in support of the efficacy of therapeutic play.

Health care play/medical play

Children with serious and/or chronic illnesses, who experience many painful procedures, will often repeatedly request medical

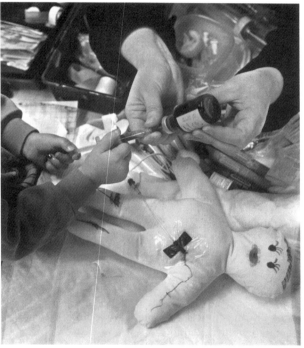

Figure 52.1 Image of a medical play session. Photographer: Copyright © Gary Yokoyama, 1999 (December 11). Making a scary world a bit safer. Republished with permission of *The Hamilton Spectator*.

play focusing on the re-enactment of interventions with the use of a body outline doll and medical supplies. This allows the exploration of the child's perception of their experiences, clarification of misconceptions or misunderstandings (Ostrenga 1980) and/or reinforcement of information previously provided during their illness (see Figure 52.1). It also permits the opportunity for the child life specialist to return and continue with this modality to reassess or debrief with the child after their experience. Requests for repeated medical play sessions will typically taper off and may resurface at stressful periods.

Medical play was used during the preparation in Carrie's case along with the provision of developmentally appropriate information. The offer of a body outline doll and an opportunity to explore the medical kit and supplies provided Carrie with a sense of control and mastery of the situation.

Thought-stopping/coping self-statements/cognitive reframing

Thought-stopping can be very effective when children find their mind repeatedly thinking the same negative statements or images. Children can recognize this and be encouraged to take control of their brain and tell it what to do. The child repeats 'stop' or a similar statement during times of distress/pain, to block out negative thoughts. Often, child life specialists will then encourage the child to choose a positive thought, strong encouraging statement such as, 'I can do this' or 'This will be over soon'. This can be easily taught and reinforced.

In reviewing Jacob's case, the child life specialist used these strategies with Jacob. Given his vivid imagination about the 'rotting flesh' it was important to use his words and re-phrase the way he perceived the healing process 'my throat tissue is healing and will keep getting better.' This became a mantra he rehearsed and his mother prompted him if he went back to his negative verbalizations.

Memory change

After a procedure is complete, it is valuable to assess the child and parents' perceptions of the experience. Sometimes, children will indicate they did not feel it went well: 'I cried' or 'I wasn't brave' or 'it hurt a lot' are common perceptions. Exploring the child's perceptions and then helping the child to reframe negative memories of the procedure into positive ones, 'Lots of boys and girls and even big people cry when something hurts (or is hard work), you stayed so still which really helped make the IV go in easier'; 'Being brave means doing something even though it's scary. You did it! You let the nurses access your Port-a-Cath™ even though it was scary and was uncomfortable', 'I noticed this time, that you didn't move your arm when the tube went in for the IV, you were able to do it, even though it was uncomfortable, I bet next time it won't bother you as much'.

The evidence

As illustrated in the clinical examples above, child life specialists frequently employ a number of evidence-based non-pharmacological pain management strategies. In a large scale survey of over 600 child life specialists in North America, Bandstra and colleagues (2008) found that over 65% of child life specialists reported providing pain management interventions for at least 50% of their patients. The most commonly reported non-pharmacological pain management strategies used by child life specialists were: providing information/preparation, comforting/reassurance, positive reinforcement, and behavioural distraction followed closely by therapeutic play, breathing exercises, and medical play (Bandstra et al., 2008). Consistent with their training and philosophy, child life specialists deliver these interventions in a developmentally appropriate manner, infused with various aspects of play. The literature indicates reassurance can increase anxiety and decrease coping responses to pain (McMurtry et al., 2010) thus further study regarding the child life specialists' use of and/or interpretation of 'reassurance' is warranted. Of note, child life specialists who were certified, those with greater involvement with children who required assistance with pain management, and those who perceived they had a greater level of knowledge

and skills in paediatric pain management were more likely to use evidence-based non-pharmacological pain management strategies (Bandstra et al., 2008). While child life specialists in this survey reported training in non-pharmacological interventions, they expressed a high degree of interest in receiving additional training in non-pharmacological pain management interventions.

There is a growing body of literature supporting the role of child life specialists in implementing non-pharmacological interventions for children and families experiencing painful interventions (Brewer et al., 2006; Eldridge and Kennedy 2010; Gursky et al., 2010; Madhok et al., 2011; Zempsky and Cravero 2004). The most significant body of evidence is found in studies of child life interventions in the ED. Gursky and colleagues' (2010) study in the ED demonstrates that non-pharmacological interventions such as preparation and distraction provided by child life specialists can decrease observed distress behaviours during suturing, that parents perceive their child is less distressed and they are more satisfied with services provided in the ED. Alcock et al. (1985) found decreased fear with child life interventions that included preparation and teaching of coping strategies and emotional support for suturing while Cavender et al. (2004) noted decreased fear with preparation, positioning for comfort, and the use of distraction strategies. Interestingly, the child's assessment of their pain during these noted procedures has not been found to be decreased with the interventions. Parent-reported perception of pain distress has been found by Sinha et al. (2006) and Gursky et al. (2010) to decrease with child life intervention of preparation and use of distraction. There is evidence to suggest that child life interventions impact satisfaction rates in the ED as well (Alcock et al., 1985; Browning and Stroud, 2008; Gursky et al., 2010). Child life specialists are in a pivotal role to teach/prepare patients, parents and staff and provide interventions to assist with pain management (Cregin et al., 2008; Zempsky and Cravero, 2004); decrease anxiety and pain perception (Alcock et al., 1985; Gursky et al., 2010); and support family participation (Cavender et al., 2004; Stephens et al., 1999)

Innovative use of technology

Children and families access the Internet for health information, prior to seeing health professionals, view videos of machinery, and watch YouTube™ videos of professionals and tests, of other families talking about procedures and what the experience will be like from an experiential and sensory perspective. Many families arrive with personal electronic devices and anticipate Internet access during health care visits. Children, youth, and families can utilize these devices to aid with coping; help minimize feelings of isolation and disconnection from family, friends and school; provide diversion from the monotony of long days and provide distraction from invasive, distressing, or painful interventions.

Child life specialists are integrating portable music devices and Wi-Fi tablets into their day-to-day practice. Closed-circuit TV is being utilized for therapeutic goal development with children/youth with the outcome of creating educational and therapeutic videos to educate and teach children/youth how to deal with worries, what to do if they have pain, how to talk to health professionals, and what happens when you have a specific test.

Tablets are replacing paper copies of preparation photos and books. The multitude of applications such as I Hear Ewe, Angry

Birds, Cookie Doodle as well as audio books, music and YouTube™ videos can provide a large repertoire of potential distraction activities (McQueen et al., 2012). Staff and families report increased success at maintaining attention for children across the age spectrum. This one tool in the child life specialists 'tool box' can provide hundreds of activities, minimizing the need to anticipate and bring a bagful of activities for any given child/youth.

Children/youth with chronic physical or mental illness are at risk of social isolation which can impact self-esteem, self-perception and overall coping with diagnosis and treatment. The advent of Starbright World® (<http://www.starbrightworld.org/default_login.aspx?ReturnURL=%2fhome.aspx>) and

Upopolis™ (<https://www.upopolis.com/webconcepteur/web/upopolis>) are examples of online Intranet support programmes that youth with chronic illness can meet others in similar situations while in a safe, closed system, on the Internet. Both programs contain health information written for children and youth in developmentally appropriate language. Studies of Starbright World® indicate improvements in mood and pain responses in children/youth and nearly significant results for anxiety (Davis et al., 2004; Rode et al., 1998).

The use of high-definition and augmentative reality will likely launch technology to a new level of interactive capacity, with growing evidence supporting the efficacy of these approaches for the management of pain in children (Kipping et al., 2012; Miller et al., 2009). This may have even more success in distracting children from distressing or painful stimuli. Research into the use of all of these devices has barely begun; however, clinically there is a great deal of excitement about the perceived success of such applications in the area of teaching, preparation, procedural support, and expressive activities.

Conclusion

Child life specialists play an important role in the assessment and management of pain in children in a variety of settings throughout the hospital as well as other health care settings. Their expertise and unique relationship with the child and family can provide a rich source of information to the interdisciplinary medical team in order to promote effective pain assessment and management and to provide the best overall collaborative and effective care for children. Child life specialists make major clinical contributions in terms of their delivery of non-pharmacological pain management strategies, with a focus on preparation, rehearsal, behavioural and cognitive distraction, and physical interventions such as positioning for comfort. Despite their considerable involvement in pain assessment and management, it has only been in recent years that empirical research on the role of child life specialists in paediatric pain had begun to emerge in the literature. Until further research emerges, the use of theoretical frameworks and evidence based literature continues to be the foundation of child life clinical practice. It is critical for the profession to continue to question the historical assumptions related to child life interventions and seek best evidence and research to ensure efficient and effective practice.

There is a need for interprofessional collaboration, training, and research in the field of paediatric pain in an effort to translate the knowledge that exists into daily practice. However, it will also be important for future studies to address the added benefit of involving child life specialists in paediatric pain care, and for studies to further our understanding of how child life specialists can provide maximum benefit to children in pain and their families.

References

Alcock, D. S., Feldman, W., Goodman, J. T., McGrath, P. J., and Park, J. M. (1985). Evaluation of child life intervention in emergency department suturing. *Pediatr Emerg Care*, 1, 111–115.

American Academy of Pediatrics Child Life Council and Committee on Hospital Care. (2006). Child life services. *Pediatrics*, 118, 1757–1763.

Anonymous. (1959). The welfare of children in hospital. *Br Med J*, 1, 166–169.

Bandstra, N. F., Skinner, L., LeBlanc, C., Chambers, C. T., Hollon, E. C., Brennan, D., *et al.* (2008). The role of child life in pediatric pain management: a survey of child life specialists. *J Pain*, 9, 320–329.

Barnes, P. (1995). Thirty years of play in hospital. *Int J Early Child*, 48–53.

Blount, R. L., and Loiselle, K. A. (2009). Behavioural assessment of pediatric pain. *Pain Res Manag*, 14, 47–52.

Bowlby, J. (1952). *Maternal care and mental health*. Geneva: World Health Organization.

Breiner, S. (2003). An evidence-based eating disorder program. *J Pediatr Nurs*, 18, 75–80.

Brewer, S., Gleditsch, S. L., Syblik, D., Tietjens, M. E., and Vacik, H. W. (2006). Pediatric anxiety: child life intervention in day surgery. *J Pediatr Nurs*, 21, 13–22.

Browning, D. and Stroud, M. A. (2008). Pediatric ED seeks to touch all the bases: advanced courses prepare staff. *ED Manage*, 20, 77–79.

Campbell, L. A., Kirkpatrick, S. E., Berry, C. C., and Lamberti, J. J. (1995). Preparing children with congenital heart disease for cardiac surgery. *J Pediatric Psychol*, 20, 313–328.

Cavender, K., Goff, M. D., Hollon, E. C., and Guzzetta, C. E. (2004). Parents' positioning and distracting children during venipuncture: effects on children's pain, fear, and distress. *J Holist Nurs*, 22, 32–56.

Chernoff, R. G., Ireys, H. T., DeVet, K. A., and Kim, Y. J. (2002). A randomized, controlled trial of a community-based support program for families of children with chronic illness: pediatric outcomes. *Arch Pediatr Adolesc Med*, 156, 533–539.

Child Life Council. (2002). *Official documents of the child life council*. Rockville, MD: Child Life Council.

Child Life Council. (2012a). *The child life profession*. Available at: <http://www.childlife.org/The%20Child%20Life%20Profession/> (accessed 17 April 2012).

Child Life Council. (2012b). *CCLS directory*. Available at: <http://ams.childlife.org/members_online/members/CCLS_Directory.asp> (accessed 17 April 2012).

Cregin, R., Rappaport, A. S., Montagnino, G., Sabogal, G., Moreau, H., and Abularrage, J. J. (2008). Improving pain management for pediatric patients undergoing nonurgent painful procedures. *Am J Heath Syst Pharm*, 65, 723–727.

Davis, M. A., Quittner, A. L., Stack, C. M., and Yang, M. C. (2004). Controlled evaluation of the STARBRIGHT CD-ROM program for children and adolescents with Cystic Fibrosis. *J Pediatr Psychol*, 29, 259–267.

Davitt, K. A., and Munn, E. K. (2008). Child life in pediatric healthcare. *J Pediatr Rehabil Med*, 1, 33–34.

Eldridge, C. and Kennedy, R. (2010). Nonpharmacologic techniques for distress reduction during emergency medical care: a review. *Clin Pediatr Emerg Med*, 11, 244–250.

Gaynard, L., Goldberger, J., Thompson, R., Redburn, L. & Laidley, L. (1990). *Psychosocial care of children in hospitals: a clinical practice manual from the ACCH Child Life Research Project*. Bethesda, MD: Association for the Care of Children's Health.

Glasrud, P. H., and Feigal, R. J. (1984). Child life and children's dentistry: broadening our scope of concern. *Child Health Care*, 12, 143–147.

Gursky, B., Kestler, L. P., and Lewis, M. (2010). Psychosocial intervention on procedure-related distress in children being treated for laceration repair. *J Dev Behav Pediatr*, 31, 217–222.

Hicks, M. (2008). *Child life beyond the hospital*. Rockville, MD: Child Life Council Inc.

Hospital Play Specialist Association of Aotearoal/New Zealand. (2012).*Official Documents and forms*. Available at: <http://www.hospitalplay.org.nz/online/official_documents.csn> (accessed 17 April 2012).

Jaaniste, T., Hayes, B., and von Baeyer, C. L. (2007). Providing children with information about forthcoming medical procedures: a review and synthesis. *Clin Psychol Sci Pract*, 14, 124–143.

Jessee, P. and Gaynard, L. (2009). Paradigm of play. In R. W. Thompson, (ed.) *The handbook of child life: a guide for pediatric psychosocial care*, pp. 136–159. Springfield, IL: Charles C. Thomas.

Jun-Tai, N. (2008). Play in hospital. *Paediatr Child Health*, 18, 233–237.

Kipping, B., Rodger, S., Miller, K., Kimble, R. M. (2012). Virtual reality for acute pain reduction in adolescents undergoing burn wound care: a prospective randomized controlled trial. *Burns*, 38, 650–657.

Kleiber, C., McCarthy, A. M., Hanrahan, K., Myers, L., and Weathers, N. (2007). Development of the distraction coaching index. *Child Health Care*, 36, 219–235.

Koller, D. (2007). *Child Life Council evidence-based practice statement: preparing children and adolescents for medical procedures*. Rockville, MD: Child Life Council.

Koller, D. (2008a). *Child Life Council evidence-based practice statement. child life assessment: variables associated with a child's ability to cope with hospitalization*. Rockville, MD: Child Life Council.

Koller, D. (2008b).*Child Life Council evidence-based practice statement: therapeutic play in pediatric health care: the essence of child life practice*. Rockville, MD: Child Life Council.

Kuttner, L. (2010). *A child in pain: what health professionals can do to help*. Bethel, CT: Crown House Publishing Ltd.

LaMontagne, L., Hepworth, J. T., Salisbury, M. H., and Cohen, F. (2003a). Effects of coping instruction in reducing young adolescents' pain after major spinal surgery. *Orthopaedic Nurs*, 22, 398–403.

LaMontagne, L. L., Hepworth, J. T., Cohen, F., and Salisbury, M. H. (2003b). Cognitive-behavioral intervention effects on adolescents' anxiety and pain following spinal fusion surgery. *Nurs Res*, 52, 183–190.

Lindeke, L., Nakai, M., and Johnson, L. (2006). Capturing children's voices for quality improvement. *Am J Matern Child Nurs*, 31, 290–297.

Madhok, M., Scribner-O'Prey, M., and Teele, M. (2011). No needless pain: Managing pediatric pain in minor injuries. *Contemp Pediatr*, 24–31.

Mahaffy, P. R. Jr (1965). The effects of hospitalization on children admitted for tonsillectomy and adenoidectomy. *Nurs Res*, 14, 12–19.

McCue, K. and Hicks, M. (2007). From vision to reality: the expansion of the child life role. *Child Life Council*, 25, 2–8.

McGee, K. (2003). The role of a child life specialist in a pediatric radiology department. *Pediatr Radiol*, 467–474.

McMurtry, C. M., Chambers, C. T., McGrath, P. J., and Asp, E. (2010). When 'don't worry' communicates fear: children's perceptions of parental reassurance and distraction during a painful medical procedure. *Pain*, 150, 52–58.

McQueen, A., Cress, C., and Tothy, A. (2012). Using a tablet computer during pediatric procedures: A case series and review of the 'apps.' *Pediatr Emerg Care*, 7, 712–714.

Miller, K., Rodger, S., Bucolo, S., Greer, R., and Kimble, R. M. (2009). Multi-modal distraction. Using technology to combat pain in young children with burn injuries. *Burns*, 36, 647–658.

Ostrenga, M. A. (1980). *Guidelines for medical play*. Evanson, IL: Hospital Play Equipment.

Patterson, K. L., and Ware, L. L. (1988). Coping skills for children undergoing painful medical procedures. *Issues Compr Pediatr Nurs*, 11, 113–143.

Plank, E. (1962). *Working with children in hospitals: a guide for the professional team* (3rd edn). Cleveland, OH: Western Reserve University.

Prugh, D. G., Staub, E. M., Sands, H. H., Kirschbaum, R. M., and Lenihan, E. A. (1953). A study of the emotional reactions of children and families to hospitalization and illness. *Am J Orthopsychiatry*, 23, 70–106.

Rode, D., Capitulo, K. L., Fishman, M., and Holden, G. (1998). The therapeutic use of technology. *Am J Nurs*, 98, 32–35.

Rubin, S. (1992). What's in a name? Child life and the play lady legacy. *Child Health Care*, 21, 4.

Shelton, T. and Stepanek, J. (1994). *Family-centred care for children needing specialized health and development services* (3rd edn). Rockville, MD: Child Life Council Inc.

Sinha, M., Christopher, N. C., Fenn, R., and Reeves, L. (2006). Evaluation of nonpharmacologic methods of pain and anxiety management for laceration repair in the pediatric emergency department. *Pediatrics*, 117, 1162–1168.

Skinner, L. and LeBlanc, C. (2002). *Child life assessment intervention plan (CLAIP). 2nd version*. Halifax, NS: Child Life Services, IWK Health Centre.

Spafford, P. A., von Baeyer, C. L., and Hicks, C. L. (2002). Expected and reported pain in children undergoing earpiercing: a randomized trial of preparation by parents. *Behaviour Res Ther*, 40, 253–266.

Sparks, L. A., Setlik, J., and Luhman, J. (2007). Parental holding and positioning to decrease IV distress in young children: a randomized controlled trial. *J Pediatr Nurs*, 22, 440–447.

Spitz, R. A. (1945). Hospitalism; an inquiry into the genesis of psychiatric conditions in early childhood. *Psychoanal Study Child*, 1, 53–74.

Stephens, B. K., Barkey, M. E., and Hall, H. R. (1999). Techniques to comfort children during stressful procedures. *Accid Emerg Nurs*, 7, 226–236.

Stevens, B. J., Abbott, L. K., Yamada, J., Harrison, D., Stinson, J., Taddio, A., et al. (2011). Epidemiology and management of painful procedures in children in Canadian hospitals. *CMAJ*, 183, E403–410.

Stevenson, M. D., Bivins, C. M., O'Brien, K., and Gonzalez del Rey, J. A. (2005). Child life intervention during angiocatheter insertion in the pediatric emergency department. *Pediatr Emerg Care*, 21, 712–718.

Suls, J. and Wan, C. K. (1989). Effects of sensory and procedural information on coping with stressful medical procedures and pain: a meta-analysis. *J Consult Clin Psychol*, 57, 372–379.

Tak, J. H., and van Bon, W. H. (2006). Pain- and distress-reducing interventions for venipuncture in children. *Child Care Health Dev*, 32, 257–268.

Thompson, R. H. (1989). Child life programs in pediatric settings. *Infant Young Child*, 2, 75–82.

Thompson, R. H., and Snow, C. W. (2009). Research in child life. In R.W. Thompson, (ed.) *The handbook of child life: a guide for pediatric psychosocial care*, pp. 36–56. Springfield, IL: Charles C. Thomas.

Uman, L. S., Chambers, C. T., McGrath, P. J., and Kisely, S. (2006). Psychological interventions for needle-related procedural pain and distress in children and adolescents. *Cochrane Database Syst Rev*, 4, CD005179.

Visintainer, M. A., and Wolfer, J. A. (1975). Psychological preparation for surgical pediatric patients: the effect on children's and parent's stress responses and adjustment. *Pediatrics*, 56, 187–202.

Wojtasik, S. and White, C. (2009). The story of child life. In R.W. Thompson, (ed.) *The handbook of child life: a guide for pediatric psychosocial care*, pp. 3–32. Springfield, IL: Charles C. Thomas.

Young, K. D. (2005). Pediatric procedural pain. *Ann Emerg Med*, 45, 160–171.

Zempsky, W. T., and Cravero, J. P. (2004). Clinical report: relief of pain and anxiety in pediatric patients in emergency medical systems. *Pediatrics*, 114, 1348–1356.

CHAPTER 53

Procedural pain distraction

Lindsey L. Cohen, Laura A. Cousins, and Sarah R. Martin

Summary

This chapter provides a brief overview of paediatric procedural pain, highlighting some of the negative repercussions of untreated pain. The behavioural approach of distraction is covered in depth, starting with the theoretical underpinnings of this pain management intervention and then summarizing the distraction literature across children's pain during immunizations, venous access, burn debridement and treatment, and cancer treatments. The chapter concludes with a discussion of some of the other reviews of this literature as well as clinical and research considerations when examining distraction for paediatric pain management.

Overview of paediatric procedural pain

Starting at birth and continuing through development, children will undergo a host of routine as well as unplanned invasive medical procedures. As an example, the World Health Organization (WHO) recommends approximately 20 to 30 vaccinations by 6 years of age (WHO, 2012). Additional vaccines for encephalitis, yellow fever, typhoid, cholera, meningococcal, rabies, mumps, and influenza are recommended for certain geographic locations and high-risk populations (WHO, 2012). The majority of these vaccinations are administered via intramuscular injections. Beyond routine procedures, roughly 78% of children admitted to hospitals will undergo at least one medical procedure, typically involving needles (e.g. venous access; Stevens et al., 2011). Although immunizations, venous access, and other invasive medical events are critical for children's health, children find needle procedures anxiety-provoking and painful (e.g. Jacobsen et al., 2001; Schechter et al., 2007). For example, data suggest that over half of children require physical restraint during routine immunizations (Blount et al., 1992).

Although invasive events are a necessary aspect of appropriate health care, there can be a host of sequelae. First, the high pain intensity associated with routine and unplanned procedures can contribute to immediate fear and anxiety, in turn heightening the pain experience in a cyclical fashion (McGrath, 1994; Rhudy and Meagher, 2003). The child's negative physical and affective reactions might lead to disruptive behaviour (e.g. Bijttebier and Vertommen, 1998; Broome et al., 1990) and contribute to parents' anxiety (e.g. Kuppenheimer and Brown, 2002). Second, these negative sensations and emotions associated with medical care are likely to influence long-term health care attitudes and behaviour (Chen et al., 2000; Jones et al., 2008; Kennedy et al., 2008; Pate et al., 1996; Taddio et al., 2009). On a physiological level, early pain might alter the pain-processing neuronal circuitry leading to heightened pain perception in the future (e.g. Hermann et al., 2006; Ruda et al., 2000; Taddio et al., 1997).

Behavioural treatment of paediatric procedural pain

Given the immediate and delayed negative effects of acute paediatric procedures, analgesics and sedatives have been used to provide some pain relief; however, these approaches have failed to consistently eliminate pain and often do little to decrease fear or anxiety. In addition, pharmacological approaches are less frequently employed for venous access and immunization injections, likely due to the brevity of the procedure. Fortunately, researchers and clinicians have employed behavioural approaches to minimize the negative physical and emotional aspects of routine invasive medical procedures. Reviews of the literature suggest that—generally speaking—behavioural approaches are beneficial to children facing distressing and painful medical events (e.g. Pillai Riddell et al., 2011; Powers, 1999; Uman et al., 2010). Unpacking these reviews quickly reveals that the 'devil is in the details'; there are many different behavioural approaches used with a variety of acute medical procedures to help a diversity of children. Behavioural interventions range from fairly circumscribed approaches (e.g. having children cough during venous access; Wallace et al., 2010) to multicomponent packages (e.g. imagery, physical vibration stimulation, distraction; Berberich and Landman, 2009); the acute pain literature spans experimental analogous approaches (e.g. cold-pressor; Dahlquist et al., 2007) to routine brief procedures (e.g. venous access; Cohen, 2008) to more invasive and severe medical events (e.g. burn debridement; Hoffman et al., 2000); and patients are diverse in a number of important ways (e.g. age, gender, culture, temperament, prior experience). In an attempt to provide some depth in this broad topic, this chapter will focus only on the use of distraction for a sample of children's acute invasive medical procedures. Other psychological interventions (e.g. cognitive behavioural therapies (Logan et al., Chapter 50), operant based treatment (Slifer et al., Chapter 51), biofeedback (Stinson and Jibb, Chapter 55)) and physical interventions (e.g. physical therapy (Tupper et al., Chapter 56), occupational therapy (Holsti et al., Chapter 57)) are fully described in other chapters in this volume.

Distraction for paediatric procedural pain

Theories of distraction mechanisms

Distraction is generally defined as shifting attention from one source onto the new one, whether it be internal (e.g. imagery) or external (e.g. watching a movie). Within the field of paediatric procedural pain management, distraction has been described as redirecting a child's attention away from anxiety-provoking painful medical stimuli, such as needles, to engaging or enjoyable stimuli (Kleiber and McCarthy, 2006; Sander et al., 2002).

Physiologically, theorists propose that distraction or selective attention may enhance electrical activity in the brain in response to a distraction task (i.e. the attended-to stimulus) as compared to the noxious or painful stimulus (i.e. the ignored stimuli). Several studies have shown that distraction tasks reduce the activity of brain areas known to process pain stimuli (Bantick et al., 2002; Frankenstein et al., 2001; Petrovic et al., 2000). According to the gate control theory of pain (Melzack and Wall, 1965; Wall, 1978), the substantia gelatinosa serves as a gate control system by modulating ascending impulses from peripheral nerves before they are perceived as pain by the cerebral cortex. When external (e.g. massage) and internal non-nociceptive input (e.g. anxiety) surpass nociceptive (pain) input, the gate may partially or entirely shut, blocking the pain signal. A distraction intervention is thus hypothesized to mitigate pain through descending non-nociceptive impulses that inhibit the chief nociceptive signal, altering nociceptive responses (Melzack and Wall, 1965), although it remains unknown how specific characteristics of distraction stimuli may alter gate modulation.

Attention can also be operationalized and assessed cognitively. A prominent cognitive theory, limited attentional capacity theory (LCT; McCaul and Malott, 1984), relies on two assumptions to support the analgesic effect of distraction. The first assumption defines nociception as an intentional process that requires effort and attentional focus on the eliciting stimulus. The second assumption posits that attentional capacity is limited and nociceptive stimuli will not be perceived if an individual's attentional focus is completely diverted to a specific task. Since undivided attention is difficult to achieve, distraction is less effective with a noxious stimulus of greater intensity (e.g. burn debridement) or with a distraction stimulus of lesser intensity (e.g. conversation on a topic that is not unique, such as school activities). LCT predicts that distraction will be more effective than placebo and redefinitional strategies (e.g. cognitive restructuring of fear) at low levels of noxious stimulus intensity. Additionally, distraction will be more effective in managing mild levels of pain and distraction stimuli that require greater attentional capacity will inhibit more attention needed to perceive pain (McCaul and Malott, 1984). Due to the theory's circular assumptions and elementary reliance on one domain of information processing, a more advanced theory, multiple attentional resource theory (MRT; Wickens, 1984, 2002) developed.

MRT proposes three distinct domains of information-processing capacity, including the perceptual demands of a task, tasks requiring a spatially driven manual response or verbal response, and tasks perceived visually versus aurally. According to this theory, the level of interference when processing other stimuli is dependent upon the degree to which two competing tasks utilize the same information-processing domain (Wickens, 1984). Researchers suggest that the level of pain perception results from how information is processed according to the three domains, with detection of pain primarily occupying the perceptual and spatial resources (Johnson et al., 1998). In contrast to LCT, MRT predicts that distraction is most effective if engaging the same system as pain (i.e. perceptual). Thus, a distraction such as a vibrating device placed on the arm (e.g. Berberich and Landman, 2009; Baxter et al., 2011) is theorized to optimize interference with pain related to an injection in the same arm.

Finally, attention can be operationalized and assessed behaviourally, as visual or auditory orienting responses to external stimuli (Pavlov, 1927). Mowrer's two-factor learning theory (Mowrer, 1947) asserts that both classical conditioning and instrumental conditioning play a significant role in pain responsivity. In classical conditioning, a neutral stimulus, such as medical equipment, accompanies a pain-eliciting unconditioned stimulus (UCS), which consistently produces an unconditioned response (UCR) (e.g. pulling away). Due to this association, the neutral stimulus becomes a conditioned stimulus (CS) that elicits a conditioned response (CR) of fear or anxiety preceding the UCS. In instrumental conditioning, avoidant responding (e.g. crying) follows the CR and persists through negative reinforcement, such as a decrease in fear, as a means of avoiding the CS and UCS. Cohen (2002) suggests that distraction tasks deter attention away from painful stimuli and conditioned stimuli that also evoke distress, ultimately reducing the CR and UCR that develop from painful paediatric procedures (i.e. a conditioned fear response). Distraction may also produce behaviours incompatible with distress, such as relaxation or laughter. Despite the lack of a unifying theoretical framework for distraction mechanisms (DeMore and Cohen, 2005), distraction remains one of the most prevalent forms of behavioural pain management among health care professionals. This is likely due to its ease of use.

Efficacy of distraction for paediatric procedural pain

When reviewing the paediatric pain literature, it should be noted that there is great variability in what is described as distraction in form, function, and efficacy. For example, a cartoon shown to a child during a procedure might serve the intended purpose of inducing a positive-mood state incompatible with distress, engaging a child in mathematical computations might occupy attentional resources, and a virtual-reality head-mounted display might effectively remove all medical stimuli from the visual and auditory fields. Thus, although all of these approaches can be described as 'distraction', they might be quite different in topography and mechanism of effect. To further complicate the issues, individual characteristics of the child (e.g. age, temperament, coping style) might react with the distraction such that it assumes a different function. For example, some children might find the latest rap song to be an enjoyable distraction from the threatening sound of a dental drill, while others might prefer the drill. The variability and subsequent effectiveness of distraction is highlighted by the efforts of Kleiber and colleagues who have developed a scale that measures both the quantity and quality of parent-provided distraction (Kleiber et al., 2007; McCarthy et al., 2010a, 2010b). Given all of these caveats about distraction for acute paediatric procedural pain, it is not surprising that results in the paediatric pain literature are inconsistent (e.g. Carlson et al., 2000; Cramer-Berness, 2007). Acknowledging that there is variability in the effects of distraction within and between studies, the subsequent sections will highlight the use of distraction in different common acute paediatric procedures. In addition, given the large number of paediatric procedural pain studies that incorporate distraction, this review will highlight some of the studies that exemplify unique aspects of the approach.

Immunizations

Immunization schedules vary by country, but it is generally recommended that children receive 20 to 30 vaccinations by 6 years of age (WHO, 2012). The majority of these vaccinations are administered via intramuscular injection, which children find anxiety-providing and painful (e.g. Jacobsen et al., 2001). As paediatric intramuscular immunization injections remain the most common painful paediatric medical procedures in health care settings, distraction has been evaluated in a number of studies (Schechter et al., 2007). For example, a series of studies evaluating nurse-led movie distraction during immunizations demonstrated that distraction was generally beneficial to infants (Cohen, 2002; Cohen et al., 2006), pre-schoolers (Cohen et al., 1997), and preadolescents (Cohen et al., 1999). However, findings were not consistent across all measures or all phases of the procedure. Wallace et al. (2010) evaluated the efficacy of the 'cough trick', requiring 4- to 5-year-olds and 11- to 13-year-olds to provide several coughs prior to and coinciding with immunization injections. This technique is thought to distract children from the immunization by focusing on coughing when prompted and possibly creating antagonistic sensations developed from the noise and feeling of the cough. Of note, the cough trick was effective for Hispanic white or non-Hispanic white children ($t_{33} = -2.86$, $p < 0.01$), but did not prove beneficial to non-Hispanic black children.

Berberich and Landman (2009) included distraction in a package to reduce pain in pre-schoolers receiving immunizations. The intervention included a multipronged arm gripper, topical analgesic, and a vibrating instrument on the opposite arm. The children were encouraged to guess when the vibrating device reached their arm. Results supported the intervention across measures (self-report scores, $p < 0.0013$; parent report scores, $p < 0.0002$; observational coding scores comparing baseline to completion of immunization series, $p < 0.0001$), but it is unclear which are the critical ingredients in package interventions such as this (Cohen, 2010).

In a systematic review of 20 randomized controlled trials (RCTs), Chambers et al. (2009) determined that both child-directed (e.g. cartoons, music) and nurse-led (e.g. trained to distraction with movies or toys) distraction were effective in mitigating pain and distress during child immunizations, whereas evidence remained inconclusive for parent-led (e.g. trained to distract with movies or toys) distraction. Chambers et al. noted that distraction with age-appropriate toys was the only psychological intervention examined in the review that can be applied to all age groups due to the ability to select toys suitable for infants, children, or adolescents. A review by DeMore and Cohen (2005) concluded that distraction is both a time- and cost-efficient strategy for immunizations and that it effectively reduces children's injection pain. Although a variety of distracters were used in the studies evaluated, the most commonly employed distraction stimuli were playing cartoon movies, non-procedural talk, and having the child listen to music. Distraction strategies that either required an overt response from the child or involved multiple sensory modalities were most effective.

To date, the immunization pain literature has predominantly focused on preschool-aged children due to the numerous vaccinations needed for school entry and their high level of reported distress. Although a few studies support the use of distraction for infant (Cohen, 2002; Cohen et al., 2006; Felt et al., 2000) and pre-adolescent participant samples (e.g. Cohen et al., 1999), further research tailored to these age groups is warranted (Cramer-Berness, 2007; Schechter et al., 2007). Additionally, most participant samples have consisted of Caucasian mother–child dyads, limiting the generalizability of findings to other races, ethnicities, and caregivers (DeMore and Cohen, 2005). Unfortunately, parents and health care professionals still exhibit a poor understanding of the value in employing distraction for immunization pain relief (Chambers et al., 2009).

Venous access

Venous access has been identified as one of the medical procedures most feared by children (Carlson et al., 2000). In one of the few studies comparing distraction interventions, MacLaren and Cohen (2005) found that passive distraction (viewing movies) was more effective than active distraction (responding to games on an electronic toy) during paediatric venous access. Bellieni et al. (2006) also found that passive distraction (watching a TV cartoon) was more effective than active distraction during venepuncture. That said, a study evaluating children's pain tolerance during a cold pressor suggests that active distraction (playing a videogame) might be more effective than passive distraction (watching a videogame) (Wohlheiter and Dahlquist, in press).

Several studies support the efficacy of audiovisual distraction techniques, through the form of animated cartoons, in diverting children's attention from venepuncture pain. Yoo et al. (2011) found an animation distraction intervention effective in reducing self-reported pain, behavioural pain responses, and serum cortisol and glucose levels in preschool-aged children during venepuncture in Seoul, Korea. Wang et al. (2008) found cartoon videos equally effective as other routine psychological interventions (i.e. explaining, therapeutic touch, encouragement, and guided imagery) in reducing self-reported pain, enhancing patient cooperation, and heightening the success rate of venepuncture procedures. Researchers also suggest that animation distraction is both simple to administer and could be easily integrated into health care settings.

Although studies remain less conclusive about caregiver participation, some suggest that distraction education for parents prior to venepuncture may be valuable (Kleiber et al., 2001). Kleiber et al. (2001) compared parent–child dyads in a control group to those in a distraction education group across two phases of venepuncture, procedural preparation and needle insertion. Parents in the distraction education group employed significantly more distraction during both phases compared to parents in the control group and children in the distraction condition exhibited less distress during the two procedural phases than children in the control condition. In a review of the literature, Cohen (2008) suggested that distraction is recommended for paediatric venous access, particularly for children aged 7 years or younger, due to its empirical support, minimal risks, and cost- and time-effectiveness.

Burn debridement and treatment

Childhood burns represent one of the most physically and emotionally traumatic injuries (Benjamin and Herndon, 2002; Hettiaratchy and Dziewulski, 2004), which often result in long-standing pain and distress (Fitzgerald, 2005; Passaretti and Billmire, 2003;

Schechter et al., 1993). Increasing research has focused on evaluating behavioural approaches for pain management for burn treatment procedures (e.g. skin debridement; de Jong et al., 2007) given that pharmacological analgesic methods often prove inadequate (e.g. Hoffman et al., 2004; for a review, see Morris et al., 2009).

The distraction literature for burn treatment procedures often involves sophisticated—and potentially highly engaging—interventions (e.g. virtual reality; Hoffman et al., 2004). This is likely related to the rationale that it is challenging to distract a child from the severe pain that is associated with burn treatment pain. To exemplify, in comparison to standard distraction and hand-held video game distraction, multi-modal distraction used for procedural preparation and distraction during dressing changes significantly reduced pain and the duration of three dressing changes among children in a paediatric burns outpatient clinic (Miller et al., 2010). This hand-held device effectively engaged children in an interactive procedural preparation story or a touch and find interactive distraction story during the dressing change procedure. In a study of children's distress related to burn-dressing changes, Mott et al. (2008) compared 'augmented reality' (akin to virtual reality although uses overlays of virtual images onto the actual world) to basic cognitive therapy. Parents' ratings and children's self-reports indicated that the augmented reality distraction was superior to control for burn treatment pain relief.

Distraction, in the form of immersive virtual reality, has also been shown effective as an adjunctive analgesic for paediatric burn patients (Schmitt et al., 2011). Participants randomly assigned to the immersive virtual reality group (i.e. SnowWorld virtual environment) reported significant decreases in pain ($p <0.05$) and improved affect when performing range-of-motion exercises on the first day of the study, which persisted across the 5 days of physical therapy sessions. Similar positive results were demonstrated by Das et al. (2005) in a study of virtual reality distraction for 5- to 18-year-olds undergoing burn treatment. Similarly, Hoffman et al. (2000) showed that virtual reality distraction reduced pain scores, anxiety, and time spent thinking about pain for two adolescents undergoing wound care for severe burns. Researchers in this area suggest that distraction should be tailored to individual patient needs, that the potency or engaging quality of the distraction should match the severity of the procedural pain, and lower cost and greater portability would provide more widespread dissemination of the interventions (Hoffman et al., 2011).

Cancer treatments

During cancer treatment, children undergo multiple invasive medical procedures including venous port access, lumbar puncture, and venepuncture; the treatments are often described as the most distressing part of the disease (Hedstrom et al., 2003). Despite advances in pharmacological approaches for pain management, there continues to be a need for additional pain and anxiety relief (e.g. Varni et al., 2004). A number of distraction interventions have been effective for the procedures faced by this population. For example, Gershon et al. (2004) found that a virtual gorilla distraction exhibit effectively lowered distress in a small sample of 7- to 19-year-olds with cancer undergoing port access procedures. Windich-Biermeier et al. (2007) had 5- to 18-year-old oncology patients select from a variety of distraction stimuli (e.g. books, bubbles, hand-held games) and showed that distraction lowered their fear and distress during port access and venous access procedures.

In a study of music distraction, researchers found this treatment effective in lowering anxiety in children with cancer receiving lumbar punctures (Nhan Nguyen et al., 2010). Although not described as distraction, commonly used hypnosis and imagery techniques are arguably forms of internally shifting attention from a noxious stimulus to another stimulus. As an example, in a study of 6- to 16-year-olds receiving venepuncture as part of their cancer care, Liossi et al. (2009) found self-hypnosis superior for pain and anxiety relief as compared to control and attention conditions. A systematic review of the literature indicated that hypnosis is a viable intervention for procedural pain in paediatric oncology patients (Richardson et al., 2006). Further discussion on hypnosis can be found elsewhere in this volume (Liossi et al., Chapter 54).

Conclusion

Given the vast array of distraction techniques and study methodology reported, meta-analyses and review studies present an integrated overview of strengths and limitations in the literature, providing direction for future research. Koller and Goldman (2011) critically assessed studies evaluating distraction for children ranging from infant to young adults undergoing medical procedures and found support for such interventions, while also addressing important gaps in the literature. A systematic review of RCTs employing psychological interventions for children and adolescents during needle-related procedures found distraction to have one of the largest effect sizes in managing procedural pain and distress compared to control conditions (Uman et al., 2008). Specifically, studies sufficiently support the use of distraction for self-reported pain, a combination of distraction and suggestion for self-reported pain, a combination of nurse coaching and distraction for distress assessed behaviourally, and a combination of parent positioning (e.g. instructing the parent where to sit and how to hold the child) and distraction for distress using observer reports. A meta-analysis examining the mean effect sizes of distraction on children's distress behaviour and self-reported pain during medical procedures concluded that although distraction had a positive effect on children's distress behaviour, moderator variables influenced the effect of distraction on children's self-reported pain intensity. Specifically, the amount of explained variance significantly increased after controlling for child age and type of procedure, suggesting that other potential moderators may also influence this relation (Kleiber and Harper, 1999).

Although most reviews support distraction as an efficacious psychological intervention for paediatric procedural pain, study limitations and recommendations for future research are also presented. Many researchers fail to elaborate on the randomization procedure used or the nature of participant attrition, which limits the value of any significant results (Uman et al., 2006). Due to the minimal number of RCTs directly comparing distraction methods, it remains challenging to discern which interventions are most effective, particularly given their varying degrees of patient engagement. Moreover, many researchers also incorporate multiple distraction approaches in the intervention design, which makes it difficult to uniquely assess specific unique distraction techniques. Established methods must also be evaluated against novel interventions longitudinally, as the novel interventions may become less efficacious as child habituation gradually increases. In addition to accounting for a child's prior exposure to a particular form of distraction, future research should also address patient preferences and other child-specific variables (e.g. temperament, past medical experience). Other areas of improvement include the incorporation of data to assess patients' and health care providers' personal experiences with distraction, recruiting larger sample sizes, examining both the short- and long-term effects of distraction, and using pain measures that have established validity. Finally, the paucity of objective measures of time spent actively engaged in distraction may also influence findings deemed significant (Koller and Goldman, 2011). Whereas distraction appears to be effective for pre-schoolers and school-age children, sufficient evidence to support the efficacy of distraction for procedural pain in infants has not been established (Cramer-Berness, 2007; Pillai Riddell et al., 2011).

In summary, there are ample data to support the general argument that distraction is an effective intervention for children's acute painful medical procedures (e.g. Kleiber and Harper, 1999). The literature supports a variety of distraction approaches used across routine (e.g. immunizations) and more invasive (e.g. burn debridement) paediatric procedures and with a range of patient populations. However, a closer inspection of the data reveals a complicated story with a number of variables (e.g. age, distraction technique, type of procedure) influencing the success of distraction for children's anxiety and pain mitigation. Future studies in distraction for paediatric procedural pain might more closely identify the mechanism of action. For example, it remains unclear as to whether the induction of a positive mood, the involvement of multiple sensory modalities, or other aspects (e.g. developmentally appropriate technique, engagement in distraction, parental attention during distraction) is critical. In fact, data suggest that mood and attention each might influence pain, but these two avenues do so in different ways (Villemure and Bushnell, 2002). In addition, the literature remains largely equivocal about matching distraction to patient characteristics, which is becoming increasingly important as pressure mounts to provide tailored treatment (Department of Health and Human Services, n.d.). For example, a handful of studies a number of years ago explored matching distraction to avoidance, blunter, or repressor coping style, but the findings were inconsistent (e.g. Christiano and Russ, 1998; Fanurik et al., 1993; Smith et al., 1989). Other fine-grained studies might identify individual patient characteristics and preferences useful in determining not only whether distraction might be beneficial to the paediatric patient, but what type of distraction would be optimal.

Case example

A case example allows an opportunity to exemplify some of the research recommendations. Taking an evidence-based practice in psychology perspective, it is important to use clinical skills to tailor the scientific findings to the patient's characteristics, culture, and preferences (American Psychological Association, 2005). In this example, 'Johnnie' is an 8-year-old who is returning for an oncology port-access procedure. The staff have noted in his medical chart that Johnnie is consistently distressed for these procedures (sensitization is not uncommon for repeated procedures; Katz et al., 1980), his parents are opposed to any pharmacological intervention, and Johnnie enjoys Anime comics and movies. Thus, topical anaesthetics are not employed to minimize pain, and the nurse has secured an age-appropriate Anime video

and several Anime comic books. The nurse begins playback of the movie and engages Johnnie in conversation about the film in advance of the medical procedure to decrease anticipatory anxiety (e.g. Cohen, 2008). Johnnie's parents join the conversation and further encourage distraction, which is expected (e.g. Cohen et al., 1997). Given that Johnnie has undergone numerous port-access procedures, information about the procedure is minimized (for a review, see Jaaniste et al., 2007). When Johnnie displays or reports distress or pain, the nurse and parents briefly and neutrally acknowledge it but immediately re-engage him in the movie; and when the port-access procedure is complete, the nurse will continue to employ distraction strategies in order to minimize post-procedure distress. Consistent with recommendations in the literature (Cohen et al., 2001), Johnnie's hopefully low to moderate anxiety and pain ratings might be retained in his medical chart so that he might review them at his next port-access procedure in order to decrease potentially distorted anticipatory anxiety.

References

APA Presidential Task Force on Evidence-Based Practice. (2006). Evidence-based practice in psychology. *Am Psychol*, 61, 271–285.

Bantick, S. J., Wise, R. G., Ploghaus, A., Clare, S., Smith, S. M., and Tracey, I. (2002). Imaging how attention modulates pain in humans using functional MRI. *Brain*, 125, 310–319.

Baxter, A. L., Cohen, L. L., Lawson, M. L., and von Baeyer, C. L. (2011). An integration of vibration and cold relieves venipuncture pain in a pediatric emergency department. *Pediatr Emerg Care*, 27, 1151–1156.

Bellieni, C. V., Cordelli, D. M., Raffaelli, M., Ricci, B., Morgese, G., and Buonocore, G. (2006). Analgesic effect of watching TV during venipuncture. *Arch Dis Child*, 91, 1015–1017.

Benjamin, D. and Herndon, D. N. (2002). Special considerations of age: the pediatric burned patient. In D. N. Herndon, (ed.) *Total Burn Care*, pp. 427–438. London: WB Saunders.

Berberich, F. R., and Landman, Z. (2009). Reducing immunization discomfort in 4- to 6-year-old children: a randomized clinical trial. *Pediatrics*, 124, e203–209.

Bijttebier, P. and Vertommen, H. (1998). The impact of previous experience on children's reactions to venipunctures. *J Health Psychol*, 3, 39–46.

Blount, R. L., Bachanas, P. J., Powers, S. W., Cotter, M. W., Franklin, A., Chaplin, W., *et al.* (1992). Training children to cope and parents to coach them during routine immunizations: effects on child, parent, and staff behaviors. *Behav Ther*, 23, 689–705.

Broome, M. E., Bates, T. A., Lillis, P. P., and McGahee, T. W. (1990). Children's medical fears, coping behaviors, and pain perceptions during a lumbar puncture. *Oncol Nurs Forum*, 17, 361–367.

Carlson, K. L., Broome, M., and Vessey, J. A., (2000). Using distraction to reduce reported pain, fear, and behavioral distress in children and adolescents: a multisite study. *J Spec Pediatr Nurs*, 5, 75–85.

Chambers, C. T., Taddio, A., Uman, L. S., and McMurty, C. M. (2009). Psychological interventions for reducing pain and distress during routine childhood immunizations: a systematic review. *Clin Ther*, 31, S77–107.

Chen, E., Zeltzer, L. K., Craske, M. G., and Katz, E. R. (2000). Children's memories for painful cancer treatment procedures: implications for distress. *Child Dev*, 71, 933–947.

Cohen, L. L. (2002). Reducing infant immunization distress through distraction. *Health Psychol*, 21, 207–211.

Cohen, L. L. (2008). Behavioral approaches to anxiety and pain management for pediatric venous access. *Pediatrics*, 122, S134–139.

Cohen, L. L. (2010). A multifaceted distraction intervention may reduce pain and discomfort in children 4–6 years of age receiving immunisation. *Evid Based Nurs*, 13, 15–16.

Cohen, L. L., Bernard, R. S., McClellan, C. B., Piazza-Waggoner, C., Taylor, B. K., and MacLaren, J. E. (2006). Topical anesthesia versus distraction for infants' immunization distress: evaluation with 6-month follow-up. *Child Health Care*, 35, 103–121.

Cohen, L. L., Blount, R. L., Cohen, R. J., Ball, C. M., McClellan, C. B., and Bernard, R. S. (2001). Children's expectations and memories of acute distress: short- and long-term efficacy of pain management interventions. *J Pediatr Psychol*, 26, 367–374.

Cohen, L. L., Blount, R. L., Cohen, R. J., Schaen, E. R., and Zaff, J. F. (1999). Comparative study of distraction versus topical anesthesia for pediatric pain management during immunizations. *Health Psychol*, 18, 591–598.

Cohen, L. L., Blount, R. L., and Panopoulos, G. (1997). Nurse coaching and cartoon distraction: an effective and practical intervention to reduce child, parent, and nurse distress during immunizations. *J Pediatr Psychol*, 22, 355–370.

Christiano, B. and Russ, S. W. (1998). Matching preparatory intervention to coping style: the effects on children's distress in the dental setting. *J Pediatr Psychol*, 23, 17–27.

Cramer-Berness, L. J. (2007). Development of the distraction for infant immunizations: the progress and challenges. *Child Health Care*, 36, 203–217.

Dahlquist, L. M., McKenna, K. D., Jones, K. K., Dillinger, L., Weiss, K. E., and Ackerman, C. S. (2007). Active and passive distraction using a head-mounted display helmet: effects on cold pressor pain in children. *Health Psychol*, 26, 794–801.

Das, D. A., Grimmer, K. A., Sparnon, A. L., McRae, S. E., and Thomas, B. H. (2005). The efficacy of playing a virtual reality game in modulating pain for children with acute burn injuries: a randomized controlled trial. *BMC Pediatrics*, 5(1), 1.

De Jong, A. E. E., Middelkoop, E., Faber, A. W., and Van Loey, N. E. E. (2007). Non-pharmacological nursing interventions for procedural pain relief in adults with burns: a systematic literature review. *Burns*, 33, 811–827.

DeMore, M. and Cohen, L. L. (2005). Distraction for pediatric immunization pain: a critical review. *J Clin Psychol Med Settings*, 12, 281–291.

Department of Health and Human Services (n.d.). *Personalized health care*. Available at: <http://www.hhs.gov/myhealthcare/> (accessed 27 January 2012).

Fanurik, D., Zeltzer, L. K., Roberts, M. C., and Blount, R. L. (1993). The relationship between children's coping styles and psychological interventions for cold pressor pain. *Pain*, 53, 213–222.

Felt, B. T., Mollen, E., Diaz, S., Renaud, E., Zeglis, M., Wheatcroft, G., et al. (2000). Behavioral interventions reduce infant distress at immunization. *Arch Pediatr Adolesc Med*, 154, 719–730.

Fitzgerald, M. (2005). The development of nociceptive circuits. *Nat Rev Neurosci*, 6, 507–520.

Frankenstein, U. N., Richter, W., McIntyre, M. C., and Rémy, F. (2001). Distraction modulates anterior cingulate gyrus activations during the cold pressor test. *NeuroImage*, 14, 827–836.

Gershon, J., Zimand, E., Pickering, M., Rothbaum, B. O., and Hodges, L. (2004). A pilot and feasibility study of virtual reality as a distraction for children with cancer. *J Am Acad Child Adolesc Psychiatry*, 43, 1243–1249.

Hedstrom, M., Haglund, K., Skolin, I., and von Essen, L. (2003). Distressing events for children and adolescents with cancer: child, parent, and nurse perceptions. *J Pediatr Oncol Nurs*, 20, 120–132.

Hermann, C., Hohmeister, J., Demirakça, S., Zohsel, K., and Flor, H. (2006). Long-term alteration of pain sensitivity in school-aged children with early pain experiences. *Pain*, 125, 278–285.

Hettiaratchy, S. and Dziewulski, P. (2004). ABC of burns: pathophysiology and types of burns. *Br Med J*, 329, 1427–1429.

Hoffman, H. G., Chambers, G. T., Meyer, W. J., Arceneaux, L. L., Russell, W. J., Seibel, E. J., et al. (2011). Virtual reality as an adjunctive non-pharmacologic analgesic for acute burn pain during medical procedures. *Ann Behav Med*, 41, 183–191.

Hoffman, H. G., Doctor, J. N., Patterson, D. R., Carrougher, G. J., and Furness, T. A. (2000). Virtual reality as an adjunctive pain control during burn wound care in adolescent patients. *Pain*, 85, 305–309.

Hoffman, H. G., Patterson, D. R., Magula, J., Carrougher, G. J., Zeltzer, K., Dagadakis, S., et al. (2004). Water-friendly virtual reality pain control during wound care. *J Clin Psychol*, 60, 189–195.

Jaaniste, T., Hayes, B., and von Baeyer, C. L. (2007). Providing children with information about forthcoming medical procedures: a review and synthesis. *Clin Psychol Sci Pract*, 15, 124–143.

Jacobsen, R. M., Swan, A., Adegbenro, A., Ludington, S. L., Wollan, P. C., Poland, G. A., and Vaccine Research Group. (2001). Making vaccines more acceptable—methods to prevent and minimize pain and other common adverse events associated with vaccines. *Vaccine*, 19, 2418–2427.

Johnson, M. H., Breakwell, G., Douglas, W., and Humphries, S. (1998). The effects of imagery and sensory detection distracters on different measures of pain: how does distraction work? *Br J Clin Psychol*, 37, 141–154.

Jones, T., DeMore, M., Cohen, L. L., O'Connell, C., and Jones, D. J. (2008). Childhood healthcare experience, healthcare attitudes, and optimism as predictors of adolescents' healthcare behavior. *J Clin Psychol Medical Settings*, 15, 234–240.

Kennedy, R. M., Luhmann, J., and Zempsky, W. T. (2008). Clinical implications of unmanaged needle-insertion pain and distress in children. *Pediatrics*, 122, S130–S133.

Kleiber, C., Craft-Rosenberg, M., and Harper, D. C. (2001). Parents as distraction coaches during IV insertion: a randomized study. *J Pain Symptom Manage*, 22, 851–861.

Kleiber, C., and Harper, D. C. (1999). Effects of distraction on children's pain and distress during medical procedures: a meta-analysis. *Nurs Res*, 48, 44–49.

Kleiber, C., and McCarthy, A. M. (2006). Evaluating instruments for a study on children's responses to a painful procedure when parents are distraction coaches. *J Pediatr Nurs Nurs Care Child Famil*, 21, 99–107.

Kleiber, C., McCarthy, A. M., Hanrahan, K., Myers, L., Weathers, N. (2007). Development of the distraction coaching index. *Child Health Care*, 36, 219–235.

Koller, D., and Goldman, R. D. (2011). Distraction techniques for children undergoing procedures: a critical review of pediatric research. *J Pediatr Nurs*. 27, 652–681.

Kuppenheimer, W. G., and Brown, R. T. (2002). Painful procedures in pediatric cancer: a comparison of interventions. *Clin Psychol Rev*, 22, 753–786.

Liossi, C., White, P., and Hatira, P. (2009). A randomized clinical trial of a brief hypnosis intervention to control venepuncture-related pain of paediatric cancer patients. *Pain*, 142, 255–263.

MacLaren, J. E., and Cohen, L. L. (2005). A comparison of distraction strategies for venipuncture distress in children. *J Pediatr Psychol*, 30, 387–396.

McCaul, K. D., and Malott, J. M. (1984). Distraction and coping with pain. *Psychol Bull*, 95, 516–533.

McCarthy, A. M., Kleiber, C., Hanrahan, K., Zimmerman, M. B., Westhus, N., and Allen, S. (2010a). Impact of parent-provided distraction on child responses to an IV insertion. *Child Health Care*, 39, 125–141.

McCarthy, A. M., Kleiber, C., Hanrahan, K., Zimmerman, M. B., Westhus, N., and Allen, S. (2010b). Factors explaining children's responses to intravenous needle insertions. *Nurs Res*, 59, 407–415.

McGrath, P. A. (1994). Psychological aspects of pain perception. *Arch Oral Biol*, 39, 55–62.

Melzack, R. and Wall, P. D. (1965). Pain mechanisms: a new theory. *Science*, 150, 971–979.

Miller, K., Rodger, S., Bucolo, S., Greer, R., and Kimble, R. M. (2010). Multi-modal distraction. Using technology to combat pain in young children with burn injuries. *Burns*, 36, 647–658.

Morris, L. D., Louw, Q. A., and Grimmer-Somers, K. (2009). The effectiveness of virtual reality on reducing pain and anxiety in burn injury patients: a systematic review. *Clin J Pain*, 25, 815–826.

Mott, J., Bucolo, S., Cuttle, L., Mill, J., Hilder, M., Miller, K., et al. (2008). The efficacy of an augmented virtual reality system to alleviate pain in children undergoing burns dressing changes: a randomised controlled trial. *Burns*, 34, 803–808.

Mowrer, O. H. (1947). On the dual nature of learning—a reinterpretation of 'conditioning' and 'problem-solving.' *Harv Education Rev*, 17, 102–148.

Nguyen, T. N., Nilsson, S., Hellström, A. L., Bengtson, A. (2010). Music therapy to reduce pain and anxiety in children with cancer undergoing lumbar puncture: a randomized clinical trial. *J Pediatr Oncol Nurs*, 27, 146–155.

Passaretti, D. and Billmire, D. A. (2003). Management of pediatric burns. *J Craniofac Surg*, 14, 713–718.

Pate, J. T., Blount, R. L., Cohen, L. L., and Smith, A. J. (1996). Childhood medical experience and temperament as predictors of adult functioning in medical situations. *Children's Health Care*, 25, 281–298.

Pavlov, I. P. (1927). *Conditioned reflexes: an investigation of the physiological activity of the cerebral cortex.* Oxford: Oxford University Press.

Petrovic, P., Petersson, K. M., Ghatan, P. H., Stone-Elander, S., and Ingvar, M. (2000). Pain-related cerebral activation is altered by a distracting cognitive task. *Pain*, 85, 19–30.

Pillai Riddell, R., Racine, N., Turcotte, K., Uman, L. S., Horton, R., Din Osmun, L., *et al.* (2011). Nonpharmacological management of procedural pain in infants and young children: an abridged cochrane review. *Pain Res Manage*, 16, 321–330.

Richardson, J., Smith, J. E., McCall, G., and Pilkington, K. (2006). Hypnosis for procedure-related pain and distress in pediatric cancer patients: a systematic review of effectiveness and methodology related to hypnosis interventions. *J Pain Symptom Manage*, 31, 70–84.

Ruda, M. A., Ling, Q., Hohmann, A. G., Peng, Y., and Tachibana, T. (2000). Altered nociceptive neuronal circuits after neonatal peripheral inflammation. *Science*, 289, 628–630.

Sander, W. S., Eshelman, D., Steele, J., and Guzzetta, C. E. (2002). Effects of distraction using virtual reality glasses during lumbar punctures in adolescents with cancer. *Oncol Nurs Forum*, 29, E8–E15.

Schechter, N., Berde, C., and Yaster, M. (1993). *Pain in infants, children and adolescents: an overview.* Baltimore, MD: Williams and Wilkins.

Schechter, N. L., Zempsky, W. T., Cohen, L. L., McGrath, P. J., Meghan McMurtry, C., and Bright, N. S. (2007). Pain reduction during pediatric immunizations: evidence-based review and recommendations. *Pediatrics*, 119, e1184–e1198.

Schmitt, Y. S., Hoffman, H. G., Blough, D. K., Patterson, D. R., Jensen, M. P., Soltani, M., *et al.* (2011). A randomized, controlled trial of immersive virtual reality analgesia, during physical therapy for pediatric burns. *Burns*, 37, 61–68.

Smith, K. E., Ackerson, J. D., and Blotcky, A. D. (1989). Reducing distress during invasive medical procedures: relating behavioral interventions to preferred coping style in pediatric cancer patients. *J Pediatr Psychol*, 14, 405–419.

Stevens, B. J., Abbott, L. K., Yamada, J., Harrison, D., Stinson, J., Taddio, A., *et al.* (2011). Epidemiology and management of painful procedures in children in Canadian hospitals. *CMAJ*, 183, E403–E410.

Taddio, A., Chambers, C. T., Halperin, S. A., Ipp, M., Lockett, D., Rieder, M. J., and Shah, V. (2009). Inadequate pain management during childhood immunizations: the nerve of it. *Clin Ther*, 31, S152–167.

Taddio, A., Katz, J., Ilersich, A. L., and Koren, G. (1997). Effect of neonatal circumcision on pain response during subsequent routine vaccination. *Lancet*, 349, 599–603.

Uman, L. S., Chambers, C. T., McGrath, P. J., and Kisely, S. (2006). Psychological interventions for needle-related procedural pain and distress in children and adolescents. *Cochrane Database Syst Rev*, 4, CD005179.

Uman, L. S., Chambers, C. T., McGrath, P. J., and Kisely, S. (2008). A systematic review of randomized controlled trials examining psychological interventions for needle-related procedural pain and distress in children and adolescents: an abbreviated cochrane review. *J Pediatr Psychol*, 33, 842–854.

Uman, L. S., Chambers, C. T., McGrath, P. J., Kisely, S., Matthews, D., and Hayton, K. (2010). Assessing the quality of randomized controlled trials examining psychological interventions for pediatric procedural pain: recommendations for quality improvement. *J Pediatr Psychol*, 35, 693–703.

Varni, J. W., Burwinkle, T. M., and Katz, E. R. (2004). The PedsQL in pediatric cancer pain: a prospective longitudinal analysis of pain and emotional distress. *J Dev Behav Pediatr*, 25, 239–246.

Villemure, C., and Bushnell, M. C. (2002). Cognitive modulation of pain: how do attention and emotion influence pain processing? *Pain*, 95, 195–199.

Wall, P. D. (1978). The gate control theory of pain mechanisms: a re-examination and re-statement. *Brain*, 101, 1–18.

Wallace, D. P., Allen, K. D., Lacroix, A. E., and Pitner, S. L. (2010). The 'cough trick': a brief strategy to manage pediatric pain from immunization injections. *Pediatrics*, 125, e367–e373.

Wang, Z., Sun, L., and Chen, A. (2008). The efficacy of non-pharmacological methods of pain management in school age children receiving venepuncture in a paediatric department: a randomized controlled trial of audiovisual distraction and routine psychological intervention. *Swiss Med Wkly*, 138, 579–584.

Wohlheiter, K. A., and Dahlquist, L. M. (2013). Interactive versus passive distraction for acute pain management in young children: the role of selective attention and development. *J Pediatr Psychol*, 38, 202–212.

World Health Organization. (2012). Summary of WHO position papers: recommendations for routine immunization. Available at : <http://www.who.int/immunization/documents/positionpapers/en/>.

Wickens, C. D. (1984). Processing resources in attention. In R. Parasuraman, and D. R. Davies (eds.) *Varieties of attention*, pp. 63–102. Orlando, FL: Academic.

Wickens, C. D. (2002). Multiple resources and performance prediction. *Theoret Issues Ergon Sci*, 3, 159–177.

Windich-Biermeier, A., Sjoberg, I., Conkin Dale, J., Eshelman, D., and Guzzetta, C. E. (2007). Effects of distraction on pain, fear, and distress during venous port access and venipuncture in children and adolescents with cancer. *J Pediatr Oncol Nurs*, 24, 8–19.

Yoo, H., Kim, S., Hur, H., and Kim, H. (2011). The effects of an animation distraction intervention on pain response of preschool children during venipuncture. *Appl Nurs Res*, 24, 94–100.

CHAPTER 54

Hypnosis and relaxation

Christina Liossi, Leora Kuttner,
Chantal Wood, and Lonnie K. Zeltzer

Introduction

Psychological approaches to symptom management are among the oldest and are an intrinsic part of medical practice in every culture. Suggestive therapy is probably the oldest of all therapeutic methods and hypnosis under various names has been used for as long as records have been kept. Despite the fact that research on clinical hypnosis with children is still in an early stage of development and the child hypnosis literature is predominantly composed of anecdotal case histories and uncontrolled research studies, one of the best-documented uses of hypnosis is in the treatment of paediatric pain where hypnosis has achieved status as an evidenced-based/empirically supported intervention. In this chapter, the current research literature and clinical practice regarding the use of hypnosis in paediatric pain management will be discussed. First hypnosis is defined and theoretical conceptualizations are briefly discussed. Second, our current understanding of the mechanisms of hypnotic analgesia is presented. Third the research evidence for the efficacy of hypnosis in the control of acute and chronic paediatric pain is reviewed; in both sections relevant clinical techniques are discussed. Following, a description and discussion of different relaxation techniques and the evidence for their efficacy in acute and chronic pain management is presented. The chapter concludes with an attempt to summarize and evaluate the existing literature and make suggestions for future studies and clinical practice.

Hypnosis

Hypnosis is a psychological state of heightened awareness and focused attention, in which critical faculties are reduced and susceptibility and receptiveness to ideas is greatly enhanced. Hypnotic induction procedures usually consist of 'an extended initial suggestion for using one's imagination' (Green et al., 2005, p. 262), or an invitation to focus one's attention. Hypnotic inductions traditionally involve suggestions to relax, although relaxation is not necessary for hypnosis, particularly with children who respond better to more active inductions. An induction can be quite brief or longer, depending upon the hypnotic subject's responsiveness and the clinician's preferences. During hypnosis the health care professional makes suggestions for changes in subjective experience, alterations in perception, sensation, emotion, thought or behaviour (Green et al., 2005; Liossi., 2011) (see Box 54.1 for examples of hypnotic

---

> **Box 54.1** Hypnotic induction and deepening techniques for young people
>
> **Favourite activity**
>
> Imagine building a Lego house at home; just let yourself feel that way now.
>
> **Arm levitation**
>
> Pay special attention to your hand and arm. Something interesting and strange is going to happen to them ... you become aware of how warm or cold your arm is, of little muscles in your hand and arm that twitch ever so slightly ... and now perhaps you would like to imagine ... that I am fastening a string around your wrist ... fastened to the other end of the string ... over there on the ground ... lies a balloon that is not yet blown up ... what colour is it? ... that's right it is bright yellow ... now the balloon is being filled with helium ... you can see the balloon lift off the ground and rise, rise higher and higher ... the string around your wrist becomes taut ... watch what happens to the arm ... yes, it is pulling the hand and arm up ...
>
> **Ascending cloud**
>
> You are relaxing on a warm sunny day, looking at a clear blue sky ... you see a fluffy white cloud floating gently down towards you ... Hop on the cloud ... the cloud starts going up again ... you feel yourself relaxing and drifting deeper and deeper into tranquillity as you remain immersed in the cloud ... that goes higher and higher ... you float at a comfortable height.

---

inductions and supplementary online materials for video clips). Hypnosis is a natural state of aroused, attentive focal concentration coupled with relative suspension of peripheral awareness. Because hypnotic capacity is a normal and widely distributed trait, and because entry into hypnotic states occurs spontaneously, hypnotic phenomena occur frequently. Even therapists who make no formal use of hypnosis can enhance their effectiveness by learning to recognize and take advantage of hypnotic mental states.

Children have blurred boundaries between fantasy and reality, a factor that makes them ideal candidates for hypnotic interventions. They are open to new experiences, find hypnosis interesting and have few if any preconceived ideas and reservations about hypnosis. Unlike adults, children usually move and talk during hypnosis without this meaning that they are disengaging from the intervention. Young patients can also easily be taught and learn self-hypnosis, which is the act of administering hypnotic procedures on one's own (Gardner and Olness, 1981). As the therapist guides the individual to experience the hypnotic suggestions as they develop, this promotes a feeling of being active and creative in the therapeutic process and facilitates a kind of 'playful' engagement between the therapist and the child (Kuttner, 1988; Liossi and Mystakidou, 1996) which is one of the cornerstones of pain management. This engagement, while challenging, is a necessary first step in building a therapeutic alliance in which the patient, family, and therapist work together to achieve a common goal.

In paediatric practice, working with children and adolescents means working with parents from the very beginning, when evaluating the problem and throughout the treatment process. Guiding the parents to focus on and actively facilitate the use of coping strategies such as hypnosis by the young patient helps the patient and family gain a sense of control over the pain. Successful parenting strategies often strike a balance between protection and acting as a 'life coach'. In many cases parents can serve as 'life coaches' and guide, especially younger patients, to use hypnosis (see supplementary online materials for video clips).

Theoretical conceptualizations of hypnosis can be loosely classified under state and non-state, intrapersonal and interpersonal, or single and multifactor theories (Yapko, 2003) (it is beyond the scope of this chapter to discuss the merits and controversies surrounding each theory, see Kallio and Revonsuo (2003), for a review). State, intrapersonal, and single theorists maintain that hypnosis represents a cognitive process distinct from normal day-to-day cognitive processes and conceptualize it as a trance state or an altered state of consciousness, i.e. the neodissociative (Hilgard and Hilgard, 1994) and 'dissociative control' views (Bowers, 1992). The neodissociative model regards hypnosis as a state in which one or more forms of consciousness is split off from the rest of mental processing. Bowers and his colleagues maintained that subsystems of control in the brain can be activated directly rather than through higher level executive control. In other words, the strategies subjects used to reduce pain were evoked automatically without any type of conscious strategy (Bowers, 1990, 1992).

The non-state, interpersonal, and multifactor theorists, also known as sociocognitive theorists, suggest a social–psychological explanation of hypnosis. These theorists maintain that there is nothing unique about hypnosis and argue that most of the hypnotic phenomena can occur without a hypnotic induction or trance, that neither hypnotic induction nor the existence of an altered state of consciousness are necessary for hypnotic responding, including responses to suggestions for pain relief (Chaves, 1993). Hypnotic analgesia is thought to reduce pain instead through cognitive–behavioural mechanisms, in which changes in cognitions are thought to alter the affective states associated with pain (Chaves, 1993). The model suggests that the operative variables in hypnosis include contextual cues in the social environment, patient and subject expectancies, demand characteristics of the setting or situation, and role enactment (Kirsch and Lynn, 1995; Patterson and Jensen, 2003; Spanos and Chaves, 1989). The intrapersonal theories of hypnosis emphasize the subjective and inner states of the hypnotized person, whereas the interpersonal models attach more importance to the social context or relational aspects of the hypnotic interaction (Yapko, 2003).

Even though debates and controversies in the field of hypnosis have been dominated by the opposition between 'state' and 'non-state' theories, these two theoretical approaches are not mutually exclusive, have several lines of convergence, and none of these can satisfactorily explain all the phenomena associated with hypnosis. More recent theorists have suggested that attempting to explain the effects of hypnosis solely in terms of one school of thought presents distinctions that are too arbitrary and the different formulations have certainly broadened our understanding of the subject and informed clinical practice (Kihlstrom, 1992; Kirsch and Lynn, 1995; Lynn et al., 2000).

Although hypnotic analgesia is among the oldest treatments for pain (Elliotson, 1843), interest in its use seems to wax and wane. Currently, interest in hypnotic treatments for acute and chronic pain in general and paediatric pain in particular appears to be on the rise, possibly due to: (1) confirmation from adult imaging studies that chronic pain is largely influenced by, and may at times be primarily the result of, supraspinal neurophysiological processes (Jensen, 2009); (2) evidence that hypnosis has observable influences on the neurophysiological processes associated with pain (Jensen, 2009); (3) empirical evidence that hypnotic analgesia is effective for acute pain particularly procedure related and promising results from the use of hypnosis in chronic pain management.

Mechanisms of hypnotic analgesia

Early research on the neurophysiological underpinnings of pain focused on peripheral activity emanating from the site of injury. With the introduction of the gate control theory (Melzack and Wall, 1965) the focus shifted to the spinal cord and with recent improvements in imaging technology, there has been a dramatic increase in the study of the central neurophysiological correlates of pain. Now more than ever, we understand how multiple integrated pain networks work together to contribute to the global experience of pain and that the neurophysiological processes that underlie the experience of pain have peripheral, spinal, and supraspinal nervous system components (for more detail see Apkarian et al., 2005; Byers and Bonica, 2001; Craig, 2003; Terman and Bonica, 2001; Rainville, 2002).

Current evidence shows that hypnotic suggestions of analgesia may modulate pain processing at multiple levels and sites within the central nervous system. At the *peripheral* level, hypnosis may modulate nociceptive input by downregulating A delta and C fibres stimulation (Benhaiem et al., 2001) and reducing sympathetic arousal (De Benedittis et al., 1994). At a *spinal* level, sensory analgesia during hypnosis has been shown to be linearly related to a reduction of the nociceptive flexion (RIII) reflex, a polysynaptic spinal reflex that is not subject to voluntary control (Kiernan et al., 1995). Using a methodology similar to that of Kiernan et al. (1995), Danziger and colleagues (Danziger et al., 1998) later found two patterns of RIII reflex associated with hypnotic analgesia in 18 individuals with high levels of hypnotizability: 11 of their study participants showed clear inhibition and seven showed facilitation of the spinal nociceptive reflex following hypnotic analgesia suggestions. Although the reasons for the differences in response are not easily explained, they do indicate that highly suggestible individuals can show changes in spinal nociceptive reflex when given hypnotic analgesia suggestions.

A number of supraspinal sites have been shown to be involved in the perception of pain, but the areas that have been identified, most consistently, across different imaging studies are the thalamus, the primary and secondary somatosensory cortex (S1 and S2), the anterior cingulate cortex (ACC), the insula, and the prefrontal cortex (see also Apkarian et al., 2005; DeLeo, 2006). At *supraspinal* cortical level, neuroimaging studies have shown that hypnosis has direct effects on many supraspinal sites involved in the experience of pain and that hypnotic suggestions of analgesia can modulate directly both sensory and affective dimensions of the pain perception. Derbyshire and colleagues, for example, have shown that suggestions for feeling pain in the hand in healthy, pain-free individuals resulted in self-reports of pain and increased activity in the thalamus, ACC, insula, prefrontal, and parietal cortices (Derbyshire et al., 2004). The effects of suggestions on both pain intensity and cerebral activation were stronger when the suggestions followed a hypnotic induction than when participants were asked to simply 'imagine' pain without a hypnotic induction. In a follow-up study, Derbyshire and colleagues suggested to individuals with chronic pain that they would experience their clinical pain as being of 'low', 'medium', and 'high' intensity, both following and not following a hypnotic induction (Derbyshire et al., 2009). Suggestions for high pain resulted in increases in both pain and in cortical activity associated with the experience of pain, whereas suggestions for low pain resulted in decreases in pain and in cortical activity in these same areas. Similarly, to their earlier study (Derbyshire et al., 2004), the suggestions had larger effects following a hypnotic induction.

Hypnotic modulation of pain dramatically alters the cortical pain matrix. The hypnotic modulation of pain intensity produces changes in pain related activity mainly in the S1, while modulation of pain unpleasantness induces changes mainly in the ACC, with the anterior (mid) cingulate cortex possibly modulating both sensory and affect components of pain (Faymonville et al., 2000; Peyron et al., 2000). Two eloquent experimental studies have demonstrated that hypnotic suggestions can selectively alter the pain experience and have 'targeted' effects on different cortical areas. In the first, Rainville and colleagues demonstrated that hypnotic suggestions for decreased and increased pain unpleasantness succeeded in reducing and increasing ratings of pain unpleasantness, respectively, but did not affect ratings of pain intensity (Rainville et al., 1997). Consistent with the self-report findings, these same hypnotic suggestions resulted in decreases and increases in activity in the ACC only. In a follow-up study, Hofbauer and colleagues showed that hypnotic modulation of the intensity of the pain sensation led to significant changes in pain evoked activity within S1 (and a trend in S2), but not in the ACC (Hofbauer et al., 2001). This double dissociation of cortical modulation indicates a relative specialization of the sensory and the classical limbic cortical areas in the processing and modulation of the sensory and affective dimensions of pain.

However, it has to be noted that these are adult studies and differences exist between adult and child brains. Brain structural and functional development, throughout childhood and into adulthood, underlies the maturation of increasingly sophisticated cognitive abilities and a shift with age from the recruitment of 'bottom-up' processing regions towards 'top-down' fronto-cortical and fronto-subcortical connections, suggesting progressive functional integration and segregation with age leading to a more mature, and controlled cognition (Rubia, 2012). A review (Rubia, 2012) of the functional magnetic resonance imaging (fMRI) literature on brain

function development of typically late developing functions of cognitive and motivation control, timing and attention as well as of resting state neural networks shows that between childhood and adulthood, concurrent with cognitive maturation, there is progressively increased functional activation in task-relevant lateral and medial frontal, striatal, and parieto-temporal brain regions that mediate these higher level control functions. This is accompanied by progressively stronger functional inter-regional connectivity within task-relevant fronto-striatal and fronto-parieto-temporal networks. Negative age associations are observed in earlier developing posterior and limbic regions. This developmental maturation trajectory could explain the development of increasing pain coping abilities in adolescents vs. in children.

High-level attentional and cognitive control processes rely on the integrity of, and dynamic interactions between, core neurocognitive networks. The right fronto-insular cortex (rFIC) is a critical component of a salience network (SN) that mediates interactions between large-scale brain networks involved in externally oriented attention (central executive network (CEN)) and internally oriented cognition (default mode network (DMN)). Structural and functional maturation of the right fronto-insular cortex pathways is a critical component of the process by which human brain networks mature during development to support complex, flexible cognitive processes in adulthood (Uddin et al., 2011). Furthermore, neurons within the lateral ventromedial thalamic nucleus (VMl) convey selectively nociceptive information from all parts of the body. VMl neurons driven by 'whole-body' nociceptive receptive fields project to the rostral part of the layer I of the dorsolateral frontal cortex. The VMl comprises a homogeneous, organized subset of thalamic neurons that allow any signals of pain to modify cortical activity in a widespread manner, by interacting with the entire layer I of the dorsolateral neocortex (Monconduit and Villanueva, 2005).

Overall, in brain development a general pattern of functional and structural increases in connectivity and integrative processing, and a changing balance between limbic/subcortical and frontal lobe functions that extend well into young adulthood exist. Given the evidence for experience-driven structural plasticity (Markham and Greenough, 2004) an exciting yet untested hypothesis is that regular use of hypnosis by young people enhances this top-down pathway and strengthens cortical connectivity. Quantification of intervention-related changes in brain structure and function may provide further useful information about the neural mechanisms underlying the hypnotically induced pain reduction in young people with pain and also knowing which neural systems have been modified may, in turn, provide additional insights relevant for fine-tuning of the initial therapeutic strategy.

Hypnosis in acute pain management

There is strong support for the efficacy of hypnosis in procedure-related pain management and hypnosis has achieved status as an empirically validated, possibly efficacious intervention in the management of paediatric procedure-related pain (Liossi, 1999) according to the criteria devised by the American Psychological Association to judge the efficacy of psychological interventions (Chambless and Hollon, 1998). All studies conducted to date (Butler et al., 2005; Hawkins et al., 1998; Hilgard and LeBaron, 1982; Katz et al., 1987; Kellerman et al., 1983; Kuttner, 1988; Liossi and Hatira, 1999, 2003; Liossi et al., 2006, 2009; Smith et al., 1996; Wall and Womack, 1989;

Zeltzer and LeBaron, 1982) found hypnosis effective in reducing the pain and anxiety of young patients during painful medical procedures such as lumbar punctures, bone marrow aspirations, venepunctures and voiding cystourethrograms. A meta-analysis concluded that hypnosis is the most promising psychological intervention for needle procedures (Uman et al., 2006). Limited support is available in the paediatric literature that hypnosis significantly lowers postoperative pain and anxiety ratings and contributes to shorter hospital stays (Lambert, 1996).

In the most recent prospective controlled trial, the efficacy of self-hypnosis in combination with a local anaesthetic (EMLA®) was compared with EMLA® in the relief of venepuncture-induced pain and anxiety in 45 paediatric cancer outpatients (age 6–16 years; Liossi et al., 2009). Patients were randomized to one of three groups: local anaesthetic, local anaesthetic plus hypnosis, and local anaesthetic plus attention. Results confirmed that patients in the local anaesthetic plus hypnosis group reported less anticipatory anxiety, and less procedure-related pain and anxiety, and were rated as demonstrating less behavioural distress during the procedure than patients in the other two groups. The therapeutic benefit of the brief hypnotic intervention was maintained in the follow-up. Moreover, parents whose children were randomized to the EMLA plus hypnosis condition experienced less anxiety during their child's procedure than parents whose children had been randomized to the other two conditions. These findings are particularly important in that this study was a randomized, controlled trial conducted in a naturalistic medical setting.

Different hypnotic analgesic techniques can be used for acute pain management including direct suggestions such as pain displacement, symptom substitution, time distortion, topical anaesthesia, glove anaesthesia (see supplementary online materials for video clip), dissociation (see Liossi, 2002), and indirect suggestions such as therapeutic stories and metaphors. Direct and indirect suggestions have been found to be equally effective (Liossi and Hatira, 2003) (Box 54.2 provides examples of hypnotic techniques). Four out of five studies (Hilgard and LeBaron, 1982; Liossi and Hatira, 2003; Liossi et al., 2006, 2009; Wall and Womack, 1989) that have examined the relationship between the child's hypnotizability and pain relief during painful medical procedures reported a significant positive relationship between hypnotizability and clinical benefit following hypnosis treatment although the majority of children received some benefit from the intervention. In all randomized trials conducted so far, the role of the parents was critical and only their direct involvement in the intervention secured the maintenance of the therapeutic effect in when children were using self-hypnosis (Liossi et al., 2006, 2009).

Hypnosis in chronic pain management

Well-designed clinical trials and accumulated clinical experience (Banez, 2008; Galili et al., 2009) support the view that hypnosis is the most efficacious treatment for chronic abdominal pain improving pain and disability outcomes and needs to be an integral part of the biobehavioural approach to management. Chronic abdominal pain (CAP) is long lasting, intermittent, or constant pain affecting 15% to 30% of children ages 4 to 18 and presents a diagnostic and treatment challenge to the physician. Most children with this disorder are found to have no specific organic aetiology (functional abdominal pain), the predictive value of diagnostic tests is questionable, and studies of the treatment of chronic abdominal pain show inconclusive

---

Box 54.2 Hypnotic analgesic techniques for acute pain management

Switchbox

The therapist explains to the child the idea that pain is transmitted by nerves from various parts of the body to the brain, which then sends a 'pain message' back to the body (coloured drawings can be used to facilitate this explanation). The patient is asked to choose a switch that can turn off or modulate incoming nerve signals situated whenever they want (e.g. in the brain or near the site of pain). Patients are asked to practise turning the switches progressively down for defined periods of time starting with 10 to 15 secs and working up to longer periods.

Topical anaesthesia

Imagine painting numbing medicine or cream onto that part of your body and make it go deep into your skin to protect you …

Moving pain away from the self

Imagine for a while that that arm (or other body part) doesn't belong to you, isn't part of you … see it just floating out there by itself, taking all the pain away …

Directing attention to pain itself

Imagine that you have come from another planet far deep in the Universe where there is no pain … you have never experienced pain before … notice the discomfort very carefully … be curious about what sensations you have … how does it make you feel …

---

evidence regarding diet regimens as well as medical and surgical treatments (Di Lorenzo et al., 2005).

In a randomized controlled trial of 53 paediatric patients Vlieger and colleagues (Vlieger et al., 2007) compared clinical effectiveness of hypnotherapy (HT) with standard medical therapy (SMT) in children with functional abdominal pain (FAP) or irritable bowel syndrome (IBS). Patients were randomized to either HT or SMT. Hypnotherapy consisted of six sessions over a 3-month period. Patients in the SMT group received standard medical care and six sessions of supportive therapy. After 3 months of therapy, 59% of the patients in the HT group were in clinical remission with another 26% significantly improved. In the control group, receiving standard medical treatment (SMT), only 12% was in remission and 32% improved. One year after treatment, 85% of the patients treated with HT were asymptomatic versus 25% of the children who received SMT. Clinical remission was defined as greater than 80% improvement in pain scores compared with baseline.

In a follow-up study, the same investigators (Vlieger et al., 2012) explored the long-term effects of HT versus standard medical treatment plus supportive therapy (SMT). All 52 participants of their previous randomized controlled trial (RCT) were invited to complete a standardized abdominal pain diary, on which pain frequency and pain intensity were scored. All 27 HT patients and 22 out of 25 SMT patients participated in this study. After a mean duration of 4.8 years' follow-up, HT was still highly superior to conventional therapy with 68 versus 20% of the patients in remission after treatment. Also, somatization scores were lower in the HT group. However, no differences were found in quality of life, doctors' visits, and missed days of school or work between the two groups.

Vlieger and colleagues further concluded that the clinical success achieved with HT in their studies cannot be explained by improvement in rectal sensitivity (Vlieger et al., 2010). In one study they randomized 46 patients with FAP (n = 28) or IBS (n = 18) to either 12 weeks of SMT or HT. To assess rectal sensitivity, a pressure-controlled intermittent distension protocol (barostat) was performed before and after the therapy. Interestingly, no relationship was established between treatment success and rectal pain thresholds. Rectal sensitivity scores at baseline were not correlated with intensity, frequency, or duration of abdominal pain.

The multifaceted and complex nature of chronic pain requires elaborate and comprehensive hypnotic interventions delivered in a number of sessions and regular and consistent use of self-hypnosis by the patient (Wood and Bioy, 2008). Especially, when considering biopsychosocial and neuropsychological models of pain, using a combination of pain-specific and non-pain-related suggestions maybe particularly effective because these suggestions can target not only pain itself, but emotional (e.g. suggestions for improved mood), cognitive (e.g. suggestions for increased self-efficacy), and behavioural (e.g. suggestions for improved sleep) factors that play an important role in the pain experience (Dillworth and Jensen, 2010). Details of the interventions will differ depending on the exact nature of the problem, the purposes of the clinical endeavour, the goals of the health care professional, and the abilities and preferences of the young patient and their family (Liossi., 2011). Box 54.3 shows an example of a hypnotic session for chronic pain management and the case example illustrates a hypnosis based therapeutic approach across time.

Hypnotic strategies and techniques for managing chronic pain, among others, include: creating anaesthesia or analgesia, a decrease in pain, an increase in comfort and relaxation, changes in sensations from unpleasant (burning) to more pleasant (warm) ones, feeling less bothered by sensations, or changes in the meaning of pain, unconscious exploration to enhance insight or resolve conflict, cognitive-perceptual alteration of pain (and pain behaviour), and decreasing awareness of pain (distraction techniques). Other useful hypnotic approaches to pain management include self-suggestions for relaxation and a sense of global calmness, ego strengthening, being in a 'special place' (that is, a place that is beautiful, safe, relaxing, and calming to the young patient; see supplementary online material for video clip), decreased tension and emotional suffering, maintaining an appropriate level of activity, focusing on life goals other than just pain reduction, increasing participation in distracting and healthy activities, appropriate activity pacing and Rossi's (Rossi et al., 2010) mind–body healing approach. In this latter approach, hypnotic suggestions can be given during the treatment session for the patient to regress and access past learning, memory, and experience and use them as therapeutic resources for pain management.

However, it needs to be acknowledged that chronic pain in children is a multifactorial condition not easily addressed by one technique only. Multidisciplinary management is required and hypnosis should be part of a cognitive-behavioural treatment framework (see also Zeltzer and Blackett-Schlank, 2005, Kuttner, 2010).

Box 54.3 Example of a hypnotic treatment session for chronic pain management

Induction and deepening suggestions

Get ready to go aboard a submarine for an extraordinary journey under the sea! Dive deeper and deeper until the water is dark blue … look through your periscope, peek under flaps, put your scuba diving equipment on … open an airlock … and dive into the ocean …

Analgesic suggestions

The water temperature is pleasant … your body relaxes … you float happily … any discomfort that you may be experiencing is leaving your body … dissolving into the water … meet ocean animals … look at the bottom of the sea …

Imagine going back in time … to a time some time ago, before any pain or discomfort, when you were full of energy and had a sense of complete well-being … when you come back to the here and now you will feel again the same sense of well-being …

Now see the pain … what shape is it? … see its colour? … feel its texture? … now change the shape, colour and texture …

Ego-strengthening

You are going to feel physically stronger and fitter in every way … you will be surprised how enthusiastically you find yourself working on your physio exercises … you will notice feeling more alert … more wide awake … every day … you'll be more curious and interested in school and extracurricular activities … in your friends and family … in whatever is going on around you … so that your mind will become completely distracted away from yourself and your difficulties … you will be able to think more clearly … and notice how you become emotionally calmer … every day … you will feel more and more independent … every day … you will feel a greater feeling of well-being …

Post-hypnotic suggestion

From now, each and every time you feel these sensations (pain) in your muscles and bones you will immediately take in a deep breath, and as you breathe out your whole body will relax …

Termination

Now I would like you to count backwards from 5 to 1 …1 you are feeling refreshed and alert and ready to continue with whatever you were doing before…

Case example

AB, a 17-year-old athlete sustained a severe injury to her shoulder in an unexpected fall. She had several months of physiotherapy with little progress and surgery was recommended to stabilize her shoulder joint. Following surgery she developed a frozen shoulder complication resulting in a severely restricted range of motion and exquisitely tender shoulder capsule. She continued with physiotherapy but now had significant limitations in her capacity to care for herself.

Daily pain became part of her life. As a result of continuous pain, she walked protecting her shoulder from accidental bumps, avoiding crowded places and became increasingly anxious about incurring further pain. After almost 2 years of living with daily pain, physical limitations, and increasing despair, she was referred for pain management.

She presented as an organized, motivated teen, who tearfully stated that pain was a steady part of her life. Despite pain and mobility restrictions, she successfully passed her exams. She complained of continual exhaustion and difficulty sleeping. She experienced secondary neck and back pain and presented as emotionally vulnerable and mildly depressed.

Treatment

Combined with ongoing physiotherapy and pharmacotherapy, hypnosis, and relaxation were used to repattern her brain-body connection so that she could learn to:

* Successfully release tension and relax more effectively.

* Develop an awareness of well-being.

* Experience her body as capable of healing.

* Decrease intensity and areas of pain.

* Sleep and wake refreshed.

* Take accurate physical inventory.

First hypnosis session—therapeutic focus: use breath to release learned physical constrictions.

Using her breath as induction, AB was coached into slow rhythmic diaphragmatic breathing to track sensory changes: 'Notice how easily your chest opens and how this invites more comfort into … and throughout your body …' 'You can do this effortlessly and experience the softening throughout your body' (this a more effective way of saying, 'don't try so hard!').

AB reported: 'experiencing a huge weight lifted from me. I feel free and so relaxed. For the first time in many months, or maybe years, I'm breathing properly. I hadn't realized I wasn't breathing properly!'.

She undertook to practise this daily

Second hypnosis session—therapeutic focus: targeting release of her secondary neck and back pain.

Using a helium balloon as hypnotic metaphor, AB was invited to focus her attention and experience her head 'floating freely and light, so that her neck was freed of any needless holding, and her shoulders could hang-down like an ordinary well-functioning coat-hanger'

AB reported: becoming more aware of her body and wondering if 'this protection could be contributing to my pain!'. This focus helped her stop guarding her arm. *Third hypnosis session—therapeutic focus:* recreating a stable reliable sleep pattern AB closed her eyes and focused on experiencing the physiological process of falling asleep. She was given the suggestion that she could rely on this occurring each night and her body would restore itself while her mind drifted easily into dreams. In the morning she would wake refreshed, getting out of bed with a sense of purpose knowing what needs to be done and doing it comfortably.

AB reported improved sleep patterns and as a result, increased energy.

Forth hypnosis session—therapeutic focus: empowering her to assess her physical status. Using the 'body scan' hypnotic technique, AB was invited to shrink herself and travel inside her body checking out her shoulder, neck, and back and take an inventory and adjust herself for comfort. At termination AB was still using this technique. Her pain has diminished over time, range of motion greatly increased, and her mood improved.

Relaxation

McCaffery and Beebe (1994, p. 188) define relaxation as 'a state of relative freedom from both anxiety and skeletal muscle tension, a quieting or calming of the mind and muscles'. This situation is characterized by decreased intake of oxygen, decreased muscle tone, lower heart and respiratory rates, normal blood pressure, decreased skin resistance and intense, slow alpha-waves in the brain (Bulechek, 1992; McCaffery and Beebe, 1994; Watt-Watson, 1992).

There are different types of relaxation including tension-release (Jacobson, 1938), autogenic (Schultz and Luthe, 1969) and meditation (Perez-De-Albeniz and Holmes, 2000). Tension–release relaxation involves slowly tensing and then releasing each muscle group individually, starting either with the muscles in the toes and finishing with those in the head or visa verse. In autogenic training both visual imagery and body awareness are used to move a person into a deep state of relaxation. The person imagines a peaceful place and then focuses on different physical sensations, moving from the feet to the head. For example, one might focus on warmth and heaviness in the limbs, easy, natural breathing, or a calm heartbeat. Box 54.4 describes a simple autogenic relaxation exercise. The two most popular forms of meditation include transcendental meditation where the patient repeats a mantra, i.e. a single

Box 54.4 Autogenic relaxation technique

1. Choose a quiet place where you won't be interrupted.

2. Before you start, do a few gentle stretching exercises to relieve muscular tension.

3. Make yourself comfortable, either sitting or lying down.

4. Start to breathe slowly and deeply, in a calm and effortless way.

5. Focus on each part of your body, starting with your feet and working your way up to your face and head.

6. As you focus on each area, think of warmth, heaviness (or lightness) and relaxation.

7. Imagine any distracting thoughts floating away like the bubbles in a fizzy drink.

8. Stay like this for about 20 min, then take some deep breaths and open your eyes, but stay sitting or lying for a few moments before you get up.

word or phrase and mindfulness meditation. Mindfulness refers to a particular way of paying attention, that is purposefully paying attention to moment-to-moment experience in a non-judgemental and accepting manner (Kabat-Zinn, 1996). As yet, research within child and adolescent populations is in its initial stages, although preliminary results of a clinical trial have evidenced the ability of children and adolescents with chronic pain to engage with the mindfulness material and adhere to regular home practice of the techniques and apply them to presenting problems (Golianu and Waelde, 2012). After successful implementation in adult health practice, mindfulness meditation groups are beginning to gain traction in paediatric settings.

Although, approximately 43% to 58% of paediatric hospitals in the US use relaxation across a variety of acute pain situations (O'Byrne et al., 1997) doubt exists in the paediatric pain literature regarding the efficacy of relaxation as an analgesic in acute pain management. Similarly relaxation in chronic pain is usually part of a multicomponent cognitive-behavioural intervention, and can be used as a first step to establish changes in muscle tension release and some personal competency.

There is a large body of related therapies with conceptual and practical similarities that are grouped together under the term 'relaxation therapies' (NIH Technology Assessment Panel, 1996) and a corresponding large body of literature examining the effectiveness of these treatments in children with headache. Overall, even though most of these studies include children with poorly defined or several different types of headaches, this literature indicates that these techniques are effective. Two meta-analyses (Palermo et al., 2010; Trautmann et al., 2006) have provided evidence for the efficacy of relaxation training as an important treatment option for recurrent headache in childhood and adolescence although conflicting evidence exists about the effectiveness of relaxation therapy when compared with no treatment or other treatments in children with tension-type headaches (Verhagen et al., 2005). Meta-analytic findings have demonstrated a large positive effect of relaxation on pain reduction at immediate post-treatment and follow-up in youth with

headache, whereas small and non-significant effects were found for improvements in disability and emotional functioning. Long-term improvements over more than 3 years after treatment with relaxation, for tension-type as well as migraine headaches, have also been shown. Recently, applied relaxation has been presented via the Internet to children and adolescents with recurrent headache with positive effects recorded in headache frequency and duration and pain catastrophizing (Trautmann and Kroner-Herwig, 2010).

The choice of relaxation technique depends on the pain problem, the patient's preferences and abilities, professional availability, and available time. Patterson (Patterson, 1992) points out that progressive muscle relaxation generally requires lengthy and frequent training before the technique is sufficiently mastered. Certain patient populations, burned children for example, are often too exhausted and ill to invest the time or have the discipline required to learn these techniques. Taal (1998) expresses further objections to this technique because the muscles must be tensed before they can be relaxed. Muscle tension in burned parts of the body can further increase pain during wound care. In other words, even a simple technique such as progressive muscle relaxation can be inappropriate for specific pain conditions. More benefit for these patients can be expected from the use of alternative techniques such as meditation, hypnosis, or autogenic relaxation (Patterson, 1992; Taal, 1998).

Conclusion

Hypnosis and relaxation are useful therapeutic techniques for the management of acute and chronic paediatric pain, although evidence for their efficacy varies depending on the type of pain. Hypnosis is an evidence-based intervention for procedure-related pain, and appears promising in the management of chronic pain with large, well-designed studies with robust methodologies, adopting standardized formats for interventions, needed to develop a firm research evidence base. There is strong evidence that relaxation can reduce pain in children with headache both in the short and long term and some evidence that it can reduce pain outcomes in both acute and chronic non-headache pain, but in these cases relaxation is better utilized as a part of multicomponent intervention rather than a standalone treatment.

References

Apkarian, A. V., Bushnell, M. C., Treede, R. D., and Zubieta, J. K. (2005). Human brain mechanisms of pain perception and regulation in health and disease. *Eur J Pain*, 9, 463–484.

Banez, G. A. (2008). Chronic abdominal pain in children: what to do following the medical evaluation. *Curr Opin Pediatr*, 20, 571–575.

Benhaiem, J. M., Attal, N., Chauvin, M., Brasseur, L., and Bouhassira, D. (2001). Local and remote effects of hypnotic suggestions of analgesia. *Pain*, 89, 167–173.

Bowers, K. S. (1990). Unconscious influences and hypnosis. In J. L. Singer, (ed.) *Repression and disocciation: implications for personality theory, psychopathology and health*, pp. 143–178. Chicago, IL: University of Chicago Press.

Bowers, K. S. (1992). Imagination and dissociation in hypnotic responding. *Int J Clin Exp Hypn*, 40, 253–275.

Bulechek, G. and McCloskey, J. C. (1992). *Nursing interventions, essential nursing treatments*. Philadelphia, PA: W.B. Saunders Company.

Butler, L. D., Symons, B. K., Henderson, S. L., Shortliffe, L. D., and Spiegel, D. (2005). Hypnosis reduces distress and duration of an invasive medical procedure for children. *Pediatrics*, 115, e77–85.

Byers, M. and Bonica, J. (2001). Peripheral pain mechanisms and nociceptor plasticity. In J. D. Loeser, S. H. Butler, C. R. Chapman, and D. C. Turk (eds) *Bonica's management of pain* (3rd edn), pp. 26–72. Philadelphia, PA: Lippincott Williams & Wilkins.

Chambless, D. L., and Hollon, S. D. (1998). Defining empirically supported therapies. *J Consult Clin Psychol*, 66, 7–18.

Chaves, J. F. (1993). Hypnosis in pain management. In J. W. Rhue, and S. J. Lynn (eds) *Handbook of clinical hypnosis*, pp. 511–532. Washington, DC: American Psychological Association.

Craig, A. D. (2003). Pain mechanisms: labeled lines versus convergence in central processing. *Annu Rev Neurosci*, 26, 1–30.

Danziger, N., Fournier, E., Bouhassira, D., Michaud, D., De Broucker, T., Santarcangelo, E., et al. (1998). Different strategies of modulation can be operative during hypnotic analgesia: a neurophysiological study. *Pain*, 75, 85–92.

De Benedittis, G., Cigada, M., Bianchi, A., Signorini, M., and Cerutti, S. (1994). Autonomic changes during hypnosis: a heart rate variability power spectrum analysis as a marker of sympathovagal balance. *Int J Clin Exp Hypn*, 42, 141–153.

Derbyshire, S. W., Whalley, M. G., and Oakley, D. A. (2009). Fibromyalgia pain and its modulation by hypnotic and non-hypnotic suggestion: an fMRI analysis. *Eur J Pain*, 13, 542–550.

Derbyshire, S. W., Whalley, M. G., Stenger, V. A., and Oakley, D. A. (2004). Cerebral activation during hypnotically induced and imagined pain. *Neuroimage*, 23, 392–401.

Di Lorenzo, C., Colletti, R. B., Lehmann, H. P., Boyle, J. T., Gerson, W. T., Hyams, J. S., et al. (2005). Chronic abdominal pain in children: a clinical report of the American Academy of Pediatrics and the North American Society for Pediatric Gastroenterology, Hepatology and Nutrition. *J Pediatr Gastroenterol Nutr*, 40, 245–248.

Dillworth, T. and Jensen, M. P. (2010). The role of suggestions in hypnosis for chronic pain: a review of the literature. *Open Pain J*, 3, 39–51.

Elliotson, J. 1843. *Numerous cases of surgical operations without pain in the mesmeric state*. Philadelphia, PA: Lea and Blanchard.

Faymonville, M. E., Laureys, S., Degueldre, C., Delfiore, G., Luxen, A., Franck, G., et al. (2000). Neural mechanisms of antinociceptive effects of hypnosis. *Anesthesiology*, 92, 1257–1267.

Galili, O., Shaoul, R., and Mogilner, J. (2009). Treatment of chronic recurrent abdominal pain: laparoscopy or hypnosis? *J Laparoendosc Adv Surg Tech A*, 19, 93–96.

Gardner, G. G., and Olness, K. (1981). *Hypnosis and hypnotherapy with children*. New York: Grune & Stratton.

Golianu, B. and Waelde, L. (2012). Mindfulness meditation for pediatric chronic pain: effects and precautions. *BMC Complement Altern Med*, 12, 178.

Green, J. P., Barabasz, A. F., Barrett, D., and Montgomery, G. H. (2005). Forging ahead: the 2003 APA Division 30 definition of hypnosis. *Int J Clin ExpHypn*, 53, 259–264.

Hawkins, P., Liossi, C., Ewart, B., and Hatira, P. (1998). Hypnosis in the alleviation of procedure related pain and distress in paediatric oncolgy patients. *Contemporary Hypnosis* 15, 199–207.

Hilgard, E. R., and Hilgard, J. R. (1994). *Hypnosis in the relief of pain*. New York: Brunner/Mazel.

Hilgard, J. R., and Lebaron, S. (1982). Relief of anxiety and pain in children and adolescents with cancer: quantitative measures and clinical observations. *Int J Clin Exp Hypn*, 30, 417–442.

Hofbauer, R. K., Rainville, P., Duncan, G. H., and Bushnell, M. C. (2001). Cortical representation of the sensory dimension of pain. *J Neurophysiol*, 86, 402–411.

Jacobson, E. (1938). *Progressive relaxation*. Chicago, IL: Chicago University Press.

Jensen, M. P. (2009). Hypnosis for chronic pain management: a new hope. *Pain*, 146, 235–237.

Kabat-Zinn, J. (1996). *Full catastrophe living: how to cope with stress, pain and illness using mindfulness meditation*. London: Piatkus.

Kallio, S. and Revonsuo, A. (2003). Hypnotic phenomena and altered states of consciousness: a multilevel framework of description and explanation. *Contemp Hypn*, 20, 111–164.

Katz, E. R., Kellerman, J., and Ellenberg, L. (1987). Hypnosis in the reduction of acute pain and distress in children with cancer. *J Pediatr Psychol*, 12, 379–394.

Kellerman, J., Zeltzer, L., Ellenberg, L., and Dash, J. (1983). Adolescents with cancer. Hypnosis for the reduction of the acute pain and anxiety associated with medical procedures. *J Adolesc Health Care*, 4, 85–90.

Kiernan, B. D., Dane, J. R., Phillips, L. H., and Price, D. D. (1995). Hypnotic analgesia reduces r-iii nociceptive reflex—further evidence concerning the multifactorial nature of hypnotic analgesia. *Pain*, 60, 39–47.

Kihlstrom, J. F. (1992). Hypnosis: a sesquicentennial essay. *Int J Clin Exp Hypn*, 40, 301–314.

Kirsch, I. and Lynn, S. J. (1995). The altered state of hypnosis—changes in the theoretical landscape. *Am Psychol*, 50, 846–858.

Kuttner, L. (1988). Favorite stories: a hypnotic pain-reduction technique for children in acute pain. *Am J Clin Hypn*, 30, 289–295.

Kuttner, L. (2010). *A child in pain: what health professionals can do to help*. Bethel, CT: Crown House Publishing.

Lambert, S. A. (1996). The effects of hypnosis/guided imagery on the postoperative course of children. *J Dev Behav Pediatr*, 17(5), 307–310.

Liossi, C. (1999). Management of paediatric procedure-related cancer pain. *Pain Rev*, 6, 279–302.

Liossi, C. (2002). *Procedure-related cancer pain in children*. Oxford: Radcliffe Medical Press Ltd.

Liossi, C. and Hatira, P. (1999). Clinical hypnosis versus cognitive behavioral training for pain management with pediatric cancer patients undergoing bone marrow aspirations. *Int J Clin Exp Hypn*, 47, 104–116.

Liossi, C. and Hatira, P. (2003). Clinical hypnosis in the alleviation of procedure-related pain in pediatric oncology patients. *Int J Clin Exp Hypn*, 51, 4–28.

Liossi, C. and Mystakidou, K. (1996). Clinical hypnosis in palliative care. *Eur J Palliat Care*, 3, 56–58.

Liossi, C., White, P., and Hatira, P. (2006). Randomized clinical trial of local anesthetic versus a combination of local anesthetic with self-hypnosis in the management of pediatric procedure-related pain. *Health Psychol*, 25, 307–315.

Liossi, C., White, P., and Hatira, P. (2009). A randomized clinical trial of a brief hypnosis intervention to control venepuncture-related pain of paediatric cancer patients. *Pain*, 142, 255–263.

Liossi. C. (2011). Hypnosis in chronic pain management. In P. Brook, T. Pickering, and J. Connell (eds) *Oxford handbook of pain management.*, pp. 266–268. Oxford: Oxford University Press.

Lynn, S., Kirsch, I., Barabasz, A., Cardeña, E., and Patterson, D. (2000). Hypnosis as an empirically supported clinical intervention. The state of evidence and a look to the future. *Int J Clin Exp Hypn* 48, 239–259.

Markham, J. A., and Greenough, W. T. (2004). Experience-driven brain plasticity: beyond the synapse. *Neuron Glia Biol*, 1, 351–363.

McCaffery, M. and Beebe, A. (1994). *Pain, clinical manual for nursing practice*. London: Mosby.

Melzack, R. and Wall, P. D. (1965). Pain mechanisms: a new theory. *Science*, 150, 971–979.

Monconduit, L. and Villanueva, L. (2005). The lateral ventromedial thalamic nucleus spreads nociceptive signals from the whole body surface to layer I of the frontal cortex. *Eur J Neurosci*, 21, 3395–3402.

NIH Technology Assessment Panel on Integration of Behavioral and Relaxation Approaches into the Treatment of Chronic Pain and Insomnia. (1996). Integration of behavioral and relaxation approaches into the treatment of chronic pain and insomnia. *JAMA*, 276, 313–318.

O'Byrne, K. K., Peterson, L., and Saldana, L. (1997). Survey of pediatric hospitals' preparation programs: Evidence of the impact of health psychology research. *Health Psychol*, 16(2), 147–154. doi: 10.1037/0278-6133.16.2.147.

Palermo, T. M., Eccleston, C., Lewandowski, A. S., Williams, A. C., and Morley, S. (2010). Randomized controlled trials of psychological therapies for management of chronic pain in children and adolescents: an updated meta-analytic review. *Pain*, 148, 387–397.

Patterson, D. R. (1992). Practical applications of psychological techniques in controlling burn pain. *J Burn Care Rehabil*, 13, 13–18.

Patterson, D. R., and Jensen, M. P. (2003). Hypnosis and clinical pain. *Psychol Bull*, 129, 495–521.

Perez-De-Albeniz, A. and Holmes, J. (2000). Meditation: concepts, effects and uses in therapy. *Int J Psychother*, 5, 49–59.

Peyron, R., Laurent, B., and Garcia-Larrea, L. (2000). Functional imaging of brain responses to pain. A review and meta-analysis. *Neurophysiol Clin*, 30, 263–288.

Rainville, P. (2002). Brain mechanisms of pain affect and pain modulation. *Curr Opin Neurobiol*, 12, 195–204.

Rainville, P., Duncan, G. H., Price, D. D., Carrier, B., and Bushnell, M. C. (1997). Pain affect encoded in human anterior cingulate but not somatosensory cortex. *Science*, 277, 968–971.

Rossi, E. L., Erickson-Klein, R., and Rossi, K. (2010). *Mind-body healing and rehabilitation*. Phoenix, AZ: The Milton H. Erickson Foundation Press.

Rubia, K. (2012). Functional brain imaging across development. *Eur Child Adolesc Psychiatry*, 24 June. [Epub ahead of print.]

Schultz, J. H., and Luthe, W. (1969). *Autogenic methods*. New York: Grune & Stratton.

Smith, J. T., Barabasz, A., and Barabasz, M. (1996). Comparison of hypnosis and distraction in severely ill children undergoing painful medical procedures. *J Counsel Psychol*, 43, 187–195.

Spanos, N. and Chaves, J. (1989). *Hypnosis: the cognitive-behavioral perspective*. Buffalo, NY: Prometheus Books.

Taal, L. A. (1998). *The psychological aspects of burn injuries*. Maastricht: Shaker Publishing B.V.

Terman, G. and Bonica, J. (2001). Spinal mechanisms and their modulation. *Bonica's management of pain* (3rd edn). Philadelphia, PA: Lippincott Williams & Wilkins.

Trautmann, E. and Kroner-Herwig, B. (2010). A randomized controlled trial of Internet-based self-help training for recurrent headache in childhood and adolescence. *Behav Res Ther*, 48, 28–37.

Trautmann, E., Lackschewitz, H., and Kroner-Herwig, B. (2006). Psychological treatment of recurrent headache in children and adolescents—a meta-analysis. *Cephalalgia*, 26, 1411–1426.

Uddin, L. Q., Supekar, K. S., Ryali, S., and Menon, V. (2011). Dynamic reconfiguration of structural and functional connectivity across core neurocognitive brain networks with development. *J Neurosci*, 31, 18578–18589.

Uman, L. S., Chambers, C. T., McGrath, P. J., and Kisely, S. (2006). Psychological interventions for needle-related procedural pain and distress in children and adolescents. *Cochrane Database Syst Rev*, 4, CD005179.

Verhagen, A. P., Damen, L., Berger, M. Y., Passchier, J., Merlijn, V., and Koes, B. W. (2005). Conservative treatments of children with episodic tension-type headache. A systematic review. *J Neurol*, 252, 1147–1154.

Vlieger, A. M., Menko-Frankenhuis, C., Wolfkamp, S. C., Tromp, E., and Benninga, M. A. (2007). Hypnotherapy for children with functional abdominal pain or irritable bowel syndrome: a randomized controlled trial. *Gastroenterology*, 133, 1430–1436.

Vlieger, A. M., Rutten, J. M., Govers, A. M., Frankenhuis, C., and Benninga, M. A. (2012). Long-term follow-up of gut-directed hypnotherapy vs. standard care in children with functional abdominal pain or irritable bowel syndrome. *Am J Gastroenterol*, 107, 627–631.

Vlieger, A. M., Van Den Berg, M. M., Menko-Frankenhuis, C., Bongers, M. E., Tromp, E., and Benninga, M. A. (2010). No change in rectal sensitivity after gut-directed hypnotherapy in children with functional abdominal pain or irritable bowel syndrome. *Am J Gastroenterol*, 105, 213–218.

Wall, V. J., and Womack, W. (1989). Hypnotic versus active cognitive strategies for alleviation of procedural distress in pediatric oncology patients. *Am J Clin Hypn*, 31, 181–191.

Watt-Watson, J. and Donovan, M. (eds) (1992). *Pain management, nursing perspective*. St Louis, MO: Mosby-Year Book Inc.

Wood, C. and Bioy, A. (2008). Hypnosis and pain in children. *J Pain Symptom Manage*, 35, 437–446.

Yapko, M. (2003). *Trancework: an introduction to the practice of clinical hypnosis*. New York: Brunner-Routledge.

Zeltzer, L. and Blackett-Schlank, C. (2005). *Conquering your child's chronic pain: a pediatrician's guide for reclaiming a normal childhood*. New York: HarperCollins.

Zeltzer, L. and Lebaron, S. (1982). Hypnosis and nonhypnotic techniques for reduction of pain and anxiety during painful procedures in children and adolescents with cancer. *J Pediatr*, 101, 1032–1035.

Online supplementary materials

Video 54.1 Hypnosis for procedural pain management: "Favourite Place". Reproduced with permission from Leora Kuttner (dir.), *No Fears No Tears*, Copyright © 1985.

Video 54.2 Hypnosis for procedural pain management: "The Magic Glove". Reproduced with permission from Leora Kuttner (dir.), *No Fears No Tears*, Copyright © 1985.

Video 54.3 Hypnosis for acute pain management: Focussed breathing. Reproduced with permission from Leora Kuttner (dir.), *No Fears No Tears*, Copyright © 1985.

Video 54.4 Hypnosis for persistent pain management: Dissociation Imagery. Reproduced with permission from Leora Kuttner (dir.), *No Fears No Tears*, Copyright © 1985.

CHAPTER 55

New information and communication technologies for pain

Jennifer Stinson and Lindsay Jibb

Summary

The rapid growth in the amount and availability of information and communication technology (ICT) in the last decade means that several new tools have become available to monitor and manage chronic pain. These tools include the Internet (and associated social support networks), mobile phones, and telemedicine and they are being used to enable self-management by people suffering from persistent pain. The benefits of ICT-based pain therapies are many and include improved treatment accessibility and satisfaction, as well as potential decreases in therapy cost. ICT therapies for people in pain represent exciting treatment possibilities. Future, rigorous research into the design and effectiveness of these therapies will shed more light on how ICT might improve the quality of life for people with chronic pain.

Introduction

Over the past decade there has been tremendous growth in the development and evaluation of ICT to deliver health care interventions including those for the treatment of chronic pain. Results from a 2010 telephone survey of 3001 American adults showed that 80% of Internet users accessed health information online and 14% accessed information specific to managing chronic pain (Fox, 2011). From a public health perspective, there is great potential for self-administered treatments to improve the health of individuals who suffer from chronic pain but are unable to access services. ICT-based programmes offer an innovative approach to improve the availability, accessibility, and acceptability of these programmes. This chapter will review ICT for pain by: defining chronic pain self-management, discussing barriers to the provision of pain self-management and psycho-educational interventions, and discussing methods by which ICT can overcome these barriers. The theories, processes, and content elements of ICT-based chronic pain programmes are defined and described. The evidence, where available, from treatment intervention trials and the advantages and disadvantages of telehealth, internet-based programmes, and mobile-health (m-health) or

Smartphone applications (apps) for the management of chronic pain are reviewed. Future directions for theory, research, and clinical practice are also described.

Chronic pain self-management

Chronic pain is common in adults (Johannes et al., 2010) as well as children and adolescents (King et al., 2011) and can negatively impact all aspects of life including physical, emotional, social, and role functioning (Law et al., 2012; Palermo, 2000; Reid et al., 2011). Chronic pain may include varying amounts of disability and may be independent of the amount of tissue damage and perceived severity of injury (Huguet and Miro, 2008; Melzack and Wall 1965). In the likely absence of a cure or total pain relief, the prevention of pain-related disability and the improvement of quality of life through better chronic pain self-management are critical (Ritterband et al., 2003). Self-management can be defined as 'the individual's ability to manage the symptoms, treatment, physical, and psychological consequences and lifestyle changes inherent in living with a chronic illness' (Barlow et al., 2002).

Self-management interventions that provide individuals with knowledge about pain, strategies to manage pain (cognitive-behavioural therapies or CBT), and social support are needed to promote optimal health outcomes. Studies in adult chronic illnesses (Foster et al., 2007; Lorig and Holman, 1993; Smith et al., 2005) have shown that comprehensive interactive face-to-face psycho-educational interventions lead to symptom reduction and improved quality of life compared with care that is strictly medication focused. The proposed mechanism of effect for this phenomenon is presumed to be enhanced self-efficacy (i.e. belief in one's ability to successfully perform a behaviour) and empowerment over disease and symptom management (Marks et al., 2005a, 2005b). For example, Lefort and colleagues (1998) found that a 12-h community-based, chronic pain psycho-educational programme led to significant short-term improvements in pain, independence, vitality, aspects of role functioning, life satisfaction, self-efficacy and resourcefulness compared to a wait-list control group in adults with chronic pain.

Variations in pain-related disability exist in young people and adults with chronic pain. However, the majority of the variance is related to several physical, psychological, and social variables (Bargiel-Matusiewicz and Krzyszkowska, 2009; Lynch et al., 2007). Thus, intervening in the pain experiences of young people and adults with chronic pain requires a broad framework that comprehensively addresses the physical and psychosocial precipitants, as well as modifiers and consequences, of chronic pain (Rapoff and Lindsley, 2000). The most successful interventions in improving pain and associated impairments in adults with chronic health conditions (including pain) are based on CBT (LeFort et al., 1998). CBT incorporate normalization of the patient's experience through education about the condition and its impact, training in specific strategies, including managing disease-related and other stressors, and guidance on developing and implementing a long-term plan for self-managing the condition (Palermo et al., 2010).

Barriers to the provision of pain psychosocial interventions

There is a solid empirical foundation supporting CBT interventions to equip individuals with the necessary coping skills to reduce chronic pain and pain-related disability (Barlow et al., 1999; Jensen, 2010; Lineker et al., 1996; Stinson et al., 2012). Historically, barriers to accessing comprehensive chronic pain-specific education and cognitive behavioural coping skills training have included: (1) limited access to services in many geographic areas (including rural and remote regions), (2) language barriers (programs offered only in English), (3) and long-wait times (Elgar and McGrath et al., 2003; Peng et al., 2006; Stinson et al., 2008; Stinson et al., 2010); (4) limited availability of trained professionals such as psychologists, particularly in non-urban centres; (5) time restrictions limiting the amount of content reviewed during regular chronic pain clinic or primary care visits; and (6) additional costs (direct and indirect) including costs of CBT and time off work and/or school associated with these therapies (Barlow and Ellard, 2006; Barlow et al., 1999; Elgar and McGrath, 2003; Lineker et al., 1996; Stinson et al., 2012).

New technologies as an intervention medium to overcome barriers to pain care

With emerging ICT (e.g. telehealth, Internet, smartphone apps), new media for the delivery of health interventions are now available (Ritterband et al., 2003). For example, the Internet has emerged as one of the top health information resources and modes of social communication, especially for youths and young adults, and continues to be increasingly integrated into the provision of health care services (Drotar et al., 2006; Gray et al., 2005; Griffiths et al., 2006). In developed countries, the vast majority of people have Internet access at home, work, school, or through the use of mobile technology (Fox, 2011; Klasnja and Pratt, 2012). ICT provides patients, families, and health care professionals with unparalleled opportunities to: (1) learn, inform, and communicate with one another; (2) receive meaningful social support; (3) fulfil the rising demand for expedient access to evidence-based health information; and (4) achieve greater involvement in health care decision-making

(Griffiths et al., 2006; Ritterband et al., 2003). Using ICT to deliver health interventions dramatically reduces geographic constraints, provides opportunities for access regardless of language spoken and travel constraints (financial or due to physical disability) and provides more immediate access to information that can help patients feel less isolated and more in control of managing their chronic condition (Griffiths et al., 2006; Nguyen et al., 2004).

Research into ICT-based psycho-educational and disease self-management interventions for adults has rapidly increased over the past decade, with results from systematic and meta-analytic reviews suggesting excellent efficacy for symptom reduction, knowledge attainment, and improved health behaviours across a wide range of chronic conditions including chronic pain (Cuijpers et al., 2008; Lorig et al., 2008; Murray et al., 2005; Nguyen et al., 2004; Palmqvist et al., 2007; Spek et al., 2007; Wantland et al., 2004). However, there is less empirical data on the availability and effectiveness of ICT-based psycho-educational and disease self-management interventions for children and adolescents with chronic health conditions (Cushing and Steele, 2010; Lelieveld et al., 2010; March et al., 2009; Palermo et al., 2010; Ritterband et al., 2003; Runge et al., 2006; Stinson et al., 2009). In the following sections, the evidence from treatment intervention trials and the advantages and disadvantages of telehealth, Internet-based programmes, and m-health (including smartphone apps) for management of chronic pain will be described.

Theoretical frameworks for ICT-based pain self-management programmes

Murray and colleagues (2005) have developed a theoretical pathway to explain changes in health outcomes mediated by ICT (primarily Internet-based programmes). According to this pathway, ICT work by combining information with peer, decision-making, and behavioural change supports to allow internalization and interpretation of the information by the user. A combination of enhanced self-efficacy with motivation and knowledge, enables users to change their health behaviours leading to changes in clinical outcomes (Murray et al., 2005).

Ritterband and colleagues (2009) have built upon this postulated pathway of change by including characteristics of the end-users (i.e. demographic, disease, cognitive and physiological factors; personality traits; beliefs and attitudes; self-efficacy and skills), the environment, and the Web-based programme (see Figure 55.1) (Ritterband et al., 2009). While this model was based on Internet-based programmes, the key concepts are applicable to other ICTs as well. The model purports that programme users are influenced by environmental factors (i.e. family, friends, significant others, employers/school, health care system, community, and societal influences) which affect website use and adherence. Website use and adherence is also influenced by the type of support provided (e.g. email, phone, face-to-face) and characteristics of the website (e.g. appearance, behavioural prescriptions (e.g. contracts, prompts), content, burden (e.g. difficulty of use, length), delivery (e.g. animations, audio, illustrations, text, testimonials), message (e.g. source and style), participation (e.g. interaction, reinforcement, testing) and assessment (e.g. personalized or tailoring)). Finally, website use leads to changes in behaviour that results in symptom improvement through various mechanisms of change such as gaining knowledge, changing attitudes and beliefs, motivation, and skill building.

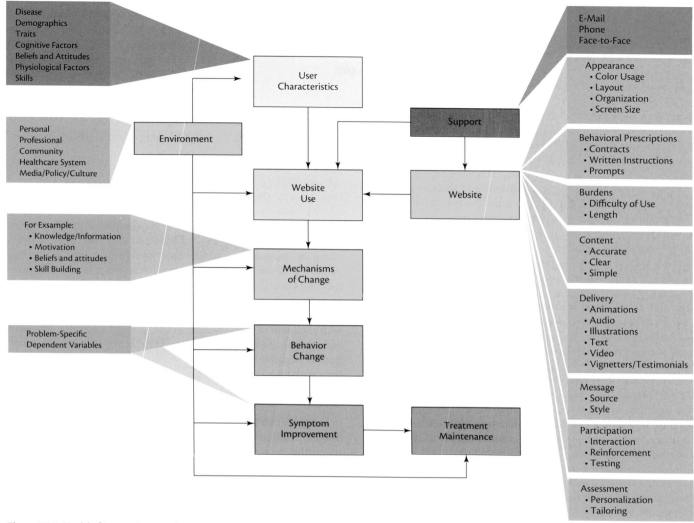

Figure 55.1 Model of Internet interventions.
Reproduced from Lee M. Ritterband et al., A behavior change model for internet interventions, *Annals of Behavioral Medicine*, Volume 38, No. 1, pp. 18–27, Copyright © The Society of Behavioural Medicine 2009, with kind permission from Springer Science and Business Media, http://www.springer.com/medicine/journal/12160.

Internet-based chronic pain interventions

Improvements in Internet access and broadband speeds have led to an increase in Web-based treatments for chronic pain. Therapeutic Internet-based interventions are treatments based on effective face-to-face interventions (e.g. psycho-educational and CBT) that are transformed for delivery via the Internet with the goal of improved health outcomes (symptom reduction (pain and pain-related disability; decreased anxiety and depression) and improved health-related quality of life). Usually, Internet-based interventions are highly structured, self-guided or partly self-guided (i.e. minimal therapist support through regular brief telephone and or email contact), tailored to the user's needs and interactive (Ritterband et al., 2003). While this is a burgeoning field, the Internet remains a relatively new medium for delivery of psychosocial health interventions. Formal evaluations of the impact of Internet health interventions on health outcomes, level of resource utilization and user satisfaction have lagged far behind intervention development (Danaher and Seeley, 2009; Nguyen et al., 2004).

The literature on Internet-based chronic pain interventions is rapidly growing with studies on feasibility and utility, as well as evidence of efficacy in improving clinical health outcomes being conducted (Lorig et al., 2008, Macea et al., 2010). Macea and colleagues recently conducted a meta-analysis of the efficacy of Web-based self-guided cognitive-behavioural interventions (4–7 weeks in length) with minimal therapist involvement (emails and/or telephone contact) for chronic pain. The primary outcome in this analysis was pain intensity. Eleven RCTs, including 2953 participants (67.5% women with mean age 41.32 (range: 7–91) years), with ten different pain-related disorders (low back pain and arthritis typically) were included. The pooled effect size (standardized mean difference between intervention and wait-list control group means) from a random effects model was 0.28 (95% confidence interval: 0.14, 0.42). Internet-based interventions resulted in significant changes favouring the experimental group in variables including medication use, health care visits, return to work capacity and pain reduction. In summary, the authors showed small treatment effects for improvement of pain, greater improvements in pain-related conditions such as work disability and that CBT interventions are effective. All studies in this review used wait-list controls instead of placebo control, thus placebo effects remain to be examined in future trials.

More recently, Bender and colleagues conducted a systematic review of 17 RCTs of Internet-based pain interventions; however, this review incorporated both acute and chronic pain conditions (Bender et al., 2011). The 17 studies included interventions providing either CBT (n = 11), moderated peer support programmes (n = 3), or clinical visit preparation/follow-up support (n = 3) to 2503 individuals in pain. Most Internet-based CBT trials (72.2%) used wait-list control conditions and three used comparable Internet-based control conditions. Interventions consisted of structured, self-administered therapy programmes offered in weekly modules that ranged in length from 6 to 20 weeks. All interventions included support from a clinical or research staff person via telephone, email, asynchronous or synchronous message boards. Minimal support typically included providing feedback on weekly reports, reminders to complete programme activities and administrative or technical assistance. Seven of eleven studies evaluated outcomes in adults and four evaluated outcomes in children and adolescents. The majority of studies showed improvements in pain (n = 7; 77.8%), activity limitation (n = 4; 57.1%) and costs associated with treatment (n = 3; 100%), whereas effects on depression (n = 2, 28.6%) and anxiety (n = 2, 50%) were less consistent.

In addition, a review and meta-analysis of computerized CBT programmes for pain, aimed specifically at children and adolescents was conducted by Velleman and colleagues (2010). Four studies met the inclusion criteria and all demonstrated 50% reduction in pain compared to control groups that was maintained out to 3 months. Meta-analysis results suggested a pooled medium effect size of −0.41 for reduction of pain intensity post-treatment with mean odds ratio of 0.63 for achieving clinically significant reductions in pain. These three systematic reviews provide growing evidence that Internet-based interventions reduce pain and pain-related disability. However, evidence on other important outcomes such as emotional functioning and cost-effectiveness compared to traditional face-to-face therapies remains to be determined.

While there are many advantages of Internet-based pain therapies; the current evidence suggests several limitations as well. For instance, given the self-guided nature and relative anonymity of this medium high trial dropout rates compared to traditional face-to-face therapies have been observed (Bender et al., 2011). However, adding human support via brief telephone/email contact with a therapist, or lay peers, and/or including social networking opportunities for intervention participants has improved motivation and adherence to online health care services, thereby optimizing the achievement of desired outcomes (Nguyen et al., 2004; Palmqvist et al., 2007; Rosser et al., 2011; Spek et al., 2007; Stinson et al., 2009). It is important that future studies collect information on reasons for dropout to inform the development of strategies to improve the adherence and efficacy of these interventions. In addition, motivational interviewing regarding readiness to change pain behaviours represents another promising method to help reduce dropout rates (Duff and Latchford, 2010; Vong et al., 2011).

Social support in the age of the Internet

Social support is a multidimensional concept, which describes the formal and informal relationships developed to provide for the needs of individuals. Social support has been identified as a key factor in aiding patients in managing painful conditions and coping with related diagnoses (Rodham et al., 2009). Social support may take the form of peer education and peer networks fostering identity, empathy, and empowerment (Polomano et al., 2007); making it an important factor in establishing effective self-management behaviours.

Several positive health outcomes from social support have been identified in people with chronic pain. For instance, von Weiss and colleagues (2002) found that in children with painful rheumatic diseases, high levels of social support predicted lower levels of depression regardless of the level of daily hassle perceived to be due to the disease. Supportive social networks may also result in facilitating self-management behaviours and smoother transitions from paediatric to adult health care for adolescents with chronic painful conditions (Stinson et al., 2008; van Staa et al., 2011). Engaging in supportive and understanding social networks also results in improvements in long-term functional disability and pain in adults with rheumatoid arthritis (Evers et al., 2003). In addition, in adults with chronic pain, supportive social interactions resulted in reductions in negative mood feelings and improved perceived abilities to cope with their diagnosis (Feldman et al., 1999).

Modern social networking

In recent years, the advent of the Internet and associated technologies has resulted in new means by which people may engage in socially supportive networks. Technology-based social networks have been used to connect people with members of existing communities, to build new communities and as modalities to disseminate and transfer knowledge (Henderson et al., 2012; Polomano et al., 2007; Scanfeld et al., 2010; Subrahmanyam et al., 2008). At present, social networking is amongst the most common reasons people access the Internet (Henderson et al., 2012). Technology-based social networking may take the form of electronic peer feedback generated from thoughts and experiences published on personal blogs and short Twitter messages or through more interactive discussion forums, online support groups and listservs (Barak et al., 2009).

The advantages of technology-based social networking opportunities for individuals with pain are many. Participating in blogging is postulated to act as an adjunct to other psychological and behavioural therapies by enabling self-reflection, debate and knowledge-exchange (Barak et al., 2009; Tan, 2008). Furthermore, the skills required to engage in online networking are relatively easy to learn and, in the case of children and young adults who have lived their entire lives in the age of the Internet (Henderson et al., 2012), are typically already possessed. Networks established via ICT have the added advantage of increasing accessibility to social support for people with pain. Online communication may act as a means to create social support networks, which would otherwise be difficult to build for persons with stigmatizing health conditions (Bargh et al., 2002; Henderson et al., 2012). Virtual communities can also facilitate interactions between people with chronic pain conditions. Peer–peer interactions may be problematic for those with rare medical presentations or those living in more remote communities. Research suggests that people with chronic and life-limiting health conditions desire the ability to make social connections and seek social support from their peers with the same condition (Bender et al., 2011; Kearney et al., 2009; Stinson et al., 2008). ICT may circumvent this issue and increase accessibility to social support networks for all people with painful health conditions.

Online social networking for people with pain

The limited number of studies (n = 2) examining peer social support in adults with chronic pain show preliminary but positive effects on pain outcomes. These studies include a 2002 investigation by Lorig and colleagues into the use of an email-based listserv to connect people with pain. Peer support was provided in a second study through the use of an Internet-based asynchronous discussion forum (Lorig et al., 2008). Chronic pain conditions in these studies were recurrent lower back pain (Lorig et al., 2002) and arthritis (Lorig et al., 2008). Both of the interventions included group moderation by either peers or health care providers and in both cases, study sample sizes were large (range: 580–855). Peer support provided by the e-mail based listserv resulted in significant reductions in pain intensity, disability, and distress in the intervention group (Lorig et al., 2002). Use of the peer moderated discussion forum by people with arthritis resulted in significant reductions in pain intensity, distress, activity limitation, and improvements in health status (Lorig et al., 2008). However, neither study was able to show a reduction in health care utilization. In addition, clinically significant changes in health outcomes were not described in either study. A third study examined the effectiveness of using email-based peer support by adults with chronic low back pain to enhance the use of complementary and alternative medicine (CAM) modalities (Bruce et al., 2005). This study showed that participants in the intervention group did not differ from those in the control group, suggesting that peer support may be ineffective in enhancing the use of CAM therapies for pain.

Despite increasing interest in the prevalence and effectiveness of social support networking by people with pain, very little is known about how this group uses the most common social networking sites (although pain-related Facebook groups and Twitter handles do exist at present). Facebook, Twitter, and MySpace are some of the most widely accessed websites in use today. Facebook alone reports over 800 million members, with 400 million logging on to the site daily (Facebook, 2012). Social support networks for people with health issues have been established on these widely-used communication platforms often by patients or their family and friends (as opposed to health care providers; Bender et al., 2011). Created groups are typically informally moderated by more active group members and lack formal hierarchical organization.

In its early stages, Internet-based social networking appears to be a promising avenue to elicit accessible social support for people with pain; it is, however, not without inherent limitations. For instance, the majority of current social support networks are unmoderated and operate with little or no input from clinical or research experts. Given the sensitive nature of the information, opinions, and beliefs being expressed through these networks, monitoring by health care professionals or disease-specific organisations is warranted. In addition, support group websites should clearly present authorship details and disclaimers related to use. Health care professionals must also engage in conversations with patients about the benefits and drawbacks of participating Internet-based social support groups.

m-Health technologies and pain

Mobile devices such as cellular phones and personal digital assistants (PDAs) represent another novel pain modality for monitoring and managing pain. In addition, the widespread use of mobile devices (85% of surveyed Americans) with increasing technical capabilities (Raine, 2010) increases the number of people electronic health interventions can reach. At present, several different mobile technology applications are being developed and tested for use in health care (Klasnja and Pratt, 2012).

The most basic of the mobile technology interventions is text messaging (short messaging service or SMS), a service allowing messages of 160 characters to be sent between mobile phones. Because the vast majority of mobile phones are capable of sending and receiving SMS, this service does not suffer from the potential drawbacks of more expensive devices (e.g. iPhones, BlackBerrys, devices with Android-based operating systems) and is commonly used in the developing world (Klasnja and Pratt, 2012). Potential health intervention uses of SMS technology include: (1) the logging of symptom data, (2) communication with health care providers and (3) the ability for patients to receive remote reminders to engage in health behaviours (Klasnja and Pratt, 2012).

A more complex use of mobile technologies for health condition management comes in the form of automated clinical decision support systems (CDSSs). The number of CDSS has increased greatly in the last two decades and CDSSs currently under development vary in their purpose and their intended user-groups (Moxey et al., 2010). Some are intended to provide health care professionals with evidence-based advice on how to proceed with patient care (Garg et al., 2005; Trafton et al., 2010). Others are designed in a 'shared-care' tradition and are intended to inform management strategies through direct use by patients (Gibson et al., 2010; Kearney et al., 2009). Because of the technical programming intricacies of these systems, they are typically available only on mobile devices that support more complex platforms, such as the iPhone or Android-operating system phones. At this time however, only a few evidence-based mobile technology-based interventions for pain management exist.

Recently, a review of 111 smartphone apps for the management of pain due to a wide variety of conditions was conducted (Rosser and Eccleston, 2011). Apps were targeted at a range of health conditions known to cause pain with the most common conditions targeted being headache or migraine (39%), followed by back pain (16%). The content of apps available at the time of review varied with 54% including education related to pain and its management, 24% including pain diary capabilities, and 17% including relaxation or meditation leading capabilities. Importantly, 86% of the apps did not report the involvement of health care professionals in content development and none have undergone rigorous evaluation using RCTs.

m-Health technologies under development

A mobile phone-delivered, and Web-based chronic pain intervention

A mobile phone-based intervention for people with chronic widespread pain has recently been developed and is in the pre-trial stages of effectiveness testing (Kristjansdottir et al., 2011). This intervention involves the remote delivery of CBT using SMS. The study involved six participants (23–48 years) with chronic wide-spread pain who completed multidimensional pain diary entries for 4 weeks on phones. A therapist then remotely logged on to a secure website, viewed the diary entries, and provided individualized feedback aimed at stimulating patient self-management of the current pain situation. This intervention received high participant acceptability and usability ratings. In addition, compliance with diary entries was high (78–94% of entries completed) and technical problems with the intervention were infrequent and minor.

In developing mobile phone-based pain management interventions, researchers and developers should seek the expertise of health care professionals in the design and implementation of mobile pain management programmes to help ensure usefulness and safety. Rigorous testing of these interventions (i.e. via randomised controlled trials or RCTs) is also needed to determine their effectiveness. Successful evidence-based development of m-health interventions for people with pain may result in accessible care and improved outcomes, making research exploration in this area important.

Telemedicine/telehealth

Telemedicine or telehealth refers to telecommunication systems in the broadest sense and includes the use of technology to help deliver and support health services (e.g. call centres, cell phones, video-conferencing, and web-based platforms). Telemedicine methods have been proposed as a means to improve access to pain management programming provided that appropriate therapists and remuneration policies are in place (MacDonald et al., 2011). A recent systematic review of telehealth for pain management found that only a limited number of RCT examinations of telemedicine versus traditional therapies exist (McGeary et al., 2012). However, based on currently available literature, there is good preliminary evidence to believe that telemedicine is an effective and viable means of managing pain (McGeary et al., 2012). The costing of telemedicine methods for pain management in adults with chronic pain has also been compared to traditional face-to-face therapies in a RCT (Pronovost et al., 2009). Results showed that direct patient costs were significantly lower in the telemedicine group than the face-to-face group and that more participants in the telemedicine group were satisfied with their consultation.

Future directions for theory, research, and clinical practice

There is great excitement and opportunity associated with new ICT for the management of long-term health conditions such as chronic pain. While there is enthusiasm, there are a number of theoretical, research and clinical issues that need further consideration. First, consensus and standards on methods of development and metrics for evaluation of ICT-based health care treatments need to be developed. There is currently little guidance on how to develop or translate therapy from traditional human face-to-face to ICT-based delivery system. To this end, user-centred designs must be the starting point. The needs and perspectives of people in pain regarding ICT-based therapies (i.e. when and under what conditions ICT therapy is preferred to face-to-face) needs to be the first step guiding development of these interventions.

Despite the rapid adoption of these therapies, a technological divide does still exist in terms of age-related differences in technology confidence, skill, and use and the unequal provision of costly infrastructure (broadband computing) in different communities. The extent to which these interventions can be independent of any human support (lay person, trained non-health care professionals, health care professionals) is not known. There is evidence that self-guided or minimal human involvement is associated with greater patient dropout compared to face-to-face therapy. Determination of the minimum amount of support required to improve outcomes and the most appropriate person to provide that support is needed.

The essential ingredients that are needed in ICT-based programmes are also largely unknown and should be determined by conducting dismantling studies. We need to determine what types of patients are best served by these programmes and when in the pain trajectory, programmes are the most effective. In addition, the cost effectiveness of these programmes compared to traditional approaches needs to be determined. The cost of the development of these programmes can be reduced by developing a core set of pain coping skills that can be used across all types of chronic pain conditions. Clinicians and policy makers will need to rethink health care processes around chronic pain management to ensure funding to support the sustainability of these ICT-based therapies. Finally, we need to ensure data security, privacy, and confidentiality of personal health information.

In terms of research, standards on the reporting and evaluation of ICT have been recently established and will provide important guidance for future studies (Eysenbach and CONSORT-EHEALTH Group, 2011). Multicentred RCTs of high quality are needed to compare ICT-based treatments with active placebos as well as face-to-face CBT. Conducted trials should include the measurement of broader biopsychosocial outcomes and move beyond simple pain intensity examinations. Dismantling studies can help determine the optimal length of interventions, specific treatment components which are effective, and whether social support or therapist involvement would improve outcomes. Finally, strategies to reduce dropout rates (e.g. motivational interviewing and minimal online support) need to be evaluated.

Conclusion

ICT-based pain treatments are an innovative way to improve the access and availability of psycho-educational pain therapies for individuals with chronic pain. There is growing evidence that ICT treatments not only reduce pain but also pain-related disability in various types of chronic pain conditions and in both paediatric and adult populations. We can continue to harness the potential of these mediums by ensuring that we explore the needs and perceptions of people in pain regarding ICT-based pain treatments—including when and under what circumstances the Internet is preferred to face-to-face therapies. This will help to tailor pain management efforts to individual preferences and enhance compliance and acceptability of these programmes. Moreover, well-designed studies with placebo control groups that include diverse patient groups are needed to strengthen the growing evidence base concerning ICT-based interventions for people with pain. Finally, we need to ensure that these programmes are publically available and that when they offer therapist involvement that this is remunerated by our health care system.

References

Barak, A., Klein, B., and Proudfoot, J. G. (2009). Defining internet-supported therapeutic interventions. *Ann Behav Med*, 38(1), 4–17.

Bargh, J. A., McKenna, K. Y. A., and Fitzsimons, G. M. (2002). Can you see the real me? Activation and expression of the "true self" on the internet. *J Soc Issues*, 58(1), 33–48.

Bargiel-Matusiewicz, K. and Krzyszkowska, A. (2009). Dispositional optimism and coping with pain. *Eur J Med Res*, 14(Suppl 4), 271–274.

Barlow, J. H., and Ellard, D. R. (2006). The psychosocial well-being of children with chronic disease, their parents and siblings: an overview of the research evidence base. *Child Care Health Dev*, 32(1), 19–31.

Barlow, J. H., Shaw, K. L., and Harrison, K. (1999). Consulting the 'experts': children's and parents' perceptions of psycho-educational interventions in the context of juvenile chronic arthritis. *Health Educ Res*, 14(5), 597–610.

Barlow, J., Wright, C., Sheasby, J., Turner, A., and Hainsworth, J. (2002). Self-management approaches for people with chronic conditions: a review. *Patient Educ Couns*, 48(2), 177–187.

Bender, J. L., Jimenez-Marroquin, M. C., and Jadad, A. R. (2011). Seeking support on Facebook: a content analysis of breast cancer groups. *J Med Internet Res*, 13(1), e16.

Bender, J. L., Radhakrishnan, A., Diorio, C., Englesakis, M., and Jadad, A. R. (2011). Can pain be managed through the Internet? A systematic review of randomized controlled trials. *Pain*, 152(8), 1740–1750.

Bruce, B., Lorig, K., Laurent, D., and Ritter, P. (2005). The impact of a moderated e-mail discussion group on use of complementary and alternative therapies in subjects with recurrent back pain. *Patient Educ Couns*, 58(3), 305–311.

Cuijpers, P., van Straten, A., and Andersson, G. (2008). Internet-administered cognitive behavior therapy for health problems: a systematic review. *J Behav Med*, 31(2), 169–177.

Cushing, C. C., and Steele, R. G. (2010). A meta-analytic review of eHealth interventions for pediatric health promoting and maintaining behaviors. *J Pediatr Psychol*, 35(9), 937–949.

Danaher, B. G., and Seeley, J. R. (2009). Methodological issues in research on web-based behavioral interventions. *Ann Behav Med*, 38(1), 28–39.

Drotar, D., Greenley, R., Hoff, A., Johnson, C., Lewandowski, A., Moore, M., *et al.* (2006). Summary of issues and challenges in the use of new technologies in clinical care and with children and adolescents with chronic Illness. *Child Health Care*, 35(1), 91–102.

Duff, A. J., and Latchford, G. J. (2010). Motivational interviewing for adherence problems in cystic fibrosis. *Pediatr Pulmonol*, 45(3), 211–220.

Elgar, F. J., and McGrath, P. J. (2003). Self-administered psychosocial treatments for children and families. *J Clin Psychol*, 59(3), 321–339.

Evers, A. W., Kraaimaat, F. W., Geenen, R., Jacobs, J. W., and Bijlsma, J. W. (2003). Pain coping and social support as predictors of long-term functional disability and pain in early rheumatoid arthritis. *Behav Res Ther*, 41(11), 1295–1310.

Eysenbach, G., and CONSORT-EHEALTH Group. (2011). CONSORT-EHEALTH: improving and standardizing evaluation reports of Web-based and mobile health interventions. *J Med Internet Res*, 13(4), e126.

Facebook. (2012). [Homepage of Facebook] [Online]. Available at: <http://www.facebook.com/press/info.php?statistics> (accessed 10 January 2012).

Feldman, S. I., Downey, G., and Schaffer-Neitz, R. (1999). Pain, negative mood, and perceived support in chronic pain patients: a daily diary study of people with reflex sympathetic dystrophy syndrome. *J Consult Clin Psychol*, 67(5), 776–785.

Foster, G., Taylor, S. J., Eldridge, S. E., Ramsay, J., and Griffiths, C. J. (2007). Self-management education programmes by lay leaders for people with chronic conditions. *Cochrane Database Syst Rev*, 4, CD005108.

Fox, S. (2011). *Health, digital divide: Health topics*. Pew Internet and American Life Project. Available at: <http://www.pewinternet.org/Reports/2011/HealthTopics.aspx>.

Garg, A. X., Adhikari, N. K., McDonald, H., Rosas-Arellano, M. P., Devereaux, P. J., Beyene, J., *et al.* (2005). Effects of computerized clinical decision support systems on practitioner performance and patient outcomes: a systematic review. *JAMA*, 293(10), 1223–1238.

Gibson, F., Aldiss, S., Taylor, R. M., Maguire, R., McCann, L., Sage, M., *et al.* (2010). Utilization of the Medical Research Council evaluation framework in the development of technology for symptom management: the ASyMS-YG Study. *Cancer Nurs*, 33(5), 343–352.

Gray, N. J., Klein, J. D., Noyce, P. R., Sesselberg, T. S., and Cantrill, J. A. (2005). Health information-seeking behaviour in adolescence: the place of the internet. *Soc Sci Med*, 60(7), 1467–1478.

Griffiths, F., Lindenmeyer, A., Powell, J., Lowe, P., and Thorogood, M. (2006). Why are health care interventions delivered over the internet? A systematic review of the published literature. *J Med Internet Res*, 8(2), e10.

Henderson, E. M., Rosser, B. A., Keogh, E., and Eccleston, C. (2012). Internet sites offering adolescents help with headache, abdominal pain, and dysmenorrhoea: a description of content, quality, and peer interactions. *J Pediatr Psychol*, 37(3), 262–271.

Huguet, A. and Miro, J. (2008). The severity of chronic pediatric pain: an epidemiological study. *J Pain*, 9(3), 226–236.

Jensen, M. P. (2010). A neuropsychological model of pain: research and clinical implications. *J Pain*, 11(1), 2–12.

Johannes, C. B., Le, T. K., Zhou, X., Johnston, J. A., and Dworkin, R. H. (2010). The prevalence of chronic pain in United States adults: results of an Internet-based survey. *J Pain*, 11(11), 1230–1239.

Kearney, N., McCann, L., Norrie, J., Taylor, L., Gray, P., McGee-Lennon, M., *et al.* (2009). Evaluation of a mobile phone-based, advanced symptom management system (ASyMS) in the management of chemotherapy-related toxicity. *Support Care Cancer*, 17(4), 437–444.

King, S., Chambers, C. T., Huguet, A., MacNevin, R. C., McGrath, P. J., *et al.* (2011). The epidemiology of chronic pain in children and adolescents revisited: a systematic review. *Pain*, 152(12), 2729–2738.

Klasnja, P. and Pratt, W. (2012). Healthcare in the pocket: mapping the space of mobile-phone health interventions. *J Biomed Informat*, 45(1), 184–198.

Kristjansdottir, O. B., Fors, E. A., Eide, E., Finset, A., van Dulmen, S., Wigers, S. H., *et al.* (2011). Written online situational feedback via mobile phone to support self-management of chronic widespread pain: a usability study of a Web-based intervention. *BMC Musculoskelet Disord*, 12, 51.

Law, E. F., Dufton, L., and Palermo, T. M. (2012). Daytime and nighttime sleep patterns in adolescents with and without chronic pain. *Health Psychol*, 31(6), 830–833.

LeFort, S. M., Gray-Donald, K., Rowat, K. M., and Jeans, M. E. (1998). Randomized controlled trial of a community-based psychoeducation program for the self-management of chronic pain. *Pain*, 74(2–3), 297–306.

Lelieveld, O. T., Armbrust, W., Geertzen, J. H., de Graaf, I., van Leeuwen, M. A., Sauer, P. J., *et al.*(2010). Promoting physical activity in children with juvenile idiopathic arthritis through an internet-based program: results of a pilot randomized controlled trial. *Arthritis Care Res*, 62(5), 697–703.

Lineker, S. C., Badley, E. M., and Dalby, D. M. (1996). Unmet service needs of children with rheumatic diseases and their parents in a metropolitan area. *J Rheumatol*, 23(6), 1054–1058.

Lorig, K. and Holman, H. (1993). Arthritis self-management studies: a twelve-year review. *Health Educ Q*, 20(1), 17–28.

Lorig, K. R., Laurent, D. D., Deyo, R. A., Marnell, M. E., Minor, M. A., Ritter, P. L. (2002). Can a back pain e-mail discussion group improve health status and lower health care costs? A randomized study. *Arch Internal Med*, 162(7), 792–796.

Lorig, K. R., Ritter, P. L., Laurent, D. D., and Plant, K. (2008). The internet-based arthritis self-management program: a one-year randomized trial for patients with arthritis or fibromyalgia. *Arthritis Rheum*, 59(7), 1009–1017.

Lynch, A. M., Kashikar-Zuck, S., Goldschneider, K. R., and Jones, B. A. (2007). Sex and age differences in coping styles among children with chronic pain. *J Pain Symptom Manage*, 33(2), 208–216.

MacDonald, N. E., Flegel, K., Hebert, P. C., and Stanbrook, M. B. (2011). Better management of chronic pain care for all. *Can Med Assoc J*, 183(16), 1815.

Macea, D. D., Gajos, K., Daglia Calil, Y. A., and Fregni, F. (2010). The efficacy of Web-based cognitive behavioral interventions for chronic pain: a systematic review and meta-analysis. *J Pain*, 11(10), 917–929.

March, S., Spence, S. H., and Donovan, C. L. (2009). The efficacy of an internet-based cognitive-behavioral therapy intervention for child anxiety disorders. *J Pediatr Psychol*, 34(5), 474–487.

Marks, R., Allegrante, J. P., and Lorig, K. (2005a). A review and synthesis of research evidence for self-efficacy-enhancing interventions for reducing chronic disability: implications for health education practice (part I). *Health Promot Pract*, 6(1), 37–43.

Marks, R., Allegrante, J. P., and Lorig, K. (2005b). A review and synthesis of research evidence for self-efficacy-enhancing interventions for reducing chronic disability: implications for health education practice (part II). *Health Promot Pract*, 6(2), 148–156.

McGeary, D. D., McGeary, C. A., and Gatchel, R. J. (2012). A comprehensive review of telehealth for pain management: where we are and the way ahead. *Pain Practice*, 12(7), 570–577.

Melzack, R. and Wall, P. D. (1965). Pain mechanisms: a new theory. *Science*, 150(699), 971–979.

Moxey, A., Robertson, J., Newby, D., Hains, I., Williamson, M., and Pearson, S. A. (2010). Computerized clinical decision support for prescribing: provision does not guarantee uptake. *J Am Med Inform Assoc*, 17(1), 25–33.

Murray, E., Burns, J., See, T. S., Lai, R., and Nazareth, I. (2005). Interactive Health Communication Applications for people with chronic disease. *Cochrane Database Syst Rev*, 4, CD004274.

Nguyen, H. Q., Carrieri-Kohlman, V., Rankin, S. H., Slaughter, R., and Stulbarg, M. S. (2004). Internet-based patient education and support interventions: a review of evaluation studies and directions for future research. *Comput Biol Med*, 34(2), 95–112.

Palermo, T. M., Eccleston, C., Lewandowski, A. S., Williams, A. C. C., and Morley, S. (2010). Randomized controlled trials of psychological therapies for management of chronic pain in children and adolescents: an updated meta-analytic review. *Pain*, 148(3), 387–397.

Palermo, T. M. (2000). Impact of recurrent and chronic pain on child and family daily functioning: a critical review of the literature. *J Dev Behav Pediatr*, 21(1), 58–69.

Palermo, T. M., Eccleston, C., Lewandowski, A. S., Williams, A. C., and Morley, S. (2010). Randomized controlled trials of psychological therapies for management of chronic pain in children and adolescents: an updated meta-analytic review. *Pain*, 148(3), 387–397.

Palmqvist, B., Carlbring, P., and Andersson, G. (2007). Internet-delivered treatments with or without therapist input: does the therapist factor have implications for efficacy and cost? *Expert Rev Pharmacoecon Outcomes Res*, 7(3), 291–297.

Peng, P. W., Stafford, M. A., Wong, D. T., and Salenieks, M. E. (2006). Use of telemedicine in chronic pain consultation: a pilot study. *Clin J Pain*, 22(4), 350–352.

Polomano, R. C., Droog, N., Purinton, M. C., and Cohen, A. S. (2007). Social support web-based resources for patients with chronic pain. *J Pain Palliat Care Pharmacotherapy*, 21(3), 49–55.

Pronovost, A., Peng, P., and Kern, R. (2009). Telemedicine in the management of chronic pain: a cost analysis study. *Can J Anaesth*, 56(8), 590–596.

Raine, L. (2010). *Internet, broadband, and cell phone statistics*. Pew Internet and American Life Project, California. Available at: <http://www.pewinternet.org/Reports/2010/Internet-broadband-and-cell-phone-statistics.aspx>.

Rapoff, M. A., and Lindsley, C. B. (2000). The pain puzzle: a visual and conceptual metaphor for understanding and treating pain in pediatric rheumatic disease. *J Rheumatol*, 58, 29–33.

Reid, K. J., Harker, J., Bala, M. M., Truyers, C., Kellen, E., Bekkering, G. E., *et al.* (2011). Epidemiology of chronic non-cancer pain in Europe: narrative review of prevalence, pain treatments and pain impact. *Curr Med Res Opin*, 27(2), 449–462.

Ritterband, L. M., Cox, D. J., Walker, L. S., Kovatchev, B., McKnight, L., Patel, K., *et al.* (2003). An Internet intervention as adjunctive therapy for pediatric encopresis. *J Consult Clin Psychol*, 71(5), 910–917.

Ritterband, L. M., Gonder-Frederick, L. A., Cox, D. J., Clifton, A. D., West, R. W., and Borowitz, S. M. (2003). Internet interventions: in review, in use, and into the future. *Prof Psychol Res Pract*, 34(5), 527–534.

Ritterband, L. M., Thorndike, F. P., Cox, D. J., Kovatchev, B. P., and Gonder-Frederick, L. A. (2009). A behavior change model for internet interventions. *Ann Behav Med*, 38(1), 18–27.

Rodham, K., McCabe, C., and Blake, D. (2009). Seeking support: An interpretative phenomenological analysis of an internet message board for people with complex regional pain syndrome. *Psychol Health*, 24(6), 619–634.

Rosser, B. A., and Eccleston, C. (2011). Smartphone applications for pain management. *J Telemed Telecare*, 17(6), 308–312.

Rosser, B. A., McCullagh, P., Davies, R., Mountain, G. A., McCracken, L., and Eccleston, C. (2011). Technology-mediated therapy for chronic pain management: the challenges of adapting behavior change interventions for delivery with pervasive communication technology. *Telemed J e-Health*, 17(3), 211–216.

Runge, C., Lecheler, J., Horn, M., Tews, J. T., and Schaefer, M. (2006). Outcomes of a Web-based patient education program for asthmatic children and adolescents. *Chest*, 129(3), 581–593.

Scanfeld, D., Scanfeld, V., and Larson, E. L. (2010). Dissemination of health information through social networks: twitter and antibiotics. *Am J Infect Control*, 38(3), 182–188.

Smith, J. R., Mugford, M., Holland, R., Candy, B., Noble, M. J., Harrison, B. D., *et al.* (2005). A systematic review to examine the impact of psycho-educational interventions on health outcomes and costs in adults and children with difficult asthma. *Health Technol Assess*, 9(23), iii–iv, 1–167.

Spek, V., Cuijpers, P., Nyklicek, I., Riper, H., Keyzer, J., and Pop, V. (2007). Internet-based cognitive behaviour therapy for symptoms of depression and anxiety: a meta-analysis. *Psychol Med*, 37(3), 319–328.

Stinson, J., McGrath, P., Hodnett, E., Feldman, B., Duffy, C., Huber, A., *et al.* (2010). Usability testing of an online self-management program for adolescents with juvenile idiopathic arthritis. *J Med Internet Res*, 12(3), e30.

Stinson, J., Wilson, R., Gill, N., Yamada, J., and Holt, J. (2009). A systematic review of internet-based self-management interventions for youth with health conditions. *J Pediatr Psychol*, 34(5), 495–510.

Stinson, J. N., Feldman, B. M., Duffy, C. M., Huber, A. M., Tucker, L. B., McGrath, P. J., *et al.* (2012). Jointly managing arthritis: Information needs of children with juvenile idiopathic arthritis (JIA) and their parents. *J Child Health Care*, 16(2), 124–140.

Stinson, J. N., Toomey, P. C., Stevens, B. J., Kagan, S., Duffy, C. M., Huber, A., *et al.* (2008). Asking the experts: exploring the self-management needs of adolescents with arthritis. *Arthritis Rheum*, 59(1), 65–72.

Subrahmanyam, K., Reich, S. M., Waechter, N., and Espinoza, G. (2008). Online and offline social networks: use of social networking sites by emerging adults. *J Appl Dev Psychol*, 29(6), 420–433.

Tan, L. (2008). Psychotherapy 2.0: MySpace blogging as self-therapy. *Am J Psychother*, 62(2), 143–163.

Trafton, J. A., Martins, S. B., Michel, M. C., Wang, D., Tu, S. W., Clark, D. J., *et al.* (2010). Designing an automated clinical decision support system to match clinical practice guidelines for opioid therapy for chronic pain. *Implementation Science*, 5, 26.

van Staa, A. L., Jedeloo, S., van Meeteren, J., and Latour, J. M. (2011). Crossing the transition chasm: experiences and recommendations for improving transitional care of young adults, parents and providers. *Child Care Health Dev*, 37(6), 821–832.

Velleman, S., Stallard, P., and Richardson, T. (2010). A review and meta-analysis of computerized cognitive behaviour therapy for the treatment of pain in children and adolescents. *Child Care Health Dev*, 36(4), 465–472.

von Weiss, R. T., Rapoff, M. A., Varni, J. W., Lindsley, C. B., Olson, N. Y., Madson, K. L., *et al.* (2002). Daily hassles and social support as predictors of adjustment in children with pediatric rheumatic disease. *J Pediatr Psychol*, 27(2), 155–165.

Vong, S. K., Cheing, G. L., Chan, F., So, E. M., and Chan, C. C. (2011). Motivational enhancement therapy in addition to physical therapy improves motivational factors and treatment outcomes in people with low back pain: a randomized controlled trial. *Arch Phys Med Rehabil*, 92(2), 176–183.

Wantland, D. J., Portillo, C. J., Holzemer, W. L., Slaughter, R., and McGhee, E. M. (2004). The effectiveness of Web-based vs. non-Web-based interventions: a meta-analysis of behavioral change outcomes. *J Med Internet Res*, 6(4), e40.

SECTION 8

Physical interventions

Physical interventions

Physical therapy interventions for pain in childhood and adolescence

Susan M. Tupper, Mary S. Swiggum, Deborah O'Rourke, and Michael L. Sangster

Introduction: physical therapist perspectives on pain

Physical therapists (PTs) consider pain in young patients from three perspectives. First, pain is recognized as a symptom of an injury or disease, or the primary manifestation of the disease itself. From this perspective, pain is monitored over the treatment course and treatment effectiveness may be examined by the overall reduction in pain. Second, pain may be provoked during physical assessment. From this perspective, pain is a dichotomous event which is either elicited with a provocation test, or not elicited. Pain from this perspective is useful to support diagnosis and identify tissue structures that may be contributing to the symptoms, or to identify hypersensitivity or allodynia resulting from peripheral or central nervous system sensitization. Finally, pain may be an unpleasant consequence of treatment procedures. Discomfort that arises from the manual therapy, modalities, or prescribed therapeutic exercises (procedural pain) may be considered an adverse event (Chorney et al., 2010). From this perspective, PTs must be equipped to monitor for this reaction, and minimize or eliminate pain from treatment. This chapter will focus on interventions which are aimed at minimizing or eliminating pain from two of these perspectives: pain as a component of injury or disease and procedural pain.

The chapter is divided into four sections. The first section will provide an overview of the theoretical foundations that can be used as a framework for possible mechanisms of effect for physical therapy (PT) interventions and identification of PT interventions oriented towards maximizing participation of children with pain in valued roles and life activities. The second will review the literature on active therapies as interventions for children with pain. The third section will review the literature on passive therapies and safety and efficacy for manual therapy or therapeutic modalities for pain. The importance of the therapeutic relationship and pain education will also be discussed. The final section will review the literature on procedural pain from a PT perspective and provide recommendations on procedural pain management. Although PT practice settings and the treatment needs of infants, children and adolescents with pain vary widely, this chapter will provide a structure for development of a theoretical and evidence-based physical therapeutic approach for all children with pain.

Theoretical foundations in treatment planning

Knowledge of pain mechanisms has evolved from the notion of pain as a uni-directional consequence of peripheral nociception, to that of a complex physical and emotional experience with biological, psychological, social, environmental and behavioural influences. Similarly, PT treatment of pain is evolving from a tissue-oriented, bio-medical approach to both active and passive therapies with potential to modify nociception and pain through peripheral and central nervous systems (Flor and Diers, 2009).

Theoretical models of pain and function enable the therapist to conceptualize causal mechanisms of effect and to consider a comprehensive approach to management of pain. It is particularly important that PTs use a theoretical framework for selecting treatments in the absence of high-quality evidence to guide the treatment approach. Although evidence-based practice should be the paradigm for PTs, in many cases because of lack of research, treatments do not have strong evidence for effectiveness. Although future research may lead to more effective PT treatments and the development of treatment guidelines, a theory-based approach guided by regular evaluation of outcomes will serve in design and delivery of appropriate care. However, a treatment approach based only on theory does not necessarily ensure that the treatments provided are effective. Clinicians need the knowledge of the latest research, combined with frequent evaluation of the effectiveness of their treatments with each patient (Jewell 2011).

Conceptual framework for pain

The neuromatrix theory will be briefly reviewed and discussed in terms of how it applies to PT treatment planning. The neuromatrix theory (Melzack, 1999) is a conceptual model for the genesis of pain that builds on the gate control (GC) theory (Melzack and Wall, 1970). The GC theory was revolutionary because it presented physiological mechanisms for bi-directional influences on pain and began to explain how competing peripheral afferent input (i.e. mechanoreceptor activity) and descending efferent activity from the central nervous system (i.e. emotional states or cognitions) could influence pain perception (Melzack and Wall, 1970).

The neuromatrix theory further reconceptualized pain as an output, or a 'neurosignature' which is generated by a complex neural network, the 'neuromatrix', as a noxious motivator to stimulate voluntary and involuntary actions that return the body to a state of homeostasis (Melzack, 1999). Melzack hypothesized that a pain neurosignature may be produced in the absence of identifiable tissue damage or disease and that the threat value assigned to the sensory information through conscious and unconscious cognitive and emotional appraisal will influence the sensory, affective, and cognitive dimensions of the pain neurosignature produced (Melzack, 1999).

Using this model as a framework, PT interventions for children with pain have three possible effects: (1) modification of the sensory afferent information, (2) modification of the cognitive and emotional evaluation (threat value) of the sensory information and (3) modification of the threshold for generation of the pain neurosignature by providing treatments that return the body to a state of homeostasis or regulate the stress-response systems (Figure 56.1). Because of the lack of specific research, PTs treating paediatric patients rely on knowledge of general neurophysiology or extrapolations from adult research to explain treatment effects. Research with children is needed to identify the mechanisms by which PT treatments have an impact on pain in young patients.

Based on what is known about the neurophysiology of nociception, it is hypothesized that sensory afferent information may be modified either by reducing activity in peripheral or central nociceptive pathways, increasing competing sensory information, such as mechanoreceptor input, or increasing central nervous system descending inhibition of pain (Woolf, 2011). The goals of treatment with therapeutic exercises, manual therapies, and modalities are to alter nociceptive afferent activity either directly (e.g. transcutaneous electrical nerve stimulation (TENS)) or indirectly by reducing inflammation (e.g. cryotherapy) or modifying structural impairments and the biomechanical stresses on tissues (e.g. mobilization of scar tissue).

Education and change in knowledge and beliefs are hypothesized to modify cognitive and emotional evaluation of sensory input. Graded exposure to sensory stimuli that provoke fear or distress, in combination with development of coping skills may also alter the patient's evaluation of feared movements (Woods and Asmundson, 2008). For example, an adolescent with idiopathic persistent pain may avoid walking long distances with the misunderstanding that she is damaging tissues when she feels increased pain with activity. PT treatment for this patient may include education to address her beliefs and fear of pain with activity as well as a graded physical activity programme. Although the ultimate goal of the activity programme would be to increase muscle strength and cardiovascular conditioning, in the initial stages the exercises could be considered a form of systematic desensitization with gradual exposure to the movements or positions that she fears (Woods and Asmundson, 2008). These exposures, if paired with development of coping strategies to manage pain, may contribute to increased function and reduction of fear-avoidance behaviours

PT treatments that aim to regulate the stress response would include general cardiovascular conditioning exercises, relaxation training, and education on sleep hygiene, diet, and healthy lifestyles. Management of acute or persistent pain must be conceptualized as one component of therapy oriented towards maximizing the child's participation in meaningful life roles and activities.

International Classification of Functioning Disability and Health as a framework for treatment planning

PT treatment for the child with pain is typically one component of a broad interdisciplinary continuum of care. Use of a common classification framework for evaluation and treatment planning will facilitate communication between professions and ensure that evaluation, goal setting and interventions are comprehensive and oriented towards improving the child's participation in valued activities (Goldstein et al., 2004).

The World Health Organization's (2007) International Classification Framework for Children and Youth (ICF-CY) is a framework used to describe health as a state of maximum engagement in desired activities within a continuum of health states (Goldstein et al., 2004). The ICF-CY identifies two main categories for assessment: functioning and disability, and contextual factors. Functioning and disability are further subdivided into body functions and structures, activities, and participation (Figure 56.2).Contextual factors are an interrelated construct that can be subdivided into environmental or personal factors.

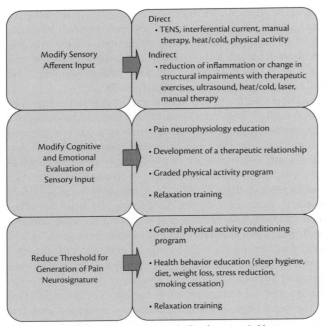

Figure 56.1 Hypothesized mechanism of effect for pain relief from PT interventions.

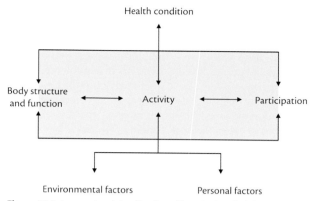

Health condition

Body structure and function   Activity   Participation

Environmental factors   Personal factors

Figure 56.2 International classification of functioning disability and health model. Reproduced with permission from World Health Organization, *ICF-CY: International Classification of Functioning, Disability and Health Children and Youth Version,* Copyright © World Health Organization 2007.

Disability is an interaction between impairments in body structures and functions and environmental and social contextual factors experienced throughout life. For example, a school-aged child with juvenile idiopathic arthritis with impaired lower extremity function resulting from inflammation, pain, and loss of muscle strength at the knee may be limited in the ability to run or walk for long distances. This may restrict participation in after school activities such as a community basketball team.

The traditional approach to PT treatment focused on strengthening exercises and modalities to reduce pain and inflammation. A participation focused approach also includes an evaluation of the specific activities and may include evaluation within the specific environment where the child experiences the participation restrictions to determine if the environment or activities could be adapted to improve participation. Treatment planning would include traditional therapies to address the impairments in body functions and structures, but may consist of specific functional activities aimed towards improved participation and performance of the desired activities. For example, rather that providing a quadriceps strengthening exercise in isolation, the child may be provided with basketball drills that build quadriceps strength. This approach addresses the impairment in the context in which it is needed, and improves the child's motivation to participate in the intervention.

Treatment may also include modifications to the activities or environments in which they are performed, including prescription of adaptive equipment such as supportive braces as well as discussions with parents, teachers, and coaches to facilitate modifications that enable the child to fully and safely participate.

Active therapies for pain in children

Across diverse health conditions, treatment adherence, health outcomes, and satisfaction with care are improved when children and adolescents are treated as partners and are actively engaged in making decisions about managing their health (Levetown, 2008). Active therapies include therapeutic exercises and general conditioning activities. Therapeutic exercises address specific impairments of body structures or functions such as limited range of motion of a joint or muscle, limited strength, impaired proprioception or balance or impaired cardiovascular conditioning. Therapeutic

exercises have been shown to be particularly beneficial for maintenance of functional outcomes and are recommended as part of a comprehensive treatment regimen for the management of patients with complex regional pain syndrome (CRPS; Bialocerkowski and Daly, 2012).

Even in the absence of impairments, children are encouraged to be regularly physically active (Tremblay et al., 2011). General cardiovascular conditioning is important for short- and long-term health (Tremblay et al., 2011). International guidelines on physical activity for children (World Health Organization, 2012) recommend participation in 1 h or more of moderate (e.g. brisk walking) to vigorous (e.g. running) physical activity daily and aerobic activity should make up most of that hour. Children living with pain tend to be less physically active and have lower cardiovascular conditioning compared to their healthy peers (Maggio et al. 2010). Improvements in cardiovascular fitness will support the child's return to participation in activities of daily living and physical and social activities.

Many children living with persistent pain present with significant mobility limitations due, in part, to the belief that movement will cause further tissue damage. Fear-avoidance behaviours can affect all domains of the child's health and functioning and result in disability (McCarthy et al., 2003). It is essential to elicit parents' and children's beliefs about the causes of pain, factors they believe exacerbate and relieve the pain, and fears related to movement and physical activity and to addresses specific and erroneous pain beliefs with education and graded activity programmes (Ayling-Campos et al., 2011). Active PT interventions for children with persistent pain may require a significant change in movement-related behaviour. An assessment of the child's readiness to change and to participate in PT is important to include in the initial evaluation.

Motivational interviewing may be used to explore a youth's thoughts and feelings about the present functional abilities, discrepancies between the current state and wishes for the future, readiness to change, and confidence in the ability to make changes (Suarez and Mullins, 2008). Information gathered from the interview is used to design a PT programme that is individualized and tailored to the child's functional goals and reflects their interests and values (Ayling-Campos et al., 2011). By focusing on the child's goals, their motivation and self-efficacy is enhanced and their role as an active and capable partner in their health and functioning is acknowledged. Using the ICF-CY framework, this approach shifts the focus of therapy towards age appropriate activity and participation goals and away from the impairment of pain or other functional limitations.

Graded physical activity programmes are a primary component of PT interventions that are effective in reducing pain and improving physical functioning and participation (Woods and Asmundson, 2008). The following guideline has been used in prescribing graded exercise programmes for children with chronic pain. For each form of activity or exercise, the therapist determines the child's baseline, which represents 50% of that activity or exercise performed to tolerance (Eccleston and Eccleston, 2004). Tolerance can be determined either through the subjective history, or a physical performance test. For example, if a child's tolerance for walking is 10 min, their baseline for walking would be 5 min. Targets for increasing activity, both physical activity interventions and activities of daily living, should be negotiated between the therapist and the patient, and performance of activity each day should be based on these goals, not based on the pain experienced

(Eccleston and Eccleston, 2004). This 'pacing' approach provides a clear plan for progression with specific physical activity targets for each day. The probable mechanism of reduction of pain by activity pacing is through modification of the threshold for generation of pain neurosignatures by re-establishing homeostasis. However, it is also possible that graded activity reduces fear of movement through successful participation in gentle activities. As the child performs movements and activities without eliciting feared responses (e.g. flares of pain or incapacitation) the child may alter his or her cognitive evaluation of the sensory information from the movement or position as non-threatening.

Graded motor imagery (GMI) may be a helpful strategy to use early in the rehabilitation process for children who experience such severe pain that movement of the affected body part is not tolerable (see case example at the end of the chapter) (Moseley et al., 2012). GMI consists of three components that are introduced in a specific sequence: (1) laterality reconstruction where the child simply looks at pictures of hands or feet and identifies them as being left or right, (2) motor imagery training where the child is asked to imagine moving the painful limb and (3) mirror therapy which requires the child to place the painful limb inside a mirror box and watch the reflection of the unaffected limb as it appears to be the affected limb moving. Mirror therapy relies on a visual illusion to 'trick the brain' into assuming the painful limb is moving. GMI improved function and reduced pain in adults with chronic pain (Moseley et al., 2012).

Passive therapies for pain in children

PTs are trained in the use of manual therapy and therapeutic modalities for treatment of pain and other functional and structural impairments in the body. There is currently limited evidence to support or refute the effectiveness or safety of these treatments for use with children. Passive therapies may have a place in the management of pain, particularly acute or procedural pain as they have the potential to modify sensory input and alter the production of a pain neurosignature; however, evidence is needed to support this hypothesis. In this section, the more commonly used passive therapies will be reviewed.

Manual therapy

Mobilization and manipulation of the spine and extremities

The therapeutic effect of joint mobilization or manipulation for pain in adults has been reported in several randomized controlled trials (RCTs) and systematic reviews (Bronfort et al., 2010). Findings indicate generally favourable support for joint mobilizations or manipulation for acute or chronic non-specific low back pain without peripheral radiation, acute or chronic neck pain (when combined with exercise), migraine or cervicogenic headache, and several disease or injuries of the upper or lower extremities (Brantingham et al., 2009; Posadzki and Ernst, 2011). Studies on the effectiveness of joint manipulations or mobilizations in children have been primarily limited to non-pain conditions such as asthma (Bronfort et al., 2010). An RCT comparing spinal manipulations to sham manipulations in children with cervicogenic headache showed no difference between groups for days with headache, headache duration, school absence, analgesic consumption, or pain intensity (Borusiak et al., 2010).

Evidence to support the safety of PT manipulations and mobilizations of the spine and extremities for pain in children is lacking (Bronfort et al. 2010); therefore literature on the incidence of adverse events from osteopathic and chiropractic manipulations will be discussed. Serious adverse events such as permanent neurological impairments have been reported (Humphreys 2010). Retrospective file reviews reported incidence rates of adverse events with spinal manipulations in children ranging from 0.53% to 9% for minor adverse events such as temporary increase in signs or symptoms (Hayes and Bezilla, 2006; Miller and Benfield, 2008). No serious adverse events were reported in these three studies; however, retrospective chart reviews are prone to biases since there is not a rigorous standardized protocol or surveillance system, and results of these reports should be interpreted with these limitations in mind. Adverse events may be underreported by children, given that the incidence of adverse events reported in the adult literature is much higher, and underreporting of symptoms is typical of children (Morrow et al., 2012). The risk of serious adverse events in adults is estimated to be approximately 0.01% (Thiel et al., 2007). Skeletal immaturity at the growth plates results in a relative structural laxity and reduced resilience of the bone to withstand trauma in children (Scheuer and Black, 2004). The developing spine and soft-tissue structures should not be considered equivalent to adults for risk of adverse events.

Massage

There is limited evidence to support the use of massage for the treatment of pain in children. Massage has shown moderate effectiveness for treatment of pain from burns (Parlak Gurol et al., 2010), headache (von Stulpnagel et al., 2009), juvenile idiopathic arthritis (Field et al., 1997), and in children attending an outpatient chronic pain clinic (Suresh et al., 2008). None of these studies were blinded and are therefore prone to biases. No studies were found that examined incidence of adverse events from massage therapy for the treatment of pain in children; however, based on the adult literature on adverse events, the rate is expected to be low (Ernst, 2003).

Therapeutic modalities

Therapeutic modalities most commonly applied for pain relief include TENS, thermal agents (heat and cold), therapeutic ultrasound, and low-level laser.

Transcutaneous electrical nerve stimulation

TENS is an easy to use therapy that delivers an electrical current through a stimulation unit with electrodes attached to the skin. TENS is thought to decrease pain by delivering a competing sensation through stimulation of A-beta nerve fibres that reduce afferent nociceptive activity of A-delta and C nerve fibres if the stimulus is below pain threshold (conventional, or high-frequency TENS), or through stimulation of endogenous opiate production and descending endogenous neural pathways if the stimulus exceeds pain threshold (low-frequency, or motor-level TENS; Prentice, 2011). Settings for type of current, waveform shape, amplitude, duration, rate of rise and decay, and frequency can be modified to produce various physiological and therapeutic effects. Electrode size and placement can be altered to affect the depth and density of tissue stimulation.

TENS is effective in reducing acute and chronic nociceptive and neuropathic pain in adults (Nnoaham and Kumbang, 2008; Yameen et al., 2011) and procedural pain in children (Lander and Fowler-Kerry, 1993). For pain relief, electrodes should be placed over or around the painful area or over the appropriate corresponding dermatome corresponding (Prentice, 2011). Alternatively, electrodes may be placed over muscle trigger points, acupuncture points, or superficial peripheral nerves. Since there is wide interindividual variability in response to TENS, several trials of electrode placement and nature of the current applied may be necessary to find the greatest pain relief for each client.

Many patients can be taught to apply this therapy with a pre-programmed light-weight, portable, battery operated unit at home. Pain relief with conventional TENS has a rapid onset (<1 h) for the majority of patients; however, pain levels typically return to pre-treatment levels within 1 h of discontinuation of the stimulation (Johnson et al., 1991).

Thermal agents

PTs use heat and cold to reduce pain and inflammation through the use of warm or cold whirlpools, contrast baths, hot-packs (hydrocollator packs) or ice packs, ice massage, cryospray, warm paraffin baths, or fluidotherapy. Pain relief with the application of heat or cold is thought to occur through stimulation of the cutaneous nerve receptors and activation of A-beta nerve fibres with both heat and cold and reduction of rate of firing of nociceptive A-delta nerve fibres with tissue cooling (Prentice 2011). Physiological effects of increased superficial circulation with the application of heat, or decreased circulation with the application of cold can have indirect effects on pain through the reduction of muscle spasm or inflammation (Prentice 2011). Hot and cold packs, warm or cold baths and ice massage are inexpensive treatments that can be taught to patients for home use as a component of the PT regimen for management of pain.

Therapeutic ultrasound

Therapeutic ultrasound delivers high-frequency sound waves (1–3 MHz) which produce thermal and non-thermal physiological effects with deeper tissue penetration than superficial thermal agents or electromagnetic radiation (Prentice, 2011). Ultrasound intensity, frequency, and pulse duration can be modified to alter the depth of penetration, and clinical effects. Ultrasound is thought to increase local blood circulation and tissue metabolism, thereby promoting soft-tissue healing, tissue remodelling, improved tissue mobility, and reduction of inflammation (Prentice, 2011). Pain relief is thought to occur through thermal effects.

Many studies reporting reduction of pain with ultrasound treatment have been criticized for methodological quality (Rutjes et al. 2010). However, there is evidence to support use of ultrasound for pain relief in adults with lower extremity osteoarthritis (Rutjes et al. 2010) and upper extremity musculoskeletal injuries (Green et al., 2003). No studies were found that examined ultrasound use for treatment of pain in children.

Low-level laser

Low-level laser is a form of electromagnetic energy that produces little or no thermal energy with outputs of less than 1 milliwatt (Prentice 2011). Laser has been used for wound healing, reduction of oedema, scar tissue, and bone remodelling, and pain reduction with lateral epicondylitis, acute and chronic neck pain, osteoarthritis, and myofascial pain syndrome (Chung et al., 2012). Pain reduction is

thought to occur as a result of reduced nerve conduction velocities, anti-inflammatory or tissue healing effects (Prentice, 2011).

Precautions and limitations of passive therapies

There are specific precautions and contraindications for the use of all thermal and electrophysical agents (Houghton et al., 2010). A qualified health professional such as a PT should be consulted for appropriate home use of modalities such as TENS. Therapeutic modalities may not be appropriate for children with vascular impairments, active infection, malignancy, recently radiated tissue, impaired sensation of the treatment area, and inability to communicate discomfort from the treatment (Houghton et al., 2010).

Therapists are urged to carefully weigh the benefits and limitations of passive therapies for children with persistent pain conditions. Given the limited empirical support and lack of evidence for safety for use with children and adolescents, passive therapies should only be used as part of a comprehensive, goal-oriented programme and not as a substitute for active therapies. Further research is needed to examine safety and effectiveness of these therapeutic approaches for pain in childhood. Although passive therapies may have a place in temporarily reducing symptoms, and may be particularly useful for treatment of acute or procedural pain, PTs are urged to use caution in the application of these therapies with children with persistent pain conditions. Injudicious use of passive therapies can provide false hope to patients for a 'cure' and foster dependence on passive therapies as a means of coping with pain.

Therapeutic relationship and pain education

The relationship between the patient and the PT is integral to the therapeutic process and a predictor of outcome. PTs are uniquely positioned to develop a positive therapeutic relationship by virtue of the frequency and duration of interventions with children and their families. The provision of pain education through a family centred lens which is individualized to the patient is a vital component towards the development of a therapeutic relationship.

In a systematic review of 13 studies involving adults with several pathologies, the therapeutic alliance between patients and the PT was positively associated with improved treatment adherence, treatment satisfaction, physical function, and reduced pain (Hall et al. 2010). No studies were found that examined the impact of the therapeutic relationship between the PT and child with chronic pain on treatment outcomes during rehabilitation. However, children with chronic pain often report difficulties in encounters with health care providers such as a perceived lack of understanding of their pain experience, judgement, and disbelief. These unsuccessful healthcare interactions can lead children and their families to become disillusioned, develop a guarded approach and a tenuous relationship in dealing with healthcare professionals (Dell'Api et al., 2007).

Three main components of the therapeutic relationship have been identified patient and PT agreement on treatment goals, agreement on the intervention, and the affective bond between patient and PT (Daniels and Wearden, 2011). In a qualitative study involving 53 children ages 10 to 17 living with chronic pain, Meldrum et al. (2009) reported that solicitation of a pain narrative is an important part of the therapeutic process and that clinicians who were willing to listen to the child's story about his or her pain condition would be in a position to assist the child in making positive therapeutic changes.

This reinforces the importance of identifying patients' functional, structural, and participation goals, and their expectations regarding the outcome of active and passive therapies. Agreement on the therapeutic goals and interventions can only be achieved with the provision of appropriate education about what are realistic expectations of therapy, and what actions on the part of the PT and patient are required in order to attain these goals.

Pain education should not be considered a one-way delivery of information from the therapist to the patient; rather, it is an opportunity to build the therapeutic relationship (Van Oosterwijck et al., 2011). PT specific pain education should address gaps between the child's beliefs about the expected outcome of PT and the types of PT needed to achieve the child's goals. It is essential to address misconceptions early in therapy and provide appropriate information to the child and his or her family on realistic outcomes from therapy regarding changes in pain, structural or functional impairments and return to participation in activities. It is also essential to address any misconceptions about the types of therapy that would be required to achieve the set goals. By providing information on pain neurophysiology and the expected outcomes form various therapies the PT can address these misconceptions and work with the child to develop a mutually agreeable plan for therapy.

Procedural pain management in children

Physical therapy procedures are increasingly being recognized as a source of pain for children receiving therapy services. Adults with cerebral palsy (CP) report that the pain related to PT interventions of stretching and bracing were the most salient negative memories of childhood (Kibele, 1989). The activity most frequently identified as painful by parents of children with CP was assisted stretching (Hadden and von Baeyer, 2002). Additional painful activities included independent standing, assisted walking, assisted sitting, and donning splints. Fifty-eight per cent of children with developmental disabilities reported pain during physical or occupational

therapy (McKearnan et al. 2004). Fifty-three per cent reported pain during a therapeutic home programme. Almost one-third of children with cystic fibrosis complain of pain during PT (Sermet-Gaudelus et al. 2009). The management of burn injuries is a source of pain and fear for children and their caregivers (Ratcliff et al. 2006). Clearly, there is evidence that the procedures commonly used by PTs to address impairments that accompany multiple childhood diagnoses are a source of stress and pain to the children and their caregivers.

Research is urgently needed to identify the prevalence and consequences of procedural pain from PT treatments, and pain-minimizing interventions that can be used during PT. This research is necessary to support the development of PT-specific guidelines towards eliminating unnecessary pain producing procedures and employment of prophylactic pain management techniques during procedures that are deemed necessary. As an example, this section will discuss pain management during stretching exercises with suggested strategies for reducing pain.

Pain management during stretching exercises

Stretching exercises are necessary for improvement of joint, muscle, and scar tissue range of motion for a variety of painful conditions such as CP, burns, muscular dystrophy, and juvenile idiopathic arthritis (Tecklin, 2008). Stretches may be performed independently (active), or with full (passive) or partial assistance (active-assisted) from a care-giver or health care provider such as a PT or PT aide. Interventions for pain management occur before, during and after the actual procedure. Table 56.1 provides an overview of examples at each stage.

Caregivers should be provided with information regarding the necessity and goals of the exercise, what will occur, and expectations of them during the stretches. Parents should be taught to avoid distress promoting behaviours, such as reassurance, apologies, or being overly empathic about the child's pain (Chambers et al., 2002).

Table 56.1 Strategies for procedural pain management during stretching exercises

Timing	Strategy	Example
Before procedure	Prepare environment to facilitate relaxation	Private space for stretching in school to avoid unwanted peer attention
	Prepare child or caregiver for procedure with age appropriate language.	Sensory information: 'Some people say this feels like a pinch, others say it feels like a pull. I want you to tell me what it feels like for you'
		Procedural information: 'For this stretch you will reach up with both hands to touch that mark on the wall, like this (demonstrate). We'll count backwards slowly from 20 and we'll do that 3 times with a rest between each stretch'
	Pair non-pharmacological and pharmacological strategies	Time therapy with maximum pharmacological effectiveness or breakthrough medications
During procedure	Coping-promoting therapist behaviours	Prompt to use coping skill, non-procedural talk
	Cognitive-behavioural methods	Distraction (e.g. blowing bubbles, toys, storytelling, books, music, television, virtual reality), guided imagery, relaxation, breathing exercises, thought stopping
	Positions of comfort	Young child sitting in parent's lap reading a book during manual therapy
After procedure	Reinforce use of coping strategies	Reinforcement: 'You did great using your deep breathing during that stretch'
	Evaluate pain-relieving strategies	Was child able to tolerate procedure? Can procedure or coping strategies be modified to improve effectiveness or pain relief?

Source: data from von Baeyer, C.L. and Tupper, S.M, Procedural pain management for children receiving physiotherapy, *Physiotherapy Canada*, Volume 62, Number 4, pp.327–337, Copyright © 2010 University of Toronto Press.

Therapist behaviours also influence pain and distress responses during painful procedures. Miller et al. (2001) found that when PTs promoted use of coping strategies, there was reduced distress and increased coping in children with CP, whereas reassuring comments such as 'it's almost over' and criticism increased distress and reduced coping during rehabilitation.

Cognitive behavioural methods that may be appropriate to lessen pain experiences of children during PT procedures include distraction, guided imagery, relaxation, breathing exercises, and thought stopping (von Baeyer and Tupper, 2010). The PT or caregiver may reinforce the child's use of coping strategies by providing positive statements or tangible rewards, such as stickers, prizes, or praise.

The PT should reflect upon the procedure and evaluate the measures that were used to alleviate distress and pain responses. Questions to be considered include:

◆ Was the strategy appropriate for the child's developmental level?

◆ Are the parent and child satisfied with the strategy for prevention of pain?

◆ Was the strategy adequately effective in preventing or alleviating the child's pain?

◆ Was it paired with pharmaceutical interventions if appropriate (i.e. burn care or post-surgical rehabilitation)?

◆ If the procedure was experienced as painful despite appropriate measures, is there research to justify continuing with this procedure or can an alternative treatment be implemented?

Recommendations

PTs are an integral component of multidisciplinary management of pain in children. However, in view of the paucity of evidence supporting the use of passive therapies for pain management in this population, therapists are encouraged to consider a comprehensive theory-based approach to treatment with an emphasis on active therapies. Treatment planning must be focused on returning children to patient or care-giver identified participation goals. Therapists are encouraged to provide opportunities early in the therapeutic process for the child to tell in their own words the story about their pain experience in order to identify treatment goals and establish a beneficial therapeutic alliance. Inactivity and fear of movement should be addressed through motivational interviewing, education, and graded activity programmes. Many PT procedures are painful for young patients, and therapists are recommended to consider applying a wide range of procedural pain management techniques to minimize or eliminate pain during therapy.

Case example: mirror therapy for unilateral upper extremity pain

Patient history: Will, a 17-year-old male, was referred to PT by his palliative care physician, diagnosed with a nasopharyngeal rhadomyosarcoma with an abdominal recurrence of metastatic disease. He received radical abdominal surgery including a nephrectomy, splenectomy, and distal pancreatectomy (see Box 56.1).

Medications: fentanyl and morphine as a part of abdominal surgery pain management. Gabapentin at 300 mg three times daily was added at the same time as the consult to PT.

Physical therapy initial assessment: On observation, Will displayed a left resting claw-hand deformity, wasting of the thenar eminence and first interosseous muscles, oedema, and significant colour changes (purple/blue skin colour over the dorsal and palmar surface of the left hand and all digits to the distal third of the forearm). Active and passive range of motion, resisted tests, and strength testing could not be performed due to intense pain. Sensory examination revealed left hand and forearm light touch allodynia with temporal summation, decreased sensation and increased pain in response to cold stimulus, and pin prick hyperalgesia. There was a positive modified upper limb neurodynamic test 1. Will's overall presentation was consistent with the Budapest clinical diagnostic criteria for CRPS probable type I (Harden et al., 2007).

Physical therapy management: PT management consisted of a 2-week trial of daily mirror therapy. CRPS is considered a central nervous system condition with changes to the primary motor and sensory maps that represent the painful body part (McCabe, 2011). Mirror visual feedback may correct sensory and motor remapping through short term cortical plasticity, thereby relieving pain. The mirror therapy approach involved Will placing his left hand behind a mirror which was situated in front of his chest in a sagittal plane. This positioning hid his affected hand from view, allowing him to view the reflection of his asymptomatic hand as if it were the affected side. Will performed a series of hand exercises with his right (asymptomatic) hand while observing this hand reflected in the mirror. Movement activities were structured according to difficulty and were tailored to simulate his treatment goals. Each session began with cardinal hand and wrist active range or motion followed by more complex functional tasks requiring more upper extremity dexterity. Mirror therapy was performed twice daily for 30 min each session.

Outcomes: Will reported immediate pain reduction following each mirror therapy session by 2 to 4 points on a 10-point scale which was maintained for an increased amount of time with each successive session. In addition, Will reported a significant decrease in the burning sensation and a 'more normal feeling' in his left hand following each session. After 2 weeks of daily mirror therapy, the distribution of his symptoms was reduced and Will reported his baseline pain at 5/10 which he now characterized as 'tingling' over the palmar aspect of the third digit. On physical re-assessment, Will displayed persistent wasting of the left thenar eminence and first interosseous, however the vasomotor and sudomotor changes observed on initial assessment were resolved. Full active range of motion of the hand, wrist, and forearm was observed. Sensory examination revealed the presence of residual pin prick hyperalgesia over the palmar aspect of the left third digit only. No allodynia and normal sensation to cold stimuli was noted. Despite persistent baseline pain at 5/10, Will was able to successfully return to playing video games after the 2-week PT mirror therapy.

Acknowledgement

Susan Tupper is the Coordinator of Integrated Pain Strategy and Research for the Saskatoon Health Region, and Clinical Assistant Professor at the School of Physical Therapy, University of Saskatchewan.

Box 56.1 Patient history for case example

7-day history of acute left hand pain and decreased sensation following routine, uncomplicated arterial line insertion.

Initially located in thumb, spread to palmar aspect of his index and middle fingers within 24 h of onset, on removal of arterial line, pain spread through entire hand and was described as a 'glove' that extended to distal third of forearm.

9/10 (constant) on a 0 to 10 numeric rating scale, with 10 being maximum pain.

Burning, cutting, numbness, and tingling with spontaneous intolerable pain episodes characterized as 'lightning for no reason.'

Colour changes reported, unable to tolerate weight of bed sheet on hand due to intense pain.

Reported having no left hand function which limited ability to play video games; primary goal was to be able to return to playing video games.

References

Ayling-Campos, A., Amaria, K., Campbell, F., and McGrath, P.A. (2011). Clinical impact and evidence base for physiotherapy in treating childhood chronic pain. *Physiother Can*, 63(1), 21–33.

Bialocerkowski, A. E. and Daly, A. (2012). Is physiotherapy effective for children with complex regional pain syndrome type 1? *Clin J Pain*, 28(1), 81–91.

Borusiak, P., Biedermann, H., Bosserhoff, S., and Opp, J. (2010). Lack of efficacy of manual therapy in children and adolescents with suspected cervicogenic headache: results of a prospective, randomized, placebo-controlled, and blinded trial. *Headache*, 50(2), 224–230.

Brantingham, J. W., Globe, G., Pollard, H., Hicks, M., Korporaal, C., and Hoskins, W. (2009). Manipulative therapy for lower extremity conditions: expansion of literature review. *J Manipulative Physiol Ther*, 32(1), 53–71.

Bronfort, G., Haas, M., Evans, R., Leininger, B., and Triano, J. (2010). Effectiveness of manual therapies: the UK evidence report. *Chiropract Osteopath*, 18(3). [Online] Available at: <http://www.chiroandosteo.com/content/18/1/3>.

Chambers, C. T., Craig, K. D., and Bennett, S. M. (2002). The impact of maternal behavior on children's pain experiences: an experimental analysis. *J Pediatr Psychol*, 27(3), 293–301.

Chorney, J. M., McGrath, P., and Finley, G. A. (2010). Pain as the neglected adverse event. *Can Med Assoc J*, 182(7), 732.

Chung, H., Dai, T., Sharma, S. K., Huang, Y. Y., Carroll, J. D., and Hamblin, M. R. (2012). The nuts and bolts of low-level laser (light) therapy. *Ann Biomed Eng*, 40(2), 516–533.

Daniels, J. and Wearden, A. J. (2011). Socialization to the model: the active component in the therapeutic alliance? A preliminary study. *Behav Cogn Psychother*, 39(2), 221–227.

Dell'Api, M., Rennick, J. E., and Rosmus, C. (2007). Childhood chronic pain and health care professional interactions: shaping the chronic pain experiences of children. *J Child Health Care*, 11(4), 269–286.

Eccleston, Z. and Eccleston, C. (2004). Interdisciplinary management of adolescent chronic pain: developing the role of physiotherapy. *Physiotherapy*, 90(2), 77–81.

Ernst, E. (2003). The safely of massage therapy. *Rheumatology*, 42(9), 1101–1106.

Field, T., Hernandez-Reif, M., Seligman, S., Rivas-Chacon, R., Schanberg, S., Kuhn, C. (1997). Juvenile rheumatoid arthritis: benefits from massage therapy. *J Pediatr Psychol*, 22(5), 607–617.

Flor, H. and Diers, M. (2009). Sensorimotor training and cortical reorganization. *Neurorehabilitation*, 25(1), 19–27.

Goldstein, D. N., Cohn, E., and Coster, W. (2004). Enhancing participation for children with disabilities: application of the ICF enablement framework to pediatric physical therapy practice. *Pediatr Phys Ther*, 16, 114–120.

Hadden, K. and von Baeyer, C. (2002). Pain in children with cerebral palsy: common triggers and expressive behaviors. *Pain*, 99(1–2), 281.

Hall, A. M., Ferreira, P. H., Maher, C. G., Latimer, J., and Ferreira, M. L. (2010). The influence of the therapist-patient relationship on treatment outcome in physical rehabilitation: a systematic review. *Phys Ther*, 90(8), 1099–1110.

Harden, R. N., Bruehl, S., Stanton-Hicks, M., and Wilson, P. R. (2007). Proposed new diagnostic criteria for complex regional pain syndrome. *Pain Med*, 8(4), 326–331.

Hayes, N. M., and Bezilla, T. A. (2006). Incidence of iatrogenesis associated with osteopathic manipulative treatment of pediatric patients. *J Am Osteopath Assoc*, 106(10), 605–608.

Houghton, P. E., Nussbaum, E. L., and Hoens, A. M. (2010). Electrophysical agents—contraindications and precautions: an evidence-based approach to clinical decision making in physical therapy. *Physiother Can*, 62(5), 1–80.

Humphreys, B. K. (2010). Possible adverse events in children treated by manual therapy: a review. *Chiropract Osteopat*, 18(12). [Online] Available at: <http://chiromt.com/content/18/1/12>.

Jewell, D. V. (2011). *Guide to evidence-based physical therapist practice* (2nd edn). Sudbury, MA: Jones & Bartlett Learning.

Johnson, M. I., Ashton, C. H., and Thompson, J. W. (1991). An in-depth study of long-term users of transcutaneous electrical nerve stimulation (TENS). Implications for clinical use of TENS. *Pain*, 44(3), 221–229.

Kibele, A. (1989). Occupational therapy's role in improving the quality of life for persons with cerebral palsy. *Am J Occup Ther*, 43(6), 371–377.

Lander, J. and Fowler-Kerry, S. (1993). TENS for children's procedural pain. *Pain*, 52(2), 209–216.

Levetown, M., and American Academy of Pediatrics Committee on Bioethics. (2008). Communicating with children and families: from everyday interactions to skill in conveying distressing information. *Pediatrics*, 121(5), 1441–1460.

Maggio, A. B., Hofer, M. F., Martin, X. E., Marchand, L. M., Beghetti, M., and Farpour-Lambert, N. J. (2010). Reduced physical activity level and cardiorespiratory fitness in children with chronic diseases. *Eur J Pediatr*, 169(10), 1187–1193.

McCabe, C. (2011). Mirror visual feedback therapy. A practical approach. *J Hand Ther*, 24(2), 170–178.

McCarthy, C. F., Shea, A. M., and Sullivan, P. (2003). Physical therapy management of pain in children. In N. L. Schechter, C. B. Berde, and M. Yaster (eds) *Pain in infants, children, and adolescents*, pp. 434–448. Philadelphia, PA: Lippincott Williams & Wilkins.

McKearnan, K. A., Kieckhefer, G. M., Engel, J. M., Jensen, M. P., and Labyak, S. (2004). Pain in children with cerebral palsy: a review. *J Neurosci Nurs*, 36(5), 252–259.

Meldrum, M. L., Tsao, J. C., and Zeltzer, L. K. (2009). 'I can't be what I want to be': children's narratives of chronic pain experiences and treatment outcomes. *Pain Med*, 10(6), 1018–1034.

Melzack, R. (1999). From the gate to the neuromatrix. *Pain*, Suppl.6, S121–126.

Melzack, R. and Wall, P. D. (1970). Evolution of pain theories. *Int Anesthesiol Clin*, 8(1), 3–34.

Miller, A. C., Johann-Murphy, M., and Zhelezniak, V. (2001). Impact of the therapist-child dyad on children's pain and coping during medical procedures. *Dev Med Child Neurol*, 43(2), 118–123.

Miller, J. E. and Benfield, K. (2008). Adverse effects of spinal manipulative therapy in children younger than 3 years: a retrospective study in a chiropractic teaching clinic. *J Manipulative Physiol Ther*, 31(6), 419–423.

Morrow, A. M., Hayen, A., Quine, S., Scheinberg, A., and Craig, J. C. (2012). A comparison of doctors', parents' and children's reports of health states and health-related quality of life in children with chronic conditions. *Child Care Health Dev*, 38(2), 186–195.

Moseley, G. L., Gallace, A., and Spence, C. (2012). Bodily illusions in health and disease: Physiological and clinical perspectives and the concept of a cortical 'body matrix'. *Neurosci Biobehav Rev*, 36(1), 34–46.

Nnoaham, K. E. and Kumbang, J. (2008). Transcutaneous electrical nerve stimulation (TENS) for chronic pain. *Cochrane Database Syst Rev*, 3, CD003222.

Parlak Gurol, A., Polat, S., and Akcay, M. N. (2010). Itching, pain, and anxiety levels are reduced with massage therapy in burned adolescents. *J Burn Care Res*, 31(3), 429–432.

Posadzki, P. and Ernst, E. (2011). Spinal manipulations for cervicogenic headaches: a systematic review of randomized clinical trials. *Headache*, 51(7), 1132–1139.

Prentice, W. E. (2011). *Therapeutic modalities in rehabilitation* (4th edn). New York: McGraw Hill Medical.

Ratcliff, S., Brown, A., Rosenberg, L., Rosenberg, M., Robert, R., Cuervo, L., *et al.* (2006). The effectiveness of a pain and anxiety protocol to treat the acute pediatric burn patient. *Burns*, 32(5), 554.

Rutjes, A. W., Nuesch, E., Sterchi, R., and Juni, P. (2010). Therapeutic ultrasound for osteoarthritis of the knee or hip. *Cochrane Database Syst Rev*, 1, CD003132.

Scheuer, L. and Black, S. M. (2004). *The juvenile skeleton*. San Diego, CA: Elsevier Academic Press.

Sermet-Gaudelus, I., De Villartay, P., de Dreuzy, P., Clairicia, M., Vrielynck, S., Canoui, P., *et al.* (2009). Pain in children and adults with cystic fibrosis: a comparative study. *J Pain Symptom Manage*, 38(2), 281–290.

Suarez, M. and Mullins, S. (2008). Motivational interviewing and pediatric health behavior interventions. *J Dev Behav Pediatr*, 29(5), 417–428.

Suresh, S., Wang, S., Porfyris, S., Kamasinski-Sol, R., and Steinhorn, D. M. (2008). Massage therapy in outpatient pediatric chronic pain patients: do they facilitate significant reductions in levels of distress, pain, tension, discomfort, and mood alterations? *Paediatr Anaesth*, 18(9), 884–887.

Tecklin, J. S. (ed) (2008). *Pediatric physical therapy* (4th edn). Philadelphia, PA: Lippincott Williams & Wilkins.

Thiel, H. W., Bolton, J. E., Docherty, S., and Portlock, J. C. (2007). Safety of chiropractic manipulation of the cervical spine: a prospective national survey. *Spine*, 32(21), 2375–2378.

Tremblay, M. S., Warburton, D. E., Janssen, I., Paterson, D. H., Latimer, A. E., Rhodes, R. E., *et al.* (2011). New Canadian physical activity guidelines. *Appl Physiol Nutr Metab*, 36(1), 36–58.

Van Oosterwijck, J., Nijs, J., Meeus, M., Truijen, S., Craps, J., Van den Keybus, N., *et al.* (2011). Pain neurophysiology education improves cognitions, pain thresholds, and movement performance in people with chronic whiplash: a pilot study. *J Rehabil Res Dev*, 48(1), 43–58.

von Baeyer, C. L. and Tupper, S. M. (2010). Procedural pain management for children receiving physiotherapy. *Physiother Can*, 62(4), 327–337.

von Stulpnagel, C., Reilich, P., Straube, A., Schafer, J., Blaschek, A., Lee, S. H., *et al.* (2009). Myofascial trigger points in children with tension-type headache: a new diagnostic and therapeutic option. *J Child Neurol*, 24(4), 406–409.

Woods, M. P. and Asmundson, G. J. (2008). Evaluating the efficacy of graded in vivo exposure for the treatment of fear in patients with chronic back pain: a randomized controlled clinical trial. *Pain*, 136(3), 271–280.

Woolf, C. J. (2011). Central sensitization: Implications for the diagnosis and treatment of pain. *Pain*, 152(Suppl 3), S2–S15.

World Health Organization. (2012). *Global strategy on diet, physical activity and health: Physical activity and young people* [Online]. Available at: <http://www.who.int/dietphysicalactivity/factsheet_young_people/en/index.html>.

World Health Organization. (2007). *ICF-CY: International classification of functioning, disability and health children and youth version*. Geneva: World Health Organization.

Yameen, F., Shahbaz, N. N., Hasan, Y., Fauz, R., and Abdullah, M. (2011). Efficacy of transcutaneous electrical nerve stimulation and its different modes in patients with trigeminal neuralgia. *J Pak Med Assoc*, 61(5), 437–439.

CHAPTER 57

Occupational therapy

Liisa Holsti, Catherine L. Backman, and Joyce M. Engel

Summary

Occupational therapists specialize in how pain impacts the development and maintenance of the occupations (self-care, productivity, leisure) of the daily lives of infants and youth in pain. Occupational therapists, working with families and other members of the health care team, use both generic and specific theoretical frameworks and models to guide clinical practice. These models ensure that a client-centred approach is used. In the everyday settings of the child, and using evidence-based practice, occupational therapists facilitate the treatment goals of children and families by integrating specific strategies, such as feeding, positioning, energy conservation, and adaptive equipment.

Introduction

Infants born as early as 24 weeks of gestation respond peripherally, centrally, and cortically to nociceptive stimulation (Bartocci et al., 2006; Beggs and Fitzgerald, 2007; Fabrizi et al., 2011). Pain experienced early in life is associated with significant long-term consequences including functional alterations in pain processing, in stress-response systems, and in development (Grunau and Tu, 2007; Hohmeister et al., 2010). Not only is it unethical to let pain and suffering in infants and youths go untreated (Johnston, 2011), but failure to treat pain places this population at greater risk for negative health outcomes as they mature (Koupil, 2007; Sullivan et al., 2008).

As in adults, infants and youths can experience acute and chronic pain in a number of ways. Undergoing painful, medical diagnostic and therapeutic procedures may be necessary to sustain life for infants or those who are born critically ill, preterm, or who have an acute trauma requiring emergency care (Stevens et al., 2011). In addition, paediatric clients may experience pain associated with preventative health care (immunizations); with trauma, such as from burns or physical abuse; with disease processes (e.g. arthritis); or with physical disabilities (Engel and Kartin, 2004; Engel, 2011; Parkinson et al., 2010). Moreover, pain may be a primary reason for seeking health care services (e.g. over-use syndromes associated with computer use; Siu et al., 2009), or may occur as a result of rehabilitative procedures, such as stretching. Finally, pain may arise and continue without a readily identifiable cause, such as

with headaches. The most current reports estimate rates of pain in the general population of youths as high as 70% (Du et al., 2011), and self-reported pain in adolescents can be as high as 40% (Dunn et al., 2011) or higher (King et al., 2011). A more detailed review of the epidemiology of pain in children can be found in this volume in Chapter 2 by Stevens and Zempsky. Irrespective of the underlying cause, pain may limit an infant's, child's or youth's ability to perform everyday occupations necessary to maintain health and well-being.

Background

The goals of occupational therapy for paediatric clients in pain are to develop, to maintain, and/or to restore their ability to participate in the occupations of their daily lives. Occupation has a broad meaning; it is everything people do to occupy themselves including activities related to self-care, to productivity, and to leisure (Townsend and Polatajko, 2007). For infants, the earliest occupations include changes in behavioural states and movements which indicate self-regulation and purposeful engagement with the environment (Holsti and Grunau, 2007a). For older infants and youths, self-care activities include engaging in their environment, feeding, sleeping, bathing, dressing, and mobility. Activities related to productivity are playing, participating in daycare and school, and in household, volunteer, or paid work. Leisure activities may also include play along with other tasks, such as social and recreational activities.

Early referral to occupational therapy services can prevent further disability and can provide critical support to family members. In order to understand more fully the unique contributions that occupational therapists make in restoring function and in mitigating pain in infants and youths, the purposes of this chapter are the following:

(1) To describe occupational therapy theory and common practice frameworks.

(2) To describe the impact/influence of pain on daily activities/occupational performance.

(3) To describe the occupational therapy practice process for infants and youths with pain including assessment, goal-setting, intervention, monitoring and modifying treatment, and evaluation.

(4) To describe occupational therapy intervention strategies used to treat pain in infants and youth.

The occupational therapy perspective

Occupational therapy theory

Theory is a tool for thinking about clinical practice. McColl and colleagues (2003) have classified occupational therapy theory, identifying generic and specific theories pertaining to everyday occupation, and a range of theories from 'small t' theory, such as theoretical ideas or propositions to 'big T' theory, encompassing more formal, well-articulated, and researched theoretical models (McColl et al., 2003). Occupational therapy professional organizations promote generic occupational therapy theoretical frameworks that identify occupational therapy's domain of concern and foster communication and professional unity. For example, both the Canadian Association of Occupational Therapists (CAOT) and the American Occupational Therapy Association (AOTA) have published general theoretical references that form a basis for the education of occupational therapists and serve as national guidelines for practice. The Canadian Model of Occupational Performance and Engagement (CMOP-E; Polatajko et al., 2007) and the Occupational Therapy Practice Framework: Domain and Process (Framework-II; AOTA Commission on Practice, 2008) outline an occupation-based domain of concern. These models/frameworks provide the building blocks for thinking about the concepts that occupational therapists address in practice. They are generic models, applicable to any practice setting.

The CMOP-E, for example, explains three occupational performance areas—self-care, productivity, and leisure—as a way of classifying what people do in everyday life (Polatajko et al., 2007). Furthermore, the characteristics a person possesses are conceptualized as spiritual, affective, cognitive, and physical. Thus, this generic theoretical model guides an occupational therapist to consider assessing what is important to a child and what motivates that child to act (spirituality), their feelings and mood, (affective component), their capacity to learn and solve problems, (cognitive component), and their ability to move, (physical component), all in the context of their usual self-care, productive, and leisure occupations (bathing, dressing, eating; school or lessons; and play). Additionally, everyday occupations are performed in context—a social, cultural, institutional, and physical environment. Using CMOP-E, occupational therapy intervention can then focus on modifying the environment, the demands of the occupation, or the child's skills in order to maintain or improve performance.

Similarly, the AOTA Framework-II describes how occupational therapy supports health and participation in life through occupational engagement. The concepts comprising occupational therapy's domain of concern are client factors, performance skills and patterns, activity demands and areas of occupation, and context and environment (AOTA Commission on Education, 2008). These concepts provide a common language for thinking and learning about the way a child (or anyone) engages in the occupations they need and want to do throughout their lives, and the impact of individual and environmental conditions on that performance. In this framework, areas of occupation are defined as activities of daily living (ADLs, such as bathing and dressing), instrumental activities of daily living (IADLs, such as community mobility and safety), rest and sleep, education, work, play, leisure, and social

participation. Collectively, the conceptual framework guides the therapist to consider all areas of occupation as topics for assessment and intervention, together with the child's performance skills and characteristics of the environment in which the child performs those occupations.

Both the CAOT and AOTA documents cited briefly offer generic models for thinking about practice with any client or client group. In contrast to generic occupational therapy theories, specific theories are those that explain particular concepts and the relationships among them that apply to a more targeted population, issue, or problem. Examples of these include sensory integration theories (e.g. Ayres, 1979), motor planning theories (e.g. Zwicker and Harris, 2009), neurodevelopmental theories (e.g. Wilson, 2005), and the gate control theory (Melzack and Wall, 1965) or the biopsychosocial model (Loeser and Fordyce, 1983). For neonates or infants, the synactive theory of development (Als, 1982) or the early life stress model (Loman and Gunnar, 2010) may also be used to inform assessment and treatment. Like other health professionals, occupational therapists often draw upon several theories simultaneously to inform thinking and action. In conjunction with process models, which provide a framework for action or problem-solving, generic and specific conceptual models guide professional reasoning.

The Occupational Performance Process Model (OPPM; Fearing and Clark, 2000) and Canadian Practice Process Framework (CPPF; Davis et al., 2007) are two process models that were designed to be compatible with the CMOP/CMOP-E and other conceptual theories. Both are step-by-step problem-solving processes to guide the identification of occupational performance issues or problems, the assessment or gathering of data about occupational performance areas, the child's personal and environmental characteristics, the development of intervention plans, and the monitoring of the effect of interventions. The AOTA Framework-II illustrates how the concepts defining the domain of occupational therapy are inextricably linked to its problem-solving process, which centres on collaboration between the practitioner and the client/family (AOTA Commission on Education, 2008). This practice process has three defining operations: evaluation, intervention, and outcomes. Evaluation requires that the therapist identify the client's occupational profile (what the child needs and wants to do) and an occupational analysis (the demands of the child's occupations and the extent to which the child can engage in them). Intervention involves developing goals and plans, then implementing and monitoring the plan. The outcomes stage refers to selecting appropriate outcome measures and applying them to determine whether or not occupational therapy achieved the intended goals and contributed to the child's health and participation in life (AOTA Commission on Education, 2008).

Importantly, occupational therapists working with children in pain are part of a team that includes other professionals, the infant or youth, and the family. Thus, other theories and process models may inform how the team works together to assess the situation and to develop an intervention plan. Occupational therapists may draw upon occupation-based theory to inform their specific contribution, as well as the team's specific philosophy or interdisciplinary theoretical approach. For example, collaborative teams working with children and families in health, educational, or community settings may use biopsychosocial, developmental, social, and/or ecological theories of human development to ensure the needs of the child are met. Bronfenbrenner and Ceci (1994) introduced a bio-ecological model of human development to explain environmental influences on the individual that crosses disciplinary boundaries. It has been tested, adapted, and applied to supporting children of all ages, and cited widely. Occupation-based theories are not only compatible with such approaches, but help to make the occupational therapist's role explicit to the team and to the family. Hickman and colleagues review empirical evidence on applying developmental and movement science theories to early intervention practices (Hickman et al., 2011). They indicate the importance of transdisciplinary approaches that support collaborative goal setting with the child and family as both a contributor to effective care and a challenge to maintain in complex care settings.

How pain affects occupation

Children engage in a range of roles aligned with their developmental stage. For example, one of the roles of an infant is to engage in the environment purposefully to ensure its survival. Roles are supported by occupational engagement. Pain may prevent children from engaging in the occupations that contribute to, or are essential for, their life roles. One way to understand the potential impact of pain is to consider a basic occupational taxonomy (such as presented by Crepeau and Schell (2009) or Polatajko et al. (2004)) and how pain may interfere at any level of that hierarchy (see Figure 57.1).

Pain may inhibit an *action*: pinching a button; a *task*: buttoning a shirt; an *activity*: getting dressed; an *occupation*: completing morning self-care. As a result, pain at any level of occupational performance may limit the child's roles in life; in this example, the occupational therapist is concerned with supporting the child to develop independence in self care because it is a natural developmental milestone, and effective and appropriate dress contributes to participation in other roles, such as playing dress-up, being in uniform for a sporting team, or being dressed for school or church. Therefore, an occupational therapy assessment will identify which aspects of occupation are affected by pain; the strengths and resources the child has; and provide direction for selecting interventions that will overcome the effect of pain on the occupations the child needs and wants to do.

Assessment

Overall purpose and process

The purpose of the assessment is to establish a baseline that in turn informs goal setting and an intervention plan, and provides

a comparator for later outcome evaluation to determine if goals were achieved. The process begins by screening for occupational performance issues—there is no need for more detailed assessment procedures unless the child's health status or symptoms, including pain, have an impact on or threaten occupational performance. An initial observation of an infant or an interview with the child and/or caregiver helps to identify specific problems and factors contributing to those problems, as well as resources to be considered in formulating an intervention plan. The assessment process may include observation, self-report, and performance-based tests in order to document baseline performance or identify individual strengths and limitations for choosing particular treatment modalities. In the presence of pain, it may not be appropriate or possible to conduct a complete evaluation in a single session or at all; priorities need to be established in light of the presenting circumstances. Although discussed as a discrete step, assessment is often ongoing and integrated into the intervention process.

Infant assessment

Assessing pain in infants is complex for a number of reasons, the most obvious one being that infants are not able to self-report. Thus, occupational therapists must first assess the context in which pain may be present (e.g. as in postoperative pain or related to a disease process) and then rely upon a combination of behavioural and physiological indices shown to be the most reliable and valid measures of pain. For infants, these indices usually include specific, anatomically defined facial and body movements, changes in sleep/wake states, and changes in heart rate. Many of these indices have been included in a number of reliable and valid tools available for assessing acute pain in infants, such as the Behavioral Indicators of Infant Pain (BIIP; Holsti and Grunau, 2007b), the Premature Infant Pain Profile (PIPP; Stevens et al., 1996), the Neonatal Facial Coding System (NFCS; Grunau and Craig, 1987), the Comfort Scale (Ambuel et al., 1992) and the FLACC scale (face, legs, activity, cry consolability; Merkel et al., 1997). The psychometric properties of neonatal and infant pain tools have been reviewed extensively in this volume by Lee and Stevens (Chapter 35) and elsewhere (Stevens et al., 2007). Most recently, technologies, such as near infrared spectroscopy (NIRS) and electroencephalography (EEG) are providing researchers and clinicians with important complementary information regarding evaluating pain responses in infants at a cortical level (as reviewed by Holsti et al., 2011).

An important consideration for occupational therapists' assessment of pain is whether or not to use a tool that combines behavioural and physiological indices into a single score (a multidimensional approach) or to evaluate these categories of indicators separately (a unidimensional approach). This choice is important because in both infants and in children, dissociation between behavioural and physiological indicators is common (e.g. Morison et al., 2001). Including both behavioural and physiological indices is critical; however, if a multidimensional tool is used, and the effects of any applied treatments are not evaluated as to their effects on *both* the behavioural and physiological components, caregivers and researchers may miss important information as to the overall efficacy of the treatment. For example, sucrose is an oral solution given to infants to reduce acute procedural pain (Stevens et al., 2010). Although sucrose consistently reduces the behavioural component

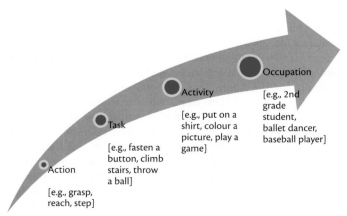

Figure 57.1 The influence of pain on childrens' occupational roles.

of the pain response, its effects on physiological responses can be variable (Stevens et al., 2010). This type of 'split' response to a treatment raises the concern that failing to reduce the physiological response leaves infants vulnerable to the destabilizing physiological effects of pain.

To begin to address this issue, one study using NIRS examined the relationship between cortical pain responses and behavioural and physiological indices (Slater et al. 2008). High correlations were found between facial actions and cerebral blood flow; adding physiological indices did not improve the relationship. Although this research strategy shows promise for finding more accurate ways of assessing pain in infants, the fact that heart rate and oxygen saturation had only a modest relationship with cortical blood flow requires further exploration. Thus, more work is needed to determine which indices applied either in combination or individually will provide the most accurate reflection of pain processing in infants.

In addition to using standardized pain-related tools, occupational therapists can perform observational evaluations of the influence that pain may have on the infant's ability to engage in the environment, with their caregivers, during self-care activities and during play (Pierce et al., 2009). For example in a home setting, formal testing can be used to evaluate function and/or development, e.g. Peabody Developmental Motor Scales-2 (Folio and Fewell, 2000), The Test of Playfulness (Bundy et al., 2001), and combined with it, either through the use of a valid scale or by using parent report or informal observation, the contribution of pain-related behaviours as potential contributors to delayed or atypical development. Once the assessment is complete, goal setting with the caregivers can commence and treatment implemented.

Infants and youth

One tool that assists more specifically with identifying occupational performance issues, goal-setting, and allows for both baseline measurement and subsequent outcome evaluation, is the Canadian Occupational Performance Measure (COPM; Law et al., 2005). The COPM is applicable to children of all ages; the parent or caregiver can be the informant for children not able to speak for themselves. It consists of a semistructured interview and rating scale. Up to five priority occupational performance issues are identified as intervention targets. After rating an issue's importance (on a 1 to 10 scale, 10 = extremely important), each one is rated in terms of the child's ability to perform it, and their current satisfaction with that level of performance, also on 1 to 10 scale (10 = able to do it very well; 10 = extremely satisfied). For example, Elly, age 6, chose jumping rope at recess, changing into a swimsuit independently for swimming lessons, and printing faster at school as important occupational performance issues. With some guidance from her mother and the occupational therapist to interpret the terms, Elly's baseline COPM ratings (see Table 57.1).

Subsequently, more detailed assessment techniques may be used to assess Elly's motor skills, the impact of pain on performance, and environmental conditions that might help or hinder performance. For other children, the issues and ratings may be from the parent's perspective (e.g. with an infant's parents, where the issues may be feeding, dressing, bathing, and playing with their child). Satisfactory psychometrical properties were reported in a clinical trial where the COPM was used with parents/caregivers of 42 children, ages 2 to 8, with cerebral palsy (Cusick et al., 2007), and in an interrater reliability study with the parents of 80 children, ages 1 to 7.5, with a range of disabilities (Verkerk et al., 2006). The latter study also found that the COPM identified individualized problems that were not captured by other standardized assessment tools (Verkerk et al., 2006). Using a tool like the COPM may facilitate assessment by identifying individual, functionally relevant goals to guide intervention and provide a concurrent outcome measure process. Skilfully conducted, the interview may also identify contributing factors to occupational performance problems that require additional assessment. It does not measure pain, but does provide a context for assessing the impact of pain.

A final example of an occupation-specific pain assessment tool is one which examines how pain interference impacts routine daily activities and participation. The Brief Pain Inventory Pain Interference (BPI) scale (Cleeland and Ryan, 1994) is a reliable and valid scale on which children or their caregivers rate on an ordinal scale of 0 (no interference) to 10 (complete interference) how much their pain has interfered with general activity, mood, walking ability, normal work, relations with other people, sleep, and enjoyment of life. Importantly, the BPI has been modified slightly for use with youths with physical disabilities (Tyler et al., 2002). The words 'walking ability' were changed to 'mobility (ability to get around)'. Persons who have mobility restrictions not related to pain (e.g. wheel chair users) can thereby rate the impact of pain on mobility. Self-care, recreational activities, and social activities items were added to be more inclusive of daily activities and participation that could be impacted by pain. 'Normal work' was changed to 'school or play'. The BPI can be helpful in determining baseline tolerance levels for specific occupations and participation as well as in evaluating outcomes before and after treatment (Tyler et al., 2002). In-depth discussion of behavioural pain assessment can be found in Section 5 of this volume (Chapters 35–41).

Interventions

Infants

Mitigating pain is vital to prevent the development of long-term changes in pain processing and in development associated with pain experienced in infancy. Pharmacological management, along with other forms of non-pharmacological management, is covered extensively in other chapters; thus the focus of this section will be

Table 57.1 Elly's baseline COPM ratings

Occupational performance issue	Importance	Performance	Satisfaction with performance
Jump rope	9	4	2
Change into swimsuit	9	5	2
Print faster	8	5	5

to evaluate the efficacy of those treatments for which occupational therapists have specialized knowledge, including modifying the environment, positioning, feeding and play.

Occupational therapists have specific expertise in assessing the impact of the environment on everyday occupations (Polatajko et al., 2007). For infants undergoing procedural pain, occupational therapists can evaluate the infant's environment to ensure stimulation is modified to minimize pain. For example, evidence from two trials suggests that reducing environmental noise and lighting reduces both physiological and behavioural pain indices in preterm infants (Catelin et al., 2005; Sizun et al., 2002); however, the procedures evaluated in these studies were not skin-breaking, and environmental modifications were combined with other interventions. Thus, more research is needed to determine the relative contribution of environmental modification on pain in infants.

Occupational therapists can also use positioning strategies, including swaddling and facilitated tucking for pain reduction in infants. Swaddling is a strategy whereby an infant's arms and legs are tucked inside a blanket throughout the procedure. Alternatively, facilitated tucking is done by a caregiver who contains the infant's arms and legs with their own hands during the procedure (Figure 57.2).

In the most recent systematic review, sufficient evidence was found for both strategies for reducing pain indices in preterm infants (−0.75: 95% confidence interval −1.14, −0.36; Pillai Riddell et al., 2011). Nevertheless, many of the studies evaluating these treatments did not use blind evaluators nor did they account for order effects in those using a cross-over design; therefore, further research is needed to determine the benefits of these methods. Most recently, over five blood collections, facilitated tucking did not reduce pain indices (behavioural) as effectively as did sucrose, but did have an additive effect when used with sucrose; however, no differences in physiological indices were found (Cignacco et al, 2012). Currently, no evidence evaluating swaddling or facilitated tucking for older infants is available.

In addition to specializing in modifying the environment and using therapeutic positioning for managing pain, occupational therapists have specialized knowledge in the development of oral motor control and feeding. Indeed, feeding is considered a primary self-care related occupation of infants. For the purposes of

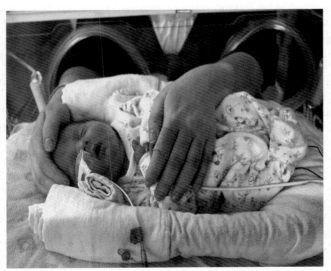

Figure 57.2 Example of a parent providing facilitated tucking.

pain management, combining sucking and ingesting oral solutions, whether sweetened solutions or the more ecologically salient and potentially potent breast milk, may stimulate multiple pain relieving pathways (Holsti et al., 2011). Oral sweeteners have been used for mitigating pain in infants; however, more recent evidence suggests that they may be inducing mild sedation rather than providing analgesia (e.g. Slater et al., 2010). Some concerns have been noted regarding the methodology of this work (e.g. Stevens et al, 2011); therefore, these results require replication. In addition, sweeteners may have unintended negative effects on development when used in very immature infants over repeated events (Johnston et al., 2002; Holsti and Grunau, 2010). For a detailed review of the use of sweet solutions, readers are directed to Harrison et al. (Chapter 49, this volume). Further work is needed to understand the mechanisms of action of sweeteners and their effects long term.

Breastfeeding provides reduction of pain-related behaviours in infants born full term (Shah et al., 2009), for infants born preterm who have mature feeding skills (Holsti et al., 2011), and for infants up to 6 months of age (Dilli et al., 2009). A clear benefit to breastfeeding is that this treatment supports mother/infant interaction. Moreover, some have found breastfeeding to be more efficacious than sucrose (Codipietro et al., 2008) and than maternal holding (Leite et al., 2009), reducing both behavioural and physiological pain indices.

The timing of the treatment and the volume of breast milk/feeding ingested is important for maximizing its pain-mitigating effects (Holsti et al., 2011). For example, the infant must feed before, during and after the painful stimulus. If breast milk is given on its own, at least 5 ml of milk must be given in combination with sucking (Upadhyay et al., 2004). To date, no studies have compared full breastfeeding with the provision of breast milk on its own. Finally, feeding as a pain-relieving treatment should be used with caution because more study is needed to examine the use of this intervention over repeated painful events, particularly in infants born preterm, and to determine the effects of feeding on cortical pain processing to ensure this treatment is not acting merely as a sedative.

Youth

For youth, occupational therapists can provide a variety of treatments aimed at mitigating or managing pain in a variety of settings, such as in hospital, in clinics, and of particular benefit is the application of treatment in the home. Indeed, home programmes are essential for transferring therapy skills from the clinic into the child's natural environments. Knowing the family's goals and activities are the first steps in determining realistic expectations for home programmes. Naturally occurring routines for teaching or reinforcing skills are sought as learning opportunities. After modelling individualized interventions, therapists should observe the family member's skill level in performing the therapeutic activity and provide guidance as needed. Written home instructions may increase the family's adherence with interventions. Therapists should strive for minimal disruption of daily routines within the child's environments. Family members' questions and concerns must be addressed. If the occupational therapist is treating an acute problem which may persist beyond a hospital stay, referrals to community resources may be needed to ensure that follow up care is maintained (Jaffe et al., 2010).

Energy conservation

When assessment findings indicate that a child experiences increased pain with more intense or longer duration activities, or their participation in such activities is precluded by pain, then some collaborative problem-solving based on energy conservation, joint protection, and/or ergonomic principles may be helpful (Backman, 2011). A critical point is to help the child (and his/her supporters) to apply the principles to the specific activities and situations that are important to them with the aim of helping to balance activity and rest so that the child can participate as long as possible without pain and fatigue. Simply providing a list of principles and examples is generally insufficient—the child needs to be encouraged to figure out how to apply and modify the principles to situations in their own occupations. Although recommended for children (Kuchta and Davidson, 2008), evidence in support of joint protection (including splints) and energy conservation principles is largely limited to studies in adults (Hammond and Freeman, 2001; Steultjens et al., 2004).

Energy conservation principles include prioritizing, planning, positioning, and pacing. Pain saps energy reserves: one may need to set clear priorities in terms of choosing the activities in which to engage during a day, week, or other period of time. When children feel well, they will engage in play and other activities that interest them (Taylor and Erlandson, 2001). Once priorities are established, plans can be made for participating in the high priority activities, such as ways to get there, preparing or practicing ahead of time, obtaining appropriate equipment or assistive devices, if applicable. Positioning refers to awareness of body posture and positioning of the tools and equipment that support the activity or occupation. Placing frequently used items within pain-free/easy reach while working on school activities, games, or crafts is one example. Setting up a computer workstation to support a well-aligned posture is another. Lastly, pacing refers to 'listening' to how one's body responds to participation in the activity—what intensity or duration is tolerable or exacerbates pain—and adapting accordingly. Children will learn how to pace, how to adjust their involvement to accommodate their pain and their interest in performing an activity concurrently. When the activities are related to school, gym, or social groups, there may also be a need to teach teachers, coaches, and leaders about the intermittent nature of pain and pacing so that further pain and fatigue is prevented whenever possible.

Joint protection principles may help prevent or reduce pain for children who have either chronic joint conditions, such as juvenile arthritis, or an acute episode of pain from a musculoskeletal condition or injury. Joint protection principles include avoiding static postures and using the largest/strongest joints possible to minimize stress on smaller joints (Niedermann et al., 2011). Kuchta and Davidson (2008) offer numerous practical examples and handouts for children with rheumatic diseases, including strategies for managing pain (e.g. how to apply heat and cold) and modifying activities (e.g. choosing a backpack, planning car or plane travel, modifying gym class). These and other handouts can be printed from the publisher's web site (<http://www.radcliffe-oxford.com/rheumaticdiseases/>), and four have been included in this text as online supplementary materials. For example, carrying books in a messenger-style shoulder bag with the strap across the body protects the smaller joints of the hands and wrists compared to gripping a book bag or lunch bag. Using an appropriate sized backpack is another alternative. In both cases, the weight carried needs to be matched to the child's size and strength. When it comes to textbooks, for those with pain, an even better alternative is to avoid carrying them back and forth to school by having a set at home and another set at school. The occupational therapist may be able to intervene with the school to justify the second set.

Play/distraction

Play is also a primary occupation of infants and children (Bundy, 1992). With respect to the paediatric pain management literature, typically, distraction is the intervention studied, and the context is for managing acute pain. A number of different distraction strategies have been studied, such as showing an infant or child a novel toy or video, some being more effective than others. More specifically, whereas showing an infant a novel toy does not appear to modify behavioural pain responses in infants and young children (e.g. Cramer-Berness and Friedman, 2005), parents showing a video do appear to reduce immunization pain in this same age group (Cohen et al., 2006). These simple strategies require limited attention and visual engagement of the infant or child. A comprehensive review of distraction techniques by Cohen et al. can be found in Chapter 53 in this volume.

Alternatively or in addition, occupational therapists and other health care providers use therapeutic play for managing pain in a number of settings (Bandstra et al., 2008). Play is a complex activity requiring more interaction with the environment and incorporating more complex cognitive and sensory-motor processes than simple distraction. When more engagement is required by the child, that is, the child actually has contact with a toy and uses it or is immersed activity in a task, such as with virtual reality, pain is reduced (e.g. Law et al., 2011; Tanabe et al., 2002). For example, in a single-subject randomized design, Melcher-McKearnan and colleagues (2000) found that in children with burn injuries, play activities were more effective in minimizing distress behaviours, maximizing activity and fun than were rote exercises. A more detailed discussion on the role of child life and recreational therapies by LeBlanc and Chambers can be found in Chapter 52 in this volume.

Instruction in body mechanics

Back pain in youths is common (Kjaer et al., 2011). Instruction in and rehearsal of proper body mechanics and postures that will not increase the risk of low back injury are essential for clients experiencing both acute and chronic back pain. Practice in using the body safely and in maximizing performance during routine tasks in natural (i.e. homework, or leisure) environments is particularly important (Grangaard, 2011; Strong, 1996). The child should be taught to avoid tasks or positions that do not allow balanced posture.

Adaptive equipment

To assist children maintain independence in routine daily activities, occupational therapists also can provide instruction for and provision of adaptive equipment (Howard, 2002). In particular, adaptive equipment is often needed for children with disabilities and to supplement therapy. Adaptive equipment includes such things as bathtub seats, high chairs, wheelchairs, car seats, and hydraulic lifts. The equipment is used to prevent abnormal movement patterns, muscle tone, positioning, and postures or support more independent function. Adaptive equipment also prevents or facilitates correct positioning when the child is not being handled. Moreover, the equipment can be used to reinforce postures and movements introduced in treatment which can then be used in home programmes. Motor, sensory, perceptual, cognitive, and psychosocial development are also promoted with its use. Equipment should be restricted in its use as much as possible so as to allow the child's free exploration of the environment. Furthermore, any equipment should be monitored regularly to ensure the child's and family's needs and therapeutic goals are met (Aubert, 2008).

Relaxation strategies

A variety of methods for inducing a relaxation response are available for managing pain. Progressive muscle relaxation (e.g. Barsky et al., 2010) or autogenic training (Payne, 2000), whereby clients are instructed in use of silently repeating seven standardized relaxation themes, are methods by which children can self-manage pain (for further details see Engel, 2011). These strategies should be integrated into the youth's daily routine, and the occupational therapist can help determine when the timing of these strategies might be most effective.

Conclusion

Pain in infants and children interferes with their ability to engage in essential interactions with caregivers, with the acquisition of developmental milestones, and with participation in activities related to self-care, leisure, play, school, and work. Using occupation-based theoretical models, such as the CMOP-E and the Occupational Therapy Practice Framework: Domain and Process, provides a foundation for the provision of occupational therapy services to infants and youth. Through an iterative and continuous problem-solving process, occupational therapists provide standardized assessment of the infant's or youth's performance problems and along with the integration of the child's environmental context, develop and monitor the effects of interventions. Occupational therapists use specific treatment strategies such as feeding, positioning, splinting, and instructing in energy conservation and joint protection strategies, and the use of adaptive equipment. While some of the effects of these strategies have been evaluated rigorously in infants and children, as happens often in other areas of paediatric rehabilitation, some techniques have been applied based solely upon research conducted in adults. Thus, much more research is needed on assessing the benefits of occupational therapy interventions for mitigating both acute and chronic pain in children.

Case example

Patricia is the consulting occupational therapist for the local hospital neonatal intensive care unit (NICU) 2 days per week and for a community school 3 days per week. At the hospital, a new infant is admitted overnight who has a significant brain bleed and will require ongoing blood tests. The nurse asked that Patricia help teach the parents ways in which they can modify the infant's environment to support the infant's development and to help with pain management. Using the synactive theory of development (Als, 1982), Patricia describes how the environment in the NICU is developmentally unexpected and shows the parents how

to cover the isolette with a blanket to shade the infant's eyes. She explains how lowered lighting and noise can help stabilize the baby. She also describes how promoting flexed positioning will support the infant's motor development, and keep the baby calm. She shows them how they can work with their nurse to use facilitated tucking for providing treatment during blood tests. She begins educating the parents regarding infant behavioural cues which can be signs of stress and stability and how these signs are integrated into the unit standardized pain assessment scale so they can evaluate how well their facilitated tucking is working.

The following day at the school, Patricia receives a referral to see Ben, a 13-year-old student who has mild spastic hemiplegia cerebral palsy, but no cognitive impairment. Ben complains of daily, 30 to 90 min episodes of mild-to-moderate intensity leg pain exacerbated by prolonged ambulation, fatigue, and situational stress. The pain interferes mildly with mobility, stress management, and sleep as indicated by his importance ratings on the COPM of 8, 7, and 9 respectively. Ben rates his performance as 6 (mobility), 6 (stress management), and 4 (sleep), moderate satisfaction in these areas.

Ben received eight autogenic relaxation training sessions in his home for stress management and sleep difficulties. Importantly, this training does not require gross motor movement or muscle contractions, both problematic for Ben. Each 45 min weekly session consisted of information on stress and relaxation rehearsal. Ben was also given a relaxation tape to guide him through practice at home and school. Pain intensity (0 equals 'no pain'; 10 equals 'pain as bad as it could be') and tension levels (0 = 'completely relaxed'; 10 equals 'uptight/tense as you can be') were rated in a diary pre and post relaxation practice. Ben was weaned from relaxation tape use, and integration of relaxation and stress management strategies into daily routines emphasized. He was also instructed in strategies to promote restful sleep. Ben's family was instructed to encourage and praise his relaxation practice. Ben reported moderate improvement in reducing pain interference, especially with stress management and sleep.

Patricia's work in these two cases was guided by a practice process of assessment, intervention, and outcome evaluation; her clinical reasoning was informed by theory. By assessing the interaction between the infant's developmental stage and the NICU environment, with an occupation focus, Patricia's recommendations enable the parents to engage with their baby (parenting role, nurturing occupation). Drawing on a specific theory related to infant development, Patricia's intervention plan minimizes threats to the infant's future occupational performance.

Into Ben's routine at home and school, Patricia integrated specific pain-relieving modalities thus facilitating his occupational roles. An outcome measure at baseline allowed for later outcome evaluation, showing progress toward achieving Ben's goals.

References

Als, H. (1982). Toward a synactive theory of development: promise for the assessment and support of infant individuality. *Infant Mental Health J*, 3, 229–243.

American Occupational Therapy Association Commission on Education. (2008). Occupational therapy practice framework: domain and process (2nd edn). *Am J Occ Ther*, 62, 625–683.

Ambuel, B., Hamlett, K. W., Marx, C. M., and Blumer, J. L. (1992). Assessing distress in pediatric intensive care environments. *J Pediatr Psychol*, 17(1), 95–109.

Aubert, E. J. (2008). Adaptive equipment and environmental aids for children with disabilities. In J. S. Tecklin (ed.) *Pediatric physical therapy* (4th edn), pp. 389–414. Baltimore MD: Lippincott Williams & Wilkins.

Ayres, A. J. (1979). *Sensory integration and the child.* Los Angeles, CA: Western Psychological Service.

Backman, C. L. (2011). Enabling performance and participation for persons with rheumatic diseases. In C. H. Christiansen and K. M. Matuska (eds) *Ways of living: intervention strategies to enable participation* (4th edn), pp. 213–238. Bethesda, MD: AOTA Press.

Bandstra, N. F., Skinner, L., LaBlanc, C., Chambers, C. T., Hollon, E. C., Brennan, D., *et al.* (2008). The role of child life in pediatric pain management: a survey of child life specialists. *J Pain*, 9, 320–329.

Barsky, A. J., Ahern, D. K., Orav, E. J., Nestoriuc, Y., Liang, M. H., Berman, I. T. *et al.* (2010). A randomized trial of three psychosocial treatments for the symptoms of rheumatoid arthritis. *Sem Arthritis Rheum*, 40(3), 222–232.

Bartocci, M., Bergqvist, L. L., Lagercrantz, H., and Anand, K. J. (2006). Pain activates cortical areas in the preterm newborn brain. *Pain*, 122, 109–117.

Beggs, S. and Fitzgerald, M. (2007). Development of peripheral and spinal nociceptive systems. In K. J. S. Anand, B. J. Stevens and P.J. McGrath (eds) *Pain in neonates and infants: pain research and clinical management* (3rd edn), pp. 11–24. Toronto: Elsevier.

Bundy, A. C. (1992). Play: the most important occupation of children. *Sensory Integration Special Interest Section Newsletter*, 15, 1–2.

Buysee, V., Bailey, D. and Bundy, A. (2001). Validity and reliability of a test of playfulness. *Occupat Ther J Res*, 21, 276–292.

Catelin, C., Tordjman, S. and Morin, V., Oger, E., and Sizun, J. (2005). Clinical, physiologic and biologic impact of environmental and behavioral interventions in neonates during a routine nursing procedure. *J Pain*, 6, 791–797.

Cignacco, E. L., Sellam, G., Stoffel, L., Gerull, R., Nelle, M., Anand, K. J., *et al.* (2012). Oral sucrose and 'facilitated tucking' for repeated pain relief in preterms: a randomized controlled trial. *Pediatrics*, 129(2), 1–10.

Cleeland, C. S. and Ryan, K. M. (1994). Pain assessment: global use of the Brief Pain Inventory. *Ann Acad Med Singapore*, 23, 129–138.

Cramer-Berness, L. J. and Friedman, A. G. (2005). Behavioral interventions for infant immunizations. *Child Health Care*, 34, 95–111.

Crepeau, E. B. and Schell, B. A. B. (2009). Analyzing occupations and activity. In E. B. Crepeau, E. S. Cohn and B. A. B. Schell (eds) *Willard & Spackman's occupational therapy* (11th edn), pp. 359–374. Philadelphia, PA: Wolters Kluwer Lippincott Williams & Wilkins.

Cohen, L. L., MacLarin, J. E., Fortson, B. L., Friedman, A., DeMore, M., Lim, C. S., *et al.* (2006). Randomized clinical trial of distraction for infant immunization pain. *Pain*, 125, 165–171.

Codipietro, L., Ceccarelli, M. and Ponzone, A. (2008). Breastfeeding or oral sucrose solution in term neonates receiving heel lance: a randomized, controlled trial. *Pediatrics*, 122, e716–e721.

Cusick, A., Lannin, N. A. and Lowe, K. (2007). Adapting the Canadian Occupational Performance Measure for use in a paediatric clinical trial. *Disabil Rehabil*, 29(10), 761–766.

Davis, J., Craik, J. and Polatajko, H. J. (2007). Using the Canadian process practice framework: amplifying the process. In E. A. Townsend and H. J. Polatajko (eds) *Enabling occupation II: advancing an occupational therapy vision for health, well-being, and justice through occupation*, pp. 247–272. Ottawa: CAOT Publications.

Dilli, D., Kucuk, I. G. and Dallar, Y. (2009). Interventions to reduce pain during vaccination in infancy. *J Pediatr*, 154(3), 385–390.

Dunn, K. M., Jordan, K. P., Manci, L., Drangsholt, M. T., and Le Resche, L. (2011). Trajectories of pain in adolescents: a prospective cohort study. *Pain*, 152(1), 66–73.

Du, Y., Knopf, H., Zhuang, W., and Elert, U. (2011). Pain perceived in a national community sample of German children and adolescents. *Eur J Pain*, 15(6), 649–657.

Engel, J. M. (2011). Pain in persons with developmental disabilities. *OT Practice*, 16(21), CE1–CE8.

Engel, J, M. and Kartin, D. (2004). Pain in youth: a primer for current practice. *Crit Rev Phys Med Rehabil Med*, 16, 53–76.

Fabrizi, L., Slater, R., Worley, A., Meek, J., Boyd, S., Olhede, S., *et al.* (2011). A shift in sensory processing that enables the developing human brain to discriminate touch from pain. *Curr Biol*, 21, 1–7.

Fearing, V. G. and Clark, J. (eds) (2000). *Individuals in context: a practical guide to client-centred practice.* Thorofare, NJ: Slack.

Folio, M. R. and Fewell, R. R. (2000). *Peabody developmental motor scales: examiner's manual* (2nd edn). Austin, TX: PRO-ED, Inc.

Grangaard, L. (2011). Low back pain. In H. M. Pendleton and W. Schultz-Krohn (eds) *Pedretti's occupational therapy: practice skills for physical dysfunction* (7th edn), pp. 1091–1109. St. Louis, MO: Elsevier Mosby.

Grunau, R. E. and Tu, M. T. (2007). Long-term consequences of pain in human neonates. In K. J. S. Anand, B. J. Stevens, and P. J. McGrath (eds) *Pain in neonates and infants: pain research and clinical management* (3rd edn), pp. 45–55. Toronto: Elsevier.

Grunau, R. V. E. and Craig, K. D. (1987). Pain expression in neonates: facial action and cry. *Pain*, 28, 395–410.

Hammond, A. and Freeman, K. (2001). One-year outcomes of a randomized controlled trial of an educational-behavioural joint protection programme for people with rheumatoid arthritis. *Rheumatology*, 40, 1044–1051.

Hickman, R., McCoy, S. W., Long, T. M. and Rauh, M. J. (2011). Applying contemporary developmental and movement science theories and evidence to early intervention practice. *Infants Young Child*, 24, 29–41.

Hohmeister, J., Kroll, A., Wollgarten-Hadamek I, Zohsel, K., Demirakça, S., Flor, H., *et al.* (2010). Cerebral processing of pain in school-aged children with neonatal nociceptive input-an exploratory fMFRI study. *Pain*, 150, 257–267.

Holsti, L. and Grunau, R. (2007a). Extremity movements help occupational therapists identify stress responses in preterm infants in the neonatal intensive care nursery: a systematic review. *Can J Occ Ther*, 74, 183–194.

Holsti, L. and Grunau, R. E. (2007b). Initial validation of the Behavioral Indicators of Infant Pain (BIIP). *Pain*, 132, 264–272.

Holsti, L. and Grunau, R. (2010). Is sucrose the solution? Considerations for using sucrose for reducing procedural pain in preterm infants. *Pediatrics*, 125, 1042–1047.

Holsti, L. Oberlander, T. and Brant R. (2011). Does breastfeeding reduce acute pain in preterm infants in the NICU. A randomized clinical trial. *Pain*, 152, 2575–2581.

Howard, L. (2002). A survey of paediatric occupational therapists in the United Kingdom. *Occup Ther Int*, 9 (4), 326–343.

Jaffe, L., Humphry, R., and Case-Smith, J. (2010). Working with families. In J. Case-Smith and J. C. O'Brien (eds) *Occupational therapy for children* (6th edn), pp. 108–145. Maryland Heights, MO: Mosby Elsevier.

Johnston, C. C. (2011). Pain control in infants and young children. *Pain Res Manag*, 16, 320.

Johnston, C. C., Filion, F., Snider, L., Majnemer, A., Limperopoulos, C., Walker, C. D., *et al.* (2002). Routine sucrose analgesia during the first week of life in neonates younger than 31 weeks' postconceptional age. *Pediatrics*, 110, 523–528.

King, S., Chambers, C. T., Huguet, A., MacNevin, R. C., McGrath, P. J., Parker, L., *et al.* (2001). The epidemiology of chronic pain in children and adolescents revisited: a systematic review. *Pain*, 152, 2729–2738.

Kjaer, P., Wedderkopp, N., Korhsholm, L., and Leboeuf-Yde C. (2011). Prevalence and tracking of back pain from childhood to adolescence. *BMC Musculoskelet Disord*, 12, 98. Available at: <http://www.biomedicalcentral.com/1471–2474/12–98> (accessed 12 January 2012).

Koupil, I. (2007). The Uppsala studies on developmental origins of health and disease. *J Int Med*, 261, 426–436.

Kuchta, G. and Davidson, I. (eds) (2008). *Occupational and physical therapy for children with rheumatic diseases: a clinical handbook*. Oxford: Radcliffe Publishing.

Law, M., Baptiste, S., Carswell, A., Opzooner, A., Polatajko, H., and Pollock, N. (2005). *Canadian occupational performance measure* (4th edn). Ottawa ON: CAOT Publications.

Law, E. F., Dahlquist, L. M., Sil, S., Weiss, K. E., Herbert, L. J., Wohlheiter, K., *et al.* (2011). Videogame distraction using virtual reality technology for children experiencing cold pressor pain: the role of cognitive processing. *J Pediatr Psychol*, 36, 84–94.

Leite, A. M., Linhares, M. B. M., Lander, J., Castral, T. C., dos Santos, C. B., and Silvan Scochi, C. G. (2009). Effects of breastfeeding on pain relief in full-term infants. *Clin J Pain*, 25, 827–832.

Loeser, J. D. and Fordyce, W. E. (1983). Chronic pain. In J. E. Carr, H. A. Dengerink, (eds) *Behavioral science in the practice of medicine*, pp. 331–345. New York: Elsevier.

Loman, M. M. and Gunnar, M. R. (2010). Early experience and the development of stress reactivity and regulation in children. *Neurosci Biobehav Rev*, 34, 867–876.

McColl, M. A., Law, M., Stewart, D., Doubt, L., Pollack, N., and Krupa, T. (2003). *Theoretical basis of occupational therapy* (2nd edn). Thorofare, NJ: Slack.

Melchert-McKearnan, K., Deitz, J., Engel, J. M., and White, O. (2000). Children with burn injuries: purposeful activity versus rote exercise. *Am J Occ Ther*, 54, 381–390.

Melzack, R. and Wall, P. (1965). Pain mechanisms: a new theory. *Science*, 50, 971–979.

Merkel, S. I., Voepel-Lewis, T., Shayevitz, J. R., and Malviya, S. (1997). The FLACC: a behavioral scale for scoring postoperative pain in young children. *Pediatr Nurs*, 23(3), 293–297.

Morison, S. J., Grunau, R. E., Oberlander, T. F., and Whitfield, M. (2001). Relationships between behavioural and cardiac autonomic reactivity to acute pain in preterm neonates. *Clin J Pain*, 17, 350–358.

Niedermann, K., de Bie, R. A., Kubli R., Ciurea, A., Steurer-Stey, C., Villiger, P. M. *et al.* (2011). Effectiveness of individual resource-oriented joint protection education in people with rheumatoid arthritis. A randomized controlled trial. *Patient Educ Couns*, 82, 42–48.

Parkinson, K. N., Gibson, L., Dickinson, H. O., and Colver, A. F. (2010). Pain in children with cerebral palsy: a cross-sectional multicentre European study. *Acta Paediatr*, 99, 446–451.

Payne, R. A. (2000). *Relaxation techniques: a practical handbook for healthcare professionals* (2nd edn). New York: Churchill Livingstone.

Pierce, D., Munier, V., and Myers, C. T. (2009). Informing early intervention through an occupational science description of infant-toddler interactions within home space. *Am J Occ Ther*, 63, 273–287.

Pillai Riddell, R., Racine, N., Turcotte, K., Uman, L., Horton, R., Din Osmun, L., *et al.* (2011). Nonpharmacological management of procedural pain in infants and young children: an abridged Cochrane review. *Pain Res Manag*, 16, 321–330.

Polatajko, H. J., Davis, J. A., Hobson, S. J. G., Landry, J. E., Mandich, A., Street, S. L., *et al.* (2004). Meeting the responsibility that comes with privilege: introducing a taxonomic code for understanding occupation. *Can J Occ Ther*, 71, 261–268.

Polatajko, H., Davis, J., Stewart D., Cantin, N., Amoroso, B., Purdie, L., *et al.* (2007). Specifying the domain of concern: occupation as core. In E. A. Townsend, and H. J. Polatajko (eds) *Enabling occupation II: advancing an occupational therapy vision for health, well-being, & justice through occupation*, pp. 9–36. Ottawa ON: CAOT Publications ACE.

Shah, P. S., Aliwalas, L. L., and Shah, V. (2009). Breastfeeding or breast milk for procedural pain in neonates. Cochrane Neonatal Group. *Cochrane Database of Syst Rev*, 3, CD004950.

Siu, D. C., Tse, L. A., Yu, I. T., and Griffiths, S. F. (2009). Computer products usage and prevalence of computer related musculoskeletal discomfort among adolescents. *Work*, 34(4), 449–54.

Sizun, J., Ansquer, H., Browne J., Tordjman, S., and Morin, J. F. (2002). Developmental care decreases physiological and behavioral pain expression in preterm neonates. *J Pain*, 3, 446–450.

Slater, R., Cornelissen, L., Fabrizi, L., Patten, D., Yoxen, J., Worley, A., *et al.* (2010). Oral sucrose as an analgesic drug for procedural pain in newborn infants: a randomized controlled trial. *Lancet*, 376, 1225–1232.

Slater, R., Cantarella, A., Franck, L., Meek, J., and Fitzgerald, M. (2008). How well do clinical pain assessment tools reflect pain in infants? *PLoS Medicine*, 5, e129.

Stevens, B., Craig, K., Johnston., C., Standish, J., Munro, J., Takacs, L., *et al.* (2011). Oral sucrose for procedural pain. *Lancet*, 377(9759), 25–26.

Stevens, B., Johnston, C. C., Petryshen, P., and Taddio, A. (1996). Premature infant pain profile: development and initial validation. *Clin J Pain*, 12, 13–22.

Steultjens, E. E. M. J., Dekker, J., Bouter, L. M., van Schaardenburg, D., van Kuyk, M. A., and van den Ende, C. H. (2004). Occupational therapy for rheumatoid arthritis. *Cochrane Database Syst Rev*, 1, CD003114.

Stevens, B. J., Pillai Riddell, R. R., Oberlander, T. E., and Gibbins, S. (2007). Assessment of pain in neonates and infants. In K. J. S. Anand, B. J. Stevens and P. J. McGrath (eds) *Pain in neonates and infants: pain research and clinical management* (3rd edn), pp. 67–90. Toronto: Elsevier.

Stevens, B., Yamada, J., and Ohlsson, A. (2010). Sucrose for analgesia in newborn infants undergoing painful procedures (Cochrane review). *Cochrane Database Syst Rev*, 1, CD001069.

Strong, J. (1996). *Chronic pain: the occupational therapist's perspective*. New York: Churchill Livingstone.

Sullivan, M. C., Hawes K., Winchester, S. B., and Miller, R. J. (2008). Developmental origins theory from prematurity to adult disease. *J Obstet Gynecol Nurs*, 37, 158–164.

Tanabe P., Ferket, K., Thomas, R., Paice, J., and Marcantonio, R. (2002). The effect of standard care, ibuprofen, and distraction on pain relief and patient satisfaction in children with musculoskeletal trauma. *J Emerg Nurs*, 28, 118–125

Taylor, J. and Erlandson, D. M. (2001). Pediatric rheumatic diseases. In L. Robbins, C. S. Burckhart, M. T. Hannan, and R. J. DeHoratius (eds) *Clinical care in the rheumatic diseases* (2nd edn), pp. 81–88. Atlanta, GA: Association of Rheumatology Health Professionals.

Townsend, E. A. and Polatajko, H. J. (2007). *Enabling occupation II: advancing an occupational therapy vision for health, well-being, & justice through occupation*. Ottawa: CAOT Publications ACE.

Tyler, E. J., Jensen, M. P., Engel, J. M., and Schwartz, L. (2002). The reliability and validity of pain interference measures in persons with cerebral palsy. *Arch Phys Med Rehabil*, 83, 236–239.

Upadhyay, A., Aggarwal, R., Narayan, S., Joshi, M., Paul, V. K., and Deorari, A. K. (2004). Analgesic effect of expressed breast milk in procedural pain in term neonates: a randomized, placebo-controlled, double blind trial. *Acta Paediatr*, 93, 518–522.

Verkerk, G. J. Q., Wolf, M. J., Louwers, A. M., Meester-Delver, A., and Nollet, F. (2006). The reproducibility and validity of the Canadian Occupational Performance Measure in parents of children with disabilities. *Clin Rehabil*, 20, 980–988.

Wilson, P. H. (2005). Practitioner review: approaches to assessment and treatment of children with DCD: an evaluative review. *J Child Psychol Psychiatry*, 46(8), 806–823.

Zwicker, J. G. and Harris, S. R. (2009). A reflection on motor learning theory in pediatric occupational therapy. *Can J Occ Ther*, 76(1), 29–37.

Supplementary online materials

Figure 57.3 Handout—recognizing pain behaviour in your child.
Reproduced from Kuchta, G. and Davidson, I. (eds) *Occupational and Physical Therapy for Children with Rheumatic Diseases: a clinical handbook*, Radcliffe

Publishing, Oxford, Copyright © Gay Kuchta and Iris Davidson 2008, with permission from Radcliffe Publishing.

Figure 57.4 Handout—what to do when your child is in pain.
Reproduced from Kuchta, G. and Davidson, I. (eds) *Occupational and Physical Therapy for Children with Rheumatic Diseases: a clinical handbook*, Radcliffe Publishing, Oxford, Copyright © Gay Kuchta and Iris Davidson 2008, with permission from Radcliffe Publishing.

Figure 57.5 Handout—managing your child's pain with heat or cold.
Reproduced from Kuchta, G. and Davidson, I. (eds) *Occupational and Physical*

Therapy for Children with Rheumatic Diseases: a clinical handbook, Radcliffe Publishing, Oxford, Copyright © Gay Kuchta and Iris Davidson 2008, with permission from Radcliffe Publishing.

Figure 57.6 Handout—fatigue management.
Reproduced from Kuchta, G. and Davidson, I. (eds) *Occupational and Physical Therapy for Children with Rheumatic Diseases: a clinical handbook*, Radcliffe Publishing, Oxford, Copyright © Gay Kuchta and Iris Davidson 2008, with permission from Radcliffe Publishing.

CHAPTER 58

Mother care for procedural pain in infants

Celeste Johnston and Marsha Campbell-Yeo

Summary

A major role of maternal care is to protect their infant from harm, including pain. The aim of this chapter is to review the evidence on the effectiveness of maternal strategies that are efficacious in managing procedural pain including breastfeeding, kangaroo mother care, and facsimiles of maternal presence such as voice recordings, odour, and other care providers. The mechanisms, as currently understood, underlying the efficacy of maternal care, will be presented. Finally, pragmatic issues, such as feasibility, will be discussed.

Introduction

Mammalian mothers almost universally take care of their young. This includes providing nourishment and protection from harm. Protection from harm, in the event of tissue damage, encompasses providing comfort to assist the infant to return to a pre-injured state. In modern human history, particularly in developed countries, ill or very preterm infants are separated from their mothers, who then lose the nurturing and protective roles that are inherent in motherhood. Even well babies undergoing routine medical care are often separated from their mothers. Infants are often removed from their mother's arms and placed in a bassinet to undergo a painful procedure. This separation is executed in the belief that health care professionals can care for the infant without the mother, and, in fact, that the mother may interfere with their ability to give the most efficient care to the infant (Campbell-Yeo et al., 2008b). As paediatric hospitals and units move towards family centred care, this separation is being questioned (Franck et al., 2011). Recent reports from the literature can be used to support the inclusion of parents, especially mothers, in the care of hospitalized infants including the role of providing comfort during painful events.

Background

Breast milk, breastfeeding

Breast milk and breastfeeding are often considered together for obvious reasons: you cannot have breastfeeding without breast milk or its precursor, colostrum. In full-term neonates, Gray and colleagues reported there was significant reduction in pain scores with breastfeeding compared to standard care (Gray et al., 2002). Other studies, compared breastfeeding to sweet taste with mixed results. Bilgen found 25% sucrose more effective in decreasing heart rate change, crying, and recovery time (Bilgen et al., 2001). Carbajal et al. (2003) reported equivalent reduction in composite pain scores between breastfeeding and glucose plus pacifier. Codipietro et al. (2008) reported significant differences on pain scores favouring breastfeeding over sucrose. Finally, Gradin et al. (2004) reported that in combination, there were synergistic effects between 30% glucose plus breastfeeding. Results from a systematic meta-analysis of breastfeeding support its use as a comforting measure for procedural pain in full-term infants (Shah et al., 2007). Pain scores measured using the Premature Infant Pain Profile (PIPP; Stevens et al., 1996, 2010) composite pain measure were significantly different between the breastfeeding group and the placebo group (weighted mean difference: -6 (range -7 to -4)), but these scores were not different when compared with the glucose plus pacifier group (weighted mean difference: 1.30 (range: 0.05 to 2.56)) (Shah et al., 2007).

Breast milk delivered by syringe alone (i.e. without a pacifier or being held) is, in all but one study (Upadhyay et al., 2004), ineffective in reducing pain (Bilgen et al., 2001; Blass, 1997; Blass and Miller, 2001; Ors et al., 1999). This finding is hypothesized to be relative to the sweetness of sugars; where lactose in breast milk is much less sweet than sucrose (Joesten et al., 2007; McDaniel et al., 1989).

These results raise certain questions about why breastfeeding is effective, since breast milk administered alone is not. Sucking could be one component since sucking alone has been reported to have a pain reducing effect (Bo and Callaghan, 2000). Maternal closeness could be another factor. Holding by the mother was more effective in reducing crying than both holding and sucrose alone but facial actions of pain were decreased only by holding (Gormally et al., 2001). However, in another study, holding by mother was not as effective as glucose on pacifier or breastfeeding (Carbajal et al., 2003).

The evidence to support breastfeeding as a comfort measure is strong (Campbell-Yeo et al., 2011). At its weakest, breastfeeding is marginally less effective than sweet taste, but the results are mixed. The underlying mechanisms are likely synergistic since neither holding, breast milk alone, nor sucking alone can explain its effectiveness. For a more in-depth discussion on sucrose and sweet taste in relieving pain in infants, please see Harrison et al. (Chapter 49, this volume).

Skin-to-skin contact, or kangaroo mother care

Skin-to-skin contact (SSC) between infant and mother is commonly referred to as kangaroo mother care (KMC), due to its similarity to marsupial maternal care. Among behavioural and physical interventions for procedural pain in the neonatal intensive care unit (NICU), SSC is of interest both because of its effectiveness, but also in its centrality to family centred care. Currently, the comforting role of mothers is lost in the typical NICU setting (Montirosso et al., 2012). Yet, pain their child experiences and the loss of that comforting parental role are among the highest sources of stress for mothers as well as fathers (Franck et al., 2005; Miles et al., 1989, 1993). By giving mothers an opportunity to take on the comforting role of parenthood, they feel they are effective and closer to their infant (Campbell-Yeo et al., 2008a).

KMC was implemented in the modern era as an alternative to the incubator to maintain preterm infants' body temperature and increase survival rate in South America where incubators were in short supply (Charpak et al., 1994). During this time, it was serendipitously noted that infants spent more time in quiet sleep state (Ludington-Hoe et al., 2006). More recently, analysis using electroencephalogram (EEG) sleep studies demonstrated that preterm infants exposed to KMC daily for 8 weeks had fewer rapid eye movements, more quiet sleep, and less spectral beta when compared to full-term infants, delivered at term or delivered preterm and corrected to term equivalent who did not receive KMC (Scher and Loparo, 2009). Since quiet state is associated with decreased pain response (Grunau and Craig, 1987; Stevens et al., 1996) the idea developed to use KMC for procedural pain management.

The first study examining the effect of KMC and pain response was conducted by Gray in 2000, in full-term neonates where decreased crying and a lower heart rate acceleration were observed (Gray et al., 2000). Three years later, Johnston, in the first study examining KMC with preterm neonates undergoing heel lance, reported a decrease in composite pain scores, as well as the individual components of decreased facial action, lower heart rate acceleration, and increased oxygen saturations for neonates receiving KMC compared to incubator care (Johnston et al., 2003). A 2-point reduction as measured using the PIPP (Stevens et al., 1996) was found at 30, 60, and 90 sec after heel lance (Johnston et al., 2003) and at 90 sec (p <0.001) in a similar study by Johnston examining the pain response of very preterm infants (Johnston et al., 2008). An even larger difference was found by Akcan et al. (2009) at 1, 2, and 3 min after heel lance or venepuncture (mean PIPP score of 7, 4, and 4 in the SSC group and 15, p <0.001, 15.5, p = 0.001 and 15, p = 0.047 in the control group). In a Cochrane review on SSC for procedural pain in infants, 15 studies that meet the inclusion criteria all showed positive results (Johnston et al., 2010) when compared to usual care (see Table 58.1). Two studies (Chermont et al., 2009; Freire et al., 2008) showed that KMC/SSC was more efficacious than sweet taste.

Auditory facsimiles of maternal presence

While infants are *in utero*, sensory learning is taking place, so that following birth, they have some knowledge of their mother's identification, notably auditory and olfactory (see later sections). During the third trimester (≥27 weeks GA) fetuses are able to hear and respond behaviourally to sound and auditory stimuli (DeCasper and Fifer, 1980; Ockleford et al., 1988). DeCasper and Spence (1986) studied pregnant women at 30 weeks of gestation who had recited a target story aloud to their fetuses twice daily until birth. At birth, the target story had greater reinforcing value (measured by sucking bursts) to the novel story and was independent of who recited the story. In another study, pregnant women at 33 weeks of gestation recited a target rhyme three times daily for a succession of 4 weeks which the fetuses differentially responded to with a brief decrease in fetal heart rate (DeCasper et al., 1994). DeCasper and Fifer (1980) examined full-term newborns within 3 days of life, and found that they preferred their mother's voice more than a female stranger's voice. In addition, the newborn, up to 8 months in age, can discriminate and show preference for their mother's voice compared to a female stranger's voice (Standley and Masen, 1990). Fifer et al. (1995) found that newborns suck a non-nutritive nipple significantly more often when syllables are paired with the maternal voice to syllables paired with another woman's voice or silence. When presented with a choice of hearing their own mother's voice in speech or a filtered version in such a way as to mimic womblike sounds, newborns suck more often to the signal predicting the '*in utero*' versions of their own mother's voice.

Based on these data of infant auditory memory of their mother's voice, as well as memory of maternal heartbeat, auditory recordings compared THE EFFECTS OF recordings of maternal sounds have been tested on pain response in infants. The first study with full-term neonates compared recordings of maternal heartbeat to Japanese drum (the study was conducted in Japan and the Japanese drum is soft and rhythmic) on salivary and serum cortiso response following heel stick (Kurihara et al., 1996). Maternal heartbeat was more effective in decreasing behavioural indicators of stress, measured using facial and vocal response during heel lance as well as cortisol levels measured 20 min post lance. More recently, maternal voice recordings of babytalk, nursery rhymes, or songs, played to preterm neonates during quiet time and then during a heel lance procedure was no more effective than usual care with no sound (Johnston et al., 2007). In this study, the decibel levels of the recordings were above the recommended levels, as was the ambient noise of the study NICU, which may have interfered with the infant's ability to process the actual sounds.

Maternal olfactory effects on pain response

There is similar olfactory as well as auditory learning of mother *in utero*. When newborn infants, separated from their mothers, were exposed to amniotic fluid, their mothers' breast odour, or no odour, the ones who were exposed to amniotic fluid calmed more quickly and cried less (Varendi et al., 1998). Furthermore, in another study of infant preference measured through head turning towards odour, infants showed recognition of their own mother's amniotic fluid, versus amniotic fluid from other women (Schaal et al., 1998). Full-term infants also preferred the smell of human milk, not necessarily their own mother's milk, over formula milk (Marlier and Schaal, 2005). Thus, the potential use of the familiar maternal odour was tested as an intervention for procedural pain in newborns.

Goubet and colleagues conducted three studies on familiar odours versus non-familiar odours on pain response in full-term infants (Goubet et al., 2003, 2007; Rattaz et al., 2005). All studies demonstrated the effectiveness of a familiar smell, be it from mother or from conditioning the infant to the smell of vanillan. One study compared odours of mother's own milk, another woman's milk, formula milk, or no odour control on grimacing, crying,

Table 58.1 Studies examining the effect of kangaroo care (KC) on pain response

Study	Sample N, GA	Design and intervention	Provider	Procedure	Outcome measures	Results in KMC
(Gray et al., 2000)	30, full term	RCT, 10–15 min, KC vs swaddled in cot	Mother	Heel lance	Duration of cry, grimacing, HR	Cry ↓ by 82%, grimacing ↓ by 65%, smaller ↑ in beats/minute during blood collection (8–10 vs 36–38)
(Johnston et al., 2003)	74, 32–36 weeks GA	RCT, crossover 30 min KC vs swaddled in incubator	Mother	Heel lance	PIPP: facial actions, heart rate, oxygen saturation, gestational age, behavioural state	PIPP scores significantly ↓ at 30 sec (MD, 1.5 points; P = 0.04), 60 sec (MD, 2.2 points; P = 0.002), and 90 sec (MD, 0.6 point; P = 0.37) after heel-lancing procedure. Heart rate and oxygen saturation similar in both conditions. Facial actions contributed significantly to total pain score (0.000 <P <0.005), with facial actions averaging 20% greater in control vs KC condition.
(Ludington-Hoe et al., 2005)	23, mean 31 weeks GA	RCT, crossover 3 h of KC vs incubator	Mother	Heel lance	HR, respiratory rate, oxygen saturation, ↓ crying, length of crying, behavioural state	Mean rise in heart rate (F(1,32) = 3.01, P = 0.047) from baseline to heel lance was less in the KC condition than in the warmer condition Crying length during KC heel lance significantly less than during warmer heel lance (F(1,32) = 7.38, P = 0.003) and post-lance period (P = 0.02).
(Kashaninia et al., 2008; Sajedi et al., 2007)[a]	100 full term	RCT, 10 min KC vs cot	Mother	IM injection	Duration of cry, NIPS score	Mean duration of crying post injection was longer, 24.61 in the control group vs 14.55 sec in the KC group p = 0.001. NIPS scores significantly ↓ immediately following injection in KC, p <0.001
(Castral et al., 2008)	59, 30–37 weeks GA	RCT, 15 min KMC vs swaddled in incubator	Mother	Heel lance	Facial action, NFCS score, behavioural state, duration of cry, HR	NFCS score significantly ↓ at heel lance (−1.140; p = 0.23) and squeeze phase (−1.872; p <0.001). Cry ↓ by 37.4%. No difference in HR
(Freire et al., 2008)	95, 28–36 weeks GA	RCT. 15 min KC vs oral glucose vs prone position in incubator	Mother	Heel lance	Behavioural state, HR variation, Oxygen saturation, PIPP scores for facial actions	No difference in behavioural state, ↓ variation in (p<0.0001) and HR in oxygen saturation (p <0.0012), ↓ scores for facial actions (p <0.0001)
(Johnston et al., 2008)	61, 28–31 weeks GA	RCT cross-over 15 min KC versus swaddled in incubator	Mother	Heel lance	PIPP, time to recover (heart rate return to baseline), facial actions, HR, oxygen saturation	PIPP scores ↓ at 90 sec (8.871 versus 10.677; p <0.001). Time to recover ↓ in KC (123 sec (95%CI 103–142)) vs 193 sec for incubator (95% CI 158–227) (F (61,1) = 13.6, p <0.000)
(Kostandy et al., 2008)	10 Preterm 30–32 weeks GA	RCT, crossover, 30 min KC vs nested in incubator	Mother	Heel lance	Audible and inaudible crying (Anderson Behavioural State Scoring system)	↓ combined crying time during heel stick (55 vs 96.2 sec; p = 0.001) and during recovery (5.8 vs 25.5 sec; p <0.01). Inaudible cry was minimal in each phase, in both conditions 0–1.34 sec
(Akcan et al., 2009)	50, Preterm 26–36 weeks GA	RCT, 45 min KC × 5 days-procedure on 5th day.	Mother	Heel stick/ venepuncture	PIPP score at 60, 90, 120 seconds following procedure	PIPP scores were ↓ in the KC group, at the 1st, 2nd and 3rd min of the painful procedure, 7.0, 4 and 4 in infants in KC group vs 15.0, 15.5 and 15.0 (p <0.001, p = 0.001, p = 0.047, respectively)

(Continued)

Table 58.1 (Continued)

Study	Sample N, GA	Design and intervention	Provider	Procedure	Outcome measures	Results in KMC
Chermont (Chermont et al., 2009)	640 Full term	RCT. 2 min KC vs standard care vs 25% dextrose vs KC/dextrose	Mother	IM injection	PIPP score. NFCS and NIPS	Mean PIPP scores for the 4 groups were standard care, 6.9±2.3; KC, 6.2±2.0; 25% dextrose treatment, 6.8±1.6; KC plus 25% dextrose treatment, 5.9±2.1
(Cong et al., 2009)	14 Preterm 30–32 weeks	RCT, crossover 60 min KC vs incubator (IC)	Mother	Heel lance	Infant behavioural state, HR, HRV	HR significantly lower in the KC condition (146±9 bpm) than in IC (152±13 bpm) during baseline period ($p < 0.05$) and Heel Stick period (KC 159 ± bpm vs IC 165 ± 14 bpm, $p < 0.05$). HRV ↑ stable in KC at baseline ($p < 01$) and at heel lance ($p < 0.001$)
(Ferber and Makhoul, 2008)	30 Preterm 28–34 weeks	RCT Crossover, 10 min KC vs incubator	Mother	Heel lance	NIDCAP	↓ motor disorganization $F(129) = 6.716$, $p = 0.002$; extension movements ($F(1, 29) = 8.554$, $p < 0.0001$); and an ↑ in attention signs negative attention signs ($F(1.29) = 27.000$, $p = 0.018$) and positive attention signs ([$F(1,29) = 3.077$, $p < 0.05$) during KC
(Johnston et al., 2009)	90 32–36 weeks GA	RCT, crossover, 30 min KC with additional rocking, singing, and sucking vs KC without additional stimulation	Mother	Heel lance	PIPP, time to recover	No significant differences in PIPP scores or time to recover significant, differences across sites
(Cong et al., 2011)	28 Preterm 30–32 weeks	RCT, crossover 14 infants, 80 min KC (Study 1); 10 infants, 30 min KC (Study 2) vs incubator	Mother	Heel lance	PIPP salivary and serum cortisol at baseline, heel warming, heel stick and recovery	Study 1: no differences Study 2: ↓ PIPP during recovery ($p < 0.05$ to $p < 0.001$), ↓ salivary cortisol at the end of recovery ($p < 0.05$) and ↓ serum cortisol during heel lance condition during heel lance
(Johnston et al., 2011)	62 Preterm 28–36 weeks	RCT, crossover 30 min MKC vs FKC	Mother Father	Heel lance	PIPP, time to recover	↓ PIPP in MKC, mean difference 1.4 at 30 sec, 1.5 at 60 sec. No difference at 90 sec and 120s sec. ↓ time to recover (204 sec MKC, 246 sec FKC). PIPP scores ↓ in both groups vs historical controls

a Same study

bpm = beats per minute; FKC =father kangaroo care; GA = gestational age; HR = heart rate; HRV = heart rate variability; IM = intramuscular injection; KC = kangaroo care; MD = mean difference; MKC = mother kangaroo care; NFCS = Neonatal Facial Coding System; NIDCAP = Newborn Individualized Developmental Care and Assessment Program; NIPS = Neonatal Infant Pain Scale; PIPP = Premature Infant Pain Profile; RCT = randomized controlled trial.

motor activity, and salivary cortisol levels in full-term neonates undergoing heel lance (Nishitani et al., 2009). Infants exposed to mothers' own milk odour had significantly lower scores and values for all outcome measures when compared to controls. There were no significant differences noted in the other groups for any of the outcomes compared to the controls.

Facilitated tucking

Facilitated tucking consists of a care provider or parent using their hands to provide containment and a supportive boundary to an infant undergoing a stressful or painful procedure. While typically performed by nurses, it has been used by mothers (Axelin et al., 2006, 2010). The infant is generally held in a side-lying, flexed fetal-type position (Axelin et al., 2006, 2009b; see Holstii et al., Chapter 57, this volume, for a more detailed description of facilitated tucking). Facilitated tucking alone, studied in both preterm and very preterm infants, has been associated with diminished pain scores following heel lance and endotracheal suctioning (Axelin et al., 2006; Ward-Larson et al., 2004) when compared to placebo. Similarly, when used in combination with non-nutritive sucking,

34 preterm infants receiving facilitated tucking during heel lance had significantly lower mean (standard deviation) pain scores during heel-stick procedures (6.39 (3.35) and 7.15 (3.88), respectively) than those receiving routine care (9.52 (4.95)) (Liaw et al., 2012). Facilitated tucking is also more beneficial when compared to oxycodone (Axelin et al., 2009b). Following endotracheal suctioning, facilitated tucking by parents was equivalent to glucose (Axelin et al., 2009a); however, this was not the case following repeated heel lance. In a study examining preterm infants between 24 and 32 weeks GA randomized to receive facilitated tucking, sucrose or combination of sucrose and facilitated tucking following over time for repeated heel lances, facilitated tucking alone was less effective than sucrose; however, Bernese Pain Scale for Neonates (Cignacco et al., 2004) scores were lowest when combined with the sweet taste (Cignacco et al., 2012).

Sensorial saturation

Combining strategies, including talking to the infant, massaging or stroking the infant as well as giving a sweet solution, has been coined sensorial saturation by Bellieni and his group (Bellieni et al., 2001, 2002). Typically, sensorial saturation is performed by nursing staff; however, in one study with full-term neonates, mothers did the sensorial saturation (Bellieni et al., 2007). Both mothers doing it for the first time and experienced nurses doing sensorial saturation were more effective than glucose and pacifier, but there were no significant differences between the two. It could be that the experience of the nurses waived differences or it could be that, it did not matter who did the intervention.

Maternal–infant interactions related to pain experience

As infants develop and have more interactions with their mothers, patterns of interactions become established. Healthy infants who do not experience hospitalization beyond normal nursery care in the first few days of life, are subjected to immunization pain. Mothers, perhaps as a reflection of the stress associated with their infant experiencing pain from an elective procedure, will intuitively apologize, empathize, and give reassurance such as 'don't worry' or 'it will be okay' (McMurtry et al., 2010). These actions, have been found to be less effective than distraction approaches that might include singing, offering a toy in reducing both intensity and duration of pain response (Blount et al., 2008, 2009; also see Cohen et al., Chapter 53, this volume). Similar to the effect in preterm neonates, proximal strategies, such as the mother rocking (Campos, 1994) also reduced pain response. Furthermore, controlling for factors such as age, previous pain exposure, medical history, in a sample of 4- and 6-month-old infants, mothers and fathers made more proximal coping promoting behaviours prior to the immunization than health care professionals which significantly decreased facial actions of their infants during the immunization (Piira et al., 2007).

It is perhaps less the specific behaviours that mothers use as opposed to maternal sensitivity to the infant cues that is important. This only becomes strongly associated with decreased pain response as mother and infant have longer time together. For example, in Sweet's prospective study of 6- and 18-month-old infants undergoing immunization, maternal sensitivity was a significant predictor of lower distress only at the 18-month visit (Sweet et al., 1999). Similarly, Pillai Riddell following a cohort of infants across the first year of life, found that maternal availability/sensitivity was

a significant predictor across all phases of the immunization procedure (Pillai Riddell et al., 2011). Pillai Riddell and colleagues suggested that this ability of the mother to accurately use the infant cues, as well as the infant's ability to display learned cues resulting in maternal caring response, is directly related to maternal-infant attachment, which typically peaks at 1 year of age (Ainsworth, 1969). For an in-depth discussion on psychological theories and models, see Pillai Riddell et al. (Chapter 9, this volume).

Other providers

KMC or SSC provides a multisensorial context encompassing tactile, olfactory, and relational systems (Campbell-Yeo et al., 2011). Consistent findings from numerous studies clearly support the comforting role of a mother. What is less known, is whether this comfort relates only to a mother or whether other providers, (e.g. an adult who cares for you or someone familiar) could provide a similar comforting effect. In the first study to address this question, alternate women (n = 22), biologically unrelated to the mother, were compared to infants' own mothers using a cross-over design (Johnston et al., 2012). PIPP scores were lower in the infant's own mother group (8.3 versus 6.0 at 90 sec post-lance) although this difference was not statistically significant due to the small pilot sample, but effect size was greater than other studies at 90 and 120 sec supporting the effectiveness of the biological mother. Although highly plausible, these findings need to be interpreted with caution due to the small sample size.

Using a similar crossover design, comparison between fathers or mothers who provided KMC for 30 min was made prior to and during heel lance (Johnston et al., 2011). Although PIPP scores were lower in both groups compared to historical controls, mothers provided more analgesic effect and infants recovered faster than when with fathers (mean difference of 1.4 at 30 sec, 1.5 at 60 sec; no difference at 90 sec and 120 sec; time to recover 204 sec versus 246 sec), respectively.

Interestingly, the PIPP scores were very low but not statistically different between preterm twins who were co-bedding (being cared for together in the same incubator allowing skin contact between them) prior and during heel lance and provided sucrose compared to a similar population receiving sucrose alone, considered standard care (SC) in the first minute post heel lance (7.1(SD2.8), 6.1(SD3.0) versus 7.2 (SD3.4), 5.2 (2.0)) (Campbell-Yeo et al., 2012). At 90 sec, PIPP scores were higher in the co-bedding group 6.0 (SD 3.0) compared to 5.0 (SD1.8) (p <0.05), in the SC group. Although higher, the clinical significance of this difference at 90 sec post lance is uncertain. Reasons for the lack of analgesic effect may be due to the lack of full ventral contact and the upright position present during kangaroo care which is not possible during co-bedding. Or, it may be that mother's ability to effectively provide pain relief is unique. Further research is needed to elucidate these findings. Nevertheless, co-bedding was associated with the twins' ability to better regulate the pain associated with heel lance. The co-bedding twins recovered more than a minute faster than the SC group, mean time of 75.6 sec, compared to 142.1 sec during SC. Further analysis using generalized estimating equation modelling (GEE) and including corrected GA less than 32 weeks at heel lance did not change these findings and resulted in a p value of 0.005. Salivary cortisol levels, a reliable biomarker of stress, were significantly lower, mean levels 0.28 mcg/dL (SD 0.25) versus 0.50 mcg/dL (SD 0.73), in the co-bedding twins (see Table 58.2).

Table 58.2 The effectiveness of maternal- or family-driven non-pharmacological strategies for reduction of procedural pain

Intervention	Gestational age	Procedure	Findings	Effect
Breastfeeding and expressed breast milk (Codipietro et al., 2008; Efe and Ozer, 2007; Gray et al., 2002; Osinaike et al., 2007; Shah et al., 2008)	Full term Preterm	Venepuncture Heel stick	↓ crying time and smaller increase in HR with breastfeeding compared to swaddling ↓ PIPP scores with breastfeeding compared to placebo. Mixed results when comparing breastfeeding to sweet solutions	Breastfeeding is effective; conflicting results regarding expressed breast milk
Kangaroo care (or skin-to-skin contact) (Akcan et al., 2009; Castral et al., 2008; Cong et al., 2009, 2011; de Sousa Freire et al., 2008; Ferber and Makhoul, 2008; Gray et al., 2000; Johnston et al., 2008; Kashaninia et al., 2008; Kostandy et al., 2008; Ludington-Hoe et al., 2005)	Full term Preterm Very preterm	Heel stick Venepuncture Intramuscular injection	↓ crying, less variation in HR ↓ PIPP scores Better results when combined with breastfeeding or sweet taste	Kangaroo care or skin-to-skin care is effective
Containment/facilitated tucking (Axelin et al., 2006, 2009b; Cignacco et al., 2012; Corff et al., 1995, Obeidat et al., 2009; Ward-Larson et al., 2004)	Term Preterm	Endotracheal/ pharyngeal suctioning/ heel Lance	↓ physiological and behavioural pain responses. Less efficacious than sucrose	Containment and swaddling are effective for single procedures. May be optimal as adjuvant strategy for repeated procedures
Auditory recognition: maternal heart rate (Kurihara et al., 1996) recorded maternal voice (Johnston et al., 2007)	Full term Preterm	Heel stick	↓ HR, ↑ oxygenation and quicker recovery Strongest effect combined with NNS	Maternal heart beat effective but not recorded maternal voice
Olfactory recognition: own mother's milk or familiar odour (Goubet et al., 2003, 2007; Nishitani et al., 2009; Rattaz et al., 2005)	Full term Preterm	Heel stick Venepuncture	↓crying and grimacing during venepuncture	Mothers own milk or familiar odour was effective during venepuncture but not heel lance

HR = heart rate; NNS = non-nutritive sucking; PIPP = Premature Infant Pain Profile.

Mechanisms underlying maternal comforting effectiveness

There are likely several underlying mechanisms for the effectiveness of maternal comfort on infant pain. The two mechanisms with the most compelling data related to endogenous opiates and oxytocin.

In the animal literature, there is a strong relationship between endogenous opiates and social affiliation (Panksepp et al., 1980, 1994), including mother–infant bonding. Endorphins are excreted in milk and the levels are augmented by suckling. Young animals, of several species, removed from their mothers display distress behaviours including specific crying, or distress vocalizations. When given opiates exogenously, the number of these distress behaviours decrease, as when they are reunited with the mother. Furthermore, naloxone, in many experiments, though not all, decreases the number of distress vocalizations when the young are separated. There is congruence of areas in the brain responsible for distress behaviours and opiate receptors. The important point is that the behaviours and the opiate excretion are mediated by maternal presence. The opiate-affiliative system is also bi-directional: dams (mother rats) given naloxone are slower to retrieve their young scattered about the nest.

The second hypothesized mechanism is related to oxytocin. Oxytocin is thought to be of major importance in mother–infant bonding; being released at delivery, with the commencement of suckling, with touch, and is found in breast milk (Carter, 1998;

Carter et al., 1992; Insel, 1997; Konner, 2004). The role of oxytocin in the mediation of pain has been tested in animals. Based on the knowledge that gentle stroking has a pleasurable anti-nociceptive function, the injection of an oxytocin antagonist blocked that function (Agren et al., 1995). Further studies revealed that: (1) stroking did increase the latency withdrawal to mechanical or thermal noxious stimulation; (2) there were increased levels of circulating oxytocin and oxytocin in the periaqueductal grey (PAG), an area important in pain processing, following stroking sessions; and (3) an *opiate* antagonist, naloxone, injected directly into the PAG, decreased the withdrawal latency. In adults, the administration of oxytocin has decreased pain (Madrazo et al., 1987; Yang, 1994).

Recommendations for practice

Given the current evidence regarding the comforting role of mothers and families in the NICU and the lack of reported adverse events, we recommend that for healthy full-term and preterm infants, KMC and breastfeeding should be considered as the behavioural pain strategy of choice for single painful events. Where possible, breastfeeding infants should establish an effective latch prior to the procedure and have as much direct skin contact with the mother as possible.

In infants who are unable to breastfeed, KMC is beneficial. Infants should be placed diaper clad in an upright position with full ventral contact with their mother prior to and during the painful procedure. The optimal duration of SSC prior to a procedure remains unknown. The majority of studies used 15 to 30 min and had positive results, and as little as 10 min seems to be effective.

In the situations where it is impossible to hold the infant, alternative strategies emphasising maternal presence such as olfactory or auditory stimuli, or facilitated tucking may be used as adjuvant therapy in conjunction with sweet taste or in combination as more holistic sensorial saturation. Further studies are required to determine the efficacy of these strategies for repeated procedures over time.

Some benefit is derived from KMC with other providers who are not the mother; however, until further studies are conducted, additional strategies in combination should be considered. For infants undergoing multiple painful procedures or those who demonstrate high behavioural pain response, adjuvant strategies used in combination specifically sweet taste, non-nutritive sucking, swaddling or containment in addition to breastfeeding or SSC are likely to be beneficial, although there remains a paucity of evidence regarding an optimal combination.

Feasibility

Some outstanding issues remain regarding the implementation of KMC during painful procedures. We know that the uptake of any clinical practice change generally lags behind dissemination of the research findings (Graham et al., 2006; also see Yamada and Hutchinson, Chapter 61, this volume). Using mothers and families as providers of comfort presents several additional several challenges, requiring a paradigm shift. Health care providers will need to further relinquish their traditional care model to consider parents as partners in provision of care rather than bystanders; thus placing increased emphasis and time for the coordination of care, scheduling, and timing of procedures to enhance parental involvement. The skill of the health care providers conducting the procedure also needs to be considered in relation to feasibility. Issues regarding safety and ergonomic needs of the care providers have also been reported (Campbell-Yeo et al., 2008b) and require further research.

Conclusion

Mothers have a unique relationship with their infant and a special role in comforting their infant in the face of pain. Data exist to support that mothers are better than others at comforting their infant, either through some biological mechanism or because of the profound caring they have for their infant, normally stronger than others. Given their effectiveness, it is highly recommended that mothers be included in comforting their infant during painful procedures whenever possible.

Case example

Madeline is a 7-day-old preterm neonate who was delivered 11 weeks early at 29 weeks gestational age. Madeline undergoes numerous painful procedures, as part of her medical care in the NICU. For example, heel lance for blood collection, the most common, occurs one to two times a day.

Madeline becomes very distressed during the heel lance as exhibited by her facial actions and changes in her physiological stability. She often requires additional supplemental oxygen during the heel lance.

Madeline's mother, Sarah, also becomes visibly upset when she watches during these procedures and describes, 'feeling helpless'. Madeline's nurse discusses the comforting benefits of SSC with Sarah and asks if she would like to hold Madeline in this way before and during her next heel lance. Sarah agrees and her nurse tells explains to her this would mean holding Madeline, while her baby wears only a diaper, and placing her upright in a ventral position on her bare chest, than covering them both with a blanket (for an example see Figure 58.1). The nurse also told her that even a small amount of SSC before the heel lance can be helpful, as little as 10 to 15 min, but that it is important to allow Madeline to recover from the transfer from the incubator to her mother's chest which may take a few extra minutes.

The next day, Sarah held Madeline in SSC during her heel lance. Sarah displayed only minimal facial response during the procedure and did not require additional oxygen. Both the nurse and Sarah felt that Madeline benefited from the SSC. Sarah also expressed that she 'truly felt like a parent since she was able to actively help her daughter' that she 'would like to be able to continue helping Madeleine in this way'.

The nurse shares with the neonatal team that Sarah would like to be an active participant in Madeleine's pain management and the team agrees that all non-emergent blood collections and procedures can be scheduled around Sarah's availability.

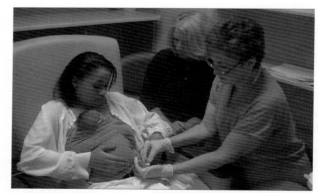

Figure 58.1 Skin-to-skin contact during a heel lance.

References

Agren, G., Lundeberg, T., Uvnas-Moberg, K., and Sato, A. (1995). The oxytocin antagonist 1-deamino-2-D-Tyr-(Oet)-4-Thr-8-Orn-oxytocin reverses the increase in the withdrawal response latency to thermal, but not mechanical nociceptive stimuli following oxytocin administration or massage-like stroking in rats. *Neurosci Lett*, 187, 49–52.

Ainsworth, M. D. (1969). Object relations, dependency, and attachment: a theoretical review of the infant-mother relationship. *Child Dev*, 40, 969–1025.

Akcan, E., Yigit, R., and Atici, A. (2009). The effect of kangaroo care on pain in premature infants during invasive procedures. *Turk J Pediatr*, 51, 14–18.

Axelin, A., Lehtonen, L., Pelander, T., and Salantera, S. (2010). Mothers' different styles of involvement in preterm infant pain care. *J Obstet Gynecol Neonatal Nurs*, 415–424.

Axelin, A., Ojajarvi, U., Viitanen, J., and Lehtonen, L. (2009a). Promoting shorter duration of ventilator treatment decreases the number of painful procedures in preterm infants. *Acta Paediatr*, 1751–1755.

Axelin, A., Salantera, S., Kirjavainen, J., and Lehtonen, L. (2009b). Oral glucose and parental holding preferable to opioid in pain management in preterm infants. *Clin J Pain*, 25, 138–145.

Axelin, A., Salantera, S., and Lehtonen, L. (2006). 'Facilitated tucking by parents' in pain management of preterm infants – a randomized crossover trial. *Early Hum Dev*, 82, 241–247.

Bellieni, C. V., Bagnoli, F., Perrone, S., Nenci, A., Cordelli, D. M., Fusi, M., *et al.* (2002). Effect of multisensory stimulation on analgesia in term neonates: a randomized controlled trial. *Pediatr Res*, 51, 460–463.

Bellieni, C. V., Buonocore, G., Nenci, A., Franci, N., Cordelli, D. M., and Bagnoli, F. (2001). Sensorial saturation: an effective analgesic tool for heel-prick in preterm infants: a prospective randomized trial. *Biol Neonate.*, 80, 15–18.

Bellieni, C. V., Cordelli, D. M., Marchi, S., Ceccarelli, S., Perrone, S., Maffei, M., *et al.* (2007). Sensorial saturation for neonatal analgesia. *Clin J Pain*, 23, 219–221.

Bilgen, H., Ozek, E., Cebeci, D., and Ors, R. (2001). Comparison of sucrose, expressed breast milk, and breast-feeding on the neonatal response to heel prick. *J Pain*, 2(5) 301–305.

Blass, E. M. (1997). Milk induced hypoalgesia in human newborns. *Pediatrics*, 99, 825–829.

Blass, E. M. and Miller, L. W. (2001). Effects of colostrum in newborn humans: dissociation between analgesic and cardiac effects. *J Dev Behav Pediatr*, 22, 385–390.

Blount, R. L., Devine, K. A., Cheng, P. S., Simons, L. E., and Hayutin, L. (2008). The impact of adult behaviors and vocalizations on infant distress during immunizations. *J Pediatr Psychol*, 33, 1163–1174.

Blount, R. L., Zempsky, W. T., Jaaniste, T., Evans, S., Cohen, L. L., Devine, K. A., *et al.* (2009). Management of pediatric pain and distress due to medical procedures. *Handbook of pediatric psychology* (4th edn). New York: Guilford Press; US.

Bo, L. K. and Callaghan, P. (2000). Soothing pain-elicited distress in Chinese neonates. *Pediatrics*, 105, E49.

Campbell-Yeo, M., Fernandes, A., and Johnston, C. (2011). Procedural pain management for neonates using nonpharmacological strategies: part 2: mother-driven interventions. *Adv Neonatal care*,11, 312–318.

Campbell-Yeo, M., Johnston, C., Filion, F., and McNaughton, K. (2008a). A comparison of nurse and mother attitudes regarding maternal skin-to-skin care as a pain relieving strategy during heel stick for preterm neonates. In K. H. Nyqvist (ed.) 1st European Conference on the Kangaroo Mothercare method & The 7th International Workshop on Kangaroo Mother Care, Uppsalla, Sweden.

Campbell-Yeo, M., Johnston, C. C., Filion, F., and McNaughton, K. (2008b). *A comparison of nurse and mother attitudes regarding maternal skin-to-skin care as a pain relieving strategy during heel lance for preterm neonates*. 1st European Conference on the Kangaroo MotherCare proceedings.

Campbell-Yeo, M. L., Johnston, C. C., Joseph, K. S., Feeley, N., Chambers, C. T., and Barrington, K. J. (2012). Cobedding and recovery time after heel lance in preterm twins: results of a randomized trial. *Pediatrics*, 130, 500–506.

Campos, R. G. (1994). Rocking and pacifiers: two comforting interventions for heelstick pain. *Res Nurs Health*, 17, 321–331.

Carbajal, R., Veerapen, S., Couderc, S., Jugie, M., and Ville, Y. (2003). Analgesic effect of breast feeding in term neonates: randomised controlled trial. *Br Med J*, 326, 13.

Carter, C. S. (1998). Neuroendocrine perspectives on social attachment and love. *Psychoneuroendocrinology*, 23, 779–818.

Carter, C. S., Williams, J. R., Witt, D. M., and Insel, T. R. (1992). Oxytocin and social bonding. *Ann N Y Acad Sci.*, 652, 204–211.

Castral, T. C., Warnock, F., Leite, A. M., Haas, V. J., and Scochi, C. G. (2008). The effects of skin-to-skin contact during acute pain in preterm newborns. *Eur J Pain*, 12, 464–471.

Charpak, N., Ruiz-Pelaez, J. G., and Charpak, Y. (1994). Rey-Martinez Kangaroo Mother Program: an alternative way of caring for low birth weight infants? One year mortality in a two cohort study. *Pediatrics*, 94, 804–810.

Chermont, A. G., Falcao, L. F., De Souza Silva, E. H., De Cassia Xavier Balda, R., and Guinsburg, R. (2009). Skin-to-skin contact and/or oral 25% dextrose for procedural pain relief for term newborn infants. *Pediatrics*, 124, e1101–1107.

Cignacco, E., Mueller, R., Hamers, J. P. H., and Gessler, P. (2004). Pain assessment in the neonate using the Bernese Pain Scale for Neonates. *Early Hum Dev*, 78, 125–131.

Cignacco, E. L., Sellam, G., Stoffel, L., Gerull, R., Nelle, M., Anand, K. J., and Engberg, S. (2012). Oral sucrose and 'facilitated tucking' for repeated pain relief in preterms: a randomized controlled trial. *Pediatrics*, 129, 299–308.

Codipietro, L., Ceccarelli, M., and Ponzone, A. (2008). Breastfeeding or oral sucrose solution in term neonates receiving heel lance: a randomized, controlled trial. *Pediatrics*, 122, e716–e721.

Cong, X., Ludington-Hoe, S. M., McCain, G., and Fu, P. (2009). Kangaroo Care modifies preterm infant heart rate variability in response to heel stick pain: pilot study. *Early Hum Dev*, 85, 561–567.

Cong, X., Ludington-Hoe, S. M., and Walsh, S. (2011). Randomized crossover trial of kangaroo care to reduce biobehavioral pain responses in preterm infants: a pilot study. *Biological Res Nurs*, 13, 204–216.

Corff, K. E., Seideman, R., Venkataraman, P. S., Lutes, L., and Yates, B. (1995). Facilitated tucking: a nonpharmacologic comfort measure for pain in preterm neonates. *J Obstet Gynecol Neonatal Nurs*, 24, 143–147.

de Sousa Freire, N. J. B., Santos Garcia, J. O. B., and Carvalho Lamy, Z. (2008). Evaluation of analgesic effect of skin-to-skin contact compared to oral glucose in preterm neonates. *Pain*, 139, 28–33.

Decasper, A. J. and Fifer, W. P. (1980). Of human bonding: newborns prefer their mothers voices. *Science*, 208, 1174–1176.

Decasper, A. J., Lecanuet, J. P., Busnel, M. C., Granier-Deferre, C., and Maugeais, R. (1994). Fetal reactions to recurrent maternal speech. *Infant Beh Devel*, 17, 159–164.

Decasper, A. J. and Spence, M. J. (1986). Prenatal maternal speech influences newborn's perception of speech sounds. *Infant Behav Dev*, 9, 133–150.

Efe, E. and Ozer, Z. C. (2007). The use of breast-feeding for pain relief during neonatal immunization injections. *Appl Nurs Res*, 20, 10–16.

Ferber, S. G. and Makhoul, I. R. (2008). Neurobehavioural assessment of skin-to-skin effects on reaction to pain in preterm infants: a randomized, controlled within-subject trial. *Acta Paediatr*, 97, 171–176.

Fifer, W. P., Moon, C., Lecanuet, J. P., Krasnegor, N., and Smotherman, W. P. (1995). *The effects of fetal experience with sound. Fetal development, a psychobiological perspective*. Hillsdale, NJ: Lawerence Erlbaum Associates.

Franck, L. S., Allen, A., Cox, S., and Winter, I. (2005). Parents' views about infant pain in neonatal intensive care. *Clin J Pain*, 21, 133–139.

Franck, L. S., Oulton, K., Nderitu, S., Lim, M., Fang, S., and Kaiser, A. (2011). Parent involvement in pain management for NICU infants: a randomized controlled trial. *Pediatrics*, 128(3), 510–518.

Freire, N. B., Garcia, J. B., and Lamy, Z. C. (2008). Evaluation of analgesic effect of skin-to-skin contact compared to oral glucose in preterm neonates. *Pain*, 139, 28–33.

Gormally, S., Barr, R. G., Wertheim, L., Alkawaf, R., Calinoiu, N., and Young, S. N. (2001). Contact and nutrient caregiving effects on newborn infant pain responses. *Dev Med Child Neurol*, 43, 28–38.

Goubet, N., Rattaz, C., Pierrat, V., Bullinger, A., and Lequien, P. (2003). Olfactory experience mediates response to pain in preterm newborns. *Dev Psychobiol*, 42, 171–180.

Goubet, N., Strasbaugh, K., and Chesney, J. (2007). Familiarity breeds content? Soothing effect of a familiar odor on full-term newborns. *J Dev Behav Pediatr*, 28, 189–194.

Gradin, M., Finnstrom, O., and Schollin, J. (2004). Feeding and oral glucose—additive effects on pain reduction in newborns. *Early Hum Dev*, 77, 57–65.

Graham, I. D., Logan, J., Harrison, M. B., Straus, S. E., Tetroe, J., Caswell, W., and Robinson, N. (2006). Lost in knowledge translation: time for a map? *J Cont Educ Health Prof*, 26, 13–24.

Gray, L., Miller, L. W., Philipp, B. L., and Blass, E. M. (2002). Breastfeeding is analgesic in healthy newborns. *Pediatrics*, 109, 590–593.

Gray, L., Watt, L., and Blass, E. M. (2000). Skin-to-skin contact is analgesic in healthy newborns. *Pediatrics*, 105, e14.

Grunau, R. V. E. and Craig, K. D. (1987). Pain expression in neonates: facial action and cry. *Pain*, 28, 395–410.

Insel, T. R. (1997). A neurobiological basis of social attachment. *Am J Psychiatry*, 154, 726–735.

Joesten, M. D., Hogg, J. L., and Castellion, M. E. (2007). *The world of chemisty: essentials*. Belmont, CA: Thomson.

Johnston, C., Byron, J., Filion, F., Campbell-Yeo, M., Gibbins, S., and NG, E. (2012). Alternative female kangaroo care for procedural pain in preterm neonates: a pilot study. *Acta Paediatr*, 101(11), 1147–1150.

Johnston, C., Campbell-Yeo, M., Fernandes, A., Inglis, D., Streiner, D., and Zee, R. (2010). Skin-to-skin care for procedural pain in neonates. *Cochrane Database Syst Rev*, 3, CD008435. doi: 10.1002/14651858.CD008435.

Johnston, C. C., Campbell-Yeo, M., and Filion, F. (2011). Paternal vs maternal kangaroo care for procedural pain in preterm neonates: a randomized crossover trial. *Arch Pediatr Adolesc Med*, 165, 792–796.

Johnston, C. C., Filion, F., Campbell-Yeo, M., Goulet, C., Bell, L., McNaughton, K., *et al.* (2009). Enhanced kangaroo mother care for heel lance in preterm neonates: a crossover trial. *J Perinatol*, 29, 51–56.

Johnston, C. C., Filion, F., Campbell-Yeo, M., Goulet, C., Bell, L., McNaughton, K., *et al.* (2008). Kangaroo mother care diminishes pain from heel lance in very preterm neonates: a crossover trial. *BMC Pediatr*, 8, 13.

Johnston, C. C., Filion, F., and Nuyt, A. M. (2007). Recorded maternal voice for preterm neonates undergoing heel lance. *Adv Neonatal care*, 7, 258–266.

Johnston, C. C., Stevens, B., Pinelli, J., Gibbins, S., Filion, F., Jack, A., *et al.* (2003). Kangaroo care is effective in diminishing pain response in preterm neonates. *Arch Pediatr Adolesc Med*, 157(11), 1084–1088.

Kashaninia, Z., Sajedi, F., Rahgozar, M., and Noghabi, F. A. (2008). The effect of Kangaroo Care on behavioral responses to pain of an intramuscular injection in neonates. *J Specialists Pediatr Nurs*, 13, 275–280.

Konner, M. (2004). The ties that bind. *Nature*, 429, 705.

Kostandy, R. R., Ludington-Hoe, S. M., Cong, X., Abouelfettoh, A., Bronson, C., Stankus, A, *et al.* (2008). Kangaroo Care (skin contact) reduces crying response to pain in preterm neonates: pilot results. *Pain Manag Nurs*, 9, 55–65.

Kurihara, H., Chiba, H., Shimizu, Y., Yanaihara, T., Takeda, M., Kawakami, K., *et al.* (1996). Behavioral and adrenocortical responses to stress in neonates and the stabilizing effects of maternal heartbeat on them. *Early Hum Dev*, 46, 117–127.

Liaw, J. J., Yang, L., Katherine Wang, K. W., Chen, C. M., Chang, Y. C., and Yin, T. (2012). Non-nutritive sucking and facilitated tucking relieve preterm infant pain during heel-stick procedures: a prospective, randomised controlled crossover trial. *Int J Nurs Stud*, 49, 300–309.

Ludington-Hoe, S. M., Hosseini, R., and Torowizc, D. L. (2005). Skin-to-skin contact (Kangaroo Care) analgesia for preterm infant heelstick. *AACN Clin Issues*, 16, 373–387.

Ludington-Hoe, S. M., Johnson, M. W., Morgan, K., Lewis, T., Gutman, J., Wilson, P. D., *et al.* (2006). Neurophysiologic assessment of neonatal sleep organization: preliminary results of a randomized, controlled trial of skin contact with preterm infants. *Pediatrics*, 117, e909–e923.

Madrazo, I., Franco-Bourland, R. E., Leon-Meza, V. M., and Mena, I. (1987). Intraventricular somatostatin-14, arginine vasopressin, and oxytocin: analgesic effect in a patient with intractable cancer pain. *Applied Neurophysiol*, 50, 427–431.

Marlier, L. and Schaal, B. (2005). Human newborns prefer human milk: conspecific milk odor is attractive without postnatal exposure. *Child Dev*, 76, 155–168.

McDaniel, M. R., Barker, E., and Lederer, C. L. (1989). Sensory characterization of human milk. *J Dairy Sci*, 72, 1149–1158.

McMurtry, C. M., Chambers, C. T., McGrath, P. J., and Asp, E. (2010). When 'don't worry' communicates fear: children's perceptions of parental reassurance and distraction during a painful medical procedure. *Pain*, 150, 52–58.

Miles, M. S., Carter, M. C., Riddle, I., Hennessey, J., and Eberly, T. W. (1989). The pediatric intensive care unit environment as a source of stress for parents. *Matern Child Nurs J*, 18(3), 199–206.

Miles, M. S., D'auria, J. P., Hart, E. M., Sedlack, D. A., and Watral, M. A. (1993). Parental role alterations experienced by mothers of children with a lifethreatening chronic illness In S. G. Funk (ed.) *Key aspects of caring for the chronically ill: hospital and home*, pp. 281–290. New York: Springer.

Montirosso, R., Provenzi, L., Calciolari, G., and Borgatti, R. (2012). Measuring maternal stress and perceived support in 25 Italian NICUs. *Acta Paediatr*, 101, 136–42.

Nishitani, S., Miyamura, T., Tagawa, M., Sumi, M., Takase, R., Doi, H., *et al.* (2009). The calming effect of a maternal breast milk odor on the human newborn infant. *Neurosci Res*, 63, 66–71.

Obeidat, H., Kahalaf, I., Callister, L. C., and Froelicher, E. S. (2009). Use of facilitated tucking for nonpharmacological pain management in preterm infants: a systematic review. *J Perinat Neonatal Nurs*, 23, 372–377.

Ockleford, E. M., Vince, M. A., Layton, C., and Reader, M. R. (1988). Response of neonates to parent's and other's voices. *Early Hum Dev*, 18, 27–36.

Ors, R., Ozek, E., Baysoy, G., Cebeci, D., Bilgen, H., Turkuner, M., and BASARAN, M. (1999). Comparison of sucrose and human milk on pain response in newborns. *Eur J Pediatrics*, 158, 63–66.

Osinaike, B. B., Oyedeji, A. O., Adeoye, O. T., Dairo, M. D., and Aderinto, D. A. (2007). Effect of breastfeeding during venepuncture in neonates. *Ann Trop Paediatr*, 27, 201–205.

Panksepp, J., Herman, B. H., Vilberg, T., Bishop, P., and Deeskinazi, F. G. (1980). Endogenous opioids and social behavior. *Neurosci Biobehav Rev*, 4, 473–487.

Panksepp, J., Nelson, E., and Siviy, S. (1994). Brain opioids and mother-infant social motivation. *Acta Paediatr Suppl*, 397, 40–46.

Piira, T., Champion, G. D., Bustos, T., Donnelly, N., and Lui, K. (2007). Factors associated with infant pain response following an immunization injection. *Early Hum Dev*, 83, 319–326.

Pillai Riddell, R., Campbell, L., Flora, D. B., Racine, N., Din Osmun, L., Garfield, H., *et al.* (2011). The relationship between caregiver sensitivity and infant pain behaviors across the first year of life. *Pain*, 152, 2819–2826.

Rattaz, C., Goubet, N., and Bullinger, A. (2005). The calming effect of a familiar odor on full-term newborns. *J Dev Behav Pediatr*, 26, 86–92.

Sajedi, F., Kashaninia, Z., Rahgozar, M., and Noghabi, F. A. (2007). The effect of Kangaroo Care on physiologic responses to pain of an intramuscular injection in neonates. *Iranian J Pediatr*, 17, 339–344.

Schaal, B., Marlier, L., and Soussignan, R. (1998). Olfactory function in the human fetus: evidence from selective neonatal responsiveness to the odor of amniotic fluid. *Behav Neurosci*, 112, 1438–1449.

Scher, M. S. and Loparo, K. A. (2009). Neonatal EEG/sleep state analyses: a complex phenotype of developmental neural plasticity. *Dev Neurosci*, 31, 259–275.

Shah, P. S., Aliwalas, L., and Shah, V. (2007). Breastfeeding or breastmilk to alleviate procedural pain in neonates: a systematic review. *Breastfeed Med*, 2, 74–82.

Shah, P. S., Aliwalas, L. L., and Shah, V. (2008). Breastfeeding or breast milk for procedural pain in neonates. *Cochrane Database Syst Rev*, 1, CD004950.

Standley, J. M., and Masen, C. K. (1990). Comparison of infant preferences and responses to auditory stimuli: music, mother, and other female voices. *J Music Ther*, 27, 54–97.

Stevens, B., Johnston, C., Taddio, A., Gibbins, S., and Yamada, J. (2010). The premature infant pain profile: evaluation 13 years after development. *Clin J Pain*, 26, 813–830.

Stevens, B. J., Johnston, C., Petryshen, P., and Taddio, A. (1996). Premature infant pain profile: development and initial validation. *Clin J Pain*, 12, 13–22.

Sweet, S. D., Mcgrath, P. J., and Symons, D. (1999). The roles of child reactivity and parenting context in infant pain response. *Pain*, 80, 655–661.

Upadhyay, A., Aggarwal, R., Narayan, S., Joshi, M., Paul, V. K., and Deorari, A. K. (2004). Analgesic effect of expressed breast milk in procedural pain in term neonates: a randomized, placebo-controlled, double-blind trial. [see comment]. *Acta Paediatr*, 93(4), 518–22.

Varendi, H., Christensson, K., Porter, R. H., and Winberg, J. (1998). Soothing effect of amniotic fluid smell in newborn infants. *Early Hum Dev*, 51, 47–55.

Ward-Larson, C., Horn, R. A., and Gosnell, F. (2004). The efficacy of facilitated tucking for relieving procedural pain of endotracheal suctioning in very low birthweight infants. *MCN Am J Matern Child Nurs*, 29, 151–156.

Yang, J. (1994). Intrathecal administration of oxytocin induces analgesia in low back pain involving the endogenous opiate peptide system. *Spine*, 19, 867–871.

SECTION 9

Special topics

CHAPTER 59

Complementary drugs—herbs, vitamins, and dietary supplements for pain and symptom management

Joy A. Weydert

Summary

Because of the interest of patients and physicians, there has been increasing research into the use of botanical agents, nutritional supplements, and diet as a means to manage pain. Pharmacological agents typically are chosen as first-line therapy for pain and symptom management; however, for some patients these agents may not work well long term or have side effects that are not tolerated. Other patients may prefer non-pharmacological therapies. Most clinicians are not trained or may not be comfortable recommending these complementary agents.

Introduction and background

The use of complementary and alternative medicine (CAM) has increased considerably in the paediatric population (Tsao and Zeltzer, 2005). Approximately 20% to 40% of healthy children seen in paediatric clinics and more than 50% of children with chronic illnesses use CAM in conjunction with conventional medical care (Kemper et al., 2008). Those groups that report higher use of CAM often have chronic disorders in which pain is a significant problem (Hagen et al., 2003; Heuschkel et al., 2002).

Families who use CAM state they do so 'not so much as a result of being dissatisfied with conventional medicine, but largely because they found these health care alternatives to be more congruent with their own values, beliefs, and philosophical orientations toward health and life' (Astin, 1998, p. 1548).

The National Center on Complementary and Alternative Medicine (NCCAM), a division of the National Institutes of Health (NIH), funds various studies on CAM. Research on the effectiveness of various CAM therapies for children is small but growing. Much of our knowledge of these therapies is extracted from adult studies, however paediatric studies will be reviewed in this chapter when available.

The herbs that will be discussed have 'Generally Recognized As Safe' status (GRAS) for use in the US. GRAS is the US Food and Drug Administration (FDA) designation that a chemical or substance is considered safe by experts, and so exempted from the usual Federal Food, Drug, and Cosmetic Act (FFDCA) food additive tolerance requirements. GRAS exemptions are granted for substances that are generally recognized, among experts qualified by scientific training and experience to evaluate their safety, as having been adequately shown through scientific procedures to be safe under the conditions of their intended use (Food and Drug Administration, 2012). Common dosages of herbs, vitamins, and dietary supplements are shown in Table 59.1.

Pain syndromes and suggested complementary drugs

Headaches

Chronic primary headaches, whether tension-type or migraine, are the most common pain problems in children affecting as many as one in five children (Perquin et al., 2000). Recent theories of headache aetiology increasingly point to similarities between migraine and tension-type headache, with both suggesting an underlying heightened central nervous system sensitivity (Peres et al., 2007). The goal for treatment, therefore, is to target the underlying problem within the nervous system to lessen reactivity.

Magnesium

Magnesium is regarded as a natural muscle relaxant and pain reliever. Its mechanism of action is through antagonizing N-type calcium-mediated channels at nerve endings. This prevents noradrenaline release, thereby depressing nerve transmission and muscle contractility (Shimosawa et al., 2004). Magnesium also has voltage-gated antagonist action at the N-methyl-D-aspartate

Table 59.1 Common dosages of herbs, vitamins, dietary supplements—please refer to text for more details on dosing, side effects, interactions

Butterbur	50–100 mg two to three times a day
Chamomile	1–3 g three to four times a day
Coenzyme Q$_{10}$	100–300 mg a day
Digestive enzymes	1 capsule before meals (25:2:25 ratio of amylase:lipase:protease)
Feverfew	50–150 mg a day
Ginger	250–500 mg three times a day
L-Carnitine	1000–2000 mg in divided doses three times a day
L-Theanine	100–200 mg one to two times a day
L-Tryptophan/5-HTP	50–300 mg a day
Lemon balm	100–200 mg three times a day
Magnesium	250–500 mg twice a day
Marshmallow	2–5 g three to four times a day
Melatonin	0.3–5 mg 30 min before bedtime
Peppermint (enteric coated)	200–400 mg three times a day
Probiotics	10–100 billion CFU one to two times a day
Slippery elm	400–500 mg 3–4 times daily
Valerian	100–300 mg before bedtime
Vitamin B complex	One tablet a day
Vitamin D$_3$	1000–4000 IU a day

(NMDA) receptors preventing excessive neuronal depolarization (Sun et al., 2005). Deficiencies in magnesium play an important role in the pathogenesis of migraine headaches by promoting cortical spreading depression, altering neurotransmitter release, promoting hyperaggregation of platelets, and causing vasoconstriction, all of which are relevant features of our current understanding of migraine pathophysiology. Magnesium deficiency also results in the generation and release of substance P, which is believed to act on sensory fibres and produce headache pain (Sun-Edelstein and Mauskop, 2009).

There have been conflicting reports in the literature regarding the actual magnesium levels in relation to reports of headache pain. Only 1% of the total body magnesium is in the measurable extracellular space, therefore the levels found on routine blood testing do not reflect total body stores. It is the serum ionized magnesium level (IMg^{2+}) that truly reflects disturbed magnesium metabolism. Patients who have low IMg^{2+} may have normal serum levels, therefore, IMg^{2+} levels provide more consistent and reliable results (Altura et al., 1992). Normal IMg^{2+} for children ranges from 1.09 to 1.51 mg/dL and typically does not vary with age (Hoshino et al., 1998). Levels of red blood cell (RBC) magnesium have also been shown to be decreased in migraineurs (Gallai et al., 1993) as well as in juvenile migraine patients with and without aura (Soriani et al., 1995). Given its commercial availability, the RBC magnesium assay may be a better way of assessing for

deficiency. Normal RBC magnesium levels for children are 4.7 to 7.0 mg/dL.

In one study, 86 children between the ages of 3 and 17 years with migraine headaches were randomly assigned to receive magnesium or placebo for 16 weeks to prevent headache pain. Baseline mean IMg^{2+} levels in both treatment and placebo groups were similar at 0.5 and 0.49 mg/dL, respectively. There was a significant reduction in both headache frequency (p = 0.0037) and severity (p = 0.0029) in the children taking magnesium oxide (9 mg elemental Mg^{2+}/kg/day) compared with those who took the placebo. The only reported side effect was loose stools—19% in magnesium oxide group and 7% in the placebo group (Wang et al., 2003). Oral magnesium supplementation has also been found to decrease pain in children due to tension-type headache (Grazzi et al., 2007). Twenty-two patients were given magnesium pidolate 2.25 g twice a day for 3 months. There was significant reduction in number of headache days (69.6% improvement, p = 0.001), analgesic consumption (65.4% improvement, p = 0.0001), and Migraine Disability Assessment scale (MIDAS) score (75.5% improvement, p = 0.001) at 12 months compared to baseline. The treatment was well tolerated and free from serious side effects.

Acute treatment with intravenous magnesium has been used in adults to abort headache pain in an outpatient clinic setting (Demirkaya et al., 2001; Mauskop et al., 1996). Of 40 patients given intravenous (IV) infusion of 1 g of magnesium sulphate, 80% had complete elimination of pain within 15 min of infusion (P <0.001). They also had complete elimination of photophobia, phonophobia, and nausea for 24 h (Mauskop et al., 1996). These patients subsequently were found to have low serum IMg^{2+} levels. There are no clinical trials using IV magnesium acutely to terminate migraine in children.

Oral magnesium's efficacy is dependent on its absorption from the gastrointestinal tract. Magnesium oxide is poorly absorbed and can cause diarrhoea. Use of the magnesium salts glycinate, aspartate, gluconate, citrate, malate, will yield better results without causing diarrhoea (Ranade and Somberg, 2001). Typical dosing for children is 250 to 500 mg orally twice a day—start with the lower dose and gradually increase the dose for effect. For acute management of migraine in a hospital or emergency department setting, 1 g of magnesium sulphate can be given IV over 15 min in patients with normal cardiovascular and renal function.

Vitamin B complex

Mitochondrial function has been found to be impaired in migraine patients (Gaby, 2011; Pieczenik and Neustad, 2007) and may be related to the B vitamins thiamin (B$_1$), riboflavin (B$_2$), niacin (B$_3$), pantothenic acid (B$_5$), pyridoxine (B$_6$), and biotin which are needed in mitochondrial energy production through synthesis of coenzyme A, transfer of amino groups, donation of methyl groups, and activation of other enzymes. In addition, elevated homocysteine levels and lower serum and red blood cell folate levels are seen in both adult and paediatric patients with migraines (Nelson et al., 2010; Oterino et al., 2010). Homocysteine accumulation leads to impaired fatty acid synthesis, inflammation, vascular damage, and nervous system dysfunction. Other B vitamins (folic acid, cobalamin (B$_{12}$), pyridoxine (B$_6$), and pantothenic acid (B$_5$)) may play a role in mitigating migraine headache by lowering homocysteine levels. Vitamin B$_6$, 100 mg given twice a day, doubled RBC magnesium levels after 4 weeks of therapy in pre-menopausal women

(Abraham et al., 1981) so could have effects in treating migraine through this mechanism as well.

Studies in children using single supplementation of riboflavin (B$_2$) at doses 50 to 200 mg have been equivocal (Bruijn et al., 2010; MacLennan et al., 2008). However, a retrospective study of 41 children given riboflavin 200 to 400 mg daily found a significant reduction in both migraine frequency and intensity (Condò et al., 2009).

In another study of 16 paediatric patients with migraine, hyperhomocysteinaemia, and methylenetetrahydrofolate reductase (MTHFR) polymorphisms, ten out of 16 patients had complete resolution of the migraine episodes using folic acid 5 mg daily for 6 months. The plasma levels of homocysteine dropped to the normal range in 100% of patients (Di Rosa et al., 2007).

Adult studies have shown efficacy in using sustained release niacin (B$_3$) 375 mg twice a day or vitamin B$_{12}$, either 1 mg intranasally daily or 1000 mcg intramuscularly every week, but these studies have not been done in children or adolescents (van der Kuy et al., 2002).

It is unlikely that any individual would have a single vitamin B deficiency. Various B vitamins share similar but not identical functions, therefore, supplementation with a daily B-50 complex formulation could be used when treating headache in children. This would provide 50 mg of vitamins B$_1$, $_{-2}$, $_{-3}$, $_{-5}$, $_{-6}$; 50 mcg of cobalamin and biotin; and 400 mcg of folic acid. All B vitamins are water-soluble, so excess amounts are readily excreted by the kidneys rather than accumulate in fatty tissue which can occur with fat-soluble vitamins—A, D, E, K.

Vitamin D—cholecalciferol (vitamin D$_3$)

Very low vitamin D levels have been found in a survey of children with migraine (O'Brien et al., 2010). Vitamin D deficiency is associated with higher levels of pro-inflammatory and pro-coagulatory biomarkers—high sensitivity C-reactive protein, homocysteine, tissue plasminogen activator antigen, and von Willebrand factor. These same biomarkers are known to be elevated in adult and paediatric patients with migraine indicative of endothelial activation and vascular reactivity caused by inflammation and oxidative stress (Nelson et al., 2010; Tietjen et al., 2009). Vitamin D, important for neurovascular stability, immune modulation, and antithrombotic effects which lessen cardiovascular and stroke risks, is likely important, too, in decreasing the incidence of migraine.

Thus far no randomized, placebo controlled studies have been conducted using vitamin D however several case reports suggest that vitamin D may indeed be effective in reducing pain in migraines and related conditions in adults. Vitamin D and calcium supplementation were used to successfully treat premenopausal and postmenopausal women with migraines who previously did not get relief with conventional therapies (Thys-Jacobs, 1994a, 1994b). Other case reports also demonstrated reduction of headache pain with vitamin D (1000–1500 IU) and calcium (1000–1500 mg) supplementation within 4 to 6 weeks. Though the role of calcium in suppressing these headaches could not be ruled out, they surmised that vitamin D was more vital for headache relief in that serum calcium levels normalized within the first week of therapy, but headache pain only abated with normalization of the 25-hydroxy vitamin D (25(OH)D) levels at 4 to 6 weeks of treatment (Prakash and Shah, 2009).

For patients with migraine or tension headaches, target a serum 25(OH) D level of 50 to 60 ng/ml. Many children may need higher than the current AAP recommendation of 400 IU daily as 100 IU of vitamin D$_3$ only raises the serum level by 1 ng/ml. It is safe to give 2000 to 4000 IU daily if levels are monitored every 6 to 8 weeks. Symptoms of vitamin D toxicity (levels >150 ng/ml) might include nausea, vomiting, poor appetite, weakness, confusion, or tingling around the mouth, and are related to hypercalcaemia and hypercalciuria. Published cases of toxicity revealed intake of greater than 40 000 IU per day (Vieth, 1999).

Butterbur (*Petasites hybridus*)

Butterbur is a perennial shrub that historically has been used to treat migraine, allergic rhinitis, chronic cough, and urinary tract spasms. The active constituents of butterbur, petasin and isopetasin, have antispasmodic effects on smooth muscle and vascular walls by non-competitive inhibition of histamine (Ko et al., 2001). They also inhibit leukotriene synthesis, and decrease the priming of mast cells, which lowers the concentration of histamine *in vitro* (Lee et al., 2003). Histamine is a key component of the neuroinflammatory process contributing to migraine acting mainly on H1 receptors which mediate inflammation and H3 receptors which serve as negative feedback to inhibit further excessive release of histamine by C-fibres (Gupta et al., 2011). Butterbur thereby impacts migraine pain via these mechanisms.

Butterbur contains hepatotoxic pyrrolizidine alkaloids (PAs) which are most concentrated in the plant roots, but may be found in all plant parts. Toxic PAs are removed from butterbur extracts. These PA-free extracts are available for use and are considered safe.

Butterbur root extract was found to be an effective and well-tolerated migraine prophylaxis for children and teenagers (Pothmann and Danesch, 2005). 108 children and adolescents between the ages of 6 and 17 were included in a multicenter prospective open-label study of butterbur. Children 6 to 9 years of age initially received 50 mg of the butterbur extract once a day and adolescents aged 10 to 17 years received 50 mg twice a day. After 2 months the dose for non-responders increased to 75 mg daily (6–9-year-olds) or 75 mg twice a day (10–17-year-olds). The number of monthly migraine attacks was reduced 63.2% for the total sample population at the end of 4 months in relation to pre-study baseline measures and the duration of pain was reduced, on average, from 10 h to 7 h. No serious adverse events occurred.

For migraine headache prophylaxis, a PA-free butterbur rhizome extract standardized to 15% petasin and isopetasin (Petadolex®) can be used in doses of 50 to 100 mg twice daily with meals. Three times daily dosing has been used in children who don't respond to the twice daily dose. The most commonly reported adverse events related to butterbur were belching, drowsiness, fatigue, nausea, and abdominal pain. These adverse events are generally considered mild and self-limiting.

Feverfew (*Tanacetum parthenium*)

Feverfew traditionally has been used for the prevention and treatment of migraine headaches, arthritis, fever and menstrual irregularities. Feverfew inhibits platelet aggregation, serotonin release from platelets and leukocytes, and the production of prostaglandins and leukotrienes in rat and human leukocytes (Sumner et al., 1992). It also has serotonin 5-HT receptor blocking effects which has relevance as serotonin dysregulation is thought to contribute to headache initiation (Shrivastava et al., 2006). One of the major active constituents in feverfew, parthenolide, inhibits the influx of extracellular calcium into vascular smooth muscle cells decreasing spasm (Pareek et al., 2011).

Randomized trials of feverfew in adult patients reduced the number and severity of migraine attacks when used singularly (Murphy et al., 1988) or in combination with ginger (Cady et al., 2011). In the 1988 study, 72 volunteers were randomly allocated to receive either dried feverfew leaves (82 mg/day) or matching placebo for 4 months with cross-over for the following 4 months. Feverfew treatment had a 24% reduction (P <0.005) in attack frequency and a significant decrease (P <0.02) in migraine-associated nausea and vomiting compared with placebo. Visual analogue scale (VAS) scores of pain also improved with feverfew.

There have been no trials of feverfew in any paediatric populations, although it is frequently recommended for paediatric headache management. No significant adverse effects have been reported with long-term use of feverfew (Pittler et al., 2000). The recommended dosing is 50 to 150 mg of feverfew extract standardized to 0.2% to 0.4% parthenolides, or two to three fresh leaves daily. Use the 50 mg dose for children 25 to 50 kg and the 150 mg dose for larger children and adults (>70 kg).

Coenzyme Q_{10} (CoQ_{10})

CoQ_{10} deficiency occurs in many paediatric patients with migraine headache (Hershey et al., 2007). There are two major factors that lead to deficiency of CoQ_{10} in humans: reduced biosynthesis and increased utilization by the body when consumed by oxygen free-radicals. Oxydative stress (indicated by low CoQ_{10} levels) with mitochondrial dysfunction (indicated by low ATP levels in blood mononuclear cells) are found in pain disorders such as migraine and fibromyalgia (Cordero et al., 2012). CoQ_{10} functions as an anti-oxidant, a membrane stabilizer, as well as a co-factor in many metabolic pathways, and is necessary for generating ATP in mitochondrial oxidative respiration (Turunen et al., 2004).

CoQ_{10} supplementation reduced headache frequency and related disability in children with migraine when CoQ_{10} blood levels were normalized. CoQ_{10} was measured in 1550 paediatric patients, aged 3 to 22 years, with migraine. Patients with low CoQ_{10} (<0.70 mcg/ml; normal levels 0.5–1.5 mcg/ml), were started on 1 to 3 mg/kg per day of CoQ_{10} in liquid gel capsule formulation. In 3 months, the total CoQ_{10} level improved to 1.20±0.59 mcg/ml (P <0.0001), while the headache frequency decreased from 19.2±10.0 to 12.5±10.8 (P <0.001) and headache disability assessed with PedMIDAS reduced from 47.4±50.6 to 22.8±30.6 (P <0.001) (Hershey et al., 2007).

CoQ_{10} is generally well tolerated and has no significant adverse effects. Small amounts are derived from dietary meats and seafood; however, the amounts ingested from foods do not approach therapeutic doses. The recommended dosing when used for migraine prevention is 100 to 300 mg daily.

Functional abdominal pain/inflammatory bowel disease

The causes of functional abdominal pain are multifactorial and often difficult to treat with only one modality. Change of diet, cognitive-behavioural therapy, and use self-regulation techniques (guided imagery, hypnosis, meditation) used concurrently can help relieve pain (Weydert, 2012). Along with these modalities, certain herbs and dietary supplements have been shown to be safe and effective in treating abdominal pain. Many of these same supplements can

also be integrated into the regimens for inflammatory bowel disease (IBD) to quell inflammation and subsequently reduce pain.

Chamomile (*Matricaria recutita*)

Chamomile traditionally has been used to treat nausea, nervous diarrhoea, gastrointestinal spasms, restlessness and insomnia. Active ingredients, alpha-bisabolol and bisabolol oxide, inhibit cyclo-oxygenase and lipo-oxygenase thereby reducing the production of inflammatory prostaglandins and leukotrienes. They also inhibit histamine release from mast cells and have antispasmodic effects on smooth muscle (Hormann and Korting, 1994). Another active ingredient, apigenin, binds to gamma-aminobutyric acid (GABA) receptors, the primary receptor sites of benzodiazepines in the central nervous system, to exert anxiolytic effects without sedation (Viola et al., 1995). In a prospective double-blind study in 33 infants with colic, an herbal preparation containing chamomile was effective in reducing colic episodes without side effects. The tea eliminated the colic in 19 (57%) of 33 infants, whereas placebo was helpful in only 9 (26%) of 35 (P <0.01) (Weizman et al., 1993).

One heaping teaspoon of dried flower heads in half a cup of boiling water steeped for 10 min yields about 3 g of chamomile extract. For infants with colic, give 1 ounce of this preparation (approximately 0.75 g) three to four times daily. Use higher doses for older children and adolescents—1 to 3 g taken three to four times daily—to reduce abdominal and/or menstrual cramps, or induce relaxation.

Ginger (*Zingiber officinale*)

Historically ginger has been used for stomach aches, headaches, nausea, and to stimulate appetite, reduce gas formation, and promote bile secretion for digestion. Its active constituent, 6-gingerol, reduces nausea and vomiting by increasing gastric motility (Ali et al., 2007). Ginger's antispasmodic effect on the visceral smooth muscle is the result of antagonism of serotonin receptor sites in the gastrointestinal tract (Murray, 1995). Twenty-four healthy volunteers were studied twice in a randomized double-blind manner and given ginger capsules (total 1200 mg) or placebo followed by a soup meal. Ginger accelerated gastric emptying (13.1±1.1 versus 26.7±3.1 min, P <0.01) and stimulated antral contractions (P <0.005) compared to placebo (Wu et al., 2008).

Ginger is well tolerated and considered safe when used in typical doses in children older than 2 years old. Ginger can be given by brewing 0.5–1 g of dried root in 150 ml boiling water for 5–10 min, then straining. Powered root in capsule form can also be used and dosed 250–500 mg 3–4 times daily up to the maximum of 4 g per day. It is generally recommended that intake not exceed 4 g per day in adults as side effects such as abdominal discomfort, heartburn, or diarrhoea may develop with doses greater than 5 g per day (Srivastava and Mustafa, 1989).

Peppermint (*Mentha piperita*)

There are over 40 different compounds found in peppermint oil. Most research has focused on menthol which decreases the influx of extracellular calcium ions through potential-dependent channels thus inhibiting smooth muscle contractions (Hills and Aaronson, 1991).

In a randomized, double-blind controlled trial, 42 children aged 8 to 17 years with irritable bowel syndrome (IBS) were given pH-dependent, enteric-coated capsules containing 187 mg of peppermint oil per capsule or placebo. Children weighing between 30 and 45 kg received one capsule three times a day whereas patients weighing more than 45 kg received two peppermint oil or placebo capsules three times a day. After 2 weeks, 75% of patients receiving peppermint oil had reduced severity of pain compared to only 19% of the placebo group (P <0.001) (Kline et al., 2001).

Peppermint is widely used as a tea. Due to its effect on calcium channels it can cause relaxation of the lower oesophageal sphincter leading to heartburn. Use of the enteric coated capsules will prevent this side effect. Typical dosage of the enteric coated capsules is 200 to 400 mg three times a day.

Slippery elm (*Ulmus fulva*)
Slippery elm inner bark, from the slippery elm or red elm tree native to North America, is known to sooth inflammation of the gastrointestinal tract. Slippery elm has demulcent and anti-oxidant properties that can protect the gastrointestinal tract from irritation. When taken internally, slippery elm causes reflex stimulation of the goblet cell nerve endings in the gastrointestinal tract producing extra mucous (Natural Medicine Comprehensive Database, 2012). It is popular among IBD patients in the UK (Langmead et al., 2000).

Significant improvement in IBS symptoms were noted with use of slippery elm. Thirty-one subjects received daily formulations of slippery elm. Twenty-one were classified as suffering from diarrhoea-predominant (DA) or alternating bowel habit IBS, and ten classified as constipation-predominant (C) IBS. In the DA group, abdominal pain scores decreased by 19% (P = 0.006), bloating scores decreased by 28% (P <0.0001), and global IBS symptoms decreased 21% (P = 0.002) during the treatment period. In the C group, there was a 14% decrease in abdominal pain scores (P = 0.032), a 13% decrease in bloating severity (P = 0.034), and a 34% reduction in global IBS symptom severity (P = 0.0005) when mean baseline scores were compared to mean scores over the treatment period (Hawrelak and Myers, 2010).

A tea can be made with adding one tablespoon of powdered inner bark to one cup of boiling water for 15 min. Use 2 to 5 ml three times a day. Capsules: 250–500 mg three to four times daily. Whole bark should not be used as it is considered an abortifacient.

Marshmallow (*Althaea officinalis*)
Marshmallow is used commonly for inflammation of the gastric mucosa, peptic ulcers, respiratory tract mucous membrane inflammation, and dry cough. Marshmallow leaf and root contain mucilage polysaccharides that form a protective layer to shield mucous membranes from local irritation. The mucilage also has antimicrobial, antispasmotic, antisecretory, and wound-healing effects (Newall et al., 1996).

The leaf tea is prepared by steeping one to two teaspoons of the dried leaf in 150 ml boiling water for 5 to 10 min and then straining. The root tea is prepared by steeping one to two teaspoons of the dried root in 150 ml cold water for 1 to 1½ h, straining, and then warming before consumption (Natural Medicine Comprehensive Database, 2012). Each preparation yields 2 to 5 g to be taken three to four times a day.

Probiotics
The human intestinal tract is populated with various microbial species that are non-pathogenic but necessary for metabolizing foods and certain drugs, absorbing nutrients, and preventing colonization by pathogenic bacteria. Probiotics produce butyrate, a short-chain fatty acid important for the health of colonocytes, particularly the epithelial cells in the rectum and left colon. Probiotics activate regulatory T cells and regulatory pathways, leading to down regulation of inflammation (Sartor, 2011).

Two recent double-blind randomized placebo-controlled trials found different types of probiotics (*Lactobacillus* GG and VSL#3®—a commercial brand containing eight different strains) reduced both the frequency and intensity of pain in children with recurrent abdominal pain/IBS (Francavilla et al., 2010; Guandalini et al., 2010). In the Francavilla study, 141 children with IBS or functional pain received either oral LGG (3×10^9 colony-forming units) or oral placebo twice per day. The number of episodes of pain per week decreased in the probiotic group from 3.7 to 1.1 (P <0.01) at 12 weeks, and to 0.9 at week 20 (P <0.02). Pain severity decreased from 4.3 to 2.3 at week 12 (P <0.01) and to 0.9 at week 20 (P <0.001). These decreases were not seen in the placebo group.

Typical dose is 10 to 100 billion colony forming units (CFU) once or twice daily. These preparations can be of a single strain (*Lactobacillis* GG, *Saccharomyces*, etc.) or made of multiple strains combined to treat both small and large intestines.

Digestive enzymes
Digestive enzymes, amylase, lipase, protease and others, are necessary to facilitate proper breakdown of foods for utilization in our bodies. Incomplete digestion of food in the gastrointestinal tract leads to gas formation, bloating, abdominal cramps and diarrhoea, and food allergies/sensitivities. Chronic hyposecretion of these enzymes not only causes maldigestion, but also malabsorption of micronutrients leading to deficiencies and increased intestinal permeability. Impaired gastric acid and pancreatic function has been reported in Crohn's disease contributing to malnutrition (Winter et al., 2004). These may also help for rehabilitation of the malnourished patient with IBD.

In one study, administration of a digestive enzyme product significantly reduced the bloating, flatulence, and abdominal pain, with a slight increase of urgency for bowel movements in patients with IBS (Ciacci et al., 2011).

A trial of a broad-spectrum digestive enzyme consisting of a ratio of 25:2:25 of amylase:lipase:protease USP units respectively, given with meals may be of benefit in those with the described symptoms. Gradually increase to the dosage recommended by the manufacturer dependant on strength.

Fibromyalgia/widespread myofacial pain
Patients with fibromyalgia (FM) frequently have musculoskeletal pain, fatigue, headache, anxiety, weakness, and IBS amongst other symptoms. Many of these symptoms can be treated with the use of herbs and dietary supplements while the underlying dysfunction is addressed for long-lasting relief.

Vitamin D—cholecalciferol (vitamin D₃)
Vitamin D deficiency is frequently seen in patients diagnosed as FM and non-specific musculoskeletal pain (Bhatty et al., 2010). Vitamin D deficiency causes muscle pain and proximal muscle weakness with reports of heaviness in the legs, rapid fatigue, and problems with climbing stairs and mobility. Vitamin D seems to increase muscle protein synthesis, possibly by activating second messengers and phosphorylation (Pfeifer et al., 2002). In paediatrics, vitamin D deficiency can present as atypical muscular pain.

The child at risk of this is typically white, breastfed, protected from the sun, and obese (Clarke and Page, 2012).

Several case reports suggest vitamin D therapy can provide prompt relief of muscle weakness and restore mobility (Prabhala et al., 2000). In a study of 61 women with FM and 25-hydroxy-vitamin D (25(OH) D) levels <20 ng/ml, significant improvement was noted when their blood level of 25(OH) D became greater than or equal to 30 ng/ml. This improvement became more significant when their blood level of 25(OH) D exceeded 50 ng/ml (Matthana, 2011).

After measuring 25(OH) D levels, dose oral vitamin D_3 to target a level of 50 to 60 ng/ml. Knowing that each 100 IU only raises the 25(OH) D level by 1 IU, doses of 2000 to 4000 IU may be needed to increase levels 20 to 40 ng/ml. Very few foods naturally contain vitamin D. Dietary sources include fortified eggs, fatty fish such as herrings, mackerel, sardines, and tuna, and some fortified foods, though these are minor sources overall.

Magnesium

As mentioned previously, magnesium is a natural muscle relaxant and pain reliever which achieves its mechanism of action by antagonizing primarily N-type calcium-mediated channels at nerve endings, reducing noradrenaline release, thereby depressing nerve transmission and muscle contractility (Shimosawa et al., 2004). It is also a cofactor driving many enzymatic reactions necessary for mitochondrial function and energy production.

Serum and RBC magnesium levels were significantly lower in patients with FM than in controls with a negative correlation between the magnesium levels and FM symptoms (Bagis et al., 2013). Supplemental magnesium has been used in its various salt forms to treat myalgias. Oral magnesium citrate treatment, 300 mg a day, was effective in reducing tender points and pain intensity of FM (Bagis et al., 2013). It was also helpful in reducing pain and tenderness in adult FM patients when taken orally as magnesium hydroxide with malic acid (Russell et al., 1995).

Typical dosing is 250 to 500 mg orally twice a day. Dietary sources of magnesium include legumes, whole grains, vegetables, seeds, and nuts, though it is difficult to get adequate amounts daily from food alone. Magnesium's efficacy is dependent on its absorption from the gastrointestinal tract. Supplement with magnesium salts, glycinate, aspartate, gluconate, citrate, or malate to promote absorption without causing diarrhoea which can occur with magnesium oxide. Epsom salts, which are 100% magnesium sulphate, can also be used as a compress or a bath soak to relieve muscle pain.

Vitamin B complex

Many of the B vitamins are cofactors in the Krebs cycle. They serve as facilitators of specific biochemical reactions, i.e. niacin→nicotinamide dinucleotide (NAD), riboflavin→flavin-adenine-dinucleotide (FAD), and therefore necessary for mitochondrial energy production. Deficiencies cause deficits of ATP leading to fatigue, reduce glutathione and nitric oxide synthesis leading to myalgias, and reduce serotonin production causing pain and mood disturbances (Eisinger, 1998).

A number of similarities exist between FM and thiamin deficiency. They include irritability, frequent headaches, unusual fatigue, muscle tenderness, muscular weakness, IBS, and sleep disturbances. Studies have demonstrated abnormalities of thiamin metabolism in FM with increased pyruvate, decreased lactate production and decreased adenosine triphosphate (ATP) (Eisinger, 1994).

Rather than supplement with separate B vitamins, it would be more effective to supplement with daily B-50 complex formulation which would provide 50 mg of vitamins B_1, $_{-2}$, $_{-3}$, $_{-5}$, $_{-6}$; 50 mcg of cobalamin and biotin; and 400 mcg of folic acid.

Coenzyme Q_{10}

CoQ_{10} deficiency, mitochondrial dysfunction, oxidative stress, and mitophagy activation in blood mononuclear cells have been observed in FM patients. CoQ_{10} transfers electrons in the mitochondrial respiratory chain and fulfils a critical role in mitochondrial ATP energy production and cellular metabolism (Cordero et al., 2010).

In a case series of five patients with a diagnosis of FM and CoQ_{10} deficiency, there was a statistically significant reduction of symptoms after receiving CoQ_{10} 300 mg daily for 9 months (Cordero et al., 2011). All patients reported an improvement in sleep, mental alertness, and a marked decrease in joint pain. There were also significant decreases in the number of tender points, the VAS for pain, the Fibromyalgia Impact Questionnaire (FIQ), the Headache Impact Test (HIT-6), and the Migraine Disability Assessment (MIDAS).

CoQ_{10} is generally well tolerated and has no significant adverse effects. The recommended dosing when used for treatment of FM is 300 mg daily.

L-Carnitine

It has been suggested that FM may be associated with mitochondrial dysfunction from a deficit of carnitine. L-carnitine plays a key role in cellular energy production. Long-chain fatty acids are too large to cross the internal mitochondrial membrane and rely on L-carnitine dependant enzymatic transportation. Once in the mitochondria, fatty acids undergo beta-oxidation to adenosine triphosphate (ATP), and L-acetyl-carnitine is excreted to begin a new transport cycle (Natural Medicine Comprehensive Database, 2012).

One multicenter randomized trial compared acetyl L-carnitine (LAC) versus placebo in patients with overt FM. A statistically significant improvement was observed for depression and musculoskeletal pain in the treatment group receiving 500 mg LAC three times daily over 10 weeks. Treatment was well-tolerated (Rossini et al., 2007).

The body obtains some carnitine from red meats and dairy products and can synthesize carnitine from the amino acids, lysine, and methionine. A typical total dose of LAC is 1000 to 2000 mg daily in three divided doses. This dose would be safe in children as doses of 100 mg/kg/day are used in children with Rett syndrome (Ellaway et al., 1999).

Sleep disorders, anxiety, restlessness

These comorbid conditions are commonly seen in patients dealing with pain and can aggravate the pain experience. There are several calming herbs and dietary supplements that may offer the desired effects to help with symptom control.

Chamomile (*Matricaria recutita*)

As discussed previously, Chamomile is used commonly to treat nausea, nervous diarrhoea, gastrointestinal spasms, restlessness, and insomnia. Its mechanism of action is through a known active ingredient, apigenin, which binds to benzodiazepine receptors in the central nervous system, to exert anxiolytic effects (Viola et al., 1995).

There were mixed results of efficacy in a double-blind, randomized trial of 34 adults with insomnia. A dose of 270 mg of chamomile given twice a day was used in this trial (Zick et al., 2011). Given that 1 to 3 g taken three to four times daily is the usual recommended dose to help induce relaxation or sleep (Robbers and Tyler, 1999), the dose in this trial may have been inadequate.

One heaping teaspoon of dried flower heads in half a cup of boiling water steeped for 10 min yields about 3 g of chamomile extract which can be taken up to four times a day. The dose suggested for children under 18 is one-half the adult dose. The essential oils of chamomile can also be used as aromatherapy to promote relaxation and reduce pain (Buckle, 1999). Theoretically, concomitant use with benzodiazepines or other sedatives might cause additive effects and side effects.

Lemon balm (*Melissa officinalis*)

Lemon balm commonly is used for anxiety, insomnia, and restlessness. As an inhalant, lemon balm is used as aroma therapy for calming patients with Alzheimer's disease. Behavioural effects are attributable to a number of possible active components of the dried leaf and essential oil of the herb. Some research suggests lemon balm has acetylcholine receptor activity with both nicotinic and muscarinic binding properties (Kennedy et al., 2002).

One RCT found significant improvements in quality of sleep during 30 days of treatment with 600 mg/day of *M. officinalis* (Cerny and Schmid, 1999).

Capsules containing 100 to 200 mg of dried herb can be taken three times daily or as needed. A tea can be made steeping ½ to 1 teaspoon of dried herb in one cup of hot water for 10 min yielding 1 to 2 g taken in divided doses four times a day. It has a long history of safe usage with no worrisome side effects (Wong et al., 1998).

Melatonin

Melatonin traditionally has been used for insomnia, delayed sleep phase syndrome (DSPS), circadian rhythm disorders in the blind, and jet lag. Melatonin is a hormone synthesized endogenously in the pineal gland produced from tryptophan →5-hydroxytryptophan→serotonin→N-acetylserotonin→melatonin. In the brain, melatonin appears to increase the binding of GABA, the primary inhibitory neurotransmitter, to its receptors (Munoz-Hoyos et al., 1998). Melatonin production is influenced by day/night cycles. Light, both natural and artificial, inhibits melatonin secretion and darkness stimulates secretion (Brzezinski, 1997).

A meta-analysis of data of randomized controlled trials which included four studies totalling 226 children showed that melatonin treatment advanced mean endogenous melatonin onset by 1.18 h (95% confidence interval (CI): 0.89–1.48 h) and clock hour of sleep onset by 0.67 h (95% CI: 0.45–0.89 h). Melatonin decreased sleep-onset latency by 23.27 min (95% CI: 4.83–41.72 min) (van Geijlswijk et al., 2010).

A typical dose for insomnia is 0.3 to 5 mg at bedtime. Start with the lowest dose and increase to higher levels if needed. Implement other sleep hygiene strategies (removal of environmental stimulants 1 to 2 h before bedtime, dusk simulation, quiet evening activities, etc.) to improve effectiveness.

L-tryptophan/5-HTP

L-tryptophan is an essential amino acid absorbed from dietary protein sources that is converted to serotonin and melatonin by the earlier described pathway. People typically use this orally for insomnia, sleep apnoea, depression, anxiety, and myofascial pain.

In clinical studies, 1 g of L-tryptophan significantly reduced sleep latency, with lower doses (0.25–0.5 g) producing a trend in the same direction (Hartmann and Spinweber, 1979). Clinical evidence suggests L-tryptophan is as helpful as light therapy in the treatment of seasonal effective disorder (Ghadirian et al., 1998).

Theoretically, concomitant use with medications that cause sedation may have additive effects. Also, combining serotonergic antidepressants with L-tryptophan/5-HTP may increase the risk of serotonin syndrome.

Consider a starting dose of 50 mg 30 min before bedtime. If not effective, increase by 50 mg each night to a maximum of 300 mg per night for children and adolescents. Occasionally individuals may feel more energized taking this at night. In that case, dose with 50 to 100 mg three times a day with meals.

Valerian (*Valeriana officinalis*)

Valerian, also known as 'nature's Valium', has been used for insomnia, anxiety-associated restlessness and sleeping disorders, mood disorders, and chronic fatigue syndrome. Valerenic acid and other constituents of valerian are GABA agonists (Natural Medicine Comprehensive Database, 2012).

An extract of valerian and lemon balm reduced restlessness and difficulties falling asleep in an open multicenter post marketing surveillance study of 918 children under age 12 with sleep disorders. Patients took one to two tablets, each containing 160 mg of valerian and 80 mg of lemon balm, twice a day. There were no significant side effects (Müller and Klement, 2006). A systematic review of the available literature suggests that valerian improves sleep quality without producing side effects (Bent et al., 2006). Some evidence shows that valerian reduces self-reported stress in social anxiety (Kohnen and Oswald, 1998).

Dosing of 100 to 300 mg 30 min before bedtime is recommended for sleep. It can also be dosed on a three-times-a-day schedule for anxiety. Valerian has been safely used in children in studies lasting 4 to 8 weeks. Use of valerian with other herbs and supplements with sedative properties might have synergistic effects, therefore caution should be used.

L-Theanine

L-Theanine is the major amino acid found in green tea and historically been used for its relaxation and anti-anxiety effects. L-theanine works to reduce anxiety by increasing levels of GABA and serotonin (Lu et al., 2004). It also antagonizes glutamate and NMDA receptors (Kakuda et al., 2000).

One study evaluated the acute effects of alprazolam and L-theanine under a relaxed and experimentally induced anxiety condition. L-theanine 200 mg was superior to alprazolam 1 mg in producing a relaxed state under resting conditions (Lu et al., 2004).

Typical dosing would be 100 to 200 mg once or twice daily.

Conclusion

The goal of this chapter is to introduce clinicians to the use of common herbs, vitamins, and dietary supplements that can be integrated into the care of children and adolescents experiencing pain. As clinicians we need to have an understanding of the benefits or potential side effects these supplements have so that we can best advise our patients in their use. The supplements outlined in this chapter, with their mechanisms of action and recommended doses, have been found to be effective and are generally regarded as safe to use in the paediatric population for various pain syndromes or symptoms associated with pain.

Case example

Suzanne presented with a 6-month history of headache, myalgias, and fatigue. This previously healthy and energetic 16-year-old developed symptoms after a prolonged viral illness. She described her headache as 'all over pressure', rated the pain as '7' on the VAS, and made worse with bright lights and noise. She stated all her muscles were achy, 'felt heavy', and worse with any physical activity. She was sleeping 12 h every night but did not feel rested when she woke and often needed to take naps during the day. Because of the fatigue and pain, she had not attended school for over 3 months and stopped all physical activity. She rarely went outside the family home. Her mother was concerned that Suzanne was becoming more depressed because she wasn't doing her normal activities nor was she able to be with her friends.

On physical examination Suzanne appeared tired and had flat affect. Her skin was pale, but she had no rashes or bruises. She had multiple tender areas with palpation of her head, neck, and upper back. She also had tenderness all along her paraspinus muscles and of the large muscle groups of her extremities. The remainder of her examination was otherwise normal.

Laboratory investigations done to assess for anaemia, infection, thyroid dysfunction, and autoimmune diseases were all normal. Her RBC magnesium level was low at 3.5 mg/dL (normal 4.7–7.0 mg/dL), homocysteine level high at 12 μmol/L (normal <8 μmol/L), 25-hydroxyvitamin D level low at 17 ng/ml (ideal 50–60 ng/ml), and coenzyme Q_{10} level was low-normal at 0.6 mcg/ml (normal 0.5–1.5 mcg/ml).

She was started on vitamin D_3 4000 IU daily, magnesium malate 500 mg twice daily, and CoQ_{10} 300 mg daily for the obvious deficiencies and for their known effects on headache pain and myalgias. She was also started on vitamin B-50 complex to provide the cofactors necessary for enzyme and energy production. She was encouraged to continue a healthy diet of lean meats, fresh fruits, and vegetables to provide other essential micronutrients. For sleep and mood, she started 5-HTP 100 mg before bedtime to boost serotonin and melatonin production, instructed on sleep hygiene strategies, encouraged to maintain a routine sleep/wake schedule every day, and asked to minimize naps to only 30 min a day. She was started on a low-intensity exercise programme of stretching followed by walking 15 min day for the first week. The time was increased only 5 min each week so as not to over-exert and trigger more fatigue/pain.

Suzanne returned for follow up 2 months later and was considerably better by her report. She was now sleeping consistently 10 h each night and felt rested when she woke in the morning. She stopped taking naps during the day, no longer had the achy muscles and was walking without fatigue about 40 min a day. She still had occasional headaches, but these were shorter in duration and intensity and could be relieved by acetaminophen. Both she and her mother reported an improved mood. Suzanne was spending more time with friends and attending school half-days with plans to return full time the following week.

Since she was clinically improved, no further laboratory tests were done. She was encouraged to continue the current regimen of supplements until she had full resolution of the symptoms and was back to her usual level of physical activity. At that time she could consider coming off the supplements and monitor for any recurrence of the symptoms.

References

Abraham, G. E., Schwartz, U. D., and Lubran, M. M. (1981). Effect of vitamin B-6 on plasma and red blood cell magnesium levels in pre-menopausal women. *Ann Clin Lab Sci*, 11(4), 333–336.

Ali, B. H., Blunden, G., Tanira, M. O., and Nemmar, A. (2007). Some phytochemical, pharmacological and toxicological properties of ginger (Zingiber officinal Roscoe): a review of recent research. *Food Chem Toxicol*, 46(2), 409–420.

Altura, B. T., Shirley, T., Young, C. C., Hiti, J., Dell'Orfano, K., Handwerker, S. M., *et al.* (1992). A new method for the rapid determination of ionized Mg2+ in whole blood, serum and plasma. *Meth Find Exp Clin Pharmacol*, 14(4), 297–304.

Astin, J. (1998). Why patients use alternative medicine: results of a national study. *JAMA*, 279(19), 1548–1553.

Bagis, S., Karabiber, M., As, I., Tamer, L., Erdogan, C., and Atalay, A. (2012). Is magnesium citrate treatment effective on pain, clinical parameters and functional status in patients with fibromyalgia? *Rheumatol Int*, 33(1), 167–172.

Bent, S., Padula, A., Moore, D., Patterson, M., and Mehling, W. (2006). Valerian for sleep: a systematic review and meta-analysis. *Am J Med*, 119(12), 1005–1012.

Bhatty, S.A., Shaikh, N.A., Irfan, M., Kashif, S. M., Vaswani, A. S., Sumbhai, A, *et al.* (2010). Vitamin D deficiency in fibromyalgia. *J Pak Med Assoc*, 60(11), 949–951.

Bruijn, J., Duivenvoorden, H., Passchier, J., Locher, H., Dijkstra, N., and Arts, W. F. (2010). Medium-dose riboflavin as a prophylactic agent in children with migraine: a preliminary placebo-controlled, randomised, double-blind, cross-over trial *Cephalalgia*, 30(12), 1426–1434.

Brzezinski, A. (1997). Melatonin in humans. *N Engl J Med*, 336, 186–195.

Buckle, J. (1999). Use of aromatherapy as a complementary treatment for chronic pain. *Altern Ther Health Med*, 5(5), 42–51.

Cady, R. K., Goldstein, J., Nett, R., Mitchell, R., Beach, M. E., and Browning, R. (2011). A double-blind placebo-controlled pilot study of sublingual feverfew and ginger (LipiGesic™ M) in the treatment of migraine. *Headache*, 51(7), 1078–1086.

Cerny, A. and Schmid, K. (1999). Tolerability and efficacy of valerian/lemon balm in healthy volunteers: a double-blind, placebo-controlled, multicentre study. *Fitoterapia*, 70(3), 221–228.

Ciacci, C., Franceschi, F., Purchiaroni, F., Capone, P., Buccelletti, F., Iacomini, P., *et al.* (2011). Effect of beta-glucan, inositol and digestive enzymes in GI symptoms of patients with IBS. *Eur Rev Med Pharmacol Sci*, 15(6), 637–643.

Clarke, N. M. and Page, J. E. (2012). Vitamin D deficiency: a paediatric orthopaedic perspective. *Curr Opin Pediatr*, 24(1), 46–49.

Condò, M., Posar, A., Arbizzani, A., and Parmeggiani, A. (2009). Riboflavin prophylaxis in pediatric and adolescent migraine. *J Headache Pain*, 10(5), 361–365.

Cordero, M. D., De Miguel, M., Moreno-Fernández, A. M., Carmona López, I. M., Garrido Maraver, J., Cotán, D., et al. (2010). Mitochondrial dysfunction and mitophagy activation in blood mononuclear cells of fibromyalgia patients: implication in the pathogenesis of the disease. Arthritis Res Ther, 12, R17.

Cordero, M. D., Alcocer-Gómez, E., de Miguel, M., Cano-García, F. J., Luque, C. M., Fernández-Riejo, P., et al. (2011). Coenzyme Q(10): a novel therapeutic approach for fibromyalgia? Case series with 5 patients. Mitochondrion, 11(4), 623–625.

Cordero, M. D., Cano-García, F. J., Alcocer-Gómez, E., De Miguel, M., and Sánchez-Alcázar, J. A. (2012) Oxidative stress correlates with headache symptoms in fibromyalgia: coenzyme Q10 effect on clinical improvement. PLoS One, 7(4), e35677. Available at: <http://www.plosone.org>.

Demirkaya, S., Vural, O., Dora, B., and Topçuoğlu, M. A. (2001). Efficacy of intravenous magnesium sulfate in the treatment of acute migraine attacks. Headache, 41(2), 171–177.

Di Rosa, G., Attina, S., Spano, M., Ingegneri, G., Sgrò, D. L., Pustorino, G., et al. (2007). Efficacy of folic acid in children with migraine, hyperhomocysteinemia and MTHFR polymorphisms. Headache, 47, 1342–1351.

Eisinger, J., Plantamura, A., and Ayavou, T. (1994). Glycolysis abnormalities in fibromyalgia. J Am Coll Nutr, 13(2), 144–148.

Eisinger, J. (1998). Alcohol, thiamin and fibromyalgia. J Am Coll Nutr, 17(3), 300–302.

Ellaway, C. M., Williams, K., Leonard, H., Higgins, G., Wilcken, B., and Christodoulou, J. (1999). Rett syndrome: randomized controlled trial of L-carnitine. J Child Neurol, 14, 162–167.

Food and Drug Administration. (2012). Generally recognized as safe (GRAS). Available at: <http://www.fda.gov/Food/IngredientsPackagingLabeling/GRAS/ucm2006850.htm>.

Francavilla, R., Miniello, V., Magistà, A. M., De Canio, A., Bucci, N., Gagliardi, F., et al. (2010). A randomized controlled trial of Lactobacillus GG in children with functional abdominal pain. Pediatrics, 126(6), e1445–1452.

Gaby, A. (2011). Migraine. In Nutritional Medicine, pp. 527–536. Concord, NH: Fritz Perlberg.

Gallai, V., Sarchielli, P., Morucci, P., and Abbritti, G. (1993). Red blood cell magnesium levels in migraine patients. Cephalalgia, 13, 94–98.

Ghadirian, A. M., Murphy, B. E., and Gendron, M. J. (1998). Efficacy of light versus tryptophan therapy in seasonal affective disorder. J Affect Disord, 50(1), 23–27.

Grazzi, L., Andrasik, F., Usai, S., and Bussone, G. (2007). Magnesium as a preventive treatment for paediatric episodic tension-type headache: results at 1-year follow-up. Neurol Sci, 28(3), 148–150.

Guandalini, S., Magazzù, G., Chiaro, A., La Balestra, V., Di Nardo, G., Gopalan, S., et al. (2010). VSL#3 improves symptoms in children with irritable bowel syndrome: a multicenter, randomized, placebo-controlled, double- blind, crossover study. J Pediatr Gastroenterol Nutr, 51(1), 24–30.

Gupta, S., Nahas, S. J., and Peterlin, B. L. (2011). Chemical mediators of migraine: preclinical and clinical observations. Headache, 51(6), 1029–1045.

Hagen, L. E., Schneider, R., Stephens, D., Modrusan, D., Feldman, B. M. (2003). Use of complementary and alternative medicine by pediatric rheumatology patients. Arthritis Rheum, 49(1), 3–6.

Hartmann, E. and Spinweber, C. L. (1979). Sleep induced by L-tryptophan. Effect of dosages within the normal dietary intake. J Nerv Ment Dis, 167, 497–499.

Hawrelak, J. A. and Myers, S. P. (2010). Effects of two natural medicine formulations on irritable bowel syndrome symptoms: a pilot study. J Altern Complement Med, 16(10), 1065–1071.

Hershey, A. D., Powers, S. W., Vockell, A. L., Lecates, S. L., Ellinor, P. L., Segers, A., et al. (2007). Coenzyme Q10 deficiency and response to supplementation in pediatric and adolescent migraine. Headache, 47(1), 73–80.

Heuschkel, R., Afzal, N., and Wuerth, A. (2002). Complementary medicine use in children and young adults with inflammatory bowel disease. Am J Gastroenterol, 97(2), 382–388

Hills, J. M. and Aaronson, P. I. (1991). The mechanism of action of peppermint oil in GI smooth muscle. Gastroenterology, 101, 55–65.

Hormann, H. P. and Korting, H. C. (1994). Evidence for the efficacy and safety of topical herbal drugs in dermatology: part I: anti-inflammatory agents. Phytomedicine, 1, 161–171.

Hoshino, K., Ogawa, K., Kitazawa, R., Nakamura, Y., and Uehara, R. (1998). Ionized magnesium level in whole blood of healthy Japanese children. Pediatrics International, 40(2), 116–121.

Kakuda, T., Yanase, H., Utsunomiya, K., Nozawa, A., Unno, T., and Kataoka, K. (2000). Protective effect of gamma-glutamylethylamide (theanine) on ischemic delayed neuronal death in gerbils. Neurosci Lett, 289, 189–192.

Kemper, K. J., Vohra, S., and Walls, R. (2008). The use of complementary and alternative medicine in Pediatrics. Pediatrics, 122, 1374–1386.

Kennedy, D. O., Scholey, A. B., Tildesley, N.T, Perry, E. K., and Wesnes, K. A. (2002). Modulation of mood and cognitive performance following acute administration of Melissa officinalis (lemon balm). Pharmacol Biochem Behav, 72, 953–964.

Kline, R. M., Kline, J. J., Di Palma, J., and Barbero, G. (2001). Enteric coated, pH-dependent peppermint oil capsules for the treatment of irritable bowel syndrome in children. J Pediatr, 138, 125–128.

Ko, W. C., Lei, C. B., Lin, Y. L., and Chen, C. F. (2001). Mechanisms of relaxant action of S-petasin and S-isopetasin, sesquiterpenes of Petasites formosanus, in isolated guinea pig trachea. Planta Med, 67(3), 224–229.

Kohnen, R. and Oswald, W. D. (1998). The effects of valerian, propranolol, and their combination on activation, performance, and mood of healthy volunteers under social stress conditions. Pharmacopsychiatry, 21(6), 447–448.

Langmead, L., Chitnis, M., and Rampton, D. (2000). Complementary therapies in GI patients: who uses them and why? Gut, 46(Suppl. II), A22 (Abstract).

Lee, D. K., Carstairs, I. J., Haggart, K., Jackson, C. M., Currie, G. P., and Lipworth, B. J. (2003). Butterbur, an herbal remedy, attenuates adenosine monophosphate induced nasal responsiveness in seasonal allergic rhinitis. Clin Exp Allergy, 33, 882–886.

Lu, K., Gray, M. A., Oliver, C., Harrison, B. J., Bartholomeusz, C. F., Phan, K. L., et al. (2004). The acute effects of L-theanine in comparison with alprazolam on anticipatory anxiety in humans. Hum Psychopharmacol, 19, 457–465.

MacLennan, S. C., Wade, F. M., Forrest, K. M., Ratanayake, P. D., Fagan, E., and Antony, J. 2008). High-dose riboflavin for migraine prophylaxis in children: a double-blind, randomized, placebo-controlled trial. J Child Neurol, 23(11), 1300–1304.

Mauskop, A., Altura, B. T., Cracco, R. Q., and Altura, B. M. (1996). Intravenous magnesium sulfate rapidly alleviates headaches of various types. Headache, 36(3), 154–160.

Matthana, M. H. (2011). The relation between vitamin D deficiency and fibromyalgia syndrome in women. Saudi Med J, 32(9), 925–929.

Müller, S. F. and Klement, S. (2006). A combination of valerian and lemon balm is effective in the treatment of restlessness and dyssomnia in children. Phytomedicine, 13(6), 383–387.

Munoz-Hoyos, A., Sanchez-Forte, M., Molina-Carballo, A., Escames, G., Martin-Medina, E., Reiter, R. J., et al. (1998). Melatonin's role as an anticonvulsant and neuronal protector: experimental and clinical evidence. J Child Neurol, 13, 501–509.

Murphy, J. J., Heptinstall, S., and Mitchell, J. R. (1988). Randomized double-blind placebo- controlled trial of feverfew in migraine prevention. Lancet, 2(8604), 189–192.

Murray, M. T. (1995). Healing power of herbs. Rocklin, CA: Prima Publishing.

Natural Medicine Comprehensive Database. (2012). Available at: <http://naturaldatabase.com>.

Nelson, K. B., Richardson, A. K., He, J., Lateef, T. M., Khoromi, S., and Merikangas, K. R. (2010). Headache and biomarkers predictive of vascular disease in a representative sample of US children. *Arch Pediatr Adolesc Med*, 164(4), 358–362.

Newall, C. A., Anderson, L. A., and Philpson, J. D. (1996). *Herbal medicine: a guide for healthcare professionals*. London: The Pharmaceutical Press.

O'Brien, H., Hershey, A. D., and Kabbouche, M. A.(2010). Prevalence of vitamin D among pediatric patients with recurrent headaches. *Headache*, 50(Suppl.1), S23.

Oterino, A., Toriello, M., Valle, N., Castillo, J., Alonso-Arranz, A., Bravo, Y., *et al.* (2010). The relationship between homocysteine and genes of folate-related enzymes in migraine patients. *Headache*, 50(1), 99–168.

Pareek, A., Suthar, M., Rathore, G. S., and Bansal, V. (2011). Feverfew (Tanacetum parthenium L.): a systematic review. *Pharmacogn Rev*, 5(9), 103–110.

Peres, M. F., Gonçalves, A. L., and Krymchantowski, A. (2007). Migraine, tension-type headache, and transformed migraine. *Curr Pain Headache Rep*, 11(6), 449–453.

Perquin, C., Hazebroek-Kampschreur, A., Hunfeld, J., Bohnen, A. M., van Suijlekom-Smit, L. W., Passchier, J., *et al.* (2000). Pain in children and adolescents: a common experience. *Pain*, 87, 51–58.

Pfeifer, M., Begerow, B., and Minne, H. W. (2002). Vitamin D and muscle function. *Osteoporos Int*, 13(3), 187–194.

Pieczenik, S. R. and Neustadt, J. (2007). Mitochondrial dysfunction and molecular pathways of disease. *Exp Mol Pathol*, 83(1), 84–92.

Pittler, M. H., Vogler, B. K., and Ernst, E. (2000). Feverfew for preventing migraine. *Cochrane Database Syst Rev*, 3, CD002286.

Pothmann, R. and Danesch, U. (2005). Migraine prevention in children and adolescents: results of an open study with a special butterbur root extract. *Headache*, 45(3), 196–203.

Prabhala, A., Garg, R., and Dandona, P. (2000). Severe myopathy associated with vitamin D deficiency in western New York. *Arch Intern Med*, 160(8), 1199–1203.

Prakash, S. and Shah, N. D. (2009). Chronic tension-type headache with vitamin D deficiency: casual or causal association? *Headache*, 49(8), 1214–1222.

Ranade, V. V. and Somberg, J.C. (2001). Bioavailability and pharmacokinetics of magnesium after administration of magnesium salts to humans. *Am J Ther*, 8(5), 345–357.

Robbers, J. E. and Tyler, V. E. (1999). *Tyler's herbs of choice: the therapeutic use of phytomedicinals* New York: The Haworth Herbal Press.

Rossini, M., Di Munno, O., Valentini, G., Bianchi, G., Biasi, G., Cacace, E., *et al.* (2007). Double-blind, multicenter trial comparing acetyl l-carnitine with placebo in the treatment of fibromyalgia patients. *Clin Exp Rheumatol*, 25(2), 182–188.

Russell, I. J., Michalek, J. E., Flechas, J. D., and Abraham, G. E. (1995). Treatment of fibromyalgia syndrome with Super Malic: a randomized, double blind, placebo controlled, crossover pilot study. *J Rheumatol*, 22, 953–958.

Sartor, R. B. (2011). Efficacy of probiotics for the management of inflammatory bowel disease. *Gastroenterol Hepatol*, 7(9), 606–608.

Shimosawa, T., Takano, K., Ando, K., and Fujita, T. (2004). Magnesium inhibits norepinephrine release by blocking N-type calcium channels at peripheral sympathetic nerve endings. *Hypertention*, 44, 897–902.

Shrivastava, R., Pechadre, J. C., and John, G. W. (2006). Tanacetum parthenium and Salix alba (Mig-RL) combination in migraine. *Clin Drug Invest*, 26(5), 287–296.

Soriani, S., Arnaldi, C., De Carlo, L., Mazzotta, D., Battistella, P. A., Sartori, S., *et al.* (1995). Serum and red blood cell magnesium levels in juvenile migraine patients. *Headache*, 35, 14–16.

Srivastava, K. C. and Mustafa, T. (1989). Ginger (Zingiber officinale) and rheumatic disorders. *Med Hypoth*, 29, 25–28.

Sumner, H., Salan, U., Knight, D. W., and Hoult, J. R. (1992). Inhibition of 5-lipoxygenase and cyclo-oxygenase in leukocytes by feverfew. Involvement of sesquiterpene lactones and other components. *Biochem Pharmacol*, 43, 2313–2320.

Sun, X., Chan, L. N., and Sucher, N. J. (2005). Magnesium as NMDA receptor blocker in the traditional Chinese medicine Danshen. *Phytomedicine*, 12(3), 173–177.

Sun-Edelstein, C. and Mauskop, A. (2009). Role of magnesium in the pathogenesis and treatment of migraine. *Expert Rev Neurother*, 9(3), 369–379.

Thys-Jacobs, S. (1994a). Alleviation of migraines with therapeutic vitamin D and calcium. *Headache*, 34(10), 590–592.

Thys-Jacobs, S. (1994b). Vitamin D and calcium in menstrual migraine. *Headache*, 34(9), 544–546.

Tietjen, G. E., Herial, N. A., White, L., Utley, C., Kosmyna, J. M., Khuder, S. A. (2009). Migraine and biomarkers of endothelial activation in young women. *Stroke*, 40(9), 2977–2982.

Tsao, J. C. I. and Zeltzer, L. K. (2005). Complementary and alternative medicine approaches for pediatric pain: a review of the state-of-the-science. *eCAM*, 2(2), 149–159.

Turunen, M., Olsson, J., and Dallner, G. (2004). Metabolism and function of coenzyme Q. *Biochimica et Biophysica Acta*, 1660, 171–199.

van der Kuy, P. H., Merkus, F. W., Lohman, J. J., ter Berg, J. W., and Hooymans, P. M. (2002). Hydroxocobalamin, a nitric oxide scavenger, in the prophylaxis of migraine: an open, pilot study. *Cephalalgia*, 22(7), 513–519.

van Geijlswijk, I. M., Korzilius, H. P., and Smits, M. G. (2010). The use of exogenous melatonin in delayed sleep phase disorder: a meta-analysis. *Sleep*, 33(12), 1605–1614.

Vieth, R. (1999). Vitamin D supplementation, 25-hydroxyvitamin D concentrations, and safety. *Am J Clin Nutr*, 69 (5), 842–856.

Viola, H., Wasowski, C., Levi de Stein, M., Wolfman, C., Silveira, R., Dajas, F., *et al.* (1995). Apigenin, a component of matricaria recutita flowers, is a central benzodiazepine receptors-ligand with anxiolytic effects. *Planta Medica*, 61, 213–216.

Wang, F., Van Den Eeden, S. K., Ackerson, L. M., Salk, S. E., Reince, R. H., and Elin, R. J. (2003). Oral magnesium oxide prophylaxis of frequent migrainous headache in children: a randomized, double-blind, placebo-controlled trial. *Headache*, 43(6), 601–610.

Weizman, Z., Alkrinawi, S., Goldfarb, D., and Bitran, C. (1993). Efficacy of herbal tea preparation in infantile colic. *J Pediatr*, 122(4), 650–652.

Weydert, J. A. (2012) Recurring abdominal pain in children. In D. Rakel (ed.) *Integrative medicine: complementary therapeutics in medical practice* (3rd edn), pp. 422–429. Philadelphia, PA: Elsevier/Saunders Company.

Winter, T. A., O'keefe, S. J., Callanan, M., and Marks, T. (2004). Impaired gastric acid and pancreatic enzyme secretion in patients with Crohn's disease may be a consequence of a poor nutritional state. *Inflamm Bowel Dis*, 10(5), 618–625.

Wong, A. H. C., Smith, M., and Boon, H. S. (1998). Herbal remedies in psychiatric practice. *Arch Gen Psychiatry*, 55, 1033–1044.

Wu, K. L., Rayner, C. K., and Chuah, S. K. (2008). Effects of ginger on gastric emptying and motility in healthy humans. *Eur J Gastroenterol Hepatol*, 20, 436–440.

Zick, S. M., Wright, B. D., Sen, A., and Arnedt, J. T. (2011). Preliminary examination of the efficacy and safety of a standardized chamomile extract for chronic primary insomnia: a randomized placebo-controlled pilot study. *BMC Complement Altern Med*, 22(11), 78.

CHAPTER 60

Complementary therapy in paediatric pain

Lonnie K. Zeltzer

Summary

There is increasing paediatric use of complementary therapies (CTs), especially for paediatric pain. This chapter reviews the key literature on studies that pertain to CTs that impact pain in children. The research is still in its infancy with few studies that have been well designed and replicated. Likely the strongest of the studies is in hypnotherapy, which will have its own chapter, and in biofeedback for headaches. Acupuncture research is growing but there are few well designed studies in children compared to those in adults. Risks in CTs mostly relate to training of the practitioner and good clinical judgement (e.g. avoiding massage in children aversive to touch). Most are safe when used with clinical judgement.

Introduction

The biopsychosocial model for understanding and treating childhood pain takes into account the many facets of and contributors to the pain experience and pain-related functional disability. Increasingly, paediatric pain programmes are incorporating complementary therapy (CT) into their existing programmes of pharmacological, physical, and psychological pain management. Typically, this quadruple of treatments is called 'integrative pain management'.

A barrier to incorporating CTs into a more traditional approach to pain treatment in children is the relatively little published science to indicate which CTs are effective and safe and for what pain conditions. The implementation of many complementary practices is often not well described.

The aim of this chapter is to present a state of the science on CTs in childhood pain, and how they would be applied to children in pain. A case of the use of complementary CTs for childhood pain is presented by an adolescent patient with discussion by the author about the choice of therapies and the integration of CTs into the total treatment plan.

The various terms for CTs, typically known collectively as complementary and alternative medicine (CAM), have been used inconsistently in the literature. Not uncommonly, the terms 'complementary', 'alternative', 'holistic', and 'integrative' have been used interchangeably. Over time there also has been a blurring of boundaries between complementary and 'traditional' therapies, as usage of CTs has become more common and the science has moved forward.

The National Center for Complementary and Alternative Medicine (NCCAM) at the National Institutes of Health has defined 'complementary therapies' as those interventional strategies used in conjunction with conventional medicine. 'Alternative therapies' are defined as treatments used in place of conventional medicine. NCCAM has divided these complementary and alternative therapies into five categories: biologically based therapies, manipulative and body-based therapies, energy therapies, mind–body interventions, and alternative medical systems. Biologically based therapies include herbal remedies that employ plant preparations for therapeutic effects, as well as vitamins and other dietary supplements. Manipulative and body-based methods include, for example, chiropractic, osteopathic manipulations, and massage. Energy therapies include Reiki and the unconventional use of electromagnetic fields. Mind–body interventions relate to techniques to increase the mind's capacity to enhance bodily function and reduce symptoms, such as hypnotherapy, biofeedback, meditation, prayer, and expressive therapies such as music, art, or dance therapy. Alternative medical systems are built upon complete systems of theory and practice and may make use of therapies from the biological, body-based, mind–body, and energy modalities. Examples are homeopathic medicine, Ayervedic healing, naturopathic medicine, and traditional Chinese medicine (TCM). An individual complementary therapy may be used in isolation from its use within an alternative medical system, such as acupuncture (TCM) and yoga (Ayervedic healing). Although CAM clearly encompasses a variety of techniques from various schools of thought, this chapter will focus on CTs that have been reported to have been used for acute or chronic pain in children.

Background

Estimates of the use of CTs range from 2% in a healthy sample of children (Davis and Darden, 2003) to as high as 73% in children with cancer (Neuhouser et al., 2001), with figures pointing to substantial increases across paediatric populations. The use of CTs in children is increasing internationally, but the reported prevalence differs by country, methodology, and populations studied

(Efe et al., 2013; Heath et al., 2012; Snyder and Brown, 2012). For example, the prevalence of CT use in the Netherlands in children with cancer was found to be about 40%, while it was 11% in a Finnish study based on a national data set of over 6000 children. In the latter study, symptom reduction was the primary reason for parents seeking complementary therapies (Singendonk et al., 2013; Siponen et al., 2012). CT use often goes unreported to physicians; as many as half of all adults using CTs do so without consulting a practitioner (Eisenberg et al., 1993) and the figure may be even higher for children (Spigelblatt et al., 1994). This practice appears to occur despite the desire of many parents to discuss their child's use of CTs with the family paediatrician (Sibinga et al., 2004).

In addition, a 2001 survey of 745 members of the American Academy of Paediatrics found that 87 % of paediatricians had been asked about CTs by a patient or a parent in the 3 months prior to the survey (Sawni-Sikand et al., 2002; Yussman et al., 2004). The paediatricians were asked most often about herbs and dietary supplements (Wilson et al., 2006; Woolf, 2003).

The 2007 National Health Interview Survey gathered information on CT use among more than 9000 children younger than 18 years (Barnes et al., 2008). Nearly 12% had used some form of CTs during the past 12 months. CT use was much more likely among children whose parents also used CTs. Adolescents aged 12 to 17 years, children with multiple health conditions, and those whose families delayed or did not use conventional medical care because of cost were also more likely to use CTs. The most common pain conditions for which CTs were used in the past 12 months included back or neck pain (8%), musculoskeletal conditions (4%), and abdominal pain (1%), with associated problems including anxiety/stress (5%), sleep problems (2%), and depression (1%). Headaches were not included in the list but related sinusitis was 2% and 'other' was (8%). Chiropractic or osteopathic manipulations were used in 3% of children, deep breathing exercises in 3%, yoga in 2%, meditation and massage in 1% each, and all other modalities were less than 1%. Integrative care including CTs is now included in major textbooks of paediatrics (Zeltzer and Krane, 2011).

Complementary therapies

Acupuncture and related techniques

Within TCM, there is a belief that an energy force flows through the body, which, if blocked, causes imbalance and sickness. Different traditions call this energy 'Qi' (pronounced 'chi'), 'prana', and 'life force'. Acupuncture is intended to restore natural energy (Qi) through the insertion of needles into points along energy pathways (meridians) in the body. The needles help stimulate the energy flow. Usually, needles are inserted into the skin from ¼ to 1 inch deep. The patient often reports light cramping, heaviness, distention, tingling, or electric sensation either around the needle or travelling up or down the energy pathway. Although the precise analgesic mechanisms have not been identified, it is likely that the body's nervous system, neurotransmitters, and endogenous substances are involved in needle stimulation (Ma 2004).

In adults, acupuncture is one of the most popular complementary therapies, yet it is less often used in children (Barnes et al., 2008). The common assumption that most children are fearful of needles may cause physicians to be averse to recommending acupuncture; yet research has found that children and adolescents find the experience acceptable (Kemper et al., 2000; Waterhouse et al., 2000; Zeltzer et al., 2002).

In treating paediatric pain, acupuncture therapy has been evaluated for its potential effectiveness in alleviating chronic headaches (Pintov et al., 1997; Pothmann et al., 2009), acute pain (Wu et al., 2009) and surgical pain (Kim et al., 2006; Lin et al., 2009). A study investigating the efficacy of laser acupuncture in 43 paediatric patients suffering with chronic headaches, randomized children to an intervention group that used low-level laser for individualized acupuncture or to a control condition of sham laser acupuncture. The intervention group had a significant decrease in headache frequency, monthly headache hours, and headache pain intensity compared to baseline but not to the sham intervention. No adverse events were observed in the study (Pothmann et al., 2009).

Pintov et al. (1997) studied acupuncture for migraine treatment in children, with12 patients randomly assigned to the true acupuncture group (TA) and ten assigned to the placebo acupuncture group (PA). The PA group received a sham acupuncture treatment by the insertion of the same size needle into the stratum corneum. Both the TA and PA groups received ten weekly sessions of intervention. The TA group had a significant reduction in both frequency and intensity of migraines and a significantly potentiated amount of panopioid activity after the acupuncture compared to that found in the PA group.

These studies (Pintov et al., 1997; Pothmann et al., 2009) provide some evidence for acupuncture effectiveness in treating chronic headaches in children, although limited by small sample sizes and the challenges of providing a sham treatment (such as the inability to double blind). The Pintov study had a biased sample by excluding children who were receiving any headache medication. Yet, these early results are promising and more randomized controlled trials (RCTs) are warranted.

A non-randomized clinical trial (Wu et al., 2009) assessed two 10 to 15 min acupuncture sessions in 11 hospitalized children with spinal fusion surgery and nine in intensive care (PICU). Both groups had a general decrease in pain scores, heart rate and systolic blood pressure after acupuncture sessions. The non-PICU group 1 had a maximal decrease of morphine PCA usage 4 to 8 h after the first acupuncture session and by the second session were placed on oral opioids. This study showed acceptance and tolerance for acupuncture for postoperative pain management within a hospital setting, although efficacy was not determined.

Lin et al. (2009) randomized 66 children aged 2.2±1.4 years undergoing bilateral myringotomy/tympanostomy tube (BMT) placement into a post-anaesthesia preoperative acupuncture or control condition without the acupuncture. The intervention group had significantly lower pain and agitation scores across the different observed time points and a lower need for postoperative acetaminophen. No adverse events were observed. Long-term effects have yet to be determined.

A study (Kim et al., 2006) of capsicum plaster placed at the Zusanli (Z:ST-36) points after a unilateral hernia repair for postoperative pain control in 108 children (4 months to 9 years) randomly assigned patient to three groups. The intervention group (Z) received capsicum plaster at Z acupoints and placebo tape at a non-acupoint in the shoulder. The sham group (S) received plaster at shoulder points and placebo tape at the Z acupoint. The control group (C) received placebo tape at both shoulder and Z points. Outcome measures were postoperative pain scores, as well as the analgesic opioid requirements during the 24 h postoperative time frame. A significantly lower use of meperidine (the postoperative opioid used in the study) was found in group The Z group had less opioid use and lower pain scores compared to the other two groups. No side effects from capsicum plaster were observed.

These studies (Kim et al., 2006; Lin et al., 2009) suggest a potentially safe complementary therapy for reduction of opioid analgesic dosage for paediatric post-operative pain management. Replication of the studies and improved study designs are warranted.

Acupuncture practitioners are licensed and regulated health care professionals in about half the states in the US. In states that do not currently require licensing, the acupuncture practitioner should be asked if he/she is certified by the National Commission for the Certification of Acupuncturists. The acupuncturist should be asked to communicate with the child's paediatrician or pain specialist for optimal integrative care. Acupuncture in Canada developed in the late 1800's primarily in Chinese communities but gradually spread to the communities until it was incorporated into the Governmental health care system. For example, in the province of Ontario, it became part of the 'Traditional Chinese Medicine Act' in 2006 (Wang and Wu 2012). Across Asia, acupuncture has been accepted and used for hundreds of years. The governmental regulations for practising acupuncture differ by country worldwide but in most places few restrictions are in place.

Biofeedback

Biofeedback uses a computer or other bodily feedback tool to help children to reduce pain or other symptoms by noticing and then learning strategies to control physiological changes associated with the stress response. These monitored changes (Evans and Zeltzer 2008) may include muscle tension, peripheral skin temperature, sweat gland response, brain wave activity, or breathing rate, with the goal of increasing the body's relaxation response. Using biofeedback helps children learn about their body's responses to stress and become aware of their own abilities to alter those responses. Biofeedback is especially popular for the treatment of migraine and headaches in children (Evans and Zeltzer, 2008).

Biofeedback has been evaluated in its effectiveness for treating paediatric headaches (Arndorfer and Allen, 2001; Bussone et al., 1998; Fentress et al., 1986; Grazzi et al., 1990, 2001; Kroner-Herwig et al.1998; Scharff et al., 2002) and abdominal pain (Schurman et al., 2010; Sowder et al., 2010). Fentress et al. (1986) randomized 18 children, ages 8 to 12 years, who had recurrent intermittent headaches and were not on preventive medication, to a biofeedback with or without a relaxation response (RR) condition or to a control wait-list group for seven weekly then two bi-weekly sessions. Headache diaries were evaluated throughout the study and at a 1-year follow-up assessment. Outcome measures included frequency of headaches, total of hours of headache, and severity of headaches. Compared to control group, both treatment groups had improvement in their headache diary measures compared to baseline and at the end of the 15-week study period. However, no differences were found between baseline and the 1 year assessment. No differences in the RR groups were found with or without biofeedback. The study was limited by small sample size, no reporting of missing data, and other design problems.

Bussone et al. (1998) randomized 30 children, ages 11 to 15 years, with episodic tension-type headache to either a biofeedback- relaxation

(BFB-REL) intervention or a relaxation placebo (REL-PLAC) control condition for ten sessions, two per week. Both groups had a 55% improvement in headache severity at the one month assessment, but only the BFB-REL group had improvement at the 6- and 12-month follow-ups, with an 85% improvement by the last assessment.

Kroner-Herwig et al. (1998) randomized 40 children, ages 8 to 14 years, with tension-type or combined headaches to an electromyographic (EMG)-frontalis biofeedback or progressive relaxation (PR) condition with and without parental involvement (PI) or to a wait list control group. There were12 bi-weekly sessions and the parent condition included three 1 h parent sessions. All four intervention groups had significant main effects in all outcome domains post-intervention. Yet, at the 6-month assessment, the biofeedback group without PI showing the greatest changes, followed by biofeedback with PI, PR alone, PR with PI, and then the control group. The biofeedback group without PI had the highest mean effect size for headache outcomes. Adding parents did not appear to improve the intervention effects.

Grazzi et al. (1990) provided EMG biofeedback to ten children, ages 12 to 15 years, with tension headache twice weekly for 6 weeks. Pain Total Index collected with a headache diary and muscular tension scores decreased in all patients from baseline to treatment completion. Grazzi et al. (2001) provided an EMG biofeedback-assisted relaxation programme in 54 children, mean 12 years, with episodic tension-type headaches with two treatment sessions per week for 5 weeks. Pain Total Index via daily diaries were significant at treatment termination but not at the 1-year follow-up. At the 3-year assessment, 84% of the participants were symptom-free. Given the lack of a control condition, the percentage of children who would have been headache free even without intervention at 3 years is unknown. Other study design weaknesses limit strength of the findings.

Arndorfer and Allen (2001) conducted a within-subject, multiple baseline, time-lagged study to evaluate thermal biofeedback therapy in five children, aged 8 to 14 years, with tension-type headaches. Baseline data over 4 to 7 weeks were followed by six thermal biofeedback treatments. All participants showed clinical improvement via daily headache diaries and four of the five were headache-free at 6 months. Lack of a control condition and small sample size limited the importance of the findings.

Scharff et al.'s (2002) study randomized children (7–17 years) with migraines to a stress management with thermal biofeedback (TB), hand-cooling biofeedback (HCB) without stress management, and an assessment control condition to reduce pain, anxiety, and depression. At the 6-week post-treatment assessment, no one in the control condition had headache improvement, while one child (10%) in the HCB and seven (54%) in TB group had significant reduction in headache severity. In a combined analysis, both treatment groups had reduced headache severity and frequency. No changes were in anxiety or depression measures. The same findings held for the 6-month follow-up. While this study is often cited as evidence of thermal biofeedback for migraines in children and despite its promising title, caution is warranted because of the many confounds that limit generalizability of the findings.

Sowder et al. (2010) provided six sessions of heart rate variability (HRV) biofeedback to restore vagal tone in 20 children, 5 to 17 years, with functional abdominal pain (FAP) and compared outcomes to ten children without FAP. The significant decrease in low frequency/high frequency (LF/HF) ratio after intervention suggested an improvement in cardiac vagal tone, along with a decrease in pain frequency and a significant correlation between the decrease in LF/HF ratios and pain frequency. This novel study of heart rate variability biofeedback in FAP was limited by the study design (no randomized trial with a control condition).

Schurman et al. (2010) randomized 20 children, ages 8 to 17 years, with functional abdominal pain (FAP) to a ten-session biofeedback-assisted relaxation training (BART) or control condition. Children in the intervention group demonstrated significantly improved pain intensity, duration of pain episodes, and overall clinical improvement in comparison to the control group. A good review of biofeedback for children's headache is found in Hermann and Blanchard (2002).

Does the discussed literature suggest strong support for the clinical utility of biofeedback for pain reduction in children? The data are suggestive but not strong. That being said, there are many individual children who report great benefit and report that biofeedback enables them to cope, attend school, and sleep well at night. Since the primary downside is cost in those countries where families have to pay out of pocket for this treatment, providing targeted biofeedback to children who need self-management tools to cope with pain and become more functional and less distressed by the pain is recommended. Targeted biofeedback means tools for learning muscle tension reduction in those body areas where muscle tension is a primary cause or contributor to the pain. Skin temperature warming might be appropriate for children with migraines, while adding EMG biofeedback would be useful if there were myofascial contributors to the headaches. Biofeedback seems to be especially useful for the child who seems to enjoy and learn best from computers and other 'gadgets'. The biofeedback clinician should be well trained in his/her craft and not promise 'amazing' results so that children who do not find it useful will not feel like they failed.

Yoga

There are many types of yoga, often named after the lineage of the school of yoga or founder of a certain tradition (the guru). In Iyengar yoga, developed by B. K. S. Iyengar (Evans et al., 2010, 2011c; Woolery et al., 2004), therapeutics provides a series of poses matched to the symptom and medical needs of the child and the pose series changes as the child improves. The poses ('asanas') are intended to correct health-related problems, both in body structure and in internal organ function. The goal is to enhance mindfulness of the body, feelings of centeredness and calm, and a sense of self-control. The poses are intended to address underlying causes of symptoms and poor postural habits that may contribute to the child's pain. The goal of treatment is to help children to learn how to change these bodily contributors to pain.

Yoga has been studied in with irritable bowel syndrome (IBS; Brands et al., 2011; Kuttner et al., 2006) and in cancer (Geyer et al., 2011). Kuttner et al. (2006) randomly assigned 25 adolescents, 11 to 18 years, with IBS to a yoga or wait-list control group. The yoga group had a single yoga session in person followed by 4 weeks of expected home practice with video guidance. The yoga group reported lower levels of emotion-focused avoidance, functional disability, and anxiety compared to the control group. Evaluating pre- and postintervention effects, merging yoga groups including those who had yoga after being in the control condition found a significant reduction in gastrointestinal symptoms. This study was limited by no monitoring for home practice adherence and small sample size.

Brands et al. (2011) evaluated the effects of ten sessions of yoga in 20 children, 8 to 18 years, with functional abdominal pain (FAP), dividing participants into groups of 8 to 11 or 12 to 18 years. Pain frequency was significantly reduced for children in both age groups at the end of the treatment, but only the younger group maintained reduced pain frequency at 3-month follow-up. This single arm study had multiple design problems.

Geyer et al. (2011) carried out five-weekly yoga sessions to determine feasibility in six hospitalized children with cancer, ages 6 to 19 years. Study feasibility with this population was supported.

Most yoga studies lack a manualized intervention where poses for the study are shown so the study could be replicated, even with individualized adjustments based on children's needs during the sessions (Evans et al., 2009). More studies of yoga for children's pain are needed and should include mechanisms and outcomes (Evans et al., 2011b).

That being said, safe types of yoga, such as hatha yoga and Iyengar yoga in which practitioners have extensive training and certification processes, can be extremely beneficial for stretching, relaxation, and body balance. Also the yoga poses give children a tool that they can use independent of requiring a clinician to 'do something' to them. In our programme we have been studying Iyengar yoga for young people with arthritis, irritable bowel syndrome, and fatigue in young survivors of childhood cancer. Across studies, participants overall feel better and want to continue with the yoga (Evans et al., 2009, 2010, 2011a, 2011b, 2011c; Woolery et al., 2004).

Chiropractic

There is limited research in chiropractic care to treat paediatric pain. Hayden et al. (2003) randomly selected 15 chiropractors from four cities in Canada to provide data on their paediatric patients with low back pain. The response was positive and there were no reported complications. Roberts and Wolfe (2009) describe complete resolution of pain after chiropractic treatment with a 6-year-old girl with multiple sites of pain following an injury with persistent long-term outcomes. Hewitt (1994) describes complete resolution of head and neck pain in a 13-year-old girl whose symptoms had persisted for the previous year after four chiropractic treatments. The data on chiropractic care for children's pain are lacking. A recent literature review of studies of spinal manipulation in children found limited studies of paediatric chiropractic overall, and nothing on spinal manipulation for back pain (Gleberzon et al., 2012). The most positive findings in this review were for asthma.

Another review found through analyses of a national data set in the US that neck and back pain were the most common reasons for chiropractic or osteopathic spinal manipulation, and that teens were more likely to use these therapies than were children (Ndetan et al., 2012). As Gilmour et al. (2011) note, practitioners should have training in the care of chiropractic with children before practising this therapy on them.

Aromatherapy

There are very few studies evaluating the effects of aromatherapy as a complementary tool in alleviating pain in paediatric patients. The few studies conducted (de Jong et al., 2012; Ndao et al., 2012) have concluded little or no significant benefits. In an observer blinded, randomized, controlled trial, de Jong et al. (2012) randomized to one of two intervention conditions (massage with or without mandarin oil) or to a usual treatment control group 60 infants, ages 3 to 36 months, for improvement in postoperative pain after major craniofacial surgery. No significant differences were found in pain or distress after intervention in any of the three groups. Only heart rate and mean arterial blood pressure were reduced in the two intervention conditions. Limitations were lack of assessment of treatment adherence, no delayed outcome evaluations, and other design flaws.

Ndao et al. (2012) randomly assigned to an aromatherapy (bergamot essential oil) or placebo group 37 children, ages 5 to 21 years, undergoing stem cell transplantation (SCT). The control group had an aromatherapy diffuser with a non-essential oil-based scented shampoo during SCT. The intervention group had significantly higher anxiety and more nausea than did the control group. The findings suggest that bergamot essential oil may increase rather than reduce symptoms in children undergoing SCT.

In summary, the studies are weak or do not support specific benefits of aromatherapy on symptoms in children's pain. More studies are needed and clinically, unless requested by the child or adolescent, it should not be automatically used.

Pet therapy

Dogs have been trained to help distressed children in a process called pet therapy, animal-assisted therapy (AAT), or canine visitation therapy (CVT). Braun et al. (2009) evaluated AAT to reduce pain in 18 children, ages 3 to 17 years, in an acute care setting with an established AAT programme. Outcomes were compared to those in 39 children without AAT. Group assignment was not described. AAT was described as having the dog match the child's breathing pattern by sitting next to the child. How this was done or measured is not described. The AAT group had significantly less pain but higher respiratory rates than did the comparison group without AAT. Blood pressure, heart, and respiratory rates did not differ between groups.

Sobo et al. (2006) found reduced pain after a single CVT for 25 children, ages 5 to 18 years, with acute postoperative pain in a hospital already with an existing CVT. The children reported that the dog provided distraction from pain, entertainment, pleasure/happiness, contact/snuggling, was calming, and eased the pain. Study limitations are clear in this descriptive study.

Overall, the studies of AAT have covered horse-assisted therapy (hippotherapy), which has been used most commonly for children with cerebral palsy, and dogs as pet therapy. Many children's hospitals now have trained pets spend time with children. Dogs are also trained in special programmes to be of eye, hearing, limb extender, and other services to children with specific disabilities. A recent study, while not in children, concludes after reviewing the literature that, while encouraging, study findings for specific significant symptom effects are weak (Muñoz et al., 2011).

Massage and touch therapies

Massage and various forms of touch have been reported clinically to be helpful and soothing, at least in adults. The effectiveness of massage has been studied in children with chronic pain (Suresh et al., 2008), rheumatoid arthritis (Field et al., 1997), sickle-cell disease (Lemanek et al., 2009), burns (Gurol et al., 2010; Hernandez-Reif et al., 2001), cancer (Post-White et al., 2009), haematopoietic cell transplant (Ackerman et al., 2012; Wolf et al., 2012), and cerebral palsy (Nilsson et al., 2011).

Suresh et al. (2008) compared symptom outcomes after 80 massage sessions with 57 children, mean 13.9 years, in an outpatient chronic pain clinic. Pain and other symptoms were reported to have improved after the massage while no symptom improvements were found in a comparison group of 25 children who did not receive massage. The study has many design flaws.

Field et al. (1997) randomized 20 children, ages 5 to 15 years, with juvenile idiopathic arthritis to a massage or relaxation group. Parents were trained to provide their child with a 15 min bedtime massage for a month, while the parents in the comparison condition guided their child in 15 min of relaxation. Outcome assessments were made pre/post intervention on the first and last treatment sessions. Parent and child reported decreased anxiety and pain and lower salivary cortisol levels were found in the massage versus the relaxation groups. Methodological problems included no assessment of treatment adherence or integrity.

Lemanek et al. (2009) randomly assigned 34 children with sickle cell disease to a massage or attention control condition. Parents were trained and asked to provide a 20 min daily massage to their child for 30 days, while the massage therapist made weekly home visits to provide massages. Parents and children in the control condition completed weekly assessments. Parents in the intervention group had significantly higher anxiety and depression than did those in the control group. Children in the intervention group reported higher functional status and lower depression, anxiety, and pain than did those in the control children. No significant group differences were found in health care utilization. Limitations were lack of measures of treatment integrity and adherence, and a control group that was not truly an attention control condition.

Hernandez-Reif et al. (2001) randomly assigned 24 children, mean age 29.3 months, who were getting dressing changes for severe burns to a massage or standard care control condition. The massage group received a 15 min massage from a trained therapist before a dressing change, while the therapist talked with the control group for 15 min before the dressing change. Children in the massage group had significantly less behavioural distress, less nurse-reported difficulty with dressing changes, and less therapist-reported child distress and less self-reported stress compared to the children in the control condition. While a good attention control condition was provided within the study design, child behaviour was the only blinded assessment, and there was no assessment of treatment integrity.

Gurol et al. (2010) compared 5 weeks of twice weekly massage to usual care in 63 burned adolescents, 12 to 18 years of age, using convenience sampling method for group assignment. Adolescents receiving massage reported lower itching, pain and anxiety pre/post intervention while only itching was reduced in the control group. Lack of randomization and no measures of treatment integrity weakened the findings.

Post-White et al. (2009) conducted a randomized crossover pilot study evaluating massage therapy (MT) or quiet-time (QT) in 23 children, ages 1 to 18 years, with cancer receiving chemotherapy. The MT group had four weekly sessions of parents receiving massage followed by child massage by massage therapists. The QT group had matched quiet rest or quite toy time. Heart rate was significantly lower in the MT children but no significant differences were found in respiratory rate, systolic or diastolic blood pressure, nausea, fatigue, anxiety or salivary cortisol. Parental anxiety was significantly less in the MT group, but parental fatigue was significantly reduced only in the QT group. The study design was excellent but other weaknesses, including the wide age range of children weakened the generalizability of the findings.

Wolf et al. (2012) compared thrice weekly Swedish/acupressure massage to usual care in 23 children, ages 5 to 18 years, receiving haematopoietic cell transplant (HCT). Lack of significant findings were likely related to insufficient power, but children receiving the massage-acupressure had fewer days of mucositis (ES 0.63), lower overall burden of symptoms (ES 0.26), improved fatigue (ES 0.86) and fewer symptoms of pain (ES 0.42), and nausea (ES 0.62). There was no difference in hospital stay between the groups.

Ackerman et al. (2012) randomized 23 children, 5 to 18 years of age, who were undergoing stem cell transplantation to a three week parent-provided massage or control condition. Parent interviews were positive about the massage effects on their child but coordination with clinical hospital routine was difficult. During acute pain episodes, children did not want the massage. Nilsson et al. (2011) studied effects of massage in orthopaedic postoperative pain management of six children with cerebral palsy. The massage therapists noted that it was important to assess the child's response to touch since some children have touch aversion. Other touch therapies, such as therapeutic touch and Reiki, are illustrated by the pilot study by Kemper et al. (2009).

The state of the science suggests that massage and other touch therapies may be beneficial for pain control in children and useful clinically. Certainly children with any form of myofascial pain, unless they are hyperalgesic to light skin touch, would likely benefit from massage therapy. Children with headaches and even those with abdominal pain may also benefit. Massage should not be offered to children with a history of sexual abuse or who are otherwise averse to touch, such as some children with autism spectrum disorders. The problem to be studied is that we don't know how to match the child with the type of massage to get the most therapeutic effects with the least negative effects. Variables to be tested include child characteristic, relevant past history, and type and location of pain. Therapist variables include training, experience with children, and sensitivity to children's body language. Massage variables include amount of pressure, muscle versus skin massage, over clothes or with direct bodily contact, use of lotions or aromatic oils, and duration, frequency, and total length of therapy. Context variables include location of massage, timing, and others' presence.

Art therapy

Art therapy is the use of various art media forms for both distraction and for self-expression, sometimes with therapist/child interpretation, to help children to cope with distress and pain. There are early reports of the value of art therapy in the paediatric hospital setting (Sundaram 1995).

Favara-Scacco et al. (2001) compared art therapy in 32 leukaemic children leukaemia undergoing painful procedures with 17 previously hospitalized children, and found more positive behaviours in the art therapy group. Madden et al. (2010) randomized 16 children with brain tumours, ages 2 to 18 years, to six weekly creative art therapy (CAT) sessions or a reading control condition. The CAT group was found to have greater parent-reported improvement in child pain and nausea. A single CAT session in a cohort of 32 children was found to reduce pain and anxiety. Further study of art therapy for reduction or prevention of pain in children is still needed.

While art therapy may be therapeutic for some children with chronic pain, more quality research is needed before this modality as a complementary therapy for pain can be recommended broadly. Art therapy may be used within psychotherapeutic treatment for coping, anxiety, or depression in children with pain, but art therapy specifically for pain control is not yet supported by research findings.

Music therapy

Music can be considered as a distractor from pain and studies have looked at the use of music during acute pain settings. In music as a distractor, little is known about the effects of type of music, child choice, duration of the music, or music volume, pitch, rhythm, or impact of instruments with or without vocals. Music as a distractor or relaxation tool is different than music therapy. Unfortunately, there are few studies of music therapy for paediatric pain. A descriptive study suggests benefits in paediatric palliative care (Lindenfelser et al., 2012). Robb et al. (2011) report on fidelity strategies in a Children's Oncology Group clinical trial of a therapeutic music video intervention for oncology patients, ages 11 to 24 years undergoing stem cell transplant.

While not a study in children, Tan et al. (2010) randomized 29 burn unit inpatients to music therapy or a control condition in randomized, crossover design for dressing changes in which patients were randomized to receive music therapy on the first or second of two consecutive days. During intervention days, patients carried out music-assisted relaxation with self-guided imagery before and after dressing changes, while creating music during dressing changes. Pain before ($P < 0.025$), during ($P < 0.05$), and after ($P < 0.025$) dressing changes were found to be reduced on music therapy in contrast to control days, with a decrease in anxiety and muscle tension during ($P < 0.05$) and muscle tension after dressing changes ($P < 0.025$). The study needs replication in children. Austin (2010) reviewed evidence and encouraged research on music therapy with children on mechanical ventilation in a paediatric intensive care unit.

Kristjánsdóttir and Kristjánsdóttir (2011) randomly assigned 118 adolescents, aged 14 years, to one of three groups receiving polio immunization: musical distraction with (n = 38) or without headphones (n = 41) and standard care (n = 39). Music therapy without headphones emerged as a significant predictor of no pain. Nilsson et al. (2009) randomized 80 children, ages 7 to 18 years, undergoing day surgery to a 45 min music distraction at entry into the postoperative care unit or to usual care. The music group had fewer children receiving morphine, lower total morphine dose, and a greater decrease in facial action coding scores than did the control group but no differences in vital signs, behavioural measures, or anxiety.

Nguyen et al. (2010) randomized 40 children with cancer, ages 7 to 12 years, to music distraction or usual care for lumbar puncture (LP) pain. Both groups had earphones beginning 10 min before the LP, but self-selected music was provided only to the music group. Pain during and after procedures, anticipatory anxiety, heart and respiratory rates during and respiratory rate after the LP were significantly decreased in the music group. Young et al. (2010) provided music distraction to 50 children during an emergency room visit, with 86% reporting that listening to music was 'helpful' or 'very helpful'.

Others have also reported on music as a distraction in various paediatric settings to reduce pain (Aitken et al., 2002; Arts et al., 1994; Malone 1996; Megel et al., 1999). One recent review of music therapy in paediatrics did not include pain as an outcome (Naylor et al., 2011).

Case example introduction

In the following paragraphs, GH, a 17-year-old girl, describes her pain experiences and her use of complementary therapies. She was first evaluated in the pain clinic when she was age 14 years with extreme leg and back pain and reduced ability to walk or sleep when the pain was severe. She had been absent from school for about 5 months because of pain. At one point she developed conversion pseudoseizures during extreme stress, although these eventually resolved. She was diagnosed with myofascial back and leg pain, an anxiety disorder, and some family-related stressors. Because she reported that she used art to express her feelings and calm herself, she was referred to our pain programme art therapist for psychotherapy through creative expression with self-interpretation and discussion. She also learned to use self-hypnosis to alter her sensory experiences, develop a sense of control over her pain, and regain control over what she described as involuntary bodily movements. She also learned an Iyengar yoga practice to strengthen and stretch key weak and contracted muscles, enhance joint flexibility within proper alignment, and to work towards maintaining emotional and musculoskeletal homeostasis within a mindful awareness paradigm. Family therapy, while needed, was not undertaken. Here is her story:

Case example

I was lost. I was depressed. I was confused. I had never been in such a dark place as I was my freshman year of high school, experiencing pain that was strong enough to make me drop out of school and sports. While I was in bed crying, alone and scared, doctors were telling me there was no reason for my pain. The ones who had more pride than passion would guess how to fix me with treatments ranging from pills to a full body cast. I went to thirty of the top doctors in my state and they all eventually threw up their hands. I told them my back and leg hurt so they took X-rays, MRIs, and bone scans of my back and leg—nothing showed up. They ran nerve tests on me and got into fights with my dad when he wouldn't let them try an epidural on me or give me morphine. It was the most frustrating experience because with every doctor who gave up and every method that failed, my pain increased and fewer people believed me. It was an endless

inner struggle between what people were telling me and what I was really feeling. I doubted my own sanity and felt myself slowly slipping away from the hours in waiting rooms, heavy medications, and maddening pain. I started passing out and having seizures. I did not feel like a 14-year-old girl anymore. I was depressed beyond belief and I was utterly and completely alone. No one knew that the cause of the pain wasn't an injury—it was an overactive nervous system. It was stress.

When I reached the Paediatric Pain Clinic I had already lost everything. I honestly thought I was going crazy and those negative feelings only increased as I was abandoned by my closest friends. I was as low as I could get when I met the pain doctor I thought I knew everything about doctors and 'the system', but she completely surprised me. She took me off the drugs and threw away my body cast. She told me to start doing hypnotherapy, art therapy, and Iyengar yoga. At first I felt like she wasn't taking me seriously. I thought there was no possible way that drawing or painting pictures could stop my pain. I had never heard about anything like this before. My family and I were as sceptical as could be, but we really had nothing to lose at that point.

In the beginning of the process I just viewed my appointments as fun ways to relax, but those three alternative treatments ended up saving my life. They felt so easy and I enjoyed them so much that it didn't feel like therapy and they didn't make me feel like a sick kid. The hypnotherapy taught me how to force myself to relax and to respect my personality. The art therapy gave me an easy and healthy way to express myself that I'd never even considered. The Iyengar yoga helped me balance my body but also, surprisingly, to balance my mind. The stress was being resolved and the pain was finally going away.

I don't feel like either one of the therapies helped me drastically more than the others. I think it took the combination to heal and regain my health. I used to be embarrassed about my weird therapies, but now I wish I could get everyone to try them. The interesting part about these alternative therapies is that they are so personalized it really depends on what works for you. Just because hypnotherapy, art therapy, and Iyengar yoga worked for me doesn't mean they will work for everyone. Other kids might need music therapy and biofeedback to feel better. That is the best part about this method—it's whatever works for you. It doesn't just address your body—it includes your mind—your brain.

These unique therapies gave me the tools I needed to take back control of my life. When I am about to have a panic attack at a party I say I am going to use the bathroom, close the door, and do my hypnotherapy. When I come out, I feel as good as new. When I am feeling really stressed and overwhelmed but don't necessarily know specifically what is wrong, I draw about it. That usually helps me realize the problem so I can address it. When I'm shopping and I start to feel pain, I go in a dressing room, lock the door, and do Iyengar yoga on the floor. Then I can keep walking around and not have to worry about going home early.

Even though I still have pain I feel confident that it will no longer inhibit my life or restrict what I do. I have taken back control of my body and I am happy with my health. These alternative methods work and I am the proof. They didn't mask the symptoms like medication, but they didn't solve them right away either. They just gave me the tools I needed to be successful. I will forever be grateful to these therapies because I have my life back.

Conclusion

Research in complementary therapies for paediatric pain is still in its infancy. While families turn to complementary therapies, there are reports of some cautions to be applied (Adams et al., 2011; Anonymous, 2011). Study designs are often not optimal because of lack of randomized controlled trials, appropriate controls, blinded assessors, use of standardized measures, intervention and assessment fidelity checks, and insufficient sample size for appropriate power to test the study outcomes. Age ranges are often so wide that they cross developmental stages and standardized norms for a specific measure. With small sample sizes, puberty, age and sex effects of the intervention cannot be assessed. As an example of a report intended to improve such studies, an assessment of the quality of measures in studies of complementary therapies was reviewed by Toupin et al. (2012).

Investigators who are knowledgeable about the populations that they are studying are necessary to move the field forward. This process could start with clinical experience in n = 1 studies or ABA designs (where there is baseline assessment, intervention, and then assessment again after removal of the intervention), case series to determine feasibility, measurement and intervention issues, and effect size in pre/post format. Such data will help in the development and implementation of appropriate randomized clinical trials with careful attention to the control condition. One example of a control condition would be to control for social support and other group effects if the therapeutic effects of a complementary modality are being tested in a group format, such as a yoga programme. In this case the control condition might be a group education programme or group light exercise. Another study factor warranting attention is the need for appropriate placebos for the intervention, such as placebo needling without skin puncture for acupuncture studies. Appropriate statistical methods, with intention to treat analyses, descriptions of methods used for addressing missing data, treatment fidelity and data integrity checks, recruitment methods, and attrition are needed. Collaborations between the complementary therapy practitioners and the clinician/research scientists are optimal. Manualized intervention protocols, while allowing for needed individualization, will allow replication of the study and generalizability of the findings. Mixed methodologies that include both quantitative and qualitative data will provide, through patient narratives, a fuller understanding of potential reasons for effectiveness or barriers to implementation and will guide future studies.

Most clinical programmes that serve children who have chronic pain use the biopsychosocial method for evaluation and treatment. Within this model, complementary therapies play an important role within the entire treatment plan. While studies are stronger for some modalities compared to others, as noted, the lack of research does not mean that these modalities are not effective. For example, our programme includes clinicians in Iyengar yoga, hypnotherapy, acupuncture, biofeedback, craniosacral therapy, art and music therapy, physiotherapy, psychotherapy, and psychopharmacology. The team mostly resides in community practice and we meet weekly as a team for an integrative approach to treatment. Determining the specific therapy to incorporate into the child's treatment plan depends upon the type of child and the needs of the child therapeutically (e.g. complex regional pain syndrome = physiotherapy and a mind therapy such as psychotherapy, biofeedback, hypnotherapy, or mindfulness, with family psycho-education). Working with complementary clinicians in an integrative, team format is the best way to insure safety and maximize efficacy of the treatment plan, even if the communication with these clinicians is via telephone or email. Depending upon the country, cost to the family might dictate or limit the options of therapies available to the child. Complementary therapy integrated into the traditional biopsychosocial model of evaluation and treatment for the child with chronic pain provides, in this author's opinion, optimal care for the child with pain.

References

Ackerman, S. L., Lown, A., Dvorak, C.C., Dunn, E.A., Abrams, D.I., Horn, B.N., *et al.* (2012). Massage for children undergoing hematopoietic cell transplantation: a qualitative report. *Evid Based Complement Alternat Med*, 2012, Art. 792042.

Adams, D., Cheng, F., Jou, H., Aung, S., Yasui, Y., and Vohra, S. (2011). The safety of pediatric acupuncture: a systematic review. *Pediatrics*, 128(6), 1575–1587.

Aitken, J. C., Wilson, S., Coury, D., and Moursi, A. M. (2002). The effect of music distraction on pain, anxiety and behavior in pediatric dental patients. *Pediatr Dent*, 24, 114–118.

Anonymous. (2011). Supplement. *Pediatrics*, 128(Suppl.4),149–212.

Arndorfer, R. E., and Allen, K. D. (2001). Extending the efficacy of a thermal biofeedback treatment package to the management of tension-type headaches in children. *Headache*, 4, 183–192.

Arts, S. E., Abu-Saad, H. H., Champion, G. D., Crawford, M. R., Fisher, R. J., Juniper, K. H., *et al.* (1994). Age-related response to lidocaine-prilocaine (EMLA) emulsion and effect of music distraction on the pain of intravenous cannulation. *Pediatrics*, 93(5), 797–801.

Austin, D. (2010). The psychophysiological effects of music therapy in intensive care units. *Paediatr Nurs*, 22(3), 14–20.

Barnes, P. M., Bloom, B., and Nahin, R. (2008). Complementary and alternative medicine use among adults and children: United States 2007. *Natl Health Stat Report*, 12, 1–23.

Brands, M. M. M. G., Purperhart, H., and Deckers-Kocken, J. M. (2011). A pilot study of yoga treatment in children with functional abdominal pain and irritable bowel syndrome. *Complement Ther Med*, 19(3), 109–114.

Braun, C., Stangler, T., Narveson, J., and Pettingell, S. (2009). Animal-assisted therapy as a pain relief intervention for children. *Complement Ther Clin Pract*, 15(2), 105–109.

Bussone, G., Grazzi, L., D'Amico, D., Leone, M., and Andrasik, F. (1998). Biofeedback-assisted relaxation training for young adolescents with tension-type headache: a controlled study. *Cephalalgia*, 18, 463–467.

Davis, M. P., and Darden, P. M. (2003). Use of complementary and alternative medicine by children in the United States. *Arch Pediatr Adolesc Med*, 157(4), 393–396.

de Jong, M., Lucas, C., Bredero, H., van, A. L., Tibboel, D., and van, D. M. (2012). Does postoperative 'M' technique® massage with or without mandarin oil reduce infants' distress after major craniofacial surgery? *J Adv Nurs*, 68(8), 1748–1757.

Efe, E., Işler, A., Sarvan, S., Başer, H., and Yeşilipek, A. (2013). Complementary and alternative medicine use in children with thalassaemia. *J Clin Nurs*, 22(5–6), 760–769.

Eisenberg, D. M., Kessler, R. C., Foster, C., Norlock, F. E., Calkins, D. R., and Delbanco, T. L. (1993). Unconventional medicine in the United States. Prevalence, costs, and patterns of use. *N Engl J Med*, 328(4), 246–252.

Evans, S., Cousins, L., Tsao, J. C., Sternlieb, B., and Zeltzer, L. K. (2011a). Protocol for a randomized controlled study of Iyengar yoga for youth with irritable bowel syndrome. *Trials*, 12(15).

Evans, S., Cousins, L., Tsao, J. C., Subramanian, S., Sternlieb, B., and Zeltzer, L. K. (2011b). A randomized controlled trial examining Iyengar yoga for young adults with rheumatoid arthritis: a study protocol. *Trials*, 12(19).

Evans, S., Moieni, M., Subramanian, S. K., Tsao, J. C. I., Sternlieb, B., Zeltzer, L. K. (2011c). Now I see a brighter day: expectations and perceived benefits of an Iyengar yoga intervention for young patients with rheumatoid arthritis. *J Yoga Phys Ther*, 1(1).

Evans, S., Moieni, M., Taub, R., Subramanian, S. K., Tsao, J. C., Sternlieb, B., Zeltzer, L. K. (2010). Iyengar yoga for young adults with rheumatoid arthritis: results from a mixed-methods pilot study. *J Pain Symptom Manage*, 39(5), 904–913.

Evans, S., Tsao, J. C., Sternlieb, B., Zeltzer, L. K. (2009). Using the biopsychosocial model to understand the health benefits of yoga. *J Comp Integ Med*, 6(1), 15.

Evans, S. and Zeltzer, L. K. (2008). Complementary and alternative approaches for chronic pain. In G. A. Walco and K. R. Goldschneider (eds) *Pediatric pain management in primary care: a practical guide*, pp. 153–60. Totowa, NJ: The Humana Press.

Favara-Scacco, C., Smirne, G., Schiliro, G., Di Cataldo, A. (2001). Art therapy as support for children with leukemia during painful procedures. *Med Pediatr Oncol*, 36, 474–480.

Fentress, D. W., Masek, B. J., Mehegan, J. E., and Benson, H. (1986). Biofeedback and relaxation-response training in the treatment of pediatric migraine. *Dev Med Child Neurol*, 28, 139–146.

Field, T., Hernandez-Reif, M., Seligman, S., Krasnegor, J., Sunshine, W., Rivas- Chacon, R., *et al.* (1997). Juvenile rheumatoid arthritis: benefits from massage therapy. *J PediatrPsychol*, 22, 607–617.

Geyer, R., Lyons, A., Amazeen, L., Alishio, L., and Cooks, L. (2011). Feasibility study: the effect of therapeutic yoga on quality of life in children hospitalized with cancer. *Pediatr Phys Ther*, 23(4), 375–379.

Gilmour, J., Harrison, C., Asadi, L., Cohen, M. H., Vohra, S. (2011). Complementary and alternative medicine practitioners' standard of care: responsibilities to patients and parents. *Pediatrics*, 128(Suppl.4), S200–205.

Gleberzon, B. J., Arts, J., Mei, A., McManus, E. L. (2012). The use of spinal manipulative therapy for pediatric health conditions: a systematic review of the literature. *J Can Chiropr Assoc*, 56(2), 128–141.

Grazzi, L., Andrasik, F., D'Amico, D., Leone, M., Moschiano, F., and Bussone, G. (2001). Electromyographic biofeedback-assisted relaxation training in juvenile episodic tension-type headache: clinical outcome at three year follow-up. *Cephalalgia*, 21, 798–803.

Grazzi, L., Leone, M., Frediani, F., and Bussone, G. (1990). A therapeutic alternative for tension headache in children: treatment and 1-year follow-up results. *Biofeedback Self-Regulat*, 15, 1–7.

Gurol, A. P., Polat, S., and Akcay, M. N. (2010). Itching, pain, and anxiety levels are reduced with massage therapy in burned adolescents. *J Burn Care Res*, 31(3), 429.

Hayden, J. A., Mior, S. A., and Verhoef, M. J. (2003). Evaluation of chiropractic management of pediatric patients with low back pain: a prospective cohort study. *J Manipulative Physiol Ther*, 26(1), 1–8.

Heath, J. A., Oh, L. J., Clarke, N. E., and Wolfe, J. (2012). Complementary and alternative medicine use in children with cancer at the end of life. *J Palliat Med*, 15(11), 1218–1221.

Hermann, C., and Blanchard, E. B. (2002). Biofeedback in the treatment of headache and other childhood pain. *Appl Psychophysiol Biofeedback*, 27, 143–162.

Hernandez-Reif, M., Field,T., Largie, S., Hart, S., Redzepi, M., Nierenberg, B., *et al.* (2001). Childrens' distress during burn treatment is reduced by massage therapy. *J Burn Care Rehabil*, 22, 191–195.

Hewitt, E. G. (1994). Chiropractic care of a 13-year-old with headache and neck pain: a case report. *Journal CCA*, 38, 160–162.

Kemper, K. J., Fletcher, N. B., Hamilton, C. A., and McLean, T. W. (2009). Impact of healing touch on pediatric oncology outpatients: pilot study. *J Soc Integr Oncol*, 7(1), 12–18.

Kemper, K. J., Sarah, R., Silver-Highfield, E., Xiarhos, E., Barnes, L. and Berde, C. (2000). On pins and needles? Pediatric pain patients' experience with acupuncture. *Pediatrics*, 105(4), 941–947.

Kim, K., Kim, D., and Yu, Y. (2006). The effect of capsicum plaster in pain after inguinal hernia repair in children. *Paediatr Anaesth*, 16 (10), 1036–1041.

Kristjánsdóttir, Ó., and Kristjánsdóttir, G. (2011). Randomized clinical trial of musical distraction with and without headphones for adolescents' immunization pain. *Scand J Caring Sci*, 25(1), 19–26.

Kroner-Herwig, B., Mohn, U., and Pothmann, R. (1998). Comparison of biofeedback and relaxation in the treatment of pediatric headache and the influence of parent involvement on outcome. *Appl Psychophysiol Biofeedback*, 23, 143–157.

Kuttner, L., Chambers, C.T., Hardial, J., Israel, D.M., Jacobson, K., and Evans, K. (2006). A randomized trial of yoga for adolescents with irritable bowel syndrome. *Pain Res Manag*, 11(4), 217–223.

Lemanek, K. L., Ranalli, M., and Lukens, C. (2009). A randomized controlled trial of massage therapy in children with sickle cell disease. *J Pediatr Psychol*, 34(10), 1091–1096.

Lin, Y., Tassone, R., Jahng, S., Rahbar, R., Holzman, R., Zurakowski, D., and Sethna, N. (2009). Acupuncture management of pain and emergence agitation in children after bilateral myringotomy and tympanostomy tube insertion. *Paediatr Anaesth*, 19(11), 1096–1101.

Lindenfelser, K. J., Hense, C., McFerran, K. (2012). Music therapy in pediatric palliative care: family-centered care to enhance quality of life. *Am J Hosp Palliat Care*, 29(3), 219–226.

Ma, S. X. (2004). Neurobiology of acupuncture: toward CAM. *Evid Based Complement Alternat Med*, 1(1), 41–47.

Madden, J. R., Mowry, P., Gao, D., Foreman, N. K., and McGuire, C. P. (2010). Creative arts therapy improves quality of life for pediatric brain tumor patients receiving outpatient chemotherapy. *J Pediatr Oncol Nurs*, 27(3), 133–145.

Malone, A. B. (1996). The effects of live music on the distress of pediatric patients receiving intravenous starts, venipunctures, injections, and heel sticks. *J Music Ther*, 33, 19–33.

Megel, M. E., Houser, C. W., and Gleaves, L. S. (1999). Children's responses to immunizations: lullabies as a distraction. *Issues Compr Pediatr Nurs*, 2, 129–145.

Muñoz, Lasa S., Ferriero, G., Brigatti, E., Valero, R., Franchignoni, F. (2011). Animal-assisted interventions in internal and rehabilitation medicine: a review of the recent literature. *Panminerva Med*, 53(2), 129–136.

Naylor, K. T., Kingsnorth, S., Lamont, A., McKeever, P., and Macarthur, C. (2011). The effectiveness of music in pediatric healthcare: a systematic review of randomized controlled trials. *Evid Based Complement Alternat Med*, Art. 464759.

Ndao, D. H., Ladas, E. J., Sands, S. A., Garvin, J. J. H., Kelly, K. M., Cheng, B., and Snyder, K. T. (2012). Inhalation aromatherapy in children and adolescents undergoing stem cell infusion: results of a placebo-controlled double-blind trial. *Psycho-oncology*, 21(3), 247–254.

Ndetan, H., Evans, M. W. Jr., Hawk, C., and Walker, C. (2012). Chiropractic or osteopathic manipulation for children in the United States: an analysis of data from the 2007 National Health Interview Survey. *J Altern Complement Med*, 18(4), 347–353.

Neuhouser, M. L., Patterson, R. E., Schwartz, S. M., Hedderson, M. M., Bowen, D. J., and Standish, L.J. (2001). Use of alternative medicine by children with cancer in Washington state. *Prev Med*, 33(5), 347–354.

Nguyen, T. N., Nilsson, S., Hellstrom, A.-L., and Bengtson, A. (2010). Music therapy to reduce pain and anxiety in children with cancer undergoing lumbar puncture: a randomized clinical trial. *J Pediatr Oncol Nurs*, 27(3), 146–155.

Nilsson, S., Johansson, G., Enskar, K., Himmelmann, K. (2011). Massage therapy in post-operative rehabilitation of children and adolescents with cerebral palsy—a pilot study. *Complement Ther Clin Prac*, 17(3), 127–131.

Nilsson, S., Kokinsky, E., Sidenvall, B., EnskAr, K., and Nilsson, U. (2009). School-aged children's experiences of postoperative music medicine on pain, distress, and anxiety. *Paediatr Anaesth*, 19(12), 1184–1190.

Pintov, S., Lahat, E., Alstein, M., Vogel, Z., and Barg, J. (1997). Acupuncture and the opioid system: implications in management of migraine. *Pediatr Neurol*, 17(2), 129–33.

Post-White, J., Fitzgerald, M., Savik, K., Hooke, M. C., Hannahan, A. B., and Sencer, S.F. (2009). Massage therapy for children with cancer. *J Pediatr Oncol Nurs*, 26, 16–28.

Pothmann, R., Gottschling, S., Meyer, S., Gribova, I., Distler, L., Berrang, J., et al. (2009). Laser acupuncture in children with headache: a double-blind, randomized, bicenter, placebo-controlled trial. *Deutsche Zeitschrift Fur Akupunktur*, 52(1).

Robb, S. L., Burns, D. S., Docherty, S. L., and Haase, J. E. (2011). Insuring treatment fidelity in a multi-site behavioral intervention study: implementing NIH Behavior Change Consortium recommendations in the SMART trial. *Psychooncology*, 20(11), 1193–2011.

Roberts, J. and Wolfe, T. (2009). Chiropractic care of a 6-year-old girl with neck pain; headaches; hand, leg, and foot pain; and other nonmusculoskeletal symptoms. *J Chiropract Med*, 8(3), 131–136.

Sawni-Sikand, A., Schubiner, H., and Thomas, R. L. (2002). Use of complementary/alternative therapies among children in primary care pediatrics. *Ambulat Pediatr*, 2(2), 99–103.

Scharff, L., Marcus, D. A., and Masek, B. J. (2002). A controlled study of minimal contact thermal biofeedback treatment in children with migraine. *J Pediatr Psychol*, 27(2), 109–119.

Schurman, J. V., Grayson, P., Friesen, C. A., and Wu, Y. P. (2010). A pilot study to assess the efficacy of biofeedback-assisted relaxation training as an adjunct treatment for pediatric functional dyspepsia associated with duodenal eosinophilia. *J Pediatr Psychol*, 35(8), 837–847.

Sibinga, E. M., Ottolini, M. C., Duggan, A. K., and Wilson, M. H. (2004). Parent-pediatrician communication about complementary and alternative medicine use for children. *Clin Pediatr (Phila)*, 43(4), 367–373.

Singendonk, M., Kaspers, G. J., Naafs-Wilstra, M., Meeteren, A. S., Loeffen, J., Vlieger, A. (2013). High prevalence of complementary and alternative medicine use in the Dutch pediatric oncology population: a multicenter survey. *Eur J Pediatr*, 172(1), 31–37.

Siponen, S. M., Ahonen, R. S., Kettis, A., and Hämeen-Anttila, K. P. (2012). Complementary or alternative? Patterns of complementary and alternative medicine (CAM) use among Finnish children. *Eur J Clin Pharmacol*, 68(12), 1639–1645.

Snyder, J. and Brown, P. (2012). Complementary and alternative medicine in children: an analysis of the recent literature. *Curr Opin Pediatr*, 24(4), 539–546.

Sobo, E. J., Eng, B., and Kassity-Krich, N. (2006). Canine visitation (pet) therapy: pilot data on decreases in child pain perception. *J Holist Nurs*, 24(1), 51–57.

Sowder, E., Gevirtz, R., Ebert, C., and Shapiro, W. (2010). Restoration of vagal tone: a possible mechanism for functional abdominal pain. *Appl Psychophysiol Biofeedback*, 35(3), 199–206.

Spigelblatt, L., Laine-Ammara, G., Pless, I. B., and Guyver, A. (1994). The use of alternative medicine by children. *Pediatrics*, 94(6 Pt 1), 811–814.

Sundaram, R. (1995). Art therapy with a hospitalized child. *Am J Art Ther*, 34, 2–8.

Suresh, S., Wang, S, Porfyris, S, Kamasinski-Sol, R., and Steinhorn, D. M. (2008). Massage therapy in outpatient pediatric chronic pain patients: do they facilitate significant reductions in levels of distress, pain, tension, discomfort, and mood alterations?. *Paediatr Anaesth*, 18(9), 884–887.

Tan, X., Yowler, C. J., Super, D. M., and Fratianne, R. B. (2010). The efficacy of music therapy protocols for decreasing pain, anxiety, and muscle tension levels during burn dressing changes: a prospective randomized crossover trial. *J Burn Care Res*, 31(4), 590–597.

Toupin, K., Moher, D., Stinson, J., Byrne, A., White, M., Boon, H., et al. (2012). Measurement properties of questionnaires assessing complementary and alternative medicine use in pediatrics: a systematic review. *PLoS One*, 7(6), e39611.

Wang, F. and Wu, B. J. (2012). Overview of acupuncture development in Ontario Canada. *Zhongguo Zhen Jiu*, 32(4), 367–369.

Waterhouse, M., Stelling, C., Powers, M., Levy, S., and Zeltzer, L. (2000). Acupuncture and hypnotherapy in the treatment of chronic pain in children. *Clinical Acupuncture and Oriental Medicine*, 1, 139–150.

Wilson, K.M., Klein, J.D., Sesselberg, T.S., Yussman, S. M., Markow, D. B., Green, A. E., et al. (2006). Use of complementary medicine and dietary supplements among U.S. adolescents. *J Adolesc Health*, 38(4), 385–394.

Wolf, E., Mehling., E., Lown, A., Dvorak, C. C., Cowan, M. J., Horn, B. N., et al. (2012). Hematopoietic cell transplant and use of massage for improved symptom management: results from a pilot randomized control trial. *Evid Based Complement Alternat Med*, 2012, Art. 450150. doi:10.1155/2012/450150.

Woolery, A., Myers, H., Sternlieb, B., and Zeltzer, L. (2004). A yoga intervention for young adults with elevated symptoms of depression. *Altern Ther Health Med*, 10(2), 60–63.

Woolf, A. D. (2003). Herbal remedies and children: do they work? Are they harmful?. *Pediatrics*, 112(1 Pt 2), 240–246.

Wu, S., Sapru, A., Stewart, M. A., Milet, M. J., Hudes, M., Livermore, L. F., et al. (2009). Using acupuncture for acute pain in hospitalized children. *Pediatr Crit Care Med*, 10(3), 291.

Young, T., Griffin, E., Phillips, E., and Stanley, E. (2010). Music as distraction in a pediatric emergency department. *J Emerg Nurs*, 36(5), 472–473.

Yussman, S. M., Ryan, S. A., Auinger, P., et al. (2004). Visits to complementary and alternative medicine providers by children and adolescents in the United States. *Ambulat Pediatr*, 4 (5), 429–435.

Zeltzer, L. K., Krane, E. J. (2011). Pediatric pain management. In R. M. Kliegman, R. E. Behrman, B. F. Stanton, N. Schor, and J. St. Geme (eds) *Nelson's textbook of pediatrics* (19th edn), pp. 360–75. Philadelphia, PA: Saunders Elsevier.

Zeltzer, L. K., Tsao, J. C., Stelling, C., Powers, M., Levy, S., and Waterhouse, M. (2002). A phase I study on the feasibility and acceptability of an acupuncture/hypnosis intervention for chronic pediatric pain. *J Pain Symptom Manage*, 24(4), 437–446.

CHAPTER 61

Theory-informed approaches to translating pain evidence into practice

Janet Yamada and Alison M. Hutchinson

Summary

Despite great strides in evidence-based pain assessment and management strategies, infants and children still experience acute pain (including multiple painful procedures) and chronic pain during hospitalization. Translating best evidence on pain assessment and management into clinical practice remains a challenge. The knowledge- or evidence-to-practice gap in pain in children can be addressed by implementing strategies, underpinned by knowledge translation theories, frameworks, and models, to promote and sustain practice change. A range of factors related to the organizational context and individual behaviour play a role in the adoption of new pain assessment and management practices.

Introduction

Access to evidence-based pain guidelines, policies, standards, and consensus statements has increased over the past decade, highlighting the importance of providing appropriate procedural pain management for infants and children anonymous (2000). In particular, evidence-based recommendations have been developed for the management of procedural pain in infants and children (Lago et al., 2009; Royal Australasian College of Physicians PCHD 2005a, 2005b), post-surgical pain and sedation (Anand et al., 2006; Yamada et al., 2008). Despite strong evidence to support the effectiveness of pain assessment and management strategies, use of such strategies for infants and children remains a challenge, highlighting a knowledge-to-practice gap (Scott-Findlay and Estabrooks, 2006). In a recent audit of paediatric pain practices from 32 hospital units in eight paediatric centres across Canada, only 28% of children who had undergone a painful procedure also received a pain management intervention specifically linked to the procedure documented in their medical chart (Stevens et al., 2011). Hospitalized infants experience an average of 12 tissue damaging procedures per day (Carbajal et al., 2008). Carbajal and colleagues (2008) reported that, of 42 413 painful procedures performed on 430 infants, pharmacological interventions were provided to only 2.1% of the infants;

18.2% painful procedures were managed using non-pharmacological strategies, and 79.2% patients received no pre-procedural analgesia. Similarly, Johnston and colleagues (2011) found that 46% of infants in neonatal intensive care units (NICUs) who were exposed to tissue damaging procedures were administered opioids for 14.5% of procedures, while in 14.3% sweet tasting solutions such as sucrose or glucose were used. These findings highlight the extent of the gap between evidence for acute pain in infants and children and its translation into practice.

This research-to-practice gap is not unique to pain management or the paediatric setting. Scholars have been exploring barriers to and facilitators of research use and studying approaches to promote uptake of evidence across a range of healthcare settings. Additionally, behavioural, psychological, and social theories, frameworks, and models have been used to guide and explain health professionals' practice changes. In this chapter, knowledge translation (KT) in the context of paediatric pain assessment and management is described and discussed.

Definition of knowledge translation

Numerous terms are used to describe KT; the purpose is to promote the use of evidence to optimize outcomes for recipients of healthcare. The term *knowledge translation* is used to describe the *process* of translating evidence into practice and/or to refer to the use of research as an event or *outcome*. One comprehensive and frequently cited definition of KT is that of the Canadian Institutes of Health Research (CIHR), which is:

> A dynamic and iterative process that includes synthesis, dissemination, exchange and ethically-sound application of knowledge to improve the health of Canadians, provide more effective health services and products and strengthen the healthcare system. (Canadian Institutes of Health Research: <http://www.cihr-irsc.gc.ca/e/29418.html>)

According to Graham et al. (2006), implicit in this definition is that *knowledge* refers predominantly to research evidence. Terms used synonymously with KT include knowledge transfer, knowledge uptake, knowledge utilization, knowledge exchange, knowledge implementation, knowledge dissemination, innovation diffusion, implementation science, and research utilization. Arguably, some of these terms have a different and/or narrower meaning than that of KT.

Why use a theory-informed approach to KT?

In the field of KT, increasing emphasis has been placed on the importance of using theory to inform: (1) selection and development of strategies to promote implementation of KT interventions, and (2) evaluation of the implementation strategies (Eccles et al., 2005; Rycroft-Malone and Bucknall 2010; Sales et al., 2006). Systematic review evidence exists for the effectiveness of a number of KT interventions (Bero et al., 1998; Grimshaw et al., 2001; Oxman et al., 1995; Prior et al., 2008; Wensing et al., 2006). However, the evidence indicates that effectiveness of such interventions varies; they are effective in some situations but not all (Hrisos et al., 2008a, 2008b). A theory-informed approach can help provide an understanding of what has been described as the 'black box'; that is, theory can illuminate how, why and under what circumstances an intervention works (Hrisos et al., 2008a, 2008b; Rycroft-Malone, 2007). According to the UK Medical Research Council Framework for Developing and Evaluating Complex Interventions (2008), interventions should be underpinned by a coherent theory and the theory should be used, systematically, to develop the intervention. A theoretical understanding about how an intervention influences behaviour enables weaknesses in, and barriers to the success of the intervention, to be targeted and overcome.

What do we mean by theory, frameworks, and models?

Theory

Theories can be used to describe, explain, and predict, for example, health professionals' behaviours related to KT (Rycroft-Malone and Bucknall, 2010). Behavioural theories have been described on a knowledge continuum ranging from broad to narrow in scope. Mid-range theories, such as the theory of planned behaviour (Azjen, 1991), are less abstract and more concrete compared to macro or grand theories. Mid-range theories are used in KT activities and can focus on changing health professionals' behaviours at the level of the individual, group, or organization (Rycroft-Malone and Bucknall, 2010).

Conceptual framework

Conceptual frameworks differ from theories in that they inform or guide practice, versus predicting practice (Rycroft-Malone and Bucknall, 2010). Examples of conceptual frameworks applied to KT evaluations are the Promoting Action on Research Implementation in Health Services (PARiHS) framework (Kitson et al., 1998) and the Knowledge to Action (KTA) framework (Graham et al., 2006).

Model

Models are more specific about the relationships that should be expected between concepts in the model (Rycroft-Malone and Bucknall, 2010). The Ottawa Model of Research Use (Logan and Graham 1998) is an example of a KT model. In the following

section, five theories, frameworks, and models that can be used to guide and explain KT implementation strategies are described.

KT theories, frameworks, and models

Diffusion of innovations

In his classic and oft-cited work, first published in 1962, Rogers (2003) describes a theory that seeks to explain the process and rate of spread of an innovation (new ideas or technology) within a social system. The theory defines four main factors that are influential in the process of innovation diffusion: (1) the innovation itself (referring to the idea, the practice or the object that is new); (2) the communication channel (the method used to inform others of the innovation); (3) time (the time taken for an individual to make the transition from first knowledge of the innovation to its acceptance or dismissal); and (4) the social system (those involved in decision-making about adoption of the innovation). According to Rogers, diffusion is a process whereby '(a) an innovation (b) is communicated through certain channels (c) over time (d) among the members of a social system' (2003, p. 11). According to the theory, individuals progress through five stages in the process of decision-making about innovation adoption: (1) *knowledge*—acquiring an awareness and understanding of the innovation; (2) *persuasion*—the stage of forming an opinion about the value of the innovation; (3) *decision*—the process of making a decision about adoption or rejection of the innovation; (4) *implementation*—the act of using or applying the innovation in practice; and (5) *confirmation*—reflection upon the decision to adopt or reject the innovation, which may lead to a reversal of the decision.

Rogers (2003) suggests that individual (adopter) and setting characteristics influence the rate and extent of diffusion of an innovation. He defines five adopter categories according to the relative speed of uptake of an innovation:

1. *Innovators*, also described as venturesome, have an interest in new innovations and are responsible for introducing the new idea to the system.

2. *Early adopters* readily adopt the new idea, provide advice and information about the innovation to others within the social network, and assist in hastening the diffusion process.

3. *Early majority* adopt the new idea following a period of decision-making, and prior to the average member of the system adopting the initiative.

4. *Late majority* cautiously adopt the new idea once most other members of the system have embraced the innovation.

5. *Laggards* who possess somewhat traditional values and are suspicious of new ideas are the last members of the system to adopt the innovation.

A critical mass is achieved when enough individuals have decided to adopt the innovation that its continued adoption becomes self-sustaining.

With respect to the innovation, several characteristics are considered important to adoption, including the innovation's relative advantage (the extent to which the innovation is perceived as superior to existing practices or technologies), compatibility (the extent to which the innovation is perceived as compatible with existing values, practices and resources), complexity (perception of the ease with which the innovation can be understood and used), trialability (the ease with which the innovation can be trialed or tested), and observability (the extent to which the innovation and its effects are visible) (Rogers 2003).

In the health literature, Roger's (2003) diffusion of innovation theory has been highly influential and has generally been assumed to represent, or be synonymous with, the theoretical underpinnings of research utilization or KT. However, according to Estabrooks et al. (2006), this assumption is yet to be rigorously tested. Voepel-Lewis et al. (2008) used diffusion of innovation theory to assess the clinical utility of three tools designed to assess pain in children in order to determine which tools were more likely to be adopted in clinical practice. The attributes (complexity, compatibility and relative advantage) of the revised-Face, Legs, Activity, Cry, Consolability (r-FLACC) tool (Malviya et al., 2006) and the Nursing Assessment of Pain Intensity (NAPI) (Schade et al, 1996) instrument rated most favourably, when compared with those of the Non-Communicating Children's Pain Checklist-Postoperative Version (NCCPC-PV) (Breau et al., 2002).

Theory of planned behaviour

The theory of planned behaviour (TPB) is a social cognitive theory where certain stimuli trigger cognitive processes (thinking), which in turn influence an individual's behaviour. Thus, the TPB, which is based on the theory of reasoned action (Azjen and Fishbein, 1980; Fishbein and Azjen, 1975), seeks to predict and explain individual behaviour under certain conditions (Azjen, 1991). *Intent* of the individual to behave in a certain way is central to the TPB. Intention is assumed to reflect factors that motivate behaviour and the strength of the individual's willingness to behave in a certain way; the greater the intent the more likely it is that the behaviour will be exhibited (Azjen, 1991). However, the decision to behave in a certain way must be within the individual's *control* (i.e. opportunities for the behaviour must exist and resources, such as time and skills to enable the behaviour, must also be available). Thus, carrying out the behaviour is a function of the opportunities, resources, and the individual's intention to act. The concept, *perceived behavioural control*, refers to an individual's perception of the degree of difficulty associated with behaving in a certain way. This concept is an important element in the TPB, and differentiates it from the theory of reasoned action. The TPB proposes that intention to act and perceived behavioural control are direct predictors of an individual's behaviour (Azjen, 1991). The strength of an intention to act or behave in a certain way is determined by the individual's *attitudes towards the behaviour* (based on their beliefs about, and evaluation of, the consequences of the behaviour), *subjective norms* (beliefs about what others think about the behaviour), and *perceived behavioural control*. According to the theory, behaviour change requires a change in intentions, which in turn requires a change in the beliefs that support the intention or the introduction of new beliefs (Fishbein and Ajzen, 1975).

The TPB has been used to study the cognitive processes that motivate individual health professionals to incorporate research findings into their practice (Eccles et al., 2007; Perkins et al., 2007). Some researchers have found evidence in support of the predictive ability of the TPB constructs (Eccles et al., 2007; Perkins et al., 2007). These findings indicate that consideration of attitudes towards the behaviour, subjective norms and perceived behavioural

control in the development of interventions to promote the uptake of research evidence in practice might contribute to the success of such interventions. Edwards et al. (2001) used the TPB to identify determinants of nurses' (including paediatric nurses) intention to administer opioids for analgesia. Attitudes, subjective norms and perceived control predicted nurses' intention to administer opioids to patients experiencing pain, accounting for 39.1% of variability in intention (F(4, 441) = 708, p <0.01).

Promoting Action on Research Implementation in Health Services (PARiHS) Framework

PARiHS is an interactive, multidimensional KT framework. Successful implementation of evidence into practice is defined as a function of sources of evidence used to support a practice change, the practice context and strategies to facilitate change (Kitson et al., 1998). Successful implementation occurs when the research evidence, practice context in which the change occurs, and facilitation strategies used to promote change are 'high' on the utilization continuum (Kitson et al., 1998; Rycroft-Malone et al., 2002). Elements of the framework (i.e. evidence, context, facilitation) were identified in a theoretical analysis of four case studies (Kitson et al., 1998). Further refinements to the framework were made through concept analyses of the three PARiHS elements (Harvey et al., 2002; McCormack et al., 2002; Rycroft-Malone et al., 2004). Rigorous, relevant and generalizable quantitative and qualitative research evidence such as systematic reviews of, for example, effective pharmacological (e.g. Stevens et al., 2013) and non-pharmacological interventions for procedural pain in infants (Pillai-Riddell et al., 2011) are rated 'high' on the evidence to practice continuum (Rycroft-Malone, 2004; Rycroft-Malone et al., 2004). Knowledge from clinical or practice-based experience and patient experience is considered 'high' on the evidence continuum when it is reflected upon, and viewed as relevant (Rycroft-Malone, 2010). Local data/information collected from the practice context is considered 'high' on the evidence to practice continuum when these data are evaluated and interpreted as relevant (Rycroft-Malone, 2010).

Context refers to the environment where pain practice change occurs (Kitson et al., 1998; McCormack et al., 2002). A receptive context includes supportive networks, available resources (e.g. human, financial resources), and initiatives that are consistent with an organization's strategic plans (Kitson et al., 2008; Rycroft-Malone, 2010). Culture, leadership and evaluation are sub-elements of context. Culture is referred to as 'the way things are done around here' (Drennan, 1992). Culture is considered 'high' on the continuum within a supportive learning environment that includes collaboration/teamwork, and decentralized decision-making (McCormack et al., 2002; Rycroft-Malone, 2010; Rycroft-Malone et al., 2004).

'High' leadership occurs when transformational leaders enable, and empower health care professionals to share a common vision by establishing clear roles, and promoting teamwork and decision-making (McCormack et al., 2002). Evaluation and feedback regarding practice change at the individual, team, and system levels are effective when strategies such as performance audits or feedback from health professionals are incorporated into the practice change process (McCormack et al., 2002).

Facilitation is defined by enabling or making easier, the translation of evidence into practice (Harvey et al., 2002). The facilitation process occurs on a continuum where the purpose or role includes low intensity, episodic contact (task oriented), to high-intensity roles (holistic oriented) that enable individuals to achieve their goals or practice changes (Harvey et al., 2002). Facilitators can be internal or external to an organization and are usually appointed to their role (Harvey et al., 2002; Rycroft-Malone et al., 2002). Facilitation is considered 'high' on the knowledge to practice continuum when appropriate supports are utilized, and when task and enabling skills are applied based on the needs of the practice change (Harvey et al., 2002). Kavanagh et al. (2010) applied the three elements from the PARiHS framework to explain the effects of an organizational KT intervention, appreciative inquiry (AI) to improve nurses' pain practices in a paediatric setting. Twelve nurse facilitators focused on improving evidence-based pain assessment documentation in a paediatric surgical unit. The AI process was viewed as a positive approach to change; however, change overload, logistics, busyness of the unit, and lack of organized follow-up within the practice context were barriers to the intervention implementation. Application of the PARiHS concepts in this study provided further support for the elements of this framework (Kavanagh et al., 2010).

In a study by Stevens and colleagues (2011), three key themes described health professionals' opinions related to factors that facilitated or hindered pain practices in the neonatal intensive care unit: (1) the culture of collaboration and support for evidence-based pain practices; (2) threats to autonomy when making decisions about pain practices, and (3) complexity in delivering pain care (Stevens et al., 2011). The authors used sub-elements of context from PARiHS to explain the study results. For example, in the PARiHS framework, practice cultures that did not value individual's judgements were considered threats to autonomy and therefore were barriers to successful implementation of evidence into practice (Stevens et al., 2011).

The Knowledge to Action (KTA) Framework

The KTA framework is a systems focused framework that can be used to guide health professionals to change their practice (Graham and Tetro, 2007; Graham et al., 2006). The KTA framework includes a knowledge creation component and an action cycle (Figure 61.1). This iterative, interactive framework also includes an assessment of the local context and culture when planning the implementation of evidence into practice.

The knowledge creation process funnel includes three phases: (1) knowledge inquiry; (2) knowledge synthesis of best evidence, and (3) development of knowledge tools/products. At each phase of the knowledge creation process, knowledge or evidence is further synthesized for the knowledge user. During the knowledge creation phase, knowledge producers identify potentially relevant evidence. Synthesis of best evidence involves generation of systematic reviews and meta-analysis of existing knowledge. Evidence-based clinical practice guidelines and decision aids are examples of knowledge tools/products created during the third phase of the knowledge creation process. Knowledge tools/products such as clinical practice guidelines can then be implemented during the action cycle. All phases of the knowledge creation process can be tailored to the needs of the knowledge user. The knowledge creation process can be used to inform each step in the action cycle, as noted by the dotted lines surrounding the knowledge creation funnel.

The action cycle refers to activities required to implement knowledge or evidence into practice and is based on 31 planned action theories that focus on changing how individuals practice within a social system (Graham and Tetro, 2010). The action cycle consists of seven phases: (1) identifying the problem, identifying, reviewing and selecting knowledge to translate into practice; (2) adapting/tailoring knowledge to the practice context; (3) identifying barriers and

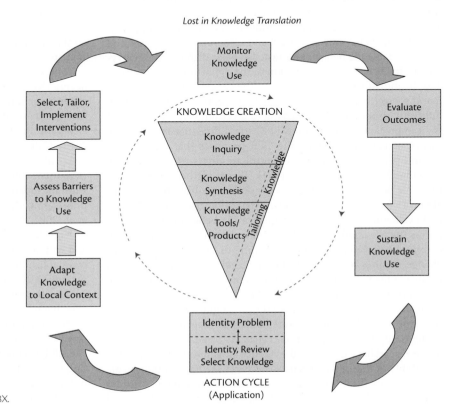

Figure 61.1 Knowledge to Action (KTA) Framework. Reprinted with permission from Ian D. Graham et al., Lost in knowledge translation: Time for a map? *Journal of Continuing Education in the Health Professions*, Volume 26, Issue 1, pp. 13–24, Copyright © 2006 Wiley Periodicals, Inc, http://onlinelibrary.wiley.com/journal/10.1002/%28ISSN%291554-558X.

facilitators to knowledge use; (4) selecting, tailoring and implementing KT interventions; (5) monitoring knowledge use such as changes in knowledge and attitudes; (6) evaluating health, health care provider and system-related outcomes, and (7) identifying strategies to sustain knowledge use or a practice change (Graham et al., 2006). The steps within the knowledge to action process are not necessarily sequential. For example, identification of new barriers to practice changes might occur, thus requiring revisions to KT strategies. To date, the KTA framework has not been cited in published paediatric pain research. However, Bandstra (2007) uses components of this framework to describe how translation of evidence-based paediatric psychological pain management interventions (e.g. distraction) could be achieved. In the knowledge creation cycle, Bandstra (2007) emphasizes the importance of developing clinically meaningful and cost-effective psychological pain management interventions. In the knowledge application or action cycle, a multidisciplinary approach to delivering psychological pain management interventions using the steps outlined in the KTA framework is recommended.

Ottawa Model of Research Use

The Ottawa Model of Research Use (OMRU) is an interactive, planned action model of change (Logan and Graham, 1998, 2010). The OMRU includes six elements that are assessed, monitored and evaluated prior to, during and after KT interventions have been implemented: (1) evidence-based innovation; (2) potential adopters; (3) practice environment; (4) knowledge translation (KT) strategies to translate evidence into practice; (5) adoption and use (both initial and sustained) of the evidence, and (6) outcomes (Logan and Graham, 1998, 2010) (Figure 61.2). The elements of this model are grounded in Rogers' (2003) diffusion of innovations theory, and health behaviour change. Barriers to and facilitators of research utilization are identified in the first three elements and are used to develop and guide the intervention. The OMRU has been applied at the level of individuals, teams, organizations, and healthcare systems (Graham and Logan, 2004).

There are several assumptions about the KT process that are inherent in the model. First, elements of the OMRU are based on an interactive approach, where KT is achieved through collaboration between individuals (i.e. researchers and health professionals; Denis et al., 2004; Graham and Logan, 2004). Secondly, patients and families are integral to the KT process. Finally, aspects of the practice environment influence the process of adopting evidence (Graham and Logan, 2004). Logan and Graham (2010) propose that additional theories could be applied to the elements of the OMRU.

The innovation refers to a new guideline, policy, or procedure that would be implemented into practice, and it should be evidence-based. The innovation attributes refer to the potential adopters' perceptions of the relative advantage, complexity, fit, and feasibility of the innovation (Logan and Graham, 2010). Potential adopters refer to health professionals, patients, and parents who may adopt the innovation. Four sub-elements include: (a) awareness of the innovation, (b) knowledge and intention to adopt the innovation, (c) knowledge and skill required to implement the innovation, and (d) concerns about the innovation or practice change (Logan and Graham, 2010). The practice environment includes four sub-elements: (a) structural factors including decision-making structure, policies, practice standards, physical structure of the practice environment, workload, and current practice; (b) culture/social factors including local politics, leadership, peer opinion; (c) patients; and (d) economic factors including available resources (Logan and Graham 2010). Interventions/KT strategies are tailored to the needs of potential adopters. Interventions are described within three sub-elements: (a) barrier management strategies to promote adoption of the innovation; (b) transfer strategies used by facilitators to train potential adopters, and (c) follow-up strategies to ensure uptake and sustainability of the innovation. A series of steps are used in the adoption process including testing the innovation and sustaining its use. Success of the innovation is measured by patient, health professionals, and system outcomes.

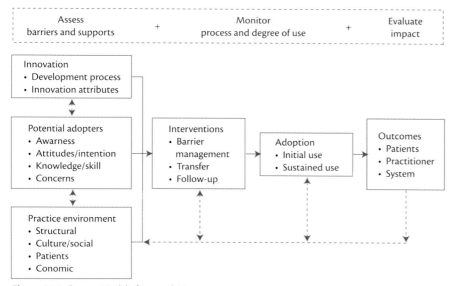

Figure 61.2 Ottawa Model of Research Use.

Case example

The following example illustrates application of the elements of the PARiHS framework to guide implementation of a KT intervention to improve pain practices in infants. The Evidence-Based Practice for Improving Quality (EPIQ), an interactive KT intervention developed by Lee et al. (2009), has been shown to improve health professional practices in relation to reducing nosocomial infection and chronic lung disease in NICUs (Lee et al., 2009). Continuous quality improvement methods that incorporate Plan-Do-Study-Act (PDSA) cycles are embedded within the EPIQ intervention. Stevens et al. (2011) recently applied a more tailored version of EPIQ to improve paediatric pain practices in medical, surgical and critical care hospital units across paediatric tertiary care centres in Canada. The EPIQ intervention consists of two phases: in the first phase of EPIQ, known as the Preparation Phase, a multidisciplinary group of health professionals known as the Research Practice Council (RPC) are identified as *facilitators* of the practice change(s). These individuals review sources of *evidence* to highlight a research or evidence-to-practice gap. The implementation and change phase is the second phase of EPIQ whereby the RPC introduces evidence-based KT strategies to encourage health professionals to modify their current practices.

Evidence

During the Preparation Phase, RPC members in a neonatal intensive care unit (NICU) evaluated the units' pain assessment and management practices by evaluating *local evidence* in the form of a chart audit. A review of medical charts prior to the intervention indicated that pain assessment using the Premature Infant Pain Profile (PIPP: Stevens et al., 1996) was documented in patient charts only 15% of the time. RPC members and health professionals confirmed a need to improve pain assessment practices in the unit. A recent systematic review supported the strong psychometric properties of the PIPP to assess procedural pain in infants (Stevens et al., 2010). Therefore, local evidence, clinical evidence and research evidence contributed to identifying gaps and supporting evidence-based pain practices. The RPC aimed to improve pain assessment documentation using the PIPP to 50% over the following 6 months.

Facilitation

In the second phase of EPIQ, the RPC, as *facilitators* of practice change, implemented evidence-based KT strategies to improve use and documentation of the PIPP. The RPC members were individuals who, in accordance with the requirements of the PARIHS framework, have the skills and ability to assist individuals, teams, and organizations to translate evidence into practice (Rycroft-Malone, 2010). The RPC engaged in task-based activities by organizing educational sessions for staff nurses on how to use and document the PIPP. Posters were situated in patient rooms to remind health professionals to assess and document pain intensity scores for their patients using the PIPP. Additionally, the RPC used a holistic approach to improving pain assessment practices by empowering unit staff to reflect on the KT strategies implemented and to participate in tailoring strategies based on the needs of the unit.

Context

During the implementation of KT strategies to improve pain assessment practices, pain became a hospital wide priority and a component of the hospitals' strategic plan. Senior medical and nursing staff in the NICU began to discuss PIPP pain intensity scores and pain management strategies during daily patient rounds. These *transformational leaders* contributed to change in pain assessment practices at the local level. Staff were updated at regularly scheduled unit workshops that included education on pain assessment. Creating an awareness of the importance of pain assessment contributes to a *receptive practice context* for change. As part of the EPIQ implementation process the RPC, supported by the unit educator, evaluated the practice change by conducting regular practice audits; the results of which were fed back to the unit. A 6-month audit showed that documentation of PIPP scores had improved from 15% to 75%. The practice aim was achieved and pain assessment using the PIPP became part of unit *culture* over time.

An initial assessment of the potential barriers and facilitators, potential adopters and the practice environment is required prior to implementing the intervention. Ongoing monitoring of the intervention implementation and degree of adoption will contribute to tailoring of the intervention to achieve the desired outcomes. The impact of the innovation is measured by evaluating patient, practitioner and system outcomes.

Ellis and colleagues (2007) implemented and evaluated a comprehensive pain management programme (CPMP) to improve paediatric nurses' pain practices with hospitalized children. A nursing management team developed a 4 h pain education workshop that focused on pain assessment and management strategies and they, along with pain resource nurse champions, implemented the CPMP components using various modes of delivery, including email, newsletters, information pegboards, and audit and feedback. The OMRU was used to guide, monitor and evaluate the implementation of the CPMP. The authors monitored nurses' adoption of pain practices by evaluating process outcomes that included aspects of the practice environment, nurses' pain assessment and management knowledge, attitudes and skill, and KT strategies used to promote pain practices. Practice outcomes were measured using pain audits pre and post intervention implementation. Focus groups were used to identify barriers, facilitators and factors that influenced implementation of the CPMP. Statistically significant improvement in nurses' perceptions about the adequacy of their pain assessment ($p < 0.004$), and management ($p < 0.017$) practices were noted as well as statistically significant improvements in use of pain measures ($p = 0.005$) and pain assessment narratives ($p < 0.01$).

Implications for practice and education, research, and theory

Evidence-based KT strategies

Evidence-based KT strategies can facilitate integration of pain evidence into practice. For example, the use of reminders to promote health professionals' use of guidelines has been shown to produce small to moderate improvements in care (Grimshaw et al., 2004; Prior et al., 2008). Audit and feedback alone or in combination with other strategies has been shown to have small but important effects in health care professionals' practices (Ivers et al., 2012). Educational strategies, specifically educational outreach, have been shown to result in small to moderate improvements in patient care (Cochrane Effective Practice and Organisation of Care Review Group, 2002; Grimshaw et al., 2004; Prior et al., 2008). Local opinion leaders (e.g. health care professionals who are members of the unit pain committee), alone or in combination with other interventions, may also facilitate the integration of evidence into practice (Flodgren et al., 2011).

Understanding the context of practice

The context of healthcare has been conceptualized in different ways, ranging from the physical environment, as the most basic conceptualization, to more complex definitions such as that proposed by French: 'the organisational environment of health care, composed of physical, social, political, and economic influences on the practical reasoning and choices of practitioners about how clinical issues are address' (2005, p. 174).

Over the past 20 years, studies conducted in several countries to examine the barriers to use of research in practice have consistently highlighted the importance of time to implement change, time to read research, the nurse's authority to change practice, reporting of understandable statistical analyses in the research literature, and accessibility of relevant literature, as the most prominent barriers to KT (Carlson and Plonczynski, 2008; Hutchinson and Johnston, 2006; Kajermo et al., 2010). KT initiatives should, therefore, take into consideration the potential for such barriers to impede uptake of pain evidence within the specific practice context and incorporate strategies to minimize or overcome them.

While much of the early work in the field of KT focused on characteristics of the individual and the research itself, it has become increasingly evident that the context in which knowledge is used is another important ingredient in the KT equation. In particular, evidence that research is adopted at different rates and with different levels of success in different contexts has highlighted the importance of context. In light of empirical evidence to indicate that context can influence the success of KT (Cummings et al., 2007, 2010), it is essential that a careful assessment is undertaken of the paediatric healthcare context in which pain evidence is to be implemented. Strengths and weaknesses in contextual characteristics can then be taken into account; capitalizing on the strengths and implementing strategies to overcome or reverse the weaknesses. As well as identification of potential barriers or challenges, an assessment of the receptiveness or readiness of the context to change is important. Meetings with key stakeholders (including health professionals, administrators, educators and children and families) may be helpful in revealing issues and concerns that should be taken into consideration.

Several measures have been developed for health professionals and researchers to evaluate the practice context. Kitson et al. (2008) developed a practical diagnostic assessment tool (which complements the PARiHS framework) to inform development of an implementation strategy. The tool is designed, to help identify aspects of the current environment or context that need to be addressed in order to optimize KT. An aggregated score can be plotted on an evaluative grid to enable visualization of the level of facilitation support required to optimize implementation. The Alberta Context Tool (ACT) (Estabrooks et al., 2009), based on elements from the PARiHS framework, consists of eight concepts that are used to measure organizational context in healthcare settings. The ACT has been validated in a sample of eight paediatric hospitals that participated in the Translating Research on Pain in Children (TROPIC) study (Stevens et al., 2008–2012) (Estabrooks et al., 2011). McCormack and colleagues (2009) have developed the Context Assessment Index (CAI), also based on the PARiHS framework, to provide health professionals with a tool to assess their practice context and readiness for use of evidence in practice. Testing of this instrument in paediatric settings has not yet been undertaken.

Promoting and sustaining behaviour change

The tendency for health professionals to adhere to tradition and rituals and to become automated in their practice (Kerfoot, 1999; Monforto et al., 2012) means that unlearning previously well-entrenched behaviour is necessary in order for them to adopt new evidence and modify their clinical practice accordingly. Documenting PIPP scores 75% of the time in patient charts is an example of a notable improvement in clinical practice. However, sustaining this practice improvement remains a challenge and should be a focus of future research

Creating opportunities for interactive sharing of new knowledge, peer review, and dialogue and debate about how evidence could be incorporated into practice, are strategies that can be used to promote and sustain behaviour change in order to facilitate KT. Additionally, promoting positive attitudes and approaches towards pain assessment practices, engaging health professionals in reflective practice, leadership that includes ongoing support, education, commitment to the practice change and performance evaluation can support and help sustain integration of evidence into practice (Davies et al., 2010).

In summary, a theory-based approach to KT research can be used to guide and plan the study design, data collection methods, and analysis. Additionally, theoretical concepts can be used to explain study results and strengthen the construct validity of the specific theory, conceptual frameworks, and models used. Further, evidence-based KT strategies (i.e. educational strategies, reminders, audit and feedback) can be used to promote pain practice changes.

References

Azjen, I. (1991). The theory of planned behavior. *Organ Behav Hum Decis Process*, 50, 179–211.

Azjen, I. and Fishbein, M. (1980). *Understanding attitudes and predicting social behavior*. Englewood Cliffs, NJ: Prentice-Hall.

American Academy of Pediatrics. (2000). Prevention and management of pain and stress in the neonate. *Pediatrics*, 105, 454–461.

Anand K.J., Aranda J. V., Berde C. B., Buckman, S., Capparelli, E. V., Carlo, W., *et al.* (2006). Summary proceedings from the neonatal pain-control group, *Pediatrics*, 117, S9–S22.

anonymous. (2000). Prevention and management of pain and stress in the neonate. American Academy of Pediatrics. Committee on Fetus and Newborn. Committee on Drugs. Section on Anesthesiology. Section on Surgery. Canadian Paediatric Society. Fetus and Newborn Committee. [Guideline Practice Guideline]. *Pediatrics*, 105(2), 454–461.

Bandstra, N. (2007). Knowledge translation in psychological interventions for pediatric pain: bridging the gap between research and practice. In C. L. von Baeyer (ed.) *Pediatric pain letter*, 9(3). Available at: <http://childpain.org/ppl/issues/v9n3_2007/v9n3_bandstra.pdf>.

Batton, D. G., Barrington, K. J., and Wallman, C. (2006). Prevention and management of pain in the neonate: an update. *Pediatrics*, 118, 2231–2241.

Bero, L. A., Grilli, R., Grimshaw, J. M., Harvey, E., Oxman, A. D., Thomson, M. A. (1998). Getting research findings into practice: closing the gap between research and practice: an overview of systematic reviews of interventions to promote the implementation of research findings. *Br Med J*, 317, 465–468.

Breau, L. M., Finley, G. A., McGrath, P. J., and Camfield, C. S. (2002). Validation of the Non-communicating Children's Pain Checklist-Postoperative Version. *Anesthesiology*, 96, 528–535.

Carbajal, R., Rousset, A., Danan, C., Coquery, S., Nolent, P., Ducrocq, S., et al. (2008). Epidemiology and treatment of painful procedures in neonates in intensive care units. *JAMA*, 300, 60–70.

Carlson, C. L. and Plonczynski, D.J. (2008). Has the BARRIERS Scale changed nursing practice? An integrative review. *J Adv Nurs*, 63, 322–333.

Cochrane Effective Practice and Organisation of Care Review Group (EPOC). (2002). *The data collection checklist 1–26*. [Online] Available at: <http://epoc.cochrane.org/sites/epoc.cochrane.org/files/uploads/datacollectionchecklist.pdf>.

Cummings, G. G., Estabrooks, C. A., Midodzi, W. K., Wallin, L., and Hayduk, L. (2007). Influence of organizational characteristics and context on research utilization. *Nurs Res*, 56(4 Suppl), S24–39.

Cummings, G. G., Hutchinson, A. M., Scott, S. D., Norton, P. G., and Estabrooks, C. A. (2010). The relationship between characteristics of context and research utilization in a pediatric setting. *BMC Health Serv Res*, 10(168). [Online] Available at: <http://www.biomedcentral.com/1472-6963/10/168/>.

Davies, B., Tremblay, D., and Edwards, N. (2010). Sustaining evidence-based practice systems and measuring the impact. In D. G. Bick and I. D. Graham (eds) *Evaluating the impact of implementing evidence-based practice*, pp. 166–188. Oxford: Wiley-Blackwell.

Denis, J. L., Lehoux, P., and Champagne, F. (2004). A knowledge utilization perspective on fine-tuning dissemination and contextualizing knowledge. In L. Lemieux-Charles and F. Champagne (eds) *Using knowledge and evidence in health care*, pp. 18–40. Toronto: University of Toronto Press.

Drennan, D. (1992). *Transforming company culture*. London: McGraw-Hill.

Eccles, M., Grimshaw, J., Walker, A., Johnston, M., and Pitts, N. (2005). Changing the behavior of healthcare professionals: the use of theory in promoting the uptake of research findings. *J Clin Epidemiol*, 58, 107–112.

Eccles, M. P., Grimshaw, J. M., Johnston, M., Steen, N., Pitts, N. B., Thomas, R., et al. (2007). Applying psychological theories to evidence-based clinical practice: identifying factors predictive of managing upper respiratory tract infections without antibiotics. *Implement Sci*, 226. [Online] Available at: <http://www.implementation science.com/content/2/1/26/>.

Eccles, M. P., Johnston, M., Hrisos, S., Francis, J., Grimshaw, J., Steen, N., et al. (2007). Translating clinicians' beliefs into implementation interventions (TRACII): a protocol for an intervention modeling experiment to change clinicians' intentions to implement evidence-based practice. *Implement Sci*, 2(27). [Online] Available at: <http://www.implementationscience.com/content/2/1/27/>.

Edwards, H. E., Nash, R. E., Najman, J., Yates, P. M., Fentiman, B. J., Dewar A., et al. (2001). Determinants of nurses' intention to administer opioids for pain relief. *Nurs Health Sci*, 3, 149–159.

Ellis, J. A., McCleary, L., Blouin, R., Rowley, B., MacNeil, M., and Cooke, C. (2007). Implementing best practice pain management in a pediatric hospital. *J Spec Pediatr Nurs*, 12, 264–277.

Estabrooks, C. A., Squires, J. E., Cummings, G. G., Birdsell, J. M., and Norton, P. G. (2009). Development and assessment of the Alberta Context Tool. *BMC Health Serv Res*, 9, 234.

Estabrooks, C. A., Squires, J. E., Hutchinson, A. M., Scott, S., Cummings, G. G., Kang, S. H., et al. (2011). Assessment of variation in the Alberta Context Tool: the contribution of unit level contextual factors and specialty in Canadian pediatric acute care settings. *BMC Health Serv Res*, 11(25). [Online] Available at: <http://www.biomedcentral.com/1472-6963/11/251/>.

Estabrooks, C.A., Thompson, D. S., Lovely, J. J., and Hofmeyer, A. (2006). A guide to knowledge translation theory. *J Contin Educ Health Prof*, 26, 25–36.

Fishbein, M. and Azjen, I. (1975). *Belief, attitude, intention and behavior. an introduction to theory and research*. Reading, MA: Addison-Wesley.

Flodgren, G., Parmelli, E., Doumit, G., Gattellari, M., O'Brien, M. A., Grimshaw, J., et al. (2011). Local opinion leaders: effects on professional practice and health care outcomes. *Cochrane Database Syst Rev*, 8, CD000125. DOI: 10.1002/14651858.CD000125.pub4.

French, B. (2005). Contextual factors influencing research use in nursing. *Worldviews Evid Based Nurs*, 2, 172–183.

Graham, K. and Logan, J. (2004). Translating research: innovations in knowledge transfer and continuity of care. *CJNR*, 36(2), 89–103.

Graham, I. D., Logan, J., Harrison, M. B., Straus, S. E., Tetroe, J., Caswell, W., et al. (2006). Lost in knowledge translation: time for a map? *J Contin Educ Health Prof*, 26, 13–24.

Graham, K. D. and Tetro, J. (2007). How to translate health research knowledge into effective healthcare action. *Healthc Q*, 10, 20–22.

Graham, I.D., Tetro, J.M. (2010). The knowledge to action framework. In J. Rycroft -Malone and T. Bucknall (eds). *Models and frameworks for implementing evidence-based practice: linking evidence to action*, pp. 207–221. Oxford : John Wiley & Sons, Ltd.

Grimshaw, J. M., Shirran, R. Thomas, G., Mowatt, G., Fraser, C., Bero, L., et al. (2001). Changing provider behaviour. An overview of systematic reviews of interventions. *Med Care*, 38, II-2–II-45.

Grimshaw, J., Thomas, R. E., MacLennan, G., Fraser, C., Ramsay, C. R., Vale, L., et al. (2004). Effectiveness and efficiency of guideline dissemination and implementation strategies. *Health Technol Asses*, 8, 1–349.

Harvey, G., Loftus-Hills, A., Rycroft-Malone, J., Titchen, A., Kitson, A., McCormack, B., et al. (2002). Getting evidence into practice: the role and function of facilitation. *J Adv Nurs*, 37, 577–588.

Hrisos, S., Eccles, M. Johnston, M., Francis, J., Kaner, E. F., Steen, N., et al. (2008a). An intervention modelling experiment to change GPs' intentions to implement evidence-based practice: using theory-based interventions to promote GP management of upper respiratory tract infection without prescribing antibiotics #2. *BMC Health Serv Res*, 8(10). [Online] Available at: <http://www.biomedcentral.com/1472-6963/8/10/>.

Hrisos, S., Eccles, M. Johnston, M., Francis, J., Kaner, E. F. S., Francis, J., Kaner, E. F., Steen, N, et al. (2008b). Developing the content of two behavioural interventions: using theory-based interventions to promote GP management of upper respiratory tract infection without prescribing antibiotics #1. *BMC Health Serv Res*, 8(11). [Online] Available at: <http://www.biomedcentral.com/1472-6963/8/11/>.

Hutchinson, A. M. and Johnstone, L. J. (2006). Beyond the BARRIERS Scale. Commonly reported barriers to research use. *J Nurs Adm*, 36, 189–199.

Ivers, N., Jamtvedt, G., Flottorp, S., Young, J. M., Odgaard-Jensen, J., French, S. D., et al. (2012). Audit and feedback: effects on professional practice and healthcare outcomes. *Cochrane Database Syst Rev*, 6, CD000259. DOI: 10.1002/14651858.CD000259.pub3

Johnston, C., Barrington, K. J., Taddio, A., Carbajal, R., and Filion, F. (2011). Pain in Canadian NICUs: have we improved over the past 12 years? *Clin J Pain*, 27, 225–232.

Kajermo, K. N., Bostrom, A.-M., Thompson, D. S., Hutchinson, A. M., Estabrooks, C. A., and Wallin, L. (2010). The BARRIERS scale—the barriers to research utilization scale: A systematic review. *Implement Sci*, 5(32). [Online] Available at: <http://www.implementationscience.com/content/5/1/32/>.

Kavanagh, T., Stevens, B., Seers, K., Sidani, S., and Watt-Watson, J. (2010). Process evaluation of appreciative inquiry to translate pain management evidence into pediatric nursing practice. *Implement Sci*, 5(90). [Online] Available at: <http://www.implementationscience.com/content/5/1/90/>.

Kerfoot, K. (1999). Creating the forgetting organization. *Pediatr Nurs*, 25, 77–78.

Kitson, A., Harvey, G., and McCormack, B. (1998). Enabling the implementation of evidence based practice: a conceptual framework. *Qual Health Care*, 7, 149–158.

Kitson, A. L., Rycroft-Malone, J., Harvey, G., McCormack, B., Seers, K., Titchen, A., et al. (2008). Evaluating the successful implementation of evidence into practice using the PARiHS framework: theoretical and practical challenges. *Implement Sci*, 3(1). [Online] Available at: <http://www.implementationscience.com/content/3/1/1>.

Lago, P., Garetti, E., Merazzi, D., Pieragostini, L., Ancora, G., Pirelli, A., et al. (2009). Guidelines for procedural pain in the newborn. *Acta Paediatr*, 98, 932–939.

Lee, S. K., Aziz, K., Singhal, N., Cronin, C. M., James, A., Lee, D. S., et al (2009). Improving the quality of care for infants: a cluster randomized controlled trial. *CMAJ*, 181, 469–76.

Logan, J., and Graham, I. D. (2010). The Ottawa Model of Research Use. In J. Rycroft-Malone and T. Bucknall (eds) *Models and frameworks for implementing evidence-based practice: linking evidence to action*, pp. 83–108. Oxford: John Wiley & Sons, Ltd.

Logan, J. and Graham, I. D. (1998). Toward a comprehensive interdisciplinary model of health care research. *Science Comm*, 20, 227–246.

Malviya, S., Voepel-Lewis, T., Burke, C., Merkel, S., and Tait, A. R. (2006). The revised FLACC observational pain tool: improved reliability and validity for pain assessment in children with cognitive impairment. *Paediatr Anaesth*, 16, 258–65.

McCormack, B., Kitson, A., Harvey, G., Rycroft-Malone, J., Titchen, A., and Seers, K. (2002). Getting evidence into practice: the meaning of 'context'. *J Adv Nurs*, 38, 94–104.

McCormack, B., McCarthy, G., Wright, J., Slater, P., and Coffey, A. (2009). Development and testing of the Context Assessment Index (CAI). *Worldviews Evid Based Nurs*, 6, 27–35.

McGrath, P. and Unruh, A. M. (2007). Neonatal and infant pain in a social context. In K. J. S. Anand, B. J. Stevens, and P. J. McGrath (eds) *Pain in neonates and infants* (3rd edn), pp.219–34. Toronto: Elsevier.

Monforto, K., Figueroa-Altmann, A., Stevens, C., Thiele, K., and Ely, E. (2012). Time for changes for scheduled nursing assessments: impact on clinical decisions and patient discharge. *J Pediatr Nurs*, 27, 26–33.

Oxman, A. D., Thomson, M. A., Davis, D. A., and Haynes, R. B. (1995). No magic bullets: A systematic review of 102 trials of interventions to help health care professionals deliver services more effectively or efficiently. *CMAJ*, 153, 1423–1431.

Perkins, M. B., Jensen, P. S., Jaccard, J., Gollwitzer, P., Oettingen, G., Pappadopulos, E., et al. (2007). Applying theory-driven approaches to understanding and modifying clinicians' behavior: what do we know? *Psychiatr Serv*, 58, 342–348.

Pillai-Riddell, R., Racine, N., Turcotte, K., Uman, L., Horton, R., Din Osmun, L., et al. (2011). Nonpharmacological management of procedural pain in infants and young children: an abridged Cochrane review. *Pain Res Manag*, 16, 321–330.

Prior, M., Guerin, M., and Grimmer-Somers, K. (2008). The effectiveness of clinical guideline implementation strategies—a synthesis of systematic review findings. *J Eval Clin Pract*, 14, 888–897.

Rogers, E. M. (2003) *Diffusion of innovations* (5th edn). New York: Free Press.

Royal Australasian College of Physicians PCHD. (2005a) *Guideline statement: management of procedure-related pain in neonates.* [Online] (Updated 19 August 2012) Available at: <http://www.racp.edu.au/page/health-policy-and-advocacy/paediatrics-and-child-health>.

Royal Australasian College of Physicians PCHD. (2005b). *Guideline statement: management of procedure-related pain in children and adolescents.*[Online] (Updated 19 August 2012) Available at: <http://www.racp.edu.au/page/health-policy-and-advocacy/paediatrics-and-child-health>.

Rycroft-Malone, J. (2004). The PARIHS framework—a framework for guiding the implementation of evidence-based practice. *J Nurs Care Qual*, 19, 297–304.

Rycroft-Malone, J. (2007). Theory and knowledge translation: setting some coordinates. *Nurs Res*, 56, S78–S85.

Rycroft-Malone, J. (2010). Promoting Action on Research Implementation in Health Services (PARIHS). In J. Rycroft-Malone and T. Bucknall (eds) *Models and frameworks for implementing evidence-based practice: linking evidence to action*, pp. 109–135. Oxford: John Wiley & Sons, Ltd.

Rycroft-Malone, J. and Bucknall, T. (2010). Theory, frameworks, and models. In J. Rycroft-Malone and T. Bucknall (eds) *Models and frameworks for implementing evidence-based practice*, pp. 23–50. Oxford: Wiley-Blackwell.

Rycroft-Malone, J., Harvey, G., Seers, K., Kitson, A., McCormack, B., and Titchen, A. (2004). An exploration of the factors that influence the implementation of evidence into practice. *J Clin Nurs*, 13, 913–924.

Rycroft-Malone, J., Kitson, A., Harvey, G., McCormack, B., Seers, K., Titchen, A., et al. (2002). Ingredients for change: revisiting a conceptual framework. *Qual Saf Health Care*, 11, 174–180.

Sales, A., Smith, J., Curran, G., and Kochevar, L. (2006). Models, strategies, and tools. Theory in implementing evidence-based findings into health care practice. *J Gen Intern Med*, 21, S21–24.

Schade, J. G., Joyce, B. A., Gerkensmeyer, J., and Keck, J. F. (1996). Comparison of three preverbal scales for postoperative pain assessment in a diverse pediatric sample. *J Pain Symptom Manage*, 12, 348–359.

Scott-Findlay, S. and Estabrooks, C. A. (2006). Knowledge translation and pain management. In G. A. Finley, P. J. McGrath, and C. Chambers (eds) *Bringing pain relief to children*, pp. 199–226. Totowa, NJ: Humana Press.

Stevens, B. J., Abbott, L. K., Yamada, J., Harrison, D., Stinson, J., Taddio, A., et al. (2011). Epidemiology and management of painful procedures in children in Canadian hospitals, *CMAJ*, 183, e 403–410.

Stevens, B., Johnston, C., Petryshen, P., and Taddio, A. (1996). Premature Infant Pain Profile: development and initial validation. *Clin J Pain*, 12, 13–22.

Stevens, B., Johnston, C., Taddio, A., Gibbins, S., and Yamada, J. (2010). The premature infant pain profile: evaluation 13 years after development. *Clin J Pain*, 26, 813–830.

Stevens, B., Barwick, M., Campbell, F., Chambers, C, Cohen, J., Cummings, G., et al. (2008–2012). *Translating Research on Pain in Children.* Canadian Institutes of Health Research (CIHR) (MOP-86605).

Stevens, B., Riahi, S., Cardoso, R., Ballantyne, M., Yamada, J., Beyene, J., et al. (2011). The influence of context on pain practices in the NICU: perceptions of health care professionals. *Qual Health Res*, 21, 757–770.

Stevens, B., Yamada, J., Lee, G. Y., and Ohlsson, A. (2013). Sucrose for analgesia in newborn infants undergoing painful procedures. *Cochrane Database Syst Rev*, 1, CD001069. DOI: 10.1002/14651858.CD001069.pub4

Voepel-Lewis, T., Malviya, S., Tait, A. R., Merkel, S., Foster, R., Krane, E. J. (2008). A comparison of the clinical utility of pain assessment tools for children with cognitive impairment. *Anesth Analg*, 106, 72–78.

Wensing, M., Wollersheim, H., and Grol, R. (2006). Organizational interventions to implement improvements in patient care: a structured review of reviews. *Implement Sci*, 1(2). [Online] Available at: <http://www.implementationscience.com/content/1/1/2>.

Yamada, J., Stinson, J., Lamba, J., Dickson, A., McGrath, P. J., Stevens, B. (2008). A review of systematic reviews on paininterventions in hospitalized infants. *Pain Res Manag*, 13, 413–420.

CHAPTER 62

Organizational systems in paediatric pain

Mark Embrett and Norman Buckley

Introduction

Over the past 20 years there has been growing recognition that paediatric pain management can be delivered in a variety of forms, and may be best delivered in a multidisciplinary setting with a shared responsibility amongst diverse health providers, who traditionally have worked independently from each other or at best in parallel. (Desparmet, 2009; Dowden et al., 2008; Weisman, 2008). The composition, size, and organization of a paediatric pain management team can differ based on the number and type of patients served, as well as the organizational structure of the health care centre (hospital, clinic, community health centre, etc.). There is no one 'right' way to organize the team, but diligence is needed when planning a multidisciplinary delivery method. This chapter presents some of the considerations relevant to organizations that are designing a new team, modifying a current arrangement, or assessing the performance/needs of an existing team.

Organizational systems should facilitate the care to be delivered. The process of patient referral and triage should be expeditious, the initial assessment process must identify the issues to be dealt with and ensure that optimal management has been carried out for medical, surgical, psychiatric, and other identifiable disorders. The business of the service or clinic (revenue sources, salary support, supplies, and materials) must be considered. The resources (personnel, supplies, programmes) necessary for the care plan must be readily available, organized, and care delivered in an effective manner with monitoring of the effect and revision as necessary.

The chapter first focuses on an overview of the similar elements to approaches of chronic pain, acute pain, and palliative care, concluding with a description of the ideal multidisciplinary pain management approach (MPMA). The chapter then proceeds to review the specific organization and operations of acute pain and chronic pain services, respectively. Finally, research about the expectation of parents when they enter a clinic and importance of accommodating and promoting positive expectations is presented. The patient flow process in acute pain differs from the chronic pain model and is described. The emphasis remains on consistent clear communication among providers and between providers and patient/family.

Acute pain, chronic pain, and palliative care: common elements of treatment and potential shared resources

All pain in children has the potential to disturb developmental processes. This section reviews the similarities and differences between experiences of and treatment options for acute pain, chronic pain, and palliative care. Acute pain is the result of an identifiable injury, an acute illness, or surgery. Many of the tenets of the multidisciplinary model of chronic pain care also apply to acute pain services; however, the usual course of acute postoperative or postinjury pain is time limited and may resolve with less overt management of the behavioural aspects. Growing awareness of the presence of 'persistent postsurgical pain' in acute care settings does suggest that there should be clearly defined mechanisms in paediatric care for appropriate treatment if pain persists beyond the expected injury resolution. Chronic pain through its persistence has the potential to greatly disrupt social and psychological processes, as the child and their family respond to the pain and their understanding (or lack thereof) of the factors contributing to it. It may be associated with persisting physiological disturbance (e.g. neuropathic pain from diabetic neuropathy or chemotherapy), or it may be a manifestation of behavioural changes arising out of a physiological event now otherwise resolved, or it may represent a behavioural manifestation of distress because of the source of the initial pain (i.e. cancer now resolved?) or a psychological/psychiatric disorder. Pain associated with terminal illness adds additional suffering to a situation already fraught with distress. Whatever the individual situation, the biopsychosocial model of pain presents a very useful theoretical framework in which to consider the organizational structure necessary to provide treatment. Each factor will be operating to a greater or lesser degree in each situation where pain is manifest, and must be considered in the treatment approach.

There are both common and unique elements of care for acute pain management, palliative care, and chronic pain management. For the acute pain situation, in the case of scheduled surgery, preparation will be helpful (child life); treatment will be directed by acute care medical providers—either surgeons or a 'pain service' usually consisting of anaesthesiology and nursing, often advised by a pharmacist, interacting with the surgical and nursing care teams. Illness and injury will benefit from the developmentally appropriate educational services of child life, well-trained nurses and in some cases technical interventions from anaesthesia. Communication with the child and their family members is important to ensure understanding of the illness or injury itself, and the meaning of pain in the process. Palliative care requires attention to the spiritual aspects of the impending death, as well as necessary and appropriate medical care, analgesia as determined by the process and impact of the pain. The family must also be cared for. When pain has become chronic, one important issue is to ensure that any responsible disease process has been definitively identified and is under optimal medical therapy (Cott, 1987). Since function may have deteriorated significantly during the 'chronification process', return to normal function may not occur without a structured treatment/recovery plan.

Any acute care paediatric treatment facility will require all of these elements—preparation, acute pain control services, counselling and spiritual support, multidisciplinary care—at least some of the time. Surgery requires preoperative preparation and postoperative analgesia. Palliative care requiring counselling, supportive care, and a wide potential range of symptom management is an unavoidable need for any facility treating serious illness and cancer. Even in the absence of a formal chronic pain programme, there will still be situations where children present with persistent pain and behavioural changes. Expertise in the form of at least some specialists with the appropriate training and a network (even if it is a virtual network of interested colleagues) will be essential to successful treatment. Our description of acute and chronic pain programmes will, it is hoped, identify the necessary elements and suggest some organizational structures and processes which will support best practice care.

MPMA refers to the practice of combining physiological, pharmaceutical, psychological, and sociological therapies at the same time to achieve improvements in outcome. These services have historically been provided in separate locations both within and outside the hospital setting. However since Dr John Bonica first described multidisciplinary treatments being provided together in one setting (Bonica, 1974), the concept has seen considerable growth in the health care arena (Howard, 2003; Reid et al., 2010; Roy, 2008; Weisman, 2008). The type of services offered in a paediatric pain facility depends on the expertise and focus of the practising professionals (McCLain, 2000; Weisman, 2008) but the goal should be to achieve a service equivalent to the Multidisciplinary Pain Clinic as defined by the International Association for the Study of Pain (IASP); teaching institutions will target the Pain Centre (International Association for the Study of Pain, 2012) (Table 62.1).

It has become standard for acute and chronic pain management in children to be performed in a multidisciplinary setting (Peng et al., 2007). Pain centres are the largest and most complex facilities and viewed as the ideal (Weisman, 2008). They also require significant resources. Quite often they focus on outpatient services

Table 62.1 Preferred characteristics of multidisciplinary pain clinics/centres

Qualifications

A variety of health care providers trained to assess and treat physical, psychosocial, medical, vocational, and social aspects of chronic pain

It is required to be able to assess and treat both the physical and the psychosocial aspects of children's complaints. Therefore, at least three medical specialties should be represented, one of which should be a psychiatrist or clinical psychologist (see below for other specialties)

Be able to deal with a wide variety of chronic pain patients, including those with pain due to cancer and pain due to other diseases

Have a consistently adequate number and variety of patients for its professional staff to maintain their skills in diagnosis and treatment

All Health care providers should be appropriately licensed and have significant knowledge of both the basic sciences and clinical practices relevant to chronic pain patients

Communication

The health care professionals should communicate with each other on a regular basis both about individual patients and the programmes which are offered in the pain treatment facility

Have established protocols for patient management and assess their efficacy periodically

Staffing essentials

Staff can include physicians, nurses, psychologists, physical therapists, occupational therapists, vocational counsellors, social workers, and neurologists

Director/Coordinator who will be responsible for monitoring of the medical services provided

Administrative/Support staff to maintain records on patients for assessment of individual treatment outcomes and evaluation of overall programme effectiveness, also to carry out additional activities

Medically trained professional available to deal with patient referrals and emergencies

Services

Diagnostic and therapeutic services which include medication management, referral for appropriate medical consultation, review of prior medical records and diagnostic tests, physical examination, psychological assessment and treatment, physical therapy, vocational assessment and counselling, and other facilities as appropriate

Facilities for inpatient services and outpatient services should be present

Research characteristics for a centre

Carry out research on chronic pain. All providers do not have to do both research and patient care but the institution should have ongoing research activities

Actively engage in educational programmes for a wide variety of health care providers, including under-graduate, graduate, and postdoctoral levels

Affiliation with a major health sciences educational or research institution

to avoid the cost of inpatient care (Weisman, 2008). There are a variety of terms used to describe multidisciplinary facilities, but the main distinctions lie between multimodal, interdisciplinary, and multidisciplinary. Multimodal treatment refers to the simultaneous application of separate and complementary therapeutic intervention performed under the supervision of a single practitioner (American Society of Anesthesiologists, 2010). The distinction between interdisciplinary and multidisciplinary treatments is less distinct. Traditionally multidisciplinary approaches have been used to describe a plan with more than one provider (usually medical specialists) delivering care without direct communication or collaboration with the other providers, and not necessarily in the same location. An interdisciplinary approach coordinates the providers in one setting (usually including several distinct disciplines including medicine, nursing, psychology, physiotherapy, etc.) so that they work together in an integrated manner and develop joint goals with the patient (Rudin, 2001). Recently, the term multidisciplinary has been used in the research literature, as an umbrella term that refers to both inter- and multidisciplinary approaches (Ospina and Harstall, 2003). This chapter will employ the term multidisciplinary pain care (MPC) to refer to the ideal setting of an interdisciplinary coordinated approach either in a pain clinic or a pain centre.

The International Association for the Study of Pain (IASP) has stated that there is significant evidence for the effectiveness of multidisciplinary treatment for chronic pain. The Canadian Pain Society (CPS) has stated the need to include both physical and psychological treatment elements into patient care. The CPS (2012) position statement states, 'Pain is not just a symptom of underlying illness or injury, but it is a disease in its own right, with significant changes in complex biological, and psychological functions'. This statement emphasizes the requirement to treat pain symptoms holistically, using a variety of providers.

Acute pain services

Acute pain services need to be available 24 h a day, 7 days a week. Services may be centralized as a formal acute pain service within a health care setting (i.e. hospital), or can be provided by surgical staff, hospitalists, and ward nurses. Either model could provide excellent care. The choice will be affected by the local situation (presence of trained and interested anaesthesiologists and nurses, acceptance by surgeons and ward nurses). Whichever model is used, there should be access to the range of strategies and techniques as described in Box 62.1.

Institutional procedures should be established for education and training, monitoring of patient outcomes, documentation, and institutional monitoring of activities, and availability of service providers (anaesthesiologists, appropriately trained nursing staff or physician assistants). Observational studies have found that education and training programmes for health care providers in pain care are correlated with lower pain levels, decreased nausea, and increased patient satisfaction (Coleman and Booker-Milburn, 1996; Harmer and Davies, 1998). Educational programmes should include content ranging from basic bedside pain assessment to sophisticated pain management techniques, and non-pharmacological interventions. Comprehensive training programmes for all new personnel are required.

There is limited evidence to suggest that monitoring of outcomes and the availability of anaesthesiologists for specialty care in pain

---

Box 62.1 Recommended established procedures for acute care models

1. The documentation of the pain history of patient, including: typical pain related behaviours, and the child's description of the pain.

2. Systematic assessment and recording of pain and all related symptoms.

3. Pharmacological management.

4. Cognitive-behavioural management.

5. Strategies to prevent pain and other symptoms.

6. Management of side effects of treatment.

7. Monitoring of pain, vital signs, and level of consciousness.

8. Ensure that all specialized services and techniques provided throughout health centre are available for treatment including: patient controlled analgesia, epidural infusions, patient controlled epidural analgesia, subarachnoid infusions, plexus infusions, implantable baclofen pumps.

9. Education and training programmes.

---

management improves outcomes, but many paediatric health practitioners agree that these are key features to be included in any acute pain service (American Society of Anesthesiologists, 2010). There is also strong agreement that in light of their expertise and training, anaesthesiologists should be involved, along with other health care providers, in the establishment of all acute pain guidelines, treatment standards and practices.

The acute pain service is a model in which a recognized group of health care providers (physicians, nurses, and pharmacists) are responsible for the development of standards for pain assessment and management throughout the health centre. There is evidence that this type of service model provides more prompt care (Miaskowski et al., 1999). This group has as its primary goal the delivery of hands on care and symptom management on a daily basis for a specific cohort of patients (Berde and Solodiuk, 2003). Advantages of this approach are that there is a dedicated team that have pain management as their sole focus not as a secondary goal. The team has expertise and a commitment to be effective and over time their experience grows and they will become a better team, able to handle a variety of situations and possible complications. There is also the potential institutional advantage of a team that the rest of the health centre can quickly contact when needed. This group is positioned to implement quality assurance strategies which contribute to improved care. Disadvantages of this model include possible inhibition of a more general development of health providers' skill beyond basic acute pain management. Providers should be aware that this may happen and develop ways to ensure professional development. In order to keep pace with innovations in other fields (new procedures, surgical techniques etc.), the pain service team should develop communication links with departments throughout the health centre. Finally, there are increased costs associated with developing a specific pain service. It may be difficult to financially justify creating a team of skilled providers for the sole purpose of acute pain treatment (Berde and Solodiuk, 2003).

The alternative to having an acute pain service model is to have primary care or health centre practice standards with educational support. In this setting pain management is implemented by the individual services using standards set by a multidisciplinary committee. Standards are for both assessment and analgesia. Regular education programmes are often provided in this setting (Berde and Solodiuk, 2003). There are several advantages to this approach but implementation requires widespread education and training. It 'empowers' providers practising throughout the health centre, intimately familiar with their patients who can evaluate pain and other symptoms within the context of their overall management. Costs are often lower than in the acute pain service model. A disadvantage is that acute pain care is no one's primary responsibility; providers may be more preoccupied with other aspects of treatment and overlook pain management. It may be unrealistic to expect busy clinicians to continually train and educate themselves on best practices in acute pain management; therefore there is a risk that treatment may not be optimal. There may be more delays in this type of treatment environment, often due to competing tasks. Finally, there may be less intensive monitoring and feedback about treatment, therefore suboptimal practices may not be identified and rectified. There is less risk that losing one or two key providers (advanced practice pain nurses, for example) will disable an entire service, but it takes longer to get all staff up to a high level of performance.

Preoperative preparation

By reducing the anxiety and distress associated with many commonly performed surgical procedures, long-term treatment outcomes can be improved (Golianu et al., 2000). Preoperative assessment and consultation around analgesic management can significant alleviate some symptoms of postoperative pain and are critical to pain management (American Society of Anesthesiologists, 2010). The MPC team will discuss with the child and family issues related to the surgical procedure, pain and expected treatment options including: expected severity of postoperative pain, pre-existing medical conditions, risk–benefit of the treatments under consideration, previous experiences with pain, and patient preferences. Preoperative establishment of a pain management protocol is associated with less overall analgesic use, shorter time to extubation, and shorter times to discharge (Susan et al., 1998).

Preparation of the patient includes continuation of usual medications (preventing abstinence syndrome) and premedication needed for the surgery. Educational sessions for the patient and family can include behavioural pain control techniques. Although it is suggested that most of the MPC team, especially the anaesthesiologist, be present during the educational components (American Society of Anesthesiologists, 2012), for practical purposes much of the transmission of information is frequently carried out by child life providers or other professionals, while the anaesthesiologist will provide their input in the context of the preoperative anaesthesia assessment. Patient and parent roles in interpreting postoperative pain should be established before surgery. This will support achieving comfort, reporting of abnormal pain patterns and proper use of analgesics.

Facilities and equipment for acute pain interventions

Table 62.2 details procedures and their associated equipment and staffing needs (Brislin and Rose, 2005; Golianu et al., 2000; Rusy

and Weisman, 2000; The Royal Australasian College of Physicians, 2006). The majority of these procedures should be available when needed. Organization of staff scheduling should bear in mind the training of available staff during each shift to maintain the availability of these procedures to be performed by highly skilled and trained staff. Several of the methods require more than one trained professional on hand; availability of such a person should be ensured. Training and education about these techniques should be routine in pain management centres.

Chronic pain management

Paediatric chronic pain has a significant impact on social, emotional, psychological, mental, and spiritual components of the life of a child and their family. The biopsychosocial model of pain provides the essential theoretical framework within which to establish a treatment programme. Delivery of care in all three areas must be provided by the organizational structure.

Three key features of the insidious development of pain from first occurrence to life changing condition have been described: impairment, disability, and handicap (Desparmet, 2009). *Impairment* is when the pain first surfaces and begins a cycle of pain–inactivity–more pain–more inactivity. This leads to *disability*, when a child is unable to physically participate in age-appropriate daily activities. Parents often identify behaviour changes and absenteeism from school and other structured activities. The physical separation from family and peers is accompanied by emotional isolation. These psychological and mental consequences often lead to *handicap*, characterized by sleep disturbance, further emotional withdrawal, and expressions of hopelessness. This may severely limit the normal development of the child. As described, chronic pain has significant far reaching negative repercussions on the child's life. Therefore treatment must address all of these concerns and should be a priority for the family. Early intervention, with the aim of limiting the duration or extent of disability, will hopefully prevent major impairment. The objective of a pain management programme may in fact be a return to normal functioning, and not resolution of pain symptoms. Paradoxically, return to function can often lead to reduction in pain (Desparmet, 2009).

Before patients enter a Paediatric Pain Centre (PPC) they have often visited a variety of other specialists over a period of 4 to 6 months and have not observed substantive positive results. This fragmentation of care exacerbates the *disability* process (Desparmet, 2009). Additionally the family is often required to restructure their daily routine and possibly their employment patterns. This disrupts the life of both the patient and their familial support system.

This paediatric MPC includes the composition of the health provider team and their individual and cumulative backgrounds as essential in developing a MPC team. Furthermore their consistent communication and progressive development is highlighted as a key to success. Paediatric chronic pain is positioned as a biopsychosocial phenomenon that requires the involvement of patient, their family, their social support, and the experiences, attitudes, and beliefs that they bring to the assessment period and through treatment. The expressed symptoms and biological determinants are considered in conjunction with medical guidelines and pathology and incorporated into the framework of the social and psychological characteristics of the family and patient. Mental health history, lifestyle, education, social patterns, stressors, and any related family

Table 62.2 Techniques and equipment for acute pain services

Technique	Personnel	Equipment
Distraction	Any health professional or family member	Materials that can capture and maintain a child's attention Kaleidoscope Stories Bubbles Counting Pop-up toys Video games
Deep breathing/muscle relaxation	Physical therapist, psychologist, nurse, or family member with some education on the process	None
Self-regulation	Nurse, psychologist	Biofeedback equipment Transcutaneous electric nerve stimulation unit
Topical anaesthesia	Anaesthesiologist, nurse, or physicians able to record the process (dose, medical history)	None
Local infiltration	Anaesthesiologist, nurse, or physicians able to record the process (dose, medical history) Must be competent in CPR	Smallest gauge needles required Correct drugs and dosage
Peripheral nerve blocks	Anaesthesiologist, nurse, or physicians able to record the process (dose, medical history) Must be competent in CPR Provider should be trained in the technique, and be familiar with it A trained assistant should be used to monitor the patient during the procedure	Short-bevelled needles or specific insulated needles for connection to a nerve stimulator Correct drug dose and volume Oxygen supply Equipment for artificial ventilation Suction equipment Defibrillator Cardiac resuscitation drugs.
Bier block (intravenous regional anaesthesia)	Anaesthesiologist, nurse, or physicians able to record the process (dose, medical history) Must be competent in CPR Staff should be trained and familiar with use and complications. A trained assistant should be used to monitor the patient during the process.	Tourniquet Proper drug dose and volume Resuscitation equipment
Nitrous oxide (N2O) analgesia	A separate person should be used to administer the N$_2$O that is not conducting procedure. Anaesthesiologist is recommended to be present especially if there are any expected complications	A means to separately delivery oxygen and N$_2$O Resuscitation equipment
Ketamine and midazolam	Staff should be trained and familiar with use, adverse effects and complications A trained assistant should be used to monitor the patient during the procedure Staff should be trained in advanced airway management	Resuscitation equipment Oxygen supply Equipment for artificial ventilation Suction Defibrillator Cardiac resuscitation drugs

history should be accounted for in order to develop the treatment with highest probability of success. Incorporating at least three health providers into an extended interview with the patient and family will allow for a variety of professional perspectives to interpret the family dynamics, communications patterns, and identify any potential threats that may arise. The team should also determine the capacity of the family to implement treatment. Factors to consider include: marital or financial stress, school absenteeism, family accommodation, school transition, high performance demands, and relationship-oriented rejection or loss (Desparmet, 2009). For example there is a surprisingly high percentage of patients that are enrolled in demanding course loads, are extremely active in extracurricular activity (sports, music, volunteerism), and have a demand placed on them to perform (Weisman, 2008).

The focus of chronic pain treatment in MPCs is rehabilitative instead of curative. The team should emphasize definable, operable

Table 62.3 Goals for a MPC paediatric patient and their family

Symptomatic improvement
Improved physical function to participate in activities appropriate for age
Reduce pain sensitivity and intensity
Regain independence appropriate for age
Family and patient master coping techniques
Master self-management skills appropriate for age
Restore individual and family productivity to a satisfactory level
Decrease inappropriate use of health care system

and realistic outcomes for the patient, rather than complete pain relief (Gardea and Gatchel, 2000). Quality of life outcomes with a focus on independence through restoration of physical, psychological, and social functioning (Table 62.3) should be the goal. The rehabilitation plan should be developed on an individual patient basis with all team members. The process of a MPC is illustrated in Figure 62.2, with further detail in the following subsections including the staff, communication, multidisciplinary integrative assessment, outcomes, patient and parent expectations and experiences and follow-up are described later in this chapter.

Staff positions and organization

The disciplines required and services offered by a PPC will be determined in part by the conditions being treated. The most commonly seen chronic pain conditions in PPCs include

headache, abdominal pain, myofascial pain, arthritis, back pain, complex regional pain syndrome, phantom limb pain, cancer pain, sickle cell pain, and cerebral palsy-related pain (Weisman, 2008). A list of staff positions will include some or all of the following: the Director, Physical therapist, Nurse, Physician(s), Anaesthesiologist, Psychologist, Pharmacist, and Child Life Specialist. Their specific roles and skill sets have been well described, as well as the contribution each makes to the overall process through their individual discipline (Berde and Solodiuk, 2003; Cravero and Blike, 2004; Eccleston, 2001; Joseph, 2007; Kingsley and Porfyris, 2011; McClain, 2000; Palermo et al., 2010; Schurman and Friesen, 2010). Each may fulfil more than one role depending upon resources and skill sets available—for example, anaesthesiologists will have a specific professional role but may also serve as the pain specialist; other physicians may serve to offer services arising out of their personal skill sets or function as speciality consultants (e.g. neurology, physical medicine, surgery, neurosurgery, psychiatry). No matter which medical or other professionals are involved in the care however, the most important overall functional issue is management of the communication process, as described next.

Staff communication/organizational relationships supporting practice

Although the specific role descriptions of the staff of a MPC team are important, they may be to some extent less relevant to the organizational systems discussion than the manner in which they relate to one another and the programmes offered. Very little specific research illuminates the issue of effective communication

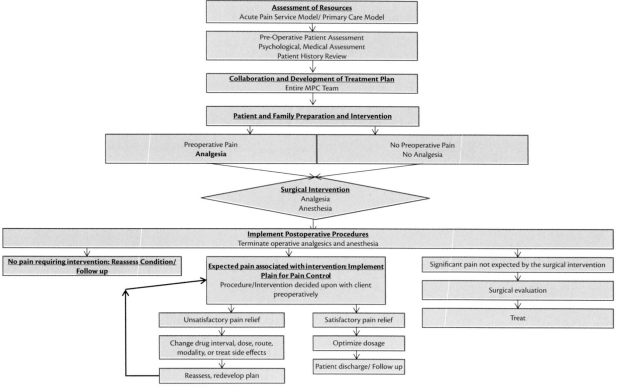

Figure 62.1 Patient flow for acute care services.

amongst MPC professionals; however consistent communication is essential to the success of the MPC team (Dowden et al., 2008). Figure 62.2 also highlights communication within the MPC team. Many of the professional roles are traditionally independent and training does not always emphasize multidisciplinary collaboration. Routines, protocols, and regularly scheduled meetings should be implemented and encouraged in order to promote effective communication and practice. Nurses, because they can have varied roles, are often the core of effective communication (Berde and Solodiuk, 2003). Nursing research examining the process of incorporating research into practice has identified those characteristics of an organization which will best support implementation of best practice. This is described as the PARIHS ('Promoting Action on Research in Health Services') framework (Rycroft-Malone, 2004). Successful implementation of best practice is best supported by: evidence itself, context, and facilitation. These three are further broken down to reflect: evidence—research evidence, clinical experience, patient experience and local data/information; context—culture, leadership, and evaluation; and facilitation—purpose, role, skills, and attributes. The organizational system thus can support this process by ensuring communication of local clinical experience and patient experience as well as providing local data and information, by providing a culture which will support/promote best practice, by selecting leaders who support these goals and putting in place communication systems to facilitate the process, and by training personnel in the skills of facilitation. It can be seen that these elements, while originally developed to address a somewhat different issue, are very relevant to the complex problems which frequently surround management of paediatric patients with chronic pain.

A paediatric chronic pain disorder such as 'functional gastrointestinal disorder' (FGID), illustrates the importance of effective communication strategies. It is associated with a complex combination of symptoms, including pain, related to biological and psychological processes. These patients have high levels of health care utilization and incur significant financial costs (Schurman and Friesen, 2010). In this type of multifaceted disorder there may not be established clinical guidelines. Treatment is thus best provided in a multidisciplinary setting in order to enhance outcomes and hopefully decrease long term health care costs. The success of treatments often depends on the integration of the recommendations of the full range of disciplines involved, especially when interventions need to be combined for these complex disorders (see Table 62.4).

Parental expectations

Unlike an adult, a child relies on the caregivers (parents) of the family to make decisions about care. Thus the family must be incorporated into the care process to an even greater extent than in adult pain management. As positive expectations for treatment and recovery on the part of both patients and their families will benefit overall outcome, it should be a goal for the MPC to initially establish an optimistic attitude towards expectations (Long and Guite, 2008). This can be a challenge because the MPC team is rarely the first service parents have sought for the child's pain. Prior to the visit to the MPC team, families with children suffering from long-term chronic pain have low expectations for MPC (Tsao et al., 2005). This is often the result of prior disappointment as previous diagnosis and treatments have failed to offer relief, which

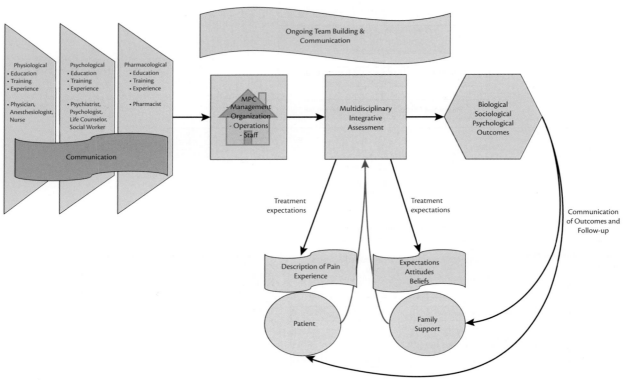

Figure 62.2 Structure and process of a MPC.

Table 62.4 Examples of biopsychosocial interventions that have been combined for complex disorders

Intervention	Primary roles
Prescription medication	Pharmacist/Physician/Nurse
Biofeedback assisted relaxation training	Psychologist/Nurse
Personalized therapy that targets: school issues, pain coping strategies, sleep hygiene	Psychologist/Life Counsellor/Nurse
Acupuncture	Physical Therapist
Massage	Physical Therapist
Physical therapy	Physical Therapist/Nurse
Family therapy	Counsellor
Sleep evaluation	Psychologist

Table 62.5 Quotes of parents' perceptions of care at a MPC

Perceptions of the MPC treating the whole body

'Knowing that they are looking at the whole picture, not just 1/4 of it'

'The mind–body connection—having both doctors meet with us together was very helpful'

'Explaining how it's all going to come together to help our son.'

Perceptions of the MPC team

'The process and desire to understand to assist and educate'

'How well the staff worked to make me and my child comfortable and how to assist my child when he has pain'

'People dedicated to getting the problem resolved.'

Text extracts reproduced from Jennifer Verrill Schurman and Craig A Friesen, Integrative treatment approaches: family satisfaction with a multidisciplinary paediatric: Abdominal Pain Clinic, *International Journal of Integrated Care*, Volume 10, p 1–9, Copyright © 2010 (CC By 3.0).

results in frustration. However, after the coordinated interdisciplinary assessment, and once treatment plans are developed, parents are often quite appreciative of the service provided in the MPC team, especially with holistic and multidisciplinary team approach (Table 62.5) (Schurman and Friesen, 2010). Many paediatric pain facilities are structured to offer a variety of health care services on the same day as the first visits. This is not only convenient for families but establishes early on that a comprehensive examination of the child's needs is being completed.

Results are not always positive, however, and it is important to recognize when MPCs do not get it right so that these situations can be planned against. If expectations are not met, mistrust and sensitivity to future advice can arise: this represents a continuation of experience of failure derived from previous visits to other single modality specialists (Weisman, 2008). Negative experiences with MPCs include the length of a visit (including time waited between meetings) waitlist times, scheduling conflicts, and complexity of the interpretation of outcomes.

Parents expect the MPC to offer coping solutions and stress management skills (Claar and Scharff, 2007). They also anticipate

receiving information about the cause of pain, treatment options, drugs, and the effects of both the pain and any underling processes associated with the pain (Reid et al., 2010). This information is expected to be provided as written information to which they can refer later. This can be very important to the parents' perceptions of successful treatment, and may be linked to better adherence. Whenever possible MPC teams should strive to meet these expectations and be aware of any lingering patient or parent doubt. When parents' expectations are not met, treatments of the child's psychological, physical, and social state may not be perceived as completed. This may lead to an extended treatment regimen or relapse of symptoms. Although it is not always the case, positive expectations for recovery are correlated with better health outcomes (Long and Guite, 2008).

Information management systems

Many centres are moving to implement electronic medical records (EMRs) which may facilitate information management programmes and help the MPC to improve transfer of information between professionals. All clinical charts must be up to date and readily available to any member of the treatment team. Towards this goal, Computerized Clinical Decision Support Systems (CCDSS or CDSS) may promote implementation of best practice care. This is somewhat complex in the sense that in order to effectively have an impact upon care, certain characteristics must be present in the CCDSS. Several systematic reviews (Kawamoto, 2005; Roshanov, 2011) have found that improvement in care could be achieved through implementation of a CCDSS. None of the trials specifically addressed pain care or paediatric pain care in particular, so the applicability and impact cannot be commented upon directly. These have also yet to demonstrate an impact on patient outcomes.

Patient flow for chronic pain services

Figure 62.3 illustrates the stages of the patient flow through a MPC. The process begins with a referral, either by the patient's general practitioner, another health care provided or health centre. Clinic intake may be defined by diagnosis, duration of the problem or presence of psychological or social comorbidities.

Initial evaluation

Organization of the data gathering process is important. Cott has argued that the initial interview for a complex problem requires the simultaneous presence of the most senior clinicians; in other programmes initial data gathering may use standardized questionnaires administered by relatively junior clinicians or non-specialists (Cott, 1987). The child should obviously be involved in all decisions (Desparmet, 2009). The evaluation of the patient should involve family members and consider the entire history and family dynamic. Parents should be prepared for the possibility of an extended meeting. A checklist of items that should be discussed during this initial evaluation is provided in Table 62.6 (adapted from National Health and Medical Research Council, 2005). The length of this extended first contact interview can be anywhere from an hour to the better part of a day (Weisman, 2008). Parents and siblings should be incorporated into the interview, which will include social history, school performance and extracurricular activities changes.

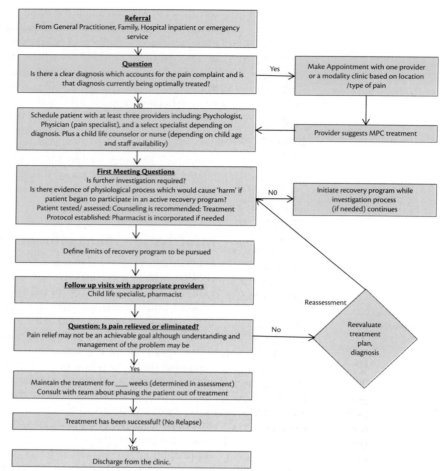

Figure 62.3 Patient flow for chronic care services.

Table 62.6 Patient assessment checklist (conducted with child and family present)

Circumstances associated with pain onset
Primary site of pain
Radiation of pain
Character of pain (throbbing, sharp, aching etc.)
Intensity of pain during movement, at rest, and at present, during last week
Highest level of intensity
Factors altering pain (what makes it worse/better?)
Associated symptoms
Temporal factors (is pain present continuously or otherwise?)
Effect of pain on activities
Effect of pain on sleep
Medications taken for pain
Additional treatments used for pain
Health professionals consulted for pain treatment

Pain history information of significance for symptomatic treatment of pain
Expectations of outcome
Patient belief around cause(s) of pain
Family belief around cause(s) of pain
Expected reduction in pain and symptoms required to resume regular activities
Patient's typical coping response for stress or pain,
Presence of anxiety or psychiatric disorders (e.g. depression or psychosis)
Family expectations and beliefs about pain, stress and postoperative course
Ways the patient describes or shows pain

Source: data from National Health and Medical Research Council, *Acute pain management: scientific evidence*, Sydney, Australia, Copyright © 2005 Commonwealth of Australia.

Physical exam, diagnosis, and feedback

The physical exam including neurological exam (Desparmet, 2009; Weisman, 2008) and the diagnosis and feedback all provide both diagnostic and communication opportunities. Ensure adequate time for understanding, and confirm comprehension (Desparmet,

2009). This is where trust between provider and patient can be reinforced. All questions should be answered thoroughly.

The plan will be multifaceted and complex, and determined by the team during evaluation of the patient's needs and capabilities.

Outcome goals are established in the feedback session, such as reintegration into various aspects of daily routine (Weisman, 2008). Families may not always accept the diagnosis and plan, follow up should be encouraged. If the family is unwilling to return then the importance of a discussion with their family doctor should be emphasized. Refer to the section on parents' perceptions about how to increase their satisfaction which has a highly positive association with adherence and good outcomes.

Conclusion

This chapter provided guidance and described options for organizations that may adopt a new or modify an existing paediatric pain centre. It focused on the importance of multidisciplinary treatment assessments and the incorporation of the entire health team through various times of the treatment plan. The information here will help identify the proper staff for a MPC, and emphasize the need for team leaders to be explicit with members about procedures and expectations from the beginning. Using options presented, multidisciplinary teams may develop such procedures; however each team may require certain customization. The emphasis should be on team cohesion, which will translate to better patient care. The sections of parental expectation and patient flow may assist teams to communicate clearly with the family about what the patient may expect from treatment and recovery options.

Case example

MacKIDS is a moderate sized paediatric hospital, contained within a large hospital corporation providing all paediatric services save solid organ transplant and cardiac surgery. It has had a robust postoperative paediatric pain service which functioned as part of the adult service until the adult inpatient surgery relocated, leaving a small paediatric service with 2 h per day of nursing time assigned from amongst the Post-Anaesthesia Care Unit nursing staff.

Recently a community foundation has offered fundraising support directed to establishment of an interdisciplinary pain programme. The community foundation has coordinated a meeting of Canadian paediatric pain experts to identify best practice in a chronic pain programme for paediatrics. They have created a 'made in Canada' approach to the problem intended to be a template for a knowledge translation effort into multiple jurisdictions supporting best practice complex pain care for children, adolescents and young adults transitioning between paediatric and adult care systems. This information is providing a model to guide programme development at MacKIDS.

The question of how to best provide paediatric chronic pain services, acute pain services and possibly also support palliative care services has arisen during a time of health care budget contraction. Awareness of the need for paediatric chronic pain care is growing. It is becoming clear that although the volume might be small, there is a need for an organized institutional approach to paediatric chronic pain care.

The challenge is to identify those elements which can be provided either through re-allocation of existing resources or at the least possible incremental cost.

References

American Society of Anesthesiologists. (2010). Practice guidelines for chronic pain management. *Anesthesiology*, 112(4), 1–24.

American Society of Anesthesiologists. (2012). Practice guidelines for acute pain management in the perioperative setting: an updated report by the American Society of Anesthesiologists Task Force on Acute Pain Management. *Anesthesiology*, 116(2), 248–273.

Berde, C. and Solodiuk, J. (2003). Multidisciplinary programs for management of acute and chronic pain in children. In N. Schechter, C. Berde, and M. Yaster (eds), *Pain in infants, children and adolescents* (2nd edn), pp. 471–488. New York: Lippincott Williams & Wilkins.

Bonica, J. (1974). Organization and function of a pain clinic. In J. Bonica (ed.) *Advances in neurology: international symposium on pain*, pp. 433–443. New York: Raven.

Brislin, R. P. and Rose, J. B. (2005). Pediatric acute pain management. *Anesthesiol Clin North Am*, 23(4), 789–814. doi:10.1016/j.atc.2005.07.002.

Claar, R. L. and Scharff, L. (2007). Parent and child perceptions of chronic pain treatments. *Child Health Care*, 36(3), 285–301. doi:10.1080/02739610701377962.

Coleman, S. A. and Booker-Milburn, J. (1996). Audit of postoperative pain control. Influence of a dedicated acute pain nurse. *Anaesthesia*, 51(12), 1093–1096. Available at: <http://www.ncbi.nlm.nih.gov/pubmed/9038438>.

Cott, A. (1987). Illness behavior: a multidisciplinary model. In S. McHugh and T. M. Vallis (eds) *The disease-illness distinction: a model for effective and practical integration of behavioural and medical sciences*, pp. 87–99. New York: Plenum Press.

Cravero, J. P. and Blike, G. T. (2004). Review of pediatric sedation. *Anesth Analg*, 99(5), 1355–1364. doi:10.1213/01.ANE.0000134810.60270.E8.

Desparmet, J. (2009). Chronic pain management: organization, techniques and guidelines. In M. Astuto (ed.) *Basics, anesthesia, intensive care and pain in neonates and children*, pp. 241–253. Milan: Springer-Verlag.

Dowden, S., McCarthy, M., and Chalkiadis, G. (2008). Achieving organizational change in pediatric pain management. *Pain Res Manage*, 13(4), 321–326. Available at: <http://www.pubmedcentral.nih.gov/articlerender.fcgi?artid=2671318&tool=pmcentrez&rendertype=abstract>.

Gardea, M. A. and Gatchel, R. J. (2000). Interdisciplinary treatment of chronic pain. *Current Rev Pain*, 4(1), 18–23. Available at: <http://www.ncbi.nlm.nih.gov/pubmed/10998711>.

Golianu, B., Krane, E. J., Galloway, K. S., and Yaster, M. (2000). Pediatric acute pain management. *Pediatr Clini North Am*, 47(3), 559–87. Available at: <http://www.ncbi.nlm.nih.gov/pubmed/20185654>.

Harmer, M., and Davies, K. A. (1998). The effect of education, assessment and a standardised prescription on postoperative pain management. The value of clinical audit in the establishment of acute pain services. *Anaesthesia*, 53(5), 424–430. Available at: <http://www.ncbi.nlm.nih.gov/pubmed/9659013>.

Howard, R. F. (2003). Current status of pain management in children. *JAMA*, 290(18), 2464–2469. doi:10.1001/jama.290.18.2464.

Joseph, M. H. (2007). Selected topics in perioperative multimodal pediatric pain management. *Semin Anesth Periop Med Pain*, 26(3), 141–148. doi:10.1053/j.sane.2007.06.006.

Kingsley, R. A. and Porfyris, S. (2011). The role of nurse practitioner in chronic pain management. In B. C. McClain and S. Suresh (eds) *Handbook of pediatric chronic pain*, pp. 375–408. New York: Springer. doi:10.1007/978-1-4419-0350-1.

Kawamoto, K., Houlihan, C. A., Balas, E. A., and Lobach, D. F. (2005). Improving clinical practice using clinical decision support systems: a systematic review of trials to identify features critical to success. *Br Med J*, 330(7494), 765.

Long, A. C. and Guite, J. W. (2008). Treatment-related expectations in pediatric chronic pain. *Pain Child*, 10(3), 18–22.

McClain, B. C. (2000). Organization of pain management services for children. In T. Benzon, J. Rathmell, C. Wu, D. Turk, and C. Argoff (eds) *Practical management of pain* (3rd edn), pp. 59–67. New York: Mosby.

Miaskowski, C., Crews, J., Ready, L. B., Paul, S. M., and Ginsberg, B. (1999). Anesthesia-based pain services improve the quality of postoperative pain management. *Pain*, 80(1–2), 23–29. Available at: <http://www.ncbi.nlm.nih.gov/pubmed/10204714>.

National Health and Medical Research Council. (2005). *Acute pain management: scientific evidence*. Sydney: National Health and Medical Research Council.

Ospina, M. and Harstall, C. (2003). *Multidisciplinary pain programs for chronic pain : evidence from systematic reviews*. Edmonton: Alberta Heritage Foundation for Medical Research.

Palermo, T. M., Eccleston, C., Lewandowski, A. S., Williams, A. C., and Morley, S. (2010). Randomized controlled trials of psychological therapies for management of chronic pain in children and adolescents: an updated meta-analytic review. *Pain*, 148(3), 387–397. doi:10.1016/j.pain.2009.10.004.Randomized.

Peng, P., Stinson, J. N., Choiniere, M., Dion, D., Intrater, H., Lefort, S., Lynch, M., *et al.* (2007). Dedicated multidisciplinary pain management centres for children in Canada: the current status. *Can J Anaesth*, 54(12), 985–91. doi:10.1007/BF03016632.

Reid, K., Lander, J., Scott, S., and Dick, B. (2010). What do the parents of children who have chronic pain expect from their first visit to a pediatric chronic pain clinic? *Pain Res Manag*, 15(3), 158–162. Available at: <http://www.pubmedcentral.nih.gov/articlerender.fcgi?artid=2912615&tool=pmcentrez&rendertype=abstract>.

Roshanov, P. S., Misra, S., Gerstein, H. C., Garg, A. X., Sebaldt, R. J., Mackay, J. A., *et al.* (2011). Computerized clinical decision support systems for chronic disease management: a decision-maker-researcher partnership systematic review. *Implement Sci*, 6(1), 92.

Roy, R. (2008). Multidisciplinary approach and chronic pain. In *Pyschosocial interventions for chronic pain*, pp. 147–164. New York: Springer. doi:10.1007/978-0-387-76296-8.

Rudin, N. J. (2001). Chronic pain rehabilitation: principles and practice. *WMJ*, 100(5), 36–43, 66. Available at: <http://www.ncbi.nlm.nih.gov/pubmed/11579799>

Rusy, L. M. and Weisman, S. J. (2000). Complementary therapies for acute pediatric pain management. *Pediatr Clin North Am*, 47(3), 589–99. Available at: <http://www.ncbi.nlm.nih.gov/pubmed/10835992>.

Rycroft-Malone, J. (2004). The PARIHS framework – a framework for guiding the implementation of evidence-based practice. *J Nurs Care Qual*, 19(4), 297–304.

Schurman, J. V. and Friesen, C. A. (2010). Integrative treatment approaches: family satisfaction with a multidisciplinary paediatric abdominal pain clinic. *Int J Integr Care*, 10, 1–9. Available at: <http://www.pubmedcentral.nih.gov/articlerender.fcgi?artid=2948677&tool=pmcentrez&rendertype=abstract>

Susan, A. F., Eastman, M., Benjamin, K., and Horgan, M. J. (1998). Outcome measures after standardized pain management strategies in postoperative patients in the neonatal intensive care unit. *J Perinat Neonatal Nurs*, 12(1), 58–69.

The Royal Australasian College of Physicians. (2006). Management of procedure-related pain in children and adolescents. *J Paediatr Child Health*, 105(2), 1–29.

Tsao, J. C. I., Meldrum, M., Bursch, B., Jacob, M. C., Kim, S. C., and Zeltzer, L. K. (2005). Treatment expectations for CAM interventions in pediatric chronic pain patients and their parents. *Evid Based Complement Alternat Med*, 2(4), 521–527. doi:10.1093/ecam/neh132.

Weisman, S. J. (2008). Multidisciplinary approaches to chronic pain. In G. A. Walco and K. R. Goldschneider (eds.), *Pain in children: a practical guide for primary care*, pp. 133–143. Totowa, NJ: Humana Press.

CHAPTER 63

Education for paediatric pain

Alison Twycross and Susan O'Conner-Von

Summary

This chapter focuses on educating children, parents, and health care professionals about pain management. The first half of the chapter examines issues related to children and parents while the second half concentrates on health care professionals. The current state of knowledge will be explored and strategies for educating each group discussed. The Promoting Action on Research Implementation in Health Services (PARiHS) model (see also Yamada and Hutchinson, Chapter 61, this volume) is used to help explain why healthcare professionals do not always use their knowledge in practice. Implications for practice, education and future research are also outlined.

Children and parental knowledge about paediatric pain

Children's knowledge about pain

It is well established that a child's cognitive development affects their perception of pain, behavioural response to pain, and ability to communicate about pain (Harbeck and Peterson, 1992). A child's view of pain tends to follow a consistent developmental pattern (McGrath, 1990). Children learn about pain and how to cope with pain through their own and their family's experiences with pain. Moreover, the significance of what children learn about pain is a direct result of their stage of cognitive development (Wood, 1993). For example, school-aged children in Piaget's concrete operational stage are able to perform cognitive operations and apply new skills when thinking about events. These children can use their past experiences to understand the reasons for administration of an analgesic drug.

Most paediatric pain research exploring the educational needs of children has focused on procedural pain. Children often consider procedures to be worse than the health issue initiating the need for the procedure (Finley and Schechter, 2003). The most commonly studied needle procedures are immunizations and injections. A systematic review of psychological interventions for needle-related procedural pain in children (28 randomized controlled trials with 1951 participants) included children aged 2 to 19 years (Uman et al., 2010). Distraction, hypnosis, and combined cognitive-behavioural interventions were found to be the most effective in terms of decreasing pain and distress (for further discussion see Cohen et al., Chapter 53; Liossi et al., Chapter 54; Logan et al., Chapter 50, this volume). There is promising but limited evidence for the efficacy of providing information and preparation (Uman et al., 2010).

Some studies have focused on developing techniques for preparing preschool and school-aged children for surgery. Educational programmes including a variety of coping models, sensory and procedural information, and structured medical play, have resulted in less situational anxiety and increased knowledge in children undergoing surgery in hospital settings (O'Conner-Von, 2000). A variety of interventions have been examined in terms of preparing children for surgery, such as individual and group preparation, videotapes, websites, and stress point preparation. Pre-surgery preparation strategies for children have been shown to be effective in reducing situational anxiety and increasing knowledge (O'Conner-Von, 2000). However, there is a paucity of research addressing educational needs of children and families of diverse cultural backgrounds, those undergoing emergency procedures and families of infants. Moreover, most research was conducted with children receiving inpatient care, yet the number of outpatient and day case procedures continues to rise placing increased responsibility on parents for pain assessment and management at home.

Parents' knowledge about pain

Regardless of culture or socioeconomic background, children find parents are their greatest source of support during a painful procedure (Jones et al., 2005). Unfortunately, little is known about parental perceptions and understanding of the information they receive about managing their child's pain (Oakes, 2011). Studies exploring parents' management of children's postoperative pain at home have found that even if they recognize their child is in pain, they often give inadequate doses of pain medication (Finley et al., 1996; Fortier et al., 2009). This is perhaps attributable to parental attitudes towards pain medications. Indeed, two studies conducted in the US found parents fear the negative side effects of analgesic drugs; consider analgesics to be addictive; and believe children should receive as little pain medication as possible (Zisk et al., 2007,

2010). Further, studies in the UK and Canada have found parents are satisfied with pain care, even if their child experiences moderate to severe pain during the postoperative period (Twycross and Collis, 2012; Twycross and Finley, 2013). Parents may not be aware of the harmful consequences of unrelieved pain. There is a need for health care professionals to educate parents about pain assessment and management.

Parents have indicated they would like more information about their child's pain management (Franck et al., 2005; Simons and Roberson, 2002; Simons et al., 2001). There is evidence of a wide variability in the amount of information, type of pain content, and clarity of pain information given to parents regarding their child's postoperative pain management (Tait et al., 2008). In Tait's study, parents (n = 187) of children scheduled for surgery completed questionnaires about their perceptions, understanding, and satisfaction with the information they received regarding their child's postoperative pain management. Of note, parents whose child received patient-controlled analgesia were given significantly more information than those receiving nurse controlled analgesia (p <0.025). However, approximately one-third of parents had no understanding of the risks of pain management postoperatively. This reinforces the importance of providing pain management education to parents.

Several studies in North America have explored the effect of providing parents with an educational booklet about pain management following day surgery (Chambers et al., 1997), cardiac surgery (Huth et al., 2003), and in the emergency department (LeMay et al., 2010). There was some evidence parental knowledge increased following the educational intervention but limited improvements in pain management were found. However, in LeMay et al.'s study, the investigators found the use of an educational booklet was not effective in reducing pain and unpleasantness related to pain, nor did it improve pain beliefs held by parents (n = 195). These investigators suggested having parents actively participate in their child's pain management would be more effective than a passive educational intervention such as a booklet. Similar results were noted in a study by Greenberg et al. (1999) using a videotape to increase parental (n = 100) knowledge. Providing parents with information about pain is not sufficient; there is also a need to empower parents to take a more active role in advocating and caring for their child in pain. For a further discussion of pain and the family, see Birnie et al. (Chapter 12, this volume).

Strategies for educating children and parents about paediatric pain

Strategies for educating children about pain

Nurses have an obligation to educate patients about their health and to assess the patient and family's comprehension of the health care information (American Nurses Association, 2001, 2008; Association of Pediatric Hematology/Oncology Nurses, 2007; US Department of Health and Human Services, 1992). Nurses are usually the health care professionals responsible for educating children about pain (American Nurses Association, 2005; Kotzer et al., 1998), yet these guidelines and standards do not provide specific strategies for educating children about pain.

A variety of methods have been used to educate children about pain. Early educational strategies for children consisted of providing information through print materials, such as My Book for Kids

with Cansur by Jason Gaes (1987) and The Berenstain Bears Go to The Doctor (Berenstain, 1981). For younger children, puppets and dolls can be effective in explaining procedures (Child Life Council, 2007; Li et al., 2006). A variety of strategies have been used to educate children about pain, including print materials, therapeutic play, and cognitive-behavioural methods (Idvall et al., 2005). For younger children, puppets and dolls can be effective in explaining procedures, whereas older children and adolescents may prefer peer group or technology-based education (Child Life Council, 2007; Li et al., 2006). However, there is a lack of research addressing the importance of development in terms of designing educational interventions for children. In addition to cognitive development, the child's psychosocial development must be considered. For example, educational strategies for a younger child should involve parents, whereas involving peer mentors may be more effective for adolescents.

Web-based interventions

Computers have changed the way we live, work, play, and learn (McGrath et al., 2010). Many children use technology in their educational and home settings using Web-based programmes is an obvious choice when designing strategies to educate children and adolescents about pain. Web-based technology has many advantages over the use of printed material. It is easy to individualize, update when new information is available, and can be interactive. Web-based education can provide information and guidance for patients without geographic or time restrictions (Brillhart, 2007). Technology has been used to educate children dealing with chronic pain (Palermo and Valenzuela, 2003), functional abdominal pain (Sato et al., 2009), cancer pain (O'Conner-Von, 2009), and arthritis pain (Stinson et al., 2012). However, more research is needed to evaluate the effectiveness of these educational interventions in terms of decreased pain intensity scores, increased knowledge of pain management strategies and improved functioning (i.e. school attendance and peer interaction). The relevant child population should be involved in the creation and critique of these programmes (O'Conner-Von, 2009).

The effectiveness of a Web-based programme designed to educate adolescents (aged 10–16 years) about tonsillectomy was tested by O'Conner-Von (2008). Children (n = 66) were randomly assigned to a Web-based educational programme or to attend the standard educational programme at the hospital prior to the day of surgery. The Web-based programme contained the same educational content as the standard hospital-based educational programme. A script was created in conversational format with early and middle adolescents teaching each other about the surgical experience, pain assessment and management, and non-pharmacological ways to cope before and after surgery. To determine content accuracy and validity of the information provided in the programme, five adult experts who care for patients in this age group reviewed the script. Next, 40 healthy adolescents read the script to determine readability and age appropriateness. Lastly, two focus groups of six adolescents (n = 12) who had undergone a tonsillectomy within the past year reviewed the Web-based programme and completed a questionnaire to rate the programme on ease of navigation, clarity of content, and age appropriateness. After completing the questionnaire, adolescents in the focus group sessions discussed their health care experience of having a tonsillectomy and their pain management during hospitalisation and at home. Then participants discussed the programme in terms of what was most helpful, not helpful and how the programme could be improved.

Seventy per cent (n = 46/66) of the patients had no prior surgical experience. On enrolment to the study, 70% of the participants reported fears related to surgery, the most frequent being fear of pain. Patients in the Web-based educational programme showed a statistically significant increase in knowledge acquisition (p = 0.0005) compared to those assigned to the standard pre-surgery educational programme as well as increased satisfaction with the method of education (p = 0.004). Although not statistically significant, pain intensity scores obtained 2-h and 24-h postoperatively were clinically significant; pain scores for patients who did not use the Web-based programme increased (mean score of 4.71 two hours after surgery, and a mean score of 6.09 twenty-four hours after surgery while at home). Patients using the Web-based programme reported advantages of this type of education such as the ability to view the programme as often as needed, when it was convenient, at their own pace, and in private.

Strategies for educating parents about pain

An essential component of educating children about pain is to educate their parents. Just as children require age-appropriate explanations of pain, it is critical to assess parents' cognitive ability, understanding of pain, experience with pain, and readiness to learn, in order to provide appropriate education. The goals of educating parents about their child's pain are to improve knowledge and awareness of pain, to decrease misconceptions about pain, to provide pain relief, and to facilitate effective communication with the health care team (Curtiss, 2010; DiMaggio et al., 2010).

Over the past three decades, a variety of strategies to educate parents about pain have been used. Earliest materials consisted of providing information through print materials such as Children's Cancer Pain can be Relieved (Wisconsin Cancer Pain Initiative, 1989), Making Cancer Less Painful (McGrath et al., 1992) and Pain, Pain, Go Away: Helping Children with Pain (McGrath et al., 1994). A randomized trial (Chambers et al., 1997) evaluating the effects of educating parents (n = 82) with the later booklet (a 15-page general guide to teach parents about assessment and management of pain) revealed that parents in the pain education group had fewer concerns about the use of paracetamol (acetaminophen) for their child undergoing day surgery and expressed more positive attitudes toward children's pain medications. However, there were no group differences in medication administration or pain assessment on the first 2 days after surgery. As a result of this study, the investigators concluded that simply providing print materials about pain is not enough to change parental behaviour, more targeted educational strategies are needed to improve parental pain assessment and management.

A recent exemplar of this type of targeted parental educational programme is the Pediatric PRO-SELF Pain Control Program which includes a comprehensive teaching booklet to increase parent's knowledge, pain management diary to track analgesic dosing, a timer to insure adherence with analgesic regimen, and interactive nurse coaching (Sutters et al., 2011). Further advances in technology provide pain education through real time telehealth (videoconferencing), social media (blogs), Web-based modules, and email or text messaging with pain professionals. For example, the Arthritis Foundation website includes specific education on parenting a child with juvenile arthritis and interactive capabilities with medical experts to answer questions about treatment, easing pain, and coping strategies. Moreover, parents have noted that activities such as blogging to track their child's pain can be an invaluable coping tool (Kuttner, 2010). Technology provides new opportunities to educate parents about their child's pain. However, much research is needed in the methodological development of these strategies and to test their effectiveness. (See also Stinson and Jibb, Chapter 55, this volume.)

Health care professionals' knowledge about paediatric pain

Nurses' knowledge about paediatric pain

Over the past 15 years, seven studies have examined nurses' knowledge about paediatric pain (Table 63.1). The results of these studies suggest gaps remain in nurses' knowledge. These studies have not all used the same questionnaire, thus precluding precise comparisons. However, the results provide an indication of where gaps in knowledge are; there seem to be particular issues in relation to pain assessment, analgesic drugs, and non-pharmacological methods. The one study that took place in the developing world (Ekim et al., in press) suggests there are greater gaps in knowledge than in other countries. Further research is needed to explore this in other developing countries and to identify effective ways of providing required education.

Other health care professionals' knowledge about paediatric pain

Little research has been carried out in relation to medical staffs' knowledge about paediatric pain. One study suggests paediatric residents (registrars) have gaps in knowledge similar to those identified with nurses (Saroyan et al., 2008). This pilot study tested the hypothesis that there are differences in residents' paediatric pain knowledge across different specialities (paediatrics (n = 26), orthopaedics (n = 19) and anaesthesiology (n = 15)). Paediatric residents had statistically significantly higher knowledge than those working in orthopaedics (p = 0.006) and anaesthesiology (p <0.001). The paediatric residents on average answered 60% or fewer questions correctly. Questions relating to pain assessment for preverbal and cognitively impaired children were particularly poorly answered. There were also gaps in knowledge about the maximum daily dose of paracetamol (acetaminophen) and equianalgesic doses of different opioids.

Kolarik and colleagues, in one US hospital, explored paediatric residents' (n = 49) perceptions about their educational needs in palliative care (Kolarik et al., 2006). Residents indicated they had little training, experience, or knowledge in most areas of paediatric palliative care and wanted more education regarding pain management. Similarly, a study amongst paediatric occupational therapists (n = 129) found only a moderate awareness of issues relating to pain in children (Turnquist and Engel, 1994). Participants thought the education received prior to qualification was limited and their current knowledge was inadequate.

There is a paucity of research in this area but from the studies carried out we can surmise that knowledge deficits exist across all professional groups. Recent reviews of curricula content in the

Table 63.1 Summary of studies examining nurses' knowledge

Author	Sample and questionnaire	Gaps in knowledge and mean score
Salantera et al. (1999)	Paediatric nurses (n=265) in Finland Completed a knowledge and attitudes questionnaire.	◆ Analgesic drugs ◆ Non-pharmacological methods Mean score: 63%
Twycross (2004)	Paediatric nurses (n=12) Used a modified version of Salantera's questionnaire	◆ Analgesic drugs ◆ Non-pharmacological methods ◆ Physiology of pain ◆ Psychology and sociology of pain Mean score: 78%
Manworren (2000)	Paediatric nurses (n=274) Pediatric Nurses' Knowledge and Attitudes Regarding Pain Survey	◆ Pain assessment ◆ Pharmacology of analgesic drugs ◆ Use of analgesic drugs ◆ Non-pharmacological methods Mean score: 66%
Vincent (2005)	Paediatric nurses (n=67) Adapted version of the Nurses' Knowledge and Attitudes Regarding Pain Survey	◆ Non-pharmacological methods ◆ Analgesic drugs ◆ Incidence of respiratory depression Mean score: 76%
Rieman and Gordon (2007)	Paediatric nurses (n=295) working in Shriner's Hospitals in the USA Revised version of the Pediatric Nurses' Knowledge and Attitudes Regarding Pain Survey.	◆ Pharmacology ◆ Incidence of respiratory depression Mean score: 74%
Tierman (2009)	Paediatric nurses (n=292) in Ireland Pediatric Nurses' Knowledge and Attitudes Regarding Pain Survey	◆ Pharmacology (particularly opioids) ◆ Pharmacokinetics ◆ Non-pharmacological methods Mean score: 62%
Ekim et al. 2012	Paediatric nurses (n=224) from five paediatric hospitals in Turkey Pediatric Nurses' Knowledge and Attitudes Regarding Pain Survey	◆ Pharmacology and the use of opioid analgesia ◆ Addiction ◆ Accuracy of child's self-report of pain Mean score: 38%

UK and Canada suggest limited input about pain within pre-qualification curricula (Briggs et al., 2011; Twycross and Roderique, 2011; Watt-Watson et al., 2009). This is despite the International Association for the Study of Pain (IASP) (2005) having published a Core Curriculum for Professional Education in Pain. The lack of pain content may impact on the quality of care provided to children and indicate a need for post-qualification training.

Is knowledge used in practice?

For many years it was assumed that educating health care professionals about pain management would result in better care and clinical outcomes. More recently it has been acknowledged that while knowledge is necessary, it is not sufficient for better pain care. An additional consideration must, therefore, be whether health care professionals use their knowledge in practice (see also Yamada and Hutchinson, Chapter 61, this volume). Limited research has been carried out in this area but two studies have explored the relationship between paediatric nurses' theoretical knowledge and the quality of their pain management practices.

Vincent and Denyes (2004) examined the relationship between knowledge and nurses' (n = 67) analgesic administration practices.

They observed the care of children (n = 132), aged 3½ to 17 years, and found nurses with a better knowledge about pain were not more likely to administer pain medications. In the second study, the researcher shadowed nurses (n = 12) to collect data about their postoperative pain management practices (Twycross, 2007). Participants also completed a modified version of Salantera's paediatric pain knowledge questionnaire (Table 63.1). When questionnaire scores were compared to observational data no relationship between individual nurse's level of knowledge and how well they managed pain was found. Even when nurses had a good level of knowledge, this was not reflected in their pain management practices. This study had a small sample size but, along with the results of Vincent and Denyes' study, suggests nurses may not apply knowledge in practice consistently. Research relating to other health care professionals' use of pain knowledge in practice has not been carried out. Future research should explore whether similar findings occur across professional groups.

Why isn't knowledge used in practice?

The Promoting Action on Research Implementation in Health Services (PARiHS) model was developed as a way of understanding

Table 63.2 Elements of PARiHS model

Element	Sub-element
Evidence	Research
	Clinical experience
	Patient experience
	Local data/information
Context	Culture
	Leadership
	Evaluation
Facilitation	Low inappropriate facilitation
	High appropriate facilitation

Source: data from Rycroft-Malone, J, Promoting Action of Research Implementation in Health Services (PARIHS), in Rycroft-Malone, J and Bucknall, T (eds.), *Models and Frameworks for Implementing Evidence-Based Practice: Linking Evidence to Action,* Wiley-Blackwell, Oxford, UK, pp. 109–136, Copyright © 2010.

the complexity of implementing evidence (and knowledge) into practice (Rycroft-Malone, 2010). The model provides a structure to support behaviour change and consists of three elements (Table 63.2), focusing on the interaction of the quality of the evidence with the context, and methods of facilitating knowledge translation. All three elements impact on health care professionals' readiness to change their pain practices thus providing an explanation for why education alone is not enough.

Gaps in knowledge about the pharmacology of analgesic drugs and the anatomy and physiology of pain may mean the rationale for implementing pain-relieving interventions is not understood. If health care professionals lack knowledge about pain assessment they may lack confidence, or be unable, to assess children's pain. Similarly if knowledge deficits exist in relation to non-pharmacological methods of pain-relief health care professionals may not feel confident using these strategies. If the PARiHS model is applied, gaps in knowledge may mean health care professionals do not have access to the evidence to use in practice.

Beliefs and attitudes are related to individual's knowledge and clinical experience and thus link to the PARiHS model. Nurses appear to believe some pain is to be expected (and accepted) during hospitalization (Hamers et al., 1994; Woodgate and Kristjanson, 1996). Further, nurses may see pain management as synonymous with administering analgesic drugs (Twycross, 2004; Twycross et al., 2013). Nurses may not attribute as much priority to pain management as they do to other aspects of their role (Twycross, 1999; Vincent, 2005). Although it should be noted the importance nurses attribute to pain management tasks does not necessarily reflect the likelihood of the task being undertaken in practice (Twycross, 2008).

Context is one of the elements of the PARiHS model. Over the past decade there has been a growing awareness that a ward/unit has a set of informal rules that determine how pain is managed. This was demonstrated by the results of Lauzon-Clabo's (2008) ethnographic study on two (adult) wards in one hospital in the US. Participants described a clear but different pattern of pain assessment on each ward. The social context of the ward appeared to influence practices. Further, in one Canadian study, paediatric nurses described the unit's pain management culture as giving pain medications regularly even if they are prescribed

prn; this appeared to be the factor that impacted most on practice (Twycross et al., 2013. Context clearly has a place in ensuring knowledge is used in practice. Indeed, it has been postulated that pain management practices remain poor because contextual factors are not taken into account (Bucknall et al., 2001; Craig, 2009). Future research should explore strategies that facilitate sustainable changes in unit culture.

The PARiHS model describes facilitators as having a key role in changing practice (Harvey et al., 2002). Indeed, a systematic review concluded that the use of local opinion leaders was an effective way of promoting evidence-based practice (Flodgren et al., 2011). As part of an action research project, Williams et al. (2010) evaluated the impact of pain resource nurses (PRNs; link nurses) acting as local opinion leaders (n = 30) in two Australian hospitals. Results demonstrated that 11 months after the introduction of PRNs:

◆ More patients had a pain score recorded on the daily observational chart ($\chi^2 = 6.038$, p = 0.014) and in the nursing care plan ($\chi^2 = 5.11$, p = 0.024).

◆ An increase in the number of patients with a pain score documented each nursing shift (morning shift: $\chi^2 = 35.146$, p <0.001; afternoon shift: $\chi^2 = 11.717$, p <0.001; night shift: $\chi^2 = 10.700$, p <0.001).

◆ No differences were noted in other areas.

PRNs may be a useful strategy for improving documentation practices. Further evaluation is needed to explore the impact on patient outcomes.

Some of the reasons knowledge is not used in practice have been explored using the PARiHS model. As well as helping us understand why knowledge is not always used in practice it also helps to identify which interventions may help to address this.

Strategies for educating health care professionals about paediatric pain

Educational strategies

A literature review carried out in 2002 concluded that not all educational interventions designed to improve health care professionals' knowledge about pain actually did so (Twycross, 2002). Successful programmes used a variety of teaching methods (interactive and didactic) and encouraged students to reflect on practice. Francke et al. (1995) had some success using confluent education methods that emphasize the importance of integrating left-brain knowledge with right brain creativity. This is similar to a stance adopted by Murinson et al. (2011). These teaching methods help ensure the integration of theory and practice, and acknowledge learner's feelings and experiences (Francke and Erkens, 1994). Examples of these teaching methods can be seen in Box 63.1.

Using a variety of teaching strategies to enhance learning is supported by the results of a systematic review, exploring the effectiveness of continuing medical education in changing practice and health outcomes (Foresetlund et al., 2009). Educational meetings alone are unlikely to change complex behaviours. Two factors were found to increase the likelihood of behaviour change and improved patient outcomes: using a mixture of interactive and didactic teaching methods, and focusing on outcomes perceived as serious. However, the effect is likely to be small

> **Box 63.1** Examples of confluent education methods
>
> ◆ Using students' clinical experiences within group discussions
> ◆ Role play
> ◆ Clinical simulations
> ◆ Gaming
> ◆ Case studies
> ◆ Reflection on what individuals have learnt from the sessions
> ◆ Reflection on how this learning will be applied in practice
> ◆ Students sharing how will apply learning in practice (with the group).

Educational outreach visits

Educational outreach visits (EOVs) involve people visiting clinicians where they practise and providing them with information to change how they practise (Soumerai and Avorn, 1990). EOVs can take many forms. Some examples of the strategies used are provided in Box 63.2. A systematic review of 69 studies examined the effectiveness of EOVs on changing practices and health care outcomes (O'Brien et al., 2008). EOVs alone, or combined with other interventions, have a relatively consistent but small impact on prescribing practice. Their effect in other areas varied from small to modest improvements.

The impact of EOVs on pain management practices in primary care has been explored in one study (Schechter et al., 2010). A 1 h teaching session on pain reduction strategies during childhood immunizations was provided to staff in 13 practices in one state in the US. At 1 month parents were: more likely to report receiving information (p = 0.04); using strategies to reduce pain (p <0.01); learning something new (p <0.01); using a Shotblocker® (p <0.01); and higher levels of satisfaction (p = 0.015). Rates all remained higher at 6 months (p <0.01) except for satisfaction. Clinician surveys at 6 months revealed significant increases in the use of longer needles (infants: p = 0.34; toddlers: p <0.001; adolescents: p = 0.002), sucrose (p = 0.003), pinwheels (p <0.001), focused breathing (p = 0.021), and Shotblockers® (p <0.001). There was no statistical difference in the use of topical anaesthetics. EOVs may be a useful strategy for changing pain management practices but further research is needed.

Individual feedback

Audit and feedback can be a useful method for changing practices within clinical areas but the effects are variable and are particularly effective where there is low compliance with a given standard (Jamtvedt et al., 2006). The effect of individual feedback

> **Box 63.2** Examples of EOV activities
>
> ◆ Feedback about performance
> ◆ Feedback on previously identified obstacles to change
> ◆ Mini-education sessions
> ◆ Roving education rounds
> ◆ Teaching moments.

on paediatric pain management practices has been explored in a clustered randomized trial in six Canadian paediatric hospitals (Johnston et al., 2007). Coaching with individual audit feedback from a chart review was provided every 2 weeks, for 6 months, by an opinion leader. Some changes were found between the experimental and control groups although there were inconsistencies across sites. For example:

◆ Documented pain assessments increased in the coaching group (from 15% to 58%, χ^2 = 138.34, p <0.0001) and decreased in the control group (from 24% to 9%, χ^2 = 34.86, p <0.001).

◆ The use of non-pharmacological interventions increased in the coaching group (from 5% to 16%, χ^2 = 28.48, p <0.0001) and decreased in the control group (from 1.5% to 0.3%, χ^2 = 2.23, p = not significant).

◆ Nurses' knowledge increased in the coaching group but decreased in the control group ($F_{(1, 791)}$ = 106.3, p< 0.0001).

Coaching has also been used successfully with nurses caring for (adult) patients undergoing an arthroscopy (Duncan and Pozehl, 2001). However, providing individual feedback is resource intensive; an economic evaluation needs undertaking before implementing this strategy more widely.

Web-based interventions

Web-based educational courses are becoming more common partly because in today's health service there is a need to ensure health care professionals receive education in as cost-effective way as possible. The English Department of Health advocate the use of e-learning as one way of addressing this issue (Department of Health, 2008). One paediatric pain e-learning product was launched in February 2012 and is made up of six units that can be purchased together or individually covering:

◆ Pharmacology of analgesic drugs

◆ Anatomy and physiology of pain

◆ Pain assessment

◆ Non-pharmacological methods of pain-relief

◆ Managing acute pain

◆ Managing procedure-related pain.

The course is aimed at registered health care professionals. Further information can be found at: <http://www.healthcare.ac.uk/cppd/short-courses-postgraduate/managing-pain-in-children-(elearning)/>.

Web-based courses need evaluating to ascertain their effectiveness in increasing knowledge and changing practice, as well as exploring how their impact compares to courses taught face-to-face. One randomized controlled trial has compared the effectiveness of Web-based training about the use of opioid therapy for chronic pain to being given a copy of current clinical guidelines for internal medicine residents (Sullivan et al., 2010). The Web-based group had a greater increase in knowledge (p <0.00001) and higher self-ratings of their competence in overall management (Wald χ^2 = 5.17, df = 1, p = 0.02) and in prescribing opioids (Wald χ^2 = 5.17, df = 1, p = 0.02). However, the Web-based training also covered shared decision-making (patient and doctor) and communication skills; it may have been this difference rather than the content relating to the use of opioids that was effective. Another study evaluated the effect of a Web-based palliative care module for medical residents in one US hospital (Dy et al., 2008). Knowledge about palliative care did not increase simply by completing the 4-year residency programme but undertaking the Web-based course resulted in a larger increase in knowledge.

Conclusion

Children and parents require education about pain and pain management. To date there is little research exploring the best ways to provide this education other than in relation to preparing children for surgery or painful procedures. When developing educational materials for children cognitive and psychosocial factors need taking into account. There is a need to create and test educational resources for children. Resources are needed for parents that increase knowledge as well as supporting them to advocate for their child. Technology provides new opportunities in this context.

Gaps remain in health care professionals' knowledge about pain that are greater in the developing world. Further research is needed to explore this across all professional groups. For practices to change education needs to be provided alongside other strategies promoting the use of knowledge in practice; education alone is not enough. The PARiHS model has been used to provide an explanation for why knowledge is not used in practice. This needs testing further; organizational culture and the role of facilitation need particular attention. Educational interventions should include a mixture of interactive and didactic teaching. Strategies that help link education with practice should also be encouraged such as reflection, clinical simulations, and the use of case studies. Web-based materials are available but their effectiveness needs evaluating.

References

American Nurses Association. (2001). *Code of ethics for nurses with interpretive statements*. Silver Spring, MD: American Nurses Association.

American Nurses Association. (2005). *Pain management nursing: scope and standards of practice*. Silver Spring, MD: Nurses Books.

American Nurses Association. (2008). *Pediatric nursing: scope and standards of practice*. Silver Spring, MD: Nurses Books.

Association of Pediatric Hematology/Oncology Nurses. (2007). *Pediatric oncology nursing: scope and standards of practice*. Glenview, IL: Association of Pediatric Hematology/Oncology Nurses.

Berenstain, S. (1981). *The Berenstain bears go to the doctor*. New York: Random House.

Briggs, E., Carr E. C. J., and Whittaker, M. (2011). Survey of undergraduate pain curricula for healthcare professionals in the United Kingdom. *Eur J Pain*, 15, 789–795.

Brillhart, B. (2007). Internet education for spinal cord injury patients: focus on urinary management. *Rehabil Nurs*, 32(5), 214–219.

Bucknall, T., Manias, E., and Botti, M. (2001). Acute pain management: implications of scientific evidence for nursing practice in the postoperative context. *Int J Nurs Pract*, 7(4), 266–273.

Chambers, C., Reid, G., McGrath, P. J., and Finley, G. A. (1997). A randomized trial of a pain education booklet: effects on parents' attitudes and postoperative pain management, *Child Health Care*, 26(1), 1–13.

Child Life Council. (2007). *Child Life Council evidence-based practice statement: preparing children and adolescents for medical procedures*. Rockville, MD.

Craig, K. D. (2009). The social communication module of pain. *Can Psychol*, 20, 22–32.

Curtiss, C. (2010). The pain management nurse as an educator. In B. St. Marie (ed.) *Core curriculum for pain management nursing*, pp. 659–672. Dubuque, IA: Kendall Hunt Professional.

Department of Health. (2008). *Modern healthcare training: e-learning in healthcare services*. London: The Stationery Office.

DiMaggio, T., Clark, L., and Czarnecki, M. (2010). Pediatric pain management. In B. St. Marie (ed.) *Core curriculum for pain management nursing*, pp. 481–542. Dubuque, IA: Kendall Hunt Professional.

Duncan, K. and Pozehl, B. (2001). Effects of individual performance feedback on nurses' adherence to pain management clinical guidelines. *Outcome Manage Nurs Pract*, 5, 57–62.

Dy, S. M., Hughes, M., Weiss, C., and Sisson, S. (2008). Evaluation of a web-based palliative care pain management programme for housestaff. *J Pain Symptom Manage*, 36(6), 596–603.

Ekim, A. and Ocakci, A. F. (2012). Knowledge and attitudes regarding pain management of pediatric nurses in Turkey. *Pain Manag* Nurs, 6 April. [Epub ahead of print.]

Finley, G. A., McGrath, P. J., Forward, S., McNeill, G., and Fitzgerald, P. (1996). Parents' management of children's pain following minor surgery. *Pain*, 64, 83–87.

Flodgren, G., Parmelli, E., Doumit, G., Gattellari, M., O'Brien, M. A., Grimshaw, J., et al. (2011). Local opinion leaders: Effects on professional practice and health care outcomes. *Cochrane Database Syst Rev*, 8, CD000125.

Fortier, M. A., MacLaren, J. E., Martin, S., Perret-Karimi, D., and Kain, Z. N. (2009). Pediatric pain after ambulatory surgery: where's the medication? *Pediatrics*, 134 (4), e588–e595.

Franck, L., Allen, A., Cox, S., and Winter, I. (2005). Parents' views about infant pain in neonatal intensive care. *Clin J Pain*, 21(2), 133–139.

Francke, A. L. and Erkens, T. (1994). Confluent education: an integrative method for nursing (continuing education). *J Adv Nurs*, 19, 356–361.

Francke, A. L., Garssen, B., and Abu-Saad, H. H. (1995). Determinants of changes in nurses' behaviour after continuing education: a literature review. *J Adv Nurs*, 21, 371–377.

Gaes, J. (1987). *My book for kids with cansur*. Aberdeen, SD: Melius & Peterson Publishing.

Greenberg, R. S., Billett, C, Zahurak, M., and Yaster, M. (1999). Videotape increases parental knowledge about pediatric pain management. *Pediatr Anesth*, 89, 899–903.

Harbeck, C. and Peterson, L. (1992). Elephants dancing in my head: a developmental approach to children's concepts of specific pains. *Child Dev*, 63, 138–149.

Harvey, G., Loftus-Hills, A., Rycroft-Malone, J., Titchen, A., Kitson, A., McCormack, B., et al. (2002). Getting evidence into practice: the role and function of facilitation. *J Adv Nurs*, 37(6), 577–588.

Huth, M., Broome, M., Mussatto, K., and Morgan, S. W. (2003). A study of the effectiveness of a pain management education booklet for parents of children having cardiac surgery. *Pain Manag Nurs*, 4(1), 31–39.

Idvall, E., Holm, C., and Runeson, I. (2005). Pain experiences and non-pharmacological strategies for pain management after tonsillectomy: a qualitative interview study of children and parents. *J Child Health Care*, 9, 196–207.

International Association of the Study of Pain. (2005). *Core curriculum for professional education in pain* (3rd edn). Seattle, WA: IASP Press.

Jamtvedt, G., Young J. M., Kristoffersen, D. T., O'Brien, M. A., and Oxman, A. D. (2006). Audit and feedback: effects on professional practice and healthcare outcomes. *Cochrane Database Syst Rev*, 2, CD000259.

Jones, M, Qazi, M., and Young, K. (2005). Ethnic differences in parent preference to be present for painful medical procedures. *Pediatrics*, 116 (2), e191–e197.

Kolarik, R. C., Walker, G., and Arnold, R. M. (2006). Pediatric residents in palliative care: a needs assessment. *Pediatrics*, 117(6), 1949–1954.

Kotzer, A., Coy, J., and LeClaire, A. (1998). The effectiveness of a standardized educational programme for children using patient-controlled analgesia. *J Soc Pediatr Nurs*, 3, 117–126.

Kuttner, L. (2010). *A child in pain: what health professionals can do to help*. Bethel, CT: Crown House Publishing.

LeMay, S., Johnston, C., Choiniere, M., Fortin, C., Hubert, I., Fréchette, G., et al. (2010). Pain management interventions with parents in the emergency department: a randomized trial. *J Adv Nurs*, 66(11), 2442–2449.

Li, H., Lopez, V., and Lee, T. (2006). Psychoeducational preparation of children for surgery: the importance of parental involvement. *Patient Educ Couns*, 65, 34–41.

Manworren, R. C. B. (2000). Pediatric nurses' knowledge and attitudes survey regarding pain. *Pediatr Nurs*, 26(6), 610–614.

McGrath, P. A. (1990). *Pain in children: nature, assessment and treatment.* New York: Guilford.

McGrath, P. J., Finley, G. A., and Turner, C. (1992). *Making cancer less painful: a handbook for parents.* Halifax, NS: Dalhousie University.

McGrath, P. J., Finley, G. A., and Ritchie, J. (1994). *Pain, pain, go away: helping children with pain.* Bethesda, MD: Association for the Care of Children's Health.

McGrath, P. J., Watters, C., and Moon, E. (2010). Technology in pediatric pain management. In G. A. Finley, P. J. McGrath, and C. Chambers (eds.), *Bringing pain relief to children: treatment approaches*, pp. 159–176. Totowa, NJ: Humana.

Murinson, B., Mezel, L., and Nenortes, E. (2011). Integrating cognitive and affective dimensions of pain experience into health professions education. *Pain Res Manag*, 16(6), 421–426.

Oakes, L. (2011). *Infant and child pain management.* New York: Springer Publishing Company.

O'Brien, M. A., Rogers, S., Jamtvedt, G., Oxman, A. D., Odgaard-Jensen, J., Kristoffersen, D. T., et al. (2008). Educational outreach visits: effects on professional practice and health care outcomes. *Cochrane Database Syst Rev*, 4, CD000409.

O'Conner-Von, S. (2000). Preparing children for surgery: an integrative research review. *AORN J*, 71(2), 334–343.

O'Conner-Von, S. (2008). Preparation of adolescents for outpatient surgery: using an Internet program. *AORN J*, 87(2), 374–398.

O'Conner-Von, S. (2009). Coping with cancer: a web-based educational programme for early and middle adolescents. *J Pediatr Oncol Nurs*, 26(4), 230–241.

Palermo, T. and Valenzuela, D. (2003). Use of pain diaries to assess recurrent and chronic pain in children. *Suffering Child*, 3, 1–14.

Rieman, M. T., Gordon, M., and Marvin, J. M. (2007). Pediatric nurses' knowledge and attitudes survey regrading pain: a competency tool modification. *Pediatr Nurs*, 33(4), 303–313.

Rycroft-Malone, J. (2010). Promoting Action of Research Implementation in Health Services (PARIHS). In J. Rycroft-Malone and T. Bucknall (eds.) *Models and frameworks for implementing evidence-based practice: linking evidence to action*, pp. 109–136. Oxford: Wiley-Blackwell.

Salantera, S., Lauri, S., Salmi, T. T., and Helenius, H. (1999). Nurses' knowledge about pharmacological and non-pharmacological pain management in children. *J Pain Symptom Manage*, 18(4), 289–299.

Sato, A., Clifford, L., Silverman, A., and Davies, W. H. (2009). Cognitive-behavioral interventions via telehealth; application to pediatric functional abdominal pain, *Child Health Care*, 38, 1–22.

Finley, G. A. and Schechter, N. L. (2003). Sedation. In N. Schechter, C. Berde, and M. Yaster (eds) *Pain in infants, children, and adolescents*, pp. 563–577. New York: Lippincott Williams & Wilkins,

Schechter, N. L., Bernstein, B. A., Zempsky, W., Bright, N. S., and Willard, A. K. (2010). Educational outreach to reduce immunization pain in office settings, *Pediatrics*, 126(6), e1514–e1521.

Simons, J., Franck, L., and Roberson, E (2001). Parent involvement in children's pain care: views of parents and nurses. *J Adv Nurs*, 36 (4), 591–599.

Simons, J. and Roberson, E. (2002). Poor communication and knowledge deficits: obstacles to effective management of children's postoperative pain. *J Adv Nurs*, 40 (1), 78–86.

Stinson, J., McGrath, P. J., Hodnet, E., Feldman, B. M., Duffy, C. M., Huber, A. M., et al. (2012). An internet-based self-management program with telephone support for adolescents with arthritis: a pilot randomized controlled trial. *J Rheumatol*, 37(9), 1944–1952.

Soumerai, S. B. and Avorn, J. (1990). Principles of education outreach ('academic detailing') to improve clinical decision making. *JAMA*, 263(4), 549–556.

Sullivan, M. D., Gaster, B., Russo, J., Bowlby, L., Rocco, N., Sinex, N., et al. (2010). Randomized trial of web-based training about opioid therapy for chronic pain. *Clin J Pain*, 26(6), 512–517.

Sutters, K., Savedra, M., and Miaskowski, C. (2011). The pediatric PRO-SELF Pain control program: an effective educational program for parents caring for children at home following tonsillectomy. *J Specialist Pediatr Nurs*, 16, 280–294.

Tait, A., Voepel-Lewis, T., Snyder, R., and Malviya, S. (2008). Parents' understanding of information regarding their child's postoperative pain management. *Clin J Pain*, 24(7), 572–577.

Tiernan, E. P. (2009). A survey of registered nurses' knowledge and attitudes regarding paediatric pain assessment and management: an Irish perspective. *Arch Dis Child*, 93(1002), n18.

Turnquist, K. M. and Engel, J. M. (1994). Occupational therapists' experiences and knowledge of pain in children, *Phys Occup Ther Pediatr*, 14(1), 35–52.

Twycross, A. (2002). Educating nurses about pain management: the way forward. *J Clin Nurs*, 11, 705–714.

Twycross, A. (2004). Children's nurses' pain management practices: theoretical knowledge, perceived importance and decision-making. Unpublished PhD Thesis, University of Central Lancashire.

Twycross, A. (2007). What is the impact of theoretical knowledge on children's nurses' postoperative pain management practices? An exploratory study. *Nurse Educ Today*, 27(7), 697–707.

Twycross, A. (2008). Does the perceived importance of a pain management task affect the quality of children's nurses' post-operative pain management practices? *J Clin Nurs*, 17(23), 3205–3216.

Twycross, A. and Collis, S. (2012). How well is acute pain in children managed? A snapshot in one English hospital. *Pain Manag Nurs*. 29 March. [Epub ahead of print.]

Twycross, A. and Finley, G. A. (in press). Parents' and children's views about pain management. *J Clin Nurs*.

Twycross, A., Finley, G. A. and Latimer, M. (2013). An in-depth study of pediatric post-operative pain management practices. *J Specialist Pediatr Nurs*. 24 March. [Epub ahead of print.]

Twycross, A. and Roderique, L. (2011). Review of pain content in three-year preregistration pediatric nursing courses in the United Kingdom. *Pain Manag Nurs*. 11 July. [Epub ahead of print.]

Uman, L., Chambers, C., McGrath, P. J., and Kisely, S. (2010). Psychological interventions for needle-related procedural pain and distress in children and adolescents. *Cochrane Database Syst Rev*, 11, CD005179. Available at <http://www.thecochranelibrary.com>.

US Department of Health and Human Services (1992). *Acute pain management in infants, children, and adolescents: operative and medical procedure. Quick reference guide for clinicians.* AHCPR Pub. No. 92–0020. Rockville, MD: Agency for Health Care Policy and Research.

Vincent, C. V. H. (2005). Nurses' knowledge, attitudes, and practices regarding children's pain. *MCN*, 30(3), 177–183.

Vincent, C. V. H. and Denyes, M. J. (2004). Relieving children's pain: nurses' abilities and analgesic administration practices. *J Pediatr Nurs*, 19(1), 40–50.

Watt-Watson, J, McGillon, M., Hunter, J., Choiniere, M., Clark, A. J., Dewar, A., et al. (2009). A survey of prelicensure pain curricula in health science faculties in Canadian universities. *Pain Res Manag*, 14(4), 439–444.

Wisconsin Cancer Pain Initiative. (1989). *Children's cancer pain can be relieved.* Madison, WI: University of Wisconsin.

Wood, D. (1993). *How children think and learn.* Cambridge, MA: Blackwell Publishers.

Zisk, R, Grey, M., Medoff-Cooper, B., and Kain, Z. N. (2007). Accuracy of parental-globe-impression of children's acute pain. *Pain Manag Nurs*, 8(2), 72–76.

Zisk-Rony, R., Fortier, M., Chorney, J., Perret, D., and Kain, Z. N. (2010). Parental postoperative pain management: attitudes, assessment, and management. *Pediatrics*, 125(8), 1372–1378.

Online supplementary materials

Figure 63.1 Additional resources

CHAPTER 64

The ethics of pain control in infants and children

Gary A. Walco and Maureen C. Kelley

Introduction

A common theme throughout writings in paediatric medicine is that 'children are not little adults', often referring to physiological and psychological differences related to maturation and development that must be taken into account in providing care. Similarly, in considering ethical challenges related to pain, it is important not to simply extrapolate from our ethical approach to pain management for adults who typically can describe their experience of pain, are fully responsible for themselves, and can represent their own interests in making treatment decisions. Unlike adults, younger children and certainly infants cannot speak for themselves and require parents and clinicians to assess their pain, determine what is in their best interest, and advocate for their well-being. However, in paediatrics, these assessments occur in the context of a child's evolving developmental capacities: as older children and adolescents mature, they begin to understand and participate more in decisions affecting their health, to report symptoms, and to communicate their wishes. In addition, as with other areas of clinical ethics, determination of the best ethical practice must be considered against the backdrop of evolving data and evidence. Recent advances in the science of pain assessment can help inform the balance of competing ethical values related to pain in infants and children.

In this chapter we will offer a way of framing the ethical balance of competing considerations in pain treatment in infants and children, distinguishing between analyses of harms and benefits, from other more pragmatic, contextual, and cultural considerations. We begin with the ethical foundations behind good pain management for any patient, and especially children: the ethical duty to prevent harm by alleviating pain or suffering, and the importance of assuring equal access to pain treatment. Historically, the driving ethical concern in paediatric pain has been the pervasive undertreatment of pain in children. In the second and main section of the chapter, we offer a detailed analysis of the practical ethical challenges involved in weighing the harms and benefits of pain relief against untreated or undertreated pain. In the third section, we will discuss the more specific concerns of socioeconomic and cultural determinants to paediatric pain treatment. Finally, in the last section, we will address concerns in conducting research on pain

interventions in infants and children, as clearly many of the modal methodologies traditionally used for clinical trials in adults (e.g. placebo control designs) pose unjustifiable risk to younger individuals. We will also discuss the importance of considering local context as it impacts standards of care to guide ethical paediatric pain research.

Ethical foundations of clinical pain control in paediatrics

The starting point in thinking about the ethics of pain control in paediatrics is relatively uncontroversial at first glance. Few would disagree that alleviating suffering is fundamentally a good thing, especially among the youngest and most vulnerable human beings, and should thus be pursued universally. Failure to address pain in any patient would constitute a straightforward violation of the Hippocratic harm principle: 'First, do no harm' (Adams, 1891). Further, failure to address pain, when we have the means to do so, violates an important and basic human right to dignity and prevention of suffering (James, 1993). While the harm principle is an effective argument against undertreatment of pain, the rights argument lends a more powerful universal appeal to the case for expanding access to pain treatment to all children, regardless of background, socioeconomic status, or geographical location (Southall et al., 2000). Such a perspective shapes the position of the World Health Organization on pain in children (World Health Organization, 1998), and the recent International Association for the Study of Pain, the Declaration of Montreal (Cousins and Lynch, 2011), which states:

Recognizing the intrinsic dignity of all persons and that withholding of pain treatment is profoundly wrong, leading to unnecessary suffering which is harmful; we declare that the following human rights must be recognized throughout the world:
Article 1. The right of all people to have access to pain management without discrimination.
Article 2. The right of people in pain to acknowledgment of their pain and to be informed about how it can be assessed and managed.
Article 3. The right of all people with pain to have access to appropriate assessment and treatment of the pain by adequately trained health care professionals.

Because pain is very common in hospitalized children, the International Association for the Study of Pain, Special Interest Group on Pain in Childhood supported the Bellagio Declaration (ChildKind International, 2010), calling for all health care facilities to commit to the developmentally appropriate prevention, assessment, and management of pain in children and adolescents aged 0 to 18 years. Lack of knowledge and subjective biases often have influenced decision-making about pain treatment in children, leaving the deleterious effects of untreated pain minimized or ignored. Such deleterious outcomes violate the principle of do no harm and a comprehensive and balanced analysis, relying on data rather than personal bias or speculation, is required.

For addressing pain in older children and adolescents, developmental appropriateness in clinical assessment and interventions also tracks to the involvement of the more mature paediatric patient in pain management decisions. The growing literature in child development over the past two decades has helped shape a much more nuanced approach to ethical decision-making with adolescent patients. The now standard ethical model calls for the increasing respect for the developing autonomy of teens and young adults as they develop the capacities to understand medical information, appreciate the implications of various health decisions, and develop the ability to weigh the risks and benefits of immediate and long-term consequences (American Academy of Pediatrics Committee on Bioethics, 1995). These decisions are ideally made with parental permission and support, not in isolation, but as paediatric patients are increasingly able to participate in important health decisions, they should be encouraged to do so, and their questions, concerns, and decisions should be increasingly respected (Ross, 1998). In the context of pain, this requires listening carefully and principally to the voice of the patient, since even the most well-meaning parents may err in interpreting the symptoms of suffering or pain in their own children. Beyond the very important principle of respecting the adolescent patient's emerging voice and autonomy, so much of good pain management depends on quality communication with the patient. Actively involving more mature patients becomes particularly important in addressing recurrent or chronic pain and in palliative settings, where ongoing relationships with patients are so important to providing the best care.

Balancing harm and benefit of paediatric pain control in clinical practice

Withholding pain treatment without further justification constitutes a violation of the harm principle in medicine, and may, as well, constitute unjust suffering and violation of the basic human right to dignity and non-discrimination in health treatment. However, as is often the case in practical clinical ethics, the apparent 'no brainer' of alleviating pain and suffering in an unqualified manner becomes a bit less straightforward in clinical practice (Lantos and Meadow, 2007). While the ethical foundation driving improved pain treatment and control in children provides strong impetus for addressing undertreatment or unequal access to treatment, we need a more nuanced approach to guide actual clinical decisions at the bedside. The balance of harm and benefit in alleviating pain in infants and children needs to be evidence based and requires appreciation of context. As the evidence evolves, preventing or minimizing present and long-term harm in children can become a more challenging balancing act. The expression and meaning of pain are subject

to cultural influences; it is a significantly subjective experience. Because we do not have undisputed data to guide us on many of the decisions we make, individuals' perspectives come into play.

Walco et al. (1994) argued that because pain and related suffering seem harmful to patients, and because caregivers are categorically committed to preventing harm in their patients, not using all available means of relieving pain must be justified. Both sides of this balance, however, have shifted a great deal over time. As outlined by Olmstead et al. (2010), our thinking on this topic has evolved. Until about four decades ago, the general lore was that young children, in particular, did not experience pain and certainly had no lasting memory of it if they did. Thus, the harm of untreated pain was not recognized. In the late 1970s and onward, there was increasing recognition that pain was undertreated in children compared to adults and that even very young premature infants have nociceptive systems in place and thus have capacity for pain perception. The work of developmental physiologists provided even greater insights and by the turn of the century, there were ample data to show that untreated or undertreated pain in young children was associated with lasting deleterious effects (Fitzgerald, 2005) (see Grunau, Chapter 4, this volume).

Three potential justifications have been proposed for not adequately treating pain in children, namely revisionist, comparative, and pragmatic justifications (Walco et al., 1994).

First, because pain is fundamentally a private, subjective experience, it is difficult to assess with validity, especially in the youngest patients who do not express themselves verbally. A *revisionist* justification focused principally on aspects of pain assessment in the young and involves a tendency for care providers to 'overrule' or 'revise' evidence of pain based on a number of preconceived notions, such as believing there is a 'correct' amount of pain associated with a given degree of tissue damage or pathophysiological condition, as well as attributions to other more benign factors (the infant is cold or hungry as opposed to in pain). In the last two decades, the field has come a long way in demonstrating reliable, valid, and clinically sensitive means of assessing pain in children of all ages (see Lee and Stevens, Chapter 35; von Baeyer, Chapter 36, this volume). Because many of the existing measures are based on physiological indicators that may be non-specific to pain, as well as observed behavioural indicators that are dependent on the expertise and knowledge of the observer, there is still risk of care providers revising or minimizing the significance of pain responses. Developing more objective indicators with enhanced reliability and validity would be most helpful (see Lee and Stevens, Chapter 35, this volume). However, to minimize or discount available data because we lack ideal assessment methods does not justify undertreating pain in the interim.

In revising children's pain complaints, care providers make implicit judgements about the validity of those responses. Such judgement and invalidation is most obvious in the use of placebos to treat pain. The clinical use of placebos to treat pain may fulfil patient and family expectations to receive *some medication* to treat the condition as well as a clinician's aim to promote a desired clinical outcome using 'inert' substances (Miller and Colloca, 2009). Consider an instance in which a child or adolescent continues to complain of pain despite being administered what is deemed by the practitioner to be sufficient quantities of analgesic medication. Especially when observed pain behaviour is inconsistent or does not match up with verbal reports, there is a tendency to attribute the pain to other than nociception, which may be 'proven' by the patient experiencing pain relief with a placebo.

Using placebos in this setting is problematic for a number of reasons. First, there is a great deal of literature to show that placebo effects operate across circumstances, including when there is little or no doubt of the pathophysiological basis of the pain (Foddy, 2009). Thus, the presumed purpose of using placebo, to determine if the pain is 'real' cannot be achieved. Second, once the patient becomes aware of the clinician's intentional deception, trust is lost not only in that provider, but in providers throughout the medical system in general (Cahana and Romagnioli, 2007; Foddy, 2009). Third, and related, if the clinician uses placebo to acquiesce to the desires of parents or family members, the threat of trust being violated extends beyond the immediate clinician-patient relationship as generalization to healthcare providers in general is possible. As a result, there is consensus, including a strong statement from the American Medical Association (Bostick et al., 2008), that the clinical use of placebos without informed consent is categorically unethical (Cahana and Romagnioli, 2007; Foddy, 2009).

A *comparative* justification focuses on weighing the benefits and risks of unrelieved pain against those of pain relief. In some circumstances, a responsible conclusion may be that the harm of unrelieved pain is less severe than the harm of pain relief. Many of the traditional concerns have focused on fears of addiction and dangerous side effects of analgesic medications, neither of which may be taken lightly. With regard to the former, certainly there is concern for misuse and addiction of opioids among children and adolescents, especially those prescribed to others and subsequently scavenged by adolescents (Bailey et al., 2009). There is little to show, however, that there is risk of addiction when these medications are appropriately prescribed and administered in paediatrics settings (Yaster et al., 2003). Thus, if one is careful about prescribing appropriate dosages and, in particular, the amount of medication prescribed in ambulatory settings, withholding opioids for pain management due to fear of addiction is not justified—this is true for all ages.

The second concern, deleterious effects of analgesic medications, requires careful cost–benefit analysis when weighing efficacy against adverse events. A common concern of opioids focuses on significant sedation and respiratory depression and, more recently, questions about long-term deleterious effects of opioid administration on cognitive development in the young have arisen.

A recent prospective study reported on the incidence, nature, and severity of serious clinical incidents (SCIs) associated with continuous opioid infusion, patient-controlled analgesia, and nurse-controlled analgesia in neonates, infants, and children under the care of paediatric acute pain teams in the UK and Eire (Morton and Errera, 2010). Predefined SCIs fell into three grades: (1) death/permanent harm; (2) harm but full recovery, technique stopped or changed, intervention required; and (3) potential harm but no actual harm. With a denominator of 10 726 opioid infusions, there were one Grade 1 SCI (cardiac arrest associated with aspiration pneumonitis and an underlying neurological condition), 28 Grade 2 SCIs, half of which were respiratory depression, and 17 Grade 3 SCIs (all of these last category occurred in a single centre related to programming or prescribing errors). It is noteworthy that of the 14 cases of respiratory depression, half of the children were less than 1 year of age. The authors emphasized the need for heightened monitoring for children posing increased risk factors, including

very young age as well as neurodevelopmental, respiratory, or cardiac comorbidities.

In children over the age of 2 years, there is consensus that the data on the safety and efficacy of opioid medications parallel findings in adults (Berde et al., 2012). However, based on developmental factors, the pharmacokinetics and pharmacodynamics of opioids are more variable in younger children. Clinically, this means that, especially in preterm and younger infants, the risk of deleterious effects, such as respiratory depression, may be greater (Simons and Anand, 2006). Thus, increased scrutiny in prescribing and administering opioid medications is needed, with special attention to aspects of the patient's status that may place them at increased risk for such complications. However, once again, these concerns should not automatically deter the use of methods to alleviate pain, recognizing that such adverse outcomes may be mitigated by proper monitoring.

A review of the literature conducted under the auspices of the American Society for Pain Management Nursing showed that there are no universally accepted guidelines to direct effective and safe assessment and monitoring practices for patients receiving opioid analgesia (Jarzyna et al., 2011). Furthermore, there have been very limited carefully controlled studies to show the actual benefits of specific monitoring methods, including pulse oximetry and capnography, in hospitalized patients receiving opioids for pain. With this as background, a position paper was generated highlighting the need to evaluate the individual patient for risk factors, including age, anatomic anomalies, physical characteristics, primary and comorbid medical conditions, psychological states, and functional status; of note risk associated with age was focused only at the upper end of the spectrum (>65 years). Based on these risk factors and the nature of the intervention, monitoring to detect difficulties early on, before serious adverse events, is deemed essential. With these safeguards, patients are not denied access to pain relieving strategies but risks of respiratory depression may be minimized. In addition, in the unfortunate circumstance when respiratory depression is of clinical significance, effective reversal agents may be used (American Academy of Pediatrics Committee on Drugs 1990). It should be noted that the guidelines espoused by Jarzyna et al. do not focus at all on paediatric populations and our review yielded no similar documents addressing the needs of children. Certainly patient safety may be enhanced with evidence-based monitoring practices for children, thereby better addressing concerns about untoward side effects of opioids used to reduce pain.

There is some question as to whether prolonged use of opioids, especially in very young infants, may have deleterious long-term effects. Specifically, opioids have often been used on an ongoing basis in an attempt to maintain the comfort of neonates who were receiving mechanical ventilation. A 5-year follow-up study indicated, however, that there may be some significant effects on intellectual functioning associated with this practice (de Graaf et al., 2011). While these data certainly serve as an alert, it is difficult to attribute deleterious outcomes specifically to opioids as there is an array of developmental, medical, and environmental factors that may impact the relatively unstable physiological systems of premature neonates (Grunau et al., 2006; see also Grunau, Chapter 4, this volume). Thus, a simple concept of 'the more the better' in utilizing agents to reduce pain and distress may need to be tempered as more data emerge (Lantos and Meadow, 2007; Mancuso and Burns, 2009).

The *pragmatic* justification focuses on the potential benefits of pain persisting. In other words, while it is acknowledged that unrelieved pain is bad, such pain may be deemed necessary to achieve a greater goal. Two general areas may be cited here, the value of pain to provide diagnostic information and the utility of pain to help build character. In the former, pain may be seen as useful to monitor an illness (cf. Bromberg and Goldman, 2007) or to indicate the ineffectiveness or limits of treatment, such as discomfort during rehabilitation after orthopaedic surgery. Eliminating or masking such pain could actually harm the patient and therefore one must weigh the benefit of immediate relief against that of long-term recovery. In such circumstances, the clinician is deemed to be operating in the patient's best interest by maintaining a degree of pain or discomfort. To assure that is the case, three specific tests should be applied. First, is the pain useful—is it the means to achieving an important goal? Second, is the pain necessary or are there other, less hurtful means of achieving that goal? Third, is the pain at the lowest possible level? Because it is not acceptable to allow children to suffer if there is any other means of achieving outcome data, if there is a therapeutic benefit from a child's pain, one must be exquisitely economical with it.

A second potential pragmatic justification derives from moral views held by some that champion traits such as courage, self-discipline, independence, and self-sacrifice. Such cultural or family views about pain may also track beliefs about gender differences: for example, that a young girl should learn to tolerate severe menstrual pain, or that a boy ought to 'tough it out' through a sports injury. Although in principle encouraging such virtues as bravery and stoicism may be ethically defensible, imposing the burden of character development on a child already encumbered by distress, sickness, or suffering reflects a lack of compassion and is ethically questionable, at best. When the total eradication of pain is not possible (as in the case of chronic pain associated with chronic illness), strengthening the child's capacity to cope with the pain is beneficial and may be justifiable. However, to intentionally allow a child to suffer in the hope of influencing character development disregards the child and the real and present need for pain relief. The scope of parental discretion, including refusals of pain treatment for reasons of character building, should be constrained by appeals to the harm principle (Diekema, 2004).

A fairly pervasive example of this phenomenon may be seen in the failure of broad-scale efforts to treat needle pain. Often statements reflecting the view that pain is a part of life and children need to cope with it serve as justification for failing to treat pain associated with needles (Taddio et al., 2009). The unfortunate outcome is that immunization rates are lowered by individuals who avoid needles and an estimated 10% of adults avoid contact with medical institutions, even when indicated, due to fear of needles (Hamilton, 1995).

Nearly 20 years ago, Walco et al. (1994, p. 543) concluded, 'All health professionals should provide care that reflects the technological growth of the field. The assessment and treatment of pain in children are important parts of paediatric practice, and failure to provide adequate control of pain amounts to substandard and unethical medical practice'. Unfortunately recent data on required and optional coursework indicate that medical school education in North America falls well short of the mark in preparing practitioners to make these informed decisions (Mezei and Murinson, 2011).

In many ways, as the knowledge base for the assessment and management of pain grows and medical education fails to keep pace, problematic outcomes appear even more amplified. A recent report from the Institute of Medicine (2011) focuses specifically on how lack of education and the overgeneralization of management principles related to acute pain have contributed to epidemic concerns about chronic pain. Certainly children are not immune from these same issues (McGrath and Ruskin 2007) and the problem is compounded by data indicating that untreated chronic pain in children and adolescents predisposes individuals to ongoing chronic pain problems well into adulthood (Dengler-Crish et al., 2011; Walker et al., 2010).

Armed with data on the poor treatment of pain in infants and children, there have been a number of initiatives advocating for improvement. Included here is a policy statement jointly issued by the American Academy of Pediatrics and the American Pain Society (American Academy of Pediatrics Committee on Psychosocial Aspects of Child and Family Health, American Pain Society Task Force on Pain in Infants, Children, and Adolescents 2001), a position statement of the International Association for the Study of Pain (IASP SIG on Pain in Childhood 2005), and a monograph by the World Health Organization (1998), all of which highlight the undertreatment of pain in infants and children and the need for improvements in the assessment and treatment of pain and suffering.

Recognizing socioeconomic and cultural determinants to pain control

As paediatric pain medicine has improved drastically in developed countries and for families with good access to health care, the next frontier in improving access to better paediatric pain treatment is to address the inequalities of paediatric pain management for underserved patients and families. If untreated pain is an unjust suffering, on either the rights argument or the basic requirement of the harm principle, we have reason to address disparities in access to pain control in children between high-resource and low-resource communities. Included among such communities are not only low-income countries, but also low-income neighbourhoods and regions in middle-to-high-income countries. Just as with adults, children the world over experience acute and chronic pain, and yet we still lack robust epidemiological data on childhood and adolescent pain prevalence (Berde et al., 2012; King et al., 2011). Accurately mapping the global burden of any disease is the first step in recognizing suffering, and a necessary step toward addressing a need in sometimes marginalized populations.

As our understanding of the global burden of paediatric chronic and acute pain prevalence and causes improves, we can more effectively target the scale-up of pain treatment regimens in underserved areas. The most pressing immediate need is for pain medicines and supplies, and improved clinical training for pain diagnosis and treatment among medical care providers. Implementation of pain programs require evidence-based advocacy from professional organizations, and an appeal to the arguments from ethics and social justice presented above.

Those advocating for better access to pain control in resource-poor communities also face a perception that there are more dire needs to be met first—for example, malaria, childhood vaccination, clean water, or nutrition. Because a child's pain left untreated is an unjust suffering, except in the cases where the pain treatment would cause more harm than the pain itself, pain treatment cannot be viewed as a luxury. It should be viewed as equally critical, alongside the provision of preventive care, such as vaccinations, and the treatment of acute infections and other endemic diseases that disproportionately affect children living in poverty. For health professionals serving children and families in poor communities, greater effort may be required to advocate for coverage of good pain management and of palliative care when resources are not readily available.

As we expand efforts to improve access to effective pain management for all families across socioeconomic and political borders, we will also encounter a wider array of cultural beliefs about pain. Pain is a subjective experience imbued with social and cultural meaning, and this known variation in the experiences of pain has three significant ethical implications for practice in diverse patient populations (Craig and Pillai Riddell, 2003).

First, social and cultural factors may impact whether and to what degree parents pursue or have adequate access to information and resources for addressing their child's pain. Given that there is variation in parents' acceptance of exposures to pain, injury, or risk in children (Goodman and McGrath, 1991), children from some communities may be at greater risk for injury and pain, and less likely to have access to treatment. In this case, undertreatment of paediatric pain may be consonant with other socioeconomic determinants of health care access for children from marginalized groups or communities and could be embraced as part of a more general effort to address health disparities in child health.

Second, specific cultural beliefs may discourage the expression or reporting of pain as a weakness, making it more difficult to assess pain in a child patient. For example, one study of Somali families reported a belief that adults and children, especially men and boys, are expected to be stoic when in pain and not openly express pain (Finnstrom and Soderhamn, 2006). For providers treating children from culturally diverse communities, approaching families with cultural humility—asking questions to help understand beliefs about a child's pain—can help inform a respectful approach to these patients, while also being alert to the potential underreporting of pain. In approaches to treating chronic pain and end of life care, it is also important to distinguish cultural beliefs and practices of a particular family from lack of knowledge about the nature of pain in a child or unfamiliarity with available treatments (Zalon et al., 2008). In such circumstances providers have an opportunity to educate parents about the biological and sensory nature of pain in children, ultimately to help them understand when pain treatment is necessary for alleviating a child's physical suffering.

Third, perceptions or beliefs among providers and other systemic factors may lead to disparities in the treatment of pain for some minority families and communities. For example, a review of pain studies in adult patients in the United States demonstrated that blacks and Hispanics are more likely to be undertreated for pain than white patients (Bonham 2001). More data are needed to understand the exact causes of such patterns of undertreatment, but a first step is to be alert to patterns of discrimination and to highlight the importance of correcting such disparities in pain management training and practice by emphasizing the universally experienced phenomena of pain across ethnic populations (Edwards et al., 2005).

In those cases where a parent's cultural beliefs discount a child's pain—for example, 'in our culture it is important for a boy to be strong; my son does not need morphine'—a provider's fundamental ethical duty is to minimize harm and suffering for the patient, but this can be managed with cultural sensitivity. As argued earlier in considering pragmatic appeals to non-treatment of pain, the duty to prevent harm and the rights argument ought to outweigh any cultural appeal to allowing pain in children. Where adults may be free to martyr themselves or choose to undergo suffering and pain for a greater good or for deeply held spiritual or cultural beliefs, they are not free to martyr their children (*Prince* v *Massachusetts*, 1944). In practice, there are more sensitive and effective ways to navigate cultural beliefs in a family. Understanding cultural perceptions of pain can help shape care providers' conversations with families about pain management; introducing current models of pain mechanisms and processing may counter cultural beliefs that mitigate adequate pain treatment. In the end, awareness of cultural underpinnings for undertreatment of pain can help shape clinical strategies but does not alter the basic moral obligation to treat a child or infant's pain. (Please see Clemente, Chapter 11, this volume.)

Ethical considerations in paediatric pain research

As already discussed, optimal clinical decision-making is based on evidence. The more data we have on the safety and effectiveness of available treatments for the population to which they will be administered, the better. If, for example, we wish to understand the safety and efficacy parameters of using a specific analgesic medication for pain relief in premature neonates, ideally we would have data from pharmacokinetic and pharmacodynamic studies, as well as from efficacy trials conducted in that population at our disposal (Anand et al., 2006). However, there are some significant ethical and pragmatic challenges to be addressed in order to do so.

The US government enacted a series of laws seeking to improve knowledge of the safety and efficacy of specific drug preparations as applied in paediatric population. These included the Food and Drug Administration Modernization Act (FDAMA) of 1997, the Best Pharmaceuticals for Children Act (BPCA) in 2002, and the Pediatric Research Equity Act (PREA) in 2003 (Sachs et al. 2008). As a function of these initiatives, as of 4 January, 2012, there have been 426 labelling changes, including 388 trials involving children. Although these results are certainly encouraging there have been very few labelling changes for medications specifically indicated for pain.

Thus, in our current state, for children under 6 months of age, there are no medications labelled for pain relief. For children between 6 and 24 months, only ibuprofen has been approved for analgesia, and for those older than 2 years, the list expands to include oral acetaminophen, aspirin, meperidine, hydrocodone, tolmetin, the combination product of acetaminophen and codeine (for age >3 years), intravenous acetaminophen, buprenorphine, meperidine, and fentanyl citrate; epidural chloroprocaine, lidocaine, and mepivacaine, continuous epidural clonidine (for intractable cancer pain), and transdermal fentanyl. A handful of other non-steroidal anti-inflammatory medications are approved for the treatment of arthritis and have analgesic effects, including celecoxib, naproxen for children over 2 years, and etodolac and oxaprozin for those over 6 years (Sachs et al., 2008; United States Food and Drug Administration, 2012). It should be noted that of these, aspirin is not used due to concerns for Reye syndrome, meperidine due to concern about normeperidine induced central nervous system excitation and seizures, and codeine due to its variable metabolism.

Recognizing the slow progress, in 2009, the United States Food and Drug Administration convened a panel of experts to examine the design of analgesic trials in children, including an examination of the propriety of extrapolating safety and efficacy data from adult studies and to recommend the best validated outcome measures for assessing pain (Berde et al., 2012). The standard paradigm used to show the clinical efficacy of analgesic medications is a placebo controlled trial. However, administration of placebos may involve additional exposure to pain by the child participant and therefore constitutes an ethical violation as it exposes the research participant to greater than minimal risk (Shaddy and Denne, 2010). It is not acceptable for a minor research participant to experience untreated pain, even for a very brief period, as that presents increased risk over standard care. While such risk may be deemed acceptable to adults who may evaluate their plights after fully informed consent, this process is not reasonable for minors, especially those who are preverbal and cannot possibly understand the risk–benefit analysis involved. It was concluded that when extrapolation from adult studies is deemed inadequate to demonstrate safety and efficacy in younger patients, alternative research paradigms are to be invoked that eliminate exposure to untreated pain.

Thus, research participation by minors in such a trial is ethically defensible only if (1) there is true equipoise and thus it is not clear that the experimental conditions pose more risk or less benefit than the current standard of care or (2) if the child participant stands to benefit directly by participating in the research. There is broad consensus on this issue, as affirmed by the most recent documents of Declaration of Helsinki (World Medical Association, 2008), the European Union Clinical Trial Directive (European Union, 2008), the Good Clinical Practice Guidelines of the United States FDA (United States Food and Drug Administration, 2011), the International Conference on Harmonisation (International Conference on Harmonisation of Technical Requirements for Registration of Pharmaceuticals for Human Use, 2000), the National Commission for the Protection of Human Subjects of Biomedical and Behavioral Research (United States Department of Health and Human Services, 2009), and the Canadian Tri-Council ethical guidelines (Canadian Institutes of Health Research, Natural Sciences and Engineering Research Council of Canada, 2010).

A critical element in evaluating the potential risk of research participation by infants and children focuses on a comparison to the 'standard of care'. How the latter is defined, however, is quite difficult to determine, as rarely are there published standards and in only some instances are there published guidelines. Even when such guidelines exist, the degree to which there is adherence may vary dramatically. For example, in 2001 the American Academy of Pediatrics and the American Pain Society jointly issued a guideline on the assessment and management of acute pain in infants, children, and adolescents (American Academy of Pediatrics Committee on Psychosocial Aspects of Child and Family Health and American Pain Society Task Force on Pain in Infants, Children, and Adolescents, 2001). To date there is little evidence, however, that the espoused elements have been adopted as a 'standard of care'.

The issue becomes even more complicated when one invokes local standards. Consider a study of venepuncture in newborns. In Institution A, the local standard is to provide a topical anaesthetic and sucrose. In Institution B, there are no standard interventions for needle pain. A placebo controlled trial is clearly not acceptable in the former setting, but is it acceptable in the latter? What constitutes 'local' to define standards, the institution, the immediate geographic area, the region, the country? What if the latter setting is in a less developed nation where innovation in pain medicine has been slow to emerge or almost non-existent? There is no consensus on these important issues at present.

When we consider paediatric pain research in the global context, it is important to take great care in determining the current 'standard of care' for the purposes of deciding whether a new intervention warrants study, or for the purposes of instituting adequate controls in a clinical trial (Lavery et al., 2007). The overriding ethical concern is to protect against exploitation of children in communities where the standard of care in pain management is very low or non-existent. For example, it would not be ethically appropriate to investigate a new drug for the management of cancer pain in children in a rural hospital where there are no available drugs for treatment of pain, and include a control arm where children receive no pain treatment because no pain treatment is the current standard of care. However, if the question under investigation is to test improved delivery of an intravenous analgesic in a refugee camp setting, and what is being tested is a low-cost, temperature-resistant bag and line placement kit, one which would not be used in a large urban hospital in a developed country, but would be highly useful in a rural clinic in a developing country, then attention to local context is highly appropriate. In fact, failing to approve such a study on the grounds that the study team is not providing the highest standard of paediatric pain treatment available would deny a specially designed pain intervention which is desperately needed in conflict zones. For this reason, the current thinking on the standard of care question in international research is to adhere to rigorous international principles of research ethics, while allowing some appeal to local standards where a study may be the only means of delivering a targeted, context-specific intervention (Bhutta, 2002).

Conclusion

'Above all, do no harm.' 'It is a human right to have access to pain management without discrimination, for people in pain to acknowledgment of their pain and to be informed about how it can be assessed and managed, of all people with pain to have access to appropriate assessment and treatment of the pain by adequately trained health care professionals' (Cousins and Lynch, 2011, p. 2674). These ethical principles form the foundation of the ethical approach to pain in infants and children. Because children are the most vulnerable of people and because they are at the greatest risk for deleterious effects of untreated pain, these issues become heightened. Whether the focus is the provision of pain relief, inclusion in research, or considerations of pain in broad societal and cultural contexts, we must constantly weigh the benefits and risks of our actions. We owe it to the children under our care to rely on science, not personal bias or speculation, in evaluating and treating pain. Failure to do so is a threat to basic ethical standards.

Case example

Nancy was a 17-year-old girl with advanced leukaemia. She was on the inpatient oncology unit, following a second failed bone marrow transplant with multiple complications, including intestinal graft-versus-host disease (GVHD). Patients in Nancy's situation can often be expected to experience deep somatic pain related to the bone marrow expansion and/or sensitization to engraftment, superficial somatic pain related to chemotherapy or radiation therapy-induced oral mucositis, oral ulcers and skin lesions associated with GVHD, visceral pain related to intestinal GVHD or neutropenic enterocolitis, and neuropathic pain related to drug-induced neuropathies (Niscola, 2008). Nancy had made it clear to providers that she would prefer comfort care to further aggressive chemotherapy regimens, unambiguously demonstrating understanding that she would die. Her mother, however, wanted to pursue experimental treatments in an attempt to prolong Nancy's life, and refused to give parental consent for comfort care, including aggressive pain management, fearing that this might compromise her daughter's response to possible disease modifying agents.

Ethical questions for consideration: the primary issue in this context was whether or not opioid analgesics should be reduced in response to parental wishes. Secondary issues for consideration included whether the patient should be given chemotherapy, even though she made it clear she did not want it; including enrolment in a trial of an experimental agent. What would be the best approach for navigating the disagreement between Nancy and her mother?

Approach: an ethics committee consultation was sought to identify an optimal approach for the oncology team. While Nancy was not an emancipated or mature minor by legal standards, being several months shy of her eighteenth birthday, she was sufficiently mature to have a voice in even life and death decisions with support from her mother and the medical team. Her wishes to move towards comfort care should be heard and respected. This would include ensuring that everything was done to help Nancy make this decision with support. Patients who are severely depressed and/or in severe pain can have trouble making difficult decisions. The team could ensure that she was as comfortable as possible when making the decision, given adequate social support, and then try re-approaching her to make sure she understands the option of experimental treatment.

Outcome: the team tried the described communication approach, and Nancy's mother remained adamant that she wanted to continue fighting for her daughter, not yielding on her stance regarding opioid analgesics. When the psychologist spoke to Nancy in private, she said that she would rather endure pain than spend her final time with her mother in a state of conflict. She decided to go along with the experimental treatment and succumbed to her illness about 8 weeks later.

References

Adams, F. (1891). *The genuine works of Hippocrates*. New York: William Wood and Company.

American Academy of Pediatrics Committee on Bioethics. (1995). Informed consent, parental permission, and assent in pediatric practice. *Pediatrics*, 95, 314–317.

American Academy of Pediatrics Committee on Drugs. (1990). Policy Statement: Naloxone dosage and route administration for infants and children: Addendum to Emeregency Drug Doses for Infants and Children. *Pediatrics*, 86, 484–485.

American Academy of Pediatrics Committee on Psychosocial Aspects of Child and Family Health and American Pain Society Task Force on Pain in Infants, Children, and Adolescents. (2001). The assessment and management of acute pain in infants, children, and adolescents. *Pediatrics*, 108,793–797.

Anand, K. J., Aranda, J. V., Berde, C. B., Buckman, S., Capparelli, E. V., Carlo, W., *et al.* (2006). Summary proceedings from the neonatal pain-control group. *Pediatrics*, 117, S9–S22.

Bailey, J. E., Campagna, E., and Dart, R. C. (2009). The underrecognized toll of prescription opioid abuse on young children. *Ann Emerg Med*, 53, 419–24.

Berde, C. B., Walco, G. A., Krane, E. J., Anand, K. J., Aranda, J. V., Craig, K. D., *et al.* (2012). Pediatric analgesic clinical trial designs, measures, and extrapolation: Report of an FDA scientific workshop. *Pediatrics*, 129(2), 354–364.

Bhutta, Z. A. (2002). Ethics in international health research: a perspective from the developing world. *Bull World Health Organ*, 80, 114–20.

Bonham, V. L. (2001). Race, ethnicity, and pain treatment: striving to understand the causes and solutions to the disparities in pain treatment. *J Law Med Ethics*, 29:52–68.

Bostick, N. A., Sade, R., Levine, M. A., and Stewart, D. Jr. (2008). Placebo use in clinical practice: report of the American Medical Association Council on Ethical and Judicial Affairs. *J Clin Ethics*, 19, 58–61.

Bromberg, R. and Goldman, R. D. (2007). Does analgesia mask diagnosis of appendicitis among children? *Can Fam Physician*, 53, 39–41.

Cahana, A. and Romagnioli, S. (2007). Not all placebos are the same: a debate on the ethics of placebo use in clinical trials versus clinical practice. *J Anesth*, 21, 102–5.

Canadian Institutes of Health Research, Natural Sciences and Engineering Research Council of Canada. (2010). *Tri-Council Policy Statement: ethical conduct for research involving humans*. Available at: <http://www.pre.ethics.gc.ca/pdf/eng/tcps2/TCPS_2_FINAL_Web.pdf> (accessed 15 January 2012).

ChildKind International. (2010). *The ChildKind Initiative: a program to reduce pain in child health facilities worldwide* [Online]. Available at: <http://www.iasp-pain.org/PainSummit/ChildKind_Initiative2010.pdf> (accessed 2 January 2012).

Cousins, M. J. and Lynch, M. E. (2011). The Declaration Montreal: access to pain management is a fundamental human right. *Pain*, 152, 2673–74.

Craig, K. D. and Pillai Riddell, R. R. (2003). Social influences, culture, and ethnicity. In P. J. McGrath and G. A. Finley (eds) *Pediatric pain: biological and social context*, pp. 159–82. Seattle, WA: IASP Press.

De Graaf, J., van Lingen, R. A., Simons, S. H., Anand, K. J., Duivenvoorden, H. J., Weisglas-Kuperus, N., *et al.* (2011). Long-term effects of routine morphine infusion in mechanically ventilated neonates on children's functioning: five-year follow-up of a randomized controlled trial. *Pain*, 152, 1391–1397.

Dengler-Crish, C. M., Horst, S. N. and Walker, L. S. (2011). Somatic complaints in childhood functional abdominal pain are associated with functional gastrointestinal disorders in adolescence and adulthood. *J Pediatr Gastroenterol Nutr*, 52, 162–65.

Diekema, D. S. (2004). Parental refusals of medical treatment: the harm principle as threshold for state intervention. *Theor Med Bioeth*, 25, 243–264.

Edwards, R. R., Moric, M., Husfeldt, B., Buvanendran, A. and Ivankovich, O. (2005). Ethnic similarities and differences in the chronic pain experience: a comparison of african american, Hispanic, and white patients. *Pain Med*, 6, 88–98.

European Union. (2008). Ethical considerations for clinical trials on medicinal products conducted with the paediatric population. *Eur J Health Law*, 15, 223–250.

Finnstrom, B. and Soderhamn, O. (2006). Conceptions of pain among Somali women. J Adv Nurs, 54, 418–425.

Fitzgerald, M. (2005). The development of nociceptive circuits. Nat Rev Neurosci, 6, 507–520.

Foddy, B. (2009). A duty to deceive: placebos in clinical practice. Am J Bioeth, 9, 4–12.

Goodman, J. E. and McGrath, P. J. (1991). The epidemiology of pain in children and adolescents: a review. Pain, 46, 247–264.

Grunau, R. E., Holsti, L. and Peters, J. W. (2006). Long-term consequences of pain in human neonates. Semin Fetal Neonatal Med, 11, 268–75.

Hamilton, J. G. (1995). Needle phobia: a neglected diagnosis. J Fam Pract, 41, 169–75.

IASP SIG on Pain in Childhood. (2005). Homepage of International Association for the Study of Pain [Online]. Available at: <http://childpain.org/> (accessed 2 January 2012).

Institute of Medicine. (2011). Relieving pain in America: a blueprint for transforming prevention, care, education, and research. Washington DC: Institute of Medicine.

International Conference on Harmonisation of Technical Requirements for Registraiton of Pharmaceuticals for Human Use. (2000). ICH harmonised tripartite: clinical investigation of medicinal products in the pediatric population. Available at: <http://www.ich.org/fileadmin/Public_Web_Site/ICH_Products/Guidelines/Efficacy/E11/Step4/E11_Guideline.pdf> (accessed 15 January 2012).

James, A. (1993). Painless human right. Lancet, 342, 567–568.

Jarzyna, D., Jungquist, C. R., Pasero, C., Willens, J. S., Nisbet, A., Oakes, L., et al. (2011). American Society for Pain Management Nursing guidelines on monitoring for opioid-induced sedation and respiratory depression. Pain Manag Nurs, 12, 118–145.

King, S., Chambers, C. T., Huguet, A., MacNevin, R. C., McGrath, P. J., Parker, L., et al. The epidemiology of chronic pain in children and adolescents revisited: a systematic review. Pain, 152, 2729–2738.

Lantos, J. and Meadow, W. (2007). Ethical issues in the treatment of neonatal and infant pain. In K. J. S. Anand, B. J. Stevens, and P. J. McGrath (eds) Pain in neonates and infants (3rd edn), pp. 211–217. Edinburgh: Elsevier.

Lavery, J., Grady C., Wahl, E. R. and Emanuel, E. J. (eds) (2007). Ethical issues in international biomedical research: a casebook. New York: Oxford University Press.

Mancuso, T. and Burns, J. (2009). Ethical concerns in the management of pain in the neonate. Paediatr Anaesth, 19, 953–957.

McGrath, P. A. and Ruskin, D. A. (2007). Caring for children with chronic pain: ethical considerations. Paediatr Anaesth, 17, 505–508.

Mezei, L. and Murinson, B. B. (2011). Pain education in North American medical schools. J Pain, 12, 1199–1208.

Miller, F. G. and Colloca, L. (2009). The legitimacy of placebo treatments in clinical practice: evidence and ethics. Am J Bioeth, 9, 39–47.

Morton, N. S. and Errera, A. (2010). APA national audit of pediatric opioid infusions. Paediatr Anaesth, 20, 119–125.

Niscola, P., Romani, C., Scaramucci, L., Dentamaro, T., Cupelli, L., Tendas, A., et al. (2008). Pain syndromes in the setting of haematopoietic stem cell transplantation for haematological malignancies. Bone Marrow Transplant, 41, 757–764.

Olmstead, D. L., Scott, S. D. and Austin, W. J. (2010). Unresolved pain in children: a relational ethics perspective. Nurs Ethics, 17, 695–704.

Prince v Massachusetts. (1944). 321 U.S. 158, 64 S. Ct. 438, 88 L. Ed. 645 edn, US.

Ross, L. F. (1998). Children, families, and health care decision-making. New York: Oxford University Press.

Sachs, H. C., Avant, D. and Rodriguez, W. J. (2008). Labeling of pediatric pain medications. In G. A. Walco and K. R. Goldschneider (eds) Pain in children: a practical guide for primary care, pp. 233–255. Totowa, NJ: Humana Press.

Shaddy, R. E. and Denne, S. C. (2010). Clinical report—guidelines for the ethical conduct of studies to evaluate drugs in pediatric populations. Pediatrics, 125, 850–860.

Simons, S. H. and Anand, K. J. (2006). Pain control: opioid dosing, population kinetics and side-effects. Semin Fetal Neonatal Med, 11, 260–267.

Southall, D. P., Burr. S., Smith, R. D., Bull, D. N., Radford, A., Williams, A., et al. (2000). The Child-Friendly Healthcare Initiative (CFHI): Healthcare provision in accordance with the UN Convention on the Rights of the Child. Child Advocacy International. Department of Child and Adolescent Health and Development of the World Health Organization (WHO). Royal College of Nursing (UK). Royal College of Paediatrics and Child Health (UK). United Nations Children's Fund (UNICEF). Pediatrics, 106, 1054–1064.

Taddio, A., Chambers, C. T., Halperin, S. A., Ipp, M., Lockett, D., Rieder, M. J., et al. (2009). Inadequate pain management during routine childhood immunizations: the nerve of it. Clin Ther, 31(Suppl 2), S152–167.

United States Department of Health and Human Services (2009). Code of Federal Regulations; Title 45; Public Welfare; Department of Health and Human Services; Part 46: Protection of Human Subjects. Available at: <http://www.hhs.gov/ohrp/humansubjects/guidance/45cfr46.html> (accessed 15 January 2012).

United States Food and Drug Administration (2011). Good clinical practice: guidance for industry [Online]. Available at: <http://www.fda.gov/downloads/AnimalVeterinary/GuidanceComplianceEnforcement/GuidanceforIndustry/UCM052417.pdf> (accessed 15 January 2012).

United States Food and Drug Administration (2012). Pediatric labeling changes table through Wednesday, January 04, 2012 [Online]. Available at: <http://www.fda.gov/downloads/ScienceResearch/SpecialTopics/PediatricTherapeuticsResearch/UCM163159.pdf> (accessed 15 January 2012).

Walco, G. A., Cassidy, R. C. and Schechter, N. L. (1994). Pain, hurt, and harm. The ethics of pain control in infants and children. N Engl J Med, 331, 541–544.

Walker, L. S., Dengler-Crish, C. M., Rippel, S. and Bruehl, S. (2010). Functional abdominal pain in childhood and adolescence increases risk for chronic pain in adulthood. Pain, 150, 568–572.

World Health Organization. (1998). Pain in children with cancer: the World Health Organization–IASP guidelines. Geneva: World Health Organization.

World Medical Association. (2008). WMA Declaration of Helsinki—ethical principles for medical research involving human subjects [Online]. Available at: <http://www.wma.net/en/30publications/10policies/b3/> (accessed 15 January 2012).

Yaster, M., Kost-Byerly, S., and Maxwell, L. (2003). Opioid agonists and antagonists. In N. L. Schechter (ed) Pain in infants, children, and adolescents (2nd edn), pp. 181–224. Philadelphia, PA: Lippincott, Williams & Wilkins.

Zalon, M. L., Constantino, R. E., and Andrews, K. L. (2008). The right to pain treatment: a reminder for nurses. Dimens Crit Care Nurs, 27, 93–101.

CHAPTER 65

Sociodemographic disparities in paediatric pain management: relationships and predictors

Miriam O. Ezenwa and Anna Huguet

Summary

The purpose of this chapter is to present a narrative review of research studies examining sociodemographic predictors of disparities in pain management in children and adolescents. Findings from this review are conflicting. In the majority of the studies, sociodemographic variables were not statistically significant predictors of disparities in pain management. However, some gaps remain. For the studies in which evidence of sociodemographic disparities exist, it is: (1) not clear whether the statistically significant sociodemographic disparities were also clinically meaningful and (2) in all of the studies reviewed, the goal was to determine predictors of disparities in pain management. Future studies need to focus on determining the clinical meaningfulness of other findings and systematically testing explanatory models for possible sociodemographic disparities in paediatric pain management. Adequately addressing these gaps will help to move forward the science of sociodemographic disparities in paediatric pain management.

Introduction

Over two decades of research in adults with pain show evidence of racial disparities in pain management. Racial and ethnic minority patients are more likely to receive poor pain management than Caucasians (Cintron and Morrison, 2006; Ezenwa and Fleming, 2012; Ezenwa et al., 2006; Meghani et al., 2012). Much research on the health disparities literature has focused on race/ethnicity as the explanatory factors for the health disparities in pain management. This focus is underscored by the definition of health care disparities provided by the Institute of Medicine (IOM). The IOM defined health disparities as 'Racial or ethnic differences in the quality of health care that are not due to access-related factors or clinical needs, preferences, and appropriateness of intervention' (Smedley et al., 2003, p. 3). While this definition is pertinent and has provided a springboard for honing in on explanatory factors for racial

disparities in pain research, there are important sociodemographic factors, other than race/ethnicity, that could be potential predictors of disparities in pain management both independently and in combination. These factors include age, sex, educational level, geographic location, and income level. Most of the studies reviewed in the IOM report on racial and ethnic disparities in health care were conducted with adults (Smedley et al., 2003). The pioneering work of scholars on pain experiences in children reporting inadequacy of pain control in children (Beyer et al., 1984; Eland and Anderson 1977; Schechter et al., 1986) set the stage for more studies focusing on paediatric pain management, including studies focused on sociodemographic disparities in paediatric pain management. However, there is still limited research.

In this chapter, a non-systematic review aimed to explore several sociodemographic factors (including age, sex, race/ethnicity, insurance status, and residential area) as potential predictors of disparities in pain management in children and adolescents is presented. Pain management is a multidimensional and global construct encompassing concepts such as pain intensity, prescription for pain medication, pain medication used, and satisfaction with pain control. For the purpose of this chapter, we define pain management as receiving pain medications or prescriptions for pain medications. Included in the review were original studies conducted in the US and Europe, in which investigators compared groups on disparities in pain management based on the following sociodemographic factors: age, sex, race/ethnicity, health insurance status, and residential region. The database searched was Medline (PubMed and Ovid Medline). We identified 12 studies that met our inclusion criteria and analysed them using a descriptive analytic approach (see Table 65.1).

Age-related factors

We identified six studies that examined age-related disparities in pain management. The findings are conflicting. In three

Table 65.1 Summary of findings on sociodemographic disparities in paediatric pain management

Authors	Design	Sample	Setting	Major findings	Statistics used
Age-related factors					
Zuppa et al. (2005)	Retrospective chart review	2348 children aged between 1-month and 16 years old hospitalized at the PICU in 2002	USA, paediatric intensive care unit (PICU)	The utilization of the most frequently administered drugs (e.g. nalbuphine, morphine, vancomycin, and cefotaxime) differed by age	Univariate (Chi-square) analysis
VanderBeek et al. (2006)	Retrospective cohort study	503 patients 18 years of age or younger with a diagnosis of fractured radius or ulna	USA, tertiary care children's hospital	No statistical age differences were found between those who use conscious sedation and those who didn't; however, younger age of the patient was a significant predictor of conscious sedation use	Univariate (t-test) and multivariate statistical (logistic regression) analysis
Stevens et al. (2010)	Retrospective survey	847 children aged between 3 and 17 years old that receive an headache diagnosis	USA, outpatient setting (including primary and secondary care)	Age was not found to be related with the likelihood of being prescribed an evidence-based medication once a diagnosis is given	Univariate logistic regression
Boyd et al. (2006)	Survey	1017 students in 5th–10th grades (ages ranged from 10 to 18 years)	USA, Detroit-area public school district	No significant age differences in were found in the reporting of use of medical use of pain medications	Univariate (Chi-square) analysis
Ellis et al. (2002)	Survey and chart review	273 children ranging in age from 10 days to 17 years who were on the inpatient unit during the 8-h study period (patients on the psychiatric and the intensive care unit were excluded)	Canada, paediatric teaching hospital	There was no significant correlation between age and the amount of opioid or non-opioid analgesia administered	Correlations
Fein et al. (2010)	Retrospective chart review	363 children younger than 21 years that had lumbar punctures performed in 2003	USA, children's tertiary care hospital	Younger patients received pain management less often than did older patients: ◆ 16 (6.5%) of 246 neonates (0–2 months), 4 (14.3%) of 28 infants (3–18 months), 9 (60%) of 15 preschoolers (19–59 months), and 55 (85.9%) of 64 older children (60 months to 21 years). ◆ 7.2% of children younger than 18 months; 82% of children 19 months or older.	Univariate (Chi-square) analysis
Gender-related factors					
Logan and Rose (2004)	Survey and chart review	102 adolescents aged between 12 and 18 years undergoing surgeries with overnight hospital stay that are typically associated with moderate to severe postoperative pain	USA, large urban paediatric hospital	Patterns of controlled analgesic (PCA) usage, PCA demands or PCA injections did not vary by sex on postoperative days	Univariate analysis (t-test)
VanderBeek et al. (2006)	Retrospective cohort study	503 patients 18 years of age or younger with a diagnosis of fractured radius or ulna	USA, tertiary care children's hospital	Gender was not found to be associated with use of conscious sedation	Univariate (Chi-square analysis) and multivariate (logistic regression) analysis
Boyd et al. (2006)	Survey	1017 students in 5th–10th grades (ages ranged from 10 to 18 years)	USA, Detroit-area public school district	Significant gender differences were found in reporting medical use of prescription pain medication. Girls (17%) were more likely to report medical use of prescription pain medication in the past year than boys (7%)	Univariate (Chi-square) analysis

(Continued)

Table 65.1 (*Continued*)

Authors	Design	Sample	Setting	Major findings	Statistics used
Ellis et al. (2002)	Survey and chart review	273 children ranging in age from 10 days to 17 years who were on the inpatient unit during the 8-h study period (patients on the psychiatric and the intensive care unit were excluded)	Canada, paediatric teaching hospital	There was no significant correlation between sex and the amount of opioid or non-opioid analgesia administered	Correlations
Taylor et al. (2008)	Survey and chart review	241 medical and surgical patients hospitalized on the day of the audit (no age limits, mean age for boys = 5.9 years, mean age for girls = 4.2 years)	Canada, tertiary and quaternary paediatric hospital	There was no sex difference in the analgesia received	Univariate (Chi-square) analysis
Race/ethnicity-related factors					
Jimenez et al. (2010)	Retrospective cohort study	94 children younger than 18 years old admitted for ambulatory surgery, 47 = Caucasians, mean age = 8.30; 47 = Latinos, mean age = 8.59	USA, ambulatory surgical paediatric hospital	There were racial differences in the receipt of postoperative opioids after tonsillectomy and adenoidectomy surgery	Mann-Whitney U tests, Univariate (Chi-square) and Fisher's exact tests
Sabin and Greenwald (2012)	Online survey	86 academic paediatricians who are faculty, residents, or fellows	USA, large urban research university's primary care, ambulatory, and acute care	Paediatricians' implicit bias was related to prescribing less opioid pain medication for African American children than for Caucasian children after surgery	Pearson's correlations, hierarchical linear regression analysis
Yen et al. (2003)[a]	Retrospective chart review	1030 records representing 3.9 million children younger than 19 years old who presented to emergency department for isolated long bone fracture, 792 records = Caucasians, 111 records = African Americans, 127 records = Hispanics	USA, emergency department	Race did not predict use of analgesics and opioid analgesics	Multivariate logistic regression analysis
VanderBeek et al., (2006)[a]	Retrospective cohort study	503 patients 18 years of age or younger with a diagnosis of fractured radius or ulna, 418 = Caucasians, 85 = African Americans	USA, Tertiary care children's hospital	Race was not associated with receiving conscious sedation	Univariate (t-test) and multivariate statistical (logistic regression) analysis
Taylor et al. (2008)	Survey and chart review	241 medical and surgical patients hospitalized on the day of the audit (no age limits, mean age for boys = 5.9 years, mean age for girls = 4.2 years)	Canada, tertiary and quaternary paediatric hospital	There was no racial difference in the analgesia received by children	Univariate (Chi-square) analysis
Stevens et al. (2010)[a]	Retrospective survey	847 children aged between 3 and 17 years old that receive a headache diagnosis. Sample size for racial groups not provided	USA, outpatient setting (including primary and secondary care)	Race was not related to the likelihood of being prescribed an evidence-based medication once a diagnosis is given	Univariate logistic regression

(Continued)

Table 65.1 (*Continued*)

Authors	Design	Sample	Setting	Major findings	Statistics used
Brodzinski et al. (2010)[a]	Retrospective chart review	3554 children who underwent laceration repair, mean age = 6.7 years, 2128 = Caucasian, and 1428 = Minority	USA, urban tertiary-care children's hospital emergency department	Race was not associated with receiving pharmacological procedural sedation	Fisher's exact tests, multivariate logistic regression analysis
Health insurance-related factors					
Brodzinski et al. (2010)[a]	Retrospective chart review	3554 children who underwent laceration repair, mean age = 6.7 years	USA, urban tertiary-care children's hospital emergency department	Health insurance status was not associated with receiving pharmacological procedural sedation	Fisher's exact tests, multivariate logistic regression analysis
Stevens (2010)[a]	Retrospective survey	847 children aged between 3 and 17 years old that receive an headache diagnosis	USA, outpatient setting (including primary and secondary care)	Health insurance status was not related to the likelihood of being prescribed an evidence-based medication once a diagnosis is given	Univariate logistic regression
Residential region-related factors					
Yen et al. (2003)[a]	Retrospective chart review	1030 records representing 3.9 million children younger than 19 years old who presented to emergency department for isolated long-bone fracture, 792 records = Caucasians, 111 records = African Americans, 127 records = Hispanics	USA, emergency department	Residential region did not predict use of analgesics and opioid analgesics	Multivariate logistic regression analysis

[a] The same study. A study can fit into more than one category. n/a = not available from original study.

studies, results support age as a predictor of disparities in pain management. In three studies, investigators did not report similar findings.

Studies where age was related to disparities in pain management

Zuppa et al. (2005) examined whether age was associated with trends in prescription for pain medication in children in the intensive care unit (ICU). All children hospitalized to Child's Hospital of Philadelphia paediatric ICU during the 2002 year were considered (n = 2348); data was obtained from the pharmacy database of the hospital. Age was significantly associated with prescription for morphine for children in the ICU (Zuppa et al., 2005). Morphine was prescribed less often for infants (1 month to <2 year) than for older children (2 to <12 years) and adolescents (12 to 16 years) (Zuppa et al., 2005). Similarly, VanderBeek et al. (2006) investigated whether age was associated with the receipt of conscious sedation for pain control for fracture reduction surgery in 503 patients aged 18 years and under. These patients were recruited from a university-affiliated tertiary care children's hospital emergency department (ED). In a multivariate statistical analysis, younger age of the patient was a statistically significant predictor of use of conscious sedation for pain management for forearm fracture reduction (VanderBeek et al., 2006). Likewise, Fein et al. (2010) examined the relationship between age and pain management (local anaesthetics and sedation) received during the lumbar puncture procedure.

They retrospectively reviewed the records of all patients younger than 21 years who had received this procedure during the year 2003 at a large urban children's hospital. Their sample included 363 children. They found that younger patients received pain management less often than did older patients: 16 (6.5%) of 246 neonates (0–2 months), 4 (14.3%) of 28 infants (3–18 months), 9 (60%) of 15 pre-schoolers (19–59 months), and 55 (85.9%) of 64 older children (60 months to 21 years) (Fein et al., 2010).

Studies where age was not related to disparities in pain management

Ellis et al. (2002) examined the relationship between age and analgesic when surveying all children and their parents who were hospitalized in a paediatric teaching hospital in eastern Ontario during the 8-h data collection period. Children hospitalized on the psychiatric unit and the intensive care units were excluded. Their sample included 273 children aged between 10 days and 17 years old. They found that there was no statistically significant correlation between age and the amount of opioid or non-opioid analgesia administered to the children (Ellis et al., 2002). Similarly, Boyd et al. (2006) in a study conducted with 1017 students in fifth to tenth grade (ages ranged from 10 years to 18 years) examined the use of pain medication for medical and non-medical purposes. They found that as grade level increased so too did prevalence rates of medical use of pain medications, but the differences were not statistically different (Boyd et al., 2006). Finally, Stevens et al. (2010), in a retrospective study including 847 children aged between 3 and 17 years old, explored whether there were sociodemographic differences in the management of children's headache. They found that age was not related to the likelihood of being prescribed an evidence-based medication for headache (Stevens et al., 2010).

Taken together, the findings of the studies that examined age-related disparities in paediatric pain management are inconsistent. Reasons for this inconsistency could be multifaceted. The wide range of age of children included within individual studies could be problematic because developmentally, these children differ in their ability to communicate presence of pain. It was not clear whether age-appropriate pain assessment measures were used for the diverse age range of the sample. Another probable explanation for the inconsistent findings could be related to type of pain. Studies have been conducted with patients with varied types of pain (headache, menstrual cramps, urological, surgical, and other unspecified types of pain). Also, the context where the pain is experienced may explain these inconsistent findings. Studies are focused on outpatients, patients undergoing a surgical procedure, or in an ICU setting located in different institutions. Hence, the decision to administer a particular dose of pain management resides with the provider as well as the culture of the institution. Provider variables such as opioidphobia and inadequate knowledge and training about pain management or lack of supporting pain management polices contributes to poor pain management (Bashayreh 2011). Consequently, the 2011 IOM report *Relieving Pain in America* recommends more training and education of both current and future health care providers on pain management skills (Institute of Medicine, 2011). Patient and caregiver training are also needed to overcome misconceptions about use of opioids, which have been reported as barriers to adequate pain management in the adult pain populations (Ward and Hernandez 1994; Ward et al., 1993).

The age groups likely to receive disparate pain management differ. For instance, VanderBeek et al. (2006) found that younger children were more likely to receive prescription pain medication. On the other hand, in Fein et al.'s (2006) study, younger children were less likely to receive prescription pain medication. The pain management goal must be to administer or provide prescriptions for pain medications that are appropriate for patients' pain level and age. To reduce and/or prevent age-related disparities in paediatric pain management, it is necessary to use age appropriate tools, such as the Poker Chip Tool for children from age 3 to 4 by Hester et al. (1990), the Faces Pain Scale- Revised for children from age 4 to 12 by Hicks et al. (2001), or the Numerical Rating Scale for children aged 8 years or older (von Baeyer et al., 2009). See McGrath et al. (2008) for evidence-based recommendations for the use of measures and assessment strategies for pain for different age groups. It is also important to use evidence-based pain management guidelines and protocols to adequately assess and treat children's pain.

Sex-related factors

In five studies, investigators examined sex differences in pain management of paediatric patients. One study supports sex as a predictor of disparities in paediatric pain management. The other four studies did not support this finding.

Study where sex was related to disparities in pain management

We have earlier described in more details Boyd et al.'s (2006) study. Boyd and colleagues also found that sex was related to inadequate pain management. They found that there was a statistically significant sex disparity in the report of medical use of prescription pain medication. Girls (17%) were more likely to report medical use of prescription pain medication in the past year than boys (7%) (Boyd et al., 2006). Boyd and colleagues when surveying the 1071 middle and high school students did not ask them for their levels of pain, so they could not control for pain levels when comparing both sex groups.

Studies where sex was not related to disparities in pain management

Reporting on the sex-related findings in the Ellis et al. (2002) study described earlier, findings show that there was no statistically significant correlation between sex and the amount of opioid or non-opioid analgesia administered (Ellis et al., 2002). No sex differences in pain levels were reported, but findings show no significant correlations between pain intensity rating provided by children or professional and amount of opioid or non-opioid analgesia prescribed and administered (Ellis et al., 2002). In another study, Logan et al. (2004) conducted a study with 102 adolescents aged 12 to 18 years who were undergoing surgeries to examine sex differences in postoperative use of patient-controlled analgesia (PCA). Although girls reported statistically significant higher low and average pain scores than boys, boys and girls did not differ significantly on total PCA usage, PCA demands, or PCA injections after surgery (Logan and Rose, 2004). Further, in the VanderBeek et al. study described earlier, in a univariate statistical analysis, sex was not associated with use of conscious sedation for pain control (VanderBeek et al., 2006). Multivariate results also show that sex was not a significant predictor of conscious sedation use (VanderBeek et al., 2006). Finally, Taylor et al. (2008) in a study with 241 medical and surgical inpatients to determine the adequacy of pain management in a sample of hospitalized children found no sex difference in the analgesia received (Taylor et al., 2008).

In sum, although sex-based disparities have often been reported in prevalence of pain and the adjustment to the pain especially around puberty with more girls reporting more pain and its impact on daily activities (Huguet and Miro 2008; King et al., 2011; Kroner-Herwig et al., 2007; Mattila et al., 2005), sex disparities tend to be observed in use of prescribed medication. The fact that girls may be more prone to develop more frequent and severe pain but use less prescribed pain medication than boys may suggest sex differences in the response to pain management as suggested by Fillingim et al. (2009) or sex differences in attitudes to drug use.

Racial- and ethnic-related factors

We identified seven studies in which investigators examined race/ethnicity as predictors of disparities in pain management. The studies reported mixed results. We have categorized them into two rubrics: studies supporting racial disparities in pain management and studies not in support of racial/ethnic disparities in pain management.

Study where race/ethnicity was related to disparities in pain management

Jimenez et al. (2008) in a retrospective cohort study of 94 children, 47 Caucasian and 47 and Latino patients presenting to the ambulatory surgical unit in a children's hospital, examined whether racial disparities exist in use of postoperative opioids. Latino children received 30% less postoperative opioids than Caucasian children presenting for tonsillectomy and adenoidectomy (Jimenez et al., 2010). Similarly, Sabin and Greenwald examined the role of paediatricians' implicit bias on pain management recommendation for children's surgical pain with 86 academic paediatricians who are faculty, residents, or fellows in large urban research university's primary care, ambulatory, and acute care settings. Race/ethnicity was a statistically significant predictor of narcotic prescriptions (Sabin and Greenwald, 2012). Paediatricians prescribed less opioid pain medication for African Americans than for Caucasians after surgery (Sabin and Greenwald, 2012).

Study where race/ethnicity was not related to disparities in pain management

Yen et al. (2003) with a nationally representative sample of children's records who presented in the ED, Caucasian, $n = 792$, African American, $n = 111$, Hispanic, $n = 127$, determined whether race was associated with receiving analgesics to control pain related to isolated long-bone fracture. After controlling for confounding variables (health insurance type, hospital owner type, geographic region, and survey year), there was no statistically significant difference between African Americans, Hispanics, and Caucasian for using analgesics and opioid analgesics for isolated long-bone fracture (Yen et al., 2003). Likewise, VanderBeek et al. (2006) in a retrospective cohort study of children presenting in a tertiary care children's hospital, Caucasian, $n = 418$ and African American, $n = 85$, found that race/ethnicity was not associated with receiving sedation for pain management for forearm fracture reduction (VanderBeek et al., 2006). In the Taylor et al. study described earlier, there is no racial/ethnic difference in the analgesia received (Taylor et al., 2008). In the same way, Stevens et al. in a retrospective study used two nationally representative samples of 847 children from outpatient setting, including primary and secondary care settings to examine whether there were race/ethnic disparities in management of children's headache. The authors did not provide the racial breakdown of their sample. Race/ethnicity was not significantly related to receiving evidence-based medication for the management of headache (Stevens et al., 2010). Finally, Brodzinski et al. examined race/ethnic disparities in pain management of Caucasian, $n = 2128$, Minority, $n = 1426$ children who presented to the emergency department for laceration repair. After controlling for other sociodemographic (age, gender, and socioeconomic status (SES)) and clinical (triage acuity, physician type, length of laceration, complexity of repair, time of day, body site of laceration, and use of topical anaesthetics) variables, there was no significant association between race/ethnicity and receipt of pharmacological procedural sedation in children who underwent laceration repair (Brodzinski et al., 2010).

In summary, although the findings related to race/ethnic disparities in paediatric pain management studies were inconsistent, the majority found no statistically significant racial or ethnic differences in the pain management of children.

Health insurance-related factors

In two studies, investigators examined patients' health insurance status as a predictor of disparities in pain management. In both studies, patients' health insurance status was not related to disparities in pain management.

Brodzinski and colleagues, in the study described earlier, included 3554 children in research to examine health insurance status, as a predictor socioeconomic disparities in pain management of children who presented to the emergency department for laceration repair in an urban tertiary-care children's hospital emergency department. There were 1946 children with private health insurance and 1608 with public or no health insurance. After controlling for sociodemographic (age, gender, and SES) and clinical (triage acuity, physician type, length of laceration, complexity of repair, time of day, body site of laceration, and use of topical anaesthetics) variables, there was no statistically significant association between health insurance status and receiving procedural sedation in these children (Brodzinski et al., 2010). Similarly, Stevens et al.'s retrospective study, described earlier, used two nationally representative samples to examine whether there were disparities in management of children's headache based on health insurance status. The authors did not provide the breakdown of children represented in their four insurance status categories: private, Medicaid, self-pay, and other. They found that health insurance status was not statistically related to receiving evidence-based medication for the management of headache (Stevens et al., 2010).

In summary, health insurance status was not found to predict disparities in pain management. These results support the ethical standards and acceptability that all children in pain receive management regardless of health insurance status.

Residential-related factors

In only one study did investigators examine the relationship between residential region and disparities in paediatric pain management. Yen et al. (2003), with a nationally representative sample of 1030 children's records, examined disparities in the receipt of analgesics for isolated long-bone fracture pain based on residential region of children who presented in EDs. After controlling for confounding variables including age, payment method, hospital type, survey year, and metropolitan statistical area status of the hospital, children from the South and West region of the United States were significantly more likely to receive opioid analgesics than children from the Northeast for isolated long-bone fracture (Yen et al., 2003). Although there was a difference in paediatric pain management based on residential region, it's not clear what this finding from one single study represents. We cannot put any emphasis on this one study until more evidence emerges in this area.

Conclusion

There is accumulating evidence about the contribution of sociodemographic factors to disparities in paediatric pain management. However, the results are inconsistent (see Table 65.1). Unlike the findings in the adult population, in the majority of the studies that focused on children, evidence did not support sociodemographic factors as predictors of disparities in paediatric pain management. For the studies in which evidence supports sociodemographic factors as predictors of disparities in pain management, we have confidence in the interpretations of the results. Investigators controlled for several confounding variables that could have obscured the interpretation of findings, e.g. age, gender, SES, triage acuity (Brodzinski et al., 2010); health insurance type, hospital owner type, geographic region, and survey year (Yen et al., 2003). However, some gaps remain. Future studies should provide evidence of clinical significance of the sociodemographic disparities in paediatric pain management. Although, the disparities might be statistically significant, they may not be clinically meaningful. This knowledge is critical because evidence of clinically meaningful sociodemographic disparities in paediatric pain management have practice implications. For example, it could suggest medical errors on the part of the providers that require serious action. Pain relief is a fundamental human right (Brennan et al., 2007). Consequently, inadequate pain management induced by sociodemographic differences is a medical error that leads to unnecessary pain and suffering (McNeill et al., 2004). Further, all of the studies have focused simply on exploring potential sociodemographic disparities in paediatric pain management without suggesting explanations for those disparities when reported. Based on these findings, we make some recommendations that will help move forward the science of sociodemographic disparities in pain paediatric pain management. We recommend that investigators should: (1) systematically and prospectively examine factors that explain sociodemographic disparities in paediatric pain management, (2) determine whether the sociodemographic disparities in paediatric pain management are clinically meaningful, and (3) examine differences using a theoretical model that may provide information on the cause of any disparities. This approach will provide evidence to develop interventions that address both patient-related and provider-related factors that contribute to sociodemographic disparities in paediatric pain management.

Our findings have education, research, and policy implications. In order to improve paediatric pain management, there needs to be more education and training for health professionals who care for children and adolescents in pain. Provider training could focus on how to incorporate pharmacological and non-pharmacological interventions and on the invaluable skills of assessing the effectiveness of the intervention to improve pain management in children. Researchers should develop interventions that focus on eliminating sociodemographic disparities in paediatric pain management. Research that examine patient-provider variables such as communication skills, racial or sex concordance, and trust that could be barriers to adequate pain treatment are desperately needed. These patient-provider factors could moderate the relationship between sociodemographic variables and pain outcomes in this population. Finally, engaging policymakers during several aspects of research in paediatric pain management has a merit. It will serve as an impetus to policymakers to advocate for more research funding for paediatric pain management to reduce pain severity and improve quality of life for these patients.

Case example: sociodemographic issues related to paediatric pain management

BJ is a happy 13-year-old African American girl whose personality is larger than life. She lives in a subsided housing apartment in Texas with her single mother and two brothers. BJ is a typical tomboy who enjoys playing soccer with her brothers. Her love for soccer helped her to secure a position as the team captain of the girls' soccer team in her middle school. Around thanksgiving holiday, BJ started complaining of headaches that eventually increased in frequency and intensity. Currently, BJ suffers numerous headaches per month and rates them as 7 or 8 on a scale of 0 to 10, where 0 is no pain and 10 is pain as bad as it can be. Over-the-counter (OTC) pain medications do not abate her frequent headaches. Her mother feels frustrated because of loss of work days when BJ is sent home from school or she needs to take BJ to the ED, which is now increasing in frequency. She asked BJ's doctors why nothing much is done to help BJ. She learned that her public health insurance does not provide coverage for a wide range of effective interventions. BJ's prescriptions for pain medications consist of only OTC and weak opioids such as codeine. These pain medications are not strong enough to relieve the severe headaches that BJ often suffers and treatments options other than medication are not available for her. Consequently, BJ suffered in pain, became depressed, and dropped out of school and the soccer team she loved. BJ was beside herself in anger and frustration after a visit from her friend, KC, a 14-year-old Caucasian boy. KC told BJ how well triptans and biofeedback were able to reduce his migraines. His father gave him strong opioid pain medication that greatly relieved his pain. BJ wonders if the poor pain management she receives was because she is a poor African American girl who lives in a poor housing unit and her mother cannot afford better pain management resources. She thought it was unfair but at the same time feels helpless to change her situation.

References

Bashayreh, A. (2011). Opioidphobia and cancer pain management. *J Pediatr Hematol Oncol*, 33(Suppl 1), S60–61.

Beyer, J. E., Ashley, L. C., Russell, G. A., and DeGood, D. E. (1984). Pediatric pain after cardiac surgery: pharmacologic management. *Dimens Crit Care Nurs*, 3(6), 326–334.

Boyd, C. J., Esteban McCabe, S., and Teter, C. J. (2006). Medical and nonmedical use of prescription pain medication by youth in a Detroit-area public school district. *Drug Alcohol Depend*, 81(1), 37–45.

Brennan, F., Carr, D. B., and Cousins, M. (2007). Pain management: a fundamental human right. *Anesth Analg*, 105(1), 205–221.

Brodzinski, H., Iyer, S., and Grupp-Phelan, J. (2010). Assessment of disparities in the use of anxiolysis and sedation among children undergoing laceration repair. *Acad Pediatr*, 10(3), 194–199.

Cintron, A. and Morrison, R. S. (2006). Pain and ethnicity in the United States: a systematic review. *J Palliat Med*, 9(6), 1454–1473.

Eland, J. M. and Anderson, J. E. (1977). The experience of pain in children. In A. Jacox (ed.) *Pain: a source book for nurses and other health professionals*, pp. 453–473. Boston, MA: LittleBrown.

Ellis, J. A., O'Connor, B. V., Cappelli, M., Goodman, J. T., Blouin, R., and Reid, C. W. (2002). Pain in hospitalized pediatric patients: how are we doing? *Clinical J Pain*, 18(4), 262–269.

Ezenwa, M. O., Ameringer, S., Ward, S. E., and Serlin, R. C. (2006). Racial and ethnic disparities in pain management in the United States. *J Nurs Scholarsh*, 38(3), 225–233.

Ezenwa, M. O. and Fleming, M.F. (2012). Racial disparities in pain management in primary care. *J Health Disparities Res Pract*, 5(3), 1.

Fein, D., Avner, J. R., and Khine, H. (2010). Pattern of pain management during lumbar puncture in children. *Pediatr Emerg Care*, 26(5), 357–360.

Fillingim, R. B., King, C. D., Ribeiro-Dasilva, M. C., Rahim-Williams, B., and Riley, J. L. 3rd. (2009). Sex, gender, and pain: a review of recent clinical and experimental findings. *J Pain*, 10(5), 447–485.

Hester, N., Foster, R., and Kristensen, K. (1990). Measurement of pain in children: generalizability and validity of the pain ladder and poker chip tool. *Adv Pain Res Ther*, 15, 79–84.

Hicks, C. L., Hicks, C. L., von Baeyer, C. L., Spafford, P. A., van Korlaar, I., and Goodenough, B. (2001). The Faces Pain Scale-Revised: toward a common metric in pediatric pain measurement. *Pain*, 93(2), 173–183.

Huguet, A. and Miro, J. (2008). The severity of chronic pediatric pain: an epidemiological study. *J Pain*, 9(3), 226–236.

Institute of Medicine (2011). *Relieving pain in America: a blueprint for transforming prevention, care, education, and research*. Washington, DC: The National Academies Press.

Jimenez, N., Seidel, K., Martin, L. D., Rivara, F. P., and Lynn, A. M. (2010). Perioperative analgesic treatment in Latino and non-Latino pediatric patients. *J Health Care Poor Underserved*, 21(1), 229–236.

King, S., Chambers, C. T., Huguet, A., MacNevin, R. C., McGrath, P. J., Parker, L., *et al.* (2011). The epidemiology of chronic pain in children and adolescents revisited: a systematic review. *Pain*, 152(12), 2729–2738.

Kroner-Herwig, B., Heinrich, M., and Morris, L. (2007). Headache in German children and adolescents: a population-based epidemiological study. *Cephalalgia*, 27(6), 519–527.

Logan, D. E. and Rose, J.B. (2004). Gender differences in post-operative pain and patient controlled analgesia use among adolescent surgical patients. *Pain*, 109(3), 481–487.

Mattila, K., Toivonen, J., Janhunen, L., Rosenberg, P. H., and Hynynen, M. (2005). Postdischarge symptoms after ambulatory surgery: first-week incidence, intensity, and risk factors. *Anesth Analg*, 101(6), 1643–1650.

McGrath, P. J., Walco, G. A., Turk, D. C., Dworkin, R. H., Brown, M. T., Davidson, K., *et al.* (2008). Core outcome domains and measures for pediatric acute and chronic/recurrent pain clinical trials: PedIMMPACT recommendations. *J Pain*, 9(9), 771–783.

McNeill, J. A., Sherwood, G. D., and Starck, P. L. (2004). The hidden error of mismanaged pain: a systems approach. *J Pain Symptom Manage*, 28(1), 47–58.

Meghani, S. H., Byun, E., and Gallagher, R. M. (2012). Time to take stock: a meta-analysis and systematic review of analgesic treatment disparities for pain in the United States. *Pain Med*, 13(2), 150–174.

Sabin, J. A. and Greenwald, A.G. (2012). The influence of implicit bias on treatment recommendations for 4 common pediatric conditions: pain, urinary tract infection, attention deficit hyperactivity disorder, and asthma. *Am J Public Health*, 102, 988–995.

Schechter, N. L., Allen, D. A., and Hanson, K. (1986). Status of pediatric pain control: a comparison of hospital analgesic usage in children and adults. *Pediatrics*, 77(1), 11–15.

Smedley, B. D., Stith, A. Y., and Nelson, A. R. (2003). *Unequal treatment: confronting racial and ethnic disparities in healthcare*. Washington, DC: The National Academies Press.

Stevens, J., Harman, J., Pakalnis, A., Lo, W., and Prescod, J. (2010). Sociodemographic differences in diagnosis and treatment of pediatric headache. *J Child Neurol*, 25(4), 435–440.

Taylor, E. M., Boyer, K., and Campbell, F. A. (2008). Pain in hospitalized children: a prospective cross-sectional survey of pain prevalence, intensity, assessment and management in a Canadian pediatric teaching hospital. *Pain Res Manag*, 13(1), 25–32.

VanderBeek, B. L., Mehlman, C. T., Foad, S. L., Wall, E. J., and Crawford, A. H. (2006). The use of conscious sedation for pain control during forearm fracture reduction in children: does race matter? *J Pediatr Orthop*, 26(1), 53–57.

von Baeyer, C. L., Spagrud, L. J., McCormick, J. C., Choo, E., Neville, K., and Connelly, M. A. (2009). Three new datasets supporting use of the Numerical Rating Scale (NRS-11) for children's self-reports of pain intensity. *Pain*, 143(3), 223–227.

Ward, S. E., Goldberg, N., Miller-McCauley, V., Mueller, C., Nolan, A., Pawlik-Plank, D., *et al.* (1993). Patient-related barriers to management of cancer pain. *Pain*, 52(3), 319–324.

Ward, S. E. and Hernandez, L. (1994). Patient-related barriers to management of cancer pain in Puerto Rico. *Pain*, 58(2), 233–238.

Yen, K., Kim, M., Stremski, E. S., and Gorelick, M. H. (2003). Effect of ethnicity and race on the use of pain medications in children with long bone fractures in the emergency department. *Ann Emerg Med*, 42(1), 41–47.

Zuppa, A. F., Adamson, P. C., Mondick, J. T., Davis, L. A., Maka, D. A., Narayan, M., *et al.* (2005). Drug utilization in the pediatric intensive care unit: monitoring prescribing trends and establishing prioritization of pharmacotherapeutic evaluation of critically ill children. *J Clin Pharmacol*, 45(11), 1305–1312.

Index

A

ABC Scale 356
abdominal cutaneous nerve entrapment
      syndrome (ACNES) 302
abdominal pain
  assessment 259–60, 291–2
  biological factors 290–1
  case example 294–5
  emergency department management
    342
  epidemiology 15, 289
  gastrointestinal conditions presenting
    with 259, 290
    constipation 264
    inflammatory bowel disease 260
    motility disorders 264–5, 290
    pancreatitis 262–4
  history 289
  psychological factors 291
  recurrent (RAP) 42–4, 289–95, 537
  social factors 291
  treatment 292–4
    collaboration with ancillary
      services 293–4
    complementary medicines 616–17
    education 292
    hypnotherapy 563–4
    intensive outpatient/inpatient
      rehabilitation 294
    medication 292–3
    psychological treatments 293, 537
    school accommodation 293
  see also gastrointestinal tract; visceral pain
academic accommodations 124
academic achievement 122–3
acceptance and commitment therapy
    (ACT) 527
  sickle cell disease pain 250
acetaminophen (paracetamol) 436–9
  adverse effects 438–9
    case example 445
  analgesia 437
  arthritis management 220
  cancer pain management 163
  dosing 439, 440
  emergency department use 339
  mechanism of action 436

  neonatal use 276
  NSAID interaction 445
  pharmacodynamics 436
  pharmacokinetics 438
  postoperative pain management 272–3
  trauma management 175
acquired immunodeficiency syndrome (AIDS)
    see human immunodeficiency virus
    (HIV)
acupuncture 624–5
  cancer pain 166
acute otitis externa (AOE) 330
acute otitis media (AOM) 330
acute pain 12, 86, 354
  communicative context 106
  family context 111–13
  hypnotherapy 562–3
  models 87–93
  multidisciplinary pain management
    approach 642–4
  postoperative pain 269–77
  preoperative preparation 645
  prevalence 12–13
  prevention 40, 44
  prolonged 12
  services 644–5, 646
  see also procedural pain
addiction 461
adjuvant analgesics 160, 161, 164–6
  arthritis 222
  bone pain 165–6
  bowel obstruction pain 166
  musculoskeletal pain 166
  neuropathic pain 165
  persisting pain with medical illness 320
  postoperative pain 275
Adult Responses to Children's Symptoms
    questionnaire 114
Advanced Trauma Life Support (ATLS) 173
A-fibres 54–5
age-related disparities in pain
    management 669–73
alpha 2 agonists
  cancer pain 164
  trauma 177
alpha-2-delta ligands, neuropathic pain
    management 498

amantidine 165
amethocaine gel 488
amitriptyline 222, 292, 303
  topical 491
amputation 161–2
  see also phantom limb pain
anaesthesia
  complications 6
  general 195
  history 4–6
  spinal 5
  see also local anaesthetics; topical
    anaesthetics
analgesia
  administration routes 271–2
  emergency department 338–9
  metabolic considerations 433
  multimodal approach 272
  neonates 275–6
  neuraxial analgesics 275, 476–9, 480
  nurse-controlled (NCA) 176, 274
  outpatient setting 329–30
  patient-controlled (PCA) 176, 274
  pre-emptive 45
  regional 177, 274–5
  see also adjuvant analgesics; specific conditions
    and drugs
animal-assisted therapy 627
animal models
  age at time of injury 21
  extrapolation across species 20–1
  handling and maternal separation
    effects 23
  pharmacological interventions 22
  time interval before evaluation 21–2
  tissue analysis and mechanisms 22
  see also long-term effects of early pain
anticipatory guidance 328
anticonvulsants 152
  cancer pain management 165
  neuropathic pain management 503
antiretroviral therapy (ART) 320, 322
anxiety
  chronic pain and 231
  management 234
arachnoiditis 160
aromatherapy 627

arthritis
  case example 224
  classification 219
  clinical presentation 217
  diagnosis 219
  juvenile idiopathic arthritis (JIA) 16, 237, 238, 241
  juvenile rheumatoid arthritis 16
  outcomes 223
  pain management 219–23
    non-pharmacological interventions 222–3
    pharmacotherapy 220–2
    surgical interventions 222
  pain mechanisms 215–17
  pain variables 217–19
  physical function assessment 420
Arthritis Impact Measurement Scales (AIMS) 420
art therapy 628
asthma 197
  NSAID adverse effects 445
attachment theory of chronic pain 41, 42
autonomic dysregulation 231
avascular necrosis (AVN) 162
aversive conditioning 533
avoidance learning 532, 533

B
back pain 237, 240
Bath Adolescent Pain Questionnaire (BAPQ) 243, 420
Behavioral Indicators of Infant Pain (BIIP) 356, 592
behavioural coaching, abdominal pain 293
behavioural measures 379–88
  case example 387–8
  characteristics of 379–80
  cultural considerations 387
  intellectual disabilities and 386
  modification of scales 387
  pain versus distress 387
  postoperative pain 384
  procedural or brief pain episodes 380–4
  procedural distress and interactions 384–6
behavioural therapy, headaches 311–13
benzodiazepines (BDZs) 176, 180
Bernese Pain Scale for Neonates 356
beta-endorphin (BE) 395, 450
biofeedback 523, 625–6
biomarkers of pain 391–8
  case example 397–8
  characteristics of 392–3
  cortisol 355, 361–2, 394–5
  definition 391–2
  endogenous opioids 395
  genetic markers 396
  heart rate/heart rate variability 355, 362, 394
  inflammatory markers 395–6
  intellectual disabilities and 397
  neonates 355, 361–2
  neuroimaging 396
  opioid effects 396
  premature infants 396–7
  response patterns 393–4
  skin conductance 395
biopsychosocial models 41, 42, 86–93
  acute pain 87–93
  chronic pain 41, 42, 86
  critical review 92–3
bisphosphonates 165, 282

bladder pain syndrome 301–2
blood oxygen level-dependent imaging (BOLD) 403, 412
  neonatal pain assessment 403
bone marrow infiltration 158
bone pain 158, 282–3
  adjuvant analgesics 165–6
  palliative care 282–3
bowel obstruction, adjuvant analgesics 166
brachial plexus injury
  during childhood 208–9
  obstetric (OBPI) 208
brain-derived neurotrophic factor (BDNF) 69
brain development 33
  pain and 32–4
    long-term effects of early pain 32
  preterm infants 32–4
brainstem, opioid receptors 452–3
brain tumours 314
breakthrough pain 281
breastfeeding 189, 600
  opioids in breast milk 460, 461
breathing techniques 522, 547
Brief Pain Inventory (BPI) 593
bupivacaine 176
buprenorphine 462
burns 171–80
  assessment 175
  case example 171, 175, 178
  distraction therapy 555–6
  emergency department care 173–6
  long-term effects of pain 31
  operant conditioning during wound care 533–4
  pre-hospital care 171–2
  ward management 176–80
    pruritis 178
  see also trauma
butterbur 615

C
calcitonin 165
Canadian Model of Occupational Performance and Engagement (CMOP-E) 591
Canadian Occupational Performance Measure (COPM) 593
cancer pain 16, 157–66
  aetiologies 158
  bone pain 158, 282
  case example 157
  CNS tumours 159
  complementary and alternative therapies 166
  neuraxial blockade 476–7
  neuropathic pain 158–9, 209
    cancer treatment-related 209
  pain syndromes 161–2
  palliative care 283
  pharmacotherapy 162–6
    adjuvant analgesics 164–6
    non-opioid analgesics 163
    opioid analgesics 163–4
  procedure-related 161
    distraction therapy 556
  treatment-related 158, 159–61, 162
  visceral pain 159
cannabinoids, neuropathic pain management 502
capnography 198
capsaicin 491
  neuropathic pain management 499

Cardiac Analgesic Assessment Scale (CAAS) 357
Carnett's sign 302
L-carnitine 618
catastrophizing pain 95–9, 112, 114, 217
catecholamine-O-methyltransferase (COMT) gene 396
cauterization 333
central neuropathic pain 284–5
  case example 284
  management 285
central pain pathways 74–80
  ascending spinal projection pathways 75–6
  descending modulation development 78–9
  developmental anatomy 75–7
  developmental plasticity 79–80
central sensitization 229
cerebral irritability 283–5
  management 285
cerebral palsy 150, 325–6
  pain treatment 152
  physical therapy 586–7
cerumen impaction 332–3
C-fibres 54–5
  sensitization 56
chamomile 616, 618–19
chemotherapy-induced peripheral neuropathy (CIN) 162
Child Activity Limitations Interview (CALI) 40, 418, 420
Child Adult Medical Procedure Interaction Scale (CAMPIS) 105, 385–6
Child Facial Coding System (CFCS) 384
Child Health Assessment Questionnaire (CHAQ) 420
Child Health Questionnaire (CHQ) 418–19
child life interventions 543–51
  assessment 544
  breathing 547
  care plan 544–5
  case examples 545–6
  distraction 547, 548–9
  evidence for 550
  historical context 543
  memory change 550
  modelling and rehearsal 549
  positioning for comfort 549
  positive reinforcement 547–9
  preparation for procedures 546–7
  technology use 550–1
  therapeutic play 549
  thought-stopping 550
Children's Hospital of Eastern Ontario Pain Scale (CHEOPS) 373, 380
Children's and Infants' Postoperative Pain Scale (CHIPPS) 356
Child Sex Role Inventory (CSRI) 129
chiropractic 626
chloral hydrate 198
chloroform 4, 6
cholecalciferol 615, 617–18
chronic pain 12, 39, 86, 319–26, 354
  anxiety and depression management 234
  case example 234–5
  chronic disease-related 16, 319–26
  communicative context 106
  contextual factors 15
  co-occurrence of chronic pain problems 228–9
  correlates 41–2

epidemiology 13–14, 228–9
  children and adolescents 13–14
  neonates and infants 13
family context 113–16
  family distress 232
genetic contribution 230
management 232–4, 526, 645–8
  biofeedback 523
  cognitive reframing/positive self-
    statements 521–2
  distraction 521
  exposure and psychological
    desensitization 522
  feedback to families 233
  hypnotherapy 563–4
  Internet-based interventions 571–2
  multicomponent approaches 524
  multidisciplinary pain management
    approach 642–51
  operant treatment 538–40
  physical activity 234
  provider communication 234
  psychoeducation 520
  recommendations for parents 116
  relaxation techniques 522
  school reintegration 233
  self-management 569–70
  sleep 233–4
  WHO recommendations 320
models 40–1, 42, 86–7
  specificity 41
neurophysiological evaluation 413–14
persisting pain with medical illness 319–26
predictors 41, 43–4
prevention 40, 45–7
prognostic factors 41–2
school impact 232
sex differences 230
shared features 229–32
  adverse life events 230–1
  mood and affect disorders 231
  orthostatic intolerance 231
  response to centrally-acting therapies 231
  sleep dysfunction 232
  temperament/personality 231
sickle cell disease 252
social support 572–3
see also musculoskeletal pain; specific
    conditions
circumcision 332
  long-term effects of pain 30
clinical decision support systems (CDSSs) 573
clonidine
  cancer pain 164
  trauma 177
CNS tumours 159
cocaine, spinal anaesthesia 5
codeine 432, 462
  drug metabolizing enzyme
    polymorphism 432
coeliac plexus blockade 479–80
coenzyme Q_{10} 311, 616, 618
cognitive-behavioural therapy (CBT) 99, 244,
  519–28
  abdominal pain management 537
  arthritis management 222
  barriers to provision 570
  cancer pain management 166
  case example 527–8
  combination with operant treatment 536–7

developmental considerations 525–6
family role 115–16, 525
group therapy 527
physical therapy and 587
preparation for CBT 524–5
relapse prevention 526
sickle cell disease pain management 250
sleep problems and 138
techniques 520–4
  acceptance and commitment therapy 527
  biofeedback 523
  cognitive reframing/positive self-
    statements 521–2
  contextual CBT 527
  distraction 521, 533–7
  exposure and psychological
    desensitization 522
  modelling and rehearsal 521
  multicomponent approaches 523–4
  preparation for procedural pain 520
  psychoeducation for chronic pain 520
  relaxation techniques 522–3
web-based treatment 527
cognitive reframing 521, 550
  chronic pain 521–2
  evidence base 522
  procedural pain 521
colic 331
colitis 260
Comfort Ability programme 527–8
comfort-function goals 374
Comfort scale 357, 592
communicative context 106
  case example 107–8
  see also social communication model
complementary and alternative
    therapies 613–20, 623–30
  abdominal pain 616–17
  acupuncture 166, 624–5
  aromatherapy 627
  art therapy 628
  biofeedback 523, 625–6
  cancer pain 166
  case example 620, 629
  chiropractic 626
  dosages 614
  fibromyalgia 617–18
  headaches 613–16
  massage 166, 223, 251, 584, 627–8
  music therapy 628–9
  pet therapy 627
  sleep disorders 618–19
  yoga 626
complex regional pain syndrome
    (CRPS) 237–8, 239–40
  case examples 99–100, 587
  interventional pain management 475–80
  see also chronic pain; musculoskeletal pain
conceptual framework 634
constipation 264
  opioid effects 467
contextual cognitive-behavioural therapy 527
contextual variables 107
coping self-statements 550
cortical indicators 355–62
cortical pain processing 75–6
  development 77
corticosteroids
  arthritis management 220
  cancer pain management 164

inflammatory bowel disease
  management 260
corticotrophin-releasing hormone (CRH) 291
cortisol biomarker 394–5
  neonates 355, 361–2
counter irritants 491
COX-2 inhibitors 439
  arthritis management 220
  cancer pain management 163
  trauma management 176, 177
Crying Requires oxygen Increased vital signs
  Expression Sleep (CRIES) Scale 357
Critical Care Pain Observation Tool
  (CPPOT) 175
Crohn's disease (CD) 260
cultural context 103–7, 664–5
  behavioural measures 387
  observational studies 104–5
  pain perception 103
  self-report studies 104, 375–6
  understanding of pain 103–4
culture 102–3
  see also cultural context
CX3CR1 receptor 69
cyclo-oxygenase 2 (COX-2) 68
  see also COX-2 inhibitors
cyproheptadine 293
cystic fibrosis 323–4
  physical therapy 586
cystitis 301–2
cytochrome P450 (CYP) family 430, 431, 432, 459
cytokines 68
  biomarkers 395–6

D
damage-associated molecular patterns
  (DAMPs) 66
day surgery 275
dental pain 14
dependence 461
depression
  chronic pain and 231
  management 234
developmental disability 148
  see also intellectual or developmental
    disabilities (I/DD)
dexamethasone
  cancer pain management 164
  topical 491
dexmedetomidine 164, 177
  intravenous 199
dextroamphetamine 165
dextromethorphan 165
diamorphine 463
Development of Infant Acute Pain Responding
  (DIAPR) model 91–2
diathesis-stress model 41, 42
diethyl ether 4
diffuse idiopathic musculoskeletal pain
  (DIP) 237, 238–9
  see also musculoskeletal pain
diffusion of innovations 634–5
diffusion tensor imaging (DTI) 404
digestive enzyme therapy 617
disability 16, 582–3, 645
  see also intellectual or developmental
    disabilities (I/DD)
disparities in pain management see
  sociodemographic disparities in pain
  management

distraction 188, 520, 548–9, 595
　chronic pain 521
　evidence base 521
　mechanisms 554
　procedural pain 521, 547, 553–7
　　burn debridement 555–6
　　cancer treatments 556
　　case example 557
　　effectiveness 554–6
　　needle procedures 188, 555
distress, versus pain 387
dorsal horn, changing output 75
　see also superficial dorsal horn (SDH)
dorsal root ganglion (DRG) 54
　neuroimmune interactions 67
　neuronal phenotype 55
Douleur Aigue de Nouveau-ne (DAN) 357
Down syndrome 149
dressings, burns 175
drug metabolism 430–1
　see also specific drugs
duloxetine 498
dysmenorrhea 298–9
dyspepsia 290

E
ear wax removal 332–3
Echelle Douleur Inconfort Nouveau-né
　　(EDIN) 357
educational interventions 653–9
　abdominal pain 292
　body mechanics instruction 595
　children's knowledge about pain 653
　distraction techniques 547
　headaches 311–12
　health care professional education 657–9
　　educational outreach visits (EOVs) 658
　　individual feedback 658
　　knowledge about pain 655–7
　　strategies 657
　　web-based interventions 658–9
　musculoskeletal pain 244
　pain education 585–6
　　child 654–5
　　parents 293, 655
　　web-based interventions 654–5
　parents' knowledge about pain 653–4
　self-mastery promotion 329
electroencephalography (EEG) 363, 396, 412
　chronic pain assessment 413
　neonatal pain assessment 402–3
electromyography (EMG) 363
　animal models 21
　neonatal pain assessment 401–2
　see also biofeedback
electronic medical records (EMR) 376
emboli 313
emergency department (ED) care 338–45
　analgesics 173–4, 338–9
　burns 173–6
　pain management for procedures 339–44
　　abdominal pain 342
　　case example 345
　　headache 342–3
　　lacerations 340–1
　　lumbar puncture 341
　　nasogastric intubation 342
　　procedural sedation and analgesia
　　　(PSA) 343–4
　　urethral catheterization 341–2

　venous access 340
　trauma 173–5
EMLA® Cream 487–8, 563
endogenous opioids see opioid peptides
endometriosis 299–301
　gastrointestinal symptoms 300
　treatment 301
energy conservation 595
enkephalin 450
enteric nervous system 257–8
ephrins 55
epidural steroid injection (ESI) 480–1
epilepsy 152
episodic pain 281–2
　breakthrough pain 281
　incident pain 281
　muscle spasm 281–2
Epiture Easytouch™ System 489
erythromelalgia 211
ethical aspects of pain control 661–7
　balancing harm and benefit 662–4
　case example 667
　research issues 665–6
　socioeconomic and cultural issues 664–5
ethnicity 103
　disparities in pain management 673–4
EVENDOL scale 358
event-related potentials (ERPs) 402–3, 412
Evidence-Based Practice for Improving
　　Quality(EPIQ) 638
exercise programmes see physical exercise
exposure techniques 522

F
Fabry's disease 209–10
Face, Legs, Activity, Cry, and Consolability scale
　　(FLACC) 357, 380–4, 592
　revised FLACC scale (FLACC–R) 386
Faceless Acute Neonatal Pain Scale (FANS) 358
faces scales 372
facet joint pain 481
facilitated tucking 603–4
family issues 111–16
　acute pain 111–13
　　case example 111
　　parental assessment of pain 111–12
　　parental behaviour influence 112–13
　　parents' pain management roles 113
　　role of fathers 113
　chronic pain 113–16
　　case example 113
　　child pain impact on family 114
　　family functioning influence 115
　　family role in interventions 115–16, 329
　　pain aggregation in families 114
　　parental impact on child pain 114–15, 538
　　parent–child relationship role 115
　family centred care 544
　multidisciplinary pain management
　　expectations 648–9
　parental education 293, 655
　parents' knowledge about pain 653–4
　see also maternal care
fathers 113
　see also family issues
fear-avoidance beliefs 40–1, 42, 96–9
　children 40–1, 42, 96–7
　clinical implications 99
　interpersonal fear avoidance model 98–9
　parents 97–8

feedback to families 233
femoral nerve block 176
fentanyl 199–200, 463–4
　cancer pain management 163
　drug interactions 463–4
　emergency department use 339
　trauma management 177
　　intranasal (INF) 172
　　patches 178
　　pre-hospital use 172
feverfew 615–16
fibromyalgia, complementary
　　medicines 617–18
foreign body removal 333
formalin injection, long-term effects 25
fractalkine 69
friendships 119–20
　clinical recommendations 123–4
　research recommendations 124
Functional Disability Inventory (FDI) 40, 418,
　　420
functional gastrointestinal disorders
　　(FGIDs) 289–90
　see also gastrointestinal tract
functional magnetic resonance imaging
　　(fMRI) 403, 412
　neonatal pain assessment 403
fundoplication 262

G
gamma-aminobutyric acid (GABA) 59
　agonists 323
gabapentin
　neurogenic itch management 178–9
　neuropathic pain management 165, 498
ganglion impar blockade 480
gastrointestinal tract
　constipation 264
　endometriosis symptoms 300
　functional gastrointestinal disorders
　　(FGIDs) 289–90
　gastro-oesophageal reflux disease
　　(GORD) 261–2
　HIV-related pain 321
　inflammatory bowel disease 260
　innervation 257–8
　neural pathways for pain 258–9
　neuromuscular motility disorders 264–5,
　　290
　pancreatitis 262–4
　see also abdominal pain; visceral pain
gate control theory 6, 85–6, 582
gender differences 104, 113
　adult pain 127
　case examples 131
　child and adolescent pain 129–30
　　contributing factors 130
　clinical implications 131
　research recommendations 131
　see also sex differences
general anaesthesia 195
genetic markers 395–6
ginger 616
gingivostomatitis 331
glucocorticosteroids 475
glycine 59
graded motor imagery (GMI) 584
greater occipital nerve blockade 482
group therapy 527
growing pain 14, 241, 332

guided imagery 522
Guillain–Barré syndrome 325

H
handicap 645
Hartwig Score 358
headaches 307–14
  complementary medicines 613–16
  emergency department management 342–3
  epidemiology 15
  migraine 307–12, 613–16
  primary 307–13
  secondary 313–14
    HIV-related 322
    infections 314
    medical-systemic causes 313
    neoplasms 314
    substance-induced 314
    vascular disorders 313
  tension-type 312–13, 613–16
head injury 310
health insurance 674
health-related quality of life (HRQOL) 417
  evaluation 418–22
    case example 422–3
    clinical interview 418
    guidance 421–2
    HRQOL questionnaires 418–20
    outcomes measurement 421
  painful conditions and 417–18
heart rate (HR) biomarker 394
heart rate variability (HRV) biomarker 394
  neonates 355, 362
herpes simplex infection 331
high-threshold mechanoreceptors (HTMs) 56
history
  anaesthesia 4–6
  ancient times to mid-19th century 3–4
  teething pain treatments 4
5-HTP 619
human immunodeficiency virus (HIV) 320–3
  case example 323
  causes of pain 321
  gastrointestinal pain 321
  headache 322
  musculoskeletal pain 322
  neuropathic pain 321–2
  pain management 322–3
  pain prevalence 320–1
  procedural pain 322
Huntington's chorea case example 284
hydrocodone 464
hydromorphone 163, 464
hyoscine butylbromide 260–1
hyperalgesia 467
  opioid-induced (OIH) 283, 467–8
  visceral hypersensitivity 285, 290, 301
hypermobility 231–2, 237, 241–2
hyperthermia 6
hypnotherapy 560–5
  acute pain management 562–3
  analgesic mechanisms 561–2
  case example 565
  chronic pain management 563–4
hypothermia 6

I
ibuprofen
  adverse effects 442–5
  emergency department use 339

headache management 311, 312–13, 343
  see also non-steroidal anti-inflammatory
    drugs (NSAIDs)
iliohypogastric nerve blockade 482
ilioinguinal nerve blockade 482
immune challenge, long-term effects 26–7
immune system activation 67–70
  long-term priming 69–70
  postnatal differences 69–70
immunizations 555
  distraction therapy 555
  see also needle procedures
impairment 645
incident pain 281
indeterminate colitis (IC) 260
infant pain see neonatal pain; paediatric pain
infection, cancer pain and 160
inflammation 56–7
  joints 215–16
    see also arthritis
  long-term effects of early pain 23–5
  neonatal superficial dorsal horn responses 60
inflammatory bowel disease 260
  pain management 260–1
    complementary medicines 616–17
infliximab 260
information and communications technology
    (ICT) 569–74
  child education about pain 654–5
  in child life interventions 550–1
  future directions 574
  ICT-based self-management
    programmes 570–1
  Internet-based interventions 571–2
  mobile device applications 573–4
  in self-report 376
  social networking 572–3
  telemedicine/telehealth 574
Initiative on Methods, Measurement and
    Pain Assessment in Clinical Trials
    (IMMPACT) 370–1
injection pain 5, 14
  cancer treatment and 160
  see also needle procedures
insomnia 138
  see also sleep problems
intellectual or developmental disabilities (I/
    DD) 147–54
  biomarkers of pain 397
  case example 153–4
  definitions 148
  historical perspectives on pain and I/DD 149
  issues created by the definition of pain 148–9
  pain assessment 150, 151
    behavioural measures 386
  pain epidemiology 147–8, 149–50
  pain treatment 150–2
Interactional Mixed Model of Learning 535–6
interactive video games (IVGs) 180
intercostal nerve blockade 482
interdisciplinary behavioural rehabilitation
    model 538–60
interleukins (IL) 67–8, 395–6
International Classification Framework for
    Children and Youth (ICF-CY) 582–3
International Physical Activity Questionnaire
    (IPAQ) 421
Internet-based interventions 571
  child education about pain 654–5
  health care professional education 658–9

social support 572–3
  see also information and communications
    technology (ICT)
interpersonal fear avoidance model 98–9
interstitial cystitis/bladder pain syndrome (IC/
    BPS) 301–2
interventional pain management
    techniques 474–5
  cancer-related pain 476–9
  complex regional pain syndrome
    (CRPS) 475–6
  correct placement aids 475
  epidural steroid injection (ESI) 480–1
  facet joint pain 481
  neuraxial blockade 275, 476–9, 480
  peripheral nerve blockade 481–2
  plexus blockade 479–80
  sacroiliac joint injection 481
intestinal pseudo-obstruction 264–5
intra-articular facet blockade 481
intranasal fentanyl (INF) 172
intubation 342
irritable bowel syndrome 290

J
joint hypermobility see hypermobility
Juvenile Arthritis Function Assessment Report
    (JAFAR) 420
Juvenile Arthritis Quality of Life Questionnaire
    (JAQQ) 420
juvenile fibromyalgia see diffuse idiopathic
    musculoskeletal pain (DIP)
juvenile idiopathic arthritis (JIA) see arthritis
juvenile rheumatoid arthritis (RA) see arthritis

K
kangaroo mother care 189, 601, 602–3
  see also maternal care
ketamine 165, 176, 200
  continuous infusion 176, 177
  emergency department 344
  neuropathic pain management 502
  pre-hospital use 172
  topical 491
  use for ward procedures 180
ketorolac 177, 339, 343
  adverse effects 442–5
  see also non-steroidal anti-inflammatory
    drugs (NSAIDs)
Knowledge to Action (KTA) framework
    636–7
knowledge translation 633–4
  behaviour change promotion 639
  case example 638
  context of practice 639
  diffusion of innovations 634–5
  evidence-based strategies 638–9
  Knowledge to Action (KTA)
    framework 636–7
  Ottawa Model of Research Use
    (OMRU) 637–8
  Promoting Action on Research
    Implementation in Health Services
    (PARiHS) framework 635–6
  theory-informed approach 634–9
  theory of planned behaviour 635

L
lacerations 340–1
language issues 329

lateral femoral cutaneous neuropathy
      (LFCN) 482
Lawson, Jeffrey 7–8
laxative treatment 264, 265
lemon balm 619
leukaemias 158
lidocaine 488–90
   emergency department use 339
   iontophoresis 489
   liposomal 488
   neuropathic pain management 165, 498,
      502–3
lidocaine and prilocaine cream 487–8
lidocaine/tetracaine topical patch 489
limited attentional capacity theory (LCT) 554
Liverpool Infant Distress Scale (LIDS) 358
Liverpool technique 5
local anaesthetics
   emergency department use 339
   neonatal use 276
   pharmacology 475
   postoperative pain management 274–5
   techniques 275
   use during needle procedures 185–7
   see also topical anaesthetics
long-term effects of early pain 30–6
   animal studies 20–7
      evaluation 20–1
      formalin injection 25
      full-thickness skin wound 25–6
      immune challenge 26–7
      non-sensory behavioural outcomes 22
      peripheral inflammation 23–5
      peripheral nerve injury 27
      repeat needle injury 25
      surgical incision 26
      visceral injury 26
      see also animal models
   burns 31
   caregiver behaviour and 34–5
   case example 36
   circumcision 30
   conscious awareness and 35
   full-term infants 30–1
   preterm infants 31–4
      later pain thresholds 31–2
      recurrent pain 32
   sex differences 22, 34
   surgery 30–1
low back pain (LBP) 237, 240
low-level laser therapy 585
low-threshold mechanoreceptors (LTMs) 56
lumbar puncture 341
lumbar sympathetic blockade 476

M

macrophage chemo-attractant protein (MCP-1/
      CCL2) 67
magnesium 613–14, 618
magnetic resonance imaging (MRI) 363, 403
   neonatal pain assessment 403–4
magnetoencephalography (MEG) 396, 412
manipulation therapy 584
manual therapy 584
massage therapy 584, 627–8
   arthritis 223
   cancer pain 166
   sickle cell disease pain 251
maternal care 600–6
   auditory effects 601

breastfeeding 189, 600
   effectiveness 605
      mechanisms 605
   facilitated tucking 603–4
   feasibility 606
   maternal–infant interactions 604
   olfactory effects 601–3
   other providers 604
   recommendations 605–6
   sensorial saturation 604
   skin-to-skin contact 189, 601, 602–3
   see also family issues
mechanoreceptors 56
medial branch nerve blockade (MBB) 481
medication overuse headache (MOH) 314
melatonin 619
memory change 550
meperidine 464
meralgia paraesthetica 482
methadone 165, 464
   cancer pain management 163–4
   neuropathic pain management 501–2
methoxyflurane, pre-hospital use 172
methylnaltrexone 166
mexiletine 503
m-health technologies 573–4
microglia 65–7
   function during development 66–7
   long-term priming of response 69–70
   nerve injury responses 68–9
midazolam 177, 198–9
migraine 307–12
   comorbid conditions 310
   diagnostic criteria 309
   emergency department management
      342–3
   epidemiology 307–8
   evaluation 309–10
   pathophysiology 308–9
   prevention 311
   treatment 310–12
      acute migraine 310–11
      biobehavioural therapy 311–12
      complementary medicines 613–16
   see also headaches
Migraine Specific Quality of Life Questionnaire
      (MSQ) 420
mindfulness meditation 566
mirror therapy 584
   case example 587
mitochondrial neurogastrointestinal
      encephalopathy (MNGIE) 265
mobile device applications 573–4
mobilization therapy 584
modafinil 165
modelling and rehearsal 521, 549
Modified Behavioural Pain Scale (MBPS) 357
Modified Infant Pain Scale (MIPS) 358
Modified Postoperative Comfort Score 359
monoclonal antibody therapy, inflammatory
      bowel disease 260
monocyte chemoattractant peptide
      (MCP)-1 395–6
morphine 464
   cancer pain management 163
   emergency department use 339
   neuropathic pain management 499
   pancreatitis management 263
   pharmacology 433
premedication 6

trauma management 176, 177
   pre-hospital use 172
mucositis 159
Multidimensional Assessment of Pain Scale
      (MAPS) 358
Multidimensional Measure for Recurrent
      Abdominal Pain (MM-RAP) 259–60
multidimensional pain 354
multidisciplinary pain management approach
      (MPMA) 642–4
   acute care services 644–5, 646
   chronic pain management 645–8
      patient flow 649–51
      staff communication 647–8
      staff positions 647
   information management systems 649
   parental expectations 648–9
multimodal distraction (MMD) 180
multiple attentional resource theory (MRT) 554
multiple sclerosis (MS) 210
muscle relaxants 166
muscle relaxation techniques 522–3
muscle spasm 281–2
musculoskeletal pain 215, 237–45
   assessment 242
      history 242–3
      physical examination 243
      physiological measures 244
      psychometric instruments 243
   case example 245
   clinical features 238
   differential diagnoses 218, 243
   epidemiology 14–15, 237–8
   HIV-related 322
   impact 242
   management 242–5
      adjuvant analgesics 166
      education 244
      pharmacotherapy 244
      physical therapies 244–5
      psychological therapy 244
      rehabilitation 244
      self-management 244
      topical anaesthetics 490–1
   outcomes 245
   physical function assessment 420–1
   see also chronic pain; specific conditions
music therapy 628–9
myofacial pain, complementary
      medicines 617–18

N

Nepean Neonatal Intensive Care Unit Pain
      Assessment Tool (NNICUPAT) 359
nasogastric intubation 342
near-infrared spectroscopy (NIRS) 363, 402,
      412
   neonatal pain assessment 402
needle procedures 184
   clinical impact 184–5
   early repeat needle injury, long-term
      effects 25
   epidemiology 184
   pain management interventions 185–90
      distraction 188, 555
      local anaesthetics 185–7
      physical interventions 188–90
      practices and attitudes 185
      procedural interventions 185
      psychological interventions 188

topical anaesthetics 486–9
sweet solutions 187
venous access 340, 555
see also injection pain
Neonatal Facial Coding System (NFCS) 354, 356, 592
Neonatal Individualized Developmental Care and Assessment Program (NIDCAP) 34, 353–4
neonatal pain
acute pain prevalence 12–13
analgesia 275–6
local anaesthesia 276
NSAIDs 276
opioids 276
paracetamol (acetaminophen) 276
assessment 353–67, 401–4
absence of response 366
acute versus chronic pain 354
biomarkers 355, 361–2
case example 367
challenges 365–7
cortical indicators 355–62, 363
electroencephalography (EEG) 402–3
electromyography (EMG) 401–2
guidelines 362–5
magnetic resonance imaging (MRI) 403–4
measures 354–5, 356–61, 366–7
near-infrared spectroscopy (NIRS) 402
unidimensional versus multidimensional pain 354
chronic pain prevalence 13
conceptualization of 353–4
hospitalized neonates 12–13
postoperative pain 275–6
scientific approaches 7–9
sensitivity 5–6
see also long-term effects of early pain; preterm infants; *specific conditions*
nerve blocks
cancer-related pain 476–9
complex regional pain syndrome (CRPS) 475–6
complications 476
correct placement aids 475
neuraxial analgesics 275, 476–9
peripheral nerve blockade 481–2
plexus blockade 479–80
trauma management 176, 177
see also neuraxial analgesics
nerve injury
long-term effects of early pain 27
peripheral (PNI) 65
spinal microglial reactivity 68–9
neuralgia
postherpetic (PNH) 210
trigeminal 210–11
neural stimulation therapy 285
neuraxial analgesics 275, 476–9, 480
complications 479
contraindications 477
delivery systems 477–9
safety issues 477
neurofibromatosis 209, 324
neuroimaging 396, 412
neuroleptic drugs, cancer pain 164
neuromatrix theory 582
neuromuscular diseases 324–5
neuromuscular motility disorders 264–5, 290
neuropathic pain 65, 86, 205–12, 495

assessment 205–6
brachial plexus injury 208–9
during childhood 208–9
obstetric (OBPI) 208
cancer-related 158–9, 165, 209
cancer treatment-related 209
case example 212
causes 496
central neuropathic pain 284–5
children versus adults 496
clinical features 495–6
definition 205, 495
genetic disorders 211
HIV-related 321–2
management 496–505
adjuvant analgesics 165
algorithm 503, 504
case example 504–5
combination strategies 503
first-line agents 496–8
fourth-line agents 502
intravenous lidocaine infusion 502–3
second-line agents 498–9
third-line agents 499–502
topical anaesthetics 490–1
metabolic disorders 209–10
neurological disorders 210–11
palliative care 285
peripheral nerve injury 65, 209
post-surgical 206
spinal cord injury (SCI) 209
trauma patients 178–9, 206–9
neuroticism 95–6
neurotrophins 55
nitric oxide (NO) 68
nitrous oxide 5, 6, 200
emergency department 344
trauma 176
pre-hospital use 172
ward procedures 180
NMDA antagonists
cancer pain management 165
HIV-related pain management 323
neuropathic pain management 503
nociception 53
evaluation 54
peripheral pathways 53–4
sensitization 56–7
spinal processing 57
see also central pain pathways; superficial dorsal horn (SDH)
nociceptors 53
transduction 55–6
see also nociception
Non-communicating Children's Pain Checklist (NCCPC) 386
non-steroidal anti-inflammatory drugs (NSAIDs) 439–45
adverse effects 273, 442–5
asthma 445
bleeding 444–5
bone healing 444
gastrointestinal effects 444
renal effects 444
arthritis management 220
cancer pain management 163
classification 441
drug interactions 442
acetaminophen (paracetamol) 445
dysmenorrhea management 299

endometriosis management 300
headache management 311, 312–13
HIV-related pain management 322
inflammatory bowel disease management 260
mechanism of action 439
neonatal use 276
pharmacodynamics 439–41
pharmacokinetics 441–2, 443
postoperative pain management 273
sickle cell disease pain management 251, 252
topical 490
trauma management 176–7
numerical rating scale (NRS) 371–2
nurse-controlled analgesia (NCA) 176, 274

O
obesity 15
observational learning 97
Observation Scale of Behavioral Distress (OSBD) 385
obstetric brachial plexus injury (OBPI) 208
occipital nerve blockade 482
Occupational Performance Process Model (OPPM) 591
occupational therapy 590–6
assessment 592–3
goals of 590
interventions 594–6
adaptive equipment 595–6
body mechanics instruction 595
energy conservation 595
infants 593–4
play/distraction 595
relaxation strategies 596
youths 594
pain effects on occupation 592
theory 591–2
octreotide 166, 264–5
olanzapine 164
omeprazole 262
operant conditioning treatment 531
abdominal pain management 537
case example 540
combination with CBT 536–7
during burn wound care 533–4
interdisciplinary behavioural rehabilitation model 538–60
origins of 531–3
parent–child interactions 538
positive reinforcement of wellness behaviour 536–7
operant models of pain 40, 42, 86, 531–3, 534–6
aversive conditioning 533
avoidance learning 532, 533
positive reinforcement 532
systematic reviews 535–6
opioid analgesics 457–70
adverse effects 274, 465–7
constipation 467
hyperalgesia 283, 467–8
itching 465
nausea and vomiting 465
respiratory effects 465–7
arthritis management 220–2
biomarker responses to 396
cancer pain management 163–4
case example 470
clinical outcomes 457–8

opioid analgesics (*Continued*)
  clinical practice guidelines (CPGs) 457–8
  dosing 463
  drug transporter polymorphisms 432–3
  emergency department use 339
  inflammatory bowel disease
      management 261
  neonatal use 276
  neuropathic pain management 499–502
  opioid contract 500–1
  outpatient setting 329–30
  palliative care 280–1
    cerebral irritability 285
  persisting pain with medical illness 319–20
  pharmacokinetics 459–60
  postoperative pain management 273–4
  prescription monitoring programmes
      (PMP) 468–9
  sickle cell disease pain management 251–2
  tolerance 161
  topical 491
  trauma management 173, 176–8
    pre-hospital use 172
  see also specific drugs
opioid-induced hypersensitivity (OIH) 283,
    467–8
opioid peptides 449–54
  biomarkers of pain 395
  developmental expression and role 450–1
  history 449–50
  receptors 451–4
    brainstem 452–3
    developmental expression 453–4
    peripheral nervous system 451–2
    spinal cord 452
  sucrose analgesia basis 509–10
  see also opioid analgesics
opium 449, 464–5
optimism 95–6
oral pain 14
orthostatic intolerance 231
otalgia 330
otitis 330
Ottawa Model of Research Use (OMRU) 637–8
OUCH cohort 91–2
ouchless place model 44
outpatient setting 328
  analgesics 329–30
  case example 335
  pain associated with specific conditions
      330–3
oxycodone 465
  cancer pain management 163, 339
  neuropathic pain management 501
oxytocin 605

P
P2X receptors 55, 69
paediatric fear-avoidance model 41, 96–7
paediatric pain 135
  assessment 370
    domains of 370–1
      neurophysiological evaluation 411–14
      quantitative sensory testing (QST) 407–11
      see also neonatal pain; self-report; *specific
          conditions*
  developmental aspects 412–13
  indicators 3–4
  measurement 370

age-appropriate measurement 371–2
    behavioural measures 379–88
  predictors 41, 43–4
  prevalence 12–17
    community health care settings 14–15
    hospitalized infants and children 12–14
  prevention 39–40, 42–4
  scientific approaches 6–9
  sensitivity to 4–5
  sleep relationships 135–6, 137
  target level 374
  see also acute pain; chronic pain; neonatal
      pain; *specific types of pain*
Pain Assessment in Neonates Scale (PAIN) 360
Pain Assessment Tool (PAT) 360
pain-associated disability syndrome
    (PADS) 538–40
Pain Experience Questionnaire (PEQ) 420
pain-sensitive office 333–4
palliative care 280
  pain management 280–6
    bone pain 282–3
    cancer pain 283
    case example 281
    central neuropathic pain 284–5
    central pain 284–5
    cerebral irritation 283–5
    episodic pain 281–2
    intractable pain 285–6
    multidisciplinary approach 642–4
    neuropathic pain 285
    opioids 280–1
    visceral hypersensitivity 285
    WHO guidelines 280–1
pancreatitis 262–4
  clinical presentation 263
  management 263–4
  pathophysiology 262–3
paracetamol *see* acetaminophen
parents *see* family issues; fathers; maternal care
Parents' Postoperative Pain Measure
    (PPPM) 384
paroxysmal extreme pain disorder 211
patient-controlled analgesia (PCA) 176, 274
Patient Reported Outcomes Measurement
    Information System (PROMIS) 40, 421
Pediatric Quality of Life Inventory
    (PedsQL) 418–19
peer relationships 119–20, 121–2
  clinical recommendations and 123–4
  research recommendations 124
pelvic pain 298–304
  assessment 302
  case example 304
  dysmenorrhea 298–9
  endometriosis 299–301
  interstitial cystitis/bladder pain
      syndrome 301–2
  pelvic floor dysfunction 301
  prostatitis 301
  treatment 302–3
pentobarbital 199
peppermint 616–17
perceived self-efficacy model 41, 42
peripheral innervation 54–5
peripheral nerve injury (PNI) 65, 209
peripheral neuropathy 65, 209
  HIV-related 321–2
peripheral sensitization 56–7

peritoneal pain 259
persisting pain *see* chronic pain
personality 95, 231
pethidine 464
pet therapy 627
P-glycoprotein (P-gp) transporter 431–2
  polymorphisms 432–3
phantom limb pain 161–2, 206–8
  associated phenomena 207
  characteristics 206–7
  incidence 207–8
  management 480
  risk factors 207–8
  time course 208
pharmacodynamics 431–2
  see also specific drugs
pharmacogenomics/pharmacogenetics 432–3
pharmacokinetics 429–31
  see also specific drugs
pharyngitis 330–1
physical exercise 583–4
  abdominal pain 294
  arthritis 222
  chronic pain 234
  physical activity assessment 421
  stretching exercises 586–7
physical function assessment 420–1
physical therapy 152, 244–5, 581–8
  active therapies 583–4
  arthritis 222
  case examples 587
  conceptual framework for pain 582–3
  passive therapies 584–6
    low-level laser 585
    manual therapy 584
    massage 584
    precautions and limitations 585
    TENS 584–5
    therapeutic ultrasound 585
    thermal agents 585
  procedural pain 586–7
  recommendations 587
  sickle cell disease pain 251
  therapeutic relationship 585–6
Pieces of Hurt measurement tool 372
pizotifen 293
plasma beta endorphin (BE) biomarker 395
play 544–5
  see also child life interventions
plexus blockade 479–80
positioning for comfort 549
positive reinforcement 532, 547–9
positive self-statements 521–2
postherpetic neuralgia (PHN) 210
postoperative pain 269–77
  analgesia 271–5
    acetaminophen (paracetamol) 272–3
    adjuvant analgesics 275
    drug administration routes 271–2
    multimodal approach 272
    neuraxial analgesics 275
    NSAIDs 273
    opioids 273–4
    regional 274–5
  assessment 270–1
    behavioural measures 384
    measurement tools 270–1
    self-report 271
  cancer patients 160–1

case example 276–7
day surgery 275
management services 270
negative effects of 269–70
neonates 275–6
neuropathic pain 206
primary prevention 44
Postoperative Pain Score (POPS) 360
postural orthostatic tachycardia syndrome (POTS) 231
prednisolone 260
pregabalin 179, 498
Premature Infant Pain Profile (PIPP) 360
Premature Infant Pain Profile–Revised (PIPP–R) 360–1
prescription monitoring programmes (PMP) 468–9
preterm infants
    biomarkers of pain 396–7
    long-term effects of early pain 31–4
        later pain thresholds 31–2
        neurodevelopment 32
        recurrent pain 32
    pain and brain development 32–4
        brain reactivity to procedures 32–3
        programming of stress systems 34
        sleep 34
prevention 39–40, 42–7
    acute pain of iatrogenic origin 40, 44
    chronic pain 40, 45–7
    future directions 46–7
    migraine 311
    primary prevention 40, 44–6
        pre-emptive analgesia 45
        psychosocial interventions 45–6
    secondary prevention 40, 46
    sickle cell disease pain 252–3
    tension-type headaches 313
    tertiary prevention 40, 46
probiotics 617
procedural pain 553
    behavioural measures 380–6
    cancer treatment 160–1, 556
    child life intervention 546–7
    cognitive-behavioural interventions 525, 553–7
        cognitive reframing/positive self-statements 521
        distraction 521, 547, 553–7
        exposure and psychological desensitization 522
        modelling and rehearsal 521
        multicomponent approaches 523–4
        preparation for procedure 520
        relaxation techniques 522
    emergency department procedures 339–44
        lacerations 340–1
        lumbar puncture 341
        nasogastric intubation 342
        procedural sedation and analgesia (PSA) 343–4
        urethral catheterization 341–2
        venous access 340
    HIV management 322
    hypnotherapy 562–3
    models 88–9
    physical therapy 586–7
    primary prevention 44
    recommendations for parents 113

topical anaesthetics 486–90
    see also needle procedures
procedural sedation see sedation
Procedure Behavioral Rating Scale (PBRS) 384
Procedure Behavior Checklist (PBCL) 384–5
prochlorperazine 343
pro-dynophrin 450
prognostic factors 39, 41–2
pro-inflammatory cytokines 68
Promoting Action on Research Implementation in Health Services (PARiHS) framework 635–6, 656–7
    case example 638
propofol 179
    intravenous 199
prostaglandin H_2 synthetase (PFHS) 436, 437
prostaglandins 68
prostatitis/prostatic pain syndrome 301
protective factors 39
pruritis 178–9
psychological desensitization techniques 522
psychostimulants 165
pudendal nerve blockade 482
purinergic receptors 55
pyloroplasty 262

Q
Quality of Life Headache in Youth (QLH-Y) 420
quantitative sensory testing (QST) 128, 407–11
    measures 408, 409
        method of adjustment 408
        method of constant stimuli 408
        method of limits (MLI) 408
    modulating influences 410–11
        age-related differences 410–11
        contextual influences 410
        procedural influences 410
        sex-related differences 411
    normative data 409
    reliability 409–10
    sensory testing site 408–9

R
race 103
    disparities in pain management 673–4
radiofrequency nerve lesioning (RFNL) 481
radionuclide therapy 165–6, 282–3
radiotherapy 282–3
ranitidine 262
rectus abdominis sheath blockade 482
recurrent abdominal pain (RAP) see abdominal pain
regional analgesia 177, 274–5
    techniques 275
rehabilitation 646–7
    abdominal pain 294
    interdisciplinary behavioural rehabilitation model 538–60
    musculoskeletal pain 244
relaxation techniques 522–3, 565–6, 596
remifentanil 467
Riley Infant Pain Scale (RIPS) 359
risk factors 39
rostroventral medulla (RVM) 78

S
sacroiliac joint injection 481
Scale for Use in Newborns (SUN) 361

school issues 122–3
    abdominal pain and 291, 293
    academic achievement 122–3
    accommodations 124, 293
    reintegration after absence 233
    research recommendations 125
    social context 123
sedation 194–201
    case example 201
    depth monitoring 195
    discharge criteria 200–1
    drugs 198–200
        analgesics 199–200
        reversal agents 200
        sedatives 198–9
        see also specific drugs
    emergency department 343–4
    equipment requirements 198
    levels of 194–5
    opioid effects 467
    palliative 285–6
    patient factors 195–6
        airway issues 196–7
        allergies and adverse reactions 195–6
        aspiration risk 196
        developmental issues 197
        general health 196
        respiratory illness 197
    procedural factors 197–8
selective serotonin and noradrenaline re-uptake inhibitors (SSNRIs) 498
    neuropathic pain management 498
selective serotonin re-uptake inhibitors (SSRIs)
    arthritis management 222
    pelvic pain management 303
selective spinal nerve blockade (SNRB) 480
self-mastery promotion 329
self-report 370–7
    age-appropriate measurement of pain 371–2
    case example 373
    chronic versus acute pain 375
    communication impairment and 375
    cultural issues 104, 375
    desirable features of 374, 375
    future research 376
    gender issues 375
    implausible scores 373–4
    interpretation 372–6
    nature of 370
    new technologies 376
    pain interference 374
    pain location 374
    pain qualities 374
    postoperative pain 271
    temporal characteristics of pain 374
    validation 374–5
sensitization 56–7, 69
    central 229
    peripheral 56
    psychological desensitization techniques 522
sex differences 113
    adult pain 127
    child and adolescent pain 128–9
        contributing factors 130
    chronic pain 230
    clinical implications 131

sex differences (*Continued*)
  quantitative sensory testing outcomes 411
  research recommendations 131
  see also gender differences
sex-related disparities in pain management 673
siblings 114
  see also family issues
sickle cell disease (SCD) pain 16, 248–54
  assessment 249–50
  case example 254
  epidemiology 248–9
  pain syndromes other than vaso-
    occlusion 249
  pathophysiology 248, 253
  pharmacological therapies 251–2
    chronic pain 252
    home management 251–2
    in-patient management 252
  physical therapies 251
  prevention 252–3
  psychological therapies 250
skin conductance as biomarker 395
skin-to-skin contact 189, 601, 602–3
  see also maternal care
skin wound, full-thickness 25
sleep problems 135–41
  arthritis 222
  assessment 137
  case example 141
  impact of 136–7
  management 233–4
    complementary medicines 618–19
    pharmacological treatments 139–40
    psychological treatments 138
    sleep interventions 138–9, 140
    sleep optimization 137–8
  pain relationships 135–6, 137
    abdominal pain 291
    chronic pain 232
  preterm infants 34
  prevalence 136
  recommendations 140
  trauma patients 179
slippery elm 617
social communication model 89–91, 119, 354
  see also communicative context
social learning theory 41, 42, 86
social networking 572–3
sociodemographic disparities in pain
    management 669–75
  age-related factors 669–73
  case example 675
  health insurance-related factors 674
  racial- and ethnic-related factors 673
  residential-related factors 674
  sex-related factors 673
sociomedical context 105–6
sodium channels 56
sore throat 330–1
spinal anaesthesia, history 5
spinal cord
  ascending projection pathways 75–6
  descending modulation development
    78–9
  injury (SCI) 209
  nociceptive processing 57
  opioid receptors 452
spinal cord stimulation (SCS) 476

spinothalamic tract (STT) 75–6
Starbright World® 551
stellate ganglion blockade 475–6
steroids
  epidural steroid injection (ESI) 480–1
  pharmacology 475
  see also corticosteroids
stimulus–response model 88
stomatitis 331
stress response 290–1
stress system programming 34
stretching exercises 586–7
substance-induced headaches 314
subungual hematoma 333
sucrose solutions *see* sweet solutions
superficial dorsal horn (SDH) 57
  developing neuron excitability 57–8
  excitatory synapses 58–9
  long-term effects of early tissue injury 60
  primary afferent input maturation 58
  signal processing under pathological
    conditions 60
  synaptic inhibition 59
superior hypogastric plexus blockade 480
suprascapular nerve blockade 482
surgery
  anaesthesia history 4–6
  long term effects of pain 30–1
    animal studies 26
  see also postoperative pain
sutures 340–1
sweet solutions 187, 508–14
  effectiveness 510–12, 513
    childhood 512, 513
    with concurrent analgesics 513
    with non-pharmacological pain relief 513
    non-procedural pain 513
    older infants 511–12
  guidelines for use 513–14
  mechanisms 508–10, 512–13
    animal studies 508–10
    infant studies 510
    opioid basis 509–10
  systematic reviews 509
sympathetic ganglion blockade 475
synactive theory of development 353–4

T
tactile stimulation 189
tapentadol 465
technology use *see* information and
    communications technology (ICT)
teething pain 331–2
  history of treatments 4
telemedicine/telehealth 574
temperament 95, 231
tension-type headaches 312–13
  prevention 313
  treatment 312–13
    complementary medicines 613–16
  see also headaches
tetracaine gel 488
thalamocortical connection development 76–7
L-theanine 619
theory of planned behaviour (TPB) 635
therapeutic ultrasound 585
thermal therapy 585
thought-stopping 550

thrombophlebitis 160
thrombosis 313
tick removal 333
tizanidine 164
TLR4 receptor 66, 68–9
T lymphocytes 67, 69
Toll-like receptors (TLRs) 66
  TLR4 66, 68–9
tonsillitis 331
topical anaesthetics 486–92
  case example 491–2
  musculoskeletal pain 490–1
  neuropathic pain 490–1
  procedural pain 486–90
tramadol 465
  arthritis management 220
  cancer pain management 163
  neuropathic pain management 499
  trauma management 175
transcutaneous electrical nerve stimulation
    (TENS) 584–5
  pelvic pain 303
transdermal medications 486
transforming growth factor beta (TGFβ) 395–6
transient receptor potential (TRP) ion
    channels 55
trauma 171–80
  case example 171, 175, 178
  definition 173
  emergency department care 173–5
    analgesic doses 173–4
    pain assessment 175
  neuropathic pain 178–9, 206–9
  pre-hospital care 171–2
  pruritis and 178
  sleep disturbance 179
  ward management 176–8
    procedural interventions 179–80
tricyclic antidepressants
  abdominal pain management 292
  arthritis management 222
  cancer pain management 164
  neuropathic pain management 496–8
  pelvic pain management 303
trigeminal nerve blockade 481
trigeminal neuralgia 210–11, 481
triptans 311, 343
L-tryptophan 619
tumor necrosis factor alpha (TNFα) 67
tumours, intracranial 314
two-factor learning theory 554
typhlitis 160
tyrosine receptor kinase A (TrkA) 54, 55

U
ulcerative colitis (UC) 260
ultrasound, therapeutic 585
unidimensional pain 354
Upopolis™ 551
upper respiratory tract infection (URTI) 197
urethral catheterization 333, 341–2
uridine diphosphate (UDP)-
    glucuronosyltransferase (UGT) 431,
    438

V
valerian 619
vapocoolant sprays 489

vasculitis 313
venepuncture 340
    see also needle procedures
venlafaxine 498
venous access
    distraction therapy 555
    emergency department 340
    see also needle procedures
verbal numeric scale (VNS) 371
virtual reality (VR) 180, 556
visceral injury 26

visceral pain
    cancer-related 159
    neural pathways 258–9
        postnatal development 259
    visceral hypersensitivity 285, 290
        endometriosis and 301
    see also abdominal pain
visual analogue scale (VAS) 371–2
vitamin B complex 614–15, 618
vitamin D 615, 617–18
voltage-gated sodium channels 56

W
web-based cognitive-behavioural
    therapy 527

Y
yoga 626
Youth Activity Questionnaire 421

Z
zolmitriptan 311